Heart Failure in Children
and Young Adults

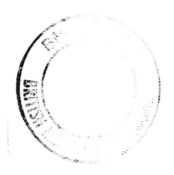

Heart Failure in Children and Young Adults

From Molecular Mechanisms to Medical and Surgical Strategies

Anthony C. Chang, MD, MBA

Director, Pediatric Cardiac Intensive Care Program
Texas Children's Hospital
Associate Professor of Cardiology—Pediatrics
Chief, Critical Care Cardiology
Baylor College of Medicine
Attending Cardiologist
Texas Heart Institute
Houston, Texas

Jeffrey A. Towbin, MD

Professor, Departments of Pediatrics (Pediatric Cardiology)
and Molecular and Human Genetics
Baylor College of Medicine
Chief, Pediatric Cardiology
Director, Heart Failure and Cardiomyopathy Service
Texas Children's Hospital
Houston, Texas

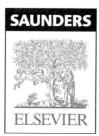

SAUNDERS

ELSEVIER

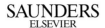

SAUNDERS
ELSEVIER

1600 John F. Kennedy Blvd.
Ste 1800
Philadelphia, PA 19103-2899

HEART FAILURE IN CHILDREN AND YOUNG ADULTS

ISBN 13: 9-7807-2160-6927
ISBN 10: 0-7216-0692-X

Library of Congress Cataloging-in-Publication Data

Heart failure in children and young adults: from molecular mechanisms to medical and
    surgical strategies/[edited by] Anthony Christopher Chang, Jeffrey A. Towbin.
        p. ; cm.
    ISBN 0-7216-0692-X
      1. Pediatric cardiology. 2. Heart failure. I. Chang, Anthony C. II. Towbin, Jeffrey A.
    [DNLM: 1. Heart Diseases—diagnosis—Adolescent. 2. Heart Diseases—diagnosis—Child.
    3. Cardiac Surgical Procedures—Adolescent. 4. Cardiac Surgical Procedures—Child.
    5. Heart Diseases—therapy—Adolescent. 6. Heart Diseases—therapy—Child. WG 210 H43479 2006]
    RJ421.H385 2006
    618.92′12—dc22
                                                                    2005042827

Acquisitions Editors: Anne Lenehan, Susan Pioli
Developmental Editor: Vera Ginsburgs
Publishing Services Manager: Frank Polizzano
Senior Project Managers: Natalie Ware, Jeff Gunning
Design Direction: Gene Harris

Printed in the United States of America

Last digit is the print number: 9 8 7 6 5 4 3 2 1

This book is dedicated to children like Joshua, Matthew, Alexandra,
and Preeta, and their eternal struggle to live with their failing hearts,
and who, with their parents, continually teach us not only about heart failure,
but also about life....

Contributors

RA-ID ABDULLA, MD
Associate Professor of Pediatrics, The University of
Chicago Pritzker School of Medicine; Director,
Pediatric Cardiology Fellowship, The University of
Chicago Hospitals and Clinics; Editor-in-Chief,
Pediatric Cardiology, Chicago, Illinois
Appendix I: Drug Formulary in Heart Failure

DEAN B. ANDROPOULOS, MD
Associate Professor of Anesthesiology and Pediatrics,
Baylor College of Medicine; Chief of Anesthesiology,
Director of the Arthur S. Keats Division of Pediatric
Cardiovascular Anesthesiology, and Kurt D. Groten, Sr.,
Family Chair in Pediatric Cardiovascular
Anesthesiology, Texas Children's Hospital, Houston,
Texas
Cardiovascular Receptors and Signaling in Heart Failure

CAROLYN A. ALTMAN, MD
Assistant Professor of Pediatrics, Baylor College of
Medicine; Associate, Department of Pediatric
Cardiology, Texas Children's Hospital, Houston, Texas
*Clinical Recognition of Congestive Heart Failure in
Children*

GAURAV ARORA, MD
Pediatric Cardiology Fellow, Baylor College of
Medicine and Texas Children's Hospital, Houston,
Texas
Cardiac Resynchronization Therapy and Heart Failure

DESMOND BOHN, MB, BCh, FRCPC
Professor of Anaesthesia and Paediatrics, University of
Toronto Faculty of Medicine; Department Chief,
Critical Care Medicine, The Hospital for Sick Children,
Toronto, Ontario, Canada
Inotropic Agents in Heart Failure

BEATRIZ BOUZAS-ZUBELDIA, MD
Cardiologist, Adult Congenital Heart Disease Unit,
Royal Brompton Hospital, London, United Kingdom
Valvular Insufficiency and Heart Failure

NEIL E. BOWLES, PhD
Assistant Professor of Pediatric Cardiology, Baylor
College of Medicine, Houston, Texas
Inflammatory Mediators in Heart Failure
Heart Failure and Mechanisms of Hypertrophy

JOHN P. BREINHOLT III, MD
Post Doctoral Fellow, Department of Pediatrics, Baylor
College of Medicine, and Division of Pediatric
Cardiology, Texas Children's Hospital, Houston, Texas
Classification of Types of Heart Failure

BRYAN C. CANNON, MD
Assistant Professor of Pediatrics, Baylor College of
Medicine; Associate, Department of Pediatric
Cardiology, Texas Children's Hospital, Houston, Texas
Dysrhythmias and Ventricular Dysfunction
*Sudden Death and Implantable Cardioverter Defibrillators in
Heart Failure*

JOSEPH A. CARCILLO, MD
Associate Professor of Critical Care Medicine and
Pediatrics, University of Pittsburgh School of Medicine;
Associate Director, Pediatric Intensive Care Unit,
Children's Hospital of Pittsburgh, Pittsburgh,
Pennsylvania
The Failing Cardiovascular System in Sepsis

ANTHONY C. CHANG, MD, MBA
Director, Pediatric Cardiac Intensive Care Program,
Texas Children's Hospital, Houston, Texas; Associate
Professor of Cardiology—Pediatrics; Chief,
Critical Care Cardiology, The Lillie Frank Abercrombie
Section of Cardiology, Baylor College of Medicine;
Attending Cardiologist, Texas Heart Institute,
Houston, Texas
*Molecular and Cellular Mechanisms in Myocardial
Dysfunction*
*Neurohumoral Axis and Natriuretic Peptides in
Heart Failure*
The Economic Aspects of Heart Failure
Right Ventricular Dysfunction in Congenital Heart Disease
Heart Failure in the Neonate
Diuretics
Phosphodiesterase Inhibitors
Catheter Device Therapy for Heart Failure
General Principles of Mechanical Cardiopulmonary Support
Long-Term Ventricular Assist Devices in Children
Appendix I: Drug Formulary in Heart Failure
*Appendix II: Selected Clinical Trials in Adult Heart Failure
Therapy*
Appendix III: Atlas of Circulatory Support Devices
Glossary of Heart Failure

MICHAEL CHEUNG, BSc(Hons), MB, ChB, MRCP
Staff Cardiologist, The Hospital for Sick Children,
Toronto, Ontario, Canada
Systolic and Diastolic Dysfunction

TAYLOR CHUNG, MD
Associate Professor of Radiology and Pediatrics, Baylor
College of Medicine; Radiologist, Edward B. Singleton
Department of Diagnostic Imaging, Texas Children's
Hospital, Houston, Texas
Magnetic Resonance Imaging Assessment in Heart Failure

SARAH K. CLUNIE, BSN, RN
Heart Transplant/Cardiomyopathy Coordinator,
Department of Pediatric Cardiology, Baylor College of
Medicine and Texas Children's Hospital, Houston, Texas
Nursing and Psychosocial Aspects of Heart Failure

GUL H. DADLANI, MD
Assistant Professor of Pediatrics, University of South
Florida School of Medicine, Tampa; Cardiologist,
Pediatric Cardiology Associates, St. Petersburg, Florida
Dilated Cardiomyopathy

SUSAN W. DENFIELD, MD
Assistant Professor of Pediatric Cardiology, Baylor
College of Medicine; Associate, Pediatric Cardiology,
and Faculty, Heart Failure and Cardiac Transplant,
Texas Children's Hospital, Houston, Texas
Restrictive Cardiomyopathy and Constrictive Pericarditis

CATHERINE L. DENT, MD
Assistant Professor of Clinical Pediatrics, University
of Cincinnati College of Medicine; Cardiologist,
Cincinnati Children's Hospital Medical Center,
Cincinnati, Ohio
Low Cardiac Output Syndrome in the Intensive Care Setting

DANIEL J. DIBARDINO, MD
Michael E. DeBakey Department of Surgery,
Baylor College of Medicine; Congenital
Heart Surgery Service Research Staff,
Texas Children's Hospital, Houston, Texas
Long-Term Ventricular Assist Devices in Children

HEATHER A. DICKERSON, MD
Senior Cardiac Intensive Care Fellow, Department of
Pediatrics, Baylor College of Medicine and Texas
Children's Hospital, Houston, Texas
Diuretics

VIVIAN DIMAS, MD
Pediatric Cardiology Fellow, Baylor College of
Medicine and Texas Children's Hospital, Houston, Texas
Catheter Device Therapy for Heart Failure

WILLIAM J. DREYER, MD
Associate Professor of Pediatric Cardiology, Baylor
College of Medicine; Medical Director, Cardiac
Transplant Program, Texas Children's Hospital,
Houston, Texas
Pediatric Heart Transplantation

BRIAN W. DUNCAN, MD
Surgical Director, Pediatric Cardiac Transplant and
Heart Failure, The Cleveland Clinic Foundation;
Associate Staff, Department of Pediatric and
Congenital Heart Surgery, The Children's Hospital
at the Cleveland Clinic, Cleveland, Ohio
*Short-Term Mechanical Cardiopulmonary
    Support Devices*

BENJAMIN W. EIDEM, MD
Assistant Professor of Pediatrics, Baylor College
of Medicine; Associate, Pediatric Cardiology,
Texas Children's Hospital, Houston, Texas
Echocardiographic Quantitation of Ventricular Function

TIMOTHY E. FELTES, MD
Chief, Pediatric Cardiology, University Hospital, The
Ohio State University Medical Center; Co-Director,
Heart Center, Columbus Children's Hospital,
Columbus, Ohio
The Alveolar-Capillary Interface and Pulmonary Edema

MARK A. FOGEL, MD, FACC, FAAP
Associate Professor of Pediatrics and Radiology,
University of Pennsylvania School of Medicine;
Director, Cardiac MRI and MRI Research, The
Children's Hospital of Philadelphia, Philadelphia,
Pennsylvania
Single Ventricle and Ventricular Performance

WAYNE J. FRANKLIN, MD
Fellow, Adult Congenital Cardiology, Department
of Adult Cardiovascular Medicine and Pediatric
Cardiology, Baylor College of Medicine; Fellow,
Adult Cardiology, St. Luke's Episcopal Hospital, and
Pediatric Cardiology, Texas Children's Hospital,
Houston, Texas
Heart Failure in Adults with Congenital Heart Disease

CHARLES D. FRASER, Jr., MD
Professor of Surgery and Pediatrics, Baylor College
of Medicine; Chief, Congenital Heart Surgery
Service, Texas Children's Hospital, Houston,
Texas
Surgical Strategies for the Failing Systemic Ventricle

O. H. FRAZIER, MD
Professor of Surgery, Department of Thoracic Surgery, University of Texas Medical School at Houston; Chief, Transplant Service, St. Luke's Episcopal Hospital; Director, Cardiovascular Surgical Research, Texas Heart Institute, Houston, Texas
Future of Mechanical Support Devices in Children and Young Adults

RICHARD FRIEDMAN, MD, MBA
Associate Professor of Pediatrics, Baylor College of Medicine; Director of Electrophysiology and Pacing, Texas Children's Hospital, Houston, Texas
Cardiac Resynchronization Therapy and Heart Failure

MICHAEL A. GATZOULIS, MD, PhD, FACC, FESC
Reader in Cardiology, National Heart and Lung Institute, Imperial College; Director, Adult Congenital Heart Unit, and Consultant Cardiologist, Royal Brompton Hospital, London, United Kingdom
Valvular Insufficiency and Heart Failure

TAL GEVA, MD
Associate Professor of Pediatric Radiology, Harvard Medical School; Senior Associate and Director, Cardiovascular MRI, Department of Cardiology, Children's Hospital, Boston, Massachusetts
Magnetic Resonance Imaging Assessment in Heart Failure

RONALD GRIFKA, MD, FAAP, FACC, FSCAI
Associate Professor of Pediatrics, Baylor College of Medicine; Director, Cardiac Catheterization Laboratories, and Clinical Director, Cardiology Division, Texas Children's Hospital, Houston, Texas
Assessment of Heart Failure by Cardiac Catheterization

HORDUR H. HARDARSON, MD
Pediatric Infectious Disease Fellow, Baylor College of Medicine and Texas Children's Hospital, Houston, Texas
Inflammatory Mediators in Heart Failure

WILLIAM G. HARMON, MD
Assistant Professor of Pediatrics, Division of Pediatric Cardiology and Critical Care Medicine, University of Rochester School of Medicine and Dentistry, Rochester, New York
Dilated Cardiomyopathy

MATTHEW T. HARTING, MD, MS
Resident, Department of Surgery, University of Texas Medical School at Houston, Houston, Texas
Future of Mechanical Support Devices in Children and Young Adults

JEFFREY S. HEINLE, MD
Assistant Professor of Surgery, Baylor College of Medicine; Associate Surgeon, Department of Congenital Heart Surgery, Texas Children's Hospital, Houston, Texas
Surgical Valve Intervention for Valve Failure

STEPHEN B. HORTON, PhD
Cardiologist, Cardiac Surgical Unit, The Royal Children's Hospital, Melbourne, Australia
Ventricular Assist Device Support in Pediatric Patients

JAMES C. HUHTA, MD
Professor and Daicoff-Andrews Chair in Perinatal Cardiology, Department of Pediatrics, and Professor, Department of Obstetrics and Gynecology, University of South Florida School of Medicine; Medical Director, Noninvasive Laboratory, All Children's Hospital, St. Petersburg, Florida
Heart Failure in the Fetus

JOHN LYNN JEFFERIES, MD, MPH
Fellow, Adult and Pediatric Cardiology, Baylor College of Medicine; Fellow, Pediatric Cardiology, Texas Children's Hospital; Fellow, Adult Cardiology, Texas Heart Institute and St. Luke's Episcopal Hospital, Houston, Texas
Neurohumoral Axis and Natriuretic Peptides in Heart Failure

RAJA JOSHI, MD
Clinical Fellow, Pediatric and Congenital Heart Surgery, The Children's Hospital at the Cleveland Clinic, Cleveland, Ohio
Short-Term Mechanical Cardiopulmonary Support Devices

HENRI JUSTINO, MD, CM, FRCPC, FACC
Assistant Professor of Pediatrics, Baylor College of Medicine; Associate in Cardiology, Texas Children's Hospital, Houston, Texas
Assessment of Heart Failure by Cardiac Catheterization

TOM R. KARL, MD
Professor of Surgery, University of California School of Medicine; Director of Pediatric Cardiothoracic Surgery, UCSF Children's Hospital, San Francisco, California
Ventricular Assist Device Support in Pediatric Patients

NAOMI J. KERTESZ, MD
Assistant Professor of Pediatrics, Baylor College of Medicine; Pediatrics, Section of Pediatric Cardiology, Texas Children's Hospital, Houston, Texas
Dysrhythmias and Ventricular Dysfunction
Sudden Death and Implantable Cardioverter Defibrillators in Heart Failure

JEFFREY KIM, MD
Pediatric Cardiology Fellow, Baylor College of Medicine
and Texas Children's Hospital, Houston, Texas
Glossary of Heart Failure

GRACE C. KUNG, MD
Assistant Professor of Pediatric Cardiology, David
Geffen School of Medicine at UCLA; Cardiologist,
Children's Hospital, Los Angeles, California
Clinical Recognition of Congestive Heart Failure in Children

GLENN T. LEONARD, Jr., MD
Interventional Fellow, Department of Pediatrics, Baylor
College of Medicine and Texas Children's Hospital,
Houston, Texas
Assessment of Heart Failure by Cardiac Catheterization

ALAN B. LEWIS, MD
Professor of Pediatrics, Keck School of Medicine of
USC; Attending Cardiologist, Children's Hospital, Los
Angeles, California
Acute Myocarditis

STEVEN E. LIPSHULTZ, MD
Professor and Chairman, Department of Pediatrics, and
Professor of Epidemiology and Public Health, and
Professor of Medicine (Oncology), University of Miami
Miller School of Medicine; Chief of Staff, Holtz
Children's Hospital of University of Miami-Jackson
Memorial Medical Center; Director, Batchelor
Children's Research Institute; Associate Director,
Mailman Institute for Child Development; Member,
Sylvester Comprehensive Cancer Center, Miami,
Florida
Dilated Cardiomyopathy

MATTHIAS LOEBE, MD, PhD
Associate Professor of Surgery, Michael E. DeBakey
Department of Surgery, Baylor College of Medicine;
Director, Perfusion Services, and Attending Surgeon,
Methodist DeBakey Heart Center, The Methodist
Hospital; Attending Transplant Surgeon, St. Luke's
Episcopal Hospital/Texas Heart Institute, Houston,
Texas
Appendix III: Atlas of Circulatory Support Devices

TARUN MAHAJAN, MD
Fellow, Department of Cardiology, Children's Hospital,
Boston, Boston, Massachusetts
Heart Failure in the Neonate

E. DEAN McKENZIE, MD, FACS
Assistant Professor of Surgery, Baylor College
of Medicine; Associate Surgeon, Department
of Congenital Heart Surgery, Texas Children's
Hospital, Houston, Texas
Long-Term Ventricular Assist Devices in Children
General Principles of Mechanical Cardiopulmonary Support

COLIN J. McMAHON, MD
Assistant Professor of Clinical Medicine and Pediatrics,
Department of Pediatrics, Baylor College of Medicine
and Texas Children's Hospital, Houston, Texas
Phosphodiesterase Inhibitors

WANDA C. MILLER-HANCE, MD
Associate Professor of Anesthesiology and Pediatrics,
Baylor College of Medicine; Pediatric Cardiovascular
Anesthesiologist and Pediatric Cardiologist, Texas
Children's Hospital, Houston, Texas
Valvular Stenosis and Heart Failure

BRADY S. MOFFETT, PharmD
Clinical Pharmacy Specialist, Pediatric Cardiology,
Texas Children's Hospital, Houston, Texas
New Drugs for Heart Failure
Appendix I: Drug Formulary in Heart Failure

DAVID L. S. MORALES, MD
Instructor of Surgery, Congenital Heart Surgery,
Baylor College of Medicine; Associate Surgeon,
Congenital Heart Surgery, Texas Children's Hospital,
Houston, Texas
Surgical Strategies for the Failing Systemic Ventricle

ANTONIO R. MOTT, MD
Assistant Professor of Pediatrics, Baylor College of
Medicine; Associate, Pediatric Cardiology, Texas
Children's Hospital, Houston, Texas
Classification of Types of Heart Failure

JONATHAN MYNARD, MD
Research Fellow, Department of Heart Research,
Murdoch Children's Research Institute,
Melbourne, Australia
The Pressure-Volume Relationship in Heart Failure

DAVID P. NELSON, MD, PhD
Associate Professor of Clinical Pediatrics, University of
Cincinnati College of Medicine; Co-Medical Director,
Cardiac Intensive Care Unit, Cincinnati Children's
Hospital Medical Center, Cincinnati, Ohio
Low Cardiac Output Syndrome in the Intensive
Care Setting

GEORGE P. NOON, MD
Chief, Division of Transplant and Assist Devices,
Department of Surgery, Methodist DeBakey Heart
Center, the Methodist Hospital; Executive Director,
Multi-Organ Transplant Center, The Methodist
Hospital, Houston, Texas
The Adult Experience with Long-Term Ventricular
Assist Devices

MONIQUE L. OGLETREE, PhD
Assistant Professor of Anesthesiology and Pediatrics,
Baylor College of Medicine; Director, Pediatric
Cardiovascular Anesthesiology Research Laboratory,
Texas Children's Hospital, Houston, Texas
Cardiovascular Receptors and Signaling in Heart Failure

DANIEL J. PENNY, MD, PhD
Professor of Pediatrics, University of Melbourne
Faculty of Medicine; Director of Cardiology, The Royal
Children's Hospital, Melbourne, Australia
The Pressure-Volume Relationship in Heart Failure

ANDREW J. POWELL, MD
Associate, Department of Cardiology, Children's
Hospital Boston, Boston, Massachusetts
Magnetic Resonance Imaging Assessment in Heart Failure

JACK F. PRICE, MD
Assistant Professor of Pediatric Cardiology, Baylor
College of Medicine; Attending Physician, Cardiac
Critical Care and Heart Failure/Transplantation
Services, Texas
Children's Hospital, Houston, Texas
Outpatient Management of Pediatric Heart Failure

BRANISLAV RADOVANCEVIC, MD
Associate Director, Cardiovascular Surgery and
Transplant Research, Texas Heart Institute,
Houston, Texas
*The Adult Experience with Long-Term Ventricular
   Assist Devices*

ANDREW N. REDINGTON, MD, FRCP
Professor of Pediatrics, Department of Medicine,
University of Toronto Faculty of Medicine; Head of
Cardiology, Department of Pediatrics, The Hospital
for Sick Children, Toronto, Ontario, Canada
Systolic and Diastolic Dysfunction

ROBERT E. SHADDY, MD
L. George Veasy Professor of Pediatrics, University of
Utah School of Medicine; Division Chief, Pediatric
Cardiology, University of Utah Hospital; Medical
Director, Heart Failure and Heart Transplant Program,
Department of Pediatric Cardiology, Primary Children's
Medical Center, Salt Lake City, Utah
β-Adrenergic Receptor Blockade

FELIX R. SHARDONOFSKY, MD
Associate Professor of Pediatrics, Department of
Pediatrics, UT Southwestern Medical School; Associate,
Pediatric Respiratory Medicine Division, University
of Texas Southwestern Medical Center at Dallas,
and Children's Medical Center, Dallas, Texas
Heart Failure in Pediatric Pulmonary Diseases

TIMOTHY C. SLESNICK, MD
Pediatric Cardiology Fellow, Baylor College
of Medicine and Texas Children's Hospital,
Houston, Texas
Right Ventricular Dysfunction in Congenital Heart Disease

FRANK W. SMART, MD
Director, Advanced Heart Failure/Cardiac
Transplantation, Texas Heart Institute, Houston, Texas
*Appendix II: Selected Clinical Trials in Adult Heart Failure
   Therapy*

THOMAS L. SPRAY, MD
Chief, Cardiothoracic Surgery, The Children's Hospital
of Philadelphia, Philadelphia, Pennsylvania
Valvular Stenosis and Heart Failure

STEPHEN A. STAYER, MD
Professor of Anesthesiology and Pediatrics, Baylor
College of Medicine; Associate Director, Pediatric
Anesthesiology, Texas Children's Hospital, Houston,
Texas
Use of Vasodilators in Heart Failure

TIA A. TORTORIELLO, MD
Assistant Professor of Pediatrics, University of Texas
Southwestern Medical School; Cardiologist,
Children's Medical Center of Dallas,
Dallas, Texas
Hemodynamic Adaptive Mechanisms in Heart Failure

JEFFREY A. TOWBIN, MD, FAAP, FACC, FAHA
Professor, Departments of Pediatrics (Pediatric
Cardiology) and Molecular and Human Genetics,
Baylor College of Medicine; Chief, Pediatric
Cardiology; Director, Phoebe Willingham Muzzy
Pediatric Molecular Cardiology Laboratory,
Heart Failure and Cardiomyopathy Service, Texas
Children's Hospital, Houston, Texas
Hypertrophic Cardiomyopathy

GERALD TULZER, MD, PhD
Head, Department of Pediatric Cardiology, Children's
Heart Center Linz, Linz, Austria
Heart Failure in the Fetus

JESUS G. VALLEJO, MD
Assistant Professor of Pediatrics and Medicine, Winters
Center for Heart Failure Research, Baylor College of
Medicine; Attending Physician, Department of
Pediatric Infectious Diseases, Texas Children's
Hospital, Houston, Texas
Inflammatory Mediators in Heart Failure
Heart Failure and Mechanisms of Hypertrophy

MATTEO VATTA, PhD
Assistant Professor of Pediatric Cardiology, Baylor
College of Medicine; Attending, Department of
Cardiology, Texas Children's Hospital, Houston, Texas;
Department of Reproductive and Developmental
Science, University of Trieste School of Medicine,
Trieste, Italy
Molecular and Cellular Mechanisms in Myocardial
   Dysfunction
Heart Failure and Mechanisms of Hypertrophy

BOJAN VRTOVEC, MD, PhD
Associate Professor of Internal Medicine, University
of Ljubljana Faculty of Medicine; Clinical Cardiologist
and Medical Director, Cardiac Transplantation
Program, Ljubljana University Medical Center,
Ljubljana, Slovenia
The Adult Experience with Long-Term Ventricular
   Assist Devices

WEI WANG, MD, PhD
Professor of Pediatrics, Shanghai Second Medical
University; Attending, Department of Pediatric
Thoracic and Cardiovascular Surgery, Shanghai
Children's Medical Center, Shanghai, People's Republic
of China
Appendix III: Atlas of Circulatory Support Devices

GARY D. WEBB, MD, FRCPC, FACC
Professor of Medicine, University of Toronto Faculty of
Medicine; Director, Toronto Congenital Cardiac Centre
and The Bitove Family Professor of Adult Congenital
Heart Disease, Toronto General Hospital, Toronto,
Ontario, Canada
Heart Failure in Adults with Congenital Heart Disease

STEVEN A. WEBBER, MBChB
Medical Director, Pediatric Heart and Heart-Lung
Transplantation, Division of Cardiology,
Children's Hospital; Associate Professor of Pediatrics,
University of Pittsburgh, Pittsburgh, Pennsylvania
Pediatric Heart Transplantation

Foreword

Section 1: Basic Science of Heart Failure

Although tremendous strides have been made in terms of our understanding of the basic mechanisms and management of adult heart failure, comparatively less is known about the pathophysiology and management of heart failure in children and young adults. In an effort to address this critical deficiency, Chang and Towbin have assembled a talented group of clinicians and scientists who, for the first time, summarize the state of the art in the field of heart failure in children and young adults. Section 1 of their splendid textbook begins with a careful and thoughtful overview of the basic science of heart failure. The section begins logically with a chapter on the molecular mechanisms of heart failure, followed by insightful chapters on receptor signaling and inflammatory cascades in heart failure. Following this, a series of three chapters delineate the adaptive responses of the failing heart, including cellular adaptations and neurohormonal responses. Section 1 then segues naturally into the consequences of heart failure, including two incisive chapters on left ventricular mechanics and a chapter on mechanisms of pulmonary edema. The remaining chapters of Section 1 focus on how clinicians and scientists assess heart failure invasively and noninvasively. The chapters are well written and are masterfully edited. Section 1 of Chang and Towbin's *Heart Failure in Children and Young Adults: From Molecular Mechanisms to Medical and Surgical Strategies* goes beyond what we have learned about heart failure in adults and provides important new insights into elucidation of the pathogenesis and recognition of heart failure in children and young adults. Accordingly, this textbook is essential reading for the trainees, clinicians, and scientists who are involved in understanding and treating this important group of patients.

DOUGLAS L. MANN, MD
Mary and Gordon Chair and Professor
Department of Medicine
Director
Winters Center for Heart Failure
  Research
Baylor College of Medicine
Staff Physician
Michael E. DeBakey Veterans Affairs
  Medical Center

Foreword

Section 2: Clinical Diagnosis and Management of Pediatric Heart Failure

Heart failure is now well recognized as a leading cause of death and morbidity in adults. Surprisingly, there is still no agreement on how best to define the condition, despite the fact that pragmatic definitions such as that offered by the great British practitioner Mackenzie*—namely, "the condition in which the heart is unable to meet the efforts necessary to the daily life of the individual"—have now existed for almost a century. Despite the burgeoning interest in the condition in adults, appreciably less concern has been shown for the syndrome as it exists in children.

All of this has now changed, since we now have this splendid compilation edited by Anthony Chang and Jeffrey Towbin. The approach taken by Chang and Towbin is encyclopedic. They have been kind enough to ask me to prepare the foreword to their second section, concerned with "Clinical Diagnosis and Management." I am unsure why a morphologist should be accorded this signal honor, since the anatomic signs of the failing myocardium remain stubbornly hidden. It is of interest that their introductory section, concerned with "Basic Science," has no chapter devoted specifically to morphology, albeit that cellular changes receive appropriate emphasis. It also may be of interest to remember that, when Sunao Tawara came from Japan to study with Ludwig Aschoff at the turn of the twentieth century, his task was to discover the anatomic substrate for the failing heart! In this, he admitted his total lack of success. But since his discoveries uncovered the existence of the atrioventricular conduction axis, there was suitable recompense. It should be mentioned that Anthony invited me to prepare a purely anatomic chapter for the first section of the book, but I did not consider that I could do the topic justice. When I now review the overall scope, I can see that my decision was correct, but I am pleased to have the opportunity of penning this short foreword.

The initial section of Chang and Towbin's book is a summary of the huge advances that have now been made in our understanding of the molecular and cellular aspects of the failing myocardium. In this second section, an equally impressive number of chapters have been solicited from virtually all of the authorities who have investigated this growing area. Thus, we move from epidemiologic and economic aspects, through detailed coverage of the various conditions associated with the failing heart, to the information needed to appreciate the condition as seen in the outpatient setting, or by the nursing profession. There is, therefore, something in this section for everyone. And that is not all! The book itself then continues with further sections, each with its own introduction, devoted first to medical and then to surgical aspects of treatment.

Anthony and Jeffrey deserve all our thanks for embarking on this ambitious project. I know from long experience how difficult it is to prise worthwhile chapters from busy authors. All of the authors writing for this book will be very busy, since they represent the cutting edge of research into this increasingly important area of pediatric cardiology. The chapters I have been able to read in their draft forms are truly authoritative. I cannot wait to see the whole project in its completed version. I predict that this will become the classic textbook in the field and should pass through several editions. It is my privilege and pleasure to have been asked to make my own small contribution. On behalf of all the future readers, I thank Anthony, Jeffrey, and all of their contributors for their hard work. It is much needed, and greatly appreciated.

Robert H. Anderson
Joseph Levy Professor of Paediatric
  Cardiac Morphology
Cardiac Unit
Institute of Child Health
University College, London
United Kingdom

*Mackenzie J: Disease of the Heart. London, Oxford Medical Publications, 1913.

Foreword

Section 3: Medical Treatment for Pediatric Heart Failure

Heart failure is the major problem in cardiovascular disease generally. Great progress has been made in elucidating basic mechanisms and in developing clinical therapies for adults with heart failure, although there are still great needs. Several of the etiologies for heart failure in children are now understood, but the treatment of heart failure is considerably more difficult. In Section 3, Drs. Chang and Towbin have brought together physician-scientist experts to discuss the state of the art in the medical treatment of heart failure in children. A broad spectrum of topics is reviewed, including the use of vasodilators and ACE inhibitors, beta blockers, inotropic agents, diuretics, and phosphodiesterase inhibitors. New drugs that are in the future for treatment of heart failure in children also are reviewed, as are transcatheter therapies for heart failure.

The medical treatment of heart failure in children is an area in which major advances need to occur in the future. One expects these advances to be based on improved insight into basic mechanisms that lead to heart failure, the development of new drugs that are specifically targeted to correct fundamental abnormalities in cellular and subcellular functions, and new and improved therapies for conditions due to infectious agents, including viruses, that lead to heart failure in children. One also anticipates a continuing development of interventional therapies that will include left ventricular assist devices and cardiac transplantation procedures that are adapted for use in children and that become progressively safer and more effective. One also anticipates the development of cell-based transplantation procedures in the future, including stem cell therapies, that will be an integral part of the medical treatment of heart failure in the coming years.

Section 3 identifies the state-of-the-art practice in the medical treatment of heart failure in children, with each of the chapters written by experts in their fields. This review will be of interest to all who care for children with cardiovascular disease and deal with this most difficult problem of heart failure.

JAMES T. WILLERSON, MD
President, The University of Texas
   Health Science Center at Houston
President-Elect, Texas Heart Institute
Alkek-Williams Distinguished
   Professor, The University of Texas
   Health Science Center at Houston

Foreword

Section 4: Cardiac Surgery and Pediatric Heart Failure

Heart failure in adults has long been recognized as a major clinical problem, requiring the establishment in many major academic health institutions and clinics of heart failure centers. With about a half-million new cases occurring annually in the United States, this condition assumes increasing importance. Great strides have been made in a better understanding of the pathophysiology and molecular mechanism, leading to considerable improvement in the clinical care of these patients. Despite these advances, the problem remains a serious clinical challenge in effective management.

In children, this problem is even more difficult. For this reason, this textbook by Anthony Chang and Jeffrey Towbin is of signal importance in providing all medical professionals interested in this field with comprehensive state-of-the-art knowledge on this topic, ranging from the underlying molecular mechanisms of heart failure to clinical management.

The final Section 4 of the textbook brings together the most up-to-date version of the surgical treatment of pediatric heart failure patients, ranging from valvuloplasty to heart transplantation. Particularly significant are the chapters dealing with both short-term and long-term mechanical support of the failing heart. This field of growing interest and importance, clearly of clinical significance, has lagged behind the adult experience. In addition to the chapters contributed by Dr. Chang himself, he has gathered experts in other fields to make this section one of the most useful and comprehensively up to date in this more recent endeavor in the management of heart failure in children and young adults. This excellent and useful textbook covers a relatively new and important clinical problem in an authoritative and comprehensive manner.

MICHAEL E. DeBAKEY, MD
Chancellor Emeritus
Olga Keith Wiess and Distinguished
   Service Professor
Michael E. DeBakey Department of
   Surgery
Director, DeBakey Heart Center
Baylor College of Medicine
Houston, Texas

Preface

As we successfully manage, not cure, patients with heart disease, the damage to their heart muscle persists....The stage is now set for a large increase in heart failure, the last great battleground of cardiac disease.
Eugene Braunwald
2003

These words of the preeminent adult cardiologist Eugene Braunwald portend the oncoming clinical paradigm shift in pediatric cardiology. After decades of heralded success in palliative and corrective surgery, accompanied by concomitant advances in interventional catheterization and cardiac intensive care, children no longer routinely succumb to lethal congenital heart defects. As in adults, however, there is a growing epidemic of chronic heart failure in children and young adults worldwide. It is now the dawn of a new field of heart failure in children and young adults, and time for learning a new lexicon (such as phospholamban and apoptosis, B-type natriuretic peptide and strain rate imaging, levosimendan and the MUSTIC trial, and Acorn device and DeBakey VAD) for the pediatric practitioners.

For the first time, heart failure in children and young adults is focused in a single volume. This textbook gathers the world's leading experts in the diagnosis and treatment of heart failure in neonates, children, and adolescents. The content provides a current state-of-the-art overview and new developments on diagnosis and management of children and young adults with heart failure, from molecular mechanisms in research to medical and surgical treatment strategies in both the intensive care and outpatient settings.

This comprehensive and balanced textbook of 50 chapters is especially designed for all cardiac surgeons, intensivists, anesthesiologists, neonatologists, perfusionists, physician assistants, and nurses who care for fetuses, neonates, children, and young adults with heart failure, as well as pediatric and adult cardiologists. The first International Conference on Heart Failure in Children and Young Adults, held in December 2003 in Houston, with over 500 international attendees, provided the essential beginnings of many of the key topics covered in this book. The distinguished contributing authors are from the diverse specialties of pediatric and adult cardiology and cardiac surgery, pediatric critical care medicine, pediatric cardiac anesthesia, pediatric pulmonary, pediatric nursing, and the disciplines of molecular biology and cardiac pharmacology. The authors were first asked to submit detailed outlines before their completed works, in order to minimize overlap of material among chapters. In addition, we realize that heart failure is a rapidly growing discipline, and the body of knowledge is evolving at an accelerating pace, so we have continually included the most current references of seminal importance, as well as additional discussions even at the final proof stage.

The first section of the book focuses on the basic science aspects of heart failure. Chapters on molecular biology, neurohormonal alterations, receptor physiology, remodeling and hypertrophy, and pressure-volume loops, as well as state-of-the-art evaluation methodologies of heart failure, provide an in-depth primer for the later sections on clinical and therapeutic aspects of heart failure. The role of molecular biology in the 21st century understanding of heart failure is becoming increasingly obvious; accordingly, a substantial proportion of the text is focused on this area. Dr. Douglas L. Mann, an adult heart failure and molecular cardiologist with a textbook of his own on heart failure in adults, penned an inspiring foreword for this section.

The second section, with a generous foreword by the scholarly Professor Robert H. Anderson, describes the clinical aspects of heart failure in all types of patients, from the fetus to the adult with congenital heart disease. This section completes a bench-to-bedside unity with the preceding section, and consolidates the essential underpinnings of the clinical aspects of heart failure in children and young adults.

The third and fourth sections focus on the medical and surgical strategies, respectively. Dr. James T. Willerson is a venerable authority on adult cardiology and heart failure and kindly provided an insightful introduction for the medical therapy section. Much of the material in this section was strongly influenced by pioneering work on heart failure by adult cardiologists.

Dr. Michael E. DeBakey, with his invaluable wisdom and academic vitality, inspired the fourth section, on the surgical strategies for heart failure. This section brings an emphasis on the myriad of mechanical support devices that will be a crucial part of the management strategy in the future for children and young adults with end-stage heart failure.

Last, we have provided three key appendices—a heart failure drug formulary, a summary of adult clinical trials, a mechanical assist device atlas, and a glossary of heart failure vocabulary—to supplement the main text as particularly useful references for the reader.

Through the millennia, Hippocrates, Galen, Harvey, and Starling all elucidated and described heart failure in the adult. There remains an alarming paucity of writing and data, however, in the clinical area of heart failure in children and young adults. We hope that this textbook will provide a substantive intellectual nascence for this field.

One of the most urgent challenges for the field of pediatric heart failure is to organize investigative trials in children, as has already been achieved in adults. Pediatric health care practitioners all must unite and learn from the successful adult trials that have wisely utilized government funding, data coordination centers, and office of human research protection. Another critical challenge is to identify and support physician and nurse champions for surgical assist devices, to overcome the innate bias in the small market of device therapy in children.

The aforementioned challenges are supremely daunting, and in the memorable words of Gene Krantz, the famed NASA director of flight command at the time of the Apollo 13 flight disaster, our ongoing and future quest to care for and cure children and young adults with heart failure should share the same mantra:

"Failure is not an option."

ANTHONY C. CHANG, MD
JEFFREY A. TOWBIN, MD

Acknowledgments

A textbook of this scope would not be possible without the ardent support of the numerous authors and colleagues at Texas Children's Hospital, as well as other collaborating pediatric and adult institutions. We would be remiss not to express our deep gratitude to our adult colleagues here at the Texas Medical Center who have provided a collective guiding light for our intellectual curiosity about heart failure. The authoritative experts all have provided their special insights and intellectual capital in this book, despite their busy schedules and numerous commitments, and for this we are grateful.

We would like to thank Elsevier and its exemplary cast of editors, assistants, and project managers, especially Anne Lenehan, Susan Pioli, Vera Ginsburgs, Natalie Ware, and Jeffrey Gunning for their utmost patience and exceptional collaboration. We also would like to acknowledge the tireless dedication of Cristina Chilton, who provided much of the administrative support throughout this process.

ANTHONY C. CHANG, MD, MBA

JEFFREY A. TOWBIN, MD

Contents

Color section immediately follows frontmatter.

SECTION 3

Medical Treatment for Pediatric Heart Failure

SECTION 4

Cardiac Surgery and Pediatric Heart Failure

Heart Failure in Children
and Young Adults

Color Figures

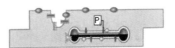

Decreased in SERCA2 activity
Decrease SERCA2 protein
Altered SERCA2 Ca sensitivity/regulation

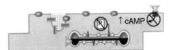

Increased PLB inhibition of SERCA
Increased PLB abundance
Decrease PLB modulation
  • Decreased b-signaling/cAMP
  • Prevention of phosphorylation by
    residue mutations
Abnormal targeting to cAMP anchoring
  proteins

A

B

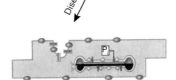

Normal cardiac myocyte with the proper abundance
of calcium regulatory molecules and normal activity.
This allows for highly regulated cardiac function and
contractile reserve.

▧▨ L-type Ca²⁺ channel
◉ NCX
† PLB
▷ RYR
◌ SERCA2

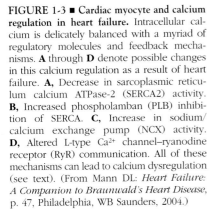

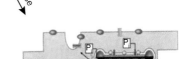

Increase in NCX activity
Increase NCX
Altered NCX distribution
Altered [Na⁺]ᵢ
Abnormalities in Na⁺/K⁺ ATPase activity
Altered NCX Na⁺/Ca²⁺ sensitivity/
  regulation

C

Altered I$_{Ca,L}$-RYR communication
Increase SL-SR membrane distance
Altered distribution of I$_{Ca,L}$ channels
  in the t-tubule
Deranged I$_{Ca,L}$ regulation
RYR phosphorylation

D

FIGURE 1-3 ■ **Cardiac myocyte and calcium regulation in heart failure.** Intracellular calcium is delicately balanced with a myriad of regulatory molecules and feedback mechanisms. **A** through **D** denote possible changes in this calcium regulation as a result of heart failure. **A,** Decrease in sarcoplasmic reticulum calcium ATPase-2 (SERCA2) activity. **B,** Increased phospholamban (PLB) inhibition of SERCA. **C,** Increase in sodium/calcium exchange pump (NCX) activity. **D,** Altered L-type Ca²⁺ channel–ryanodine receptor (RyR) communication. All of these mechanisms can lead to calcium dysregulation (see text). (From Mann DL: *Heart Failure: A Companion to Braunwald's Heart Disease,* p. 47, Philadelphia, WB Saunders, 2004.)

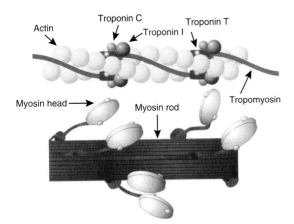

FIGURE 1-5 ■ **Essential contractile proteins.** The thick filament comprises the myosin heavy chains. The globular heads of the myosin molecules project outward to form cross-bridges. The thin filament is made of actin, but tropomyosin binds to troponin T at various sites along the thin filament. This interaction inhibits the actin-myosin interaction. (From Sprito P, Seidman CE, McKenna WJ, et al: *The management of hypertrophic cardiomyopathy.* N Engl J Med 1997; 336:775-785.)

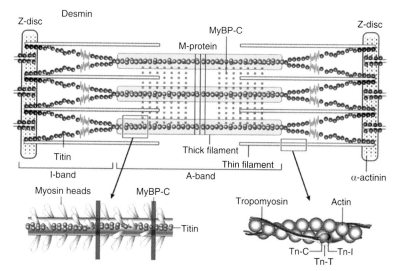

FIGURE 1-6 ■ Contractile apparatus. In addition to thin and thick filaments, the sarcomere has several other important proteins, such as titin, desmin, myosin binding protein C (*MyBP-C*), and α-actinin, which provide stability and flexibility to the sarcomere (see text for details). Tn-C, troponin C; Tn-I, troponin I; Tn-T, troponin T. (From Mann DL: *Heart Failure: A Companion to Braunwald's Heart Disease.* Philadelphia, WB Saunders, 2004.)

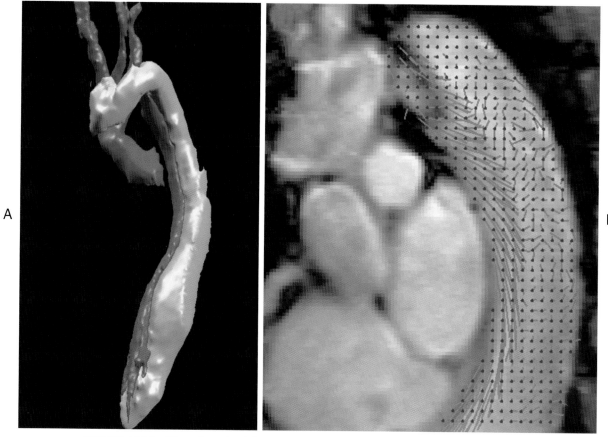

FIGURE 11-10 ■ Three-dimensional flow vector mapping. Aortic dissection in a patient with Marfan syndrome. **A,** Color-coded reconstruction of gadolinium-enhanced three-dimensional magnetic resonance angiography of the aorta. The true aortic lumen is coded in red and the false lumen in yellow. **B,** Systolic frame of three-dimensional flow vector mapping in the descending aorta. Note the streamline flow vectors in the true lumen and the low-velocity (shorter vectors) swirling flow (vectors oriented in different directions) in the false lumen.

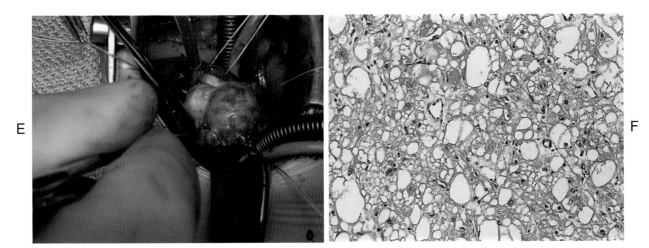

FIGURE 11-11 ■ E, Intraoperative photograph of the tumor confirms the MRI characterization of the tumor location, size, and morphology. F, Histology of the tumor shows features of rhabdomyoma (hematoxylin-eosin stain).

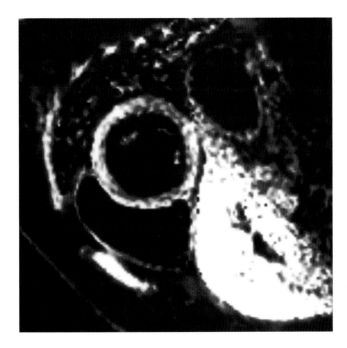

FIGURE 11-14 ■ MRI tissue characterization. Color-coded T2* map of myocardial iron load in a patient with thalassemia. Signal is brighter in the liver compared with the myocardium, indicating higher iron concentration in the liver (see text for discussion).

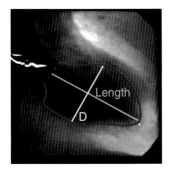

$$V = \pi/6 \, LD^2$$

FIGURE 12-1 ■ Ventricular volume determination: area-length method. On the left, a right anterior oblique view of the left ventriculogram at end diastole, with manually traced endocardial outline and calculated axial length and diameter (D). On the right, left ventricular volume represented as an ellipsoid with major diameter (L) and minor diameter (D). In this example, only one plane is used. (From Sheehan FH: http:/www.avnrt.com/docs/arealen.jpg.)

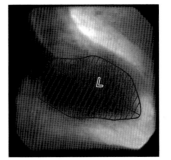

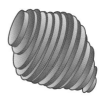

$$V = \Sigma_{i=1}^{n} \, \pi/4 \, D_i^2 \, \Delta L$$

FIGURE 12-2 ■ Simpson rule method for left ventricular volume. On the left, a right anterior oblique view of the left ventriculogram at end diastole, with manually traced endocardial outline and calculated axial length (L) subdivided into segments. On the right, representation of left ventricular volume as the summed volumes of graduated discs with diameter (D_i) and thickness ΔL_i. The Riemann sum of the disc volumes is processed according to the Simpson rule, allowing for a smooth (not stepped) endocardial curvature. (From Sheehan FH: http:/www.avnrt.com/docs/arealen.jpg.)

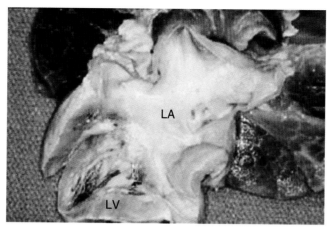

FIGURE 19-1 ■ **Restrictive cardiomyopathy.** The left atrium (LA) is massively dilated, dwarfing the size of the left ventricle (LV), in this autopsy specimen from a patient with restrictive cardiomyopathy.

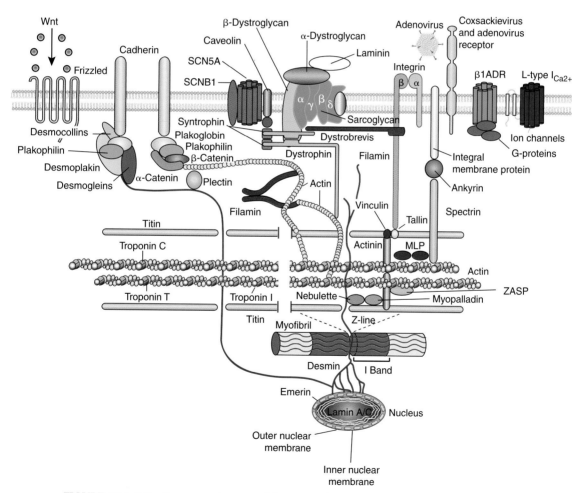

FIGURE 20-1 ■ **Cardiac myocyte cytoarchitecture.** Schematic of the interactions between dystrophin and the dystrophin-associated proteins in the sarcolemma and intracellular cytoplasm (dystroglycans, sarcoglycans, syntrophins, dystrobrevin, sarcospan) at the carboxy-terminal end of the dystrophin. The integral membrane proteins interact with the extracellular matrix via α-dystroglycan-laminin α2 connections. The amino-terminus of dystrophin binds actin and connects dystrophin with the sarcomere intracellularly, the sarcolemma, and the extracellular matrix. Additional sarcolemmal proteins include ion channels, adrenergic receptors, integrins, and the coxsackie and adenoviral receptors. Cell-cell junctions, including cadherins and the plakin and other desmosomal family proteins, also are notable. Also shown is the interaction between intermediate filament proteins (i.e., desmin) with the nucleus. MLP, muscle LIM protein.

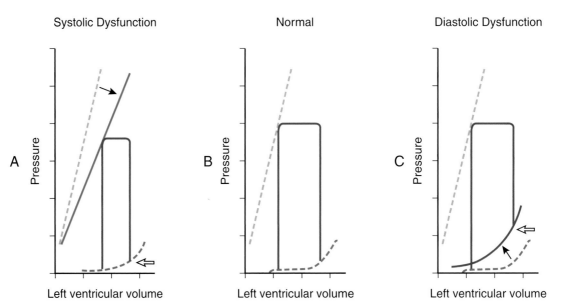

Sarcomeric Assembly

Z-Disc
alpha-Actinin Ankyrin
Desmin
Capz Obscurin
S100
Myopalladin
Troponin
Tropomyosin Actin
CARP MLP

Titin Myosin Non-muscle Nebulette Myopodin
myosin II ALP
43 nm T-Cap Mink
gamma-Filamin Calsarcin Cypher
Calcineurin PKC Myostatin

FIGURE 20-2 ▪ Z-disc architecture. The Z-disc of the sarcomere comprises multiple interacting proteins that anchor the sarcomere. The proteins involved in the Z-disc structure include α-actinin, MLP, Cypher (ZASP), and others. ALP, actinin-associated LIM protein; CapZ, actin capping protein; MLP, muscle LIM protein; T-Cap, telethonin. (From Pyle WG, Solaro RJ: At the crossroads of myocardial signaling: The role of Z-discs in intracellular signaling and cardiac function. Circ Res 2004;94:296-305.)

Systolic Dysfunction   Normal   Diastolic Dysfunction

A   B   C

Pressure   Pressure   Pressure

Left ventricular volume   Left ventricular volume   Left ventricular volume

FIGURE 20-4 ▪ Left ventricular pressure volume loops in systolic and diastolic dysfunction. In systolic dysfunction, left ventricular contractility is depressed, and the end-systolic pressure volume line is displaced downward and to the right (*black arrow* in **A**); as a result, there is a diminished capacity to eject blood into the high-pressure aorta. **B** is the pressure-volume loop in normal hearts. In diastolic dysfunction, the diastolic pressure volume line is displaced upward and to the left (*black arrow* in **C**), and the end-diastolic pressure is normal (*open arrow* in **A**); in diastolic dysfunction, the ejection fraction is normal, and the end-diastolic pressure is elevated (*open arrow* in **C**).

Hypertrophic Cardiomyopathy:
A Disease of the Sarcomere

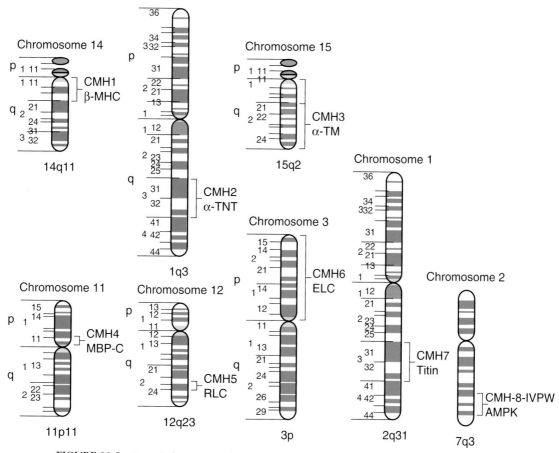

FIGURE 20-5 ■ **Genetic location of hypertrophic cardiomyopathy–causing genes.**

LV Noncompaction

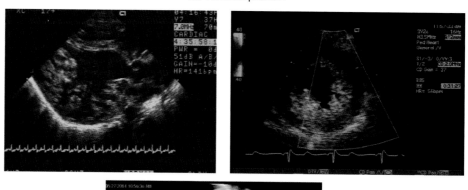

FIGURE 20-7 ■ **Echocardiographic features of left ventricular noncompaction.** *Top left panel,* Parasternal long-axis view shows a hypertrophic posterior left ventricular wall with a moth-eaten pattern. The left ventricular chamber is small. *Top right panel,* Parasternal short-axis view with color Doppler shows hypertrophy of the left ventricular apex with deep trabeculations filled with blood (red flow). *Bottom panel,* Subxiphoid view.

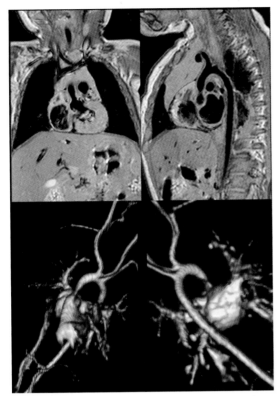

FIGURE 22-3 ■ Supravalvar aortic stenosis. *Top panel,* Coronal *(left)* and sagittal *(right)* spin MRI scans show the characteristic area of narrowing above the sinuses of Valsalva in supravalvar aortic stenosis. The discrete area of obstruction, just distal to the origin of the coronary arteries, is shown. *Bottom panel,* Three-dimensional rendered MRI scans from gadolinium-enhanced contrast injection in two different long-axis projections further define the aortic pathology and the anatomy of surrounding structures.

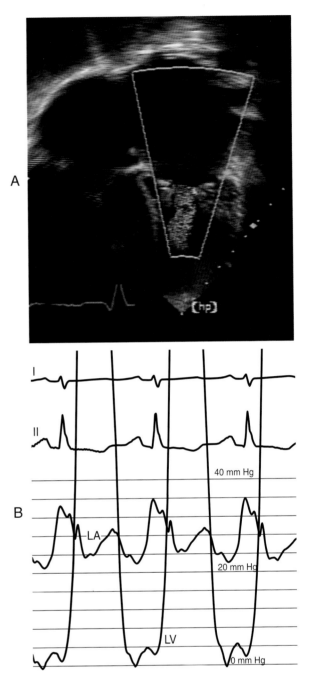

FIGURE 22-5 ■ Mitral stenosis. A, Four-chamber transthoracic echocardiogram in a child with rheumatic mitral stenosis displaying aliased, disturbed flow across the restrictive valvar orifice by color Doppler interrogation. **B,** Pressure tracings obtained at cardiac catheterization during transcatheter intervention. A large diastolic pressure gradient is identified between the left atrium (LA) and left ventricle (LV).

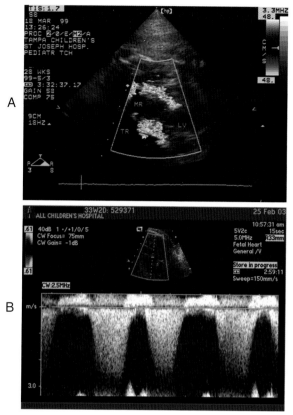

FIGURE 25-5 ■ **Mitral regurgitation (MR) and tricuspid regurgitation (TR) result in a massively enlarged heart. A,** The atrioventricular valve regurgitation fills the entire chest. **B,** The slow upstroke of the MR jet is shown by continuous-wave Doppler in an apical view. LV, left ventricle.

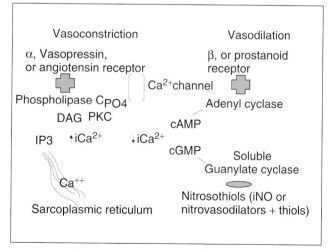

FIGURE 29-3 ■ **Vasoconstrictors and vasodilators stimulate opposing second messenger systems.** α-Adrenergic agonists, angiotensin, and vasopressin stimulate different receptors, which stimulate the production of inositol triphosphate (IP3) and diacylglycerol (DAG), leading to increased inducible calcium (iCa²⁺) and contraction. β₂-Agonists and vasodilator prostanoids stimulate cAMP production, and nitroso-vasodilators and inducible nitric oxide (iNO) stimulate GMP production. These second messengers decrease iCa²⁺ and induce vasodilation. Type III and type V phosphodiesterase inhibitors can potentiate the effect of vasodilators

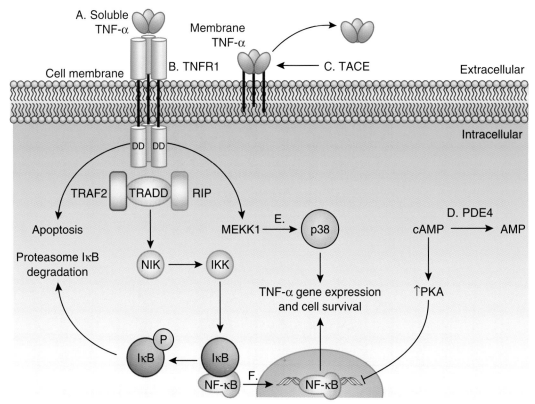

FIGURE 38-4 ■ **Potential targets for the inhibition of tumor necrosis factor (TNF)-α signaling pathways or protein expression.** Given the complexity of TNF-α signaling and the various mechanisms associated with the regulation of TNF expression, there are many potential targets for the inhibition of TNF-related activities. Some protein-based inhibitors target the TNF-α molecule or its receptor (**A** and **B**), which prevents the resultant signaling pathways. Additional targets include TNF-converting enzyme (TACE) (**C**), which processes the 26-κDa membrane form of TNF-α to the soluble 17-κDa form, preventing its release into the circulation. Molecules targeting intracellular TNF-related signaling pathways also have been identified, including inhibitors of phosphodiesterase 4 (PDE4) (**D**) and p38 (**E**). Additionally, nuclear factor-κB (NF-κB) inhibitors include molecules targeting the activities of upstream signaling events involved in the initial activation of NF-κB (NF-κB-inducing kinase [NIK], inhibitor of NF-κB [IB] kinase [IKK], IB degradation). Inhibition of the activation of NF-κB (**F**) prevents the synthesis of NF-κB inducible genes, which include many proinflammatory cytokines and other important inflammation-related proteins. NF-κB inhibition also can promote cell death in certain sensitive cell types, including cancers, suggesting the use of NF-κB inhibitors as potential cancer therapeutics. DD, death domain; MEKK1, mitogen-activated protein kinase 1; PKA, protein kinase A; RIP, receptor-interacting protein; TNFR1, TNF receptor 1; TRADD, TNFR1-associated death domain–containing protein; TRAF2, TNFR-associated factor 2. (From Palladino MA, Bahjat FR, Theodorakis EA, Moldawer LL: *Anti-TNF-alpha therapies: The next generation. Nat Rev Drug Discov* 2003;2:736-746.)

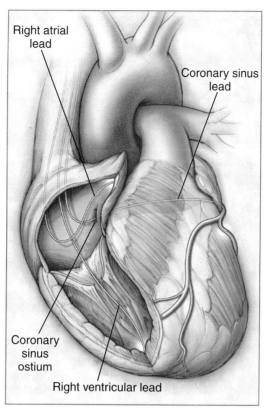

FIGURE 39-2 ■ **Cardiac resynchronization therapy with leads in place.** The three leads of cardiac resynchronization therapy are seen in the right atrium, right ventricle, and coronary sinus (to function as the left ventricle pacing lead). (Courtesy of Guidant, Indianapolis, IN.)

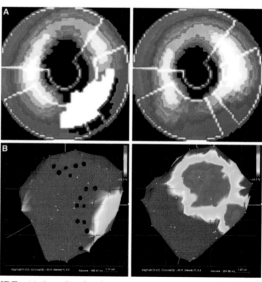

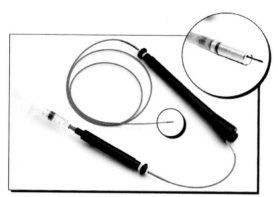

FIGURE 40-4 ■ **The NOGA Myostar injection catheter.** The catheter is seen with the needle in the extended position *(inset)*. The catheter is advanced into the left ventricle, and the catheter tip is placed against the endocardial surface with the needle extended into the myocardium to deliver the cells. (From Perin EC, Dohmann HF, Borojevic R, et al: *Transendocardial autologous bone marrow cell transplantation in severe, chronic ischemic heart failure. Circulation* 2003;107:2294-2302.)

FIGURE 40-5 ■ **Single-photon emission computed tomography (SPECT) polar maps and electromechanical maps. A,** SPECT polar map at baseline shows an inferolateral ischemic area in white and non-reversible stress defect in black *(left)*. Follow-up SPECT at 2 months *(right)* after autologous bone marrow cell transplantation shows complete resolution of ischemic defect. **B,** Electromechanical map from the inferior position. Mechanical map at the time of the injection procedure *(left)*. shows the 15 injection sites in black. Follow-up mechanical map at 4 months *(right)* shows marked improvement in contractile function in the injected area. (From Perin EC, Dohmann HF, Borojevic R, et al: *Transendocardial autologous bone marrow cell transplantation in severe, chronic ischemic heart failure. Circulation* 2003;107:2294-2302.)

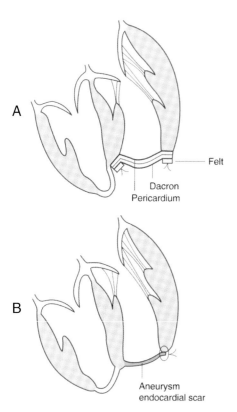

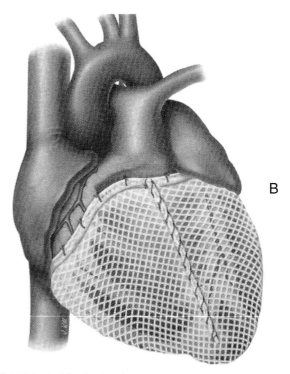

Felt

Dacron
Pericardium

Aneurysm
endocardial scar

FIGURE 42-5 ■ **The Dor procedure.** The procedure includes a looped stitch around the aneurysm to shrink the area. An endoventricular Dacron patch is used to exclude the areas that are akinetic or dyskinetic. The operation transforms the failing ventricle from a spherical to its original elliptical shape. **A,** A pericardial covered Dacron patch is used. **B,** An autogenous endocardium from septal scar is seen. (From Westaby S, Katsumata T, Frazier OH: *Surgical restoration of the failing left ventricle.* In Narula J, Virmani R, Ballester M, et al, [eds]: *Heart Failure: Pathogenesis and Treatment,* p. 625. London, Martin Kunitz, 2002.)

FIGURE 42-6 ■ **The CorCap device.** This fabric mesh implant device is designed to reduce wall stress by passive support to reverse the progression of ventricular dilation. Several sizes are available. **B,** The device is seen wrapped around the ventricles to arrest progressive dilation of the ventricles. (From Westaby S, Katsumata T, Frazier OH: *Surgical restoration of the failing left ventricle.* In Narula J, Virmani R, Ballester M, et al [eds]: *Heart Failure: Pathogenesis and Treatment,* p. 643. London, Martin Kunitz, 2002.)

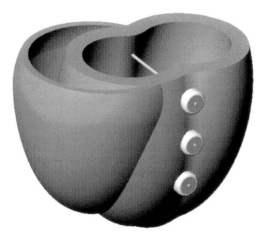

FIGURE 42-7 ■ **The Myosplint device.** This transcavitary tensioning device consists of three rods with wide buttons at either end. The pads at either end of the rod are made of high-strength polymer with polyester velour to encourage tissue incorporation. The rods are inserted in such a way as to change the left ventricle shape from globular to bilobular, reducing the radius of the left ventricular dimension. (From Westaby S, Katsumata T, Frazier OH: *Surgical restoration of the failing left ventricle.* In Narula J, Virmani R, Ballester M, et al [eds]: *Heart Failure: Pathogenesis and Treatment,* p. 645. London, Martin Kunitz, 2002.)

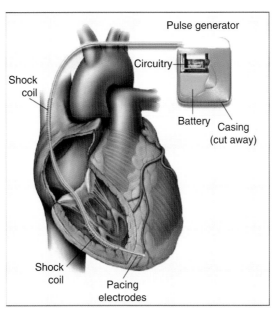

FIGURE 43-1 ■ **Implantable cardioverter defibrillator.** The implantable cardioverter defibrillator system is shown with the pulse generator and the lead that is used for pacing and defibrillation. (From DiMarco JP: Implantable cardioverter-defibrillators. N Engl J Med 2003;349:1836-1847.)

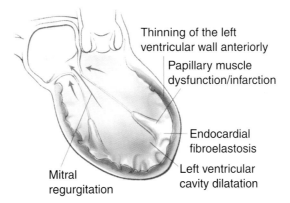

FIGURE 47-2 ■ **Anatomic and physiologic derangements seen with anomalous origin of the left coronary artery from the pulmonary artery.** As a result of myocardial ischemia from decreased coronary circulation, anatomic changes occur and require time for recovery. A ventricular assist device is ideal for this to occur after surgical correction of the coronary supply.

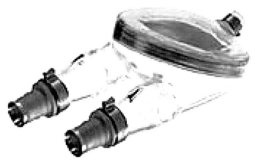

FIGURE 48-1 ■ Berlin Heart ventricular assist system. Pulsatile ventricular assist system from the Berlin Heart Institute, Berlin, Germany. This paracorporeal pulsatile device has a pediatric miniaturized version. The polyurethane pumps, with two different valve systems made of either mechanical tilting discs or polyurethane leaflets, have a wide range of stroke volumes of 10 mL, 25 mL, 30 mL, 50 mL, and 60 mL designed for pediatric use, but can go up to 80 mL for adults. (Courtesy of Berlin Heart AG, Berlin, Germany.)

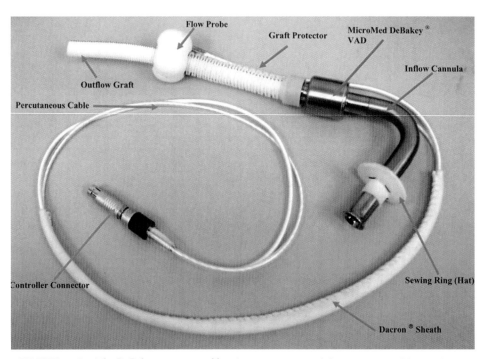

FIGURE 48-5 ■ The DeBakey pump assembly. The various parts of the pump assembly are shown and labeled (see text for details). (From MicroMed Technology, Houston, TX.)

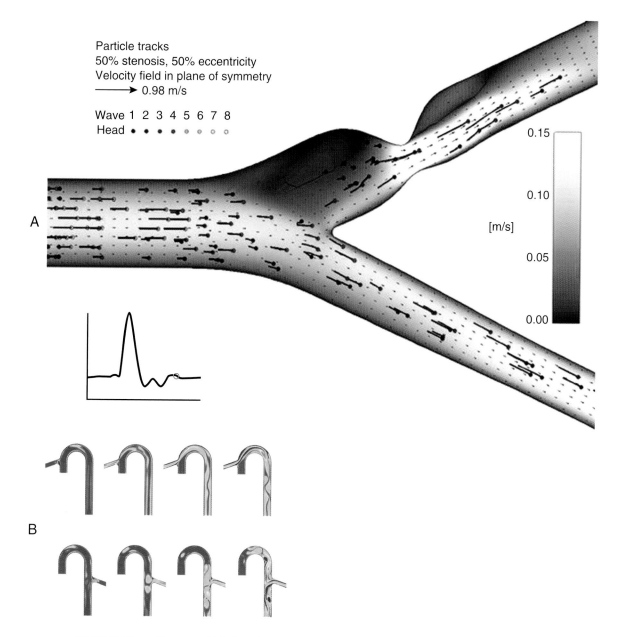

Particle tracks
50% stenosis, 50% eccentricity
Velocity field in plane of symmetry
$\longrightarrow$ 0.98 m/s

Wave 1 2 3 4 5 6 7 8
Head ● ● ● ● ● ○ ○ ○

A

0.15

0.10

[m/s]

0.05

0.00

B

FIGURE 50-1 ■ Computer-aided flow designs. **A,** Continuous flow throughout the cardiac cycle, converting diastolic flow from passive to active, is being studied by means of computer-aided design, computational fluid dynamics, and flow simulation studies. **B,** Computer-aided design studies, comparing flows in ascending *(top)* versus descending *(bottom)* aortic anastomoses. The flow rate increases from left to right. (**A** courtesy of Ralph Metcalfe, University of Houston. For more information, see http://celsius.ifdt.uh.edu/3d/particle/index.html.)

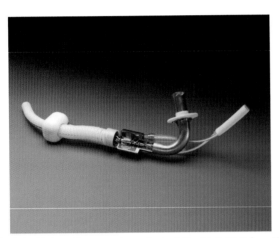

FIGURE 50-4 ■ Cutaway view of the MicroMed DeBakey VAD (MicroMed Technology, Houston, TX). (Courtesy of MicroMed Technology, Inc., Houston, TX.)

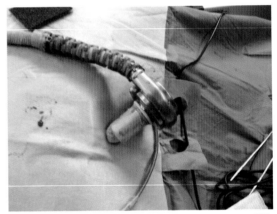

FIGURE 50-5 ■ The HeartWare (HeartWare, Inc, Miramar, FL). This device is a novel miniaturized passive magnetic-levitation centrifugal ventricular assist device.

CHAPTER 1

Molecular and Cellular Mechanisms in Myocardial Dysfunction

Matteo Vatta
Anthony C. Chang

A **myofiber** comprises a group of myocytes bound by surrounding collagen connective tissue. Each myocyte, filled with rodlike bundles called **myofibrils**, is bounded by the cell membrane **sarcolemma**. The sarcolemma is a lipid bilayer that measures 7 to 9 nm thick with a network of invaginated tubular structures called **transverse tubules**, which reach into the cell interior. These tubules reach the extensions of the intracellular membranous network **sarcoplasmic reticulum** (SR), termed the **subsarcolemmal cisternae**. The cisternae of the SR form a close union with the transverse tubules of the sarcolemma, facilitating the excitation-contraction process, and set the cellular milieu for the exquisitely choreographed process of calcium-induced calcium release. The relaxation process follows with reuptake of cytosolic calcium via another set of receptors that reside in the longitudinal portion of the SR.

Heart failure alters the structure and function of the myocardium at the molecular and the cellular levels. In more specific terms, calcium regulation and its influence on excitation-contraction coupling and the contractile apparatus undergo maladaptive changes as a result of the increased demand on the heart as it fails. Calcium is the essential second messenger that serves as the interconnecting link between myocyte depolarization and myofibril contraction, and this messenger becomes dysregulated in heart failure. This chapter focuses on these essential aspects in the normal and in the failing myocardium. Dystrophin and its glycoproteins, as an essential protein complex in the maintenance of the structural integrity of the myocardium, also are discussed.

EXCITATION-CONTRACTION COUPLING AND HEART FAILURE

Briefly, the generation and propagation of the cardiac action potential lead to a wave of cell membrane depolarization that activates the opening of L-type Ca^{2+} channels in the cardiomyocytes, leading to Ca^{2+} influx into the cytoplasm. This relatively small inflow of calcium ions triggers the larger release of Ca^{2+} from the intracellular storages, particularly from the SR via the ryanodine (RyR) calcium channels. The free calcium proceeds to the sarcomere, where it starts the contractile process. The reuptake of intracellular calcium occurs via the SR calcium/ATPase pump, which is regulated by the protein phospholamban (PLB). A complex interplay of ion channels and pumps along with proteins and enzymes works to maintain calcium regulation via a close temporal and spatial relationship between the sarcolemma and the SR (Table 1-1).

In the next sections, the factors involved in the generation of the contractile function and Ca^{2+} reuptake that determine the ability of the cardiomyocytes to undergo relaxation and restart the contractile cycle are described. Alterations in the function of these mechanisms observed with heart failure also are elucidated (calcium receptors and regulation are discussed in more detail in Chapter 2).

Calcium Movement Across the Sarcolemma

One of the first mechanisms that increase intracellular calcium is the opening of the sarcolemmal membrane **voltage-dependent L-type Ca^{2+} channel** (also termed dihydropyridine receptor because of the sensitivity to this class of calcium channel blockers) (Fig. 1-1). Other types of plasma membrane calcium channels with differing conductances and gating mechanisms exist (T, N, P, Q, and R), but the L-type channel is the most important plasma membrane calcium channel in the heart.[1,2] The L-type Ca^{2+} channel is enriched in the transverse tubule membrane, where it acts as a voltage-dependent Ca^{2+} channel and a voltage sensor for RyR opening on the SR membrane. Activation of the L-type Ca^{2+} channel depends on the depolarization wave and cytosolic $[Ca^{2+}]$ concentration.[3] The L-type Ca^{2+} channels not only contribute to the inward, depolarizing currents that sustain the membrane potential of the cardiac action potential in ventricular cells, but also maintain the plateau phase and trigger the opening of intracellular calcium channels on the SR, initiating the excitation-contraction activity.[4]

In addition to the L-type calcium channel for calcium influx, there are two essential proteins, the **sarcolemmal Na^+/Ca^{2+} exchanger (NCX)** and the **sarcolemmal calcium ATPase pump**, both of which are involved in the myocyte calcium efflux. The NCX usually exchanges

TABLE 1-1

Molecular Components in the Calcium Regulation of the Myocyte		
Structure	Role in Excitation-Contraction Coupling	Role in Relaxation
Plasma membrane		
Sarcolemma		
Sodium channel	Depolarization	
Calcium channel (dihydropyridine receptor)	Action potential plateau, calcium-triggered calcium release	
Potassium channels	Repolarization	
Calcium pump (PMCA)		Calcium removal
Sodium/calcium exchanger	Calcium entry	Calcium removal
Sodium pump		Establish sodium gradient
Transverse tubule		
Sodium channel	Action potential propagation	
Calcium channel (dihydropyridine receptor)	Calcium-triggered calcium release	
Sarcoplasmic reticulum		
Subsarcolemmal cisternae		
Calcium release channel (ryanodine receptor)	Calcium release	
Sarcotubular network		
Calcium pump (SERCA)		Calcium removal
Phospholamban		Sensitizes SERCA to calcium
Myofilaments		
Myosin	Energy transducer (ATPase site)	
Actin	Activates and binds myosin	
Troponin C	Calcium receptor	
Tropomyosin, troponins I and T	Allosteric regulation	

SERCA, Sarcoplasmic reticulum Ca^{2+}/ATPase pump.
From Katz AM: Heart Failure: Pathophysiology, Molecular Biology, and Clinical Management. Philadelphia, Lippincott Williams & Wilkins 2000.

extracellular sodium for intracellular calcium by using the osmotic energy of the sodium gradient (created by the sodium/potassium pump), but its mode can be reversed (to result in calcium influx). Although there is a high density of these exchangers near the T tubules to facilitate a calcium-induced calcium release process, the primary role for these exchangers is to extrude calcium. The sarcolemmal calcium ATPase pump acts in concert with a calcium-binding protein called **calmodulin**; this sensitivity to calmodulin does not exist with the SR-associated calcium ATPase pump. Mitochondria also act as a source of buffer against fluctuations in cytosolic calcium.

Calcium Movement Across the Sarcoplasmic Reticulum

The primary intracellular Ca^{2+} storage/release organelle in most cells is the endoplasmic reticulum; in striated muscles, it is the **sarcoplasmic reticulum (SR)**. The SR is an enclosed membranous network that surrounds the myofilaments. The SR contains specialized Ca^{2+} release channels belonging to two related families: the **ryanodine receptor (RyR)** (termed for its interaction with the plant alkaloid ryanodine) and the **inositol triphosphate receptor**,[5] although the latter has a higher presence in vascular smooth muscle cells and in myocytes under heart failure.

At least three isoforms of the RyR (RyR1, RyR2, and RyR3) have been isolated in mammals so far. The RyRs are present in other tissues, such as neuronal cells, but the main localization and highest density are in terminal cisternae of striated muscles. Tissue specificity occurs in mammals with RyR1 as the major isoform in skeletal muscle and RyR2 as the most representative isoform in cardiac muscle; RyR3 represents only a small fraction of all RyRs in striated muscle. To study the physiologic role of all three RyRs, deficient mice were generated for each of the isoforms.[6,7] Mice lacking in RyR1 and RyR2 died during embryonic development[6,7]; knockout mice for RyR3 led to viable animals with a nearly normal life span and normal striated muscle morphology.[8] Despite the lack of a clear-cut phenotype, RyR3 knockout mice seem to have impaired calcium-induced calcium release, but this does not seem to create any deficits secondary to compensatory pathways.[9]

Because the inward Ca^{2+} current from the L-type calcium channels is not nearly sufficient to drive the conformational change in troponin C needed for contraction to occur, an additional large quantum of calcium is required. This additional calcium is released by RyR localized in areas of the SR membrane adjacent to L-type voltage-dependent channels within the T tubules of the sarcolemma. A small Ca^{2+} inward current via the L-type calcium channels triggers calcium release from the SR in a process aptly termed **calcium-induced calcium release**. The immature myocardium (with its immature

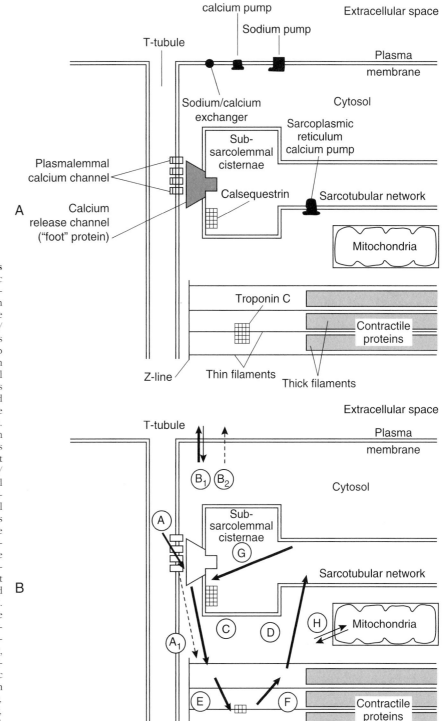

FIGURE 1-1 ■ Calcium regulatory molecules in excitation-contraction coupling. Schematic diagram shows key structures **(A)** and calcium fluxes **(B)** during excitation-contraction coupling. The arrow thickness denotes the magnitude of the calcium flux, and the up/down arrow directions indicate the energetics (down arrow is passive flux, whereas up arrow is energy-requiring transport). Calcium first enters the cell via the L-type plasmalemmal calcium channel. As shown by *arrow A*, this influx of calcium triggers the calcium-induced calcium release process via the calcium release channel (also called the *ryanodine receptor*). A small amount of the inward flux of calcium directly activates the contractile proteins (*dotted arrow A_1*). *Arrows B_1 and B_2* represent the two outward calcium fluxes via the sodium/calcium exchanger and the plasmalemmal calcium pump. As shown by *arrow C*, the calcium released from the subsarcolemmal cisternae via the calcium release channel is used for contraction. *Arrow D* represents the calcium reuptake process via the sarcoplasmic reticulum calcium pump (SERCA) of the sarcotubular network. An important regulatory protein of SERCA, phospholamban, is not seen. *Arrows E and F* denote the binding and dissociation of the calcium from troponin C. *Arrow G* represents the calcium flux inside the sarcoplasmic reticulum toward the subsarcolemmal cisternae for storage via calcium-binding proteins, such as calsequestrin. Finally, a small amount of calcium movement associated with mitochondria buffers the cytosolic calcium concentration (*arrow H*). (From Katz AM: *Heart Failure: Pathophysiology, Molecular Biology, and Clinical Management,* p. 74, Philadelphia, Lippincott Williams & Wilkins, 2000.)

SR apparatus) is more dependent on the L-type calcium channels for excitation-contraction coupling, whereas the more mature myocardium is able to generate the cytosolic calcium increase via the calcium-induced calcium release mechanism.

Although some of the Ca^{2+} stored in the SR is free, most is associated with calcium-binding proteins, such as **calsequestrin, calcireticulin,** and **histidine-rich calcium-binding protein**, which trap complex Ca^{2+} within the SR. These calcium-binding proteins are concentrated in the subsarcolemmal cisternae, which are spatially connected with the complex machinery that triggers excitation-contraction. The resultant sudden and dramatic Ca^{2+} flux interacts with sarcomeric components to activate the excitation-contraction process. It is this large (10-fold) and abrupt ion mobilization of $[Ca^{2+}]_i$ that results in the effective interaction of calcium ions with troponin C to trigger the contraction.

The phosphorylation of the RyR is the final event in a signal amplification cascade that begins with β_1-adrenergic receptor activation, either by sympathetic nerves or by circulating catecholamines. This β_1-adrenergic receptor activation subsequently leads to the activation of adenylate cyclase and the generation of cyclic AMP, which switches on phosphorylating enzymes, such as protein kinase A.[10] Sympathetic tone can modulate cardiac excitation-contraction coupling by norepinephrine release, and this process underlies the improvements in hemodynamic parameters seen with many positive inotropic drugs. The hemodynamic improvement is due to greater influx of calcium through the L-type voltage-dependent channel for any given depolarization and a greater release of SR calcium through RyR on phosphorylation of crucial channel components.

The inotropic effect is terminated by the SR calcium reuptake or resequestration mechanism during relaxation via the **SR Ca^{2+}/ATPase pump (SERCA)**, which is coupled to an inhibitory subunit, **phospholamban (PLB)**. When PLB is in an unphosphorylated state, it suppresses the calcium ATPase so that it has low affinity for calcium. When PLB is phosphorylated (via protein kinase A–mediated pathways), however, changes occur in its conformation, such that it detaches from SERCA, and Ca^{2+} transport back into the SR is triggered to initiate the resequestration process. PLB phosphorylation accelerates calcium removal and myocyte relaxation (lusitropy). By retaining Ca^{2+} within the cell, PLB also increases contractility during β-adrenergic stimulation (because sufficient SR calcium is made available for the next wave of depolarization).[11] The levels of transient intracellular Ca^{2+} required to initiate contraction depend on the level of Ca^{2+} within the SR. In short, the synchronized release of Ca^{2+} throughout the cell after depolarization creates a global intracellular Ca^{2+} transient of sufficient magnitude to bring about contraction. Myocyte relaxation results from closure of RyR and the rapid removal of cytosolic calcium, either by (1) reuptake into the SR via the SERCA system or (2) its efflux out of the cell via NCX. These two processes balance the earlier cellular influx and SR release of calcium so that there is no net gain or loss of cellular calcium with each contraction-relaxation cycle.

Although calcium is the primary modulator of excitation-contraction coupling, the cardiac muscle is capable of increased contractile force with an augmented preload or resting length in a phenomenon described as the **length dependence** of cardiac contractility. This cellular observation is correlated with the in vivo heart function phenomenon known as the *Frank-Starling relationship*. This length dependence of the myocyte

has molecular implications because calcium flux and sensitivity are modulated by the resting length.[12,13]

Calcium Movement in Heart Failure

Overall, the complex interplay of ion pumps and exchangers along with receptors and binding proteins in the regulation of calcium becomes dysregulated in the presence of heart failure. First, there is a flattened force-frequency relationship of the failing ventricular myocyte; second, the action potential is prolonged and attenuated in the failing myocyte secondary to a lower intracellular calcium level during the initial activation of the action potential (Fig. 1-2). During the late phase of the action potential, the intracellular calcium is at a higher level because clearance is less efficient than in the normal myocyte.

Among the possible excitation-contraction defects associated with the progression of heart failure, perhaps the most important is the significant reduction in SR calcium levels. When this store of calcium is relatively depleted, amplitude and duration of SR calcium release are impaired, and as a result, a reduced contractile force is generated. Of the possible causes of lowered SR calcium stores, a **decrease in SERCA2 activity**, resulting in reduced loading of the SR with calcium, seems to be the most probable (Fig. 1-3).[14,15] Decreased SERCA expression has been shown in patients with decreased ventricular filling, ventricular dysfunction, and heart failure, although no mutations have been identified so far.

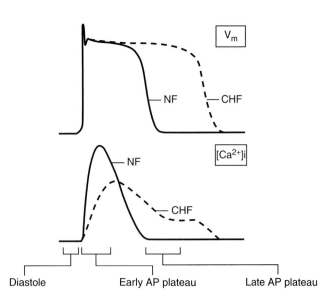

FIGURE 1-2 ■ The action potential in nonfailing (NF) myocytes and in myocytes with congestive heart failure (CHF). The action potential (AP) is prolonged and attenuated in the failing myocyte. The intracellular calcium level is lower during the initial activation in the early part of the AP. During the late phase of the AP, the intracellular calcium is at a higher level because clearance is less efficient than in the normal myocyte. (From Mann DL: *Heart Failure: A Companion to Braunwald's Heart Disease*, p. 43, Philadelphia, WB Saunders, 2004.)

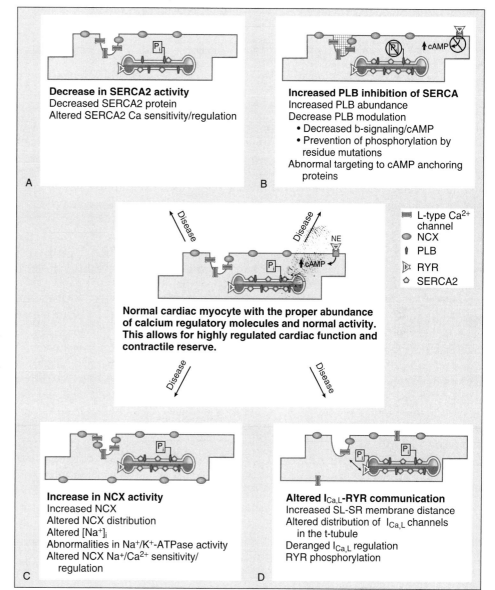

FIGURE 1-3 ■ Cardiac myocyte and calcium regulation in heart failure. Intracellular calcium is delicately balanced with a myriad of regulatory molecules and feedback mechanisms. **A** through **D** denote possible changes in this calcium regulation as a result of heart failure. **A,** Decrease in sarcoplasmic reticulum calcium ATPase-2 (SERCA2) activity. **B,** Increased phospholamban (PLB) inhibition of SERCA. **C,** Increase in sodium/calcium exchange pump (NCX) activity. **D,** Altered L-type Ca²⁺ channel–ryanodine receptor (RyR) communication. All of these mechanisms can lead to calcium dysregulation (see text). (See also Color Section) (From Mann DL: *Heart Failure: A Companion to Braunwald's Heart Disease*, p. 47, Philadelphia, WB Saunders, 2004.)

Conversely, increased SERCA expression with adenoviral infection methodologies has been shown to improve rat hearts with failure.[16,17]

An **increased PLB inhibition of SERCA** via mechanisms such as increased PLB quantity,[18] hypophosphorylation of PLB,[19] or an increased PLB/SERCA stoichiometric ratio[20] can lead to heart failure.[21] In addition, elimination of PLB expression in the mouse model has been associated with prevention of heart failure.[22] Genetic screening also has led to the identification of mutations in the PLB gene promoter in subjects with dilated or even hypertrophic cardiomyopathy.[23,24]

Significant SR calcium depletion also can result from **increase in NCX activity** (see Fig. 1-3), which occurs in heart failure. NCX plays a more prominent role in the excitation-contraction coupling during fetal and senescent

life, when it represents the more important mechanism of Ca²⁺ influx. In the overall economy of intracellular Ca²⁺, NCX accounts for about 28% of Ca²⁺ mobilization, suggesting that alterations in this protein can lead to significantly altered Ca²⁺ homeostasis, heart failure, and lethal arrhythmias. In particular, the two functional modes of NCX suggest that during heart failure, the forward mode (calcium efflux with sodium influx) balances cytosolic Ca²⁺ concentration in cases of ineffective SERCA reuptake.[25] NCX mRNA and protein overexpression have been observed in cardiac hypertrophy and ventricular remodeling leading to heart failure and malignant arrhythmias. This increased NCX expression could be a compensatory response to oppose the declining Ca²⁺ reuptake secondary to the reduction of SERCA.[26,27] A dog model of heart failure showed simultaneous decreased

SERCA levels and increased NCX activity, which only partially restores cellular Ca^{2+} homeostasis. Ca^{2+} removal from the cytosol is crucial for diastolic phase, but increased NCX activity along with decreased SERCA function create a substrate for arrhythmogenesis because Ca^{2+} efflux is associated with Na^+ influx, which can prolong depolarization and induce afterdepolarization. The existence of an NCX reverse mode of function observed in heart failure also has been suggested to provide inotropic support to the failing myocardium. So far, no mutations in NCX have been reported in human subjects with heart failure.

Altered $I_{Ca,L}$-RyR communication can reduce effectiveness of calcium handling because calcium-induced calcium release depends on this vital molecular bond. In isolated cardiomyocytes from failing human heart, single active L-type Ca^{2+} channels show a markedly increased availability compared with channels in the nonfailing myocardium; this finding suggests that the number of functionally active Ca^{2+} channels is reduced in heart failure. Ca^{2+} influx during the depolarization wave in isolated cardiomyocytes from failing rat myocardium also is reduced.[28] In the failing heart, the Ca^{2+} channel activity may be sufficient at slow pacing rates to compensate for the lower contractile ability, but when a higher pacing rate is triggered (e.g., by norepinephrine release from the sympathetic innervations), this compensatory mechanism fails, and the contraction force remains unchanged or even decreases.[29] In the failing heart, L-type Ca^{2+} channels also have been shown to trigger arrhythmogenesis when action potentials are prolonged; the use of Ca^{2+} channel blockers to inhibit arrhythmogenic early afterdepolarizations under these conditions can be justified.[30] Ca^{2+} binding abnormalities also can result in Ca^{2+} imbalance and heart failure, as shown by the calsequestrin overexpression in mice. In this model of abnormal calcium binding, the mice develop dilated cardiomyopathy and arrhythmias.

Reduced RyR activity does not seem to be a significant factor in declining SR calcium release; on the contrary, there is evidence that RyR hyperphosphorylation may be present as a compensatory mechanism. If this mechanism persists over time and becomes a chronic maladaptation, however, SR calcium depletion occurs despite any short-term compensatory pathway. In addition, RyR phosphorylation can modify its channel gating properties and induce a diastolic leak of SR calcium, triggering delayed afterdepolarizations and ventricular arrhythmias in heart failure.[31] Any compensatory gain in cardiac excitation-contraction that is mediated by sympathetic stimulation is ultimately unsuccessful in preventing the functional deterioration observed in untreated chronic heart failure. RyR hyperphosphorylation with decreased SR release of calcium observed in heart failure leads to alterations that include decreased sarcomere shortening, reduced velocity of sarcomere movement, myocardial

dysfunction, and unwanted leak of SR calcium, particularly during diastole.

The precise beneficial action of β-blockers in heart failure has never been adequately explained because these agents function also as negative effectors on myocardial contraction in the normal heart. By inhibiting the excessive compensatory phosphorylation response on RyR in heart failure, these agents may be able to restore channel function. Therapies aimed at abolishing the SR calcium diastolic leak caused by hyperphosphorylated RyR could remove the threat of arrhythmogenic-delayed afterdepolarizations, preventing sudden arrhythmogenic death and improving contraction.

CONTRACTILE APPARATUS AND HEART FAILURE

The fundamental morphologic unit **sarcomere** characterizes the contractile apparatus in striated muscle. The contractile proteins that compose the sarcomere account for more than one half of the volume of the cardiomyocyte. This extraordinary contractile machinery is characterized by an ordered structural pattern of thin (light) and thick (dark) fibers, corresponding to actin and myosin filaments. The **thin filaments** consist of monomers of α-actin that are arranged into long intertwined filaments, whereas the **thick filaments** comprise interdigitating myosin molecules. The overlapping of the filaments gives rise to the characteristic banding of the sarcomere (Fig. 1-4).

A dark strip called **Z line** (or Z band) delineates the boundaries of the sarcomeres at each side; thin filaments

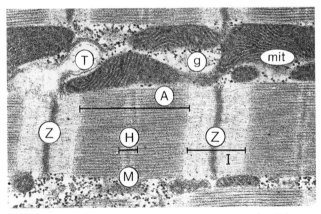

FIGURE 1-4 ■ The sarcomere. An electron micrograph of the sarcomere (×32,000 of rat papillary muscle). The H zone has only myosin filaments, the A band has actin-myosin overlap, and the I band has actin filaments and the Z-line. g, glycogen granules; mit, mitochondria; T, transverse tubules. (From Opie LH: *Mechanisms of cardiac contraction and relaxation.* In Braunwald E [ed]: *Heart Disease: A Textbook of Cardiovascular Medicine,* 6th ed. Philadelphia, WB Saunders, 2001.)

project from the Z lines. Within these limits, the central **A band** contains the thick filaments and parts of the thin filaments that overlap with the thick filaments, whereas the adjacent **I band** contains the thin filaments, titin, and the Z line. In addition, in the middle of the A band lies the **M line**, which results from the extremities or heads of the myosin light chain that do not overlap with the actin filaments. The **H zone** is the central clear zone that contains only the myosin filament bodies, including the M line. When the muscle contracts, the actin filaments move centrally and shorten the sarcomere and the distance between Z lines.

Several proteins are essential and responsible for the contractile process and its control. **Myosin** is the major protein of the thick filament, and each myosin molecule consists of six polypeptides separated into two sections: a tail section with long heavy chains and a globular head section with two sets of light chains. The myosin head section, on hydrolysis of ATP, helps to provide movement of actin filament along the thick filament and results in sarcomere shortening. The thin filaments are composed of (1) **actin** monomers with two helical strands; (2) **tropomyosin**, a support protein with double-stranded polypeptide chains that stretch along the longitudinal grooves of the actin strands in the thin filament; and (3) troponin complex.

Interactions that involve tropomyosin and the heterotrimer **troponin complex** (troponins C, I, and T) control the force generation by actin-myosin reaction; the calcium that is released from the SR directly interacts with the sarcomere to proceed with excitation-contraction. In particular, the troponin complex provides the necessary substrate for the biochemical interaction that initiates actin-myosin association via two binding sites, one for actin and the other for tropomyosin (via troponin T). **Troponin I**, in concert with tropomyosin, reversibly inhibits the interactions between actin and myosin; **troponin T** anchors the troponin complex to tropomyosin; and **troponin C** contains the high-affinity, calcium-binding sites that couple with intracellular calcium released from SR. When Ca^{2+} binds to troponin C, conformational changes occur in the proteins of the actin thin filaments that release the association of troponin I with actin. This release results in a displacement of tropomyosin, which moves between actin chains and exposes actin-binding sites that provide substrate for the mechanochemical transduction process of **myosin cross-bridge formation** (Fig. 1-5). Calcium binding to troponin C determines the number of interacting cross-bridges, and this can be negatively affected by intracellular acidosis.[32] The entire sequence of events leads to the myosin ATPase on the myosin heads undergoing hydrolysis of ATP, providing the energy needed to pull the actin thin filaments toward the middle of the A band in a ratchet motion fashion. Calcium binding to troponin C leads to conformational changes, which lead to movement of

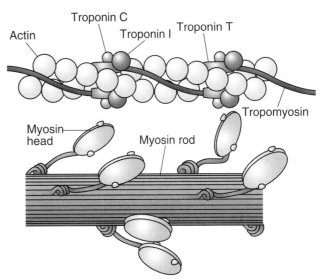

FIGURE 1-5 ■ **Essential contractile proteins.** The thick filament comprises the myosin heavy chains. The globular heads of the myosin molecules project outward to form cross-bridges. The thin filament is made of actin, but tropomyosin binds to troponin T at various sites along the thin filament. This interaction inhibits the actin-myosin interaction. (See also Color Section) (From Sprito P, Seidman CE, McKenna WJ, et al: *The management of hypertrophic cardiomyopathy. N Engl J Med* 1997;336: 775-785.)

tropomyosin, the modulator of actin-myosin cross-bridge interaction.

There are **isoforms** of actin and myosin and other contractile proteins, and these isoforms may change in expression in heart failure, resulting in depressed myocardial contractility and decreased calcium sensitivity of the contractile response. As the heart matures, there is proportionally more skeletal (versus cardiac) α-actin, but no smooth muscle α-actin. In heart failure, there is re-expression of the smooth muscle α-actin.[33] In addition, the myosin molecule, consisting of two heavy and four light chains, can have the heavy chains be either the α or β type. The α heavy chain has higher ATPase activity and is capable of higher contractility, whereas the β heavy chain, with a lower ATPase activity, possesses a weaker and slower contractility. The various myosin isoforms are based on the α and β configurations: V1 has two α chains, V2 has one α and one β chain, and V3 has two β chains. In smaller animals, the V1 isoform predominates, but the stimulus of ventricular overload could transform the ventricle to the V3 isoform.[34] The ventricle may have a different response to volume versus pressure overload, with the latter more influential in changing the myosin isoform.[35] The human ventricle is characterized predominantly by the V3 isoform throughout life. In heart failure in humans and large animals, there can be a transition to a lower α myosin heavy chain state or even a predominant β myosin heavy chain pattern.[36,37] Increased expression of the low ATPase isoform of the myosin heavy chain in heart failure reduces myocardial contractility via altered cross-bridge formation. Although troponin C usually is not associated with change in isoform expression in heart failure, troponins I and T have been reported to be capable of isoform re-expression.[38]

Mutations in any of the sarcomere proteins potentially can result in cardiomyopathies and heart failure. In particular, mutations in the myosin heavy chain gene (*α-MyHC*) result in hypertrophic cardiomyopathy. In the 1980s and 1990s, the investigation of the genetic basis of hypertrophic cardiomyopathy benefited from the application of molecular biology techniques such as linkage analysis. Subsequently, several other genes encoding sarcomere proteins have been identified, including ventricular myosin essential light chain 1 (*MLC-1s/v*), ventricular myosin regulatory light chain 2 (*MLC-2s/v*), cardiac actin, cardiac troponin T, cardiac troponin I, α-tropomyosin, myosin-binding protein C (*MyBP-C*), and titin. In addition to hypertrophic cardiomyopathy, mutations in components of the sarcomere have been identified to cause dilated cardiomyopathy, such as cardiac actin, *α-MyHC*, cardiac troponin T, α-tropomyosin, and titin. Sarcomeric mutations have been found in rare disorders, such as restrictive cardiomyopathy;[39] cardiac troponin I mutations have been associated with a familial form of restrictive cardiomyopathy.[40]

CYTOSKELETAL INTEGRITY AND THE ROLE OF DYSTROPHIN IN HEART FAILURE

In the last several years, investigators showed a role for the cytoskeletal proteins in cardiomyopathies and heart failure.[41]

Z Line and the Sarcomere-to-Sarcolemma Linkage

Although actin and myosin are the protagonists of the contractile process that occurs in the sarcomere, other components participate in the cooperative interactions that modulate the development and the intensity of the contractile process (Fig. 1-6). The **Z line** or Z disk is a specialized subsarcolemmal multifunctional protein. One of its complex functions is to cross-link overlapping actin filaments from adjacent sarcomeres.[42] More recently it became clear, however, that the Z line plays many other roles, such as an interface between the force-generating contractile apparatus, a link for other cytoskeletal components, and a signaling molecule.

One of the molecules that participate in the Z line complex is the giant protein **titin**, which creates a third filament system in striated muscle that stabilizes the myofibril and transmits contractile forces by anchoring myosin to the Z line and connecting the M line to the Z line.[43] The intermediate filament protein **desmin**, also associated with Z lines, further aids in distributing the contractile force through the sarcomeric matrix to maintain myofibril integrity. Contractile forces also are distributed through the Z line to the sarcolemma and underlying extracellular matrix via cytoskeletal structures known as **costameres**. In addition, **myosin-binding protein C** links adjacent thick filaments to one another.

Dimers of α-actinin cross-link overlapping actin filaments from adjacent sarcomeres and cross-link the amino-termini of titin molecules from adjacent sarcomeres.[44] Costameric complexes based on dystrophin/sarcoglycan, integrins, and the spectrin membrane skeleton may be linked via α-actinin in the Z line. The importance of the Z line as the interface between the contractile apparatus and the cytoskeleton suggests its

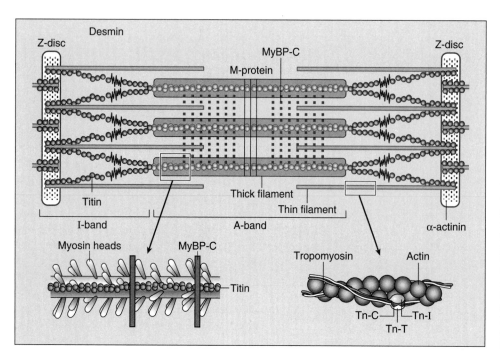

FIGURE 1-6 ■ **Contractile apparatus.** In addition to thin and thick filaments, the sarcomere has several other important proteins, such as titin, desmin, myosin binding protein C (*MyBP-C*), and α-actinin, which provide stability and flexibility to the sarcomere (see text for details). Tn-C, troponin C; Tn-I, troponin I; Tn-T, troponin T. (See also Color Section) (From Mann DL: *Heart Failure: A Companion to Braunwald's Heart Disease*. Philadelphia, WB Saunders, 2004.)

potential role in force transmission and in contractile sensing and signaling modulation. This role is noted by the observation that Z line structural or signaling function impairment leads to ventricular dilation and heart failure.[45] All these data confirm that the Z line connection is key in determining structural and functional pathways; when the Z line is disrupted, heart failure and arrhythmias can ensue.

Dystrophin Glycoprotein Complex

Muscle contraction occurs at the sarcomere level, but the force generated in the sarcomere must be transmitted to the sarcolemma to complete the mechanical contraction process. In addition, because the cardiac cell is not isolated from adjacent cardiomyocytes, the cells associate with one another through the connections that occur between the plasma membrane and the extracellular matrix.

This association between the plasma membrane and the extracellular matrix is ensured by the **dystrophin glycoprotein complex (DGC)**. **Dystrophin**, with its 420-kDa molecular weight, is one of the largest proteins in the human. The central portion of dystrophin, called the *rod domain,* has four hinge portions (H1 through H4), which determine the protein flexibility. The N-terminus of dystrophin binds to the actin filaments, connecting the sarcomere to the sarcolemmal proteins of the DGC, which is associated with the cardiomyocyte extracellular matrix. Although it has been shown that there is another actin-binding epitope in the rod domain, the role of the N-terminus domain of dystrophin is key in the interaction and should be preserved to guarantee a fully functional dystrophin. A disruption of this complex that connects the actin to the sarcolemma/extracellular matrix results in myocardial dysfunction (Fig. 1-7).

An approach aimed to use dystrophin mini-genes for gene therapy in muscular dystrophy has helped clinicians to understand the functional role of each dystrophin domain. Yue and associates[46] used a dystrophin mini-gene construct containing the N-terminus (actin-binding domain) as a vector for gene therapy and showed reconstitution of the DGC complex in dystrophin-deficient mdx mice, a model for dilated cardiomyopathy. Although dystrophin originally was identified as the gene responsible for Duchenne and Becker muscular dystrophies,[47] Towbin and colleagues[48] more recently associated dystrophin with an X-linked form of dilated cardiomyopathy. Typically, mutations in the amino-terminus (N-terminus) of dystrophin have been reported in patients with X-linked dilated cardiomyopathy, whereas patients with Duchenne and Becker muscular dystrophies have mutations scattered throughout the gene. Dystrophin not only plays a key role in the transduction of physical forces in striated muscle,[49] but also provides an anchorage for the DGC, as shown in Duchenne muscular dystrophy patients in whom primary dystrophin deficiency results in destabilization

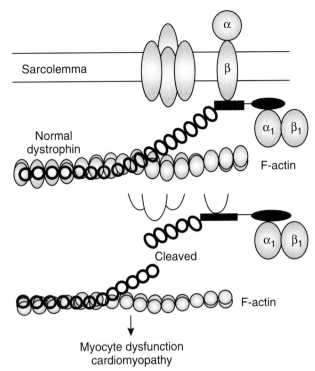

FIGURE 1-7 ■ The dystrophin protein with the glycoprotein complex in heart failure. Dystrophin is seen in the normal state above but is cleaved below. This abnormality is seen in enteroviral myocarditis, but also is seen in the cardiomyopathy associated with Duchenne dystrophy. α and β are part of the dystrophin-associated protein complex, whereas α_1 and β_1 are syntrophins. (From Bardoff C, Lee G-H, Lamphear BJ, et al: *Enteroviral protease 2A cleaves dystrophin: Evidence of cytoskeletal disruption in an acquired cardiomyopathy. Nat Med* 1999;5:320-326.)

of the entire complex.[50] Mutations in dystrophin, actin, or DGC subcomplexes all result in a wide spectrum of skeletal myopathy or cardiomyopathy or both in humans and animal models.

In addition to mutations in the dystrophin gene, a selective abnormality of the N-terminus of dystrophin in the left ventricular myocardium of patients with end-stage cardiomyopathy regardless of the underlying etiology was shown.[51] This dystrophin defect also was observed in the right ventricle, suggesting that this is a common molecular mechanism in myocardial dysfunction. Chronic mechanical unloading with left ventricular assist devices has resulted in reverse remodeling of dystrophin in the right and the left ventricles, suggesting that dystrophin is a reliable biomolecular marker for diagnosis and progression of heart failure.

In addition to its structural importance, dystrophin is important for the clustering of ion channels and affecting their functions; this phenomenon was shown in dystrophin-deficient mice when a decreased density in the voltage sodium channel SkM1 in extrajunctional sarcolemma was observed.[52] Genetic or acquired abnormalities that lead to the loss of dystrophin integrity result in progressive dysfunction, heart failure, and abnormal regulation of ion channel expression that can render the heart susceptible to malignant ventricular arrhythmias. After the identification of dystrophin as the cause of the X-linked form of DCM,[52] it became clear that all proteins directly connected to dystrophin—the entire DGC— should be considered as possible etiologic candidates for the cardiomyopathies and heart failure. The roles of proteins, such as sarcoglycans, dystroglycans, laminin, and integrins, in the pathogenesis of heart failure currently are being investigated in great detail.

CURRENT STATUS AND FUTURE TRENDS

The complex molecular biology and genetic regulation of the heart are just beginning to be unraveled. Novel exciting insights have occurred into the enormous variety of clinical presentations with possible common molecular origin, specifically that of myocardial dystrophin as a scheme for the progression of cardiac dysfunction.[53] In addition, the understanding of the mechanism through which the cytoskeleton is maintained or remodeled could lead to a much better appreciation for the intricate and complex nature of the myocyte intracellular milieu. Finally, modulation of loss or malfunction of molecular subsystems in calcium cycling and cytoskeletal integrity may provide a pharmacologic/genetic therapy against heart failure to complete the bench-to-bedside-to-bench cycle in the future.[54-57]

Key Concepts

■ The cisternae of the SR form a close union with the transverse tubules of the sarcolemma, facilitating the excitation-contraction process, and set the cellular milieu for the exquisitely choreographed process of calcium-induced calcium release. The relaxation process follows with reuptake of cytosolic calcium via another set of receptors that reside in the longitudinal portion of the SR.

■ A complex interplay of ion channels and pumps along with proteins and enzymes works to maintain calcium regulation via a close temporal and spatial relationship between the sarcolemma and the SR.

■ The L-type Ca^{2+} channel is enriched in the transverse tubule membrane, where it acts as a voltage-dependent Ca^{2+} channel and a voltage sensor for RyR opening on the SR membrane.

■ In addition to the L-type calcium channel for calcium influx, there are two essential proteins, the NCX and the sarcolemmal calcium ATPase pump, both of which are involved in the myocyte calcium efflux.

■ The SR contains specialized Ca^{2+} release channels belonging to two related families: the RyR (termed for its interaction with the plant alkaloid ryanodine) and the inositol triphosphate receptor.

■ Because the inward Ca^{2+} current from the L-type calcium channels is not nearly sufficient to drive the conformational change in troponin C needed for contraction to occur, an additional large quantum of calcium is required. This additional calcium is released by RyR localized in areas of the SR membrane adjacent to L-type voltage-dependent channels within the T tubules of the sarcolemma. A small Ca^{2+} inward current via the L-type calcium channel triggers calcium release from the SR in a process aptly termed calcium-induced calcium release.

■ The immature myocardium (with its immature SR apparatus) is more dependent on the L-type calcium channels for excitation-contraction coupling, whereas the more mature myocardium is able to generate the cytosolic calcium increase via the calcium-induced calcium release mechanism.

■ The inotropic effect is terminated by the SR calcium reuptake or resequestration mechanism during relaxation via SERCA, which is coupled to an inhibitory subunit, PLB. When PLB is in an unphosphorylated state, it suppresses the calcium ATPase so that it has low affinity for calcium. When PLB is phosphorylated (via protein kinase A–mediated pathways), however, changes occur in its conformation such that it detaches from SERCA, and Ca^{2+} transport back into the SR is triggered to initiate the resequestration process.

■ Myocyte relaxation results from closure of RyR and the rapid removal of cytosolic calcium, either by (1) reuptake into the SR via the SERCA system or (2) its efflux out of the cell via NCX. These two processes balance the earlier cellular influx and SR release of calcium so that there is no net gain or loss of cellular calcium with each contraction-relaxation cycle.

■ Overall, the complex interplay of ion pumps and exchangers along with receptors and binding proteins in the regulation of calcium becomes dysregulated in the presence of heart failure. First, there is a flattened force-frequency relationship of the failing ventricular myocyte; second, the action potential is prolonged and attenuated in the failing myocyte secondary to a lower intracellular calcium level during the initial activation of the action potential. During the late phase of the action potential, the intracellular calcium is at a higher level because clearance is less efficient than in the normal myocyte.

■ Among the possible excitation-contraction defects associated with the progression of heart failure, perhaps the most important is the significant reduction in SR calcium levels. When this store of calcium is relatively depleted, amplitude and duration of SR calcium release are impaired, and as a result, a reduced contractile force is generated. Of the possible causes of lowered SR calcium stores, a decrease in SERCA activity, resulting in reduced loading of the SR with calcium, seems to be the most probable.

■ When Ca²⁺ binds to troponin C, conformational changes occur in the proteins of the actin thin filaments that release the association of troponin I with actin. This release results in a displacement of tropomyosin, which moves between actin chains and exposes actin-binding sites that provide substrate for the mechanochemical transduction process of myosin cross-bridge formation.

■ There are isoforms of actin and myosin and other contractile proteins, and these isoforms may change in expression in heart failure, resulting in depressed myocardial contractility and decreased calcium sensitivity of the contractile response.

■ The N-terminus of dystrophin binds to the actin filaments, connecting the sarcomere to the sarcolemmal proteins of the DGC, which is associated with the cardiomyocyte extracellular matrix.

■ Mutations in dystrophin, actin, or DGC subcomplexes all result in a wide spectrum of skeletal myopathy or cardiomyopathy or both in humans and animal models.

REFERENCES

1. Zhang L, Bonev AD, Nelson MT, Mawe GM: Ionic basis of the action potential of guinea pig gallbladder smooth muscle cells. Am J Physiol 1993;265:C1552-C1561.

2. Katz AM: Protein families that mediate Ca²⁺ signaling in the cardiovascular system. Am J Cardiol 1996;78:2-6.

3. Bers DM, Ziolo MT: When is cAMP not cAMP? Effects of compartmentalization. Circ Res 2001;89:373-375.

4. Bers DM, Perez-Reyes E: Ca channels in cardiac myocytes: Structure and function in Ca influx and intracellular Ca release. Cardiovasc Res 1999;42:339-360.

5. Fill M, Copello JA: Ryanodine receptor calcium release channels. Physiol Rev 2002;82:893-922.

6. Takeshima H, Yamazawa T, Ikemoto T, et al: Ca²⁺-induced Ca²⁺ release in myocytes from dyspedic mice lacking the type-1 ryanodine receptor. EMBO J 1995;14:2999-3006.

7. Takeshima H, Komazaki S, Hirose K, et al: Embryonic lethality and abnormal cardiac myocytes in mice lacking ryanodine receptor type 2. EMBO J 1998;17:3309-3316.

8. Clancy JS, Takeshima H, Hamilton SL, Reid MB: Contractile function is unaltered in diaphragm from mice lacking calcium release channel isoform 3. Am J Physiol 1999;277:R1205-R1209.

9. Yang D, Pan Z, Takeshima H, et al: RyR3 amplifies RyR1-mediated Ca²⁺-induced Ca²⁺ release in neonatal mammalian skeletal muscle. J Biol Chem 2001;276:40210-40214.

10. Hartzell HC, Mery PF, Fischmeister R, Szabo G: Sympathetic regulation of cardiac calcium current is due exclusively to cAMP-dependent phosphorylation. Nature 1991;351:573-576.

11. Tada M, Toyofuku T: Molecular regulation of phospholamban function and expression. Trends Cardiovasc Med 1998;8:330-340.

12. Allen DG, Kurihara S: The effects of muscle length on intracellular calcium transients in mammalian cardiac muscle. J Physiol 1982; 327:79-94.

13. Hibberd MG, Jewell BR: Calcium and length dependent force production in rat ventricular muscle. J Physiol 1982;329: 527-540.

14. Hobai IA, O'Rourke B: Decreased sarcoplasmic reticulum calcium content is responsible for defective excitation-contraction coupling in canine heart failure. Circulation 2001;103:1577-1584.

15. Piacentino VR, Weber CR, Chen X, et al: Cellular basis of abnormal calcium transients of failing human ventricular myocytes. Circ Res 2003;92:651-658.

16. Miyamoto MI, del Monte F, Schmidt U, et al: Adenoviral gene transfer of SERCA2a improves left ventricular function in aortic banded rats in transition to heart failure. Proc Natl Acad Sci U S A 2000;97:793-798.

17. Schmidt U, del Monte F, Miyamoto MI, et al: Restoration of diastolic function in senescent rat hearts through adenoviral gene transfer of sarcoplasmic reticulum Ca2+-ATPase. Circulation 2000; 1:790-796.

18. Arai M, Alpert NR, MacLennan DH, et al: Alterations in sarcoplasmic reticulum gene expression in human heart failure: A possible mechanism for alterations in systolic and diastolic properties of the failing myocardium. Circ Res 1993;72:463-469.

19. Schmidt U, Hajjar RJ, Kim CS, et al: Human heart failure: cAMP stimulation of SR Ca²⁺ATPase activity and phosphorylation level of phospholamban. Am J Physiol 1999;277:H474-H480.

20. Meyer M, Bluhm WF, He H, et al: Phospholamban-to-SERCA2 ratio controls the force-frequency relationship. Am J Physiol 1999; 276:H779-H785.

21. Hasenfuss G, Pieske B: Calcium cycling in congestive heart failure. J Mol Cell Cardiol 2002;34:951-969.

22. Minamisawa S, Hoshijima M, Chu G, et al: Chronic phospholamban-sarcoplasmic reticulum calcium ATPase interaction is the critical calcium cycling defect in dilated cardiomyopathy. Cell 1999; 99:313-322.

23. Chien DR, Ross J, Hoshijima M: Calcium and heart failure: The cycle game. Nat Med 2003;69:508-509.

24. Minamisawa S, Sato Y, Tatsuguchi Y, et al: Mutation of the phospholamban promoter associated with hypertrophic cardiomyopathy. Biochem Biophys Res Commun 2003;304:1-4.

25. Bers DM, Eisner DA, Valdivia HH: Sarcoplasmic reticulum Ca²⁺ and heart failure: Roles of diastolic leak and Ca²⁺ transport. Circ Res 2003;93:487-490.

26. Hasenfuss G, Meyer M, Schillinger W, et al: Calcium handling proteins in the failing human heart. Basic Res Cardiol 1997; 92(Suppl 1):87-93.

27. Gias U, Ahmmed G, Hong Dong P, et al: Changes in Ca²⁺ cycling proteins underlie cardiac action potential prolongation in a pressure-overloaded guinea pig model with cardiac hypertrophy and failure. Circ Res 2000;86:558-570.

28. Hersel J, Jung S, Mohacsi P, Hullin R: Expression of the L-type calcium channel in human heart failure. Basic Res Cardiol 2002;97:I4-I10.

29. Pieske B, Kretschmann B, Meyer M, et al: Alterations in intracellular calcium handling associated with the inverse force-frequency relation in human dilated cardiomyopathy. Circulation 1995;92:1169-1178.

30. Marban E, Robinson SW, Wier WG: Mechanisms of arrhythmogenic delayed and early afterdepolarizations in ferret ventricular muscle. J Clin Invest 1986;78:1185-1192.

31. Shannon TR, Pogwizd SM, Bers DM: Elevated sarcoplasmic reticulum Ca²⁺ leak in intact ventricular myocytes from rabbits in heart failure. Circ Res 2003;93:592-594.

32. Jacobus WE, Pores IH, Lucas SK, et al: Intracellular acidosis and contractility in the normal and ischemic heart as examined by 31P NMR. J Mol Cell Cardiol 1982;14(Suppl 3):13-20.

33. Black FM, Packer SE, Parker TG, et al: The vascular smooth muscle alpha-actin gene is reactivated during cardiac hypertrophy provoked by load. J Clin Invest 1991;88:1581-1588.

34. Alpert NR, Hamrell BB, Halpern W: Mechanical and biochemical correlates of cardiac hypertrophy. Circ Res 1974;34-35(Suppl):71-82.

35. Imamura T, McDermott P, Kent R, et al: Acute changes in myosin heavy chain synthesis rate in pressure versus volume overload. Circ Res 1994;75:418-425.

36. Nakao K, Minobe W, Roden R, et al: Myosin heavy chain gene expression in human heart failure. J Clin Invest 1997;100:2363-2370.

37. Ojamaa K, Samarel AM, Kupfer JM, et al: Thyroid hormone effects on cardiac gene expression independent of cardiac growth and protein synthesis. Am J Physiol 1992;263:E534-E540.

38. Bodor GS, Oakeley AE, Allen PD, et al: Troponin I phosphorylation in the normal and failing adult human heart. Circulation 1997;96:1495-1500.

39. Franz WM, Muller OJ, Katus HA: Cardiomyopathies: From genetics to the prospect of treatment. Lancet 2001;358:1627-1637.

40. Mogensen J, Kubo T, Duque M, et al: Idiopathic restrictive cardiomyopathy is part of the clinical expression of cardiac troponin I mutations. J Clin Invest 2003;111:209-216.

41. Towþin JA, Bowles NE: The failing heart. Nature Vol 415: 2002;227-233.

42. Knoll R, Hoshijima M, Hoffman HM, et al: The cardiac mechanical stretch sensor machinery involves a Z disc complex that is defective in a subset of human dilated cardiomyopathy. Cell 2002;111: 943-955.

43. Ervasti JM: Costameres: The Achilles' heel of Herculean muscle. J Biol Chem 2003;278:13591-13594.

44. Faulkner G, Lanfranchi G, Valle G: Telethonin and other new proteins of the Z-disc of skeletal muscle. IUBMB Life 2001;51:275-282.

45. Chen J, Chien KR: Complexity in simplicity: Monogenic disorders and complex cardiomyopathies. J Clin Invest 1999;103:1483-1485.

46. Yue Y, Li Z, Harper SQ, et al: Microdystrophin gene therapy of cardiomyopathy restores dystrophin-glycoprotein complex and improves sarcolemma integrity in the mdx mouse heart. Circulation 2003;108:1626-1632.

47. Hoffman EP, Brown RH Jr, Kunkel LM: Dystrophin: The protein product of the Duchenne muscular dystrophy locus. Cell 1987; 51:919-928.

48. Towbin JA, Hejtmancik JF, Brink P, et al: X-linked dilated cardiomyopathy: Molecular genetic evidence of linkage to the Duchenne muscular dystrophy (dystrophin) gene at the Xp21 locus. Circulation 1993;87:1854-1865.

49. Brown SC, Lucy JA: Dystrophin as a mechanochemical transducer in skeletal muscle. Bioessays Vol 15(6): 1993;413-419.

50. Cohn RD, Campbell KP: Molecular basis of muscular dystrophies. Muscle Nerve Vol 23(10): 2000;1456-1471.

51. Vatta M, Stetson SJ, Perez-Verdia A, et al: Molecular remodeling of dystrophin in patients with end-stage cardiomyopathies and reversal in patients on assistance-device therapy. Lancet 2002;359:936-941.

52. Ribaux P, Bleicher F, Couble ML, et al: Voltage-gated sodium channel (SkM1) content in dystrophin-deficient muscle. Pflugers Arch 2001;441:746-755.

53. Toyo-Oka T, Kawada T, Nakata J, et al: Translocation and cleavage of myocardial dystrophin as a common pathway to advanced heart failure: A scheme for the progression of cardiac dysfunction. Proc Natl Acad Sci U S A 2004;101:7381-7385.

54. Strehler EE, Treiman M: Calcium pumps of plasma membrane and cell interior. Curr Mol Med 2004;4:323-335.

55. Hirsch JC, Borton AR, Albayya FP, et al: Comparative analysis of parvalbumin and SERCA2a cardiac myocyte gene transfer in a large animal model of diastolic dysfunction. Am J Physiol Heart Circ Physiol 2004;286:H2314-H2321.

56. Tang T, Gao MH, Roth DM, et al: Adenylyl cyclase type VI corrects cardiac sarcoplasmic reticulum calcium uptake defects in cardiomyopathy. Am J Physiol Heart Circ Physiol 2004;287(5): H1906-121. Jul 8 [Epub].

57. Takahashi M, Tanonaka K, Yoshida H, et al: Effects of ACE inhibitor and AT1 blocker on dystrophin-related proteins and calpain in failing heart. Cardiovasc Res. 2005 Feb 1;65(2):299-301.

CHAPTER 2

Cardiovascular Receptors and Signaling in Heart Failure

Dean B. Andropoulos
Monique L. Ogletree

Cardiovascular receptor signaling regulates beat-to-beat cardiac function and resistance in the systemic and pulmonary circulations, which is the major determinant of oxygen delivery to the tissues, the ultimate goal of the cardiovascular system. This chapter reviews normal receptor signaling and calcium cycling in the cardiac myocyte and the systemic and pulmonary circulations, including developmental changes. The changes in function of these receptor-signaling systems in acute and chronic heart failure also are discussed.

ADRENERGIC RECEPTORS

An overview of the receptors and signaling systems implicated in heart failure is presented in Table 2-1. The adrenergic receptors (ARs) mediate their biologic responses through interaction with a guanine nucleotide regulatory protein, or **G protein**.[1] The AR system is the most important component in the regulation of cardiovascular function, and its physiology is the best understood of all the receptor systems involved in heart failure. The AR superfamily of receptors shares a common structure, characterized by seven hydrophobic domains spanning the lipid bilayer (Fig. 2-1). The seven domains are interconnected by three internal loops and three external loops between the amine terminus and the cytoplasmic carboxyl terminus. A specific agonist (or ligand) binds to the receptor, which causes a conformational change. This structural change permits the interaction between the intracellular portion of the receptor and G protein.

This interaction, also referred to as **coupling**, links the activated receptor to a specific biologic response. The regulation of the biologic response is initiated by the specificity of the receptor for a particular extracellular agonist and the coupling of a specific G protein to that activated receptor. The conformational change in the β-AR triggers the interaction of the G protein with the amino acids of the third intracellular loop of the β-AR, leading to G-protein activation (Fig. 2-2).[2] There are three different classes of G proteins: stimulatory

G protein (G_s), inhibitory G protein (G_i), and the G_q. Under normal conditions, all of the β-receptors interact with G_s, α1-receptors interact with G_q, and α2-receptors interact with G_i. Each G protein consists of three subunits: α, β, and γ. The activation of the G protein–coupled receptor causes an exchange of bound GDP for GTP within the α subunit and initiates the dissociation of the β-γ subunit from the α subunit. The GTP-activated α subunit modulates the activity of a specific effector enzyme within a specific signaling pathway by catalyzing the hydrolysis of GTP to GDP and inorganic phosphate. This hydrolysis causes the transference of a high-energy phosphate group to an enzyme and causes the deactivation of the α subunit. This process eventually leads to the deactivation of the α subunit and the reassociation with the β-γ complex. This cycle is repeated continuously until the agonist becomes unbound from the receptor. Downstream from enzyme activation, the production of a second messenger regulates the biologic response.

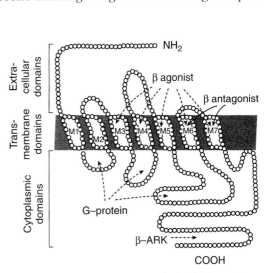

FIGURE 2-1 ■ **Molecular structure of the β-adrenergic receptor.** Molecular structure of the β-adrenergic receptor showing its three domains. The transmembrane domains serve as ligand-binding pockets for agonists (*dashed arrows*) and antagonists (*solid arrows*). The cytoplasmic domains interact with G proteins and β-adrenergic receptor kinases (β-ARK). (From Moss J, Renz CL: *The autonomic nervous system.* In Miller RD [ed]: *Anesthesia,* 5th ed. Philadelphia, Churchill Livingstone, 2000, pp 523-577.)

TABLE 2-1

Receptors and Signaling Systems Implicated in Heart Failure			
Receptor	**Tissue Distribution***	**Major Function**	**Changes in Heart Failure**
Adrenergic			
α_1	S, Cm (neonate)	Vasoconstriction, ↓ inotropy (adult), ↑ inotropy (neonate)	↓ (but may ↑ inotropy)
β_1	Cm	↑ inotropy/chronotropy	↓↓
β_2	S, P, Cm (neonate)	Vasodilation, ↑ inotropy (neonate)	↓↓
Eicosanoids			
PGE_1	P, Sm	Vasodilation	↓
PGI_2	P, Sm	Vasodilation	↓
TXA_2	P, Sm	Vasoconstriction	↑
Nitric Oxide			
NO	P, S, Ci	Vasodilation	↑↑
Cytokines			
TNF-α, IL-1β, IL-6	C, S, Pi		↑↑
Endothelins			
ET-A	P, Sm	Vasoconstriction	↑↑
ET-B	P, Sm		↑↑
Angiotensin			
Angiotensin II	Sm	Vasoconstriction	↑↑
Phosphatidylinositol			
Phospholipase C	S, Ci	↑ Ca^{2+} flux out of SR, vasoconstriction or ↑, ↓ inotropy (mature), ↑ inotropy (neonate)	↑↑
Vasopressin			
V1α	C, S, Pm	↑ Ca^{2+} flux out of SR, vasoconstriction or ↑, ↓ inotropy (mature), ↑ inotropy (neonate)	↑↑
V2	Renal	↑ free water retention	↑↑
Thyroid Hormone			
Triiodothyronine (T3)	Cm, i, n	↑ β-AR response, ↑ cardiac proteins	↓
Steroids			
	Ci, n	↑ β-AR response	– or ↑
Ca^{2+} Cycling			
Ryanodine	Ci	↑ Ca^{2+} flux out of SR	↓
Phospholamban	Ci	↓ Ca^{2+} flux into SR	↑↑
L-type Ca^{2+} channel	Cm	↑ Ca^{2+} flux into cytosol	↓
Na^+/Ca^{2+} exchanger	Cm	↑ Ca^{2+} flux out of cytosol	↓

*Tissue distribution listed in order of decreasing predominance.

C, cardiac tissue; S, systemic circulation; P, pulmonary circulation; m, membrane receptor; i, intracellular receptor; n, nuclear receptor; PGE_1, prostaglandin E_1; PGI_2, prostacyclin; TXA_2, thromboxane A_2; NO, nitric oxide; TNF-α, tumor necrosis factor-α; IL, interleukin; ET-A, endothelin-A; ET-B, endothelin-B; V1α, vasopressin 1α receptor; V2, vasopressin 2 receptor; SR, sarcoplasmic reticulum; β-AR, β-adrenoreceptor.

↑, small increase; ↑↑, moderate or large increase; ↓, small decrease; ↓↓, moderate or large decrease; –, no change.

ARs have been subdivided into two groups based on the results of binding studies using a series of selective agonists and antagonists. In 1948, Alquist[3] used the difference in rank orders of potency of a series of agonists to classify the ARs into two principal receptor groups, the α-receptor and β-receptor groups. This division has been confirmed repeatedly with the development of more selective α and β agonists and antagonists. Soon after the distinction between the α-receptor and β-receptor types was known, it became more evident that the simple separation into two broad types was not sufficient to explain pharmacologic studies using rank order of potency for antagonists. With the advent of radioligand-labeled antagonists and new molecular cloning techniques examining receptor gene expression, it became clear that the two principal receptor groups could be subdivided further into additional subtypes (Fig. 2-3).

Within the β-adrenergic receptor (β-AR) group, four different subtypes have been identified: β_1, β_2, β_3, and β_4. Pharmacologically β_1-receptors and β_2-receptors are differentiated by their affinities for different catecholamines: epinephrine, norepinephrine, and isoproterenol.

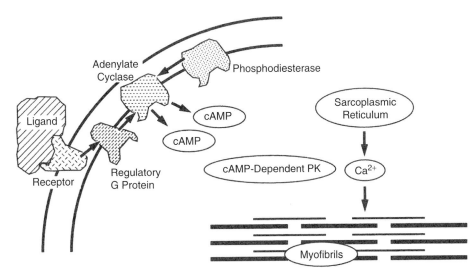

FIGURE 2-2 ■ Adrenergic receptor activation and interaction with G protein. Adrenergic receptor activation produces conformational changes in the receptor and the G protein and its subunits, which increases adenylate cyclase activity and cAMP activity. The cAMP-dependent protein kinase (PK) activity increases, which results in the phosphorylation of many intracellular proteins, the net result of which is release of calcium from the sarcoplasmic reticulum and activation of the actin-myosin complex by binding to troponin C. Phosphodiesterase breaks down cAMP and leads to the reduction of phosphorylation and all of the downstream cascade effects. (From Fisher DJ, Feltes TF, Moore JW, et al: *Management of acute congestive cardiac failure.* In Garson A, Bricker JT, Fisher DJ, et al [eds]: *The Science and Practice of Pediatric Cardiology,* 2nd ed. Baltimore, Williams & Wilkins, 1998, p 2330.)

β_1-Receptors have similar affinity for epinephrine and norepinephrine, whereas β_2-receptors have a higher affinity for epinephrine than for norepinephrine. β_1-Receptors and β_2-receptors have the same affinity for isoproterenol. β_3-Receptors and β_4-receptors have minor roles in cardiovascular function and are not discussed further.

The expression and distribution of each β-AR subtype depend on the organ, which adds another level of specificity. Distribution of a particular β-AR in two different tissue types may result in two different functions. β_1-Receptor is predominantly expressed in heart tissue. The stimulation of the receptor subtype leads to inotropic and chronotropic effects on cardiac function, resulting in an increase in the myocardial contractility, an acceleration in the velocity of relaxation, and an increase in heart rate, respectively. These effects ultimately lead to a marked increase in cardiac output. Although β_2-receptors also can be found in the heart (especially in immature hearts), they are predominantly expressed in vascular smooth muscle. The distribution and function relevance of this receptor subtype in the heart are controversial and may change with alterations in cardiac function (see later). The percentage of β_2-receptors in the nonfailing mature heart is about 20% in the ventricle[4] and 30% in the atrium; the ratio of β_1-receptors to β_2-receptors is approximately 3:1 in immature hearts.[5,6]

Each signaling pathway is specific to each AR. When the agonist binds to the β_1-receptor causing the coupling of the G protein, the G protein α subunit becomes activated followed by an increase in adenylate cyclase activity, which induces the conversion of ATP to cAMP. The second messenger, cAMP, phosphorylates protein kinase A (PKA). The function of a kinase is to phosphorylate other target proteins, which initiate a biologic response. PKA phosphorylates many effector proteins, and the phosphorylation of many of these proteins functions to increase the concentration of intracellular calcium.

The β_2-receptor also has been shown to function through the cAMP signaling pathway causing the activation of PKA, but not nearly to the extent of β_1-receptor in cardiomyocytes.[7] The response of this stimulation seems to have a larger effect on vascular smooth muscle. In this tissue type, the stimulation of β_2-receptor and the subsequent increase in cAMP promote the vasodilation of vascular smooth muscle and may lead to alterations in blood pressure. In these tissues, the effect of β_1-receptor stimulation seems to be minimal, owing to lack of β_1-receptors in the smooth muscle.

α-Adrenergic receptors (α-**AR**s) can be pharmacologically subdivided into α_1 and α_2 subtypes. The α_1-receptor is distributed in most vascular smooth muscle and to a lesser extent in the heart. The α_2-receptor is predominantly a presynaptic receptor in the central and peripheral nervous systems. Molecular techniques have identified three additional subtypes of the α_1-receptor (α_{1A}, α_{1B}, and α_{1D}) and three additional subtypes of the α_2-receptor.[1] Binding of an agonist to an α_1-receptor in the heart or vascular smooth muscle results in activation of the G_q subunit of the G protein, which activates the phospholipase C (PLC) system (see later), producing diacylglycerol and inositol 1,4,5-triphosphate, which releases Ca^{2+} from the sarcoplasmic reticulum (SR) and increases vascular smooth muscle tone or cardiac contractility.

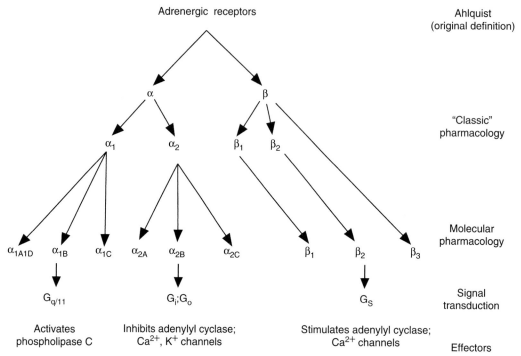

FIGURE 2-3 ■ Modern schematic classification of adrenergic receptors. (From Moss J, Renz CL: *The autonomic nervous system.* In Miller RD [ed]: *Anesthesia,* 5th ed. Philadelphia, Churchill Livingstone, 2000, pp 523-577.)

A schematic classification of ARs incorporating knowledge of molecular pharmacology and signal transduction is presented in Figure 2-3.[1]

The AR concentration in cardiac tissue is small and measured as femtomoles per milligram of protein. The response to stimulation of the receptor is subject to signal amplification, however, resulting in a greatly magnified downstream response. In rat ventricular myocytes, the ratio between the β-receptors and the next two downstream signaling components (β-receptor-to-G protein-to-adenylate cyclase) is 1:200:3.[8] The rate-limiting component that ultimately regulates intracellular production of cAMP is receptor density and the enzyme concentration of adenylate cyclase.

Developmental Changes in Adrenergic Receptor Signaling

Information concerning changes in AR function during the transition from neonatal to more mature myocardial development is limited to a few animal studies. β-AR density is higher in the ventricular myocardium of neonatal versus adult rabbits, but the inotropic response to the same concentration of isoproterenol is significantly greater in the adult tissue.[9] In the neonatal rat, the mechanism of β-adrenergic–mediated increase in contractility is entirely due to β_2-receptor stimulation, whereas in the adult rat it is due solely to β_1-receptor activation. Coupling of the β_2-receptor to G_i protein action is apparently defective in the neonatal rat because the ratio of G_i to G_s subunits is much higher in the neonate. The relative proportion of β_1-receptors and β_2-receptors is the

same in neonatal versus adult hearts (17% β_2-receptors); this approximates the ratio measured in children with mild congenital heart disease, which is about 22%.[10]

There is animal and human evidence that α-AR-mediated chronotropic and inotropic effects on the cardiac myocyte change with development. In the neonatal animal model, α_1-receptor stimulation produces positive inotropic and chronotropic effects, whereas in the adult it produces negative effects.[11,12] The chronotropic response to α_1-receptor stimulation diminishes with increasing age in children being evaluated for autonomic dysfunction after vagal and sympathetic blockade.[13]

Receptor Signaling in Disease States

A discussion of β-AR signaling in myocardial dysfunction is useful to serve as the basis for understanding many of the therapies discussed later in this text. We discuss receptor physiology in three settings: (1) acute myocardial dysfunction as seen after cardiac surgery and cardiopulmonary bypass, (2) changes seen as responses to chronic cyanotic congenital heart disease, and (3) alterations that occur with chronic congestive heart failure and cardiomyopathy.

Acute myocardial dysfunction, such as that sometimes seen after cardiopulmonary bypass, often is treated with catecholamines. These drugs can be ineffective if used in escalating doses. In children undergoing cardiac surgery with bypass, the number and subtype distribution of β-ARs in atrial tissue are not affected; however, the activation of adenylate cyclase by isoproterenol is significantly less after bypass.[14] This finding suggests uncoupling of β-receptors from the G_s protein–adenylate cyclase complex as a mechanism for the reduced sensitivity to catecholamines. Another mechanism for desensitization to moderate or high doses of catecholamines may occur after only a few minutes of administration because of increased cAMP concentrations, which result in receptor phosphorylation by PKA or protein kinase C or by G protein–coupled receptor kinases (at high catecholamine doses), which results in uncoupling from the G_s protein.[15]

Phosphorylated ARs produced by high doses of catecholamines may be inactivated by a process called **sequestration** after only a few minutes. These receptors can be sequestered by endocytosis, in a process involving a protein called **β-arrestin,** which binds to the receptor and a sarcolemmal protein called **clathrin** (Fig. 2-4). These sequestered receptors either may be recycled back to the cell membrane surface or may be destroyed by lysosomes.[16] This permanent destruction and degradation of receptors occurs after hours of exposure to catecholamines and is accompanied by decreased mRNA and receptor protein synthesis, resulting in prolonged decrease in AR concentrations, which

is reversed by decreasing exogenous catecholamines (but only as fast as new receptors can be synthesized).

Neonatal hearts may exhibit a different response to the acute or prolonged administration of catecholamines. Instead of desensitization, neonatal animal models show an enhanced β-AR response, accompanied by an increase in adenylate cyclase activity.[17] Desensitization as described previously occurs later in development, but the exact translation of these data to humans is not clear.

Treatment with catecholamines also may increase the concentration of G_i protein subunits, decreasing the sensitivity of the β-AR. This relative decrease in the ratio of G_s to G_i protein subunits has been shown in rat and dog models.[18,19]

Another possible mechanism of catecholamine-induced desensitization of the neonatal myocyte was shown in a rat model, in which prolonged exposure to norepinephrine causes an initial increase in functional L-type Ca^{2+} channels on the sarcolemmal membrane. Continued exposure causes a decrease in L-type Ca^{2+} channel mRNA to 50% of control values.[20] Sarcoplasmic reticulum Ca^{2+}-ATPase concentrations are reduced with

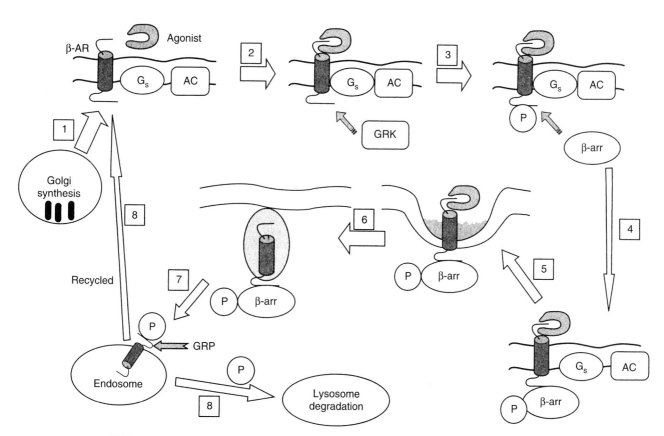

FIGURE 2-4 ■ Desensitization and down-regulation of the β-adrenoreceptor (β-AR). The sequence of desensitization and down-regulation of the β-AR is illustrated: agonist binding (1), phosphorylation of the β-AR by G protein–coupled receptor kinases (GRK) (2), β-arrestin binds to the GRK-phosphorylated β-AR, which is bound to the G_s protein (3). The receptor is sequestrated to the endosomal compartment (4–7), to be dephosphorylated, then either recycled back to the sarcolemma (8) or translocated to lysosomes for further degradation (8). AC, adenylate cyclase; GRP, G protein–coupled receptor phosphatase; P, inorganic phosphate groups; β-arr, β-arrestin. (From Booker PD: *Pharmacological support for children with myocardial dysfunction. Paediatr Anaesth* 2002;12:5-25.)

chronic norepinephrine administration in the dog.[21] Finally, exposing adult or neonatal rat myocytes to high concentrations of catecholamines for 24 hours leads to increased apoptosis of myocardial cells, a genetically programmed energy-dependent mechanism for cell death and removal.[22,23] This effect is mediated through β-ARs in the adult model, and α-ARs in the neonatal model.

All of these studies provide the theoretical basis for the argument that administration of catecholamines to patients with acute myocardial dysfunction should be as limited in dose and duration as possible; this is difficult to accomplish in the setting of acute myocardial dysfunction. Strategies that may limit catecholamine dose include administering low doses of catecholamines together with phosphodiesterase inhibitors or new therapies such as steroid rescue, which may avoid some of the aforementioned problems.[24]

In the 1990s, new information became available concerning AR signaling in patients with **congenital heart disease**. In a study of 71 infants and children undergoing cardiac surgery, the right atrial appendage was studied for β-AR density, distribution of β_1-receptor and β_2-receptor subtypes, and coupling to adenylate cyclase.[25] This study found that patients with severe or poorly compensated acyanotic (e.g., congestive heart failure) or cyanotic (e.g., severe cyanosis) heart disease have significantly reduced β-AR densities. Outside of the newborn period, this down-regulation in patients with heart failure is β_1 selective, but in newborns with critical aortic stenosis or transposition of the great arteries, there is additional significant down-regulation of the β_2-receptor subtype. Among patients with tetralogy of Fallot, patients treated with propranolol have significant increases in the number and density of β-ARs compared with untreated patients. β-AR down-regulation correlates with increased circulating norepinephrine levels. In severely affected patients, adenylate cyclase activity is reduced, showing a partial decoupling as noted previously. Other studies have determined that symptomatic tetralogy of Fallot patients (i.e., patients with cyanotic spells) have a significantly greater number of β-ARs in the right ventricular outflow tract muscle, and adenylate cyclase activity is greater compared with patients without cyanotic spells.[26]

α_1-ARs also are affected by congenital heart disease. In a study of atrial tissue excised at surgery in 17 children, α-AR versus β-AR stimulation was evaluated with pharmacologic agents, and the α component was responsible for 0% to 44% of the inotropic response, and β-AR stimulation was responsible for 56% to 100% of the response, with the degree of right ventricular hypertrophy and pressure load correlating with the amount of α-AR stimulation found.[27]

In children with **congestive heart failure** secondary to chronic left-to-right shunting and volume overload of the heart, circulating norepinephrine levels are elevated, as they are in adults with congestive heart failure. This elevation leads to a down-regulation in β-AR density.[28] The degree of elevation of pulmonary artery pressure and level of left-to-right shunting correlate with the plasma catecholamine levels and are inversely correlated with β-AR density. All of these abnormalities return to normal control levels after corrective surgery. The degree of receptor down-regulation in congestive heart failure may correlate with postoperative morbidity in infants and children. Children with a prolonged intensive care unit stay of greater than 7 days or who die during the early postoperative course (9 of the 26) have significantly less β_1 and β_2 mRNA gene expression than children who have better outcomes.[29] In addition, children receiving propranolol for treatment of congestive heart failure have higher β-AR mRNA levels and tend to have improved outcomes. Finally, children with dilated cardiomyopathy and a depressed ejection fraction of 41% show no significant increase in ejection fraction during dobutamine stress test.

α_1-ARs also have been shown to be down-regulated in chronic heart failure.[31] In models of chronic heart failure, in contrast to the normal negative inotropic response in the mature heart, α_1-AR stimulation seems to have a positive inotropic effect similar to that seen in the neonatal heart.[32]

As discussed previously, chronic β-AR stimulation in heart failure has many deleterious effects, ranging from uncoupling, desensitization, and down-regulation of the β-AR leading to decreased response to adrenergic stimulation, to increased apoptosis and switching on of fetal gene programs that lead to myocyte hypertrophy. These deleterious effects have led to the use of β**-adrenergic blockade** as a treatment for heart failure in adults, and in recent years this strategy has been extended to pediatric patients. It was hypothesized that β-adrenergic blockade would prevent down-regulation of β-ARs, and this has been shown to be true in some settings, resulting in enhanced β-adrenergic responsiveness. In preliminary studies of propranolol treatment of infants with congestive heart failure from large left-to-right intracardiac shunts, β blockade prevents down-regulation of the β_2 receptor subtype.[33] β_2 receptors are thought to play a more important role in neonates and infants (see earlier). Other beneficial changes with propranolol treatment include lower plasma levels of aldosterone and renin, and a trend toward lower levels of norepinephrine, epinephrine, and endothelin. Clinical effects include improved diastolic function and less ventricular hypertrophy.

RECEPTOR-MEDIATED REGULATION OF VASCULAR TONE

The regulation of vascular tone is an important consideration in the understanding and treatment of congenital heart disease and heart failure. The systemic and the pulmonary circulations have exceedingly complex systems to maintain appropriate vascular resistance, and a delicate balance between vasodilating and vasoconstricting mediators is seen in normal individuals. Abnormal responses may develop in response to a multitude of stimuli, however, which lead to pulmonary or systemic hypertension or, conversely, vasodilation. We summarize some of the systems involved in regulation of vascular tone, which serve as a basis for understanding some of the pathophysiologic states and the approaches to some of the treatments outlined later in this text.

A schematic representation of some of these mediators is shown in Figure 2-5. To some extent, the control mechanisms reviewed are present in the systemic and the pulmonary circulations; however, certain mechanisms are perceived to be more important in one circulation versus the other. The endothelial-mediated systems (nitric oxide [NO]–cGMP pathways) seem to predominate in the pulmonary circulation (low-resistance circulation), whereas the phospholipase systems function in the systemic circulation (high-resistance circulation).

Pulmonary Circulation

Vasoactive metabolites of arachidonic acid, called **eicosanoids**, are produced in cell membranes and via the lipoxygenase pathway form **leukotrienes** or via the cyclooxygenase pathway form **prostaglandins**. Important vasodilating prostaglandins include prostaglandin E_1, which promotes and maintains patency of

the ductus arteriosus and is lifesaving in ductus-dependent congenital heart disease, and prostacyclin, or prostaglandin I_2, which is a potent pulmonary vasodilator.[34] Prostaglandins act in vascular smooth muscle of the systemic and pulmonary circulations by binding to receptors in the smooth muscle cell membrane, activating adenylate cyclase and increasing cAMP concentrations, which lead to lower Ca^{2+} levels and to relaxation of vascular tone. Thromboxane A_2 is a potent leukotriene that has the opposite effects of the prostaglandins, producing vasoconstriction and platelet aggregation. Imbalance in this system caused by chronic hypoxia and high pulmonary artery pressures can lead to chronic pulmonary hypertension.

Nitric oxide (NO) is an endothelium-derived relaxant factor that causes relaxation of vascular smooth muscle cells by activating guanylate cyclase, increasing the concentration of cGMP, reducing the local concentration of Ca^{2+}, and reducing vascular tone.[35] The Ca^{2+}-sensitive potassium channels have been shown to contribute to the vasodilation caused by NO via a cGMP-dependent protein kinase.[36] NO is formed from L-arginine by inducible NO synthase and quickly inactivated by binding to hemoglobin. NO diffuses into the vascular smooth muscle cell and stimulates guanylate cyclase to produce cGMP, which results in vasodilation. Phosphodiesterase V breaks down cGMP, so phosphodiesterase-inhibiting drugs can potentiate NO-mediated vasodilation; this is

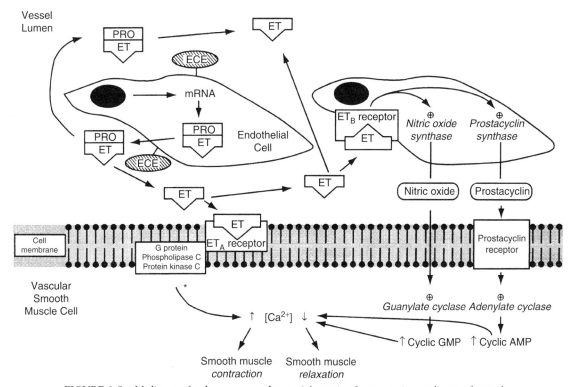

FIGURE 2-5 ■ Mediators of pulmonary vasculature. Schematic of some major mediators of vascular tone in the pulmonary circulation (e.g., nitric oxide, prostacyclin, endothelin-1) in the overall complex interplay. ET, endothelin-1; PROET, proendothelin-1; ECE, endothelin-converting enzyme. (From Haynes WG, Webb DJ: *The endothelin family of peptides: Local hormones with diverse roles in health and disease? Clin Sci (Lond)* 1993;84:485-500.)

the basis for testing drugs such as sildenafil to treat pulmonary hypertension in congenital heart disease.[37] Inducible NO synthase levels are increased in heart failure.[38] High levels of NO reduce β-adrenergic responsiveness and reduce myocyte contractile responses[39,40]; this occurs in part because of the increased cGMP levels, which reduce available Ca^{2+}. This altered NO signaling and its effects on cardiac myocytes may be distinct from NO signaling in the pulmonary vasculature, where NO has a beneficial effect on pulmonary vasodilation.[41] This increased level of NO is mediated by increased levels of inflammatory cytokines seen in heart failure, such as tumor necrosis factor-α, interleukin-1β, and interleukin-6.

Endothelin is a powerful endothelium-derived vasoactive peptide, of which endothelin-1 (ET-1) is the best characterized. ET-1 is produced from proendothelin-1 by endothelin-converting enzymes in the endothelial cells of the systemic and pulmonary vasculature. Increased pressure, shear stress, and hypoxia can lead to increased production of ET-1 in the pulmonary circulation. Two ET-1 receptors, ET-A and ET-B, mediate effects on smooth muscle vascular tone.[42] The ET-A receptor is found on the smooth muscle cell membrane and mediates vasoconstriction, whereas the ET-B receptor is located on the endothelial cell itself and results in increased NO synthase activity and increased NO and vasodilation. The primary activity of ET-1 seems to be to stimulate the ET-A receptor, and increased levels of ET-1 are found in many pulmonary hypertensive states, such as Eisenmenger syndrome and primary pulmonary hypertension.[43] ET-1 levels also are elevated in chronic heart failure in adults and children and are implicated in the pulmonary hypertension often seen in these conditions.[44] ET-A receptor antagonists now are being investigated as potential treatments for pulmonary hypertension seen in heart failure.[45,46]

Systemic Circulation

There are multiple levels of control over the peripheral circulation. **Neural regulation** by the sympathetic and parasympathetic nervous systems comprises an afferent limb consisting of receptors such as stretch receptors within the walls of the heart and baroreceptors in the walls of arteries, such as the aortic arch and carotid sinuses. Stimulation of the baroreceptors by stretch in the arterial wall leads to vasodilation and heart rate slowing mediated by the vasomotor centers of the medulla.[47] Stimulation of atrial stretch receptors inhibits secretion of vasopressin from the hypothalamus. The efferent limb of the autonomic nervous system comprises sympathetic and parasympathetic nerve fibers. The sympathetic nerves can be divided into vasoconstrictor and vasodilator fibers. The vasoconstrictor fibers release norepinephrine when stimulated, resulting in activation of α-ARs and vasoconstriction. The vasodilator fibers release acetylcholine or epinephrine and are mainly present in skeletal muscle. Parasympathetic fibers are vital in the control of

heart rate and function, but have only a minor role in controlling the peripheral circulation.[48] Hormonal control and receptor-mediated intracellular signaling are other important mechanisms and are discussed in more detail.

Norepinephrine primarily stimulates the peripheral α-receptors and causes intense vasoconstriction. It is secreted by the adrenal medulla and by sympathetic nerves in proximity to the systemic blood vessels. **Epinephrine** also is secreted by the adrenal medulla, but its primary action is to stimulate the $β_2$-receptors in the peripheral circulation, causing vasodilation through cAMP-mediated reductions in intracellular Ca^{2+} concentrations. **Angiotensin II** is produced by activation of the renin-angiotensin-aldosterone axis in response to low circulating blood volume and low blood pressure, sensed by the juxtaglomerular apparatus in the kidney. Renin produces angiotensin I by cleaving angiotensinogen, and angiotensin II is produced when angiotensin I passes through the lung by angiotensin-converting enzyme. Angiotensin II is a potent vasoconstrictor (see later) and induces the hypothalamus to secrete vasopressin (antidiuretic hormone), which also has potent vasoconstrictor properties. Angiotensin II levels often are increased in chronic heart failure.

Vasopressin is increasingly recognized as playing an important role in the regulation of vascular tone and salt and water retention in congestive heart failure.[49] Arginine vasopressin is secreted by the posterior pituitary, and levels are significantly elevated in chronic heart failure, resulting in retention of free water. Vasopressin receptors have been divided into V1α and V2 subtypes. The V1α receptors are found in myocardium and systemic and pulmonary vasculature and mediate their effects through the phospholipase C system, resulting in an increase in intracellular Ca^{2+} and pulmonary and systemic vasoconstriction.[50,51] In addition, in the mature heart, stimulation of the V1α receptor results in decreased myocardial contractility at higher agonist doses. V2 receptors are found in the kidney and act via cAMP pathways; stimulation results in retention of free water. These findings have led to the administration of vasopressin antagonists, such as conavaptan, a selective V1α and V2 receptor antagonist, and tolvaptan, a V2 receptor antagonist, to improve heart failure. Experimental data with these antagonists in animal models and in humans in heart failure show improved myocardial contractility, excretion of free water and higher serum sodium concentrations, and improvements in signs and symptoms of congestive heart failure.[52,53] In neonatal animals, V1α receptor stimulation in the myocardium results in increased intracellular Ca^{2+} concentrations via a non–SR-mediated pathway mediated by the PLC system and results in increased myocardial contractility.[54] This divergent effect in neonatal versus mature hearts seems to be similar to the response to $α_1$-adrenergic stimulation, also mediated through the PLC pathway (see earlier).

Atrial natriuretic factor is released from atrial myocytes in response to stretch (elevation of right or left atrial pressure) on the atrium. Atrial natriuretic factor has vasodilatory and cardioinhibitory effects and decreases tubular reabsorption of sodium in the kidney.[55] B-type natriuretic peptide is released by ventricular myocardium, also in response to stretch, and causes an increase in cGMP, leading to vasodilation in arterial and venous systems. In addition, it increases urinary sodium and water excretion.[56] Atrial natriuretic factor and B-type natriuretic peptide are discussed in more detail in Chapter 6.

Extensive progress has been made in elucidating the second messenger systems active in converting activation of receptors on systemic vascular cell membranes to changes in vascular tone. The **phosphoinositide signaling system** (or phospholipase C system) is the common pathway for many of these agonists (Fig. 2-6).[47] Membrane kinases phosphorylate phosphatidylinositol, which is an inositol lipid located mainly in the inner lamella of the plasma membrane. Phosphatidylinositol 4,5-biphosphate is produced. It is from this compound

that the second messenger, inositol 1,4,5-triphosphate, is produced, by the action of the enzyme PLC.[57] The sequence begins with the binding of an agonist, such as angiotensin II, vasopressin, norepinephrine, or endothelin, to a receptor with seven membrane-spanning domains. This receptor is linked to activated G_q protein subunit, which stimulates phosphatidylinositol-specific phospholipase C to produce inositol 1,4,5,-triphosphate. This substance acts to cause release of Ca^{2+} from the SR, resulting in activation of the actin-myosin system in the smooth muscle cells, resulting in contraction and an increase in vascular tone. Another second messenger, 1,2-diacylglycerol, also is produced, which goes on to activate protein kinase C, which has a role in mitogenesis and proliferation of smooth muscle cells and is implicated in producing ventricular hypertrophy. There are many isozymes of PLC; the form implicated in this series of events is the PLCβ form. The PLCγ isoform is activated when cell growth factors, such as platelet-derived growth factor, bind to their receptors on the cell surface and activate tyrosine kinases. This activity results in the production of phosphatidylinositol

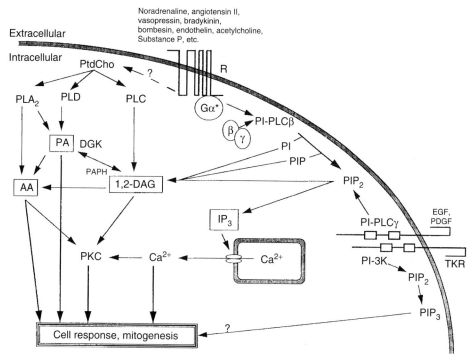

FIGURE 2-6 ■ **Phospholipase C system.** Diagram summarizing the major receptor-activated pathways for the production of inositol 1,4,5-triphosphate (IP_3) and 1,2-diacylglycerol (1,2-DAG). The binding of an agonist to a receptor R with seven membrane-spanning domains results in the activation of the phosphatidylinositol-specific phospholipase Cβ (PI-PLCβ), whereas the stimulation of tyrosine kinase receptors (TKR) by polypeptide growth factors activates PI-PLCβ. Both pathways result in the hydrolysis of phosphatidylinositol 4,5-biphosphate (PIP_2) and the formation of IP_3 and 1,2-DAG. In addition, agonists that act on the heterotrimeric receptors may stimulate phosphatidylcholine (PtdCho) hydrolysis, and activation of tyrosine kinase receptors stimulates the production of phosphatidylinositol 3,4,5-triphosphate (PIP_3). DGK, diacylglycerol kinase; PAPH, phosphatidic acid phosphohydrolase; Gα*, activated G-protein subunit, β subunits; PLD, phospholipase D; PKC, protein kinase C; PI-3K, phosphatidylinositol 3-kinase; PI, phosphatidylinositol; PIP, phosphatidylinositol 4-phosphate; EGF, epidermal growth factor; PDGF, platelet-derived growth factor; PLA₂, phospholipase A₂; AA, arachidonic acid. (From Izzard AS, Ohanian J, Tulip JR, et al: *The structure and function of the systemic circulation.* In Anderson RH, Baker EJ, MacCartney F, et al [eds]: *Paediatric Cardiology,* 2nd ed. London, Churchill Livingstone, 2002, pp 95-109.)

3,4,5-triphosphate, which also may be implicated in mitogenesis.

Vasodilation of the systemic circulation results from the formation of NO by nitrovasodilators or by activation of β_2-ARs in the peripheral vasculature, both of which result in the activation of guanylate cyclase and the production of cGMP, which reduces intracellular Ca^{2+} concentrations and results in the relaxation of vascular smooth muscle.[58] Autoregulation, or maintaining relatively constant blood flow over a wide range arterial pressures, predominates in the cerebral circulation but is not as crucial in other tissue beds. Autoregulation and carbon dioxide responsiveness are blunted in the fetal and immature brain.[59] The vascular beds in various peripheral tissues differ in the amount of local metabolic control of vascular tone; pH has much more influence on the pulmonary circuit, with low pH leading to vasoconstriction and higher pH leading to vasodilation, than in other tissues. Local carbon dioxide concentration is much more important to central nervous system vasculature, with high levels leading to vasodilation. Decrease in oxygen tension often leads to vasodilation, as adenosine is released in response to the decreased oxygen delivery.

Triiodothyronine (T$_3$) has been increasingly recognized as having a crucial role in the development of the cardiovascular system and in its acute regulation and performance. Normal T$_3$ levels are essential for normal maturation and development of the heart through expression of genes responsible for the production of the cardiac contractile proteins, elements of the calcium cycling apparatus, and development and density of β-ARs.[60] Cell nucleus–mediated effects of T$_3$ result in an increase in protein synthesis and require at least 8 hours to occur. These effects include up-regulation of β-ARs; increase in cardiac contractile protein synthesis; increases in mitochondrial density, volume, and respiration; increase in SR Ca^{2+}-ATPase mRNA; and changes in myosin heavy-chain isoforms. Acute effects of T$_3$ on cardiac myocytes occur in minutes; result from interaction with specific sarcolemmal receptors; and include stimulation of L-type Ca^{2+} pump activity, stimulation of SR Ca^{2+}-ATPase activity, increased protein kinase activity, and decrease in phospholamban.[61] Cardiac surgery and cardiopulmonary bypass interfere with the conversion of thyroxine to T$_3$, and serum levels decrease significantly after cardiac surgery in infants and children.[62] T$_3$ infusion can improve myocardial function in children after cardiac surgery and reduce intensive care unit stay.[63]

Corticosteroids seem to have a critical role in the regulation of the systemic circulation. Normal functioning of the hypothalamic-pituitary-adrenal axis is important for normal functioning of the cardiovascular system. Adrenal insufficiency has long been known to affect blood pressure and vascular volume and electrolyte regulation, but more recently it has been recognized to have a more important role in the regulation of cardiac contractility

and function in acute settings. Immature humans and animals with adrenal insufficiency exhibit myocardial dysfunction and hypotension, which responds within 6 hours to the administration of corticosteroids.[64,65] This area of research has important implications in the treatment of acute and chronic cardiac dysfunction.

CALCIUM CYCLING AND REGULATION

Calcium assumes a central role in the process of myocardial contraction and relaxation, serving as the second messenger between depolarization of the cardiac myocyte and its contraction mediated by the actin-myosin system. Calcium's role in this excitation-contraction coupling in the normal mature heart is discussed in greater detail in Chapter 1, but it is reviewed briefly here before discussions of developmental changes and changes with heart failure.[66]

Normal Heart
Cardiac muscle cell contraction depends on an increase in intracellular Ca^{2+} above a certain threshold, and relaxation ensues when intracellular Ca^{2+} falls below this threshold. Two major regions of Ca^{2+} flux occur: across the sarcolemmal membrane (slow response) and release from internal stores—the SR (rapid release and reuptake) (Fig. 2-7).[67]

The primary site of entry of Ca^{2+} through the sarcolemmal membrane is through the L-type, or low voltage dependent, Ca^{2+} channel.[68] Depolarization of the sarcolemmal membrane triggers opening of these channels, resulting in triggering of release of a large amount of Ca^{2+} from the SR—the major internal Ca^{2+} storage mechanism. Ca^{2+} entry through the slowly inactivating channels serves to fill the SR with adequate Ca^{2+} stores. Removal of Ca^{2+} from the cytoplasm to the exterior of the cell occurs via two major mechanisms: the Na^+/Ca^{2+} exchanger and the calcium/ATPase pump. The **Na^+/Ca^{2+} exchanger** usually serves to exchange three sodium ions (moving into the cell) for one Ca^{2+} (moving out of the cell), although the reverse action as well as a 1:1 exchange is possible.[69] The **Ca^{2+}/ATPase pump** actively transports Ca^{2+} (in a 1:1 Ca^{2+}-to-ATP ratio) out of the cell in an energy-dependent, high-affinity but low-capacity manner.[70] The affinity of the sarcolemmal Ca^{2+}/ATPase pump is enhanced by calmodulin, binder of free cytoplasmic Ca^{2+} (see later). An important concept concerning regulation of Ca^{2+} flux by these mechanisms is that although they do play important roles in balancing internal and external Ca^{2+} concentration, in supplying Ca^{2+} to replenish SR Ca^{2+} stores, and in initiating the Ca^{2+}-induced release of Ca^{2+} from the SR, the amount of Ca^{2+} flux is far less than across the SR, the far more important mechanism for excitation-contraction coupling in the mature heart.[71] The sarcolemmal Ca^{2+} flux mechanisms play a

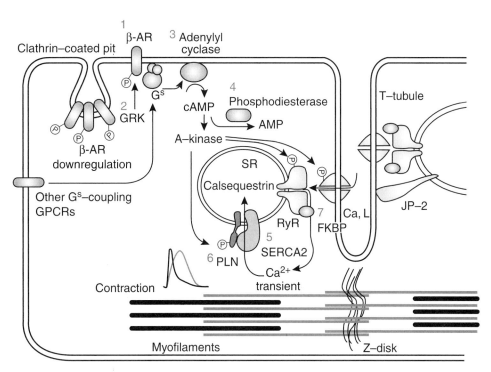

FIGURE 2-7 ■ Calcium cycling and the β-adrenergic receptor (β-AR) system. Calcium cycling and its relationship to the β-AR system and myocyte myofilaments (see text for details). G$_s$, stimulatory G protein; GRK, G-receptor kinase; A-kinase, protein kinase A; SR, sarcoplasmic reticulum; RyR, ryanodine receptor; SERCA2, sarcoplasmic reticulum Ca^{2+}-ATPase; PLN, phospholamban; Ca, L, L-type Ca^{2+} channel; FKBP, FK-506 binding protein; JP-2, junctophilin-2; GPCR, G-protein coupling receptor. Encircled P represents sites of phosphorylation by the various kinases. Numbers 1 through 7 represent targets for pharmacologic therapy in cardiac failure. (From Hoshijima M, Chien KR: *Mixed signals in heart failure: Cancer rules. J Clin Invest* 2002; 109: 849-855.)

much more important role in the excitation-contraction coupling of the neonatal (immature) heart, as is discussed subsequently.

The massive release and reuptake of Ca^{2+} responsible for activation and deactivation of the actin-myosin complex and cardiocyte contraction and relaxation occurs at the level of the SR. The SR is a closed, intracellular membranous network that is intimately related to the myofilaments responsible for contraction (Fig. 2-8).[72] The SR is connected to the sarcolemmal membrane via the transverse tubule (T tubule) system. Depolarization of the sarcolemmal membrane results in transfer of charge down the T tubules to the SR, resulting in the opening of **SR Ca^{2+} channels** (also known as the **ryanodine receptor**) and the release of large amounts of Ca^{2+} into the cytoplasm, where it can bind to troponin and initiate the actin-myosin interaction. The SR is divided into longitudinal SR and terminal cisternae; the latter connect to the T tubules. The terminal cisternae are primarily involved in the release of Ca^{2+}, and the longitudinal SR is involved in its reuptake.[73]

The primary Ca^{2+} release mechanism of the SR is the ligand-gated Ca^{2+} release channels that bind to the drug ryanodine. The channels are activated by two primary mechanisms: depolarization via the T tubules and binding of intracellular Ca^{2+} itself. The predominance of one mechanism over the other differs in cardiac versus skeletal muscle. The close proximity of the L-type sarcolemmal Ca^{2+} channels in the T tubules to the ligand-gated Ca^{2+} release channels enables the depolarization to allow Ca^{2+} rapidly into the cell and open the SR Ca^{2+} channels. These ligand-gated Ca^{2+} release channels close

when the cytosolic Ca^{2+} concentration increases—it opens at 0.6 μM of Ca^{2+} and closes at 3 μM of Ca^{2+}.[67]

The reuptake and sequestration of Ca^{2+} allows relaxation of the cardiac myocyte and is an active transport mechanism, primarily involving hydrolysis of ATP by the **SR Ca^{2+}/ATPase pump (SERCA)**, located in the longitudinal SR.[74] SERCA binds to Ca^{2+} with high affinity and rapidly transports Ca^{2+} to the inside of the SR. This transport system differs from the sarcolemmal membrane: It has higher affinity, allows for more rapid transport,

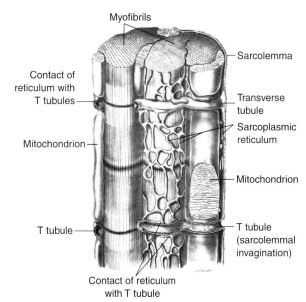

FIGURE 2-8 ■ **Normal, mature cardiac myocyte structure.** (From Bloom W, Fawcett DW: *A Textbook of Histology.* Philadelphia, WB Saunders, 1968, p 293.)

and is not sensitive to calmodulin. Ca^{2+} is stored in the SR by **calsequestrin,** a high-capacity, low-affinity protein that acts as a Ca^{2+} sink, which is reloaded, awaiting opening of the SR Ca^{2+} channels with the next cardiac cycle. There are two other proteins with essential roles in the regulation of Ca^{2+} flux: phospholamban and calmodulin.[75,76] **Phospholamban** is associated with SERCA and can be phosphorylated by at least four different protein kinases (see earlier)—cAMP dependent, Ca^{2+}/calmodulin dependent, cGMP dependent, or protein kinase C. When phosphorylated at its serine-16 residue, phospholamban changes its conformation, and this increases the affinity of SERCA for Ca^{2+}, facilitating Ca^{2+} flux back into the SR, and the inotropic and lusitropic states of the heart are enhanced. Phospholamban plays a central role in the β-adrenergic–mediated increase in the inotropic state of the heart. **Calmodulin** is a Ca^{2+} storage protein with four binding sites found in the cytoplasm; it interacts with the sarcolemmal Ca^{2+}/ATPase pump (increasing its affinity for Ca^{2+}) and the SR ligand-gated Ca^{2+} release channel (inhibiting its activity at optimal cytoplasmic Ca^{2+}) and binds to theCa^{2+}/calmodulin–dependent protein kinase.[77]

The increase in intracellular cytoplasmic Ca^{2+} initiates the contractile process through a complicated series of interactions within the contractile protein system, which is briefly reviewed. Myosin is the major component of the thick filaments that compose the microscopic structure of the myofibril, and its interaction with actin (the major component of the thin filaments) provides the mechanical basis of cardiac muscle cell contraction.[77] Actin and myosin constitute approximately 80% of the contractile apparatus and are arranged in a parallel, longitudinal fashion, projecting from a Z line or band (Fig. 2-9) to form the basic contractile unit called the **sarcomere.** A three-dimensional lattice, consisting of interdigitated thick and thin filaments in a hexagonal array with three thin filaments in close proximity to each thick filament, is formed. The actin and myosin are linked by projections on the myosin protein called **S1 cross-bridges,** which bind to actin and, via an energy-dependent hingelike mechanism, produce the sliding filament cross-bridge action that is thought to produce sarcomere shortening and lengthening. The lattice is held together by connecting proteins, such as titin, nebulin, and α-actinin.[78] The actin-myosin interaction is initiated when Ca^{2+} binds to troponin, a protein closely connected to actin that consists of three subunits: a Ca^{2+} binding subunit (troponin C), a tropomyosin binding unit (troponin T), and an inhibitory subunit (troponin I). Troponin C can bind four Ca^{2+} ions, and this produces a conformational change on the thin filament, which allows the S1 myosin head cross-bridges to attach.[79] This also changes the conformation of troponin I and allows tropomyosin, another protein integral in filament interaction, to move aside and expose the binding sites on actin, allowing the strong binding to the S1 cross-bridges.

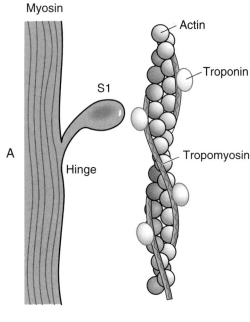

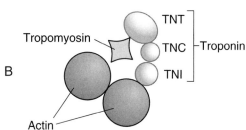

FIGURE 2-9 ■ Myosin and actin interaction. A, Single thick and thin filament showing the S1 cross-bridge and hingelike mechanism. **B,** Relationship of actin to tropomyosin and the three troponin subunits (TNT, TNC, TNI). (From Michael LH: *Cardiac contractile proteins in the normal heart: The contractile process and its regulation.* In Garson A, Bricker JT, Fisher DJ, et al [eds]: *The Science and Practice of Pediatric Cardiology,* 2nd ed. Baltimore, Williams & Wilkins, 1998, p 182.)

With Ca^{2+} present, actin causes myosin ATPase to hydrolyze one ATP molecule, providing energy that results in the S1 myosin head pulling on the thin filament, resulting in sarcomere shortening. Troponin C is the most important aspect of the regulation of cardiocyte contraction and is exquisitely sensitive with a steep response curve to local levels of Ca^{2+}. When Ca^{2+} levels decline rapidly, associated with its reuptake into the SR, the inhibitory form of the troponin, tropomyosin, and actin complex returns, and the result is reversal of the cross-bridge binding and sarcomere relaxation. Besides calcium, many other regulatory mechanisms exist to influence the interaction and sensitivity of Ca^{2+} binding to troponin, including β-adrenergic stimulation, thyroid hormone, and phosphorylation by cAMP-dependent protein kinases.

Developmental Changes

Several aspects of the excitation-contraction system are different in the immature heart. In neonatal hearts, the T tubule is not fully formed.[80] The SR in neonatal animal models has been shown to have less storage capacity and less structural organization,[81] less mRNA expression, and less functional responsiveness to chemical blockade.[82-84] There is some human evidence that the inhibitory subunit of troponin (troponin I) changes from a predominately cAMP-insensitive form to a cAMP-responsive form by 9 months of age, giving a possible explanation for the increased responsiveness seen with β-adrenergic stimulation after the neonatal period.[85] All of this information has led to the theory that the neonatal cardiac myocyte is more dependent on free cytosolic Ca^{2+} fluxes than is the mature heart and more susceptible to blockade of the L-type Ca^{2+} sarcolemmal channels as a mechanism of depression of myocardial contractility. The latter is thought to be an explanation for the greater hemodynamic depression seen with halothane in neonatal rat myocytes than with sevoflurane and an explanation for the same phenomenon seen clinically.[86] Because nearly all of this experimental evidence comes from various animal models, there is a need for studies in human tissue to determine if these explanations are valid in patients. The age of cardiac intracellular and extracellular maturity in humans is not clear because of this lack of information, but on clinical grounds it is thought to be approximately 6 months of age. The major differences in cardiac development and function between the neonatal and mature heart are summarized in Table 2-2.

Heart Failure

An increasing body of evidence points to the hypophosphorylation of phospholamban as a common pathway in many forms of heart failure.[87,88] Phosphorylation of phospholamban at its serine-16 position leads to proportional increases in the rate of reuptake of Ca^{2+} into the SR by SERCA, enhancing the efficiency of Ca^{2+} cycling and contraction and relaxation of the cardiac myocyte. Mice with genetically engineered dilated cardiomyopathy that are genetically altered further to eliminate normal phospholamban expression do not develop decreased systolic or diastolic function or dilated cardiomyopathy.[87] In addition, the phospholamban-SERCA interaction seems to have the central role in establishing normal basal cardiac contractility and relaxation, and eliminating phospholamban in otherwise normal mice greatly diminishes or eliminates the effect of β-adrenergic signaling. Other components of the calcium cycling systems (i.e., dissociation of L-type Ca^{2+} channels from ryanodine receptors or altered Na^+/Ca^{2+} exchanger function) may play roles in heart failure, but experimental evidence to this point suggests that these other changes play minor roles, and that the phospholamban-SERCA interaction is predominant.

CURRENT STATUS AND FUTURE TRENDS

More recent research has delineated the crucial role of the AR system in the regulation of cardiovascular function in heart failure, but much remains to be learned about the adrenergic system in the failing immature heart. Long-standing myocardial dysfunction and dilated cardiomyopathy, whatever the underlying etiology, lead to desensitization and down-regulation of the β-AR. This leads to less downstream phosphorylation of proteins

TABLE 2-2

Summary of the Major Differences Between Neonatal and Mature Hearts		
	Neonatal	**Mature**
Physiology		
Contractility	Limited	Normal
Heart rate dependence	High	Low
Contractile reserve	Low	High
Afterload tolerance	Low	Higher
Preload tolerance	Limited	Better
Ventricular interdependence	Significant	Less
Ca^{2+} cycling		
Predominant site of Ca^{2+} flux	Sarcolemma	SR
Dependence on normal ionized Ca^{2+}	High	Lower
Circulating catecholamines	High	Lower
Adrenergic receptors	Down-regulated, insensitive β_2, α_1 predominant	Normal, β_1
Predominant innervation	Parasympathetic predominates; sympathetic incomplete	Complete
Cytoskeleton	Higher water content	Lower water content
Cellular elements	Incomplete SR, disorganized myofibrils	Mature SR, organized myofibrils

SR, sarcoplasmic reticulum.

involved in excitation-contraction coupling, including phospholamban. An increasing body of evidence points to the hypophosphorylation of phospholamban as a common pathway in many forms of heart failure.

Other experimental data have implicated the ryanodine receptor in heart failure.[89] The opening of ryanodine-sensitive Ca^{2+} release channels in the SR causes a large Ca^{2+} flux into the cytosol, resulting in cardiac myocyte contraction. Evidence from animal models and human tissue suggests that in chronic heart failure and myocardial dysfunction, there is a diastolic "leak" of Ca^{2+} from the SR, resulting in less available Ca^{2+} for release in systole.[90,91] This altered function of the ryanodine receptor is thought to be caused by increased phosphorylation, by increased sympathetic nervous system activity, and increased β-adrenergic pathway activation, although, as discussed previously, desensitization and down-regulation of the β-AR should lead to less downstream phosphorylation. The ryanodine receptor is a large and complex molecule subject to numerous regulatory mechanisms, and undoubtedly much new information will be generated about its role in heart failure in the near future.[92-94]

Key Concepts

■ A specific agonist (or ligand) binds to the receptor,[94] which causes a conformational change. This structural change permits the interaction between the intracellular portion of the receptor and G protein. This interaction, also referred to as coupling, links the activated receptor to a specific biologic response.

■ Distribution of a particular β-AR in two different tissue types may result in two different functions. The β_1-receptor is predominantly expressed in heart tissue. The stimulation of the receptor subtype leads to inotropic and chronotropic effects on cardiac function, resulting in an increase in the myocardial contractility, an acceleration in the velocity of relaxation, and an increase in heart rate, respectively. These effects ultimately lead to a marked increase in cardiac output. Although β_2-receptors also can be found in the heart (especially in immature hearts), they are predominantly expressed in vascular smooth muscle.

■ α-ARs can be pharmacologically subdivided into α_1 and α_2 subtypes. The α_1-receptor is distributed in most vascular smooth muscle and to a lesser extent in the heart. The α_2-receptor is predominantly a presynaptic receptor in the central and peripheral nervous systems.

■ Phosphorylated adrenergic receptors produced by high doses of catecholamines may be inactivated by a process called sequestration after only a few minutes. These receptors can be sequestered by endocytosis, in a process involving a protein called β-arrestin, which binds to the receptor, and a sarcolemmal protein called clathrin.

■ Patients with severe or poorly compensated acyanotic (e.g., congestive heart failure) or cyanotic (e.g., severe cyanosis) heart disease have significantly reduced β-AR densities.

■ In children with congestive heart failure secondary to chronic left-to-right shunting and volume overload of the heart, circulating norepinephrine levels are elevated, as they are in adults with congestive heart failure. This elevation leads to a down-regulation in β-AR density.

■ Chronic β-AR stimulation in heart failure has many deleterious effects, ranging from uncoupling, desensitization, and down-regulation of the β-AR leading to decreased response to adrenergic stimulation to increased apoptosis, and switching on of fetal gene programs that lead to myocyte hypertrophy.

■ The endothelial-mediated systems (NO-cGMP pathways) seem to predominate in the pulmonary circulation (low-resistance circulation), whereas the phospholipase systems function in the systemic circulation (high-resistance circulation).

■ NO is an endothelium-derived relaxant factor that causes relaxation of vascular smooth muscle cells by activating guanylate cyclase, increasing the concentration of cGMP, reducing the local concentration of Ca^{2+}, and reducing vascular tone.

■ Vasodilation of the systemic circulation results from the formation of NO by nitrovasodilators or by activation of β_2-ARs in the peripheral vasculature, both of which result in the activation of guanylate cyclase and the production of cGMP, which reduces intracellular Ca^{2+} concentrations and results in the relaxation of vascular smooth muscle.

■ The neonatal cardiac myocyte is more dependent on free cytosolic Ca^{2+} fluxes than is the mature heart and more susceptible to blockade of the L-type Ca^{2+} sarcolemmal channels as a mechanism of depression of myocardial contractility.

REFERENCES

1. Moss J, Renz CL: The autonomic nervous system. In Miller RD [ed]: Anesthesia, 5th ed. Philadelphia, Churchill Livingstone, 2000, pp 523-577.
2. Booker PD: Pharmacological support for children with myocardial dysfunction. Paediatr Anaesth 2002;12:5-25.
3. Ahlquist RP: A study of the adrenotropic receptors. Am J Physiol 1948;153:586-600.
4. Bristow MR, Ginsburg R, Umans V, et al: Beta 1- and beta 2-adrenergic-receptor subpopulations in nonfailing and failing human ventricular myocardium: Coupling of both receptor subtypes to muscle contraction and selective beta 1-receptor down-regulation in heart failure. Circ Res 1986;59:297-309.
5. Kozlik R, Kramer HH, Wicht H, et al: Myocardial beta-adrenoreceptor density and the distribution of beta 1- and beta 2-adrenoceptor subpopulations in children with congenital heart disease. Eur J Pediatr 1991;150:388-394.
6. Sun LS, Du F, Quaegebeur JM: Right ventricular infundibular beta-adrenoceptor complex in tetralogy of Fallot patients. Pediatr Res 1997;42:12-16.
7. Xiao RP, Cheng H, Zhou YY, et al: Recent advances in cardiac beta(2)-adrenergic signal transduction. Circ Res 1999;85:1092-1100.

8. Post SR, Hilal-Dandan R, Urasawa K, et al: Quantification of signaling components and amplification in the beta-adrenergic-receptor-adenylate cyclase pathway in isolated adult rat ventricular myocytes. Biochem J 1995;311(Pt 1):75-80.

9. Sun LS: Regulation of myocardial beta-adrenergic receptor function in adult and neonatal rabbits. Biol Neonate 1999;76:181-192.

10. Kozlik R, Kramer HH, Wicht H, et al: Myocardial beta-adrenoreceptor density and the distribution of beta 1- and beta 2-adrenoceptor subpopulations in children with congenital heart disease. Eur J Pediatr 1991;150:388-394.

11. Tanaka H, Manita S, Matsuda T, et al: Sustained negative inotropism mediated by alpha-adrenoreceptors in adult mouse myocardium: Developmental conversion from positive response in the neonate. Br J Pharmacol 1995;114:673-677.

12. Sun LS, Rybin VO, Steinberg SF, Robinson RB: Characterization of the alpha-1 adrenergic chronotropic response in neuropeptide Y-treated cardiomyocytes. Eur J Pharmacol 1998;349:377-381.

13. Tanaka H, Takenaka Y, Yamaguchi H, et al: Evidence of alpha-adrenoceptor-mediated chronotropic action in children. Pediatr Cardiol 2001;22:40-43.

14. Schranz D, Droege A, Broede A, et al: Uncoupling of human cardiac beta-adrenergic receptors during cardiopulmonary bypass with cardioplegic arrest. Circulation 1993;87:422-426.

15. Smiley RM, Kwatra MM, Schwinn DA: New developments in cardiovascular adrenergic receptor pharmacology: Molecular mechanisms and clinical relevance. J Cardiothorac Vasc Anesth 1998;12:80-95.

16. Garcia-Sainz HA, Vazquez-Prado J, Carmen-Medina L: α1-adrenoceptors: function and phosphorylation. Eur J Pharmacol 2000;389:1-12.

17. Zeiders JL, Seidler FJ, Slotkin TA: Agonist-induced sensitization of β-adrenoceptor signaling in neonatal rat heart: Expression and catalytic activity of adenylyl cyclase. J Pharmacol Exp Ther 1999;291:503-510.

18. Muller FU, Boheler KR, Eschenhagen T, et al: Isoprenaline stimulates gene transcription of the inhibitory G protein alpha-subunit Gi alpha-2 in rat heart. Circ Res 1993;72:696-700.

19. Lai LP, Suematsu M, Elam H, Liang CS: Differential changes of myocardial beta-adrenoceptor subtypes and G-proteins in dogs with right-sided congestive heart failure. Eur J Pharmacol 1996;309:201-208.

20. Maki T, Gruver EJ, Davidoff AJ, et al: Regulation of calcium channel expression in neonatal myocytes by catecholamines. J Clin Invest 1996;97:656-663.

21. Lai LP, Raju VS, Delehanty JM, et al: Altered sarcoplasmic reticulum Ca^{2+}-ATPase gene expression in congestive heart failure: Effect of chronic norepinephrine infusion. J Mol Cell Cardiol 1998;30:175-185.

22. Communal C, Singh K, Pimentel DR, Colucci WS: Norepinephrine stimulates apoptosis in adult rat ventricular myocytes by activation of the beta-adrenergic pathway. Circulation 1998;98:1329-1334.

23. Iwai-Kanai E, Hasegawa K, Araki M, et al: Alpha- and beta-adrenergic pathways differentially regulate cell type-specific apoptosis in rat cardiac myocytes. Circulation 1999;100:305-311.

24. Hoffman TM, Wernovsky G, Atz A, et al: Efficacy and safety of milrinone in preventing low cardiac output syndrome in infants and children after corrective surgery for congenital heart disease. Circulation 2003;107:996-1002.

25. Kozlik-Feldmann R, Kramer HH, Wicht H, et al: Distribution of myocardial beta-adrenoceptor subtypes and coupling to the adenylate cyclase in children with congenital heart disease and implications for treatment. J Clin Pharmacol 1993;33:588-595.

26. Sun LS, Du F, Quagebeur JM: Right ventricular infundibular beta-adrenoceptor complex in tetralogy of Fallot patients. Pediatr Res 1997;42:12-16.

27. Borthne K, Haga P, Langslet A, et al: Endogenous norepinephrine stimulates both alpha 1- and beta adreceptors in myocardium from with congenital heart defects. J Mol Cell Cardiol 1995;27:693-699.

28. Wu JR, Chang HR, Chen SS, Huang TY: Circulating noradrenaline and beta-adrenergic receptors in children with congestive heart failure. Acta Paediatr 1996;85:923-927.

29. Buchhorn R, Huylpke-Wette M, Ruschewski W, et al: Beta-receptor downregulation in congenital heart disease: A risk factor for complications after surgical repair? Ann Thorac Surg 2002;73:610-613.

30. Zeng H, Li W, Li Y, et al: Evaluation of cardiac beta-adrenergic receptor function in children by dobutamine stress echocardiography. Chin Med J 1999;112:623-626.

31. Re G, Bergamasco L, Badino P, et al: Canine dilated cardiomyopathy: Lymphocyte and cardiac alpha (1)- and beta-adrenoceptor concentrations in normal and affected Great Danes. Vet J 1999;158:120-127.

32. Sjaastad I, Schiander I, Sjetnan A, et al: Increased contribution of alpha 1- vs. beta-adrenoceptor-mediated inotropic response in rats with congestive heart failure. Acta Physiol Scand 2003;177:449-458.

33. Buchhorn R, Hulpke-Wette M, Ruschewski W, et al: Effects of therapeutic beta blockade on myocardial function and cardiac remodeling in congenital cardiac disease. Cardiol Young 2003;13:36-43.

34. Christman BW, McPherson CD, Newman JH, et al: An imbalance between the excretion of thromboxane and prostacyclin metabolites in pulmonary hypertension. N Engl J Med 1992;327:70-75.

35. Palmer RM, Ferrige AG, Moncada S: Nitric oxide release accounts for the biological activity of endothelium-derived relaxing factor. Nature 1987;327:524-526.

36. Archer SL, Huang JM, Hampl V, et al: Nitric oxide and cGMP cause vasorelaxation by activation of a charybdotoxin-sensitive K channel by cGMP-dependent protein kinase. Proc Natl Acad Sci U S A 1994;91:7583-7587.

37. Atz AM, Wessel DL: Sildenafil ameliorates effects of inhaled nitric oxide withdrawal. Anesthesiology 1999;91:307-310.

38. Haywood GA, Tsao OS, con der Leyen HE, et al: Expression of inducible nitric oxide synthase in human heart failure. Circulation 1996;93:1087-1094.

39. Brady AJ, Warren JB, Poole-Wilson PA, et al: Nitric oxide attenuates cardiac myocyte contraction. Am J Physiol 1993;265:H176-H182.

40. Hare JM, Loh E, Creager MA, et al: Nitric oxide inhibits the positive inotropic response to beta-adrenergic stimulation in humans with left ventricular dysfunction. Circulation 1995;92:2198-2203.

41. Champion HC, Skaf MW, Hare JM: Role of nitric oxide in the pathophysiology of heart failure. Heart Fail Rev 2003;8:35-46.

42. Yanagisawa M, Kurihara H, Kimura S, et al: A novel potent vasoconstrictor peptide produced by vascular endothelial cells. Nature 1988;332:411-415.

43. Cacoub P, Dorent R, Maistre G, et al: Endothelin-1 in primary pulmonary hypertension and the Eisenmenger syndrome. Am J Cardiol 1993;71:448-450.

44. Galindo-Fraga A, Arrieta O, Castillo-Martinez L, et al: Elevation of plasmatic endothelin in patients with heart failure. Arch Med Res 2003;34:367-372.

45. Schultze-Nieck I, Li J, Reader JA, et al: The endothelin antagonist BQ123 reduces pulmonary vascular resistance after surgical intervention for congenital heart disease. J Thorac Cardiovasc Surg 2002;124:435-441.

46. Ram CV: Possible therapeutic role of endothelin antagonists in cardiovascular disease. Am J Ther 2003;10:396-400.

47. Izzard AS, Ohanian J, Tulip JR, Heagerty AM: The structure and function of the systemic circulation. In Anderson RH, Baker EJ, MaCartney F, et al (eds): Paediatric Cardiology, 2nd ed. London, Churchill Livingstone, 2002, pp 95-109.

48. Ebert TJ, Stowe DF: Neural and endothelial control of the peripheral circulation—implications for anesthesia: Part I. neural control of the peripheral vasculature. J Cardiothorac Vasc Anesth 1996;10:147-158.

49. Lee CR, Watkins ML, Patterson JH, et al: Vasopressin: A new target for the treatment of heart failure. Am Heart J 2003;146:9-18.

50. Leather HA, Segers P, Berends N, et al: Effects of vasopressin on right ventricular function in an experimental model of acute pulmonary hypertension. Crit Care Med 2002;30:2548-2552.

51. Liard JF: Interaction between V1 and V2 effects in hemodynamic response to vasopressin in dogs. Am J Physiol 1990;258: H482-H489.

52. Gheorghiade M, Niazi I, Ouyang J, et al: Vasopressin V2-receptor blockade with tolvaptan in patients with chronic heart failure: Results from a double-blind, randomized trial. Circulation 2003;107:2690-2696.

53. Yatsu T, Kusayama T, Tomura Y, et al: Effect of conivaptan, a combined vasopressin V(1a) and V(2) receptor antagonist, on vasopressin-induced cardiac and hemodynamic changes in anaesthetized dogs. Pharmacol Res 2002;46:375-381.

54. Liu P, Hopfner RL, Xu YJ, et al: Vasopressin-evolved [Ca2+i] responses in neonatal rat cardiomyocytes. Cardiovasc Pharmacol 1999;34:540-546.

55. Athanassopoulos G, Cokkinos DV: Atrial natriuretic factor. Prog Cardiovasc Dis 1991;33:313-328.

56. deLemos JA, McGuire DK, Drazner MH: B-type natriuretic peptide in cardiovascular disease. Lancet 2003;26:316-322.

57. Katan M, Williams RL: Phosphoinositide-specific phospholipase C: Structural basis for catalysis and regulatory interactions. Semin Cell Dev Biol 1997;8:287-296.

58. Moncada S, Higgs A: The L-arginine:nitric oxide pathway. N Engl J Med 1993;329:2002-2012.

59. Szymonowicz W, Walker AM, Cussen L, et al: Developmental changes in regional cerebral blood flow in fetal and newborn lambs. Am J Physiol 1988;254:H52-H58.

60. Davis PJ, Davis FB: Acute cellular actions of thyroid hormone and myocardial function. Ann Thorac Surg 1993;56:S16-S23.

61. Novotny J, Bourova L, Malkova O, et al: G proteins, β-adrenoceptors, and β-adrenergic responsiveness in immature and adult rat ventricular myocardium: Influence of neonatal hypo- and hyperthyroidism. J Mol Cell Cardiol 1999;31:761-772.

62. Mitchell IM, Pollock JC, Jamieson MP, et al: The effects of cardiopulmonary bypass on thyroid function in infants weighing less than five kilograms. J Thorac Cardiovasc Surg 1992;103:800-805.

63. Bettendorf M, Schmidt KG, Grulich-Henn J, et al: Tri-iodothyronine treatment in children after cardiac surgery: A double-blind, randomized, placebo-controlled study. Lancet 2000;356:529-534.

64. Seri I, Tan R, Evans J: Cardiovascular effects of hydrocortisone in preterm infants with pressor-resistant hypotension. Pediatrics 2001;107:1070-1074.

65. Yoder B, Martin H, McCurnin DC, et al: Impaired urinary cortisol excretion and early cardiopulmonary dysfunction in immature baboons. Pediatr Res 2002;51:422-424.

66. Tate CA, Taffet GE, Fisher DJ, Hyek MF: Excitation-contraction coupling: Control of normal myocardial cellular calcium movements. In Garson A, Bricker JT, Fisher DJ, Neish SR (eds): The Science and Practice of Pediatric Cardiology, 2nd ed. Baltimore, Williams & Wilkins, 1998, pp 171-180.

67. Fabiato A: Myoplasmic free calcium concentration reached during the twitch on an intact isolated cardiac cell and during calcium-induced release of calcium from the sarcoplasmic reticulum of a skinned cardiac cell from the adult rat or rabbit ventricle. J Gen Physiol 1981;78:457.

68. Bean BP: Two kinds of calcium channels in canine atrial cells: Difference in kinetic, selectivity, and pharmacology. J Gen Physiol 1985;86:1.

69. Eisner DA, Lederer WJ: Na-Ca exchange: Stoichiometry and electrogenicity. Am J Physiol 1985;248:C189.

70. Caroni P, Carafoli E: The Ca2+-pumping ATPase of heart sarcolemma. J Biol Chem 1981;256:3263.

71. Fabiato A: Time and calcium independence of activation and inactivation of calcium-induced release of calcium from the sarcoplasmic reticulum of a skinned cardiac Purkinje cell. J Gen Physiol 1985;85:247.

72. Van Winkle WB: The structure of striated muscle sarcoplasmic reticulum. In Entman M, Van Winkle WB (eds): Sarcoplasmic Reticulum in Muscle Physiology. Boca Raton, Fla, CRC Press, 1986, pp. 17-46.

73. Jones LR, Seler SM, Van Winkle WB: Regional differences in sarcoplasmic reticulum function. In Entman M, Van Winkle WB (eds): Sarcoplasmic Reticulum in Muscle Physiology. Boca Raton, Fla, CRC Press, 1986, pp. 1-20.

74. Levitsky DO, Benevolensky DS, Levchenko TS, et al: Calcium-binding rate and capacity of cardiac sarcoplasmic reticulum. J Mol Cell Cardiol 1981;13:785.

75. Jorgensen AO, Jones LR: Localization of phospholamban in slow but not fast canine skeletal muscle fibers. J Biol Chem 1986;261:3775.

76. Walsh KB, Cheng Q: Intracellular calcium regulates the responsiveness of the cardiac L-type calcium current to protein kinase A: Role of calmodulin. Am J Physiol Heart Circ Physiol 2003;286:H186-194.

77. Murray J, Weber A: The cooperative action of muscle proteins. Sci Am 1974;230:59-71.

78. Goldstein M, Michael L, Schroeter J, et al: Z band dynamics as a function of sarcomere length and the contractile state of muscle. FASEB J 1987;1:133-142.

79. Noble M, Pollack G: Molecular mechanisms of contraction. Cir Res 1977;40:333-342.

80. Chen F, Mottino G, Klitzner TS, et al: Distribution of the Na+/Ca2+ exchange protein in developing rabbit myocytes. Am J Physiol 1995;268:C1126-C1132.

81. Nakanishi T, Seguchi M, Takao A: Development of the myocardial contractile system. Experientia 1988;44:936-944.

82. Mahony L, Jones LR: Developmental changes in cardiac sarcoplasmic reticulum in sheep. J Biol Chem 1986;261:15257-15265.

83. Maylie JG: Excitation-contraction coupling in neonatal and adult myocardium of cat. Am J Physiol 1982;242:H834-H843.

84. Klitzner TS, Chen FH, Raven RR, et al: Calcium current and tension generation in immature mammalian myocardium: Effects of diltiazem. J Mol Cell Cardiol 1991;23:807-815.

85. Sasse S, Brand N, Kypreanou P, et al: Troponin I gene expression during human cardiac development and in end-stage heart failure. Circ Res 1993;72:932-938.

86. Prakash YS, Seckin I, Hunter IW, et al: Mechanisms underlying greater sensitivity of neonatal cardiac muscle to volatile anesthetics. Anesthesiology 2002;96:893-906.

87. Minamisawa S, Hoshijima M, Chu G, et al: Chronic phospholamban-sarcoplasmic reticulum calcium ATPase interaction is the critical calcium cycling defect in dilated cardiomyopathy. Cell 1999;99:313-322.

88. Hoshijima M, Chien KR: Mixed signals in heart failure: Cancer rules. J Clin Invest 2002;109:849-855.

89. Wehrens XH, Marks AR: Altered function and regulation of cardiac ryanodine receptors in cardiac disease. Trends Biochem Sci 2003;28:671-678.

90. Shannon TR, Pogwizd SM, Bers DM: Elevated sarcoplasmic reticulum Ca2+ leak in intact ventricular myocytes from rabbits in heart failure. Circ Res 2003;93:592-594.

91. Reiken S, Wehrens XH, Vest JA, et al: Beta-blockers restore calcium release channel function and improve cardiac muscle performance in human heart failure. Circulation 2003;107:2459-2466.

92. Marx SO, Marks AR: Regulation of the ryanodine receptor in heart failure. Basic Res Cardiol 2002;97(Suppl 1):I49-I51.

93. Xu L, Meissner G: Mechanisms of calmodulin inhibition of cardiac sarcoplasmic reticulum Ca2+ release channel (ryanodine receptor). Biophys J 2004;86:797-804.

94. Taur Y, Frishman WH: The cardiac ryanodine receptor (RyR2) and its role in heart disease. Cardiol Rev 2005 May-Jun;13(3): 142-146.

CHAPTER 3

Inflammatory Mediators in Heart Failure

Hordur H. Hardarson
Neil E. Bowles
Jesus G. Vallejo

Traditional concepts of heart failure have focused on the sympathetic nervous system and the renin-angiotensin system, but heart failure also results in a generalized perturbation of the inflammatory cascade and an overall disturbance of its molecular milieu. Heart failure of diverse etiologies is now recognized to have an important immunologic component, with the participation of a portfolio of proinflammatory and anti-inflammatory mediators influencing the process of myocardial function and cardiac remodeling.

Since the 1990s, this immunologic aspect of heart failure has been a clinical and an investigative focus in adult patients with heart failure. In children, acute viral infections of the heart are an important cause of cardiac dysfunction; dilated cardiomyopathy is sometimes a sequela of viral myocarditis. Children also frequently undergo cardiopulmonary bypass for palliative and corrective procedures. Overall, similar levels of interest and understanding of this inflammatory influence in heart dysfunction should be promoted in children with heart disease and heart failure.

This chapter provides an overview of the biology of proinflammatory and anti-inflammatory mediators, including cytokines, and discusses their adaptive and maladaptive effects in certain inflammatory heart diseases, especially in heart failure. Myocarditis, dilated cardiomyopathy, low cardiac output syndrome after cardiopulmonary bypass, and sepsis are discussed separately in subsequent chapters in more detail. Viral myocarditis is discussed here first as the classic inflammatory process in heart disease, followed by a more detailed presentation of the key inflammatory mediators in heart failure with adaptive and maladaptive roles. Finally, the overall effects of these mediators on myocardial function and remodeling are discussed.

INFLAMMATION AND THE HEART

Viruses are an important cause of myocarditis, with coxsackie virus being the most common viral pathogen. Adenovirus also has been implicated as a common etiologic agent of myocarditis.[1] Other viruses reported to cause myocarditis include Epstein-Barr virus,[2] human herpesvirus,[3] parvovirus B19,[4] and hepatitis C virus.[5] Coxsackieviruses B3 and B4 are the dominant viruses

detected serologically in patients with myocarditis or by direct molecular probing of myocardial tissue.

Advances in molecular biology have increased the diagnostic sensitivity of cardiac biopsy in myocarditis. Many institutions routinely use polymerase chain reaction and RNA hybridization to provide rapid, reliable, and specific detection of viral genetic material in myocardial specimens. Evidence of enteroviral infection has been found by such techniques in 30% of adult patients who have dilated cardiomyopathy.[6,7] Less invasive substrates also have been used for molecular diagnosis of viral pathogens: Polymerase chain reaction results on tracheal aspirates (in mechanically ventilated patients) for enterovirus, adenovirus, herpesvirus, cytomegalovirus, respiratory syncytial virus, and Epstein-Barr virus yielded identical results to polymerase chain reaction analysis of endomyocardial biopsy specimen.[8]

Myocarditis remains a poorly understood disease, insofar as it progresses through different phases with distinctly different mechanisms and clinical manifestations. Liu and Mason[9] elegantly summarized myocarditis as a disease continuum that comprises three separate phases: acute viral infection (phase I), autoimmunity (phase II), and dilated cardiomyopathy (phase III) (see Chapter 17). Briefly, phase I of the disease is triggered by the entry and proliferation in the myocardium of the causative virus. Phase I concludes with activation of the host immune system, which attenuates viral proliferation, but also may enhance viral entry. Ideally the immune response should down-regulate to a resting state when viral proliferation is controlled. If immune activation continues unabated despite elimination of the virus, autoimmune disease may result, initiating phase II of the disease. The continuous activation of the T cells in myocarditis is ultimately detrimental to the host because cytokine-mediated and direct T cell–mediated myocyte damage reduces the number of contractile units. The cumulative effect causes impairment of contractile function, which leads to long-term remodeling and progression to dilated cardiomyopathy (phase III).

In 1974, Woodruff and Woodruff,[10] using a murine model, showed for the first time a role for **T lymphocytes** in the pathogenesis of viral myocarditis. In this study, mice depleted of T lymphocytes had a decrease in the inflammatory response and decreased mortality. Subsequently, Opavsky and coworkers[11] defined the specific contributions of T cell subsets (CD4 and CD8) to the pathogenesis of viral myocarditis. When CD4$^{-/-}$ and CD8$^{-/-}$ mice were exposed to coxsackievirus B3, loss of CD8$^{+/+}$ immune cells did not affect survival significantly, but viral proliferation was attenuated. In contrast, CD4$^{-/-}$ mice showed a trend toward an improvement in survival. Mice deficient in CD4 and CD8 immune cells had the best outcomes in terms of viral attenuation and decreased mortality. These findings provided further support for the hypothesis that T cell responses in viral myocarditis lead to increased inflammation, myocyte destruction, and cardiac dysfunction in the host. More recent studies suggest, however, that the adaptive immune system does not function independently and that almost every aspect of the adaptive immune response may be controlled by the innate immune system.

The discovery of a family of mammalian receptors related to *Drosophila toll* has provided an explanation for how cells of the innate immune system recognize and react against a wide variety of microbial antigens through pattern recognition receptors.[12] A loss of function mutation in the *Drosophila toll* gene resulted in increased susceptibility to fungal infections in the fly, whereas it did not disrupt host defense mechanisms against bacterial pathogens. Homologues of the *Drosophila toll,* termed **toll-like receptors (TLRs)**, have been identified in higher vertebrate species, including mammals. This family of TLRs consists of 10 members that have a shared structural homology and signaling component. Medzhitov and colleagues[13] described the first human homologue of *Drosophila toll,* termed *human TLR4,* which activates the nuclear factor κ B (NF-κB) signaling pathway (see later) that is crucial for up-regulating the expression of a variety of inflammatory mediators in response to bacterial lipopolysaccharide (LPS).

Ligands for many of the TLRs have been described. The major cell wall component of gram-positive bacteria, peptidoglycan, is recognized by TLR2; TLR9 binds unmethylated bacterial CpG DNA; and TLR2 and TLR4 recognize lipoteichoic acid.[14-16] Activation of adaptive immunity is largely provided by dendritic cells (DCs). Several bacterial components, such as LPS, CpG DNA, lipoprotein, and the cell wall skeleton of *Mycobacterium,* have been shown to induce the maturation of DCs via TLRs.[14,17,18] The expressions of TLR1, TLR2, TLR4, and TLR5 have been observed in immature DCs but decrease as DCs mature.[19] In contrast, TLR3 is preferentially expressed in mature DCs, raising the intriguing possibility that this receptor may have a unique function in sensing pathogens linking the transition from innate to adaptive immunity.[20] Relevant to viral inflammatory heart disease is the finding that TLR3 recognizes double-stranded RNA (dsRNA), which is produced by most viruses at some point during their replication.[21] TLR3 may play an important role in the transition from innate to adaptive immunity.

INFLAMMATORY MEDIATORS AND THE FAILING HEART

Nuclear Factor κB

The activation of the inflammatory response requires the coordinated expression of numerous effector systems that respond to external stress. The external stimuli, which may include infection, cytokine or neurohormone receptor activation, or oxidative stress, all converge through intracellular signaling pathways on specific families of nuclear transcription factors, a prominent member being NF-κB. NF-κB is a dimeric transcription factor consisting of homodimers or heterodimers of Rel-related

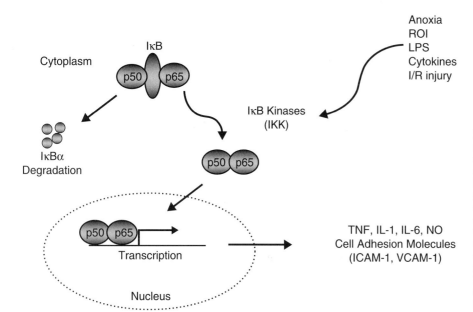

FIGURE 3-1 ■ **Activation of the transcription factor nuclear factor κB (NF-κB).** In the cytoplasm, the NF-κB dimer consists of the subunits p50/p65 bound to the inhibitory proteins known as inhibitory κ B (IκB). Stimuli activation of IκB kinases (IKK) causes translocation of NF-κB to the nucleus, and transcription of target genes begins. ROI, reactive oxygen intermediates; LPS, lipopolysaccharide; I/R, ischemia/reperfusion; TNF, tumor necrosis factor; IL-1, interleukin-1; IL-6, interleukin-6; ICAM-1, intercellular adhesion molecule 1; VCAM-1, vascular adhesion molecule 1.

proteins (Fig. 3-1). It normally resides in the cytoplasm, complexed with the **inhibitor (IκB)**, in an inactive form. On activation by external stimuli, the inflammatory signals converge on a set of regulatory control IκB kinases known as the **IKK complex**. The IKK complexes can phosphorylate IκB, leading to its ubiquitination and degradation by the proteosome. The liberated NF-κB enters the nucleus and interacts with κB elements in the promoter region of many inflammatory response genes, leading to activation of more cytokines. NF-κB plays a role in processes that range from acute myocardial injury to chronic heart failure.

In the heart, a role for NF-κB has been shown almost exclusively in ischemia-reperfusion experiments or in the early phase of myocardial infarction. Inhibition of NF-κB by in vivo introduction of a synthetic dsDNA with high affinity for NF-κB significantly reduced infarct size in ischemia and reperfusion.[22] Studies suggest that the inflammatory response participates in the development of heart failure of diverse etiologies, and NF-κB may be important in this aspect of pathologies.[23-25] Frantz and colleagues[23] showed chronic activation of NF-κB in experimental and human end-stage heart failure. These findings extend the more recent description of NF-κB activation in myocardial biopsy specimens of patients with heart failure and left ventricular (LV) assist devices.[25,26] NF-κB activation was reduced when cardiac function and remodeling improved as a result of a LV assist device.[26] NF-κB activation may have functional significance given that it is a central element in the regulation of the innate immune system, wound healing, apoptosis, and cell structure, which all play crucial roles in LV remodeling.

Evidence also exists that activation of NF-κB might be protective: NF-κB is readily activated by oxidative stress.[27] In addition, proinflammatory cytokines, such as tumor necrosis factor (TNF)-α and interleukin (IL)-1β, have been shown to activate NF-κB, leading to the up-regulation of cytoprotective genes (including *MnSOD,* the cellular inhibitors of apoptosis 1 and 2 [*c-IAP1* and *c-IAP2*], and members of the *Bcl-2* family [*Bcl-2, Bfl-1,* and *Bcl-xL*]). Inhibition of TLR2, an activator of NF-κB, inhibited hydrogen peroxide–induced NF-kB activation.[28] This reduction in NF-κB activation led to increased cytotoxicity and apoptosis of cardiac myocytes. Considering the important role of apoptosis in heart failure and the expression of TLR, especially in the border zone between viable and damaged myocardium, one might speculate that activation of NF-κB could play a role in the protection of ischemic but viable myocardium in heart failure. In addition to its role in the activation of cytokines via amplification, NF-κB regulates apoptosis and protein synthesis and increases inducible nitric oxide synthase (NOS) and cell adhesion molecules.

Tumor Necrosis Factor and Receptors

TNF is a multifunctional cytokine (a peptide with biologic function) that has local homeostatic effects in a diverse array of cells, including cardiac myocytes. TNF is initially produced as a nonglycosylated transmembrane protein of approximately 25 kDa. A fragment is proteolytically cleaved off the plasma membrane by a membrane-bound enzyme called **TNF-converting enzyme** to produce the secreted form of the cytokine. Kapadia and colleagues[29] were the first to provide direct evidence that cardiac myocytes can produce TNF endogenously in response to stresses or injury independent of the presence of inflammatory cells. Similarly, TNF expression was found to be up-regulated in the heart after experimental myocardial infarction and ischemia-reperfusion injury.[30,31] These data showed that the heart has an innate capacity to produce TNF in response to diverse pathophysiologic stimuli. Known or speculative negative effects of TNF in heart failure include myocyte changes (hypertrophy and apoptosis), ventricular dilation and dysfunction, extracellular matrix alterations (degradation of fibrillar collagen), β-adrenergic receptor uncoupling, disturbances of myocyte metabolism, endothelial dysfunction, and activation of fetal gene expression.

TNF receptors (TNFRs) signal as homotrimers and can exist either as membrane-bound or as truncated **soluble forms (STNFRs)**.[32] Two distinct surface receptors mediate the effects of TNF, TNFR1 (p55) and TNFR2 (p75).[32] Despite the conserved extracellular domains, the cytoplasmic domains of the two receptors lack homology, suggesting activation of different downstream transduction pathways (Fig. 3-2). TNFR1 is constitutively expressed in most tissues, whereas expression of TNFR2 is highly regulated. In most cells, TNFR1 seems to be the key mediator of TNF signaling, whereas in the lymphoid system, TNFR2 seems to play a major role.

Torre-Amione and associates[33] were the first to show that both receptor subtypes are expressed in human cardiac myocytes. Although the exact functional significances of TNFR1 and TNFR2 in the heart remain to be defined, the deleterious effects of TNF are coupled to TNFR1, whereas activation of TNFR2 seems to exert protective effects in the heart. The extracellular domains of both receptors can be proteolytically cleaved, yielding soluble receptor fragments with potential neutralizing capacity. Although there is a strong correlation between elevated soluble TNFRs and increased 30-day mortality in patients with severe heart failure, the precise role of soluble TNFRs remains unknown.[34] It has been suggested that soluble TNFRs may increase the bioactivity of TNF, relative to unbound TNF, by stabilizing the molecule.[35,36]

Interleukin-1 and Receptors

IL-1, which exists in two forms, **IL-1α** and **IL-1β**, and is synthesized in the myocardial cells and cardiac fibroblasts, is one of the cytokines thought to be involved in changes observed in heart failure and heart dysfunction, specifically myocyte hypertrophy and calcium homeostasis. Each IL-1 is produced by a separate gene as a 31-kDa precursor protein, termed proIL-1α and proIL-1β.[37] The proIL-1

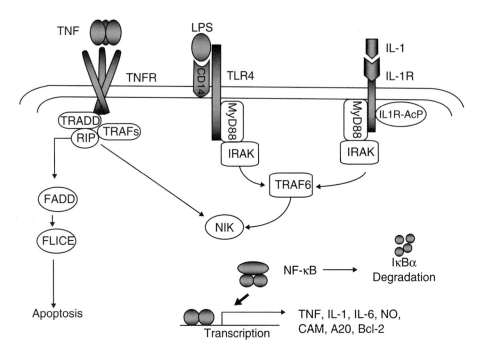

FIGURE 3-2 ■ **Tumor necrosis factor (TNF) and toll/interleukin (IL)-1 receptor signaling pathways.** Tumor necrosis factor receptor (TNFR) I activation favors induction of apoptosis through association with TNFR-associated death domain (TRADD), Fas-associated death domain (FADD), and receptor-interacting protein (RIP). Activation of TNFR II favors pathways leading to nuclear factor κ B (NF-κB) activation. The toll-like receptor and IL-1 receptor family members share several signaling components leading to the activation of NF-κB. FLICE, FADD-like IL-converting enzyme; NIK, NF-κB–inducing kinase; TLR, toll-like receptor; MyD88, myeloid differentiation factor 88; IRAK, IL receptor–associated kinase; TRAF6, TNF receptor–associated factor; IL1R-AcP, IL-1 accessory protein.

forms subsequently are cleaved by specific cellular proteases, including IL-1-converting enzyme, into mature 17-kDa proteins. IL-1α is generally located intracellularly or expressed on the cell surface. In contrast, IL-1β is released from the cell and produces its effects by acting on other cells. **IL-1R antagonist** is the third member of the IL-1 family. It is produced and secreted as a 17-kDa protein by almost all cells that express IL-1.[38]

Similar to TNF, IL-1β seems to be synthesized within the myocardium in response to stressful stimuli. In one of the first studies documenting IL-1 expression in the heart, Han and coworkers[39] reported increased expression of IL-1β mRNA in the hearts of patients with idiopathic dilated cardiomyopathy. Subsequently, Francis and associates[40] reported increased levels of this cytokine in the heart of patients with viral myocarditis.

The members of the IL-1 family bind to two distinct **IL-1 receptors, type I (IL-1RI)** and **type II (IL-1RII)**.[37] Binding to IL-1RI, but not IL-1RII, leads to receptor activation and subsequent intracellular signal transduction (see Fig. 3-2). When IL-1 binds to IL-1RI, a second component is recruited into the complex, called the IL-1 receptor accessory protein.[41,42] Signal transduction pathways activated by the approximated cytoplasmic domains of IL-1RI and IL-1R accessory protein include the NF-κB, JNK/AP-1, and p38 mitogen activated protein kinase pathways. IL-1RII is considered a decoy receptor that may serve to buffer the effects of excessive IL-1 production. In addition, the extracellular domains of both receptors are found in soluble form in the circulation, where they also may buffer the actions of IL-1. The soluble cytokine receptors are produced either by shedding via partial proteolysis of membrane-bound receptors or by de novo synthesis. In addition, IL-1R antagonist also functions as a competitive receptor antagonist

blocking IL-1RI activation and inhibiting the biologic actions of IL-1. The fact that recombinant IL-1 induces biologic effects in isolated neonatal cardiac myocytes suggests that IL-1R is present in these cells.

Interleukin-6, Interleukin-6 Receptors, and Interleukin-6-Related Cytokines

IL-6 and related cytokines, such as TNF and IL-1, are implicated in heart failure and changes such as myocyte hypertrophy; IL-6 also is thought to protect myocytes from apoptosis. IL-6 is a member of a family of cytokines that consists of leukemia inhibitory factor, IL-11, ciliary neurotropic factor, oncostatin M, and cardiotrophin 1 (CT-1).[43] Their classification is based on similarities in helical protein structure and a shared receptor subunit, transmembrane glycoprotein 130 (gp130). IL-6 is produced by many different cells, but the main sources in vivo are stimulated monocytes/macrophages, fibroblasts, and vascular endothelial cells. Typical stimuli for IL-6 production are IL-1, TNF, and bacterial LPS. Hypoxia induces IL-6 in cultured endothelial cells, and hypoxia in vivo elevates plasma IL-6 levels.[44,45] More recent studies have shown that plasma concentrations of IL-6 and IL-6-related cytokines are increased in patients with heart failure in relation to decreasing functional status.[46] Experimental studies also indicate that IL-6 and IL-6-related cytokines are elevated in patients with heart failure and may play important roles in the regulation of cardiac myocyte hypertrophy and apoptosis in the early stages of pressure overload.[46,47]

All IL-6-related cytokines signal through a multisubunit receptor complex that shares transmembrane gp130 (Fig. 3-3). Intracellular signaling is triggered either through homodimerization of gp130 (IL-6) or through heterodimerization of gp130 with a structural protein,

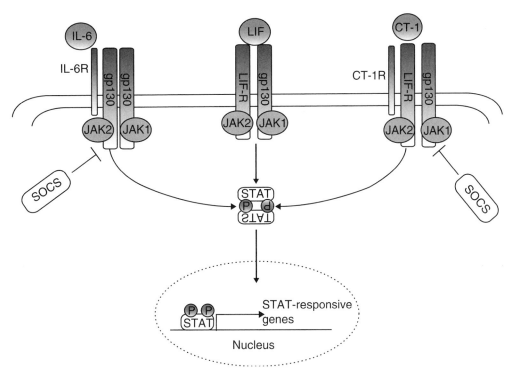

FIGURE 3-3 ■ **Interleukin (IL)-6 and IL-6 related cytokine receptor complexes.** Downstream signaling is triggered by the homodimerization of gp130 or heterodimerization of gp130 with leukemia inhibitory factor (LIF) receptor. Ligand-induced gp-130 dimerization results in the activation of several intracellular pathways, most notably the Janus kinase (JAK)–signal transducer and activator of transcription (STAT) pathway. Activation of the JAK-STAT pathway can be regulated by suppressors of cytokine signaling (SOCS).

the leukemia inhibitory factor receptor. The downstream pathways activated by the gp130 complex include the intracellular tyrosine kinases called **Janus kinase (JAK)** and several members of the transcription factor family called **signal transducer and activators of transcription (STAT)**.[48] The JAK-STAT pathway is activated by cytokine-induced phosphorylation of tyrosine and leads to STAT binding to regulatory regions of the DNA.

In addition, gp130 signaling is known to activate signaling intermediates that promote cell survival, such as **mitogen activated protein kinases** and phosphatidylinositol 3-kinase.[49,50] The activation of the JAK-STAT pathway in the heart is negatively regulated by suppression of cytokine signaling (SOCS) type 1 (SOCS1) and type 3 (SOCS3).[51] Studies have shown that signaling via the gp130-JAK-STAT pathway is profoundly disrupted in the hearts of patients with end-stage dilated cardiomyopathy.[52] A balance of the JAK-STAT-SOCS circuit may determine the overall effects of IL-6 and IL-6-related cytokines in the heart.

Nitric Oxide

Nitric oxide (NO) is a small gaseous molecule that mediates multiple signaling pathways in the heart with many effects on the myocyte, including increasing cGMP via activation of guanylate cyclase, inhibiting mitochondrial electron transport, decreasing affinity of contractile proteins for calcium, and modulating transsarcolemmal calcium flux and excitation-contraction coupling. NO is generated from L-arginine by three different isoforms of nitric oxide synthase (NOS).[53] All three NOS isoforms can be expressed in the heart. **Neuronal NOS (NOSI)** is found in nerve fibers and within cardiac myocytes. **Endothelial-type NOS (NOSIII)** is expressed constitutively in endothelial and endocardial cells and, at a much lower concentration, in cardiac myocytes. On appropriate stimulation, notably by cytokines, high-output **inducible NOS (NOSII)** can be expressed by many different cell types (e.g., infiltrating inflammatory cells, endothelial cells, and cardiac myocytes). In contrast to NOSI and NOSIII isoforms, NOSII synthesizes large NO amounts independent of calcium.

NO has a myriad of beneficial and toxic effects depending on sites of synthesis and resultant concentration (Table 3-1). Although positive effects of NO include improved relaxation and preload reserve, negative effects entail myocardial depression and β-adrenergic desensitization. In disease states associated with infection, inflammation, or cytokine activation, the expression of NOSII is clearly shown in the heart, including in the cardiac myocytes.[54-56] In human dilated cardiomyopathy and congestive heart failure, increased systemic NO production and enhanced myocardial NOSII mRNA and NOSII enzymatic activity have been reported.[56] The pathophysiologic role of NO in this context is controversial, however.

TABLE 3-1

Nitric Oxide and Differential Effects Based on Site of Action and Concentration
Cytosol (low concentration)—intracellular messenger that activates:
Guanylyl cyclase
Nuclear factor κ B
Cytokines
Antiapoptotic mechanisms
Extracellular (intermediate concentration)—autocrine and paracrine messenger that regulates:
Vasodilation (vascular endothelium to smooth muscle cells)
Amplification of nitric oxide production by tumor necrosis factor
Extracellular (high concentration)—toxic amounts produced by inducible nitric oxide leads to:
Generation of free radicals
Myocardial depression
DNA alterations
Apoptosis

Modified from Dugas B, Debre P, Moncada S, et al: Nitric oxide, a vital poison inside the immune and inflammatory network. Res Immunol 1995;146:664-670.

Heger and coworkers[57] reported that increased cardiac NOSII expression did not alter cardiac structure and function. In contrast, Mungrue and associates[58] described that conditional cardiac overexpression of NOSII in transgenic mice leads to a mild inflammatory infiltrate, cardiac fibrosis, hypertrophy, chamber dilation, and, albeit infrequently, congestive heart failure. Although the cytoskeleton of these transgenic mice was not directly assessed, the development of cardiac fibrosis suggests some degree of cytoskeletal reorganization. An important point when interpreting such studies is that NOS expression level does not reflect the amount of bioactive NO produced. In settings of increased oxidative stress, NO is inactivated by O_2^- in a reaction that can generate peroxynitrite. Not only does this reaction reduce NO concentrations, but also peroxynitrite itself is a potentially toxic species that can disrupt the function of diverse proteins through nitration and oxidation reactions.

Toll-like Receptors

There is now substantial evidence that the mediators and effectors of the innate immune response, including proinflammatory cytokines (TNF, IL-1β), NO, and chemokines, are expressed in the adult mammalian heart in response to challenge with classic agents, such as LPS and viral particles (i.e., dsRNA).[29,59] Studies have identified the presence of TLR2, TLR3, TLR4, and TLR6 in the adult mammalian myocardium.[21,28,60,61] TLR4-deficient mice have been shown to have a delayed and blunted response to LPS, with lower values of myocardial TNF, IL-1β, and inducible NOS proteins and lower NO production, suggesting that TLR4 mediates the immune response to LPS in the heart.[60]

dsRNA is produced by most viruses, and it is known to have important immunostimulatory activity partly as a result of its ability to activate the **dsRNA-dependent protein kinase, PKR**.[62] PKR-deficient cells have been shown to respond to dsRNA and its synthetic analogue, polyIC, indicating the existence of another receptor for dsRNA. Alexopoulou and colleagues[21] reported that mice deficient in TLR3 have a profound defect in their responsiveness to viral dsRNA and polyIC. As shown in Figure 3-4, activation of TLR3 by dsRNA induces the

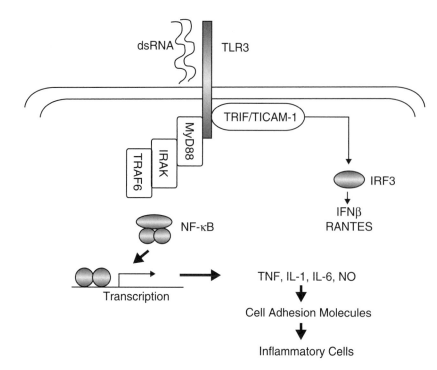

FIGURE 3-4 ■ **Toll-like 3 (TLR3) receptor.** TLR3 receptor is capable of recognizing specific pathogen-associated molecular patterns that are associated with viral infections. The recognition of double-stranded RNA (dsRNA) leads to the activation of nuclear factor κ B (NF-κB) through an MyD88 pathway, which then triggers the production of proinflammatory cytokines, interferons, cell adhesion molecules, and inflammatory cells. As shown, TLR3 also signals through a MyD88-independent pathway via toll/interleukin (IL)-1 receptor domain-containing adapter inducing interferon-β (TRIF) leading to the activation of interferon regulatory factor 3 (IRF3). TICAM-1, toll/IL-1 receptor domain-containing adapter protein.

expression of proinflammatory cytokines (e.g., TNF, IL-1β, IL-6, and interferons), all of which may have beneficial or deleterious effects on the heart or both. It is possible that TLR3 may specifically activate signaling pathways that render cells more resistant to viral infection. Challenge of TLR3-deficient mice with live viruses would be required to assess further the role of this receptor in the host's defense against viral infection.

A feature of TLR biology of particular importance in cardiovascular diseases is that extensive tissue damage may trigger endogenous TLR stimulation. Frantz and coworkers[61] showed that injured human and murine myocardium exhibits focal areas of intense TLR4 expression. The reasons for this differential expression of TLR4 and the function of TLR4 in the injured heart in the absence of infection remain to be defined. More recent studies have shown, however, that **heat-shock protein 60**, a protein released by cells undergoing necrotic cell death, and fibronectin may activate innate immune cells through a TLR4-dependent mechanism.[63,64] Necrotic, but not apoptotic, cells were shown to activate NF-κB and inflammatory gene induction in a TLR2-dependent manner.[65] When TLR2 is blocked, increased cytotoxicity is noted in cardiac myocytes exposed to hydrogen peroxide, indicating that the toll-NF-κB pathway may play an important role in the remodeling and repair process of the injured myocardium.[28] Further studies are required to define better the role of TLRs in the heart.

INFLAMMATORY MEDIATORS AND VIRAL-MEDIATED INFLAMMATORY HEART DISEASE

An overview of the key cytokines involved in heart disease and heart failure has been given; now their roles in viral-mediated inflammatory heart disease are reviewed. An important role for proinflammatory mediators in myocyte damage associated with inflammatory heart disease is suggested by the high incidence of cytokines, especially **TNF**, in patients with myocarditis and dilated cardiomyopathy.[66,67] Matsumori and coworkers[68] showed that patients with myocarditis have marked activation of cytokines, including TNF, IL-1, and IL-6. In patients with myocarditis, TNF mRNA expression levels correlated positively with LV volumes and inversely with LV systolic function.[67] TNF is thought to play an integral role in the inflammatory reaction present in myocarditis, given that administration of exogenous TNF aggravates myocarditis, and neutralization of TNF by antibodies or soluble receptors attenuates viral-induced damage.[69,70] Mice deficient in the TNF p55 receptor (TNF-R1$^{-/-}$) have milder autoimmune myocarditis compared with wild-type mice.[71] The robust overexpression of TNF in the absence of viral pathogens has been shown to result in lethal myocarditis in mice.[72,73] Less abundant expression of TNF in mice results in a lymphohistiocytic interstitial

inflammatory infiltrate, with progressive heart failure.[74] Together, these data support an adverse effect of TNF in myocarditis, and this is consistent with the proposed roles of TNF in activating endothelial cells, recruiting inflammatory cells, enhancing inflammatory cytokine production, and inducing negative inotropic effects.

In contrast to these disease-enhancing effects, TNF is thought to be important in host defense against microorganisms, a probable advantageous effect of this cytokine in response to microbial-induced myocarditis.[75] The requirement of TNF in the immunologic defense against myocarditis was shown in TNF-deficient mice exposed to encephalomyocarditis virus.[59] The TNF-deficient mice developed severe myocarditis with 100% mortality within 14 days. In contrast, 67% of the wild-type control mice were alive at 14 days. The requirement of TNF was confirmed by rescuing the TNF-deficient mice by treating them with recombinant TNF before viral infection.

The development of viral myocarditis is associated with the infiltration of the heart with inflammatory cells that secrete **IL-1,** and treatment with recombinant IL-1 has been shown to enhance coxsackievirus B3 myocarditis in partially resistant mice.[76,77] Expression of IL-1R antagonist in the mouse heart by plasmid DNA decreases acute myocardial inflammation in coxsackievirus B3 myocarditis, further suggesting a detrimental role of IL-1β in viral heart disease.[78] Shioi and associates[79] showed that IL-1 gene expression in the chronic stage of viral myocarditis is relatively high compared with other cytokines and positively correlates with the extent of fibrotic lesions. IFN-γ, IL-2, and TNF gene expressions in the chronic stage did not correlate with the extent of fibrosis. Eriksson and colleagues[80] provided the first in vivo evidence that IL-1R1 triggering is crucial for expansion of autoreactive CD4$^+$ T cells and subsequent induction of autoimmune heart disease. Mice lacking the IL-1R1 were protected from myocarditis and showed impaired priming of heart myosin-specific CD4$^+$ T cells, which resulted from defective activation of DCs. These findings suggest that IL-1 may play an important role in the three phases of viral inflammatory heart disease.

IL-6 has been shown to suppress inflammation in several animal models, an effect that is attributed to the inhibition of TNF and IL-1 production.[81,82] Kanda and associates[83] showed that exogenous IL-6, administered at the same time as viral inoculation in C3H/HeJ mice, improved survival rates, decreased cardiac viral titers, and reduced myocardial necrosis and lymphocytic infiltration in mice with viral myocarditis. The administration of IL-6 either 4 days before virus inoculation or 4 days after—the latter coincident with the peak in viremia and at the beginning of observable clinical illness—did not influence survival or myocardial destruction, however. Serum TNF levels in animals treated with IL-6 were significantly reduced in the early phase of viral myocarditis compared with control animals. These findings suggested that IL-6 might have a beneficial role in the acute phase of myocarditis. Subsequent studies by this same group have shown that mice with targeted overexpression of myocardial IL-6 have accelerated tissue injury and decreased viral clearance after infection with encephalomyocarditis virus.[84] The accelerated tissue injury was linked to decreased TNF production because administration of exogenous TNF resulted in significant improvement in viral clearance and less tissue destruction in IL-6 transgenic mice. The short-term expression of IL-6 may function as an adaptive response to modulate inflammatory and immune responses within acceptable ranges. Sustained IL-6 expression may engender adverse outcomes, however, if IL-6-induced anti-inflammatory or immunosuppressive responses or both are excessive and prevent activation of the appropriate antiviral response.

IL-6, CT-1 (gp130-related cytokines), IL-10, IL-12, IFN-α/β, and IFN-γ are induced during the early stages of viral infection and can activate JAK signaling.[79,83-85] The exogenous administration of these cytokines has been shown to ameliorate the severity of viral myocarditis in mouse models of infection. Yasukawa and coworkers[86] provided evidence for the essential role of JAK signaling in cardiac myocyte antiviral defense and a negative role of SOCS in the early stages of viral myocarditis. Cardiac myocyte–specific transgenic expression of SOCS1 inhibited enterovirus-induced signaling of **JAK-STAT**, with accompanying increases in viral replication, cardiomyopathy, and mortality in coxsackievirus B3–infected mice. The inhibition of SOCS in the cardiac myocyte through adenovirus-mediated expression of a dominant-negative SOCS1 increased the myocyte resistance to the acute cardiac injury caused by coxsackievirus B3. These data show that with enteroviral infection of the heart, the up-regulation of SOCS1 expression has a maladaptive effect in the early stages of viral replication and facilitates replication of the virus by preventing the full action of the JAK-STAT signaling pathway.

NO plays a pivotal role in the pathogenesis of viral myocarditis, mediating macrophage defense against viral infection. Because NOSII expression is regulated by cytokines, it can be postulated that viral myocarditis may result in a cytokine environment suitable for induction of this enzyme within the heart. The induced NOSII has been shown to mediate the antiviral properties of IFN-γ, and in vivo studies have confirmed the antiviral properties of NO.[87] NOSII activity appears on day 4, peaks on day 8, and can be detected for 1 month after virus inoculation in the murine model. Evidence from mice homozygous for a disrupted NOSII allele suggests that coxsackievirus-induced myocarditis is more severe when NOSII is lacking.[88] Reports by Badorff and colleagues[89,90] help to shed some additional light on these important questions by providing a potential molecular

mechanism for a protective role for NO in viral infection. These investigators showed that Coxsackievirus B3 possesses a protease (2A) that cleaves an integral membrane glycoprotein, dystrophin, in human and mouse cardiac membranes. They also provided evidence that NO donors can s-nitrosylate a cysteine residue that is essential for catalytic activity of protease 2A. More recent studies have shown that the hearts of dystrophin-deficient mice are more susceptible to enterovirus-induced cardiomyopathy, as indicated by the higher proportion of Evans blue dye–positive myocytes and higher viral titers after infection.[91] The elaboration of NO by cardiac myocytes may prevent dystrophin cleavage by inactivating viral protease 2A. The cytokine-induced elaboration of NO may have evolved as an important adaptive mechanism in preventing the development of dilated cardiomyopathy after exposure to Coxsackievirus B3. This possibility would suggest that defects in the NO-mediated host response to viral infection also could contribute to some of the variability in the natural history of idiopathic cardiomyopathy.

INFLAMMATORY MEDIATORS AND MYOCARDIAL DYSFUNCTION

The observation that proinflammatory mediators modulated LV function was first reported in a series of experimental studies showing that direct injections of **TNF** produced hypotension, metabolic acidosis, hemoconcentration, and death within minutes, mimicking the cardiac/hemodynamic response associated with LPS-induced septic shock.[92] Administration of antibodies directed against TNF attenuated the hemodynamic collapse seen in LPS shock. Similarly, TNF-induced depression of myocardial function in an ex vivo, crystalloid superperfused papillary muscle preparation was reported by Finkel and associates.[93] Experimental studies by Bozkurt and coworkers[94] showed that circulating concentrations of TNF similar to concentrations measured in patients with heart failure were sufficient to produce persistent negative inotropic effects that were detectable at the level of the cardiac myocyte. The observed negative inotropic effects of TNF were completely reversible when the infusion of TNF was discontinued. Subsequent studies in transgenic mice with targeted overexpression of TNF in the cardiac compartment showed that the overexpression of TNF results in depressed LV ejection performance.[74,95]

Calcium homeostasis is crucial to the normal myocardial contraction-relaxation, and TNF-induced disruption of calcium handling may lead to contractile dysfunction. Yokoyama and associates[96] showed that soon after the exposure to TNF, the amplitude of the calcium transient decreased during systole. TNF seems to disrupt L-type channel–induced calcium influx, thus depressing calcium transients.[97] In addition to disrupting calcium homeostasis, TNF can cause myocardial dysfunction through direct cytotoxicity, oxidant stress, and induction of other cardiac depressants, such as IL-1 and IL-6.[98] IL-1 synergistically enhances TNF-induced myocardial depression and cytotoxicity.[99,100] Although several investigators have implicated NO in TNF-induced cardiac depression, others have not been able to attribute all of the negative effects of TNF to NO.[93]

TNF seems to modulate myocardial function through at least two different mechanisms (immediate and delayed). The early phase of TNF-induced functional depression occurs within minutes, whereas the delayed phase seems to require hours of TNF exposure. Oral and colleagues[101] reported that TNF-induced sphingosine production is necessary for the negative inotropic effects of this cytokine, insofar as blocking sphingosine production through inhibition of ceramidase abrogated the negative inotropic effects of TNF. The production of myocardial sphingosine occurred within minutes of TNF exposure and correlated with myocardial dysfunction and calcium dyshomeostasis in cardiac myocytes. These data suggest that sphingosine mediates the early depression (NO independent) and that NO mediates the late dysfunction induced by TNF.

Although **IL-1** and **IL-6** have been shown to produce negative inotropic effects in various experimental models, the signal transduction pathways that are responsible for the negative inotropic effects of IL-6 have not been clearly established.[98] In contrast, the negative inotropic effects of IL-1 seem to be mediated, at least in part, through the production of NO (i.e., the delayed pathway).[102] It has been suggested that TNF and IL-1 may produce negative inotropic effects indirectly through activation or release (or both) of IL-18, which is a member of the IL-1 family of cytokines.[37] Specific blockade of IL-18 using neutralizing IL-18-binding protein leads to an improvement in myocardial contractility in atrial tissue that has been subjected to ischemia-reperfusion injury.[103] Although the signaling pathways that are responsible for the IL-18-induced negative inotropic effects have not been delineated so far, it is likely that they will overlap the effects for IL-1 and TLRs, given that the IL-18 receptor complex uses components of the IL-1/toll signaling pathway.

The role of **NO** in heart failure and precisely how it interacts with all the other cytokines remains to be elucidated further (Fig. 3-5). The discovery that the high-output isoform NOSII is expressed in the myocardium of patients with heart failure,[104] coupled with previous in vitro data that NOSII expression can induce contractile dysfunction,[105] has led to considerable interest in the potential role of NO in the pathophysiology of cardiac dysfunction in heart failure. NOSII expression or activity or both have been documented in end-stage failing heart tissue and in endomyocardial biopsy specimens obtained from patients with less severe heart failure of diverse etiology.[24,56] Direct evidence for a deleterious role of NOSII in human

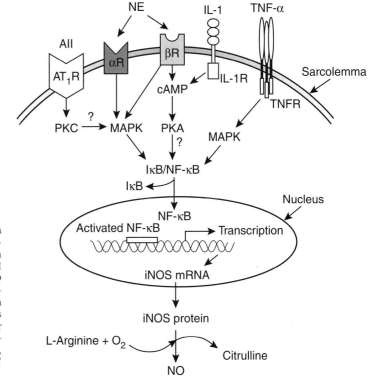

FIGURE 3-5 ■ Nitric oxide (NO) and interaction with cytokines and other molecules. Schematic diagram illustrates the complex interplay between cytokines interleukin (IL)-1 and tumor necrosis factor (TNF) with angiotensin II (AII) and norepinephrine (NE). IL-1 stimulates inducible NO synthase (iNOS) mRNA expression and subsequent NO production via cAMP, protein kinase A (PKA), and activation with nuclear translocation of nuclear factor κ B (NF-κB). This IL-1–mediated NO production is enhanced with the other mediators in the diagram. IκB, inhibitory κB; MAPK, mitogen-activated protein kinase; PKC, protein kinase C. (From Kan H, Finkel MS: *Interactions between cytokines and neurohormonal systems in the failing heart. Heart Fail Rev* 2001;6:119-127.)

heart failure is limited. The initial speculative suggestions that excessive NO production by inducible NOS has acute negative inotropic effects are too simplistic.

In patients with dilated cardiomyopathy of varying severities, intracoronary N(G)-monomethyl-L-arginine (L-NMMA) infusion had no effect either on basal contractile function or on the force-frequency relation.[106] Likewise, intracoronary L-arginine did not alter basal function.[107] It is possible that NOSII may have important chronic deleterious effects on the myocardium either caused by increased NO production or, more likely, mediated via peroxynitrite, which are reversible by acute administration of NOS inhibitors. Based on in vitro findings, such deleterious effects of NO could include cellular apoptosis, an irreversible impairment of contractile function, an irreversible decrease in myocardial oxygen consumption, and abnormal heart rate and rhythm regulation. Good evidence to support such effects of NOSII is currently lacking, however, even in experimental animal models of heart failure.

NO also is reported to modulate inotropic and chronotropic stimulation and response to β-adrenoceptor stimulation; low doses enhance and high doses reduce β-adrenergic response. In a physiologic context, these effects may be regarded as beneficial by optimizing or modulating responses to β-adrenoceptor stimulation. An effect of endogenous NO to modulate β-adrenergic inotropic responses in humans in vivo could be shown only in patients with impaired LV function and not in normal subjects.[104] Likewise, in carefully conducted studies in anesthetized pigs, there was no demonstrable effect of endogenous NO on β-adrenergic inotropic responsiveness.[108]

LV remodeling refers to the multitude of changes that occur in cardiac shape, size, and composition in response to myocardial injury. Inflammatory mediators have many important effects that may play important roles in the process of LV remodeling, including myocyte hypertrophy,[109] alterations in fetal gene expression,[74] and progressive myocyte loss through apoptosis.[110] In addition to the aforementioned effects, there is evidence suggesting that TNF may promote LV remodeling through alterations in the extracellular matrix. Bozkurt and associates[94] showed that when concentrations of TNF that overlap the concentrations observed in patients with heart failure are infused continuously in rats, there is a time-dependent change in LV dimension that is accompanied by progressive degradation of the extracellular matrix. Similar findings have been reported after a single infusion of TNF in dogs.[111] Kubota and coworkers[73] showed that a transgenic mouse line with overexpressed TNF in the cardiac compartment had progressive LV dilation over 24 weeks of observation (Fig. 3-6). Similar findings were reported by Bryant and colleagues[72] and Sivasubramanian and colleagues,[112] who observed identical findings with respect to LV dysfunction and LV dilation in transgenic mice with targeted overexpression of TNF in the heart.

Although the precise mechanisms that are involved in TNF-induced LV dilation are not fully delineated, it has been suggested that TNF-induced activation of **matrix metalloproteinases (MMPs)**, which leads to

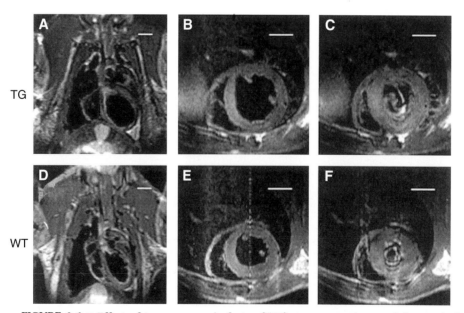

FIGURE 3-6 ■ Effect of tumor necrosis factor (TNF) overexpression on left ventricular remodeling. Magnetic resonance imaging of hearts from transgenic mice with overexpression of TNF **(A-C)** shows dilation of the left ventricle compared with control mice **(D-F)** (From Kubota T, McTiernan CF, Frye CS, et al: *Cardiac-specific overexpression of tumor necrosis factor-alpha causes lethal myocarditis in transgenic mice. J Card Fail* 1997;3:117.)

degradation of the extracellular matrix, is responsible for this effect.[112,113] The hearts of transgenic mice overexpressing TNF in the cardiac compartment with progressive loss of fibrillar collagen and increased MMP activation have been documented. In these mice, long-term stimulation (8 to 12 weeks) with TNF resulted in an increase in fibrillar collagen content that was accompanied by decreased MMP activity and increased expression of the **tissue inhibitors of MMPs (TIMPs)**.[112] Taken together, these observations suggest that sustained myocardial inflammation provokes time-dependent changes in the balance between MMP activity and TIMP activity. During the early stages of inflammation, there is an increase in the ratio of MMP activity to TIMP levels that leads to LV dilation. With chronic inflammatory signaling, however, there is a time-dependent increase in TIMP levels, leading to a decrease in the ratio of MMP activity to TIMP activity and a subsequent increase in myocardial fibrillar collagen content. Although the molecular mechanisms that are responsible for the transition between excessive degradation and excessive synthesis of the extracellular matrix are not known, studies in other experimental models of chronic injury/inflammation have shown an initial increase in MMP expression followed by increased TIMP expression and increased expression of numerous fibrogenic cytokines, most notably transforming growth factor-β.[114] Excessive activation of proinflammatory cytokines may contribute to LV remodeling through a variety of different mechanisms that involve the myocyte and nonmyocyte components of the myocardium.

NO activity in the heart also may influence its structure by exerting an antihypertrophic effect. Studies have shown that NOSI$^{-/-}$ and NOSIII$^{-/-}$ mice develop age-related hypertrophy, although only NOSIII$^{-/-}$ mice are hypertensive.[115] NOSI/III$^{-/-}$ double-knockout mice have an additional phenotype of marked LV remodeling. NOSIII$^{-/-}$ mice also have greater LV end-diastolic dimension and mass, but lower fractional shortening and greater depression of dP/dt than wild-type mice 28 days after myocardial infarction, suggesting that the effects of NO generated from NOSIII have greater effects on post–myocardial infarction LV remodeling and function.[116] Heger and coworkers[57] reported that increased cardiac NOSII expression did not alter cardiac structure and function. The independent contributions of NOS isoforms to maintain cardiac structure may have important implications in the pathophysiology of heart failure.

Patients who have congestive heart failure may develop a wasting syndrome known as *cardiac cachexia,* which is associated with a poor prognosis.[117] A suitable definition for cardiac cachexia is the presence of nonedematous weight loss of more than 7.5% compared with previous normal body weight over a period of at least 6 months.[118] This condition is a relatively common complication of congestive heart failure in adults with an estimated prevalence of approximately 15%.[117] TNF levels are markedly increased in cachectic congestive

heart failure patients, and these levels have been found to be the strongest predictors of the degree of previous weight loss.[119] Apoptosis, which is associated with an impairment of exercise capacity, frequently is found in the skeletal muscle of congestive heart failure patients.[120] TNF also is capable of inducing skeletal muscle wasting and apoptosis as shown in animal experiments.[110,121] The aforementioned properties make TNF an attractive candidate for producing many of the clinical features seen in heart failure.

CURRENT STATUS AND FUTURE TRENDS

Accumulating evidence indicates that cytokines are important mediators of cardiovascular disease. The cytokines now have been implicated in the pathogenesis of a myriad of disease states, such as viral myocarditis, dilated cardiomyopathy, cardiac allograft rejection, myocardial infarction and reperfusion, cardiopulmonary bypass, hypertrophic cardiomyopathy, sepsis-induced LV dysfunction, and, as mentioned earlier, heart failure. The complex interplay of all of these mediators is just beginning to be unraveled.[122]

Several hypotheses as to the site of inflammatory mediators in heart failure exist, including activation of the immune system, biosynthesis from myocytes, underperfusion of tissue such as the gastrointestinal tract, and stimulation of the neurohormonal system.[123,124] This chapter also has highlighted the complex interrelationship that exists between the adaptive/maladaptive immune, cytoprotective, growth, and contractile effects of the inflammatory mediators. Currently, these complexities may preclude clinicians' ability to develop comprehensive strategies to control these mediators in the diverse array of cardiovascular diseases discussed here.

The greatest opportunity for basic research regarding cytokines in the heart may be the investigation of their roles in mediating innate cardiac protection against viral myocarditis and heart failure. Much of the investigative focus up to now has been on adults and experimental animals. Understanding the mechanisms underlying this innate cytoprotection, especially in neonates and children, has the vast potential to identify new immunomodulatory strategies and targets to treat cardiac disease and heart failure in children in the future.

Key Concepts

■ The continuous activation of the T cells in myocarditis is ultimately detrimental to the host because cytokine-mediated and direct T cell–mediated myocyte damage reduces the number of contractile units. The cumulative effect causes impairment of contractile function, which leads to long-term remodeling and progression to dilated cardiomyopathy.

■ The activation of the inflammatory response requires the coordinated expression of numerous effector systems that respond to external stress. The external stimuli, which may include infection, cytokine or neurohormone receptor activation, or oxidative stress, all converge through intracellular signaling pathways on specific families of nuclear transcription factors, a prominent member being NF-κB.

■ In addition to its role in the activation of cytokines via amplification, NF-κB regulates apoptosis and protein synthesis and increases inducible NOS and cell adhesion molecules.

■ Known or speculative negative effects of TNF in heart failure include myocyte changes (hypertrophy and apoptosis), ventricular dilation and dysfunction, extracellular matrix alterations (degradation of fibrillar collagen), β-adrenergic receptor uncoupling, disturbances of myocyte metabolism, endothelial dysfunction, and activation of fetal gene expression.

■ IL-1, which exists in two forms, IL-1α and IL-1β, and is synthesized in the myocardial cells and cardiac fibroblasts, is one of the cytokines thought to be involved in changes observed in heart failure and heart dysfunction, specifically myocyte hypertrophy and calcium homeostasis.

■ IL-6 and related cytokines, such as TNF and IL-1, are implicated in heart failure and changes such as myocyte hypertrophy; IL-6 also is thought to protect myocytes from apoptosis.

■ NO is a small gaseous molecule that mediates multiple signaling pathways in the heart with many effects on the myocyte, including increasing cGMP via activation of guanylate cyclase, inhibiting mitochondrial electron transport, decreasing affinity of contractile proteins for calcium, and modulating transsarcolemmal calcium flux and excitation-contraction coupling.

■ A feature of TLR biology of particular importance in cardiovascular diseases is that extensive tissue damage may trigger endogenous TLR stimulation.

■ The short-term expression of IL-6 may function as an adaptive response to modulate inflammatory and immune responses within acceptable ranges. Sustained IL-6 expression may engender adverse outcomes, however, if IL-6-induced anti-inflammatory or immunosuppressive responses or both are excessive and prevent activation of the appropriate antiviral response.

■ In addition to disrupting calcium homeostasis, TNF can cause myocardial dysfunction through direct cytotoxicity, oxidant stress, and induction of other cardiac depressants, such as IL-1 and IL-6.

■ Deleterious effects of NO include cellular apoptosis, an irreversible impairment of contractile function, an irreversible decrease in myocardial oxygen consumption, and abnormal heart rate and rhythm regulation.

■ NO also is reported to modulate inotropic and chronotropic stimulation and response to β-adrenoceptor stimulation; low doses enhance and high doses reduce β-adrenergic response.

■ Inflammatory mediators have many important effects that may play important roles in the process of LV remodeling, including myocyte hypertrophy, alterations in fetal gene expression, and progressive myocyte loss through apoptosis.

REFERENCES

1. Grumbach IM, Heim A, Pring-Akerblom P, et al: Adenoviruses and enteroviruses as pathogens in myocarditis and dilated cardiomyopathy. Acta Cardiol 1999;54:83.
2. Fraisse A, Paut O, Zandotti C, et al: Epstein-Barr virus: An unusual cause of acute myocarditis in children. Arch Pediatr 2000;7:752.
3. Fukae S, Ashizawa N, Morikawa S, et al: A fatal case of fulminant myocarditis with human herpesvirus-6 infection. Intern Med 2000;39:632.
4. Nigro G, Bastianon V, Colloridi V, et al: Human parvovirus B19 infection in infancy associated with acute and chronic lymphocytic myocarditis and high cytokine levels: Report of 3 cases and review. Clin Infect Dis 2000;31:65.
5. Matsumori A, Yutani C, Ikeda Y, et al: Hepatitis C virus from the hearts of patients with myocarditis and cardiomyopathy. Lab Invest 2000;80:1137.
6. Kandolf R, Ameis D, Kirschner P, et al: In situ detection of enteroviral genomes in myocardial cells by nucleic acid hybridization: An approach to the diagnosis of viral heart disease. Proc Natl Acad Sci U S A 1987;84:6272.
7. Tracy S, Wiegand V, McManus B, et al: Molecular approaches to enteroviral diagnosis in idiopathic cardiomyopathy and myocarditis. J Am Coll Cardiol 1990;15:1688.
8. Akhtar N, Ni J, Stromberg D, et al: Tracheal aspirate as a substrate for polymerase chain reaction detection of viral genome in childhood pneumonia and myocarditis. Circulation 1999;99:2011.
9. Liu PP, Mason JW: Advances in the understanding of myocarditis. Circulation 2001;104:1076.
10. Woodruff JF, Woodruff JJ: Involvement of T lymphocytes in the pathogenesis of coxsackie virus B3 heart disease. J Immunol 1974;113:1726.
11. Opavsky MA, Penninger J, Aitken K, et al: Susceptibility to myocarditis is dependent on the response of alpha/beta T lymphocytes to Coxsackieviral infection. Circ Res 1999;85:551.
12. Medzhitov R, Janeway CA Jr: Innate immunity: The virtues of a nonclonal system of recognition. Cell 1997;91:295.
13. Medzhitov R, Preston-Hurlburt P, Janeway CA Jr: A human homologue of the Drosophila Toll protein signals activation of adaptive immunity. Nature 1997;388:394.
14. Hemmi H, Takeuchi O, Kawai T, et al: A Toll-like receptor recognizes bacterial DNA. Nature 2000;408:740.
15. Michelsen KS, Aicher A, Mohaupt M, et al: The role of toll-like receptors (TLRs) in bacteria-induced maturation of murine dendritic cells (DCS): Peptidoglycan and lipoteichoic acid are inducers of DC maturation and require TLR2. J Biol Chem 2001;276:25680.
16. Takeuchi O, Hoshino K, Kawai T, et al: Differential roles of TLR2 and TLR4 in recognition of gram-negative and gram-positive bacterial cell wall components. Immunity 1999;11:443.
17. Hemmi H, Kaisho T, Takeda K, et al: The roles of Toll-like receptor 9, MyD88, and DNA-dependent protein kinase catalytic subunit in the effects of two distinct CpG DNAs on dendritic cell subsets. J Immunol 2003;170:3059.
18. Tsuji S, Matsumoto M, Takeuchi O, et al: Maturation of human dendritic cells by cell wall skeleton of Mycobacterium bovis bacillus Calmette-Guerin: Involvement of toll-like receptors. Infect Immun 2000;68:6883.
19. Visintin A, Mazzoni A, Spitzer JH, et al: Regulation of Toll-like receptors in human monocytes and dendritic cells. J Immunol 2001;166:249-255.
20. Muzio M, Bosisio D, Polentarutti N, et al: Differential expression and regulation of toll-like receptors (TLR) in human leukocytes:

Selective expression of TLR3 in dendritic cells. J Immunol 2000;164:5998.

21. Alexopoulou L, Holt AC, Medzhitov R, et al: Recognition of double-stranded RNA and activation of NF-κB by Toll-like receptor 3. Nature 2001;413:732.

22. Morishita R, Sugimoto T, Aoki M, et al: In vivo transfection of cis element "decoy" against nuclear factor-κB binding site prevents myocardial infarction. Nat Med 1997;3:894.

23. Frantz S, Fraccarollo D, Wagner H, et al: Sustained activation of nuclear factor κB and activator protein 1 in chronic heart failure. Cardiovasc Res 2003;57:749.

24. Haywood GA, Tsao PS, der Leyen HE, et al: Expression of inducible nitric oxide synthase in human heart failure. Circulation 1996;93:1087.

25. Wong SC, Fukuchi M, Melnyk P, et al: Induction of cyclooxygenase-2 and activation of nuclear factor-κB in myocardium of patients with congestive heart failure. Circulation 1998;98:100.

26. Grabellus F, Levkau B, Sokoll A, et al: Reversible activation of nuclear factor-κB in human end-stage heart failure after left ventricular mechanical support. Cardiovasc Res 2002;53:124.

27. Xuan YT, Tang XL, Banerjee S, et al: Nuclear factor-κB plays an essential role in the late phase of ischemic preconditioning in conscious rabbits. Circ Res 1999;84:1095.

28. Frantz S, Kelly RA, Bourcier T: Role of TLR-2 in the activation of nuclear factor κB by oxidative stress in cardiac myocytes. J Biol Chem 2001;276:5197.

29. Kapadia S, Lee J, Torre-Amione G, et al: Tumor necrosis factor-α gene and protein expression in adult feline myocardium after endotoxin administration. J Clin Invest 1995;96:1042.

30. Gurevitch J, Frolkis I, Yuhas Y, et al: Tumor necrosis factor-α is released from the isolated heart undergoing ischemia and reperfusion. J Am Coll Cardiol 1996;28:247.

31. Meldrum DR: Tumor necrosis factor in the heart. Am J Physiol 1998;274:R577.

32. Baker SJ, Reddy EP: Transducers of life and death: TNF receptor superfamily and associated proteins. Oncogene 1996;12:1.

33. Torre-Amione G, Kapadia S, Lee J, et al: Expression and functional significance of tumor necrosis factor receptors in human myocardium. Circulation 1995;92:1487-1493.

34. Ferrari R, Bachetti T, Confortini R, et al: Tumor necrosis factor soluble receptors in patients with various degrees of congestive heart failure. Circulation 1995;92:1479.

35. Frishman JI, Edwards CK, Sonnenberg MG, et al: Tumor necrosis factor (TNF)-α-induced interleukin-8 in human blood cultures discriminates neutralization by the p55 and p75 TNF soluble receptors. J Infect Dis 2000;182:1722.

36. Klein B, Brailly H: Cytokine-binding proteins: stimulating antagonists. Immunol Today 1995;16:216.

37. Dinarello CA: Interleukin-1 β, interleukin-18, and the interleukin-1 β converting enzyme. Ann N Y Acad Sci 1998; 856:1.

38. Arend WP, Malyak M, Guthridge CJ, et al: Interleukin-1 receptor antagonist: Role in biology. Annu Rev Immunol 1998;16:27.

39. Han RO, Ray PE, Baughman KL, et al: Detection of interleukin and interleukin-receptor mRNA in human heart by polymerase chain reaction. Biochem Biophys Res Commun 1991;181:520.

40. Francis SE, Holden H, Holt CM, et al: Interleukin-1 in myocardium and coronary arteries of patients with dilated cardiomyopathy. J Mol Cell Cardiol 1998;30:215.

41. Greenfeder SA, Varnell T, Powers G, et al: Insertion of a structural domain of interleukin (IL)-1 β confers agonist activity to the IL-1 receptor antagonist: Implications for IL-1 bioactivity. J Biol Chem 1995;270:22460.

42. Greenfeder SA, Nunes P, Kwee L, et al: Molecular cloning and characterization of a second subunit of the interleukin 1 receptor complex. J Biol Chem 1995;270:13757.

43. Gadient RA, Otten UH: Interleukin-6 (IL-6)—a molecule with both beneficial and destructive potentials. Prog Neurobiol 1997;52:379.

44. Klausen T, Olsen NV, Poulsen TD, et al: Hypoxemia increases serum interleukin-6 in humans. Eur J Appl Physiol Occup Physiol 1997;76:480.

45. Mazzeo RS, Donovan D, Fleshner M, et al: Interleukin-6 response to exercise and high-altitude exposure: Influence of α-adrenergic blockade. J Appl Physiol 2001;91:2143.

46. Wollert KC, Drexler H: The role of interleukin-6 in the failing heart. Heart Fail Rev 2001;6:95.

47. Hirota H, Chen J, Betz UA, et al: Loss of a gp130 cardiac muscle cell survival pathway is a critical event in the onset of heart failure during biomechanical stress. Cell 1999;97:189.

48. Heinrich PC, Behrmann I, Haan S, et al: Principles of IL-6-type cytokine signaling and its regulation. Biochem J 2003;374:1.

49. Alonzi T, Middleton G, Wyatt S, et al: Role of STAT3 and PI 3-kinase/Akt in mediating the survival actions of cytokines on sensory neurons. Mol Cell Neurosci 2001;18:270.

50. Heinrich PC, Behrmann I, Muller-Newen G, et al: Interleukin-6-type cytokine signalling through the gp130/Jak/STAT pathway. Biochem J 1998;334:297.

51. Auernhammer CJ, Melmed S: The central role of SOCS-3 in integrating the neuro-immunoendocrine interface. J Clin Invest 2001;108:1735.

52. Podewski EK, Hilfiker-Kleiner D, Hilfiker A, et al: Alterations in Janus kinase (JAK)-signal transducers and activators of transcription (STAT) signaling in patients with end-stage dilated cardiomyopathy. Circulation 2003;107:798.

53. Moncada S, Higgs A: The L-arginine-nitric oxide pathway. N Engl J Med 1993;329:2002.

54. Cotton, JM, Kearney MT, Shah AM: Nitric oxide and myocardial function in heart failure: Friend or foe? Heart 2002;88:564.

55. de Belder AJ, Radomski MW, Why HJ, et al: Nitric oxide synthase activities in human myocardium. Lancet 1993;341:84.

56. de Belder AJ, Radomski MW, Why HJ, et al: Myocardial calcium-independent nitric oxide synthase activity is present in dilated cardiomyopathy, myocarditis, and postpartum cardiomyopathy but not in ischaemic or valvar heart disease. Br Heart J 1995; 74:426.

57. Heger J, Godecke A, Flogel U, et al: Cardiac-specific overexpression of inducible nitric oxide synthase does not result in severe cardiac dysfunction. Circ Res 2002;90:93.

58. Mungrue IN, Gros R, You X, et al: Cardiomyocyte overexpression of iNOS in mice results in peroxynitrite generation, heart block, and sudden death. J Clin Invest 2002;109:735.

59. Wada H, Saito K, Kanda T, et al: Tumor necrosis factor-α (TNF-α) plays a protective role in acute viralmyocarditis in mice: A study using mice lacking TNF-α. Circulation 2001;103:743.

60. Baumgarten G, Knuefermann P, Nozaki N, et al: In vivo expression of proinflammatory mediators in the adult heart after endotoxin administration: The role of toll-like receptor-4. J Infect Dis 2001;183:1617.

61. Frantz S, Kobzik L, Kim YD, et al: Toll-4 (TLR4) expression in cardiac myocytes in normal and failing myocardium. J Clin Invest 1999;104:271.

62. Iordanov MS, Wong J, Bell JC, et al: Activation of NF-κB by double-stranded RNA (dsRNA) in the absence of protein kinase R and RNase L demonstrates the existence of two separate dsRNA-triggered antiviral programs. Mol Cell Biol 2001;21:61.

63. Ohashi K, Burkart V, Flohe S, et al: Cutting edge: Heat shock protein 60 is a putative endogenous ligand of the toll-like receptor-4 complex. J Immunol 2000;164:558.

64. Okamura Y, Watari M, Jerud ES, et al: The EDA domain of fibronectin activates toll-like receptor 4. J Biol Chem 2001; 276:10229.

65. Li M, Carpio DF, Zheng Y, et al: An essential role of the NF-κB/Toll-like receptor pathway in induction of inflammatory and tissue-repair gene expression by necrotic cells. J Immunol 2001;166:7128.

66. Satoh M, Tamura G, Segawa I, et al: Expression of cytokine genes and presence of enteroviral genomic RNA in endomyocardial biopsy tissues of myocarditis and dilated cardiomyopathy. Virchows Arch 1996;427:503.

67. Satoh M, Nakamura M, Satoh H, et al: Expression of tumor necrosis factor-α–converting enzyme and tumor necrosis factor-α in human myocarditis. J Am Coll Cardiol 2000;36:1288.

68. Matsumori A, Yamada T, Suzuki H, et al: Increased circulating cytokines in patients with myocarditis and cardiomyopathy. Br Heart J 1994;72:561.

69. Kubota T, Bounoutas GS, Miyagishima M, et al: Soluble tumor necrosis factor receptor abrogates myocardial inflammation but not hypertrophy in cytokine-induced cardiomyopathy. Circulation 2000;101:2518.

70. Yamada T, Matsumori A, Sasayama S: Therapeutic effect of antitumor necrosis factor-α antibody on the murine model of viral myocarditis induced by encephalomyocarditis virus. Circulation 1994;89:846.

71. Bachmaier K, Pummerer C, Kozieradzki I, et al: Low-molecular-weight tumor necrosis factor receptor p55 controls induction of autoimmune heart disease. Circulation 1997;95:65.

72. Bryant D, Becker L, Richardson J, et al: Cardiac failure in transgenic mice with myocardial expression of tumor necrosis factor-α. Circulation 1998;97:1375-1381.

73. Kubota T, McTiernan CF, Frye CS, et al: Cardiac-specific overexpression of tumor necrosis factor-α causes lethal myocarditis in transgenic mice. J Card Fail 1997;3:117.

74. Kubota T, McTiernan CF, Frye CS, et al: Dilated cardiomyopathy in transgenic mice with cardiac-specific overexpression of tumor necrosis factor-α. Circ Res 1997;81:627.

75. Herzum M, Mahr P, Wietrzychowski F, et al: Left ventricular haemodynamics in murine viral myocarditis. Eur Heart J 1995; 16(Suppl):28.

76. Lane JR, Neumann DA, Lafond-Walker A, et al: Interleukin 1 or tumor necrosis factor can promote coxsackie B3-induced myocarditis in resistant B10.A mice. J Exp Med 1992;175:1123.

77. Lane JR, Neumann DA, Lafond-Walker A, et al: Role of IL-1 and tumor necrosis factor in coxsackie virus-induced autoimmune myocarditis. J Immunol 1993;151:1682.

78. Lim BK, Choe SC, Shin JO, et al: Local expression of interleukin-1 receptor antagonist by plasmid DNA improves mortality and decreases myocardial inflammation in experimental coxsackieviral myocarditis. Circulation 2002;105:1278.

79. Shioi T, Matsumori A, Sasayama S: Persistent expression of cytokine in the chronic stage of viral myocarditis in mice. Circulation 1996;94:2930.

80. Eriksson U, Kurrer MO, Sonderegger I, et al: Activation of dendritic cells through the interleukin 1 receptor 1 is critical for the induction of autoimmune myocarditis. J Exp Med 2003;197:323.

81. Fattori E, Cappelletti M, Costa P, et al: Defective inflammatory response in interleukin 6-deficient mice. J Exp Med 1994;180:1243.

82. Tilg H, Dinarello CA, Mier JW: IL-6 and APPs: Anti-inflammatory and immunosuppressive mediators. Immunol Today 1997;18:428.

83. Kanda T, McManus JE, Nagai R, et al: Modification of viral myocarditis in mice by interleukin-6. Circ Res 1996;78:848.

84. Tanaka T, Kanda T, McManus BM, et al: Overexpression of interleukin-6 aggravates viral myocarditis: Impaired increase in tumor necrosis factor-α. J Mol Cell Cardiol 2001;33:1627.

85. Okuno M, Nakagawa M, Shimada M, et al: Expressional patterns of cytokines in a murine model of acute myocarditis: Early expression of cardiotrophin-1. Lab Invest 2000;80:433.

86. Yasukawa H, Yajima T, Duplain H, et al: The suppressor of cytokine signaling-1 (SOCS1) is a novel therapeutic target for enterovirus-induced cardiac injury. J Clin Invest 2003;111:469.

87. Lowenstein CJ, Hill SL, Lafond-Walker A, et al: Nitric oxide inhibits viral replication in murine myocarditis. J Clin Invest 1996;97:1837.

88. Zaragoza C, Ocampo C, Saura M, et al: The role of inducible nitric oxide synthase in the host response to Coxsackievirus myocarditis. Proc Natl Acad Sci U S A 1998;95:2469.

89. Badorff C, Berkely N, Mehrotra S, et al: Enteroviral protease 2A directly cleaves dystrophin and is inhibited by a dystrophin-based substrate analogue. J Biol Chem 2000;275:11191.

90. Badorff C, Fichtlscherer B, Rhoads RE, et al: Nitric oxide inhibits dystrophin proteolysis by Coxsackieviral protease 2A through S-nitrosylation: A protective mechanism against enteroviral cardiomyopathy. Circulation 2000;102:2276-2281.

91. Xiong D, Lee GH, Badorff C, et al: Dystrophin deficiency markedly increases enterovirus-induced cardiomyopathy: A genetic predisposition to viral heart disease. Nat Med 2002;8:872.

92. Tracey KJ, Beutler B, Lowry SF, et al: Shock and tissue injury induced by recombinant human cachectin. Science 1986;234:470.

93. Finkel MS, Oddis CV, Jacob TD, et al: Negative inotropic effects of cytokines on the heart mediated by nitric oxide. Science 1992;257:387.

94. Bozkurt B, Kribbs S, Clubb FJ, et al: Pathophysiologically relevant concentrations of tumor necrosis factor-α promote progressive left ventricular dysfunction and remodeling in rats. Circulation 1998;97:1382.

95. Franco F, Thomas GD, Giroir B, et al: Magnetic resonance imaging and invasive evaluation of development of heart failure in transgenic mice with myocardial expression of tumor necrosis factor-α. Circulation 1999;99:448.

96. Yokoyama T, Vaca L, Rossen RD, et al: Cellular basis for the negative inotropic effects of tumor necrosis factor-α in the adult mammalian heart. J Clin Invest 1993;92:2303.

97. Krown KA, Yasui K, Brooker MJ, et al: TNF α receptor expression in rat cardiac myocytes: TNF α inhibition of L-type Ca²⁺ current and Ca²⁺ transients. FEBS Lett 1995;376:24.

98. Kinugawa K, Takahashi T, Kohmoto O, et al: Nitric oxide-mediated effects of interleukin-6 on [Ca²⁺]i and cell contraction in cultured chick ventricular myocytes. Circ Res 1994;75:285.

99. Cain BS, Meldrum DR, Dinarello CA, et al: Tumor necrosis factor-α and interleukin-1β synergistically depress human myocardial function. Crit Care Med 1999;27:1309.

100. Kumar A, Thota V, Dee L, et al: Tumor necrosis factor α and interleukin 1β are responsible for in vitro myocardial cell depression induced by human shock serum. J Exp Med 1996; 183:949.

101. Oral H, Dorn GW, Mann DL: Sphingosine mediates the immediate negative inotropic effects of tumor necrosis factor-α in the adult mammalian cardiac myocyte. J Biol Chem 1997; 272:4836.

102. Kumar A, Brar R, Wang P, et al: Role of nitric oxide and cGMP in human septic serum-induced depression of cardiac myocyte contractility. Am J Physiol 1999;276:R265.

103. Pomerantz BJ, Reznikov LL, Harken AH, et al: Inhibition of caspase 1 reduces human myocardial ischemic dysfunction via inhibition of IL-18 and IL-1β. Proc Natl Acad Sci U S A 2001;98:2871.

104. Hare JM, Givertz MM, Creager MA, et al: Increased sensitivity to nitric oxide synthase inhibition in patients with heart failure: Potentiation of β-adrenergic inotropic responsiveness. Circulation 1998;97:161.

105. Balligand JL, Ungureanu-Longrois D, Simmons WW, et al: Cytokine-inducible nitric oxide synthase (iNOS) expression in cardiac myocytes: Characterization and regulation of iNOS expression and detection of iNOS activity in single cardiac myocytes in vitro. J Biol Chem 1994;269:27580.

106. Cotton JM, Kearney MT, MacCarthy PA, et al: Effects of nitric oxide synthase inhibition on basal function and the force-frequency relationship in the normal and failing human heart in vivo. Circulation 2001;104:2318.

107. Paulus WJ, Kastner S, Pujadas P, et al: Left ventricular contractile effects of inducible nitric oxide synthase in the human allograft. Circulation 1997;96:3436.

108. Post H, Schulz R, Gres P, et al: No involvement of nitric oxide in the limitation of β-adrenergic inotropic responsiveness during ischemia. Am J Physiol Heart Circ Physiol 2001;281:H2392.

109. Yokoyama T, Nakano M, Bednarczyk JL, et al: Tumor necrosis factor-α provokes a hypertrophic growth response in adult cardiac myocytes. Circulation 1997;95:1247.

110. Krown KA, Page MT, Nguyen C, et al: Tumor necrosis factor α-induced apoptosis in cardiac myocytes: Involvement of the sphingolipid signaling cascade in cardiac cell death. J Clin Invest 1996;98:2854.

111. Pagani FD, Baker LS, Knox MA, et al: Load-insensitive assessment of myocardial performance after tumor necrosis factor-α in dogs. Surgery 1992;111:683.

112. Sivasubramanian N, Coker ML, Kurrelmeyer K, et al: Left ventricular remodeling in transgenic mice with cardiac restricted overexpression of tumor necrosis factor. Circulation 2001;104:826.

113. Li YY, Feng YQ, Kadokami T, et al: Myocardial extracellular matrix remodeling in transgenic mice overexpressing tumor necrosis factor α can be modulated by anti-tumor necrosis factor α therapy. Proc Natl Acad Sci U S A 2000;97:12746.

114. Sime PJ, Marr RA, Gauldie D, et al: Transfer of tumor necrosis factor-α to rat lung induces severe pulmonary inflammation and patchy interstitial fibrogenesis with induction of transforming growth factor-β1 and myofibroblasts. Am J Pathol 1998;153:825.

115. Barouch LA, Harrison RW, Skaf MW, et al: Nitric oxide regulates the heart by spatial confinement of nitric oxide synthase isoforms. Nature 2002;416:337.

116. Scherrer-Crosbie M, Ullrich R, Bloch KD, et al: Endothelial nitric oxide synthase limits left ventricular remodeling after myocardial infarction in mice. Circulation 2001;104:1286.

117. Anker SD, Ponikowski P, Varney S, et al: Wasting as independent risk factor for mortality in chronic heart failure. Lancet 1997;349:1050.

118. Sharma R, Coats AJ, Anker SD: The role of inflammatory mediators in chronic heart failure: Cytokines, nitric oxide, and endothelin-1. Int J Cardiol 2000;72:175.

119. Anker SD, Chua TP, Ponikowski P, et al: Hormonal changes and catabolic/anabolic imbalance in chronic heart failure and their importance for cardiac cachexia. Circulation 1997;96:526.

120. Adams V, Jiang H, Yu J, et al: Apoptosis in skeletal myocytes of patients with chronic heart failure is associated with exercise intolerance. J Am Coll Cardiol 1999;33:959.

121. Tracey, KJ, Morgello S, Koplin B, et al: Metabolic effects of cachectin/tumor necrosis factor are modified by site of production: Cachectin/tumor necrosis factor-secreting tumor in skeletal muscle induces chronic cachexia, while implantation in brain induces predominantly acute anorexia. J Clin Invest 1990;86:2014.

122. Chang AC: Inflammatory mediators in children undergoing cardiopulmonary bypass: Is there a unified field theory amidst this biomolecular chaos? Pediatr Crit Care Med 2003;4:386-387.

123. Mann DL: Activation of inflammatory mediators in heart failure. In Mann DL (ed): Heart Failure: A Companion to Braunwald's Cardiology. Philadelphia, WB Saunders, 2004, pp 159-180.

124. von Hachling S, Anker SD: Future prospects of anticytokine therapy in chronic heart failure. Expert Opin Investig Drugs. 2005 Feb;14(2):163-176.

CHAPTER 4

Heart Failure and Mechanisms
of Hypertrophy

Neil E. Bowles
Jesus G. Vallejo
Matteo Vatta

When myocardial injury or stress occurs, there is induction of the signaling pathways to restore function. This activation of signaling pathways leads to sequelae of impaired function, myocyte loss, and hypertrophy involving molecular disturbances that include sarcomeric reorganization, altered gene expression, increased protein synthesis, and increased myocyte size.[1] Cardiac hypertrophy is a crucial part of myocardial remodeling that occurs in response to stimuli, such as disruption of the myocyte structure and function owing to genetic mutations (intrinsic stimuli) or hemodynamic overload, mechanical stress, and exposure to hormones and cytokines (extrinsic stimuli). This remodeling process initially is beneficial to the restoration of cardiac function, but eventually it can lead to the development of congestive heart failure, cardiac arrhythmias, and sudden death.

The identification of genetic mutations in many components of the cardiomyocyte cytoarchitecture has revealed that familial structural heart disease is often a consequence of changes in the cytoskeleton and sarcomere. In addition, extrinsic stresses, such as hypertension and valvular disease, can result in myocardial remodeling that is similar to that observed in genetic cardiomyopathy. The stimuli for the heart to remodel result in the activation of signaling pathways and reactivation of the fetal gene program, leading to cellular growth (hypertrophy). Many of these signaling pathways have been characterized in recent years, including pathways mediated by the integrins; G protein–coupled receptors; β-adrenergic signaling; changes in calcium signaling; and activation of numerous kinases, including extracellular signal-regulated kinase (ERK), Jun N-terminal kinase (JNK), Janus-activating kinase and signal transducers and activators of transcription (JAK/STATs), and protein kinase C (PKC). In particular, many signaling pathways have been identified that may be key regulators of changes in myocardial structure and function in response to mutations in structural components of the cardiomyocytes (Fig. 4-1).

Many conditions result in the development of myocyte hypertrophy, including mechanical overload (or stretch) and exposure to numerous humoral factors, such as signal proteins and cytokines. It is likely that outside of genetic mutations affecting the integrity of the cardiomyocyte cytoarchitecture, a major stimulus for cardiac hypertrophy is mechanical stress secondary to hemodynamic overload. These mechanical forces are capable of inducing protein synthesis[2] and gene expression changes, including the induction of the fetal gene program.[3-5]

SIGNAL PROTEINS AND HYPERTROPHY

Although hemodynamic overload can induce cardiac hypertrophy directly, humoral factors likely play an essential role. These factors often are released from hypertrophied hearts, specifically from cardiac myocytes and other cell types, such as cardiac fibroblasts, endothelial cells, and vascular smooth muscle cells. These factors, which are described in greater detail subsequently, include endothelin-1, angiotensin II, transforming growth factor-β, and others. These factors may act on the cells from which they are released (autocrine mechanism) or on adjacent cells (paracrine mechanism) or both.

Endothelin-1 (ET-1), a vasoconstrictor peptide originally identified from the supernatant of cultured porcine aortic endothelial cells,[6] is a potent inducer of cardiac hypertrophy. In vitro, ET-1 stimulates cardiomyocyte hypertrophy, as shown by increases in protein synthesis and cell size.[7,8] In pressure-overloaded rat ventricles, ventricular ET-1 levels increase within 8 days of overload and correlate with the degree of cardiac hypertrophy[9]; the ET-1 is expressed within the cardiac myocytes. In addition, mechanical stretching of cultured cardiomyocytes results in the secretion and production of ET-1 and Ang II.[10] Finally, expression of skeletal α-actin and atrial natriuretic peptide are stimulated, but this phenomenon can be reversed by treatment with an ET-1 receptor antagonist.[11]

Angiotensin II (Ang II) is the effector peptide of the renin-angiotensin system. Mechanical stress induces angiotensinogen expression in cardiomyocytes and promotes Ang II release from secretory granules.[12] The peptide hormone Ang II is derived from the protein precursor angiotensinogen by the sequential actions of proteolytic enzymes. The classic pathway of Ang II synthesis includes the conversion of angiotensinogen to Ang I, catalyzed by renin, followed by the conversion of Ang I to Ang II by the action of angiotensin-converting enzyme.

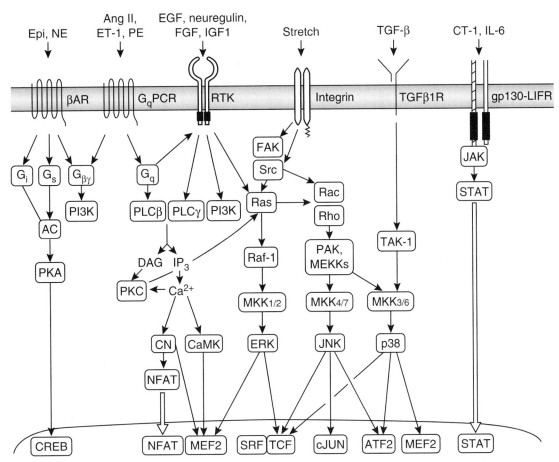

FIGURE 4-1 ■ Signaling pathways in hypertrophy. Schematic representation of signaling pathways activated during the hypertrophic response in the cardiomyocyte, including changes that involve (from left to right): (1) β-agonists (epinephrine and norepinephrine [NE]) via the β-adrenergic receptor (β-AR); (2) angiotensin II and endothelin-1 (ET-1) via G protein–coupled receptor (GqPCR); (3) the growth factors epidermal growth factor (EGF), neuregulin, and fibroblast growth factor (FGF) and insulin-like growth factor (IGF1) and their influence on the receptor tyrosine kinase (RTK); (4) stretch (and its effect on integrin); (5) transforming growth factor β (TGF-β) and its interaction with its receptor (TGF-β1R); and (6) cardiotrophin-1 (CT-1) and interleukin-6 (IL-6) with interaction with gp130 and the JAK-STAT pathway. See text for details. (From Izumo S, Pu WT: *The molecular basis of heart failure*. In Mann DL [ed]: *Heart Failure: A Companion to Braunwald's Heart Disease*, p. 17, Philadelphia, WB Saunders, 2003, p.17.)

Angiotensin binding to the Ang II type 1 (AT$_1$) receptor results in the induction of the fetal gene program.[13] Stimulation of the AT$_1$ receptor leads to the generation of the second messengers phospholipase C (PLC), PKC, and Ca^{2+}, through Gα$_{q/11}$ or via Gβγ-subunits after G$_q$ activation. This generation of second messengers results in the activation of multiple signaling proteins, including (1) mitogen-activated protein kinases (MAPKs), such as ERK 1 and 2 (ERK1/2), p38 MAPK, JNK, and stress-activated protein kinase (SAPK), and (2) JAK/STATs (see later). Activation of AT$_1$ receptors also causes activation and nuclear translocation of nuclear factor κB after stimulation by PKC or by apoptosis signal-regulating kinase 1 (ASK1, also known as MAPKKK), which is stimulated by reactive oxygen species. These signals activate target genes such as *c-fos, c-jun,* and *Elk1* in the nucleus, leading to cell growth, hypertrophy, and apoptosis.[14,15] The metalloprotease ADAM (a disintegrin and metalloprotease) also is activated by these signaling molecules, which

leads to the enzymatic conversion of proheparin-binding epidermal growth factor (proHB-EGF) to HB-EGF, which binds to, phosphorylates, and activates the EGF receptor.

Transforming growth factor-β (TGF-β) has three isoforms: TGF-β$_1$, TGF-β$_2$, and TGF-β$_3$.[16,17] TGF-β is secreted in a latent form and probably becomes activated on proteolytic cleavage by proteases. Several lines of evidence suggest that TGF-β$_1$ plays a role in cardiac hypertrophy. This evidence includes the observation that TGF-β$_1$ induces the expression of collagen mRNA in cardiac fibroblasts and β-myosin heavy chain (β-MyHC) and skeletal α-actin in cardiomyocytes.[18] In addition, in pressure-overloaded hearts, TGF-β$_1$ expression increases in cardiomyocytes along with the expression of extracellular matrix (ECM) proteins, such as fibronectin and collagen.[19] Other hypertrophic stimuli, such as stretch, result in increased synthesis of TGF-β$_1$ by cardiomyocytes.[20] TGF-β seems to have an autocrine and a paracrine role in the induction of cardiac hypertrophy.

Growth Factors

Many growth factors are agonists of tyrosine kinase, which initiate the hypertrophic response by binding to receptors that have intrinsic tyrosine kinase activity (receptor tyrosine kinase [RTK]), including fibroblast growth factor 2, insulin-like growth factor, EGF, and neuregulins.

Fibroblast growth factor 2 (FGF-2) (or basic FGF) is a peptide growth factor that can induce a fetal-like gene program in cultured rat neonatal ventricular myocytes, consistent with induction of the hypertrophic program. FGF-2 is produced by cardiomyocytes or nonmyocytes within the heart, and its receptor has an intracellular tyrosine kinase activity to elicit further signaling. Pacing of adult cardiac myocytes induced FGF-2 expression and release from cardiomyocytes, which stimulated a hypertrophic phenotype.[21] Pressure overload of FGF-2-null mice resulted in attenuation of the hypertrophic response observed in wild-type controls, indicating that this signaling pathway was a necessary regulator of cardiac hypertrophy.[22] Finally, FGF-2 seems to elicit its hypertrophic signal at least in part through an MAPK cascade.[23]

Insulin-like growth factor (IGF) I and II (IGF-I and IGF-II) are peptides that convey growth factor–like signals, which promote cellular proliferation or differentiation or both through binding to a specific heterotetrameric RTK.[24] PI3K activation is central to many important cellular processes, including protection from apoptosis, increased translation, and alteration in intracellular calcium. PI3K leads to protein kinase B/Akt activation and increases the initiation of translation via alterations in the phosphorylation state of eukaryotic initiation factor 4 binding protein and the p70 S6 kinase.[25] The activation of p70 S6 kinase increases the translation of mRNAs encoding ribosomal proteins and elongation factors, integral components of the protein synthesis machinery.

IGF-I has been implicated in the development of cardiac hypertrophy under conditions of pressure overload in rats.[26] Transgenic mice overexpressing IGF-I were reported to have cardiomyocyte hyperplasia but no hypertrophy,[27] but another model in which expression was confined to the myocardium indicated that the mice developed cardiac hypertrophy and an associated reduction in systolic performance.[28] Overexpression of an activated form of the PI3K catalytic subunit in mice resulted in cardiac hypertrophy, whereas transgenic overexpression of a dominant-negative PI3K produced smaller hearts and individual fibers.[29]

Many of the mitogenic effects of Ang II are mediated through transactivation of the **epidermal growth factor (EGF)** receptor. Activation of EGF receptors initiates an MAPK cascade through the recruitment of adaptor proteins, such as the Shc-Grb-Sos complex, which activates the small G protein Ras and subsequently Raf, MAPK kinase (MEK), and ERK1/2. EGF receptor stimulation also leads to the activation of the JAK/STAT and the PI3K and protein kinase B (Akt) pathways, culminating in cell growth and hypertrophy. Blocking EGF receptor kinase activity abolished Ang II–mediated downstream signaling, such as activation of ERK1/2 in several cell types, including vascular smooth muscle cells and cardiac myocytes.[30,31]

The receptors for the **neureglins** are Her2/neu and Her4, with RTKs implicated in hypertrophic and survival signaling pathways in cardiomyocytes.[32] The Her2/neu are up-regulated in patients undergoing left ventricular assist device therapy whose cardiac function is improving.[33] In addition, glycoprotein 130 (gp130) and Her2/neu can heterodimerize to form a receptor that has antiapoptotic activity in tumor cells and potentially in the heart.[34]

Cytokines

Numerous studies have shown that cytokines of the **interleukin-6 (IL-6)** family induce cardiomyocyte hypertrophy and inhibit apoptosis in newborn ventricular rat cardiomyocytes in culture[35] and can induce this hypertrophy through activation of gp130 in a transgenic mouse model.[36] gp130 is a signal transducing receptor that interacts with numerous cytokine receptors, including the IL-6 receptor. Constitutive gp130 inactivation induces embryonic lethality associated with hypoplastic development of embryonic hearts,[37] whereas postnatal inactivation of gp130 induces heart atrophy.[38] These data suggest that gp130 is involved in heart development by regulating hyperplasia before birth and inducing hypertrophy after birth. Adult mice with a cardiac restricted gp130 knockout have a rapid onset of dilated cardiomyopathy (DCM) and a massive induction of myocyte apoptosis during aortic pressure overload, whereas control mice display compensatory hypertrophy.[39] The cytokines of the IL-6 family may prevent heart failure by inducing compensatory hypertrophy and inhibiting apoptosis of cardiomyocytes.[40]

EXTRACELLULAR MATRIX IN HEART FAILURE AND HYPERTROPHY

The ECM is a complex network of collagens, proteoglycans, glycosaminoglycans, and glycoproteins that act as structural components and in the regulation of cell function.[41] Within the ECM, there are growth factors, cytokines, and proteases, termed *matricellular proteins,* that are important for the regulation of cell growth, migration, and apoptosis.[42] These regulate cell-matrix interactions, playing an important role in mechanical signaling. The collagens are the principal structural components of the ECM and form a complex network interconnecting myocytes, fibroblasts, and the vasculature. The development of this elastic stress-tolerant collagenous network is intimately associated with the generation and transmission of mechanical forces to and from the myocytes.[43] The ECM contains active and latent signaling components that are essential in homeostasis, remodeling in response to pathophysiologic signals (growth factors), activation of cell surface receptors (integrins), and remodeling of the collagenous network.

Exposure of the cardiomyocytes to mechanical stress results in the activation of numerous signaling pathways. This process, called *mechanotransduction,* is mediated by remodeling of the ECM and its signaling components and alterations in cell surface receptors of molecules. The induction of the hypertrophic response involves mechanisms using numerous proteins, including receptors, enzymes, and exchangers/ion channels.

Receptors

Several classes of receptors are important in the transmission of mechanical forces between cells and ECM. The **discoidin domain receptors** are transmembrane complexes that attach specifically to collagen and have tyrosine kinase motifs in the cytoplasmic domain.[44] The **cadherins,** which regulate cell-cell interaction,[45] also are believed to play a role in force transmission between myocytes. **Costameres** seem to have a crucial role in sensing and transducing mechanical stress into biochemical signals that coordinate growth responses to hypertrophic stimuli in cardiac and skeletal muscle.[46,47] The prominent location of integrins at the junction of ECM to Z-discs makes them candidates for acting as biomechanical sensors in cardiac myocytes. Mutations have been identified in many of the proteins of the costameres in patients with DCM. Costameric proteins physically interact with Z-disc or sarcolemmal proteins, many of which also have been identified to be mutated in patients with cardiac or skeletal myopathies, which also cause myopathies when missing or defective.

Integrins are a family of cell surface receptors that link the ECM to the cellular cytoskeleton.[48] Integrins are composed of α and β subunit heterodimers that consist of a large extracellular domain, a transmembrane region, and usually a short cytoplasmic domain. The extracellular domain binds to proteins of the ECM or to counter-receptors on other cells, whereas the cytoplasmic domain forms links with cytoskeletal proteins and intracellular signaling molecules, such as α-actinin and focal adhesion kinase.[49] The integrins function as sites of adhesive interactions between cells and the ECM, regulating cell adhesion, cell growth, and cell motility, and as signal transducers that regulate gene expression and cellular growth.

Stretch of cardiac fibroblasts caused activation of MAPK signal transduction pathways involved in the hypertrophic response,[50] whereas overexpression of β_1-integrin in cardiomyocytes increased atrial natriuretic peptide expression and protein synthesis.[51] In addition, β_3-integrin and the two nonreceptor kinases, focal adhesion kinase and c-Src, associate with the cytoskeleton in hypertrophic cat hearts, and on integrin-induced phosphorylation of these kinases, they become activated and initiate the Ras/ERK signal transduction pathway.[52,53]

Integrin-mediated signaling seems to involve organization of the actin cytoskeleton, through intermediary molecules including α-actinin, talin, vinculin, paxillin, and tensin.[54] This mechanism also may modulate gene expression because mechanical stress induces increases in sarcomere length, which causes concomitant changes in the desmin-laminin filament network that links Z-discs to the chromatin, altering the distribution of chromatin, which may initiate gene transcription.[55] In addition, the colocalization of signaling molecules in focal adhesion complexes may be involved in integrin signaling. Signaling proteins and their substrates are brought into close proximity, facilitating signal transduction. Integrins also can interact with growth factor receptors and their substrates to phosphorylate their receptor kinases and to activate ERKs and JNKs on ligand binding.[56] Integrins may integrate a variety of different signaling pathways that are activated by the ECM and growth factors to establish a well-coordinated response to mechanical stress and to growth factors released on mechanical stress.

Heterotrimeric G protein–coupled receptors (GPCRs) mediate between extracellular biochemical signals and intracellular effectors. These receptors are heptahelical structures with extracellular, transmembrane, and intracellular domains coupled to specific G proteins that comprise three (α, β, and γ) subunits. Four functional classes of GPCRs are identified in the cardiovascular system, and these have a significant impact on myocardial function, including the induction of myocyte hypertrophy in response to pathologic stimuli.[57]

These GPCRs correspond to several major classes of G proteins. **β-adrenergic receptors (β-ARs)**, which couple primarily to $G\alpha_s$, mediate changes in heart rate and myocardial contractility in response to epinephrine and norepinephrine stimulation.[58] The cholinergic receptors, typically coupled to $G\alpha_i$, are activated by acetylcholine, whereas the Ang II, ET-1, and α-adrenergic receptors (α-ARs) are coupled primarily to $G\alpha_q$.

Activation of $G\alpha_i$ subunits results in the attenuation of adenylate cyclase, which catalyzes the formation of cyclic AMP (cAMP). cAMP increases myocardial contractility through a protein kinase A signaling pathway, involving phospholamban inhibition and increased sarcoplasmic reticulum Ca^{2+}-ATPase 2 (SERCA2) activity, which augments calcium handling in the heart. This $G\alpha_i$-mediated inhibition of adenylate cyclase would be expected to contribute to the pathology of cardiac hypertrophy and heart failure. In two small studies, up-regulation of $G\alpha_i$ and reduction in adenylate cyclase activity were reported in patients with heart failure,[59] and these observations have been confirmed in studies.[60] In addition, increased $G\alpha_i$ content and impaired adenylate cyclase activity have been shown in animal models of hypertension characterized by cardiac hypertrophy.[61] One major cellular effect of cAMP cascade activation is the stimulation of transcription after phosphorylation of nuclear factors by the cAMP-dependent protein kinase A (PKA).

The transcription factor cAMP response element binding protein (CREB) is the best characterized nuclear protein that mediates stimulation of transcription by CAMP,[62] and CREB has been implicated in the induction of the fetal gene program associated with hypertrophy (see later).

In contrast to the $G\alpha_i$ subunit, activation of the $G\alpha_s$ subunit activates adenylate cyclase and increases cAMP levels. The roles of altered $G\alpha_s$ expression and activity in cardiac hypertrophy and heart failure are controversial. In transgenic mice overexpressing $G\alpha_s$, there were no changes in adenylate cyclase activity and basal left ventricular contractility, although enhanced isoproterenol-stimulated contractility was noted.[63] $G\alpha_s$ overexpression increased myocardial collagen content and fibrosis, however, with variable cardiomyocyte atrophy or hypertrophy associated with increased apoptosis.[64] These changes resemble the alterations in cardiac function and pathology associated with exogenously administered catecholamines in humans.[65]

$G\alpha_q$ signaling also seems to play a crucial role in cardiac hypertrophy. Stimulation of neonatal cardiomyocytes with the α-AR agonist norepinephrine, but not the β-AR agonist isoproterenol, increased cell size.[66] Subsequently, phenylephrine, Ang II, ET-1, and prostaglandin $F_{2\alpha}$ have been shown to induce similar hypertrophic effects on cultured cells; each of these agents mediated activation of PLC, suggesting G_q and PLC are hypertrophy-signaling effectors. Overexpression of G_q-coupled receptors or activated $G\alpha_q$ in cardiomyocytes promoted cellular hypertrophy,[67] whereas inhibition of $G\alpha_q$ signaling prevented α-AR-mediated cardiomyocyte hypertrophy.[68]

Transgenic mice overexpressing $G\alpha_q$ develop cardiac hypertrophy with a concomitant induction of the fetal gene program and increases in cardiomyocyte cross-sectional area.[69] In contrast to pressure-overload models of hypertrophy, however, these mice also exhibit eccentric ventricular remodeling, resting sinus bradycardia, and left ventricular contractile depression.[70] In a model of overexpression of an activated mutant of $G\alpha_q$, the mice exhibited a DCM phenotype, with progressive ventricular dilation.[71] In addition, in mice with cardiac-specific overexpression of a peptide fragment derived from the carboxy terminus of $G\alpha_q$, which can block $G\alpha_q$ receptor coupling effectively, pressure overload resulted in less cardiac hypertrophy than in wild-type controls.[72] These mice still developed some hypertrophy, however, suggesting that other signaling pathways, such as tyrosine kinase–mediated pathways, also play a role in the development of cardiac hypertrophy. In mice in which the AT_{1A} receptor was knocked out, pressure overload continued to induce cardiac hypertrophy,[73] indicating the presence of other pathways that may mediate the hypertrophic response.

Signal transduction by β-**ARs** is regulated by changes in the functional state of the receptor and the number of receptors on the cell surface. Agonist occupancy of β-ARs leads to activation of the adenylate cyclase stimulatory G protein, G_s, resulting in an increase in intracellular cAMP (see Chapter 21). The accumulation of cAMP leads to enhanced cAMP-dependent PKA activity, the predominant mechanism by which the cell surface signal is transduced inside the cell. To control the level of β-AR signaling, elaborate mechanisms exist to turn off or desensitize activated receptors.[74] Desensitization is a phenomenon of decreasing cellular responsiveness of the receptors despite continued presence of ligand. Desensitization of β-ARs is a characteristic of cardiac hypertrophy, caused in part by elevated levels of β-AR kinase 1.[75] The mechanism for the functional uncoupling of receptor from its cognate G protein is through phosphorylation of the receptor, mediated by either second messenger–activated kinases PKA and PKC, or the G protein–coupled receptor kinases.[76]

Enzymes

The **phospholipases** are enzymes that catalyze the breakdown of plasma membrane phospholipids, generating second messenger molecules. Major families of PLC include a protein kinase–regulated PLCγ family, a PLCδ family, and a G protein–regulated PLCβ family. These families all are membranecoupled, and their catalytic activity is regulated by Ca^{2+} or tyrosine phosphorylation. Phospholipase D is regulated by small G proteins and protein kinase C (PKC) and by tyrosine kinases. AT_1 receptor activation results in the PLC-dependent hydrolysis of phosphatidylinositol-4,5-biphosphate, producing 1,4,5-inositol triphosphate and diacylglycerol, which are involved in Ca^{2+} mobilization from the sarcoplasmic reticulum (SR) and stimulation of PKC.[77]

The functions of **protein kinases** A, B (Akt), and C depend on a series of ordered phosphorylations, including activation loop phosphorylation. For protein kinase B, PKC, and possibly PKA, this cascade of phosphorylations is initiated by phosphoinositide-dependent kinase-1.[78] Activation of PKC requires the removal of the autoinhibitory C1 domain from the active site. 1,4,5-Inositol triphosphate induces calcium release from the SR, resulting in the translocation of the Ca^{2+}-sensitive PKC isoforms to the sarcolemma, where the binding of diacylglycerol results in the activation of PKC.

PKC is hypothesized to modulate cardiac hypertrophy by phosphorylation of transcription factors, such as c-jun and fos, controlling expression of hypertrophic genes (Fig. 4-2).[79] Signal transduction cascades, such as MAPK pathways that lead to *c-jun* and *fos* activation, are activated by PKC in agonist-stimulated cardiomyocytes.[80] Similarly, in pressure overload–induced hypertrophy in rats, there is translocation of PKC ε, βI, and βII and increases in PKC-dependent phosphorylation activity.[81] Overexpression of PKC βII in transgenic mice results in myocyte hypertrophy and dysfunction, along with up-regulation of the fetal gene program,[82] an effect that was inhibited by an oral PKC βII inhibitor. Inhibition of

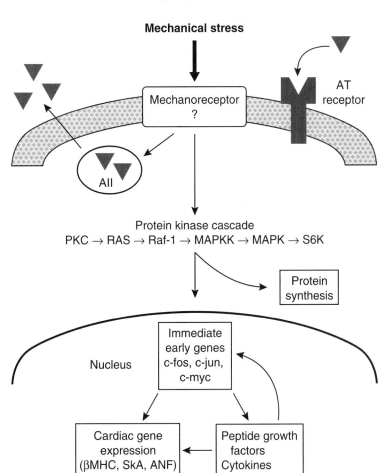

FIGURE 4-2 ■ Protein kinase cascade. The protein kinase cascade is activated by mechanical stress, and this leads to induction of the immediate early genes, such as *c-fos, d-jun,* and *c-myc.* In addition, cardiac gene expression via myosin heavy chain (βMHC), skeletal α-actin (SkA), and atrial natriuretic factor (ANF) and other factors, such as peptide growth factors and cytokines, are activated. AII, angiotensin II; AT receptor, angiotensin II receptor; MAPK, mitogen-activated protein kinase; MAPKK, mitogen-activated protein kinase kinase; PKC, protein kinase C, S6K, S6 kinase. (From MacLellan WR, Mann DL: *Basic mechanisms of adaptive and maladaptive growth of the adult mammalian heart.* In Garson A, Bricker JT, Fisher DJ, et al [eds]: *The Science and Practice of Pediatric Cardiology,* 2nd ed. Philadelphia, Williams & Wilkins, 1998.)

PKC translocation by an angiotensin-converting enzyme inhibitor improves cardiomyocyte and left ventricular function after pressure overload–induced hypertrophy.[83] In the hearts of patients with end-stage heart disease secondary to DCM or ischemic cardiomyopathy, PKC βI and βII are up-regulated, with significant translocation of PKC α, βI, and βII, and an increase in PKC activity.[84] It seems that the activation of PKC is a common pathway in the development of cardiac hypertrophy.

Exchangers and Ion Channels

The **Na+/H+ exchanger (NHE)** may play a role in mechanotransduction because its activation increases intracellular pH, which stimulates expression of hypertrophic marker genes and protein synthesis. The NHE is located in the sarcolemma; it regulates Na+ influx and H+ efflux[164] and is regulated by a variety of extracellular stimuli, most of which act through GPCRs. The hypertrophic response of adult rat ventricular myocytes to adrenergic stimulation is attenuated by NHE inhibition.[85] NHE inhibition attenuates the hypertrophic responses to sustained stimulation of either α-ARs or β-ARs, despite the fact that acute β-AR stimulation inhibits sarcolemmal NHE activity.[86] The ventricular hypertrophy that develops spontaneously in transgenic mice with cardiac-specific overexpression of the β-AR requires NHE activity.[87] NHE activity seems to play a fundamental role in the induction and evolution of myocardial hypertrophy. Nevertheless, the relative importance of increased sarcolemmal NHE activity and the molecular mechanisms through which NHE activity may regulate myocardial hypertrophy remain to be elucidated.

In the hypertrophic and failing heart, there also is up-regulation of the **Na+/Ca2+ exchanger (NCX)**. NCX catalyzes the electrogenic exchange of Na+ for Ca2+ across the cardiac sarcolemma and is reversible, operating in either forward (Ca2+-efflux) or reverse (Ca2+-influx) modes. NCX is the primary Ca2+ extrusion mechanism in the heart and is required to remove the increment of Ca2+ entering the myocyte via Ca2+ channels on each beat.[88] In humans and animal models of heart failure in which SR function is impaired, there is a compensatory increase in the levels of NCX at the mRNA and protein levels.[89,90] This increase in NCX compensates for defective SR Ca2+ removal, but depletes the releasable pool of Ca2+ and increases the depolarizing current and propensity for arrhythmias.[91] These data suggest that NCX has an important role in altered excitation contraction coupling and arrhythmogenesis in the context of cardiac hypertrophy and failure.

The activation of **stretch-sensitive (mechanosensitive) ion channels** has been proposed as the transduction mechanism between mechanical stress and protein synthesis in cardiac hypertrophy,[92] because these stretch-activated channels allow the passage of the major monovalent physiologic cations, Na^+ and K^+, and the divalent cation, Ca^{2+}.[93] Stretch induces an increase in intracellular calcium that depends partially on release of Ca^{2+} influx from intracellular stores, but primarily on Ca^{2+} extracellular sources. Calcium influx across the plasma membrane could occur through a stretch-activated channel or voltage-gated Ca^{2+} channel activation as a result of stretch-activated, channel-induced depolarization. Membrane proteins, such as ion channels and exchangers, can receive extracellular stimuli first and evoke intracellular signals.[94] The mechanisms by which Ca^{2+} influx may contribute to the development of cardiac hypertrophy include increased intracellular Ca^{2+} that may enhance PKC activity or activate the calcium/calmodulin–dependent protein kinase (CaMK) (see Chapter 21).

SIGNAL TRANSDUCTION IN HEART FAILURE AND HYPERTROPHY

As described previously, the induction of cardiac hypertrophy requires signaling through several pathways, including the MAPK signaling pathways, JAK/STAT pathways, and calcium signaling pathways.

Mitogen-Activated Protein Kinase Signaling Pathway

The MAPK signaling pathways consist of a sequence of successively acting kinases that become activated on tyrosine/threonine phosphorylation and additional modifications, then phosphorylate and activate nuclear substrates (e.g., c-myc, c-jun, and activating transcription family 2 [ATF-2]).[95] The MAPK signaling cascade is initiated in cardiac myocytes by activation of GPCRs, RTKs, IL-6-like receptors, and TGF-β receptors or by stress.[96] The MAPK superfamily has several subfamilies, of which the best known are (1) the ERKs, (2) the JNKs, and (3) the p38 MAPKs. In each case, the MAPKs are the final components of a pathway that involves a cascade of three kinases:[97] the MEK kinases (MEKKs), the MAPK/ERK kinases (MEKs or MKKs), and the MAPKs.

Of the six **extra cellular signal-regulated kinases (ERKs)** (ERK1 through ERK6), ERK1 is the most highly expressed in the heart, although expression decreases with age. The ERK pathway can be stimulated on agonist binding to GPCRs; on binding of growth factors to RTKs; or by mechanical stress, involving PKC, tyrosine kinases, and Ras.[98] There also is a signal transduction pathway leading to ERK activation that involves PKA and may be Ca^{2+} dependent.[99] MAPK pathways, including ERKs, are stimulated by activation of IL-6 cytokine receptors.[100]

The **Jun N-terminal kinases (JNKs)** and p38 MAPK pathways are cell stress-activated pathways, and their component kinases also are called *SAPKs*.[101] The JNKs are named after the first substrate identified, *c-jun*, and are encoded by three genes (*JNK-1, JNK-2,* and *JNK-3*), which are alternatively spliced to yield different isoforms[102] with molecular weights of approximately 46 kDa or 54 kDa. The two MAPKK proteins that act as upstream JNK activators are MKK7 (MEK7), which is primarily activated by cytokines (tumor necrosis factor-α, IL-1β), and MKK4 (MEK4), which is primarily activated by environmental stress. The MEKK activators of the JNK pathway are composed of a group of more than 12 intracellular proteins.[103] Four negative JNK regulatory factors have been identified: MAPK phosphatase MKP7, heat-shock protein 72, Evi1 oncoprotein, and nitric oxide.

Data suggest that positive and negative signals mediated by parallel MAPK cascades interact with Rho-dependent pathways to regulate hypertrophic gene expression. In a study in rat neonatal ventricular myocytes, activation of JNK led to inhibition of atrial natriuretic factor (ANF) expression induced by MEKK1 and hypertrophic agonists,[104] and MEKK1-induced ANF expression was negatively regulated by expression of c-jun. In MEKK1-deficient mice, pressure-overload JNK activity did not increase, in contrast to the wild-type littermates,[105] suggesting that MEKK1 mediates JNK activation by pressure overload. Even in the knockout mice, however, pressure overload caused cardiac hypertrophy and expression of ANF. It seems that MEKK1 is required for JNK activation, but is dispensable for the induction of cardiac hypertrophy.

Four genes encode the **p38 mitogen-activated protein kinases (MAPK) family**—p38 MAPKα, p38 MAPKβ, p38 MAPKδ, and p38 MAPKγ—yielding at least six isoforms.[106] The substrate of p38 MAPK is MAPK-activated protein kinase 2, which can phosphorylate and activate the human heat-shock proteins,[107] thought to be cytoprotective in the heart.[108] In a mouse model of pressure overload–induced cardiac hypertrophy, p38 MAPK activity was increased, whereas stretch of cardiomyocytes induced phosphorylation of p38 MAPK, ERKs, and JNKs.[109] In AT_{1a}-receptor knockout mice, stretch resulted in the activation of ERKs and p38 MAPK, followed by induction of c-fos expression.[110] The p38 MAPK pathway is further implicated in cardiac hypertrophy because overexpression of activated MKK3 or MKK6 in neonatal cardiomyocytes induces hypertrophy and ANF expression.[111]

Transgenic mice expressing MKK3 or MKK6 in the heart did not develop cardiac hypertrophy, despite the fact that both had marked interstitial fibrosis with expression of fetal marker genes characteristic of cardiac failure.[112] There was a similar degree of systolic contractile depression and restrictive diastolic abnormalities related to markedly increased passive chamber stiffness.

In addition, the MKK3-expressing hearts had increased end-systolic chamber volumes and a thinned ventricular wall, associated with heterogeneous myocyte atrophy, whereas MKK6 hearts had reduced end-diastolic ventricular cavity size, a modest increase in myocyte size, and no significant myocyte atrophy. In transgenic mice expressing dominant-negative mutants of p38 MAPKα, MKK3, or MKK6 in the heart, there was enhanced cardiac hypertrophy after aortic banding or infusion with Ang II, isoproterenol, or phenylephrine.[113] These data suggest that reduced p38 MAPK signaling in the heart promotes myocyte growth through a mechanism involving enhanced signaling of calcineurin and nuclear factor of activated T cells (NFAT), whereas p38 MAPK activation in ventricular myocytes has negative inotropic and restrictive diastolic effects.

A few studies report a role for the **MAP kinase phosphatases** (MKPs) in cardiac hypertrophy. In a study of transgenic mice overexpressing phospholamban, left ventricular hypertrophy/dilation developed in males concurrent with cardiac p38 MAPK activation, whereas in females there was a temporal delay in p38 MAPK activation, hypertrophy, and mortality (22 months), associated with sustained cardiac levels of MKP-1.[114] As the females aged, there was a decrease in cardiac MKP-1, accompanied by increased p38 MAPK activation. These data suggest that cardiac hypertrophy is linked with p38 MAPK activation, which is modulated by MKP-1 expression. Expressions of MKP-1 and MKP-2 were increased in failing hearts, suggesting these contribute to decreased MAPK activity in the failing human myocardium.[115]

Janus Kinases and Signal Transducers and Activators of Transcription Signaling Pathway

The JAK-STAT pathway is a signaling cascade that has been implicated in numerous cardiac cellular and pathologic events, including hypertrophy, apoptosis, cytoprotection, and angiotensin gene expression. The Janus-activating kinases are a family of receptor-associated cytosolic protein tyrosine kinases that play a crucial role in the rapid transduction of signals from the cell surface to the nucleus. These kinases have two domains: the JAK homology 1 (JH1) (kinase) domain and the JH2 (pseudokinase) domain. The JH1 domain is responsible for the catalytic activity of JAKs, whereas the function of the JH2 domain is unknown, although it may be a docking site for STAT, serving a regulatory function. The first JAK (JAK1) was described in 1989,[116] and the JAK-STAT pathway subsequently was recognized as a functional signal-transduction mechanism in the context of interferon signaling. Four JAKs (JAK1, JAK2, JAK3, and TYK2) have been identified in mammals, all of which are activated by tyrosine phosphorylation and three of which are expressed in cardiac myocytes (JAK1, JAK2, and TYK2). JAKs bind specifically to intracellular domains of cytokine receptor signaling chains, which after dimerization results in transphosphorylation and activation of two adjacent JAKs.

Signal transducers and activators of transcription are a unique class of transcription factors with seven known members (STAT1, STAT2, STAT3, STAT4, STAT5A, STAT5B, and STAT6) that play a crucial role in the transcriptional regulation of multiple genes. Phosphorylation of STATs on activating tyrosine residues by JAKs leads to STAT homodimerization and heterodimerization. STAT dimers are transported from the cytoplasm to the nucleus and bind DNA motifs resulting in increased transcription. Negative regulation of the JAK-STAT pathway is accomplished by receptor internalization and degradation and inhibition by protein tyrosine phosphatases that dephosphorylate activated STAT dimers, resulting in translocation of the STAT monomer to the cytoplasm.[117] Suppressors of cytokine signaling proteins are JAK inhibitors,[118] whereas the protein inhibitors of activated STATs bind to phosphorylated STAT dimers, preventing DNA recognition.[119]

Each member of the STAT family is expressed in the cultured cardiac myocytes. Multiple stimuli that activate hypertrophic growth of cardiac myocytes or provide cardioprotection or do both also activate JAK-STAT signaling, with increased STAT activity, as assessed by electrophoretic mobility shift assays of DNA binding activity or promoter-reporter assays of transcriptional activity. Stimuli of JAK-STAT signaling include mechanical stretch and pressure overload, Ang II, insulin, and IL-1β. The IL-6-related cytokines, cardiotrophin-1 and leukemia inhibitory factor, which are potent inducers of cardiac hypertrophy, activate the JAK-STAT pathway.[120] IL-6 activates JAK1 and JAK2, producing a phosphotyrosine docking site for STAT3, and activates STAT1, leading to homodimers and heterodimers of STAT1 and STAT3.

Calcium Signaling Pathway

The Ca²⁺-calmodulin–activated phosphatase **calcineurin** and its downstream transcriptional effector, NFAT, have been implicated in cardiac hypertrophy, linking changes in intracellular calcium handling to the hypertrophic response (Fig. 4-3). Calcineurin is a heterodimer, consisting of the calcineurin A and B subunits. Calcineurin A encodes the catalytic site of the enzyme, whereas the B subunit contains the Ca²⁺-binding regulatory domain.[121]

A variety of stimuli trigger an increase in sarcoplasmic free Ca²⁺ from resting levels. At the elevated Ca²⁺, Ca²⁺ binds to calmodulin, the ubiquitous and multifunctional Ca²⁺-binding protein. The interaction of Ca²⁺ with calmodulin induces a conformational change in this Ca²⁺-binding protein, with exposure of a site or sites of interaction with target proteins, such as calcineurin A, displacing an autoinhibitory domain and allowing access of protein substrates to the catalytic domain.[122] In addition, changes in intracellular calcium promote

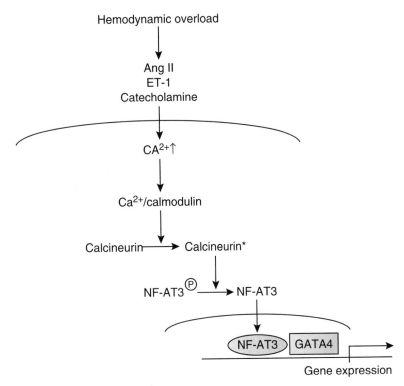

FIGURE 4-3 ■ **Calcium and calcineurin in cardiac hypertrophy.** A variety of stimuli trigger an increase in sarcoplasmic free Ca^{2+} from resting levels. At the elevated Ca^{2+}, Ca^{2+} binds to calmodulin. The interaction of Ca^{2+} with calmodulin induces a conformational change in this Ca^{2+}-binding protein, with exposure of a site or sites of interaction with target proteins, such as calcineurin A. Nuclear factor of activated T cells (NF-AT3) is shown to shuttle between the cytoplasmic and nuclear compartments under influence of a Ca^{2+} signal. Ang II, angiotensin II; ET-1, endothelin-1; GATA4, GATA binding protein 4. (From Komuro I, Yazaki Y: *Molecular basis of cardiac hypertrophy.* In Narula J, Virmani R, Ballester M, et al [eds]: *Heart Failure and Pathogenesis and Treatment.* London, Martin Dunitz, 2002, p. 182.)

binding of Ca^{2+} directly to calcineurin B. NFAT was shown to shuttle between the cytoplasmic and nuclear compartments under the influence of a Ca^{2+} signal.

The first evidence for a role of calcineurin in gene induction and cardiac hypertrophy was obtained by the observation that the interaction between the GATA4 and the DNA binding domain of NFATc4 (NFAT3) resulted in activation of a brain natriuretic peptide promoter.[123] In addition, cyclosporine prevented the response of cultured cardiomyocytes to hypertrophy-inducing factors, such as Ang II and phenylephrine. Transgenic mice expressing the calcineurin Aα subunit developed a hypertrophic response, ranging from benign forms of concentric hypertrophy to severe forms of DCM, depending on the gene copy number, which could be inhibited by cyclosporine injections.[123] Transgenic mice expressing an activated calcineurin-independent mutant developed a hypertrophic myopathy associated with re-expression of fetal genes, which was not prevented by cyclosporine administration.

Calcineurin Aβ mRNA and protein levels are up-regulated in cardiac myocytes undergoing hypertrophy,[124] and calcineurin Aβ null mice had reduced cardiac calcineurin and failed to mount a hypertrophic response induced by pressure overload, Ang II infusion, or isoproterenol infusion, with an associated defect in the induction of the fetal gene program.[125] There have been reports of varying levels of calcineurin in the heart in response to hypertrophic stimuli, including up-regulation, down-regulation, and no change, and variable calcineurin

levels and activities have been reported in failing human hearts.[126] Calcineurin also may regulate the cardiac hypertrophic response in coordination with other intracellular signal transduction pathways. It is not known how calcineurin activates kinases such as JNK and PKC, but it may initiate autocrine regulatory mechanisms, such as Ang II or ET-1 release, which promote signaling through GPCRs and RTKs leading to the secondary activation of PKC and MAPKs.

It is unclear why changes in Ca^{2+} concentration that occur during each cycle of contraction and relaxation do not activate calmodulin and the calcineurin pathway. In some cell types, NFATc remains nuclear only in response to prolonged, low-amplitude Ca^{2+} signals and is insensitive to transient, high-amplitude Ca^{2+} alterations, whereas the activity of CaMK is sensitive only to transient, high-amplitude Ca^{2+} concentration changes.[127] In addition, the source of Ca^{2+} that activates calcineurin may be important. L-type Ca^{2+} channels, which respond downstream of GPCR agonists, such as ET-1, Ang II, or phenylephrine,[128] and gp130 receptor agonists, such as leukemia inhibitory factor,[129] may play a crucial role.

TRANSCRIPTION FACTORS AND HYPERTROPHY

Cardiac hypertrophy is characterized by increases in cell size and protein synthesis, reactivation of the fetal gene program, and up-regulation of genes encoding proteins involved in signaling pathways and energy metabolism. These genes include the so-called early genes (e.g., *egr-1, hsp70, c-fos, c-jun, c-myc*) and subsequently reactivation of fetal genes, such as β-MyHC, skeletal α-actin, and ANF and up-regulation of constitutively expressed contractile proteins, such as ventricular myosin light chain 2 (MLC2) and cardiac α-actin. As noted earlier, multiple signaling pathways result in the activation of cardiac transcription factors, which regulate genes that are up-regulated in the hypertrophied myocardium.

Serine phosphorylation of **GATA-binding protein 4 (GATA4)** is induced by phenylephrine stimulation, whereas ERK2 phosphorylates GATA4 in vitro, and phenylephrine-induced phosphorylation and activation of GATA4 are inhibited by an ERK kinase (MKK1) inhibitor.[130] These data suggest GATA4 is a transcriptional effector acting downstream from the ERK signaling pathway, and GATA4 is activated through serine phosphorylation by the p38 MAPK pathway: Inhibition of p38 MAPK attenuated ET-1-induced protein synthesis and DNA binding and phosphorylation of GATA4.[131] Rho and ROCK, a target of Rho, are linked to phenylephrine-induced GATA4 activation through the ERK pathway,[132] and RhoA induces the potentiation of GATA4 transcriptional activity through p38.[133] Overexpression of GATA4 induced cardiac hypertrophy in cultured cardiomyocytes and in transgenic mice.[134] These results suggest that GATA4 is a sufficient transcriptional regulator for the generation of cardiac hypertrophy and is an effector by which divergent signaling pathways integrate during the generation of cardiac hypertrophy. GATA4 directly regulates the basal expression of numerous cardiac-specific genes, such as α-MyHC, β-MyHC, AT_{1a} receptor, MLC1/3, cardiac troponin C, cardiac troponin I, ANF, brain natriuretic peptide, cardiac-restricted ankyrin repeat protein, and NCX1, and their up-regulation in response to hypertrophic stimuli.[135]

Myocyte enhancement factor 2 (MEF2) transcription factors also are involved in the regulation of gene expression during myocardial cell hypertrophy in response to a variety of stimuli.[136] Although the pathophysiologic significance of the p38 MAPK–MEF2 pathway during cardiac hypertrophy has not been fully determined, the ERK5-MEF2 pathway participates in inducible gene expression of the immediate-early gene *c-fos,* the induction of eccentric cardiac hypertrophy, and the transduction of cytokine signals that regulate serial sarcomere assembly.[137] MEF2-binding sequences have been identified within the promoters of the cardiac genes muscle creatine kinase, α-MyHC, MLC1/3, MLC2v, skeletal α-actin, SERCA, cardiac troponin T, cardiac troponin C, cardiac troponin I, desmin, and dystrophin, among others.[138] IGF-I stimulation also activates the transcriptional activity of MEF2 through the PI3-K-Akt pathway.[139] The MEF2 factors also function as effectors

of Ca^{2+} signaling pathways, and MEF2 activity is stimulated by CaMK. Although CaMKs directly phosphorylate MEF2 in vitro,[140] the activation of MEF2 by CaMK is mediated mainly through the phosphorylation of transcriptional repressors, the histone deacetylases (HDACs).[141] The role of HDACs in cardiac hypertrophy is reinforced by the observation that HDAC9-deficient mice display spontaneous cardiac hypertrophy and are predisposed to more severe hypertrophic growth after banding of the thoracic aorta.[142] Although HDAC kinase activity is enhanced in cardiac extracts from hypertrophied hearts of mice, and CaMKs are capable of phosphorylating HDACs, it is unclear whether CaMKs are the functional HDAC kinases that are responsive to hypertrophic stimulation. MEF2, similar to GATA4, is regulated through protein-protein interactions with other transcription factors, and these factors synergistically activate the transcription of several cardiac genes, such as ANF, brain natriuretic peptide, α-MyHC, and cardiac α-actin.

Other transcription factors involved in hypertrophy are reviewed only briefly here. The **ATF/CREB** family shares a DNA-binding domain consisting of a cluster of basic amino acids and a leucine zipper region, the so-called b-ZIP. They form homodimers or heterodimers with c-jun through the leucine zipper and bind to the cAMP response element.[143] In addition, the transcription factor **serum response factor (SRF)** is a key regulator of several extracellular stimuli–regulated genes important for cell growth, hypertrophy, apoptosis, and differentiation. SRF plays a central role in the induction and maintenance of cardiac myogenic program and interacts and synergistically cooperates with other cardiac-myogenic factors, such as GATA4.[144] Transgenic mice expressing SRF in the myocardium develop cardiac hypertrophy, four-chamber dilation, collagen deposition, and interstitial fibrosis, and altered the expression of SRF-regulated genes, which resulted in cardiac muscle dysfunction and death from heart failure within 6 months of birth.[145] Lastly, **activator protein 1** regulates a wide range of cellular processes, including cell proliferation, hypertrophy, apoptosis, and differentiation.[146]

APOPTOSIS IN HEART FAILURE

Apoptosis, the process in which cells undergo programmed cell death, has been associated with tissues in processes such as separation of digits from blunt ends of fetal limbs during embryonic development. Apoptosis also is a phenomenon in which damaged or malignant cells are eliminated from the organism during adult life. Although cardiomyocytes are not replaced if injured or destroyed, these cells are capable of undergoing apoptosis under clinical situations, such as myocardial ischemia or pressure overload. There is now abundant evidence supporting cardiac apoptosis in disease states

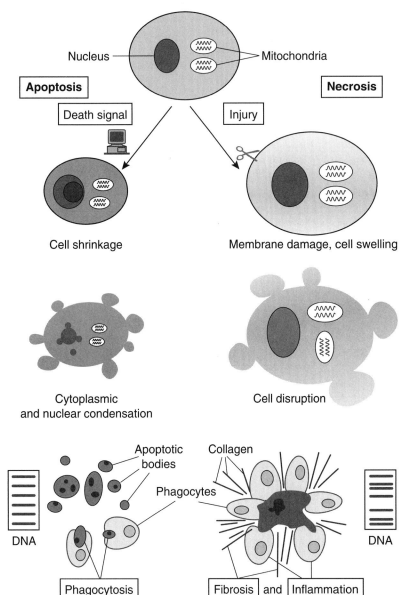

FIGURE 4-4 ■ Apoptosis versus necrosis. These processes are fundamentally different mechanisms of cell death. Apoptosis is a regulated process that includes cell shrinkage and condensation of cytoplasm and nuclear materials. The apoptotic bodies undergo phagocytosis and do not induce an inflammatory reaction. Apoptosis also yields orderly fragments of DNA. Necrosis leads to membrane damage and cell swelling with disruption of the cellular membrane. This process leads to an inflammatory reaction that leads to fibrosis. Necrosis yields fragments of DNA that are random sized, rather than the orderly fragments seen with apoptosis. (From Katz A: *Heart Failure: Pathophysiology, Molecular Biology, and Clinical Management.* Philadelphia, Lippincott, Williams & Wilkins, 2000, p. 209.)

such as ischemic and nonischemic cardiomyopathies.[147] Finally, apoptosis is a distinctly different process compared with necrosis (Fig. 4-4).

Hirota and colleagues[148] discussed in a knockout mice model that absence of the gp130 cytokine receptor does not prevent normal development. They further showed, however, that pressure overload (created surgically by constriction of the aorta) had differing effects on the mice depending on the presence or absence of the gp130 cytokine receptor: The control mice with normal levels of gp130 had compensatory left ventricular hypertrophy, whereas the knockout mice with reduced expression of gp130 had increased apoptosis and dilated cardiomyopathy.[148] With pressure overload stress and secretion of cytokines, the initiation of gp130-mediated intracellular signaling events that block these cytokines in inducing apoptosis can result in DCM. In other words,

gp130 signaling events (e.g., activation of the STAT3 transcription factor and induction of antiapoptotic proteins, such as Bcl-X1) are observed with pressure overload, and it is the failure of these events that leads to myocardial dysfunction.

CURRENT STATUS AND FUTURE TRENDS

Since the 1990s, significant progress has been made in delineating the complex array of cellular signaling pathways that transduce hypertrophic stimuli into the hypertrophic response. Many of these studies have emerged from the development of transgenic mouse models overexpressing the components of these pathways. To a large extent, these pathways are well characterized, although some contradictory data need to be resolved. It has become increasingly apparent that many cases of cardiomyopathy are familial in nature, with mutations identified in sarcomeric, cytoskeletal, and calcium channel proteins. For some of these mutations, it is apparent that they trigger the same signaling pathways identified in hypertrophy induced by extrinsic stimuli, such as pressure overload, hormone exposure, or cytokine exposure.

For mutations of the sarcomere (in patients with hypertrophic cardiomyopathy), it is likely that many result in contraction defects, which lead to pressure overload. Mutations in cytoskeletal proteins may activate signaling pathways through integrin-mediated pathways or by altering the distribution of chromatin. In addition, changes in cytoskeletal proteins may change the cellular localization and activity of ion channels. Finally, there remains much to be learned about the synergy between physiologic growth and pathologic adaptations in hypertrophy.[149] The development of mouse models of these mutations is likely to identify which of these signaling pathways is activated and may serve as targets for drugs to prevent hypertrophy and heart failure.[150,151]

Key Concepts

■ When myocardial injury or stress occurs, there is induction of the signaling pathways to restore function. This activation of signaling pathways leads to sequelae of impaired function, myocyte loss, and hypertrophy involving molecular disturbances that include sarcomeric reorganization, altered gene expression, increased protein synthesis, and increased myocyte size.

■ Cardiac hypertrophy is a crucial part of myocardial remodeling that occurs in response to stimuli, such as disruption of the myocyte structure and function owing to genetic mutations (intrinsic stimuli) or hemodynamic overload, mechanical stress, and exposure to hormones and cytokines (extrinsic stimuli).

■ The stimuli for the heart to remodel result in the activation of signaling pathways and reactivation of the fetal gene program, leading to cellular growth (hypertrophy).

■ Endothelin-1 (ET-1), a vasoconstrictor peptide originally identified from the supernatant of cultured porcine aortic endothelial cells,[6] is a potent inducer of cardiac hypertrophy.

■ TGF-β seems to have an autocrine and a paracrine role in the induction of cardiac hypertrophy.

■ Many growth factors are agonists of tyrosine kinase, which initiate the hypertrophic response by binding to receptors that have intrinsic tyrosine kinase activity receptor tyrosine kinase [RTK], including FGF-2, IGF, EGF, and neuregulins.

■ FGF-2 is a peptide growth factor that can induce a fetal-like gene program in cultured rat neonatal ventricular myocytes, consistent with induction of the hypertrophic program.

■ IGF-I and IGF-II are peptides that convey growth factor–like signals that promote cellular proliferation or differentiation or both through binding to a specific heterotetrameric RTK.

■ The cytokines of the IL-6 family may prevent heart failure by inducing compensatory hypertrophy and inhibiting apoptosis of cardiomyocytes.

■ The ECM is a complex network of collagens, proteoglycans, glycosaminoglycans, and glycoproteins that act as structural components and in the regulation of cell function.

■ The ECM contains active and latent signaling components that are essential in homeostasis, remodeling in response to pathophysiologic signals (growth factors), activation of cell surface receptors (integrins), and remodeling of the collagenous network.

■ Exposure of the cardiomyocytes to mechanical stress results in the activation of many signaling pathways. This process, called mechanotransduction, is mediated by remodeling of the ECM and its signaling components and alterations in cell surface receptors of molecules. The induction of the hypertrophic response involves mechanisms using numerous proteins, including receptors, enzymes, and exchangers/ion channels.

■ The integrins function as sites of adhesive interactions between cells and the ECM, regulating cell adhesion, cell growth, and cell motility, and as signal transducers that regulate gene expression and cellular growth.

■ Integrins may integrate a variety of different signaling pathways that are activated by the ECM and growth factors to establish a well-coordinated response to mechanical stress and to growth factors released on mechanical stress.

■ The NHE may play a role in mechanotransduction because its activation increases intracellular pH, which stimulates expression of hypertrophic marker genes and protein synthesis.

■ In the hypertrophic and failing heart, there also is up-regulation of the NCX.

■ The mechanisms by which Ca^{2+} influx may contribute to the development of cardiac hypertrophy include increased intracellular Ca^{2+} that may enhance PKC activity or activate the CaMK.

■ The induction of cardiac hypertrophy requires signaling through several pathways, including the MAPK signaling pathways, JAK/STAT pathways, and calcium signaling pathways.

■ Cardiac hypertrophy is characterized by increases in cell size and protein synthesis, reactivation of the fetal gene program, and up-regulation of genes encoding proteins involved in signaling pathways and energy metabolism. These include the so-called early genes (e.g., *egr-1, hsp70, c-fos, c-jun, c-myc*) and subsequently reactivation of fetal genes, such as β-MyHC, skeletal α-actin, and ANF, and up-regulation of constitutively expressed contractile proteins, such as ventricular MLC-2 and cardiac α-actin.

■ Although cardiomyocytes are not replaced if injured or destroyed, these cells are capable of undergoing apoptosis under clinical situations, such as myocardial ischemia or pressure overload.

REFERENCES

1. Izumo S, Pu WT: The molecular basis of heart failure. In Mann D (ed): Heart Failure: A Companion to Braunwald's Heart Disease. Philadelphia, WB Saunders, 2004.

2. Kira Y, Kochel PJ, Gordon EE, Morgan HE: Aortic perfusion pressure as a determinant of cardiac protein synthesis. Am J Physiol 1984;246:C247-C258.

3. Sadoshima J, Jahn L, Takahashi T, et al: Molecular characterization of the stretch-induced adaptation of cultured cardiac cells: An in vitro model of load-induced cardiac hypertrophy. J Biol Chem 1992;267:10551-10560.

4. Komuro I, Kaida T, Shibazaki Y, et al: Stretching cardiac myocytes stimulates protooncogene expression. J Biol Chem 1990;265:3595-3598.

5. Mann DL, Kent RL, Cooper GT: Load regulation of the properties of adult feline cardiocytes: Growth induction by cellular deformation. Circ Res 1989;64:1079-1090.

6. Yanagisawa M, Kurihara H, Kimura S, et al: A novel peptide vasoconstrictor, endothelin, is produced by vascular endothelium and modulates smooth muscle Ca^{2+} channels. J Hypertens 1988;6(Suppl):S188-S191.

7. Shubeita HE, McDonough PM, Harris AN, et al: Endothelin induction of inositol phospholipid hydrolysis, sarcomere assembly, and cardiac gene expression in ventricular myocytes: A paracrine mechanism for myocardial cell hypertrophy. J Biol Chem 1990;265:20555-20562.

8. Ito H, Hirata Y, Hiroe M, et al: Endothelin-1 induces hypertrophy with enhanced expression of muscle-specific genes in cultured neonatal rat cardiomyocytes. Circ Res 1991;69:209-215.

9. Arai M, Yoguchi A, Iso T, et al: Endothelin-1 and its binding sites are upregulated in pressure overload cardiac hypertrophy. Am J Physiol 1995;268:H2084-H2091.

10. Yamazaki T, Komuro I, Kudoh S, et al: Endothelin-1 is involved in mechanical stress-induced cardiomyocyte hypertrophy. J Biol Chem 1996;271:3221-3228.

11. Ito H, Hiroe M, Hirata Y, et al (ed): Endothelin ET(A) receptor antagonist blocks cardiac hypertrophy provoked by hemodynamic overload. Circulation 1994;89:2198-2203.

12. Sadoshima J, Xu Y, Slayter HS, Izumo S: Autocrine release of angiotensin II mediates stretch-induced hypertrophy of cardiac myocytes in vitro. Cell 1993;75:977-984.

13. Miyata S, Haneda T, Osaki J, Kikuchi K: Renin-angiotensin system in stretch-induced hypertrophy of cultured neonatal rat heart cells. Eur J Pharmacol 1996;307:81-88.

14. Shah BH, Catt KJ: A central role of EGF receptor transactivation in angiotensin II-induced cardiac hypertrophy. Trends Pharmacol Sci 2003;24:239-244.

15. Berk BC: Angiotensin II signal transduction in vascular smooth muscle: Pathways activated by specific tyrosine kinases. J Am Soc Nephrol 1999;10(Suppl 11):S62-S68.

16. Massague J, Cheifetz S, Laiho M, et al: Transforming growth factor-beta. Cancer Surv 1992;12:81-103.

17. Johnson AN, Newfeld SJ: The TGF family: Signaling pathways, developmental roles, and tumor suppressor activities. Sci World J 2002;2:892-925.

18. Parker TG, Packer SE, Schneider MD: Peptide growth factors can provoke "fetal" contractile protein gene expression in rat cardiac myocytes. J Clin Invest 1990;85:507-514.

19. Komuro I, Katoh Y, Kaida T, et al: Mechanical loading stimulates cell hypertrophy and specific gene expression in cultured rat cardiac myocytes: Possible role of protein kinase C activation. J Biol Chem 1991;266:1265-1268.

20. Takahashi N, Calderone A, Izzo NJ Jr, et al: Hypertrophic stimuli induce transforming growth factor-beta 1 expression in rat ventricular myocytes. J Clin Invest 1994;94:1470-1476.

21. Kaye D, Pimental D, Prasad S, et al: Role of transiently altered sarcolemmal membrane permeability and basic fibroblast growth factor release in the hypertrophic response of adult rat ventricular myocytes to increased mechanical activity in vitro. J Clin Invest 1996;97:281-291.

22. Schultz JE, Witt SA, Nieman ML, et al: Fibroblast growth factor-2 mediates pressure-induced hypertrophic response. J Clin Invest 1999;104:709-719.

23. Bogoyevitch MA, Glennon PE, Andersson MB, et al: Endothelin-1 and fibroblast growth factors stimulate the mitogen-activated protein kinase signaling cascade in cardiac myocytes: The potential role of the cascade in the integration of two signaling pathways leading to myocyte hypertrophy. J Biol Chem 1994;269:1110-1119.

24. Ren J, Samson WK, Sowers JR: Insulin-like growth factor I as a cardiac hormone: Physiological and pathophysiological implications in heart disease. J Mol Cell Cardiol 1999;31:2049-2061.

25. Adams GR: Exercise effects on muscle insulin signaling and action: Invited review: Autocrine/paracrine IGF-I and skeletal muscle adaptation. J Appl Physiol 2002;93:1159-1167.

26. Donohue T, Dworkin L, Lango M, et al: Induction of myocardial insulin-like growth factor-I gene expression in left ventricular hypertrophy. Circulation 1994;89:799-809.

27. Reiss K, Cheng W, Ferber A, et al: Overexpression of insulin-like growth factor-1 in the heart is coupled with myocyte proliferation in transgenic mice. Proc Natl Acad Sci U S A 1996;93:8630-8635.

28. Delaughter MC, Taffet GE, Fiorotto ML, et al: Local insulin-like growth factor I expression induces physiologic, then pathologic, cardiac hypertrophy in transgenic mice. FASEB J 1999;13:1923-1929.

29. Shioi T, Kang PM, Douglas PS, et al: The conserved phospho-inositide 3-kinase pathway determines heart size in mice. EMBO J 2000;19:2537-2548.

30. Eguchi S, Inagami T: Signal transduction of angiotensin II type 1 receptor through receptor tyrosine kinase. Regul Pept 2000;91:13-20.

31. Saito Y, Berk BC: Angiotensin II-mediated signal transduction pathways. Curr Hypertens Rep 2002;4:167-171.

32. Rohrbach S, Yan X, Weinberg EO, et al: Neuregulin in cardiac hypertrophy in rats with aortic stenosis: Differential expression of erbB2 and erbB4 receptors. Circulation 1999;100:407-412.

33. Uray IP, Connelly JH, Thomazy V, et al: Left ventricular unloading alters receptor tyrosine kinase expression in the failing human heart. J Heart Lung Transplant 2002;21:771-782.

34. Chien KR: Stress pathways and heart failure. Cell 1999;98:555-558.

35. Pennica D, King KL, Shaw KJ, et al: Expression cloning of cardiotrophin 1, a cytokine that induces cardiac myocyte hypertrophy. Proc Natl Acad Sci U S A 1995;92:1142-1146.

36. Hirota H, Yoshida K, Kishimoto T, Taga T: Continuous activation of gp130, a signal-transducing receptor component for interleukin 6-related cytokines, causes myocardial hypertrophy in mice. Proc Natl Acad Sci U S A 1995;92:4862-4866.

37. Yoshida K, Taga T, Saito M, et al: Targeted disruption of gp130, a common signal transducer for the interleukin 6 family of cytokines, leads to myocardial and hematological disorders. Proc Natl Acad Sci U S A 1996;93:407-411.

38. Betz UA, Bloch W, van den Broek M, et al: Postnatally induced inactivation of gp130 in mice results in neurological, cardiac, hematopoietic, immunological, hepatic, and pulmonary defects. J Exp Med 1998;188:1955-1965.

39. Hirota H, Chen J, Betz UA, et al: Loss of a gp130 cardiac muscle cell survival pathway is a critical event in the onset of heart failure during biomechanical stress. Cell 1999;97:189-198.

40. Hunter JJ, Chien KR: Signaling pathways for cardiac hypertrophy and failure. N Engl J Med 1999;341:1276-1283.

41. Adams JC: Cell-matrix contact structures. Cell Mol Life Sci 2001; 58:371-392.

42. Bornstein P, Sage EH: Matricellular proteins: Extracellular modulators of cell function. Curr Opin Cell Biol 2002;14:608-616.

43. Borg TK, Caulfield JB: The collagen matrix of the heart. Fed Proc 1981;40:2037-2041.

44. Vogel WF: Collagen-receptor signaling in health and disease. Eur J Dermatol 2001;11:506-514.

45. Gumbiner BM: Regulation of cadherin adhesive activity. J Cell Biol 2000;148:399-404.

46. Ross RS, Borg TK: Integrins and the myocardium. Circ Res 2001; 88:1112-1119.

47. Sussman MA, McCulloch A, Borg TK: Dance band on the Titanic: Biomechanical signaling in cardiac hypertrophy. Circ Res 2002; 91:888-898.

48. Schwartz MA, Schaller MD, Ginsberg MH: Integrins: Emerging paradigms of signal transduction. Annu Rev Cell Dev Biol 1995;11:549-599.

49. Lewis JM, Schwartz MA: Mapping in vivo associations of cytoplasmic proteins with integrin beta 1 cytoplasmic domain mutants. Mol Biol Cell 1995;6:151-160.

50. MacKenna DA, Dolfi F, Vuori K, Ruoslahti E: Extracellular signal-regulated kinase and c-Jun NH2-terminal kinase activation by mechanical stretch is integrin-dependent and matrix-specific in rat cardiac fibroblasts. J Clin Invest 1998;101:301-310.

51. Ross RS, Pham C, Shai SY, et al: Beta1 integrins participate in the hypertrophic response of rat ventricular myocytes. Circ Res 1998; 82:1160-1172.

52. Kuppuswamy D, Kerr C, Narishige T, et al: Association of tyrosine-phosphorylated c-Src with the cytoskeleton of hypertrophying myocardium. J Biol Chem 1997;272:4500-4508.

53. Parsons JT, Parsons SJ: Src family protein tyrosine kinases: Cooperating with growth factor and adhesion signaling pathways. Curr Opin Cell Biol 1997;9:187-192.

54. Ingber D: In search of cellular control: Signal transduction in context. J Cell Biochem 1998;30-31(Suppl):232-237.

55. Bloom S, Lockard VG, Bloom M: Intermediate filament-mediated stretch-induced changes in chromatin: A hypothesis for growth initiation in cardiac myocytes. J Mol Cell Cardiol 1996;28: 2123-2127.

56. Plopper GE, McNamee HP, Dike LE, et al: Convergence of integrin and growth factor receptor signaling pathways within the focal adhesion complex. Mol Biol Cell 1995;6:1349-1365.

57. Knowlton KU, Michel MC, Itani M, et al: The alpha 1A-adrenergic receptor subtype mediates biochemical, molecular, and morphologic features of cultured myocardial cell hypertrophy. J Biol Chem 1993;268:15374-15380.

58. Koch WJ, Lefkowitz RJ, Rockman HA: Functional consequences of altering myocardial adrenergic receptor signaling. Annu Rev Physiol 2000;62:237-260.

59. Hershberger RE, Feldman AM, Bristow MR: A1-adenosine receptor inhibition of adenylate cyclase in failing and nonfailing human ventricular myocardium. Circulation 1991;83:1343-1351.

60. Molkentin JD, Dorn IG 2nd: Cytoplasmic signaling pathways that regulate cardiac hypertrophy. Annu Rev Physiol 2001;63: 391-426.

61. Bohm M, Gierschik P, Knorr A, et al: Desensitization of adenylate cyclase and increase of Gi alpha in cardiac hypertrophy due to acquired hypertension. Hypertension 1992;20:103-112.

62. Rosenberg D, Groussin L, Jullian E, et al: Role of the PKA-regulated transcription factor CREB in development and tumorigenesis of endocrine tissues. Ann N Y Acad Sci 2002;968:65-74.

63. Gaudin C, Ishikawa Y, Wight DC, et al: Overexpression of Gs alpha protein in the hearts of transgenic mice. J Clin Invest 1995;95: 1676-1683.

64. Iwase M, Bishop SP, Uechi M, et al: Adverse effects of chronic endogenous sympathetic drive induced by cardiac Gs alpha overexpression. Circ Res 1996;78:517-524.

65. Sardesai SH, Mourant AJ, Sivathandon Y, et al: Phaeochromocytoma and catecholamine induced cardiomyopathy presenting as heart failure. Br Heart J 1990;63:234-237.

66. Simpson P, McGrath A, Savion S: Myocyte hypertrophy in neonatal rat heart cultures and its regulation by serum and by catecholamines. Circ Res 1982;51:787-801.

67. Adams JW, Sakata Y, Davis MG, et al: Enhanced G alpha q signaling: A common pathway mediates cardiac hypertrophy and apoptotic heart failure. Proc Natl Acad Sci U S A 1998;95: 10140-10145.

68. LaMorte VJ, Thorburn J, Absher D, et al: Gq- and ras-dependent pathways mediate hypertrophy of neonatal rat ventricular myocytes following alpha 1-adrenergic stimulation. J Biol Chem 1994;269:13490-13496.

69. D'Angelo DD, Sakata Y, Lorenz JN, et al: Transgenic Galphaq overexpression induces cardiac contractile failure in mice. Proc Natl Acad Sci U S A 1997;94:8121-8126.

70. Sakata Y, Hoit BD, Liggett SB, et al: Decompensation of pressure-overload hypertrophy in G alpha q-overexpressing mice. Circulation 1998;97:1488-1495.

71. Mende U, Kagen A, Cohen A, et al: Transient cardiac expression of constitutively active G alpha q leads to hypertrophy and dilated cardiomyopathy by calcineurin-dependent and independent pathways. Proc Natl Acad Sci U S A 1998;95: 13893-13898.

72. Akhter SA, Luttrell LM, Rockman HA, et al: Targeting the receptor-Gq interface to inhibit in vivo pressure overload myocardial hypertrophy. Science 1998;280:574-577.

73. Harada K, Komuro I, Shiojima I, et al: Pressure overload induces cardiac hypertrophy in angiotensin II type 1A receptor knockout mice. Circulation 1998;97:1952-1959.

74. Kompa AR, Gu XH, Evans BA, Summers RJ: Desensitization of cardiac beta-adrenoceptor signaling with heart failure produced by myocardial infarction in the rat: Evidence for the role of Gi but not Gs or phosphorylating proteins. J Mol Cell Cardiol 1999;31:1185-1201.

75. Choi DJ, Rockman HA: Beta-adrenergic receptor desensitization in cardiac hypertrophy and heart failure. Cell Biochem Biophys 1999;31:321-329.

76. Lefkowitz RJ: G protein-coupled receptors: III. New roles for receptor kinases and beta-arrestins in receptor signaling and desensitization. J Biol Chem 1998;273:18677-18680.

77. Lamers JM, De Jonge HW, Panagia V, Van Heugten HA: Receptor-mediated signalling pathways acting through hydrolysis of membrane phospholipids in cardiomyocytes. Cardioscience 1993;4:121-131.

78. Toker A, Newton AC: Cellular signaling: Pivoting around PDK-1. Cell 2000;103:185-188.

79. Shubeita HE, Martinson EA, Van Bilsen M, et al: Transcriptional activation of the cardiac myosin light chain 2 and atrial natriuretic factor genes by protein kinase C in neonatal rat ventricular myocytes. Proc Natl Acad Sci U S A 1992;89:1305-1309.

80. Bogoyevitch MA, Glennon PE, Sugden PH: Endothelin-1, phorbol esters and phenylephrine stimulate MAP kinase activities in ventricular cardiomyocytes. FEBS Lett 1993;317:271-275.

81. Gu X, Bishop SP: Increased protein kinase C and isozyme redistribution in pressure-overload cardiac hypertrophy in the rat. Circ Res 1994;75:926-931.

82. Wakasaki H, Koya D, Schoen FJ, et al: Targeted overexpression of protein kinase C beta 2 isoform in myocardium causes cardiomyopathy. Proc Natl Acad Sci U S A 1997;94:9320-9325.

83. Takeishi Y, Bhagwat A, Ball NA, et al: Effect of angiotensin-converting enzyme inhibition on protein kinase C and SR proteins in heart failure. Am J Physiol 1999;276:H53-H62.

84. Bowling N, Walsh RA, Song G, et al: Increased protein kinase C activity and expression of Ca²⁺-sensitive isoforms in the failing human heart. Circulation 1999;99:384-391.

85. Schluter KD, Schafer M, Balser C, et al: Influence of pHi and creatine phosphate on alpha-adrenoceptor-mediated cardiac hypertrophy. J Mol Cell Cardiol 1998;30:763-771.

86. Schafer M, Schafer C, Michael Piper H, Schluter KD: Hypertrophic responsiveness of cardiomyocytes to alpha- or beta-adrenoceptor stimulation requires sodium-proton-exchanger-1 (NHE-1) activation but not cellular alkalization. Eur J Heart Fail 2002;4:249-254.

87. Engelhardt S, Hein L, Keller U, et al: Inhibition of Na(+)-H(+) exchange prevents hypertrophy, fibrosis, and heart failure in beta(1)-adrenergic receptor transgenic mice. Circ Res 2002;90:814-819.

88. Choi HS, Trafford AW, Eisner DA: Measurement of calcium entry and exit in quiescent rat ventricular myocytes. Pflugers Arch 2000;440:600-608.

89. Studer R, Reinecke H, Vetter R, et al: Expression and function of the cardiac Na⁺/Ca²⁺ exchanger in postnatal development of the rat, in experimental-induced cardiac hypertrophy and in the failing human heart. Basic Res Cardiol 1997;92(Suppl 1):53-58.

90. Flesch M, Putz F, Schwinger RH, Bohm M: Functional relevance of an enhanced expression of the Na⁺-Ca²⁺ exchanger in the failing human heart. Ann N Y Acad Sci 1996;779:539-542.

91. Sipido KR, Volders PG, de Groot SH, et al: Enhanced Ca²⁺ release and Na/Ca exchange activity in hypertrophied canine ventricular myocytes: Potential link between contractile adaptation and arrhythmogenesis. Circulation 2000;102:2137-2144.

92. Hu H, Sachs F: Stretch-activated ion channels in the heart. J Mol Cell Cardiol 1997;29:1511-1523.

93. Ruknudin A, Sachs F, Bustamante JO: Stretch-activated ion channels in tissue-cultured chick heart. Am J Physiol 1993;264:H960-H972.

94. Yamazaki T, Komuro I, Kudoh S, et al: Role of ion channels and exchangers in mechanical stretch-induced cardiomyocyte hypertrophy. Circ Res 1998;82:430-437.

95. Widmann C, Gibson S, Jarpe MB, Johnson GL: Mitogen-activated protein kinase: Conservation of a three-kinase module from yeast to human. Physiol Rev 1999;79:143-180.

96. Sugden PH, Clerk A: "Stress-responsive" mitogen-activated protein kinases (c-Jun N-terminal kinases and p38 mitogen-activated protein kinases) in the myocardium. Circ Res 1998;83:345-352.

97. Sugden PH, Clerk A: Cellular mechanisms of cardiac hypertrophy. J Mol Med 1998;76:725-746.

98. Hefti MA, Harder BA, Eppenberger HM, Schaub MC: Signaling pathways in cardiac myocyte hypertrophy. J Mol Cell Cardiol 1997;29:2873-2892.

99. Yamazaki T, Komuro I, Zou Y, et al: Protein kinase A and protein kinase C synergistically activate the Raf-1 kinase/mitogen-activated protein kinase cascade in neonatal rat cardiomyocytes. J Mol Cell Cardiol 1997;29:2491-2501.

100. Kunisada K, Hirota H, Fujio Y, et al: Activation of JAK-STAT and MAP kinases by leukemia inhibitory factor through gp130 in cardiac myocytes. Circulation 1996;94:2626-2632.

101. Cohen JJ: Apoptosis. Immunol Today 1993;14:126-130.

102. Kyriakis JM, Banerjee P, Nikolakaki E, et al: The stress-activated protein kinase subfamily of c-Jun kinases. Nature 1994;369:156-160.

103. Weston CR, Davis RJ: The JNK signal transduction pathway. Curr Opin Genet Dev 2002;12:14-21.

104. Nemoto S, Sheng Z, Lin A: Opposing effects of Jun kinase and p38 mitogen-activated protein kinases on cardiomyocyte hypertrophy. Mol Cell Biol 1998;18:3518-3526.

105. Sadoshima J, Montagne O, Wang Q, et al: The MEKK1-JNK pathway plays a protective role in pressure overload but does not mediate cardiac hypertrophy. J Clin Invest 2002;110:271-279.

106. Ruwhof C, van Wamel JT, Noordzij LA, et al: Mechanical stress stimulates phospholipase C activity and intracellular calcium ion levels in neonatal rat cardiomyocytes. Cell Calcium 2001;29:73-83.

107. Stokoe D, Engel K, Campbell DG, et al: Identification of MAPKAP kinase 2 as a major enzyme responsible for the phosphorylation of the small mammalian heat shock proteins. FEBS Lett 1992;313:307-313.

108. Benjamin IJ, McMillan DR: Stress (heat shock) proteins: Molecular chaperones in cardiovascular biology and disease. Circ Res 1998;83:117-132.

109. Seko Y, Takahashi N, Tobe K, et al: Pulsatile stretch activates mitogen-activated protein kinase (MAPK) family members and focal adhesion kinase (p125[FAK]) in cultured rat cardiac myocytes. Biochem Biophys Res Commun 1999;259:8-14.

110. Kudoh S, Komuro I, Hiroi Y, et al: Mechanical stretch induces hypertrophic responses in cardiac myocytes of angiotensin II type 1a receptor knockout mice. J Biol Chem 1998;273:24037-24043.

111. Wang Y, Huang S, Sah VP, et al: Cardiac muscle cell hypertrophy and apoptosis induced by distinct members of the p38 mitogen-activated protein kinase family. J Biol Chem 1998;273:2161-2168.

112. Liao P, Georgakopoulos D, Kovacs A, et al: The in vivo role of p38 MAP kinases in cardiac remodeling and restrictive cardiomyopathy. Proc Natl Acad Sci U S A 2001;98:12283-12288.

113. Braz JC, Bueno OF, Liang Q, et al: Targeted inhibition of p38 MAPK promotes hypertrophic cardiomyopathy through upregulation of calcineurin-NFAT signaling. J Clin Invest 2003;111:1475-1486.

114. Dash R, Schmidt AG, Pathak A, et al: Differential regulation of p38 mitogen-activated protein kinase mediates gender-dependent catecholamine-induced hypertrophy. Cardiovasc Res 2003;57:704-714.

115. Communal C, Colucci WS, Remondino A, et al: Reciprocal modulation of mitogen-activated protein kinases and mitogen-activated protein kinase phosphatase 1 and 2 in failing human myocardium. J Card Fail 2002;8:86-92.

116. Wilks AF: Two putative protein-tyrosine kinases identified by application of the polymerase chain reaction. Proc Natl Acad Sci U S A 1989;86:1603-1607.

117. Ramana CV, Gil MP, Han Y, et al: Stat1-independent regulation of gene expression in response to IFN-gamma. Proc Natl Acad Sci U S A 2001;98:6674-6679.

118. Krebs DL, Hilton DJ: SOCS proteins: Negative regulators of cytokine signaling. Stem Cells 2001;19:378-387.

119. Shuai K: Modulation of STAT signaling by STAT-interacting proteins. Oncogene 2000;19:2638-2644.

120. Heinrich PC, Behrmann I, Haan S, et al: Principles of interleukin (IL)-6-type cytokine signalling and its regulation. Biochem J 2003;374:1-20.

121. Bueno OF, van Rooij E, Molkentin JD, et al: Calcineurin and hypertrophic heart disease: Novel insights and remaining questions. Cardiovasc Res 2002;53:806-821.

122. Rothermel BA, Vega RB, Williams RS: The role of modulatory calcineurin-interacting proteins in calcineurin signaling. Trends Cardiovasc Med 2003;13:15-21.

123. Molkentin JD, Lu JR, Antos CL, et al: A calcineurin-dependent transcriptional pathway for cardiac hypertrophy. Cell 1998;93:215-228.

124. Taigen T, De Windt LJ, Lim HW, Molkentin JD: Targeted inhibition of calcineurin prevents agonist-induced cardiomyocyte hypertrophy. Proc Natl Acad Sci U S A 2000;97:1196-201.

125. Bueno OF, Wilkins BJ, Tymitz KM, et al: Impaired cardiac hypertrophic response in calcineurin abeta-deficient mice. Proc Natl Acad Sci U S A 2002;99:4586-4591.

126. Molkentin JD, Dorn IG 2nd: Cytoplasmic signaling pathways that regulate cardiac hypertrophy. Annu Rev Physiol 2001; 63:391-426.

127. Dolmetsch RE, Lewis RS, Goodnow CC, Healy JI: Differential activation of transcription factors induced by Ca^{2+} response amplitude and duration. Nature 1997;386:855-858.

128. Zhu W, Zou Y, Shiojima I, et al: Ca^{2+}/calmodulin-dependent kinase II and calcineurin play critical roles in endothelin-1-induced cardiomyocyte hypertrophy. J Biol Chem 2000;275:15239-15245.

129. Kato T, Sano M, Miyoshi S, et al: Calmodulin kinases II and IV and calcineurin are involved in leukemia inhibitory factor-induced cardiac hypertrophy in rats. Circ Res 2000;87:937-945.

130. Morimoto T, Hasegawa K, Kaburagi S, et al: Phosphorylation of GATA-4 is involved in alpha 1-adrenergic agonist-responsive transcription of the endothelin-1 gene in cardiac myocytes. J Biol Chem 2000;275:13721-13726.

131. Kerkela R, Pikkarainen S, Majalahti-Palviainen T, et al: Distinct roles of mitogen-activated protein kinase pathways in GATA-4 transcription factor-mediated regulation of B-type natriuretic peptide gene. J Biol Chem 2002;277:13752-13760.

132. Yanazume T, Hasegawa K, Wada H, et al: Rho/ROCK pathway contributes to the activation of extracellular signal-regulated kinase/GATA-4 during myocardial cell hypertrophy. J Biol Chem 2002;277:8618-8625.

133. Charron F, Tsimiklis G, Arcand M, et al: Tissue-specific GATA factors are transcriptional effectors of the small GTPase RhoA. Genes Dev 2001;15:2702-2719.

134. Liang Q, De Windt LJ, Witt SA, et al: The transcription factors GATA4 and GATA6 regulate cardiomyocyte hypertrophy in vitro and in vivo. J Biol Chem 2001;276:30245-30253.

135. Hasegawa K, Lee SJ, Jobe SM, et al: cis-Acting sequences that mediate induction of beta-myosin heavy chain gene expression during left ventricular hypertrophy due to aortic constriction. Circulation 1997;96:3943-3953.

136. Akazawa H, Komuro I: Roles of cardiac transcription factors in cardiac hypertrophy. Circ Res 2003;92:1079-1088.

137. Nicol RL, Frey N, Pearson G, et al: Activated MEK5 induces serial assembly of sarcomeres and eccentric cardiac hypertrophy. EMBO J 2001;20:2757-2767.

138. Black BL, Olson EN: Transcriptional control of muscle development by myocyte enhancer factor-2 (MEF2) proteins. Annu Rev Cell Dev Biol 1998;14:167-196.

139. Xu Q, Wu Z: The insulin-like growth factor-phosphatidylinositol 3-kinase-Akt signaling pathway regulates myogenin expression in normal myogenic cells but not in rhabdomyosarcoma-derived RD cells. J Biol Chem 2000;275:36750-36757.

140. Blaeser F, Ho N, Prywes R, Chatila TA: Ca^{2+}-dependent gene expression mediated by MEF2 transcription factors. J Biol Chem 2000;275:197-209.

141. McKinsey TA, Zhang CL, Lu J, Olson EN: Signal-dependent nuclear export of a histone deacetylase regulates muscle differentiation. Nature 2000;408:106-111.

142. Zhang CL, McKinsey TA, Chang S, et al: Class II histone deacetylases act as signal-responsive repressors of cardiac hypertrophy. Cell 2002;110:479-488.

143. Hai T, Curran T: Cross-family dimerization of transcription factors Fos/Jun and ATF/CREB alters DNA binding specificity. Proc Natl Acad Sci U S A 1991;88:3720-3724.

144. Davis FJ, Gupta M, Camoretti-Mercado B, et al: Calcium/calmodulin-dependent protein kinase activates serum response factor transcription activity by its dissociation from histone deacetylase, HDAC4: Implications in cardiac muscle gene regulation during hypertrophy. J Biol Chem 2003;278:20047-20058.

145. Zhang X, Azhar G, Chai J, et al: Cardiomyopathy in transgenic mice with cardiac-specific overexpression of serum response factor. Am J Physiol Heart Circ Physiol 2001;280:H1782-H1792.

146. Karin M: The regulation of AP-1 activity by mitogen-activated protein kinases. Philos Trans R Soc Lond B Biol Sci 1996;351:127-134.

147. Williams RS: Apoptosis and heart failure. N Engl J Med 1999;341:759-760.

148. Hirota H, Chen J, Betz UA, et al: Loss of a gp130 cardiac muscle cell survival pathway is a critical event in the onset of heart failure during biomechanical stress. Cell 1999;97:189-198.

149. Syed F, Odley A, Hahn HS, et al: Physiological growth synergizes with pathological genes in experimental cardiomyopathy. Circ Res 2004;Nov 11 [Epub]:95, 1200-1206.

150. Liao JK: Statin therapy for cardiac hypertrophy and heart failure. J Invest Med 2004;52:248-253.

152. Gupta S, Young D, Sen S: Inhibition of NF-κB induces regression of cardiac hypertrophy, independent of blood pressure control, in spontaneously hypertensive rats. Am J Physiol Heart Circ Physiol 2005 Mar 4;

CHAPTER 5

Hemodynamic Adaptive Mechanisms in Heart Failure

Tia A. Tortoriello

Starling, credited with elucidating the first mechanism governing heart action, recognized that a reduction in cardiac output elicits compensatory homeostatic responses that are mediated by neurohumoral mechanisms.[1] Mechanoreceptors in the left ventricle, carotid sinus, aortic arch, and renal afferent arterioles all contribute to detecting arterial underfilling (Fig. 5-1). The undersensing of these receptors leads to a cascade of sympathetic system outflow (with concomitant parasympathetic withdrawal) (Fig. 5-2), renin-angiotensin-aldosterone system activation, and other mediator release (e.g., arginine vasopressin [AVP] via the supraoptic and paraventricular nuclei in the hypothalamus).

Among the homeostatic mechanisms activated when the heart fails as a pump, an increase in peripheral vascular resistance and expansion of the extracellular fluid volume secondary to salt and water retention are prominent. In healthy individuals, circulation regulatory mechanisms respond appropriately to acute reductions in circulating blood volume; these responses lead to short-term compensatory effects. In a patient with cardiac dysfunction, however, long-term effects are often deleterious and are targets of therapy.[2]

Because physicians traditionally have considered heart failure to be a hemodynamic disorder, they have described the syndrome of heart failure using hemodynamic concepts and have designed treatment strategies to correct the hemodynamic derangements of the disease. Although hemodynamic abnormalities may explain the symptoms of heart failure, these are not sufficient to

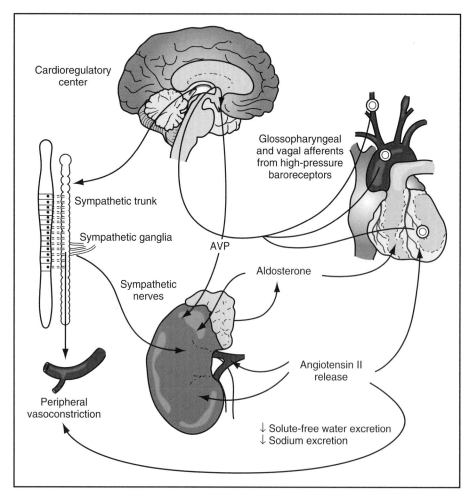

FIGURE 5-1 ■ **The sympathetic nervous system and the heart.** The left ventricle, carotid sinus, and aortic arch have receptors that respond to arterial underfilling by sending afferent signals to the regions of the brain, resulting in efferent signals via the sympathetic pathways. These signals result in release of angiotensin II and aldosterone and arginine vasopressin (AVP). The mediators released effect changes such as peripheral vasoconstriction, decreased solute-free water excretion, and decreased sodium excretion (see text for more details). (From Colucci WS, Braunwald E: *Pathophysiology of heart failure.* In Braunwald E [ed]: *Heart Disease,* 7th ed, Philadelphia, WB Saunders, 2005, p. 527.)

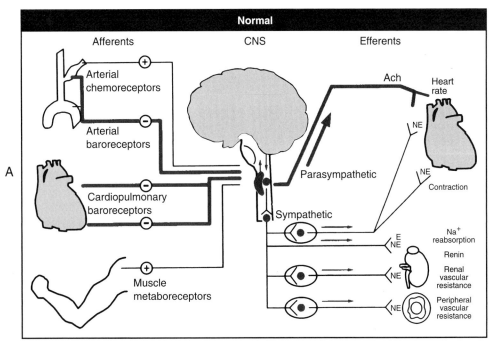

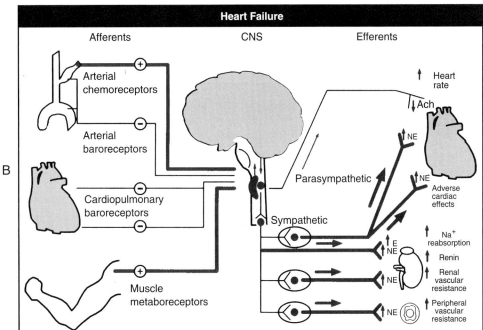

FIGURE 5-2 ■ **The sympathetic and parasympathetic nervous system in normal individuals and heart failure patients. A,** In normal individuals, negative inputs (−) from the afferent baroreceptors influence the sympathetic outflow. This results in low efferent activity to the sympathetic nerves and norepinephrine (NE) release. **B,** In patients with heart failure, the inhibitory input from the mechanoreceptors decreases, while the excitatory (+) input from the arterial chemoreceptors increases. This results in increased sympathetic drive with increased NE release, leading to increased sodium retention and renin and increased renal and peripheral vascular resistances. There is decreased parasympathetic tone in heart failure so as to create an imbalance between these two systems. CNS, central nervous system; Ach, acetylcholine; E, epinephrine. (From Floras JS: *Clinical aspects of sympathetic activation and parasympathetic withdrawal in heart failure. J Am Coll Cardiol* 1991;22:72A.)

explain the progression of heart failure and ultimately the death of the patient. The neurohumoral response predominates in the progression of chronic heart failure. Activation of the sympathetic nervous system and renin-angiotensin-aldosterone system can have adverse

hemodynamic consequences in heart failure because both of these systems enhance systemic vasoconstriction and promote the retention of sodium and water.[3,4]

According to Katz,[5] the major elements of the neurohumoral response in heart failure fall into three classes, each of which has adaptive and maladaptive consequences. The first homeostatic mechanism, the **inflammatory reaction**, includes an inflammatory response that operates systemically and locally. Mediators of the inflammatory cascade include cytokines, tumor necrosis factor-α, activation of the complement system, and the JAK-STAT pathway (see Chapter 3). The second class of homeostatic mechanisms that has been recognized to play a crucial role in the patient with heart failure is the **hypertrophic response** of the myocardium. Similar to the inflammatory response, hypertrophy of a damaged or overloaded heart is initially adaptive, but after time, maladaptive effects that accompany cardiac enlargement begin to dominate (see Chapter 4).

The focus of this chapter is on the homeostatic mechanisms that constitute the **hemodynamic defense response**. This essential hemodynamic principle is a response that enables the body to react to challenges that impair circulation, including systemic arterial underfilling or a decline in blood pressure (Table 5-1). This response is adaptive in the short-term to maintain blood pressure and cardiac output, as is shown during exercise and acute blood loss secondary to hemorrhage. Beyond hemodynamic effects alone, endogenous or exogenous neurohumoral stimulation of the cardiovascular system in chronic heart failure leads to progressive circulatory dysfunction and subsequent increased morbidity and mortality.[6]

HEMODYNAMIC DEFENSE RESPONSE

Many of the adaptations to heart failure are similar to the homeostatic mechanisms used by the body in response to circulatory failure from any cause. The overall function of the sympathetic system is coordinated in the central nervous system, where the special pattern of response, called the *defense reaction,* was first identified by Hilton and Spyer.[7] Harris[8-10] further proposed the theory that the neurohumoral response evoked during heart failure is the same that evolved to support survival of the species under two main circumstances: physical exercise and hemorrhage.

During exercise, there is an increase in heart rate, systolic blood pressure, and stroke volume with an increase in contractility that results in a redistribution of blood flow to the working muscles.[11,12] There is a complex interplay of alterations of heart rate, loading conditions, contractility, and peripheral vascular adaptations that are called on to maintain adequate perfusion during exercise in normal individuals.[13] In the setting of hemorrhagic shock, there is an abrupt decrease in cardiac output and arterial blood pressure that results from a decrease in venous return to the heart. Similar to during exercise, the challenge for the body is to maintain systemic blood pressure.

The most important difference among all of these conditions is in the duration of the condition. With heart failure, blood pressure is continuously and chronically threatened over a prolonged period, rather than the minutes to hours as occurs during exercise and hemorrhage. The hemodynamic defense response is called on to continue for as long as the threat persists. As a result, the body abnormally intensifies the hemodynamic defense response with which arterial pressure should be maintained, and a vicious cycle is established.[5,14,15]

Katz[5] elucidated that there are three major components to the hemodynamic defense response in any patient with heart failure: salt and fluid retention, vasoconstriction, and cardiac stimulation. The compensatory mechanisms initiated by the short-term decrease in cardiac output, as occurs during exercise and hemorrhage, generate an adaptive response. When sustained, however, as in chronic heart failure, these same mechanisms cause maladaptive responses that further reduce cardiac output, exacerbate symptoms, and accelerate cell death.

TABLE 5-1

Hemodynamic Defense Response in Heart Failure		
Mechanism	Short-Term, Adaptive	Long-Term, Maladaptive
Salt and water retention	↑ Preload	Pulmonary congestion, anasarca
	Maintain cardiac output	Pulmonary congestion
Vasoconstriction	↑ Afterload	↓ Cardiac output
	Maintain blood pressure	↑ Cardiac energy expenditure
	Maintain cardiac output	Cardiac necrosis
Cardiac stimulation	↑ Contractility	↑ Cytosolic calcium
	↑ Relaxation	↑ Cardiac energy expenditure
	↑ Heart rate	Cardiac necrosis
		Arrhythmias, sudden death

Modified from Katz AM (ed): The hemodynamic defense reaction. In: Heart Failure: Pathophysiology, Molecular Biology, and Clinical Management. Philadelphia, Lippincott Williams & Wilkins, 2000, p. 110.

TABLE 5-2

Mediators of the Neurohumoral Response in Heart Failure			
Mediator	Fluid Retention	Vasoconstriction	Cardiac Stimulation
Peptide and Protein			
Angiotensin II	++	++	+
Arginine vasopressin (ADH)	++	++	+
Atrial natriuretic peptide	−	−	−
Bradykinin	0	−	0
Endothelin	++	++	+
Neuropeptide Y	+	++	−
Catecholamine			
Norepinephrine			
α_1-Receptors	++	++	+
α_2-Receptors (central)	−	−	−
β-Receptors	0	−	++
Dopamine	−	−	+
Steroid			
Aldosterone	+	0	0
Fatty Acid			
Prostaglandins	+ and −	+ and −	0
Others			
Nitric oxide	−	−	−
Agmatine	−	−	−

++ = strong stimulatory effect; + = weak stimulatory effect; 0 = effect insignificant or absent; − = inhibitory effect.
ADH, antidiuretic hormone
From Katz AM (ed): The hemodynamic defense reaction. In: Heart Failure: Pathophysiology, Molecular Biology, and Clinical Management. Philadelphia, Lippincott Williams & Wilkins, 2000, p. 113.

Each of these components of the hemodynamic defense response are mediated by signaling molecules or mediators that can activate not only the heart, but also the kidneys, blood vessels, and skeletal muscle (Table 5-2). Signaling molecules that play a regulatory role in the hemodynamic defense response include the catecholamines (epinephrine and norepinephrine), angiotensin II (Ang II), AVP, and endothelin (ET). Counterregulatory effects of the hemodynamic defense response also are controlled through various mediators, including the catecholamines, natriuretic peptides, nitric oxide (NO), bradykinin, and dopamine. Whether the mediator activates a regulatory or counterregulatory effect depends on which receptor class it is stimulating.

Fluid and Sodium Retention

Traditional definitions of heart failure often highlight the clinical signs and symptoms that occur when the failing cardiac pump cannot meet the needs of the body. Many patients accumulate fluid, develop edema, and occasionally develop anasarca, a syndrome referred to as *congestive heart failure* (CHF). The clinical picture in most patients with heart failure is dominated by secondary abnormalities in end organs that are the result of a failing pump, including shortness of breath (lungs), salt and water retention (kidneys), and fatigue (skeletal muscle). The most evident clinical manifestations of heart failure depend on whether the underlying cause affects the right or the left ventricle. Right heart failure results in the accumulation of blood behind the right ventricle and results in an elevation in right atrial and systemic venous pressures. The end result is the formation of edema in the dependent portions of the body, most prominently in the legs, where gravity increases the pressure that forces fluid out of the capillaries into the soft tissues. *Anasarca* is defined as the filling of the body with fluid, which can accumulate in the abdomen (ascites), lungs (pleural effusions), and pericardium (pericardial effusion). Left heart failure results in the accumulation of blood behind the left ventricle and an elevation in left atrial and pulmonary venous pressures causing pulmonary edema. Dyspnea, orthopnea, and paroxysmal nocturnal dyspnea are the end results of left heart failure (see Chapter 15).

These fundamental features of heart failure have been known since the turn of the 20th century, when Starling[16] became aware that blood volume was increased in patients with edema; measurements made by Wollheim[17] in 1931 confirmed that this concept was correct. Soon thereafter, Starr and Rawson[18,19] showed that edema could not occur unless the venous pressure was elevated, and Warren and Stead[20] observed that during the early stages of heart failure an increase in weight precedes a rise in venous pressure. In the late 1940s, Merrill[21,22] found that weight gain in these patients was the result of salt and water retention by the kidney owing to decreased renal blood flow. For more than 50 years, it has been known that edema formation in heart failure is correlated with retention of salt and water by the kidney.

The predominant feature involved in the electrolyte and water imbalances in heart failure is renal conservation of sodium — (see Key Concepts) — a process mediated by substances such as aldosterone, Ang II, and norepinephrine and counterregulated by signaling molecules, such as prostaglandins (PGs) and natriuretic peptides. The retention of sodium, rather than of water, is the major cause of the expanded extracellular fluid volume in heart failure. The kidney functions as a compensatory mechanism to restore normal renal blood flow by promoting increased retention of sodium and water in an effort to improve cardiac output by augmenting circulatory blood volume and enhancing ventricular filling and cardiac function.[23]

The mechanisms whereby sodium is retained and concomitant edema is produced have been shown to be multifactorial. It generally has been recognized that decreased cardiac output from the failing myocardium, the underfilling hypothesis, leads to reductions in renal plasma flow (RPF) and renal glomerular filtration rate (GFR).[14,24-26] Starling[27] is credited with the first argument that implicated renal sodium retention as responsible for the edema of chronic CHF. Starling[27] elucidated the key elements to the underfilling theory: a diminished perfusion of the kidneys as a result of an inadequate cardiac output, an attempt by the kidney to retain salt and water to promote cardiac filling, and the eventual effect of such a vicious cycle. The idea of an effective circulatory volume was crucial to Starling's argument, however, and it was Peters[28] who deduced that there were mechanisms for sensing blood volume, and that these sensing mechanisms were the key factors responsible for mediating renal sodium excretion.

In 1942, Stead and Ebert[29] integrated Starling's original argument and Peters' idea of an effective circulatory volume into what we now understand about systolic pump dysfunction. Stead and Ebert[29] recognized that an inability to translocate fluid from the venous to the arterial side could result in a dramatic reduction in effective circulatory volume. Studies done by Merrill[21] in 1946 and Mokotoff and colleagues[30] in 1948 further supported the view of a decrease in sodium excretion in heart failure patients owing to a combination of low cardiac output, which would decrease renal perfusion, and an elevated venous pressure, which slowed the return of blood from the renal circulation. These investigators showed that RPF was diminished in heart failure in humans, and that in chronic CHF a reduction in RPF had no relation to the magnitude of venous pressure. Further studies began to prove that fluid retention and edema formation in heart failure involve more than a hemodynamic abnormality of diminished blood flow.[31,32] Merrill and Cargell[31] showed that some patients with fluid retention who had mild heart failure had resting GFRs that were within the normal range. Other factors were discovered that contributed to the pathogenesis of fluid retention, including various mediators acting locally on different regions of the renal vasculature that provoke abnormal blood flow distribution within the kidney.[33-35]

In patients without heart failure, extracellular volume and its intravascular (plasma volume) and extravascular (interstitial space) compartments remain remarkably constant despite alterations in dietary sodium and water intake.[36,37] Sodium comprises more than 90% of the total solute of the extracellular fluid and is largely confined to the extracellular space. Because sodium is the major component of the extracellular fluid, it is the primary determinant of oncotic pressure; control of the extracellular volume depends on the regulation of sodium balance. The regulation of sodium balance is determined by sodium intake and the excretion of sodium by the kidneys. If the extracellular volume is increased in normal subjects, the kidneys excrete extra salt and water and return the extracellular volume to normal. In patients with heart failure and edema, the retention of sodium and water by the kidney persists despite expansion of the extracellular volume and increases in total body water and total body sodium.

With regards to the integrated mechanisms of salt and water retention in CHF, three factors are considered the major determinants in the preservation of sodium (Fig. 5-3), including the reduction in RPF; the influence of the hormone aldosterone and the stimulation of the renin-angiotensin system (RAS); and the additional sodium-retaining factors, which are extra-adrenal and exert their influence on the kidney to conserve sodium.[25,26] Each of these factors has a role in the various afferent and efferent mechanisms that play a crucial role in the pathophysiology of heart failure.

Briefly, numerous receptors that monitor stretch are located in various sites in the arterial system, great veins, and cardiac chambers. In low-pressure chambers, stretch of these receptors reflects primarily volume changes, whereas in the high-pressure arterial system, stretch of these receptors monitors blood pressure.[14] Table 5-3 outlines the various afferent mechanisms responsible for detecting these changes in stretch and

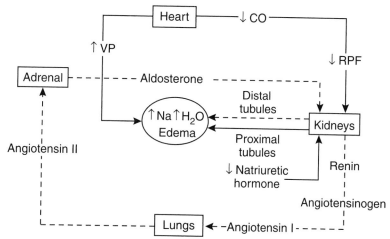

FIGURE 5-3 ■ Factors leading to sodium and water retention in congestive heart failure. Cardiac dysfunction leads to reduced cardiac output (CO), which results in a decreased renal perfusion pressure and renal plasma flow (RPF), causing increased reabsorption of Na and H_2O from the proximal renal tubules. A decreased RPF is shown by the ***solid clockwise arrows***. Reduced RPF activates the renal secretion of renin, which ultimately results in increased adrenal secretion of aldosterone, producing increased Na and H_2O reabsorption from the distal renal tubules. The events centered around aldosterone secretion are shown by ***broken clockwise arrows***. In addition, extra-adrenal Na-retaining factors exert their influence on the kidney to conserve sodium. Finally, the hemodynamic effect of elevated venous pressure (VP) on edema formation is depicted by the ***solid counterclockwise arrow***. (From Tonkin MJ, Rosen SM, Mason DT: *Renal function and edema formation in congestive heart failure.* In Mason DT [ed]: *Congestive Heart Failure: Mechanisms, Evaluation and Treatment,* pp. 169-177. New York, Dun-Donnelley Publishing Corporation, 1976, p. 170.)

TABLE 5-3

Afferent Mechanisms and Efferent Mechanisms

Afferent Mechanisms

Low-pressure or low-volume receptors
    Atrial receptors
    Neural pathways
    Hormonal factors
High-pressure baroreceptors
    Carotid sinus and aortic arch baroreceptors
    Renal sensors
        Juxtaglomerular cells
        Macula densa
        Renal parenchymal mechanoreceptors
Other receptors
    Central nervous system and liver

Efferent Mechanisms

Sympathetic nervous system
    Renal sympathetic nerves
Neurohormones
    Renin-angiotensin-aldosterone system
    Vasopressin
    Atrial natriuretic peptides
Intrarenal hormones
    Prostaglandins
    Kallikrein-kinin system
Renal responses
    Glomerular filtration
    Peritubular capillary Starling forces

From Inder SA: Pathogenesis of salt and water retention in the congestive heart failure syndrome. In Poole-Wilson PA, Colucci WS, Massie BM, et al (eds): Heart Failure. New York, Churchill Livingstone, 1997, p. 160.

their corresponding location in the body. Low-pressure receptors are located in the atria and great veins, and signals from these receptors are transmitted to the hypothalamus and medullary centers, which control renal sympathetic discharge,[38,39] systemic vascular resistance,[40] and release of AVP.[41,42] The existence of a hormonal factor in the atria became clear in 1979, when de Bold and coworkers[43,44] discovered atrial natriuretic peptide (ANP), which is stored in atrial tissue and released after atrial stretch.[45,46]

Constriction of the efferent arterioles of the glomeruli is the most important of the hemodynamic abnormalities in the kidneys of patients with CHF. This and other efferent mechanisms that are activated in CHF and that help to retain sodium and water are outlined in Table 5-3. Vasoconstriction of these efferent arterioles increases GFR by increasing intraglomerular pressure, but at the same time reduces total renal blood flow. In the kidney, sympathetic stimulation and catecholamine release increase sodium reabsorption by renal hemodynamic and tubular effects similar to Ang II.[47-49] Catecholamines also stimulate secretion of renin and antagonize the counterregulatory effects of vasodilator neurohormones.[50]

As discussed earlier, mediators of the selective vasoconstrictor responses that lead to sodium and water retention include norepinephrine, AVP, Ang II, and ET. In addition, several of these extracellular mediators also exert effects directly on the renal epithelium to cause sodium and water retention. Aldosterone, Ang II, and norepinephrine all increase tubular reabsorption of sodium, and AVP acts on the collecting ducts to promote water reabsorption. The remaining portion of this discussion focuses on these extracellular messengers generated by the neurohumoral response to sodium and water retention in CHF.

Aldosterone is a steroid hormone that is secreted by the zona glomerulosa of the adrenal cortex in response to changes in fluid and electrolyte balance and blood pressure. Aldosterone acts directly on the kidney to decrease the rate of sodium ion excretion (with accompanying retention of water) and to increase the rate of potassium and hydrogen ion excretion. In normal individuals, the secretion of aldosterone is mainly regulated by concentrations of potassium ion in the extracellular fluid, with increases in potassium ion resulting in stimulation of aldosterone secretion. In these individuals, aldosterone secretion also is controlled by adrenocorticotropic hormone (ACTH), a pituitary hormone that regulates the normal diurnal changes in aldosterone secretion. Stress also plays an important role in aldosterone secretion by further increasing ACTH secretion.

In patients with CHF, the stimulus for aldosterone secretion is controlled as a part of the neurohumoral defense reaction, promoting increased fluid retention by the kidneys. In heart failure, the most important stimulus for aldosterone release is Ang II, which is released in response to activation of the RAS as a result of decreased renal blood flow. Other mediators that influence aldosterone release include norepinephrine, ET, and vasopressin. Diuretics, the mainstay of treatment for all patients with CHF, bring about a considerable clinical improvement in patients with chronic heart failure at the expense of stimulating the RAS. Previous studies showed that before diuretic treatment, plasma renin activity and plasma Ang II concentrations were within normal ranges, but were significantly higher in patients already on diuretic therapy. Patients with acute heart failure have increased plasma concentrations of other mediators of the neurohumoral response, notably ANP, AVP, and catecholamines that stimulate the release of aldosterone.[51,52] In recent years, the understanding of the role of aldosterone has expanded beyond the known classic effects of promoting renal sodium retention and potassium loss.[53,54] Aldosterone is known to cause myocardial uptake of norepinephrine[55] and has been shown to promote cardiac fibrosis in various experimental models[56,57] and to promote adverse ventricular remodeling in humans.[58,59] In conjunction with Ang II, aldosterone causes vascular damage, endothelial dysfunction, and decreased vascular compliance.[60-63]

Several important adult studies have shown efficacy in blocking the deleterious effects of aldosterone. The Randomized Aldactone Evaluation Study (RALES) showed that the addition of a modest dose of spironolactone (Aldactone) to current standard of care treatment for severe (New York Heart Association class III) heart failure provided a 30% improvement in survival and a 35% improvement in morbidity/hospitalization.[64]

The Eplerenone Post-Acute Myocardial Infarction Heart Failure Efficacy and Survival Study (EPHESUS) has confirmed in a post–myocardial infarction population the efficacy of a selective aldosterone inhibitor, eplerenone, in reducing mortality in patients receiving angiotensin-converting enzyme (ACE) inhibitor or β-blocker.[65] Results from the Valsartan Heart Failure Trial (Val-HeFT) also confirmed that the addition of valsartan, an angiotensin receptor blocker, to background therapy for heart failure produces sustained reduction in plasma aldosterone, consistent with the observed significant reduction in the combined mortality/morbidity end point.[66]

Arginine vasopressin (AVP) is a polypeptide that is formed in the supraoptic nuclei of the hypothalamus and is stored and released by the posterior pituitary gland. AVP plays an important role in the regulation of body fluid balance through its antidiuretic action (hence its other name, *antidiuretic hormone*). AVP also is known to be a potent vasoconstrictor that regulates the cardiovascular system.[67-69] Vasopressin contributes to cardiovascular regulation by causing vasoconstriction and by stimulating renal water absorption through V_1 and V_2 receptors. V_2 receptor activation can lead to vasodilation. The classification of vasopressin receptor subtypes originally was proposed by Mitchell and coworkers[70] and was based on intracellular mechanisms: cyclic AMP (cAMP)–independent (V_{1a}) and cAMP-dependent (V_2) pathways. The V_{1a} receptors are located on vascular smooth muscle cells and cardiomyocytes and have been shown to modulate blood vessel vasoconstriction and myocardial function.[71,72] The V_2 receptors are located on renal collecting duct cells, which are coupled to aquaporin water channels and regulate volume status through stimulation of free water and urea reabsorption.[73]

AVP plays a significant role in volume homeostasis under normal physiologic conditions through continuous response to changes in plasma tonicity.[73] Changes in plasma tonicity cause stimulation of osmoreceptors in the hypothalamus that result in the release of AVP from the pituitary. After release into the circulation, AVP binds to V_2 receptors located on collecting duct principal cells in the kidney and stimulates the synthesis of aquaporin water channel proteins that allow free water to be reabsorbed across the apical membrane of the collecting duct. AVP secretion alters collecting duct permeability, increases free water reabsorption, and ultimately decreases plasma osmolality.[74]

In patients with heart failure, these adaptive mechanisms are altered and even lost.[52,75] Similar to aldosterone secretion in patients with CHF, AVP is not under physiologic control in these individuals. Rather than responding to changes in plasma osmolarity, AVP levels in heart failure are increased by the reduced arterial filling[76] and a central effect of increased Ang II.[77] AVP release does not appear to be primarily mediated through osmotic balance because systemic AVP concentrations remain elevated despite reductions in plasma osmolality and plasma serum sodium concentrations.[78,79] Numerous studies have shown that plasma AVP concentrations are significantly and chronically elevated in patients with heart failure, particularly in patients with significant cardiac decompensation and hyponatremia.[78-80] Goldsmith and associates[78] reported significantly elevated plasma AVP concentrations in patients with advanced heart failure compared with healthy age-matched controls (9.5 pg/mL versus 4.7 pg/mL; *P* < .001). In addition, a substudy of the Studies of Left Ventricular Dysfunction (SOLVD) database showed an incremental increase in plasma AVP concentrations from healthy individuals compared with asymptomatic and symptomatic patients with left ventricular dysfunction.[79]

In patients with heart failure, excess AVP activity seems to be integrally involved in the impaired excretion of free water,[79] elevations in systemic vascular resistance and pulmonary capillary wedge pressure,[80] and induction of unfavorable structural changes in the myocardium.[81-84] AVP has been shown to stimulate myocardial cell hypertrophy by enhancing protein synthesis and cellular growth without affecting cell division in neonatal rat cardiomyocytes.[81,82] Subsequent to these findings, many AVP antagonists are currently under development as potential therapeutic agents for the treatment of acute and chronic heart failure. Preliminary preclinical and clinical trials with these agents have shown hemodynamic improvements and significant water diuresis of potential clinical utility.[82-86] A current trial has shown that a decrease in body weight, normalization of serum sodium in patients with hyponatremia, and amelioration of edema can be achieved in patients with mild signs of congestion on long-term diuretic therapy in response to tolvaptan, an oral, once-a-day vasopressin V_2-receptor blocker.[86]

Natriuretic peptides are a group of naturally occurring substances that act in the body to oppose the activity of the RAS, aldosterone, ET, and vasopressin (see Chapter 6). There are three major natriuretic peptides: ANP, which is synthesized in the atria; B type natriuretic peptide (BNP), which is synthesized in the ventricles; and C-type natriuretic peptide, which is synthesized in the brain.[87] The site of synthesis for *Dendroaspis* natriuretic peptide is unknown.[88] The identification of atrial granules using electron microscopy[89] in 1956 was probably the first experiment of the natriuretic peptide system. Also in 1956, independent work from Henry and colleagues[90] showed that diuresis was induced by atrial distention. In 1981, de Bold and colleagues[44] noted, however, that the infusion of atrial, but not ventricular, extracts into rats caused natriuresis, diuresis, and hypotension. Soon thereafter, Flynn and coworkers[91] were the first to purify ANP from rat atria to homogeneity and produced the first amino acid sequence of human α-atrial natriuretic polypeptide.

ANP and BNP are released in response to atrial and ventricular stretch and cause vasorelaxation, inhibition of aldosterone secretion in the adrenal cortex, and inhibition of renin secretion in the kidney. ANP and BNP cause natriuresis and a reduction in intravascular volume, both of which are amplified by antagonism of AVP.[87] ANP inhibits renin and AVP release and inhibits Ang II–stimulated aldosterone secretion.[92,93] In addition, ANP inhibits sodium reabsorption in the medullary collecting tubules[94] and Ang II–stimulated reabsorption in the proximal tubules.[95] ANP is one of the earliest neurohormones to increase with the development of left ventricular dysfunction,[80,96] and circulating levels of ANP during heart failure correlate with atrial pressures.[97] Despite greatly increased circulating ANP, patients with heart failure retain salt and water, suggesting an attenuation of its effects in patients with this condition. The physiologic effects of C-type natriuretic peptide are different from those of ANP and BNP; C-type natriuretic peptide has a hypotensive effect, but does not alter significantly diuretic or natriuretic actions.[87] *Dendroaspis* natriuretic peptide has been described only recently, but early investigation suggests that this peptide has important natriuretic and vasodilating effects and may modulate cardiac function as well.[98]

Increased blood levels of natriuretic peptides have been found in certain disease states, suggesting a role in the pathophysiology of those diseases, including CHF, systemic hypertension, and acute myocardial infarction.[87] Current research has focused on the use of the natriuretic peptides as disease markers and indicators of prognosis in various cardiovascular conditions, including CHF.[87,99-102] In contrast to ANP, whose major storage sites include the atria and ventricles, the major source of plasma BNP is the cardiac ventricles, where it is synthesized as preproBNP and secreted as NT-proBNP and BNP.[102] This suggests that BNP and NT-proBNP may be more sensitive and specific indicators of ventricular disorders than other natriuretic peptides. Clinical experience suggests that BNP may have utility in the urgent care setting, where it has been used to discriminate accurately acute dyspnea due to CHF from other causes.[102-104] In a multinational study of men and women seen in the emergency department with acute dyspnea (Breathing Not Properly Multinational Study), BNP measurement would have added to clinical judgment in establishing a final diagnosis of CHF.[102] In patients with an intermediate probability of CHF, BNP would have clarified the diagnosis in most cases (74%).[102] Finally, in patients in whom the plasma levels of BNP are normal, other causes of dyspnea should be considered.[102]

Vasoconstriction

The second major feature of the hemodynamic defense response in heart failure is increased peripheral vascular resistance. Arterial and venous vasoconstrictor reflexes are activated initially in response to a decreasing cardiac output to maintain perfusion pressure to support cerebral and coronary flow, reduce urine flow to correct fluid

TABLE 5-4

Impact of Vascular Tone on Circulation			
Site of Vascular Smooth Muscle	Functional Effect	Effect on Ventricular Load	Effect on Hemodynamics
↑ Arterial tone	↑ Systemic vascular resistance	↑ LV afterload	↑ Mean arterial blood pressure
↑ Aortic and large artery tone	↓ Arterial capacitance	↑ LV afterload	↑ Arterial pulse pressure
↑ Venous tone	↓ Venous capacitance	↑ RV and LV preload	↑ Right atrial, pulmonary capillary wedge, and ventricular end-diastolic pressures

LV, left ventricular; RV, right ventricular.
From Jaski BE (ed): Circulation. In: Basics of Heart Failure: A Problem Solving Approach. Boston, Mass, Kluwer Academic Publishers, 2000, p. 31.

deficits, and shift blood volume centrally to augment cardiac filling. In the presence of heart failure, these vasoconstrictor mechanisms also are stimulated and are initially beneficial. Vascular tone is a determinant of preload—via venous constriction that augments blood return to the heart—and increases preload and stroke volume through the Frank-Starling mechanism as long as the ventricle is operating on the ascending portion of its ventricular performance curve. Vascular tone also is a determinant of afterload—via arteriolar constriction that increases the peripheral vascular resistance and helps to maintain blood pressure. The regional distribution of α receptors is such that during sympathetic stimulation, blood flow is redistributed to vital organs (e.g., heart and brain) at the expense of the skin, splanchnic viscera, and kidneys (Table 5-4).[105] The consequence of this response in patients with heart failure is that a negative-feedback mechanism becomes transformed into a positive-feedback mechanism that may lead to progressive cardiac failure.

Three neurohumoral vasoconstrictor systems are known to exist and may be activated in patients with heart failure: the sympathetic nervous system, the RAS, and the AVP system. The effects of AVP on vasoconstriction via V_1 receptors and the simultaneous effect on vasodilation via V_2 receptors already have been described. Many vasoconstrictors are secreted by the sympathetic nervous system in heart failure, the principal regulator being norepinephrine, which binds to α_1-adrenergic receptors on arteriolar smooth muscle, causing vasoconstriction (see later). Other vasoconstrictors include Ang II, ET, and AVP. Similar to the neurohumoral response in the kidneys, there also are counterregulatory mediators that promote vasodilation, including natriuretic peptides, bradykinin, NO, dopamine, and some PGs (PGI_2 and PGE_2). All of these mediators act directly to relax arteriolar smooth muscle, producing vasodilation. The remaining sections of this chapter focus on the effects of the sympathetic nervous system and the RAS in patients with heart failure.

The discovery of the RAS opened a new era in the research of the physiology and pathology of the cardiovascular system. Briefly, the RAS is activated during states of sodium restriction, hemorrhage or intravascular volume contraction, increased adrenergic state, or acute cardiac decompensation.[107] **Angiotensin II (Ang II)** is the effector hormone of the RAS. It is generated by a cascade of events starting with the secretion of the proteolytic enzyme, **renin**, mostly from the juxtaglomerular apparatus in the renal cortex, in response either to a decrease in intrarenal perfusion pressure or to accumulation of sodium at the site of the adjacent macula densa.[108] Renin is a proteolytic enzyme that is synthesized, stored, and released by the juxtaglomerular cells. The circulating substrate for renin is α_2-globulin—**angiotensinogen**—which is synthesized in the liver.[109,110] In the plasma, renin acts on the polypeptide, angiotensinogen, to produce **angiotensin I**, a decapeptide. Angiotensin I is the main substrate for **Angiotensin-converting enzyme (ACE)**, which cleaves off two amino acids from the C-terminal of angiotensin I to form Ang II, an octapeptide (Fig. 5-4). Ang II serves as the principal stimulus for the release of aldosterone from the adrenal gland.[111-113]

Ang II has important renal and extrarenal effects. The two main direct renal effects of Ang II occur at low concentrations: 10-fold to 100-fold lower than what produces extrarenal effects.[114,115] The first and most important renal hemodynamic effect of Ang II is vasoconstriction of efferent arterioles of the glomerulus,[114] which increases the filtration fraction and helps to preserve the GFR[116]; the hemodynamic consequences of this effect also are responsible for enhanced proximal tubular reabsorption of sodium. The second renal effect of Ang II is on the proximal tubular epithelial cells, causing a direct increase in sodium reabsorption.[115] The extrarenal actions of Ang II include systemic vasoconstriction,[117] release of norepinephrine from sympathetic nerve terminals, central stimulation of thirst, and stimulation of aldosterone production by the adrenal cortex,[117,118] all of which help to maintain arterial blood pressure. Metabolism and growth in myocyte cells also are altered by circulating angiotensin, which results in cardiac hypertrophy with ventricular diastolic dysfunction and

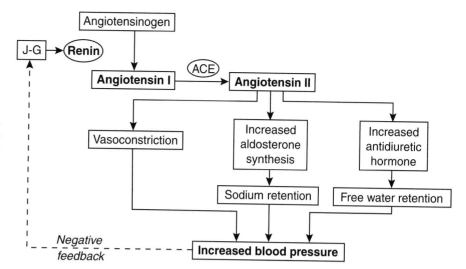

FIGURE 5-4 ■ Renin-angiotensin-aldosterone system (RAAS) and its effects on the hemodynamic stress response. Angiotensin II has multiple effects that all lead to increased blood pressure (via vasoconstriction, sodium retention, or free water retention). ACE, angiotensin-converting enzyme; J-G, juxtaglomerular cells. (From Jaski BE [ed]: *Circulation.* In: *Basics of Heart Failure: A Problem Solving Approach,* p. 31. New York, Kluwer Academic Publishers, 2000.)

impaired systolic contractile activity.[119] Ang II also has been shown to stimulate the expression of the ET-1 gene[120,121] and to induce ET-mediated proliferation[122] and hypertrophy[123] of cardiac and vascular myocytes.

Elevated systemic vascular resistance is the hallmark of decompensated CHF. It is attributed to activation of the vasoconstrictor neurohormones, including Ang II, catecholamines, AVP, and ET, in an effort to maintain circulatory hemostasis in the face of diminishing systolic function; this compensatory cascade further contributes, however, to deterioration of contractile capacity and decrease in cardiac output. The first attempt to treat heart failure with Ang II blockade[124] showed immediate hemodynamic amelioration of systemic and cardiac hemodynamics: decrease in peripheral vascular resistance, increase in cardiac output, and improved left ventricular work index with increased coronary blood flow. Improvements in symptoms, ejection fraction, and exercise capacity have been reported even with ACE inhibitors in patients with mild-to-moderate heart failure.[125-127]

There are two parallel systems that allow different ACE enzymes to produce Ang II. Renin of renal origin is the rate-limiting step in the production of circulating Ang II and has been used as a substitute for actual levels of circulating Ang II in most clinical studies.[128] More recently, the importance of circulating versus locally generated Ang II has been a matter of much debate.[129,130] Differentiated cells of various organs, including the cardiomyocytes and vascular smooth muscle cells, contain components of the RAS cascade and may possess the capability to generate Ang II. Locally produced Ang II may bind to adjacent cells or to receptors on the same cell that produces this extracellular messenger. Evidence suggests that intracardiac renin is constitutively produced by cardiomyocytes and other cardiac cells (fibroblasts) in culture,[131] and that renin mRNA is produced by cardiac tissues.[132] The renal renin and the circulating components of the RAS are produced in amounts greater by several

orders of magnitude (compared with amounts produced by extrarenal tissues) and are primarily responsible for the systemic hormonal and hemodynamic effects of Ang II. Locally generated Ang II seems to be the most important in the normal heart[133] and is activated by the failing heart (Fig. 5-5).[134]

It has been shown that there are three additional, biologically active **angiotensin metabolites** formed by further proteolytic cleavage of the octapeptide Ang II; these are Ang III(2-8), Ang IV(3-8), and Ang(1-7). Ang II is cleaved by aminopeptidase A to **Ang III(2-8)** and is metabolized further to Ang IV(3-8) by aminopeptidase M.[135,136] Ang III remains active and has an affinity for Ang II type 1 (AT$_1$) and AT$_2$ receptors similar to Ang II.[135] Injections of Ang III or aminopeptidase A into the

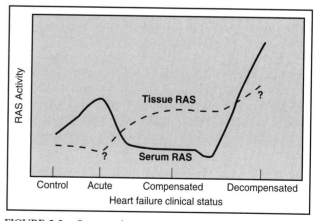

FIGURE 5-5 ■ **Serum and tissue renin-angiotensin systems (RAS) in heart failure.** The relative roles of the serum and tissue RAS in heart failure are delineated graphically. The tissue system has alternative pathways for the production of angiotensin II (e.g., chymases) that are independent of the converting enzyme; the system may not be entirely suppressible by converting enzyme inhibitors. Although tissue RAS is more activated in heart failure, circulating RAS may be diminished in activity during the compensated state of heart failure. During decompensated heart failure, serum and tissue RAS are activated. (From Dzau VJ: *Tissue renin-angiotensin system in myocardial hypertrophy and failure. Arch Intern Med* 1993;153:937-942.)

intracerebroventricular area led to increases in blood pressure, vasopressin release, and water consumption similar to those seen with Ang II injection.[137] Using an aminopeptidase A antiserum to block Ang II conversion, Song and coworkers[138] hypothesized that Ang III, rather than Ang II, is the main effector peptide in the brain. The hexapeptide, **Ang IV**, has been shown to bind preferentially to a novel Ang binding site (AT_4 receptor) in the rat kidney. Handa and colleagues[139] showed that the kidney AT_4 receptor system is localized to the proximal tubule and may have a potential role in the regulation of sodium transport by inhibiting the ouabain-sensitive component of sodium-potassium-ATP activity in the rat. The final Ang fragment, the heptapeptide **Ang(1-7)**, has been described by Ferrario and associates[140] as an additional biologically active product of the RAS. Ang(1-7) counterbalances vasoconstriction and the mitogenic, arrhythmogenic, and prothrombotic actions of Ang II. Ang(1-7) also induces a natriuresis and diuresis that oppose the water and sodium retention produced by Ang II.[141] Although a binding site with a high affinity for Ang(1-7) and Ang II has been shown in human cardiac fibroblasts,[142] no Ang(1-7) typical receptor has been cloned.[143]

Previously the peripheral and central effects of the RAS were believed to be mediated by a single Ang receptor. The actions of Ang II are now known to be mediated by highly specific and selective populations of **Ang II receptors AT_1 and AT_2.**[144,145] The characterization of Ang II receptor subtypes was made possible by the discovery and development of selective nonpeptide Ang II receptor antagonists, known as *losartan* (AT_1-selective) and *PD123319* (AT_2-selective).[146] Other compounds similar to losartan, such as candesartan, irbesartan, and valsartan, are used as antihypertensive and heart failure drugs because they block the AT_1 receptor and mediate the classic effects of the RAS related to blood pressure control and salt and water reabsorption.[143,146-148] The AT_1 receptors include at least two subsubtypes AT_{1A} and AT_{1B}, but these are likely present only in rats and mice, rather than humans.[149] The AT_2 receptor is characterized by its high affinity for PD123319, PD123177, and CGP42112 and low affinity for losartan and candesartan.[146] Ang II binds to the AT_2 receptor with the same affinity as to the AT_1 receptor.[144] The two Ang II receptor subtypes exert different effects that, in many cases, oppose one another. The AT_1 receptors exert regulatory effects, whereas the effects of the AT_2 receptor stimulation are generally counterregulatory. The function of the AT_2 receptors has been implicated in antiproliferation,[150,151] cell differentiation,[152,153] programmed cell death,[154] and neuronal regeneration.[155]

Blockade of the Ang II receptors is among the newest approaches to ameliorating neurohormonal mechanisms of heart failure related to the renin-angiotensin-aldosterone system. Ongoing large-scale studies are expected to define further the role of Ang II receptor blockers as possible first-line therapy in patients with established heart failure and in patients at risk for developing heart failure. Current studies yet to be published include (1) Candesartan in Heart Failure—Assessment of Reduction in Morbidity and Mortality (CHARM);[165] (2) a placebo-controlled trial involving 6500 patients with heart failure stratified by concurrent treatment with an ACE inhibitor; and (3) the Valsartan in Acute Myocardial Infarction Trial (VALIANT),[166] comparing valsartan alone and in combination with captopril in 14,500 post–myocardial infarction patients with heart failure or left ventricular systolic dysfunction. It seems that the Ang II receptor blockers may be the most useful in treating patients who cannot tolerate ACE inhibitor therapy or as a combination therapy with ACE inhibitors, providing a more complete blockade of the RAS.

The potential cardiac effects of **endothelin (ET)** and its isopeptides were shown some 2000 years before its discovery[167] in the death of Cleopatra. It is believed that the snake used by Cleopatra to kill herself was the Israeli burrowing snake, *Atractaspis engaddensis,* and that coronary vasospasm was the primary cause of death from the venom of this snake. One of the components of this snake venom is sarafotoxin 6c, whose human homologue is ET. In addition to the vasoconstrictor effects, ET exhibits other properties of a regulator of the hemodynamic defense reaction.

The ET system, similar to other vascular regulatory systems, consists of a parent peptide that undergoes enzymatic activation and exerts its biologic effects by modulating specific receptors. ET-1, originally termed by Yanagisawa and associates,[167] is a 12-amino acid peptide with three isopeptides (ET-2, ET-3, and ET-4) that are separate gene products with a high degree of homology. ET-1 is the predominant isoform in the cardiovascular system, which is generated through the cleavage of prepro ET-1 to big ET-1 and then to ET-1 by the action of ET-converting enzymes. ET-1 is found in endothelial cells and is released toward the vascular smooth muscle consistent with a paracrine role, but it also is produced by smooth muscle cells and cardiomyocytes.[167,168] ET-1 has vasoconstrictive and mitogenic effects, potentiates the effects of transforming growth factor-β and platelet-derived growth factor, and stimulates the production of growth factors such as vascular endothelial growth factor and fibroblast growth factor.[169-173] Endogenous inhibitors of ET-1 synthesis include NO, prostacyclin, ANP, and estrogen.[174-176]

ET-1 exerts its major effects through activation of two distinct G protein–coupled **ET receptors, ET_A and ET_B.** ET_A receptors are present in the medial smooth muscle layers of the blood vessels and in the atrial and ventricular myocardium,[177] whereas ET_B receptors are localized on endothelial cells, smooth muscle cells, and macrophages.[178] Under normal situations, the ET_B receptor mediates a balance between production and clearance so that circulating ET-1 is at a low level. ET_B receptor activation causes release of NO and prostacyclin and prevents apoptosis.[179]

Stimulation of the ET_A receptor on smooth muscle cells causes vasoconstriction, proliferation, and migration, whereas stimulation of the ET_B receptor on endothelial cells opposes these actions by stimulating NO and prostacyclin production.[180] In pathologic states, such as in CHF, up-regulation of the ET_B receptor on the vascular smooth muscle cell (and possibly down-regulation of the ET_B receptor on endothelial cells) results in a predominant effect of ET producing vasoconstriction, smooth muscle cell proliferation, and migration.[181]

Increased expression of ET-1 has been well described in experimental and human CHF and has been thought to potentiate the progression of this disorder through hemodynamic effects and vascular and cardiac remodeling.[182-183] Various studies have shown that an elevation of ET-1 in patients with heart failure correlates well with the severity of the disease, magnitude of alterations of cardiac hemodynamics, and survival.[183-186] Circulating levels of ET-1 are increased in the acute phase of myocardial infarction and CHF, and these levels correlate closely with indices of disease, such as capillary wedge pressure, left ventricular ejection fraction, cardiac index, New York Heart Association class, and 12-month survival.[187,188] The most important effects of the elevated levels of ET-1 in heart failure patients are mediated by the ET_A receptor, which causes vasoconstriction, increases myocardial contractility, stimulates aldosterone secretion, and inhibits sodium and water excretion by the kidneys.[189-194]

Early investigations of heart failure animal models[195,196] and early clinical studies[197-199] supported a potential beneficial effect of ET-1 blockade on heart failure. Intravenous and oral ET receptor antagonists have been studied for acute and chronic heart failure in larger clinical trials. These larger scale clinical trials have failed to support, however, the value of long-term ET receptor blockade in reducing symptoms or adverse clinical outcomes for patients with heart failure.[200-207] There was an initial worsening of heart failure symptoms in the Research on Endothelin Antagonism in Chronic Heart Failure (REACH-1)[206,207] and the Endothelin Antagonist Bosentan for Lowering Cardiac Events in Heart Failure (ENABLE)[204] trials, which was mediated in part through increased fluid and sodium retention. More recently, Schirgir and colleagues[208] showed that myocardial and plasma ET-1 is selectively activated before the RAS in the transition stage to overt heart failure in animals with ventricular dysfunction. They also reported that early initiation of ET_A receptor antagonism in experimental CHF has deleterious neurohormonal and renal actions, which include further activation of the RAS with continued sodium retention. It is yet to be determined what role ET receptor antagonists will have in the treatment of patients with chronic CHF.

Nitric oxide (NO) is a gaseous biologic mediator that accounts for the vasodilatory activity of endothelium-derived relaxing factor,[209,210] a non-PG vasorelaxant substance first described in the endothelial cells by Furchgott and Zawadzki.[211] NO is generated by the enzyme NO synthase (NOS) from guanidine nitrogen of L-arginine yielding citrulline[212,213] and plays an important role in controlling a variety of functions in the cardiovascular, immune, reproductive, and nervous systems.[214-216]

The three major NOS isoforms originally were identified in the brain: neuronal or epithelial NOS (nNOS),[217] macrophage or inducible NOS (iNOS),[218,219] and endothelial cell or endothelial NOS (eNOS).[220] All three isoforms (nNOS, iNOS, and eNOS) have been identified in the human heart.[221] nNOS and eNOS are considered to be constitutively expressed and activated by calcium entry into cells,[222,223] whereas iNOS is calcium independent, and its synthesis is induced in inflammatory and other cell types by stimuli such as endotoxin and proinflammatory cytokines.[224,225] In the heart, eNOS and iNOS have been involved in signaling pathways that modulate the contractile properties of cardiac myocytes. The eNOS isoform is expressed within the heart in the endothelium of the endocardium and coronary vasculature, in cardiac myocytes, and in cardiac conduction tissue; eNOS activity seems to be regulated by the contractile state of the heart.[226,227] Cytokines in cardiac myocytes, endocardial endothelium, infiltrating inflammatory cells, vascular smooth muscle, fibroblasts, and microvascular endothelium have been shown to induce iNOS expression.[227-229]

NO that is produced by any of these isoforms is a freely diffusible gas that is released from capillary endothelial cells under basal and agonist-stimulated conditions. When released from the endothelial cell, NO has paracrine actions on smooth muscle cells and cardiac myocytes (Fig. 5-6). In the cardiovascular system,

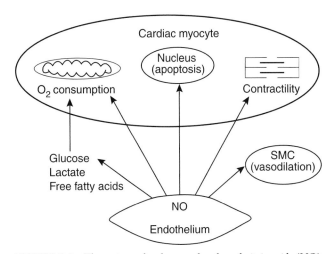

FIGURE 5-6 ■ **The actions of endogenously released nitric oxide (NO).** NO acts on capillary endothelial cells, vascular smooth muscle cells (SMC), and cardiac myocytes. NO can diffuse from the vascular endothelial cell and affect functions in the vascular SMC and myocardial cell. (From Bernstein RD, Recchia FA, Kaley G, et al: Nitric oxide and the heart. In Share L [ed]: *Hormones and the Heart in Health and Disease*, pp. 175-193. NJ, Humana Press, Totowa, New Jersey 1999, p. 175.)

NO not only causes vessel relaxation, but also inhibits platelet adhesion and aggregation, smooth muscle cell proliferation, monocyte adhesion, expression of different adhesion molecules, and ET-1 production.[231-235] Evidence has shown that the basal endogenous NO production supports myocardial contractility and heart rate, whereas the expression of iNOS has been reported to have cardiodepressive actions because of the negative inotropic effects of NO at high concentrations.[236]

The mechanisms involved in the effects of NO in heart failure are complex and not completely understood. Most experimental evidence in dogs,[237] rats,[238] and humans[239] suggests that there is a reduction in the ability of the blood vessels to synthesize NO in heart failure. More recent evidence suggests that in heart failure endothelium-derived NO could be inactivated by oxygen free radicals.[240] It is well known that heart failure is associated with an increase in circulating cytokines (see Chapter 3) and expression of iNOS in the myocardium. Animal and human models have suggested that the induction of iNOS, resulting in high NO production, exerts a negative inotropic effect in heart failure.[236] In contrast to the deleterious effects of iNOS, beneficial effects mainly attributable to NO derived from eNOS occur in clinical conditions such as ischemic or nonischemic cardiomyopathies, heart failure, and septic cardiodepression and other inflammatory diseases of the heart.[241-243]

Distinctions also must be made between acute and chronic conditions of the heart because each has different effects on NO production. In acute processes, such as acute ischemia, initial stages of heart failure, early sepsis, or myocarditis, NO production generally is increased by induction of eNOS and iNOS. During chronic diseases, such as end-stage cardiomyopathies, iNOS may be overexpressed and eNOS downregulated.[241] It is yet to be determined whether this imbalance between iNOS overexpression and eNOS down-regulation has a potential role in the pathogenesis of chronic heart failure.

Kinins are polypeptides that contain the sequence of the nonapeptide, bradykinin, in their structure. Bradykinin and related peptides, called *kallidins,* are vasoactive kinins that are liberated from the substrate kininogen by the action of kallikrein and are known to be involved in a wide range of biologic processes.[244] Similar to the RAS, the kallikrein-bradykinin system includes a circulating (plasma) and a tissue system. Kininogenases in the tissue system release kinins from low-molecular-weight kininogen and from high-molecular-weight kininogen in the plasma.[245] Kinins are rapidly hydrolyzed in various tissues and plasma by a group of enzymes called *kinases,* the most important of which are ACE and endopeptidase 24.11. Kinins release various endothelial products, including NO, endothelium-derived hyperpolarizing factor, eicosanoids, and tissue plasminogen activator. Work in experimental animals has suggested

that the kinins exert a protective effect in various pathologic states of the cardiovascular system and seem to provide cardioprotection against ischemia-reperfusion injury, ventricular hypertrophy, CHF, and thrombosis.[246-250]

The effects of kinins are mediated by stimulation of at least two known subtypes of **kinin receptors B_1 and B_2**, which have been characterized by the use of various bradykinin analogues.[244] B_1 and B_2 receptors cause the various physiologic actions of bradykinin through different second messengers and mediators (NO, PGs).[251] The B_1 receptor is the principal receptor for des-Arg[9] bradykinin and is mainly expressed under pathologic conditions, such as inflammation and sepsis.[252] Most of the cardiovascular actions of bradykinin are initiated by the binding of bradykinin or lys-bradykinin to the B_2 receptor. B_1 and B_2 receptors are transmembrane G protein–linked serpentine receptors and are divided into B_2A and B_2B subtypes.[253]

It has been shown that plasma levels of bradykinin are elevated in animal models of CHF.[254] Bradykinin, through the B_2 kinin receptor, has been shown to promote coronary and systemic vasodilation and improvement of left ventricular relaxation, filling, and contractile performance.[254] Evidence suggests that the actions of bradykinin may blunt the other neurohormonal systems in CHF, including the RAS, the adrenergic nervous system, and ET and vasopressin systems.[250,254] Kuoppala and associates[255] showed in human heart tissue from end-stage heart failure patients that the level of bradykinin type 2 receptor mRNA expression was significantly lower than that in normal hearts. The bradykinin type 2 receptor protein level was significantly reduced in end-stage heart failure patients and involved all myocardial cell types. This receptor downregulation of the type 2 bradykinin receptor also was associated with a decrease in eNOS in these heart failure patients. More recent investigational research involves the therapeutic potential of bradykinin B_2 receptor agonists in the treatment of cardiovascular disease. It is unknown, however, whether there is a sufficient safe therapeutic window between potential cardioprotective and proinflammatory effects after bradykinin B_2 receptor agonism.[255,256]

Adrenomedullin was discovered from human pheochromocytoma tissue by monitoring the elevating activity of intracellular cAMP in rat platelets in 1993.[257] Adrenomedullin acts as a circulating hormone and elicits multiple biologic activities in a paracrine and autocrine manner. Infusion of adrenomedullin has been shown to cause vasodilation, diuresis, and natriuresis in normal animals.[258,259] Plasma adrenomedullin levels are increased in patients with CHF[260,261] and have been shown to increase cardiac output and left ventricular contractility in vivo[262] and exert a direct inotropic effect in vitro.[263] Adrenomedullin inhibits ET secretion, stimulates NO synthesis, inhibits salt and water appetite, and inhibits the secretion of aldosterone and vasopressin.

Intravenous infusions of adrenomedullin in patients with CHF predominantly improved cardiac function by increasing cardiac index, lowering pulmonary capillary wedge pressure, and promoting natriuresis and diuresis.[264] Further clinical trials are needed to investigate the potential therapeutic benefit of adrenomedullin in CHF.

Prostaglandins (PGs) are one of several eicosanoids that are produced by the metabolism of arachidonic acid (5,8,11,14-cis-eicosatetraenoic acid), which is released from the breakdown of tissue phospholipids in response to neurohumoral stimulation after activation by cyclooxygenase. **PGI$_2$** is the major arachidonic acid metabolite generated in the human heart,[265,266] with the coronary vasculature being the primary site of cardiac synthesis.[267,268] Cardiac myocytes convert exogenous arachidonic acid to PGI$_2$, PGE$_2$, PGF$_2\alpha$, and PGD$_2$.[269] Stimulation of the adrenergic and cholinergic cardiac nerves or release of norepinephrine or acetylcholine stimulates the release of eicosanoids.[270-272] PGI$_2$ is the principal eicosanoid released in response to either adrenergic or cholinergic stimuli, although small amounts of other products also are detected.[272,273] Several humoral agents secreted in response to the hemodynamic defense reaction, including Ang II, vasopressin, ET, and bradykinin, stimulate PG synthesis in the intact heart, cardiac myocytes, or fibroblasts.[273-275]

Cardiac Stimulation

The third major component of the hemodynamic defense reaction is stimulation of the heart through the sympathetic adrenergic branch of the autonomic nervous system. Sympathetic activation of the heart causes an increase in heart rate and inotropy via the release of norepinephrine acting primarily on β$_1$-adrenoceptors (β$_1$-ARs). The increase in inotropy by sympathetic activation may not be sufficient, however, to restore normal inotropy, particularly in ventricles having systolic dysfunction. Inotropic responses also are blunted because of down-regulation of β$_1$-ARs. Sympathetic activation has other important effects that can be deleterious, including ventricular hypertrophy, enhanced arrhythmogenesis, and molecular and biochemical changes that lead to further dysfunction over time. Although sympathetic activation may play some compensatory role in the failing heart, there is considerable evidence that it accompanies[276-279] and, more importantly, exacerbates[280,281] the progression of chronic heart failure. For this reason, the use of β-blockers in some forms of heart failure has been gaining in popularity because of their proven efficacy.

Activation of sympathetic efferent nerves to the heart increases heart rate (positive chronotropy), contractility (positive inotropy), and conduction velocity (positive dromotropy). Parasympathetic effects are opposite: Parasympathetic effects on inotropy are weak in the ventricle, but relatively strong in the atria. Physiologically, whenever the body activates the sympathetic system, it down-regulates parasympathetic activity, and vice versa,

so that the activities of these two branches of the autonomic nervous system respond reciprocally. The overall effect of sympathetic activation is to increase cardiac output, systemic vascular resistance (arteries and veins), and arterial blood pressure. Enhanced sympathetic activity is particularly important during exercise, emotional stress, and hemorrhagic shock.

Reflex stimulation of the sympathetic nervous system may result from baroreceptor perception of a change in arterial pressure, pulse pressure, stroke volume, arterial compliance, or cardiac filling.[282] The resultant stimulation of sympathetic outflow leads to the neural release of norepinephrine and epinephrine. In hypovolemic states, such as hemorrhage or during exercise, this sympathetic increase causes several physiologic effects, as follows: (1) arterial vasoconstriction to maintain blood pressure in the face of reduced cardiac output, (2) venoconstriction to shift the depleted vascular volume centrally in an effort to maintain cardiac filling, (3) stimulation of the heart rate and contractility to maintain cardiac output despite reduced filling, and (4) renal vasoconstriction to decrease salt and water excretion and to expand the intravascular volume. In chronic CHF, stimulation of the sympathetic nervous system may lead to cardiovascular effects with deleterious consequences, as follows: (1) The increase in vascular resistance may depress cardiac output further, (2) the increase in cardiac filling may aggravate systemic and pulmonary congestion, (3) cardiac stimulation may not lead to improved cardiac performance because of intrinsic myocardial or coronary disease, and (4) the renal vasoconstriction may limit urine output despite sodium and fluid overload.[283]

Sympathetic stimulation increases the release of **catecholamines**, including epinephrine from the adrenal medulla and norepinephrine from sympathetic nerve endings on the heart and blood vessels. The sympathetic nervous system gives rise to nerve terminals that supply the entire cardiovascular system, including arteries, veins, cardiac chambers, conduction system, and myocardium. Stored in the nerve terminals are large concentrations of the neurotransmitter norepinephrine, which is released after stimulation of these nerve terminals.[284] When released, norepinephrine can bind to various receptor subtypes (adrenoceptors) that determine the norepinephrine regulatory effects. An adrenergic receptor (or adrenoceptor) is a cell membrane protein that is the target of catecholamines.

The term *adrenoceptor* first was introduced by Ahlquist to explain the different physiologic effects of catecholamines.[285] In 1948, Ahlquist[286] further differentiated α-receptors and β-receptors because of their response to epinephrine. In vascular smooth muscle, norepinephrine results in vasoconstriction, which leads to increased resistance and arterial blood pressure through the α-adrenoceptors (α-ARs). The vasodilatory effect, positive chronotropic effect, and increased inotropic effect are the results of epinephrine acting through β-ARs. Molecular biologic studies revealed further subtypes of adrenergic receptors,[287] such as the α_{1A}, α_{1B}, and α_{1D}[288,289] types of the α_1 receptors or the α_{2A}, α_{2B}, and α_{2C}[290-292] types of the α_2 receptor.

The α_1-ARs are important mediators of sympathetic nervous system responses, particularly the responses involved in cardiovascular homeostasis, such as arteriolar smooth muscle constriction and cardiac contraction.[293,294] α_1-ARs exist on mammalian myocardial cells,[295,296] and their activation produces a positive inotropic response.[296,297] α_1-ARs also have been shown to play a role in the pathogenesis of cardiac hypertrophy and protein synthesis,[298-300] in ischemia-induced cardiac arrhythmias, and in ischemic preconditioning.[293,301] Similar to other adrenergic receptors, they are members of the G protein–coupled receptor superfamily of membrane proteins that mediate the actions of the endogenous catecholamines, epinephrine and norepinephrine. Data collected from functional,[302,303] radioligand,[304] and biochemical studies[305] of α_1-ARs have shown that they are a heterogeneous group of distinct but related proteins. This idea has been confirmed with the molecular cloning of three distinct α_1-receptor subtypes, which are designated α_{1A}, α_{1B}, and α_{1D}.[306,307]

In the human heart, the presence of α_1-ARs has been shown in mRNA, protein, and functional studies. All studies have agreed that α_{1A}-AR is the most abundant in the human heart, but there is debate as to whether α_{1B}-AR and α_{1D}-AR exist in the human heart.[308-311] α_1-ARs have been shown in the human right ventricle and left ventricle[312-314]; however, their density is far less than that of β-adrenoceptors.[315] Stimulation of α_1-ARs causes positive inotropic effects in the isolated human heart, although the mechanism of the positive inotropic effect induced by α_1-AR stimulation is still a matter of debate.[316,317]

A reduction in β-ARs is well documented in heart failure,[318] but a similar reduction in α_1-ARs has not been reported in most studies[312-314]; human heart failure seems to be associated with a slightly increased cardiac α_1-AR number.[314,319-321] The lack of α_1-AR down-regulation in heart failure has led some to hypothesize that in severe heart failure, α_1-ARs might be an inotropic back-up system in the face of diminishing β-adrenergic responsiveness.[322] This hypothesis is not supported, however, by the functional data showing that positive inotropic effects of α_1-AR stimulation in vitro are unchanged[312] or even reduced in heart failure,[320] even though receptor number was increased.

Three human α2AR subtypes exist: α_{2A}, α_{2B}, and α_{2C}.[323] Several studies have reported the presence of α_2-AR subtypes in the human heart at the mRNA level, but at the protein level, data have failed to show α_2-ARs.[322] Functional studies on human cardiac α_2-ARs have focused on presynaptic inhibition of norepinephrine release. Several groups have shown the existence of presynaptic α_2-ARs mediating inhibition of norepinephrine

release in human right atrium.[324-326] The subtype of α_2-ARs that functions as the prejunctional inhibitory receptor is still a matter of debate; one author has subclassified the receptor as the α_{2C}-AR,[325] and a second author has shown in a variety of species that the presynaptic α_2-AR is of the α_{2A}-AR or the α_{2D}-AR subtype.[327] The α_2-ARs affect the cardiovascular system through central counterregulatory mechanisms that inhibit sympathetic outflow. Studies of intracoronary infusion of the α-AR antagonist phentolamine did not modify catecholamine spillover in subjects with normal left ventricular function, but enhanced it in patients with CHF.[328] These data suggest that prejunctional α_2-ARs play a functional norepinephrine release–inhibiting role in the human heart that becomes evident under conditions of enhanced sympathetic activity.

There are three different β-AR subtypes that have been cloned and identified pharmacologically: β_1-ARs, β_2-ARs, and β_3-ARs.[323,329] In the human heart, the existence of β_1-ARs and β_2-ARs has been shown at the mRNA level through RNase protection assays and reverse transcription polymerase chain reaction,[330-332] at the protein level with radioligand binding, and in functional studies in vitro and in vivo.[318,330] The β_3-receptors primarily regulate gastrointestinal motility and lipolysis, but also have a negative inotropic effect and do not interact with β_1-receptor or β_2-receptor blockers.[333] β_1-ARs and β_2-ARs in the human heart couple to G_s to activate adenylyl cyclase, and stimulation of both receptor subtypes increases the intracellular level of cAMP and enhances contraction. In human atria and ventricular myocardium, β_1-AR and β_2-AR stimulation enhances myocardial relaxation.[334] In the nonfailing heart, the β_1-AR is the primary subtype, with the β_1-AR-to-β_2-AR ratio about 60% to 70%:30% to 40% in the atria and about 70% to 80%:20% to 30% in the ventricles.[318] In contrast, in the failing heart, β_1-ARs are markedly reduced in number and density as a consequence of the process of down-regulation,[335-337] but the number and density of β_2-ARs are unchanged. As a result, the proportion of β_2-ARs increases, and their function is altered because these receptors become partially uncoupled from adenylyl cyclase,[335] possibly related to the change in concentration of G proteins that occurs in heart failure.[338-340]

It has been known since the 1960s that heart failure is frequently associated with functional alterations in the sympathetic nervous system. Chidsey and coworkers[277] showed in 1964 that the daily urinary excretion of norepinephrine is increased in most patients with heart failure, and that the presence of heart disease without failure is not associated with such an increase. Previously, Chidsey and coworkers[276] had observed that augmented plasma norepinephrine levels were present during exercise in heart failure patients, findings also consistent with increased sympathetic activity. Initially, these findings were thought to be simply a marker of heart failure, with considerably higher levels found in patients with severe symptoms than in patients with mild symptoms.[341-343] A seminal work by Cohn and associates showed,[344] however, a striking correlation between high plasma norepinephrine concentration and worse prognosis in chronic heart failure patients. To strengthen these findings, a study showed reduced norepinephrine in atrial tissue of patients with heart failure, averaging 0.49 mg/g compared with 1.77 mg/g in cardiac patients without failure. A reduction of norepinephrine also was observed in the left ventricle, and the concentrations in the ventricle were found to be lowest in the patients with the lowest atrial norepinephrine concentrations. Increased urinary excretion of norpeinephrine was observed in these same patients with markedly depressed cardiac concentrations of the neurotransmitter substance.[277]

Mechanisms of cardiac norepinephrine depletion have been studied extensively and include the possibility of abnormalities in the synthesis, uptake, binding, storage, and release of norepinephrine. The defect in neuronal binding or reuptake of norepinephrine was determined by measurement of the norepinephrine retained in the hearts and kidneys after infusion of norepinephrine in a group of normal guinea pigs and a group with CHF.[345] In the normal animals, the ventricular concentrations of norepinephrine increased with the infusions, then decreased as the infusion was completed. In contrast, the increase in ventricular concentrations of norepinephrine in the heart failure animals was minimal, whereas the renal norepinephrine in this group increased in a manner similar to that observed in the normal group. Although there has been some evidence of impairment of norepinephrine uptake in heart failure, the major abnormality seems to be the increased release of norepinephrine into the blood and urine of patients with heart failure.[346-349] Applications of newer methods, such as sympathetic nerve recordings[350,351] and the isotope dilution method[346,352] for determining organ-specific rates of norepinephrine spillover into plasma, have advanced even further the understanding of mechanisms responsible for sympathetic activation and its adverse consequences in chronic heart failure.

CURRENT STATUS AND FUTURE TRENDS

Chronic CHF is a complex multisystem disorder that is characterized by abnormalities of cardiac, skeletal muscle, and renal function; stimulation of the sympathetic nervous system; and numerous hormonal and neuroendocrine changes. Impairment in left ventricular function leads to a decline in cardiac output, peripheral hypoperfusion, and a decline in arterial blood pressure. In an effort to preserve circulatory homeostasis and maintain blood pressure, numerous compensatory mechanisms are set in motion that increase afterload, preload, and heart rate. Activation of the sympathetic nervous system is the earliest of these changes that takes place, in an effort to maintain cardiac output with an increase in heart rate, increased myocardial contractility, and peripheral vasoconstriction (increased catecholamines). Sustained sympathetic stimulation, although beneficial in the acute phase of heart failure, supports excessive vasoconstriction with increased ventricular afterload and, by stimulating the RAS, promoting fluid retention, leading to an increased ventricular preload. Under chronic conditions, this stimulation leads to further deterioration of ventricular function, activates the neuroendocrine systems, and increases systemic vascular resistance even further. The progressive spiral of chronic heart failure has now begun.

Activation of the RAS leads to increased concentrations of renin, plasma Ang II, and aldosterone. These increased concentrations are associated with further increases in peripheral vascular resistance and renal glomerular filtration pressure through vasoconstrictor mechanisms, leading to worsening fluid and sodium retention. Angiotensin also contributes to cardiac hypertrophy, further worsening ventricular diastolic dysfunction and systolic contractility. Finally, angiotensin stimulates the release of norepinephrine from sympathetic nerve terminals, inhibits vagal tone, and promotes the release of aldosterone. Aldosterone and AVP secretion further contribute to the retention of sodium and water, the excretion of potassium, and vasoconstriction.

In response to the above-mentioned vasoconstrictor, fluid-retaining, and sodium-retaining factors, numerous mediators counteract these changes by stimulating vasodilation, volume, and sodium-eliminating factors in chronic heart failure. These mediators include ANPs, PGs, bradykinins, and plasma dopamine. All of these mechanisms act together to lower systemic vascular resistance and to increase sodium excretion. Nonetheless, despite all attempts at vasodilation and natriuresis by these mediators, these agents are overwhelmed in the setting of chronic heart failure by the sodium retention and vasoconstriction caused by the sympathetic nervous system, activation of the RAS, and secretion of AVP.

The response the body mounts to chronic heart failure is not specific, but rather is a choreographed neuroendocrine response for which it has been programmed under circumstances that threaten life, such as hypovolemia, hemorrhage, and exercise. Although the neuroendocrine response may be crucial to maintaining arterial blood pressure in these acute circumstances, chronic heart failure is a lifelong process. The body abnormally intensifies the neuroendocrine responses, and a series of vicious cycles that further worsen the damaged heart are put in motion. A better understanding of the neurohumoral activation that occurs with chronic heart failure and its interaction with hemodynamic factors is essential for optimizing pharmacologic therapy, minimizing morbidity, and preventing mortality in these patients.[353-355]

Key Concepts

■ There are three major components to the hemodynamic defense response in any patient with heart failure: salt and fluid retention, vasoconstriction, and cardiac stimulation.

■ The predominant feature involved in the electrolyte and water imbalances in heart failure is renal conservation of sodium—a process mediated by substances such as aldosterone, Ang II, and norepinephrine and counterregulated by signaling molecules such as PGs and natriuretic peptides.

■ Numerous receptors that monitor stretch are located in various sites in the arterial system, great veins, and cardiac chambers. In low-pressure chambers, stretch of these receptors reflects primarily volume changes, whereas in the high-pressure arterial system, stretch of these receptors monitors blood pressure.

■ Constriction of the efferent arterioles of the glomeruli is the most important of the hemodynamic abnormalities in the kidneys of patients with CHF. Vasoconstriction of these efferent arterioles increases GFR by increasing intraglomerular pressure, but at the same time reduces total renal blood flow. In the kidney, sympathetic stimulation and catecholamine release increase sodium reabsorption by renal hemodynamic and tubular effects similar to Ang II.

■ Aldosterone, Ang II, and norepinephrine all increase tubular reabsorption of sodium, and AVP acts on the collecting ducts to promote water reabsorption.

■ In heart failure, the most important stimulus for aldosterone release is Ang II, which is released in response to activation of the RAS as a result of decreased renal blood flow.

■ Vasopressin contributes to cardiovascular regulation by causing vasoconstriction and by stimulating renal water absorption through V_1 and V_2 receptors.

■ Natriuretic peptides are a group of naturally occurring substances that act in the body to oppose the activity of the RAS, aldosterone, ET, and vasopressin.

■ There are three neurohumoral vasoconstrictor systems that are known to exist and may be activated in patients with heart failure: the sympathetic nervous system, the RAS, and the AVP system.

■ Many vasoconstrictors are secreted by the sympathetic nervous system in heart failure, the principal regulator being norepinephrine, which binds to α_1-adrenergic receptors on arteriolar smooth muscle, causing vasoconstriction. Other vasoconstrictors include Ang II, ET, and AVP. Similar to the neurohumoral response in the kidneys, there also are counterregulatory mediators that promote vasodilation; these include natriuretic peptides, bradykinin, NO, dopamine, and some PGs (PGI_2 and PGE_2).

■ The first and most important renal hemodynamic effect of Ang II is vasoconstriction of efferent arterioles of the glomerulus, which increases the filtration fraction and helps to preserve the GFR; the hemodynamic consequences of this effect also are responsible for enhanced proximal tubular reabsorption of sodium. The second renal effect of Ang II is on the proximal tubular epithelial cells, causing a direct increase in sodium reabsorption. The extrarenal actions of Ang II include systemic vasoconstriction, release of norepinephrine from sympathetic nerve terminals, central stimulation of thirst, and stimulation of aldosterone production by the adrenal cortex, all of which help to maintain arterial blood pressure.

■ Differentiated cells of various organs, including the cardiomyocytes and vascular smooth muscle cells, contain components of the RAS cascade and may possess the capability to generate Ang II. Locally produced Ang II may bind to adjacent cells or to receptors on the same cell that produces this extracellular messenger.

■ Stimulation of the ET_A receptor on smooth muscle cells causes vasoconstriction, proliferation, and migration, whereas stimulation of the ET_B receptor on endothelial cells opposes these actions by stimulating NO and prostacyclin production. In pathologic states, such as in CHF, up-regulation of the ET_B receptor on the vascular smooth muscle cell (and possibly down-regulation of the ET_B receptor on endothelial cells) results in a predominant effect of ET producing vasoconstriction, smooth muscle cell proliferation, and migration.

■ In the cardiovascular system, NO not only causes vessel relaxation, but also inhibits platelet adhesion and aggregation, smooth muscle cell proliferation, monocyte adhesion, expression of different adhesion molecules, and ET-1 production.

■ The kinins exert a protective effect in various pathologic states of the cardiovascular system and seem to provide cardioprotection against ischemia-reperfusion injury, ventricular hypertrophy, CHF, and thrombosis.

■ In chronic CHF, stimulation of the sympathetic nervous system may lead to cardiovascular effects with deleterious consequences, as follows: (1) The increase in vascular resistance may depress cardiac output further, (2) the increase in cardiac filling may aggravate systemic and pulmonary congestion, (3) cardiac stimulation may not lead to improved cardiac performance because of intrinsic myocardial or coronary disease, and (4) the renal vasoconstriction may limit urine output despite sodium and fluid overload.

REFERENCES

1. Braunwald E: The autonomic nervous system in heart failure. In Braunwald E, Selwyn A (eds): The Myocardium: Failure and Infarction. New York, HP Publishing, 1974, pp 59-69.
2. Katz AM: Heart failure. In Fozzard HA, Haber E, Jennings RB, et al (eds): The Heart and Cardiovascular System, 2nd ed. New York, Raven Press, 1991, pp 333-353.

3. Swedberg K, Hjalmarson A, Waagstein F, et al: Prolongation of survival in congestive cardiomyopathy by β-receptor blockade. Lancet 1979;2:1374-1376.

4. Tan LB, Jakil JE, Janicki JS, et al: Cardiotoxic effects of angiotensin II. J Am Coll Cardiol 1989;13(Suppl):2A.

5. Katz AM (ed): The hemodynamic defense reaction. In: Heart Failure: Pathophysiology, Molecular Biology, and Clinical Management. Philadelphia, Lippincott Williams & Wilkins, 2000, pp 109-152.

6. Packer M: The neurohormonal hypothesis: A theory to explain the mechanism of disease progression in heart failure. J Am Coll Cardiol 1992;20:248-254.

7. Hilton SM, Spyer KM: Central nervous regulation of vascular resistance. Ann Rev Physiol 1980;42:399-411.

8. Harris P: Evolution and the cardiac patient. Cardiovasc Res 1983;17:313.

9. Harris P: Congestive cardiac failure: Central role of the arterial blood pressure. Br Heart J 1987;58:190-203.

10. Harris P: Role of arterial pressure in the oedema of heart disease. Lancet 1988;1:1036-1038.

11. Francis GS, Goldsmith SR, Ziesche S, et al: Relative attenuation of sympathetic drive during exercise in patients with congestive heart failure. J Am Coll Cardiol 1985;5:832.

12. Ferrari R, Ceconi C, Rodella A, et al: Temporal relations of the endocrine response to exercise. Cardioscience 1991;2:131-139.

13. Francis GS: Hemodynamic and neurohumoral responses to dynamic exercise: Normal subjects versus patients with heart disease. Circulation 1987;76(Suppl VI):VI-11.

14. Inder SA: Pathogenesis of salt and water retention in the congestive heart failure syndrome. In Poole-Wilson PA, Colucci WS, Massie BM, et al (eds): Heart Failure. New York, Churchill Livingstone, 1997, pp 155-171.

15. Ferrari R, Ceconi C, Curello CS: Activation of the neuroendocrine response in heart failure: Adaptive or maladaptive process? Cardiovasc Drugs Ther 1996;10:623-629.

16. Starling EH: On the absorption of fluids from the connective tissue spaced. J Physiol (Lond) 1896;19:312-326.

17. Wollheim E: Die zirkulierende blutmenge und ihre bedeutung fur kompensation und dekompensation des kreislaufs. Z Klin Med 1931;116:269-397.

18. Starr I, Rawson AJ: Role of the "static blood pressure" in abnormal increments of venous pressure, especially in heart failure: I. Theoretical studies on an improved circulation schema whose pump obeys Starling's law of the heart. Am J Med Sci 1940;199:27-39.

19. Starr I: Role of the "static blood pressure" in abnormal increments of venous pressure, especially in heart failure: II. Clinical and experimental studies. Am J Med Sci 1940;199:40-55.

20. Warren JV, Stead EA Jr: Fluid dynamics in chronic congestive failure. Arch Intern Med 1944;73:138-147.

21. Merrill AJ: Edema and decreased renal blood flow in patients with chronic congestive heart failure: Evidence of "forward failure" as the primary cause of edema. J Clin Invest 1946;6:357-367.

22. Merrill AJ: Mechanism of salt and water retention in heart failure. Am J Med 1949;6:357-367.

23. Mason DT, Spann JF, Zelis R: Alterations of hemodynamics and myocardial mechanics in patients with congestive heart failure: Pathophysiologic mechanisms and assessment of cardiac function and ventricular contractility. Prog Cardiovasc Dis 1970;12:507-557.

24. Andreoli TE: Pathogenesis of renal sodium retention in congestive heart failure. Miner Electrolyte Metab 1999;25:11-20.

25. Davis JO: Mechanisms of salt and water retention in cardiac failure. In Braunwald E, Selwyn A (eds): The Myocardium: Failure and Infarction. New York, HP Publishing, 1974, pp 80-89.

26. Tonkon MJ, Rosen SM, Mason DT: Renal function and edema formation in congestive heart failure. In Mason DT (ed): Congestive Heart Failure: Mechanisms, Evaluation and Treatment. New York, Dun-Donnelley Publishing, 1976, pp 169-177.

27. Starling EH: Physiologic factors involved in the causation of dropsy. Lancet 1896;1:1407-1410.

28. Peters JP: Body Water. Springfield, Ill, Thomas, 1935.

29. Stead EA, Ebert RV: Shock syndrome produced by failure of the heart. Arch Intern Med 1942;69:75-89.

30. Mokotoff R, Ross G, Leiter L: Renal plasma flow and sodium reabsorption in congestive heart failure. J Clin Invest 1948;27:1-9.

31. Merrill AJ, Cargell WH: The effect of exercise on renal plasma flow and filtration rate of normal and cardiac subjects. J Clin Invest 1948;27:272-277.

32. Heller BI, Jacobson WE: Renal hemodynamics in heart disease. Am Heart J 1950;39:188-204.

33. Vander AJ, Marvin RL, Wilde WS, et al: Re-examination of salt and water retention in congestive heart failure. Am J Med 1958;25:497-502.

34. Kilcoyne MM, Schmidt DH, Cannon PJ: Intrarenal blood flow in congestive heart failure. Circulation 1973;47:786-797.

35. Ichikawa I, Pfeffer JM, Pfeffer MA: Role of angiotensin II in the altered renal function of congestive heart failure. Circ Res 1984;55:669-675.

36. McCance RA: Experimental sodium chloride deficiency in man. Proc R Soc Lond B 1936;119:245.

37. Luft FC, Rankin LI, Block R, et al: Cardiovascular and humoral responses to extremes of sodium intake in normal black and white men. Circulation 1979;60:697-706.

38. Sheperd JT: Intrathoracic baroreflexes. Mayo Clin Proc 1973;48:426-437.

39. Myers BD, Peterson C, Molina C, et al: Role of cardiac atria in the human renal response to changing plasma volume. Am J Physiol 1988;254:F562-F573.

40. Linden RJ, Kappagoda CT: Atrial receptors. In: Monographs of the Physiological Society No. 39. Cambridge, Cambridge University Press, 1982.

41. De Torrente A, Robertson G, McDonald KM, et al: Mechanism of diuretic response to increased left atrial pressure in the anesthetized dog. Kidney Int 1975;8:355-361.

42. Quail AW, Woods RL, Korner PI: Cardiac and arterial baroreceptor influences in release of vasopressin and renin during hemorrhage. Am J Physiol 1987;252:H1120-H1126.

43. de Bold AJ: Heart atrial granularity: Effects of changes in water-electrolyte balance. Proc Soc Exp Biol Med 1979;161:508-511.

44. de Bold AJ, Borenstein HB, Veress AT, et al: A rapid and potent natriuretic response to intravenous injection of atrial myocardial extract in rats. Life Sci 1981;28:89-94.

45. Schiebinger RJ, Linden J: The influence of resting tension on immunoreactive atrial natriuretic petide secretion by rat atria superfused in vitro. Circ Res 1986;59:105-109.

46. Agnoletti G, Rodella A, Ferrari R, et al: Release of atrial natriuretic peptide-like immunoreactive material during stretching of the rat atrium. J Mol Cell Cardiol 1987;19:217-222.

47. Myers ED, Dean WM, Brenner DM: Effects of norepinephrine and angiotensin II on the determinants of glomerular ultrafiltration and proximal tubule fluid reabsorption in the rat. Circ Res 1975;37:101-110.

48. DiBona GF: The functions of the renal nerves. Rev Physiol Biochem Pharmacol 1982;94:75-94.

49. Bello-Reuss E: Effect of catecholamines on fluid reabsorption by the isolated proximal convoluted tubule. Am J Physiol 1980;238:F347-F352.

50. Packer M: Neurohumoral interactions and adaptations in congestive heart failure. Circulation 1988;77:721-730.

51. Broqvist M, Dahlstrom U, Karlberg BE, et al: Neuroendocrine response in acute heart failure and the influence of treatment. Eur Heart J 1989;10:1075-1083.

52. Francis GS: Neuroendocrine activity in congestive heart failure. Am J Cardiol 1990;66:33D-39D.

53. Smith AGE: Spironolactone in the long-term management of patients with congestive heart failure. Curr Med Res Opin 1980;7:131-136.

54. Muller J: Spironolactone in the management of congestive heart failure: A review. Clin Ther 1986;9:63-76.

55. Sun Y, Ramires FJA, Wever KT: Fibrosis of atria and great vessels in response to angiotensin II or aldosterone infusion. Cardiovasc Res 1997;35:138-147.

56. Lijnen P, Petrov V: Antagonism of the renin-angiotensin-aldosterone system and collagen metabolism in cardiac fibroblasts. Methods Find Exp Clin Pharmacol 1999;21:215-227.

57. Delcayre C, Silvestre JS: Aldosterone and the heart: Towards a physiologic function? Cardiovasc Res 1999;43:7-12.

58. Schunkert H, Hense HW, Muscholl M, et al: Association between circulating components of the renin-angiotensin-aldosterone system and left ventricular mass. Heart 1997;77:24-31.

59. Tsutamoto T, Wada A, Maeda K, et al: Effect of spironolactone on plasma brain naturetic peptide and left ventricular remodeling in patients with congestive heart failure. J Am Coll Cardiol 2001;37: 1228-1233.

60. Barr CS, Lang CC, Hanson J, et al: Effects of adding spironolactone to an angiotensin-converting enzyme inhibitor in chronic congestive heart failure secondary to coronary artery disease. Am J Cardiol 1995;76:1259-1265.

61. Pitt B: "Escape" of aldosterone production in patients with left ventricular dysfunction treated with an angiotensin converting enzyme inhibitor: Implications for therapy. Cardiovasc Drugs Ther 1995;9:145-149.

62. Struthers AD: Why does spironolactone improve mortality over and above an ACE inhibitor in chronic congestive heart failure? Br J Clin Pharmacol 1999;47:479-482.

63. Struthers A: Aldosterone and artery compliance in heart failure. Eur Heart J 1998;19:1273.

64. Pitt B, Zannad F, Remme WJ, et al: Randomized Aldactone Evaluation Study Investigators: The effect of spironolactone on morbidity and mortality in patients with severe heart failure. N Engl J Med 1999;341:709-717.

65. Pitt B, Remme W, Zannad F, et al: Eplerenone, a selective aldosterone blocker, in patients with left ventricular dysfunction after myocardial infarction. N Engl J Med 2003;348:1309-1321.

66. Cohn JN, Anand IS, Latini R, et al: Sustained reduction of aldosterone in response to the angiotensin receptor blocker valsartan in patients with chronic heart failure: Results from the Valsartan Heart Failure Trial. Circulation 2003;108:1306-1309.

67. Walker BR, Childs ME, Adams EM: Direct cardiac effects of vasopressin: Role of V_1- and V_2-vasopressinergic receptors. Am J Physiol 1988;255:H261-H265.

68. Schoemaker IE, Meulemans AL, Andries LJ, et al: Role of endocardial endothelium in positive inotropic action of vasopressin. Am J Physiol 1990;259:H1148-H1151.

69. Cheng CP, Igarashi Y, Klopfenstein HS, et al: Effect of vasopressin on left ventricular performance. Am J Physiol 1993;264:H53-H60.

70. Mitchell RH, Kirk CJ, Billah MM: Hormonal stimulation of phosphatidylinositol breakdown with particular reference to the hepatic effects of vasopressin. Biochem Soc Trans 1979;7:861-865.

71. Penit J, Faure M, Jard S: Vasopressin and angiotensin II receptors in rat aortic smooth muscle cells in culture. Am J Physiol 1983;244: E72-E82.

72. Thibonnier M, Auzan C, Madhun Z, et al: Molecular cloning, sequencing and functional expression of a cDNA encoding the human V_{1A} vasopressor receptor. J Biol Chem 1994;269:3304-3310.

73. Nielson S, Kwon TH, Christensen BM, et al: Physiology and pathophysiology of renal aquaporins. J Am Soc Nephrol 1999;10:647-663.

74. Guyton AC: The kidneys and body fluids. In Guyton AC, Hall JE (eds): Textbook of Medical Physiology, 10th ed. Philadelphia, WB Saunders, 1996, pp 308-372.

75. Francis GS, Goldsmith SR, Levine TB, et al: The neurohumoral axis in congestive heart failure. Ann Intern Med 1984;101:370-377.

76. Schrier RW: Pathogenesis of sodium and water retention in high-output and low-output cardiac failure, nephrotic syndrome, cirrhosis, and pregnancy. N Engl J Med 1988;319:1127-1134.

77. Share L: Interrelations between angiotensin and the renin-angiotensin system. Fed Proc 1979;38:2267-2271.

78. Goldsmith SR, Francis GS, Cowley AW, et al: Increased plasma arginine vasopressin levels in patients with congestive heart failure. J Am Coll Cardiol 1983;1:1385-1390.

79. Szatalowicz VL, Arnold PE, Chaimovitz C, et al: Radioimmunoassay of plasma arginine vasopressin levels in hyponatremic patients with congestive heart failure. N Engl J Med 1981;305:263-266.

80. Francis GS, Benedict C, Johnstone DE, et al: Comparison of neuroendocrine activation on patients with and without congestive heart failure: A substudy of the Studies of Left Ventricular Dysfunction (SOLVD). Circulation 1990;82:1724-1729.

81. Goldsmith SR, Francis GS, Cowley AW, et al: Hemodynamics effects of infused arginine vasopressin in congestive heart failure. J Am Coll Cardiol 1986;8:779-783.

82. Tahara A, Tomura Y, Wada K, et al: Effect of YM087, a potent nonpeptide vasopressin antagonist, on vasopressin-induced protein synthesis in neonatal rat cardiomyocyte. Cardiovasc Res 1986;38:198-205.

83. Nakamura Y, Haneda T, Osaki J, et al: Hypertrophic growth of cultured neonatal rat heart cells mediated by vasopressin V1a receptor. Eur J Pharmacol 2000;391:39-48.

84. Fukuzawa J, Haneda T, Kikuchi K: Arginine vasopressin increases the rate of protein synthesis in isolated perfused adult rat heart via the V1 receptor. Mol Cell Biochem 1999;195: 93-98.

85. Bird E, Sasseville V, Dorso C, et al: Significant reduction in cardiac fibrosis and hypertrophy in spontaneously hypertensive rats (SHR) treated with a V1a receptor antagonist [abstract]. Circulation 2001;104(2 Suppl):186.

86. Gheorghiade M, Niazi I, Ouyang J, et al: Vasopressin V2-receptor blockade with Tolvaptan in patients with chronic heart failure: Results from a double-blind, randomized trial. Circulation 2003;107:2690-2696.

87. Cho Y, Somer BG, Amatya A: Natriuretic peptides and their therapeutic potential. Heart Dis 1999;1:305-328.

88. Richards M, Lainchbury JG, Nicholls MG, et al: Dendroaspis natriuretic peptide: Endogenous or dubious? Lancet 2002;359:5-6.

89. Kirsch B: Electron microscopy of the atrium of the heart: I. Guinea pig. Exp Med Surg 1956;14:99-112.

90. Henry JP, Gauer OH, Reeves JL: Evidence of atrial location of receptors influencing urine flow. Circ Res 1956;4:85-90.

91. Flynn TG, de Bold ML, de Bold AJ: The amino acid sequence of an atrial peptide with potent diuretic and natriuretic properties. Biochem Biophys Res Commun 1983;117:859-865.

92. Shenker Y: Atrial natriuretic hormone effect on renal function and aldosterone secretion in sodium depletion. Am J Physiol 1988;255:R867-R873.

93. Isales CM, Bollag WB, Kiernan LC, et al: Effect of ANP on sustained aldosterone secretion stimulated by angiotensin II. Am J Physiol 1989;256:C89-C95.

94. Sonnenberg H, Honrath U, Chong CK, et al: Atrial natriuretic factor inhibits sodium transport in medullary collecting duct. Am J Physiol 1986;250:F963-F966.

95. Harris PJ, Thomas D, Morgan TO: Atrial natriuretic peptide inhibits angiotensin-stimulated proximal tubular sodium and water reabsorption. Nature 1987;326:697-698.

96. Redfield MM, Aarhus LL, Wright RS, et al: Cardiorenal and neurohumoral function in a canine model of early left ventricular dysfunction. Circulation 1993;87:2016-2022.

97. Raine AEG, Erne P, Burgisser E, et al: Atrial natriuretic peptide and atrial pressure in patients with congestive heart failure. N Engl J Med 1986;315:553.

98. Chen HH, Burnett JC: The natriuretic peptides in the pathophysiology of congestive heart failure. Curr Cardiol Rep 2003;3:198-205.

99. McCullough PA, Omland T, Maisel AS: B-type natriuretic peptides: A diagnostic breakthrough for clinicians. Rev Cardiovasc Med 2003;4:72-80.

100. Adams KF, Mathur VS, Gheorghiade M, et al: B-type natri-uretic peptide: From bench to bedside. Am Heart J 2003;145:S34-S46.

101. Ruskoaho H: Cardiac hormones as diagnostic tools in heart failure. Endocr Rev 2003;24:341-356.

102. McCullough PA, Nowak RM, McCord J, et al: B-type natriuretic peptide and clinical judgement in emergency diagnosis of heart failure: Analysis from Breathing Not Properly (BNP) Multinational Study. Circulation 2002;106:416-422.

103. Dao Q, Kazenegra R, Garcia A, et al: Utility of B-type natriuretic peptide in the diagnosis of congestive heart failure in an urgent-care setting. J Am Coll Cardiol 2001;37:379-385.

104. Maisel AS, Krishnaswamy P, Nowak RM, et al: Rapid measurement of B-type natriuretic peptide in the emergency diagnosis of heart failure. N Engl J Med 2002;347:161-167.

105. Lilly LS (ed): Pathophysiology of Heart Disease: A Collaborative Project of Medical Students and Faculty, 3rd ed. Philadelphia, Lippincott Williams & Wilkins, 1998, pp 222-224.

106. Jaski BE (ed): Circulation. In: Basics of Heart Failure: A Problem Solving Approach. Boston, Mass, Kluwer Academic Publishers, 2000, p 31.

107. Hirsch AT, Pinto YM, Schunkert H, et al: Potential role of the tissue renin-angiotensin system in the pathophysiology of congestive heart failure. Am J Cardiol 1990;66:22D-32D.

108. Gavaras H, Gavras I: The renin-angiotensin system and the heart. In Share L (ed): Hormones and the Heart in Health and Disease. Totowa, New Jersey, Humana Press, 1999, pp 53-67.

109. Peart WS: Renin-angiotensin system. N Engl J Med 1975;292:302.

110. Oparil S, Haber E: The renin-angiotensin system. N Engl J Med 1974;291:389.

111. Page IH, Helmer OM: A crystalline pressor substance (angiotonin) resulting from the reaction between renin and renin activator. J Exp Med 1940;71:29-42.

112. Braun-Menendez E, Fasciolo E, Leloir JC, et al: The substance causing renal hypertension. J Physiol (Lond) 1940;98:283-298.

113. Braun-Menendez E, Page IH: Suggested revision of nomencla-ture-angiotensin. Science 1958;127:242.

114. Edwards EM: Segmental effects of norepinephrine and angiotensin II on isolated renal microvessels. Am J Physiol 1983;244:F526-F534.

115. Schuster VL, Kokko GP, Jacobson HR: Angiotensin II directly stimulates transport in rabbit proximal convoluted tubules. J Clin Invest 1984;73:507-515.

116. Hall JE, Guyton AC, Jackson TE, et al: Control of glomerular filtration rate by renin-angiotensin system. Am J Physiol 1977;233:F366-F372.

117. Laragh JH, Sealey JE: The renin-angiotensin-aldosterone hormonal system and regulation of sodium, potassium, and blood pressure homeostasis. In Orloff J, Berliner RW (eds): Handbook of Physiology: Renal Physiology. Washington, DC, American Physiological Society, 1973, pp 831-908.

118. Hall JE, Granger JP: Role of peripheral sympathetic nervous system in mediating chronic blood pressure and renal hemodynamic effects of angiotensin II [abstract]. Fed Proc 1983;42:589.

119. Weber KT, Anversa P, Armstrong PW, et al: Remodeling and reparation of the cardiovascular system. J Am Coll Cardiol 1992;20:3-16.

120. Imai T, Hirata Y, Emori T, et al: Induction of endothelin-1 gene by angiotensin and vasopressin in endothelial cells. Hypertension 1992;19:753-757.

121. Chua BH, Chua CC, Diglio CA, et al: Regulation of endothelin-1 mRNA by angiotensin II in rat heart endothelial cells. Biochem Biophys Acta 1993;1178:201-206.

122. Sung CP, Arleth AJ, Storer BL, et al: Angiotensin type I receptors mediate smooth muscle proliferation and endothelin biosynthesis in rat vascular smooth muscle. J Pharmacol Exp Ther 1994;271:429-437.

123. Ito H, Hirata Y, Adachi S, et al: Endothelin-1 is an autocrine/paracrine factor in the mechanism of angiotensin II-induced hypertrophy in cultured rat cardiac myocytes. J Clin Invest 1993;92: 398-403.

124. Gavras H, Flessas A, Ryan TJ, et al: Angiotensin II inhibition: Treatment of congestive cardiac failure in a high-renin hypertension. JAMA 1977;238:880-882.

125. The Captopril Multicenter Research Group: A placebo-controlled trial of captopril in refractory chronic congestive heart failure. J Am Coll Cardiol 1983;2:755-763.

126. Cleland JGF, Dargie HJ, Bal SG, et al: Effects of enalapril in heart failure: A double blind study of effects on exercise performance, renal function, hormones, and metabolic state. Br Heart J 1985;54:305-312.

127. Riegger GAJ: The effects of ACE inhibitors on exercise capacity in the treatment of congestive heart failure. J Cardiovasc Pharmacol 1990;15:S41-S46.

128. Lee MR: Kinetics of renin-substrate reaction. In: Renin and Hypertension. Baltimore, Williams & Wilkins, 1969, pp 25-27.

129. Campbell DJ: Circulating and tissue angiotensin systems. J Clin Invest 1987;79:1-5.

130. Laragh JH: Extrarenal tissue prorenin systems do exist: Are intrinsic vascular and cardiac tissue renins fact or fancy? Am J Hypertens 1989;2:262-265.

131. Dostal DE, Baker KM: Biochemistry, molecular biology, and potential roles of the cardiac renin-angiotensin system. In Dhalla NS, Takeda N, Nagano M (eds): The Failing Heart. Philadelphia, Lippincott-Raven, 1995, pp 275-294.

132. Dzau VJ, Ellison EK, Brody T, et al: Comparison study of the distribution of renin and angiotensin messenger ribonucleic acids in rat and mouse tissues. Endocrinology 1987;120:2334-2338.

133. van Kats JP, Danser AHJ, van Meegen JR, et al: Angiotensin production by the heart: A quantitative study in pigs with the use of radiolabeled angiotensin infusions. Circulation 1998;98:73-81.

134. Studer R, Reinecke H, Muller B, et al: Increased angiotensin-converting enzyme gene expression in failing human heart. J Clin Invest 1994;94:301-310.

135. Abhold RH, Sullivan MJ, Wright JM, et al: Binding, degradation, and pressor activity of angiotensin II and III after amino peptidase inhibition with amastatin and bestatin. J Pharmacol Exp Ther 1987;242:957-962.

136. Zini S, Fournie-Zaluski MC, Chauvel E, et al: Identification of metabolic pathways of brain angiotensin II and III using specific aminopeptidase inhibitors: Predominant role of angiotensin II in the control of vasopressin release. Proc Natl Acad Sci U S A 1996;93:11968-11973.

137. Wright JW, Harding JW: Brain angiotensin receptor subtypes in the control of physiological and behavioral responses. Pharmaceut Pharmacol Lett 1993;3:24-27.

138. Song L, Wilk S, Healy DP: Aminopeptidase A antiserum inhibits intracerebroventricular angiotensin II-induced dipsogenic and pressor responses. Brain Res 1997;744:1-6.

139. Handa RK, Krebs LT, Harding JW, et al: Angiotensin IV AT4-receptor system in the rat kidney. Am J Physiol Renal Physiol 1998;274:F290-F299.

140. Ferrario CM, Brosnihan KB, Diz DI, et al: Angiotensin(1-7): A new hormone of the angiotensin system. Hypertension 1991;18(Suppl III):III126-III133.

141. Kucharewicz I, Pawlak R, Chabielska E, et al: Angiotensin-(1-7): An active member of the renin-angiotensin system. J Physiol Pharmacol 2002;53:533-540.

142. Neuss M, Regitz-Zagrosek V, Fleck E: Human cardiac fibroblasts express an angiotensin receptor with unusual binding characteristics. Biochem Biophys Res Commun 1994;204:1334-1339.

143. Stroth U, Unger T: The renin-angiotensin system and its receptors. J Cardiovasc Pharmacol 1999;33(Suppl 1):S21-S28.

144. DeGasparo M, Husain A, Alexander W, et al: Proposed update on angiotensin receptor nomenclature. Hypertension 1995;25:924-927.

145. Unger T, Chung O, Csikos T, et al: Angiotensin receptors. J Hypertens 1996;14:S95-S103.

146. Timmermans PB, Wong PC, Chiu AT, et al: Angiotensin II receptors and angiotensin II rceptor antagonists. Pharmacol Rev 1993;45:205-251.

147. Criscone L, Bradley WA, Buhlmayer P, et al: Valsartan: Preclinical and clinical profile of an antihypertensive angiotensin-II antagonist. Cardiovasc Drug Rev 1995;13:230-250.

148. Kubo, K, Inada Y, Kohara Y, et al: Nonpeptide angiotensin II receptor antagonists: Synthesis and biological activity of benzimidazoles. J Med Chem 1993;36:1772-1784.

149. Suzuki J, Matsubara H, Urakami M, et al: Rat angiotensin II (type 1A) receptor mRNA regulation and subtype expression in myocardial growth and hypertrophy. Circ Res 1993;73:439-447.

150. Stoll, M, Stecklings UM, Paul M, et al: The angiotensin AT2-receptor mediates inhibition of cell proliferation in coronary endothelial cells. J Clin Invest 1995;95:651-657.

151. Munzenmaier DH, Greene AS: Opposing actions of angiotensin II on microvascular growth and arterial blood pressure. Hypertension 1996;27:760-765.

152. Laflamme L, DeGasparo M, Gallo JM, et al: Angiotensin II induction of neurite outgrowth by AT2 receptors in NG108-15 cells. J Biol Chem 1996;271:22729-22735.

153. Meffert S, Stoll M, Stecklings MU, et al: The angiotensin AT2 receptor inhibits cell proliferation and promotes differentiation in PC12W cells. Mol Cell Endocrinol 1996;122:59-67.

154. Yamada T, Horiuchi M, Dzau VJ: Angiotensin II type 2 receptor mediates programmed cell death. Proc Natl Acad Sci U S A 1996;93:156-160.

155. Gallinat S, Csikos T, Meffert S, et al: The angiotensin AT2 receptor mediates down-regulation of neurofilament M in PC12W cells. Neurosci Lett 1997;227:29-32.

156. Pitt B, Segal R, Martinez FA, et al: Randomized trial of losartan versus captopril in patients over 65 with heart failure (Evaluation of Losartan in the Elderly Study, ELITE). Lancet 1997;349:747-752.

157. McKelvie RS, Yusuf S, Pericak D, et al: Comparison of candesartan, enalapril, and their combination in congestive heart failure: Randomized Evaluation of Strategies for Left Ventricular Dysfunction (RESOLVD) Pilot Trial. The RESOLVD Pilot Study Investigators. Circulation 1999;100:1056-1064.

158. Pitt B, Poole-Wilson PA, Segal R, et al: Effect of losartan compared with captopril on mortality in patients with symptomatic heart failure: Randomized trial—the Losartan Heart Failure Survival Study ELITE II. Lancet 2000;355:1582-1587.

159. Dickstein K, Kjekshus J: Comparison of the effects of losartan and captopril on mortality in patients after acute myocardial infarction: The OPTIMAAL trial design. Am J Cardiol 1999;83:477-481.

160. Dickstein K, Kjekshus J: Comparison of the effects of losartan and captopril on mortality and morbidity in high-risk patients after acute-myocardial infarction: The OPTIMAAL randomized trial. Lancet 2002;360:752-760.

161. Cohn JN, Tognoni G: A randomized trial of the angiotensin-receptor blocker valsartan in chronic heart failure. N Engl J Med 2001;345:1667-1675.

162. Maggioni AP, Anand I, Gottlieb SO, et al: Effects of valsartan on morbidity and mortality in patients with heart failure not receiving angiotensin-converting enzyme inhibitors. J Am Coll Cardiol 2002;40:1414-1421.

163. Jong P, Demers C, McKelvie RS, et al: Angiotensin receptor blockers in heart failure: Meta-analysis of randomized controlled trials. J Am Coll Cardiol 2002;39:463-470.

164. DiBianco R: Update on therapy for heart failure. Am J Med 2003;115:480-488.

165. Swedberg K, Pfeffer M, Granger C, et al: Candesartan in Heart failure—Assessment of Reduction in Mortality and morbidity (CHARM): Rationale and design. J Card Fail 1999;5:276-282.

166. Pfeffer MA, McMurray J, Leizorovicz A, et al: Valsartan in Acute Myocardial Infarction Trial (VALIANT): Rationale and design. Am Heart J 2000;140:727-734.

167. Yanagisawa M, Kurihara H, Kimura S, et al: A novel potent vasoconstrictor peptide produced by vascular endothelial cells. Nature 1988;332:411-415.

168. Levin ER: Endothelins. N Engl J Med 1995;333:356-363.

169. Ito H, Hirata Y, Tiroe M, et al: Endothelin-1 induces hypertrophy with enhanced expression of muscle-specific genes in cultures neonatal rat cardiomyocytes. Circ Res 1991;69:209-215.

170. Matsuura A, Yamachi W, Hirata K, et al: Stimulatory interaction between vascular endothelial growth factor and endothelin-1 on gene expression. Hypertension 1998;32:89-95.

171. Perfley KA, Winkles JA: Angiotensin II and endothelin-1 increase fibroblast growth factor-2 mRNA expression in vascular smooth muscle cells. Biochem Biophys Res Commun 1998;242: 202-208.

172. Weissberg PZ, Witchel C, Davenport AP, et al: The endothelial peptides ET-1, ET-2, ET-3, and satafatoxin S6b are co-mitogenic with platelet derived growth factors for vascular smooth muscle cells. Atherosclerosis 1990;83:257-262.

173. Yang Z, Krasniei N, Luscher TF: Endothelin-1 potentiates human smooth muscle cell growth to PDGF: Effects of ETA and ETB receptor blockade. Circulation 1990;100:5-8.

174. Wada A, Tsutamato T, Maeda Y, et al: Endogenous atrial natriuretic peptides inhibits endothelin-1 secretion in dogs with severe congestive heart failure. Am J Physiol 1996;270: H1819-H1824.

175. Stewart D, Cernacek P, Mahamed F, et al: Role of cyclic nucleotides in the regulation of endothelial cells. Am J Physiol 1994;266:H944-H951.

176. Boulanger C, Luscher TF: Release of endothelin from porcine aorta: Inhibition by endothelium-derived nitric oxide. J Clin Invest 1990;85:587-590.

177. Hosada K, Nakao K, Arai H, et al: Cloning and expression of endothelin-1 receptor cDNA. FEBS Lett 1991;287:23-26.

178. Ogawa Y, Nakao K, Arai H, et al: Molecular cloning of a non-isopeptide-selective human endothelial receptor. Biochem Biophys Res Commun 1991;178:248-255.

179. Niwa Y, Nagata N, Oka M, et al: Production of nitric oxide from endothelial cells by 31-amino-acid length endothelin-1: A novel vasoconstrictive product by human chymase. Life Sci 2000;67: 1103-1109.

180. Rich S, McLaughlin VV: Endothelin receptor blockers in cardiovascular disease. Circulation 2003;108:2184-2190.

181. Haynes WG, Strachan FE, Webb DJ: Endothelin ETA and ETB receptors mediate vasoconstriction of human resistance and capacitance vessels in vivo. Circulation 1995;92:357-363.

182. Marguiles K, Hidebrand FLJ, Lerman A, et al: Increased endothelin in experimental heart failure. Circulation 1990;82:2226-2230.

183. Wei C, Lerman A, Rodeheffer R, et al: Endothelin in human congestive heart failure. Circulation 1994;89:1580-1586.

184. Pacher R, Stanek B, Hulsmann M, et al: Prognostic impact of big endothelin-1 plasma concentrations compared with invasive hemodynamic evaluation in severe heart failure. J Am Coll Cardiol 1996;27:633-641.

185. Cacoub P, Dorent R, Nataf P, et al: Plasma endothelin and pulmonary pressures in patients with congestive heart failure. Am Heart J 1993;126:1484-1488.

186. Stewart DJ, Cernacek P, Costello KB, et al: Elevated endothelin-1 in heart failure and loss of normal response to postural change. Circulation 1992;85:510-517.

187. Omland T, Lie RT, Aakvaag T, et al: Plasma endothelin determinations as a prognostic indication of one year mortality after acute myocardial infarction. Circulation 1994;89:1573-1579.

188. Pousset F, Isnard R, Lechat P, et al: Prognostic value of endothelin-1 in patients with chronic heart failure. Eur Heart J 1997;18: 254-258.

189. Suzuki T, Hoshi H, Mitsui Y: Endothelin stimulates hypertrophy and contractility of neonatal rat cardiac myocytes in serum-free medium. FEBS Lett 1989;268:149-151.

190. Ishikawa T, Yanagisawa M, Kurihara H, et al: Positive inotropic effects of novel potent vasoconstrictor peptide endothelin on guinea pig atria. Am J Physiol 1988;255:H970-973.

191. Cavero PG, Miller WL, Heublein DM, et al: Endothelin in experimental congestive heart failure in the anesthetized dog. Am J Physiol 1990;259:F312-317.

192. Cozza EN, Gomez-Sanchez CE, Foecking MF, et al: Endothelin binding to cultured calf adrenal zona glomerulosa cells and stimulation of aldosterone secretion. J Clin Invest 1989;84:1032-1035.

193. Brooks DP: Role of endothelin in renal function and dysfunction. Clin Exp Pharmacol Physiol 1996;23:3445-3448.

194. Karet FE: Endothelin peptides and receptors in human kidney. Clin Sci 1996;91:267-273.

195. Spinale FG, Walker JD, Mukherjee R, et al: Concomitant endothelin receptor subtype-A blockade during progression of pacing induced congestive heart failure in rabbits. Circulation 1997;95:1918-1929.

196. Borgeson DD, Grantham JA, Williamson EE, et al: Chronic endothelin type A receptor antagonism in experimental heart failure. Hypertension 1998;31:776-770.

197. Love MP, Haynes WG, Gray GA, et al: Vasodilatory effects of endothelin converting enzyme inhibition and endothelin ETA receptor blockade in chronic heart failure patients treated with ACE inhibitors. Circulation 1998;94:2131-2137.

198. Mulder P, Richard V, Derumeaux G, et al: Role of endogenous endothelin in chronic heart failure: Effect of long-term treatment with an endothelin receptor antagonist on survival, hemodynamics, and remodeling. Circulation 1997;96:1976-1982.

199. Sutsch G, Kiowski W, Yan X, et al: Short-term oral endothelin-receptor antagonist therapy in conventionally treated patients with symptomatic severe chronic heart failure. Circulation 1998;98:2262-2268.

200. Coletta AP, Cleland JG: Clinical trials update: Highlights of the Scientific Sessions of the XXIII Congress of the European Society of Cardiology—WARIS II, ESCAMI, PAFAC, RITZ-1 and TIME. Eur J Heart Fail 2001;3:747-750.

201. Louis A, Clelan JG, Crabbe S, et al: Clinical trials update: CAPRICORN, COPERNICUS, MIRACL, STAF, RITZ-2, RECOVER and RENAISSANCE and cachexia and cholesterol in heart failure. Highlights of the Scientific Sessions from the Am College of Cardiology. Eur J Heart Fail 2001;3:381-387.

202. O'Conner CM, Gattis WA, Adams KF, et al: Tezosentan in patients with acute heart failure and acute coronary syndromes. J Am Coll Cardiol 2003;41:1452-1457.

203. Kaluski E, Korbin I, Zimlichman R, et al: RITZ-5 randomized intravenous tezosentan (an endothelin-A/B antagonist) for the treatment of pulmonary edema. J Am Coll Cardiol 2003;41:204-210.

204. Packer M: Effects of the endothelin receptor antagonist bosentan on the morbidity and mortality in patients with congestive heart failure: Results of the ENABLE 1 and 2 program. Late Breaking Clinical Trials: Special Topics #412. In Congress of the American College of Cardiology, 2002.

205. Luscher TF, Enseleit F, Pacher R, et al: Hemodynamic and neurohumoral effects of selective endothelin (ET[A]) receptor blockade in chronic heart failure: The Heart Failure ET(A) Receptor Blockade Trial (HEAT). Circulation 2002;106:2666-2672.

206. Pacher M, Caspi A, Charlon V, et al: Multicenter, double-blind, placebo-controlled study of the efficacy of long-term endothelin blockade with bosentan in chronic heart failure: Results of the REACH-1 trial [abstract]. Circulation 1998;98(Suppl):12.

207. Mylona P, Cleland JG: Update of REACH-1 and MERIT-HF clinical trials in heart failure: Cardio-net Editorial Team. Eur J Heart Fail 1999;1:197-200.

208. Schirgir JA, Chen HH, Jougasaki M, et al: Endothelin A receptor antagonism in experimental congestive heart failure results in augmentation of the renin-angiotensin system and sustained sodium retention. Circulation 2004;109:249-254.

209. Palmer RM, Ferrige AG, Moncada S: Nitric oxide release accounts for the biological activity of endothelium-derived relaxing factor. Nature 1987;327:524-526.

210. Moncada S, Radomski MW, Palmer RM: Endothelium-derived relaxing factor: Identification as nitric oxide and role in the control of vascular tone and platelet function. Biochem Pharmacol 1988;37:2495-2501.

211. Furchgott RF, Zawadzki JV: The obligatory role of endothelial cells in the relaxation of arterial smooth muscle by acetycholine. Nature 1980;288:373-376.

212. Marletta MA: Nitric oxide synthase: Aspects concerning structure and catalysis. Cell 1994;78:927-930.

213. Moncada S, Higgs A: The L-arginine-nitric oxide pathway. N Engl J Med 1993;329:2002-2012.

214. Knowles RG, Palacios M, Palmer RM, et al: Formation of nitric oxide from L-arginine in the central nervous system: A transduction mechanism for stimulation of the soluble guanylate cyclase. Proc Natl Acad Sci U S A 1989;86:5159-5162.

215. Bredt DS, Snyder SH: Isolation of nitric oxide synthase, calmodulin-requiring enzyme. Proc Natl Acad Sci U S A 1990;87:682-685.

216. Moncada S, Higgs EA: Endogenous nitric oxide: Physiology, pathology, and clinical relevance. Eur J Clin Invest 1991;21:361-374.

217. Bredt DS, Hwang PM, Glatt CE, et al: Cloned and expressed nitric oxide synthase structurally resembles cytochrome P-450 reductase. Nature 1991;351:714-718.

218. Xie QW, Cho HJ, Calaycay J, et al: Cloning and characterization of inducible nitric oxide synthase from mouse macrophages. Science 1992;256:225-228.

219. Lyons CR, Orloff GJ, Cunningham JM: Molecular cloning and finctional expression of an inducible nitric oxide synthase from a murine macrophage cell line. J Biol Chem 1992;267:6370-6374.

220. Lamas S, Marsden PA, Li GK, et al: Endothelial nitric oxide synthase: Molecular cloning and characterization of a distinct constitutive enzyme isoform. Proc Natl Acad Sci U S A 1992;89:6348-6352.

221. Balligand JL: Regulation of cardiac beta-adrenergic response by nitric oxide. Cardiovasc Res 1999;43:607-620.

222. Ignarro LJ, Buga GM, Wood KS, et al: Endothelium-derived relaxing factor produced and released from artery and vein is nitric oxide. Proc Natl Acad Sci U S A 1987;84:9265-9269.

223. Palmer RM, Ashton DS, Moncada S: Vascular endothelial cells synthesize nitric oxide from L-arginine. Nature 1988;333:664-666.

224. Marletta MA, Yoon PS, Iyengar R, et al: Macrophage oxidation of L-arginine to nitrite and nitrate: Nitric oxide is the intermediate. Biochemistry 1988;27:8706-8711.

225. Szabo C, Thiemermann C: Regulation of the expression of the inducible isoform of nitric oxide synthase. Adv Pharmacol 1995;34:113-153.

226. Schulz R, Smith JA, Lewis MJ, et al: Nitric oxide synthase in cultured endocardial cells of the pig. Br J Pharmacol 1991;104: 21-24.

227. Balligand JL, Kobzik L, Han X, et al: Nitric-oxide-dependent parasympathetic signaling is due to activation of constitutive endothelial (type III) nitric oxide synthase in cardiac myocytes. J Biol Chem 1995;270:14582-14586.

228. Schulz R, Nava E, Moncada S: Induction and potential biological relevance of a Ca^{2+}-independent nitric oxide synthase in the myocardium. Br J Pharmacol 1992;105:575-580.

229. Balligand JL, Ungureanu-Longrois D, Simmons WW, et al: Cytokine-inducible nitric oxide synthase (iNOS) expression in cardiac myocytes: Characterization and regulation of iNOS expression and detection of iNOS activity in single cardiac myocytes in vitro. J Biol Chem 1994;269:27580-27588.

230. Bernstein RD, Recchia FA, Kaley G, et al: Nitric oxide and the heart. In Share L (ed): Hormones and the Heart in Health and Disease. Totowa, New Jersey, Humana Press, 1999, pp 175-193.

231. Radomski MW, Palmer RM, Moncada S: Comparative pharmacology of endothelium-derived relaxing factor, nitric oxide and prostacyclin in platelets. Br J Pharmacol 1987;92:181-187.

232. Radomski MW, Palmer RM, Moncada S: Endogenous nitric oxide inhibits human platelet adhesion to vascular endothelium. Lancet 1987;2:1057-1058.

233. Radomski MW, Palmer RM, Moncada S: The anti-aggregating properties of vascular endothelium: Interactions between prostacyclin and nitric oxide. Br J Pharmacol 1987;92:639-646.

234. Radomski MW, Palmer RM, Moncada S: The role of nitric oxide and cGMP in platelet adhesion to vascular endothelium. Biochem Biophys Res Commun 1987;148:1482-1489.

235. Taddei S, Virdis A, Ghiadoni L, et al: Relationship with cyclooxygenase-derived endothelium-dependent contracting factors and nitric oxide. J Cardiovasc Pharmacol 2000;35:S37-S40.

236. Kojda G, Kottenberg K: Regulation of basal myocardial function by NO. Cardiovasc Res 1999;41:514-523.

237. Wang J, Seyedi N, Xu X, et al: Defective endothelium-mediated control of coronary circulation in conscious dogs after heart failure. Am J Physiol Heart Circ Physiol 1994;266:H670-H680.

238. Ontkean M, Gay R, Greenberg B: Diminished endothelium-derived relaxing factor activity in an experimental model of chronic heart failure. Circ Res 1991;69:1088-1096.

239. Kubo SH, Rector TS, Bank AJ, et al: Endothelium-dependent vasodilation is attenuated in patients with heart failure. Circulation 1991;84:1589-1596.

240. Arimura K, Egashira K, Nakamura R, et al: Increased activation of nitric oxide is involved in coronary endothelial dysfunction in heart failure. Am J Physiol Heart Circ Physiol 2001;280:H68-H75.

241. Massion PB, Moniotte S, Balligand JL: Nitric oxide: Does it play a role in the heart of the critically ill? Curr Opin Crit Care 2001;7:323-336.

242. Alonso D, Radomski MW: The nitric oxide-endothelin-1 connection. Heart Fail Rev 2003;8:107-115.

243. Massion PB, Feron O, Dessy C, et al: Nitric oxide and cardiac function. Circ Res 2003;93:388-398.

244. Carretero OA, Scicli AG: The kallikrein-kinin system as a regulator of cardiovascular and renal function. In Laragh JH, Brenner BM (eds): Hypertension: Pathophysiology, Diagnosis and Management. New York, Raven Press, 1995, pp 983-999.

245. Carretero OA: Kinins in the heart. In Share L (ed): Hormones and the Heart in Health and Disease. Totowa, New Jersey, Humana Press, 1999, pp 137-158.

246. Palkhiwala SA, Frishman WH, Warshafsky S: Bradykinin for the treatment of cardiovascular disease. Heart Dis 2001;3:333-339.

247. Carretero OA: Kinins: Local hormones in regulation of blood pressure and renal function. Choices Cardiol 1993;7(Suppl 1):10.

248. Yang XP, Liu YH, Scicli GM, et al: Role of kinins in the cardioprotective effect of preconditioning: Study of myocardial ischemia/reperfusion injury in B2 receptor knockout mice and kinogen-deficient rats. Hypertension 1997;30:735-740.

249. Kitakaze M, Node K, Minamino T, et al: Inhibition of angiotensin-converting enzyme increases the nitric oxide levels in canine ischemic myocardium. J Mol Cell Cardiol 1998;30:2461-2466.

250. Su JB, Barbe F, Houel R, et al: Preserved vasodilator effect of bradykinin in dogs with heart failure. Circulation 1998;98:2911-2918.

251. Regoli D, Rhaleb NE, Drapeau G, et al: Basic pharmacology of kinins: Pharmacologic receptors and other mechanisms. Adv Exp Med Biol 1989;247:A399-A407.

252. Faussner A, Bathon JM, Proud D: Comparison of the responses of B and B2 kinin receptors to agonist stimulation. Immunopharmacology 1999;45:13-20.

253. Regoli D, Gobeil F, Nguyen QT, et al: Bradykinin receptor types and B2 subtypes. Life Sci 1994;55:735-749.

254. Cheng CP, Onishi K, Ohte N, et al: Functional effects of endogenous bradykinin in congestive heart failure. J Am Coll Cardiol 1998;31:1679-1686.

255. Kuoppala A, Shiota N, Kokkonen JO, et al: Down-regulation of cardioprotective type-2 receptors in the left ventricle of patients with end-stage heart failure. J Am Coll Cardiol 2002;40:119-125.

256. Heitsch H: The therapeutic potential of bradykinin B2 receptor agonists in the treatment of cardiovascular disease. Expert Opin Invest Drugs 2003;12:759-770.

257. Kitmaru K, Kangawa K, Kawamoto M, et al: Adrenomedullin: A novel hypotensive peptide isolated from human phechromocytoma. Biochem Biophys Res Commun 1993;200:553-560.

258. Ishizaka Y, Ishizaka Y, Tanaka M, et al: Adrenomedullin stimulates cAMP formation in rat vascular smooth muscle cells. Biochem Biophys Res Commun 1994;200:642-646.

259. Majid DSA, Kadowitz PJ, Coy DH, et al: Renal responses to intra-arterial administration of adrenomedullin in dogs. Am J Physiol 1996;270:F200-F205.

260. Jougasaki M, Wei C-M, McKinley LJ, et al: Elevation of circulating and ventricular adrenomedullin in human congestive heart failure. Circulation 1995;92:286-289.

261. Nishikimi T, Saito Y, Kitamura K, et al: Increased plasma levels of adrenomedullin in patients with heart failure. J Am Coll Cardiol 1995;26:1424-1431.

262. Parkes DG, May CN: Direct cardiac and vascular actions of adrenomedullin in conscious sheep. Br J Pharmacol 1997;120:1179-1185.

263. Szokodi I, Kinninen P, Tavi P, et al: Evidence for cAMP-independent mechanisms mediating the effects of adrenomedullin, a new inotropic peptide. Circulation 1998;97:1062-1070.

264. Nagaya N, Satoh T, Nishikimi T, et al: Hemodynamic, renal, and hormonal effects of adrenomedullin infusion in patients with congestive heart failure. Circulation 2000;101:498-503.

265. Moncada S, Vane JR: Pharmacology and endogenous role of prostaglandin endoperoxidases, thromboxane A2 and prostacyclin. Pharmacol Rev 1978;30:243-331.

266. De Decker EAM, Nugteren DH, Ten Hoor F: Prostacyclin is the major prostaglandin released from isolated perfused rabbit and rat heart. Nature 1977;268:163-168.

267. Hsueh W, Needleman P: Sites of lipase activation and prostaglandin synthesis in isolated, perfused rabbit hearts and hydronephrotic kidneys. Prostaglandins 1978;16:661-681.

268. Wennmalm A: Prostaglandin-mediated inhibition of noradrenalin release: VI. On the intra-cardiac source of prostaglandin released from isolated rabbit hearts. Acta Physiol Scand 1979;105:254-256.

269. Bolton HS, Chanderbahn R, Bryant RW, et al: Prostaglandin synthesis by adult heart myocytes. J Mol Cell Cardiol 1980;12:1287-1298.

270. Hedqvist P: Basic mechanisms of prostaglandin actions on autonomic neurotransmission. Annu Rev Pharmacol Toxicol 1977;17:259-279.

271. Junstad M, Wennmalm A: On the release of prostaglandin E_2 from rabbit heart following infusion of noradrenalin. Acta Physiol Scand 1973;87:573-574.

272. Jaiswal N, Malik KU: Prostaglandin synthesis elicited by cholinergic stimuli is mediated by activation of M2 muscarinic receptors in rabbit heart. J Pharmacol 1974;52:370-375.

273. Shaffer JE, Malik KU: Enhancement of prostaglandin output during activation of beta-1 adrenoceptors in the isolated rabbit heart. J Pharmacol Exp Ther 1982;223:729-735.

274. Needleman P, Marshall GR, Sobel BE: Hormone interactions in the isolated rabbit heart, synthesis and coronary vasomotor effects of prostaglandins, angiotensin, and bradykinin. Circ Res 1975;37:802-808.

275. Hecker M, Dambacher T, Busse R: Role of endothelin-derived bradykinin in the control of vascular tone. J Cardiovasc Pharmacol 1992;20(Suppl 9):S55-S61.

276. Chidsey CA, Harrison DC, Braunwald E: Augmentation of plasma norepinephrine response to exercise in patients with congestive heart failure. N Engl J Med 1962;267:650-654.

277. Chidsey CA, Braunwald E, Morrow AG: Catecholamine excretion and cardiac stress of congestive heart failure. Am J Med 1965;39:442-451.

278. Floras JS: Sympathetic activation in human heart failure: Diverse mechanism, therapeutic opportunities. Acta Physiol Scand 2003;177:391-398.

279. Grassi G, Seravalle G, Cattaneo BM, et al: Sympathetic activation and loss of reflex sympathetic control in mild congestive heart failure. Circulation 1995;92:3206-3211.

280. Kaye DM, Lambert GW, Lefkovits J, et al: Neurochemical evidence of cardiac sympathetic activation and increased central nervous system norepinephrine turnover in severe congestive heart failure. J Am Coll Cardiol 1994;23:570-578.

281. Kaye DM, Lefkovits J, Jennings GL, et al: Adverse consequences of high sympathetic nervous activity in the failing human heart. J Am Coll Cardiol 2001;26:1257-1263.

282. Gero J, Gerova M: The role of parameters of pulsating pressure in the stimulation of intracarotid receptors. Arch Int Pharmacodyn Ther 1962;140:35.

283. Cohn JN, Levine B, Francis GS, et al: Neurohumoral control mechanisms in congestive heart failure. Am Heart J 1981;102:509.

284. Rutenberg HL, Spann JF: Alterations of cardiac sympathetic neurotransmitter activity in congestive heart failure. In Mason DT (ed): Congestive Heart Failure: Mechanisms, Evaluation and Treatment. New York, Dun-Donnelley Publishing, 1976, pp 85-95.

285. Brodde OE: Die rolle adrenerger α- und β-rezeptoren in der pathogenese von hypertonie und herzerkrankungen. Der Internist 1988;29:397-413.

286. Ahlquist RP: A study of adrenotropic receptors. Am J Physiol 1948;153:586-600.

287. Strasser RH, Ihl-Val R, Marquetant R: Molecular review: Molecular biology of adrenergic receptors. J Hypertension 1992;10:501-506.

288. Chung FZ, Wang CD, Dotter PC, et al: Site-directed mutagenesis and continuous expression of human β-adrenergic receptors. J Biol Chem 1988;263:4052-4055.

289. Bouvier M, Hausdorff WP, Blasi AD, et al: Removal of phosphorylation sites from the β₂-adrenergic receptor delays onset of agonist-promoted desensitization. Nature 1988;33:370-373.

290. Lanier M, Homey CJ, Patenaude, et al: Identification of structurally distinct α₂ adrenergic receptors. J Biol Chem 1988;263:14491-14496.

291. Lomasney JW, Lorenz W, Allen LF, et al: Expansion of the α₂-adrenergic receptor family: Cloning and characterization of a human α₂-adrenergic receptor subtype, the gene of which is located on chromosome 2. Proc Natl Acad Sci U S A 1990;87:5094-5098.

292. Regan JW, Kobilka TS, Yang-Feng TL, et al: Cloning and expression of a human kidney cDNA for an α₂-adrenergic receptor subtype. Proc Natl Acad Sci U S A 1988;85: 6301-6305.

293. Hwa J, De Young MB, Perez DM, et al: Autonomic control of myocardium: Alpha-adrenoceptor mechanisms. In Burnstock G (ed): The Autonomic Nervous System: Vol VIII. The Nervous Control of the Heart. Amsterdam, Harwood Academic Publishers. 1996; pp 49–79.

294. Graham RM: Adrenergic receptor: Structure and function. Cleve Clin J Med 1990;57:481-491.

295. Benfey BG: Function of myocardial α-adrenoceptors. Life Sci 1990;46:743-757.

296. Li K, He H, Li C, et al: Myocardial α₁-adrenoceptors: Inotropic effect and physiologic implication. Life Sci 1997;60:1305-1308.

297. Otani H, Das DK: α₁-Adrenoceptor-mediated phosphoinositide breakdown and inotropic response in rat left ventricular papillary muscles. Circ Res 1994;62:8-17.

298. Simpson P, MeGrath A, Savio S: Myocyte hypertrophy in neonatal rat heart cell cultures and its regulation by serum and by catecholamines. Circ Res 1982;51:787-801.

299. Milano CA, Dolber PC, Rockman HA, et al: Myocardial expression of a constitutively active α₁B-adrenergic receptor in transgenic mice induces cardiac hypertrophy. Proc Natl Acad Sci U S A 1994;91:10109-10113.

300. Ramirez MT, Sah VP, Zhao XL, et al: The MEKK-JNK pathway is stimulated by α1-adrenergic receptor and Ras activation and is associated with in vitro and in vivo cardiac hypertrophy. J Biol Chem 1997;272:14057-14061.

301. Mitchell MB, Meng X, Ao L, et al: Preconditioning of isolated rat heart is mediated by protein kinase C. Circ Res 1995;76:73-81.

302. McGrath JC: Evidence of more than one type of post-junctional α-adrenoceptor. Biochem Pharmacol 1982;31:467-484.

303. Ruffolo RR: Relative agonist potency as a means of differentiating alpha-adrenoceptors and alpha-adrenergic mechanisms. Clin Sci 1985;10:9s-14s.

304. Morrow AL, Creese I: Characterization of α₁-adrenoceptor subtypes in rat brain: A reevaluation of [3H]WB4104 and [3H]prazosin binding. Mol Pharmacol 1986;29:321-330.

305. Graham RM, Perez DM, Piascik MT, et al: Characterization of α1-adrenergic receptor subtypes. Pharmacol Commun 1995;6: 15-22.

306. Hieble JP, Bylund DB, Clarke DE, et al: International Union of Pharmacology X: Recommendation for nomenclature of α₁-adrenoceptors: Consensus update. Pharmacol Rev 1995;47: 267-270.

307. Michel MC, Kenny B, Schwinn DA: Classification of α₁-adrenoceptor subtypes. Naunyn-Schmiedeberg's Arch Pharmacol 1995;352:1-10.

308. Faure C, Gouhier C, Langer SZ, et al: Quantification of α₁-adrenoceptor subtypes in human tissues by competitive RT-PCR analysis. Biochem Biophys Res Commun 1995;213:935-943.

309. Hirasawa A, Horie K, Tanaka T, et al: Cloning, functional expression and tissue distribution of human cDNA for the α₁C-adrenergic receptor. Biochem Biophys Res Commun 1993;195: 902-909.

310. Price DT, Lefkowitz RJ, Caron MG, et al: Localization of mRNA for three distinct α₁-adrenergic receptor subtypes in human tissues: Implications for human a-adrenergic physiology. Mol Pharmacol 1994;45:171-175.

311. Weinberg DH, Trivedi P, Tan CP, et al: Cloning, expression and characterization of human a-adrenergic receptors α₁A, α₁B and α₁C. Biochem Biophys Res Commun 1994;201:1296-1304.

312. Bohm M, Diet F, Feiler, et al: α-Adrenoceptors and a-adrenoceptor-mediated positive inotropic effects in failing human myocardium. J Cardiovasc Pharmacol 1988;12:357-364.

313. Bristow MR, Minobe W, Rasmussen R, et al: Alpha-1 adrenergic receptors in the nonfailing and failing human heart. J Pharmacol Exp Ther 1988;247:1039-1045.

314. Hwang K-C, Gray CD, Sweet WE, et al: α₁-Adrenergic receptor coupling with Gh in the failing human heart. Circulation 1996;94:718-726.

315. Brodde O-E, Broede A, Daul A, et al: Receptor systems in the non-failing human heart. Basic Res Cardiol 1992;87(Suppl 1):1-14.

316. Endoh M, Hiramoto T, Ishihata A, et al: Myocardial alpha-1 adrenoceptors mediate positive inotropic effect and changes in phosphatidylinositol metabolism: Species differences in receptor distribution and the intracellular process in mammalian ventricular myocardium. Circ Res 1991;68:1179-1190.

317. Terzic A, Puceat M, Vassort G, et al: Cardiac α₁-adrenoceptors: An overview. Pharmacol Rev 1993;45:147-175.

318. Brodde O-E. β₁- and β₂-adrenoceptors in the human heart: Properties, function and alterations in chronic heart failure. Pharmacol Rev 1991;43:203-242.

319. Vago T, Bevilacqua M, Norbiato G, et al: Identification of α₁-adrenergic receptors on sarcolemma from normal subjects and patients with idiopathic dilated cardiomyopathy: Characteristics and linkage to GTP-binding protein. Circ Res 1989;64:474-481.

320. Steinfath M, Danielson W, von der Leyen H, et al: Reduced α₁- and β₂-adrenoceptor mediated positive inotropic effects in human end-stage heart failure. Br J Pharmacol 1992;105: 463-469.

321. Yoshikawa T, Port JD, Asano K, et al: Cardiac adrenergic receptor effects of carvedilol. Eur Heart J 1996;17(Suppl B):8-16.

322. Brodde O-E, Michel MC: Adrenergic and muscarinic receptors in the human heart. Pharmacol Rev 1999;51:651-689.

323. Bylund DB, Eikenberg DC, Hieble JP, et al: IV. International Union of Pharmacology Nomenclature of Adrenoceptors. Pharmacol Rev 1994;46:121-136.

324. Likungu J, Molderings GJ, Gothert M: Presynaptic imadazoline receptors and α2-adrenoceptors in the human heart: Discrimination by clonidine and moxonidine. Naunyn-Schmiedeberg's Arch Pharmacol 1996;354:689-692.

325. Rump LC, Bohmann C, Schaible U, et al: $α_{2C}$-Adrenoceptor-modulated release of noradrenaline in human right atrium. Br J Pharmacol 1995;116:2617-2624.

326. Rump LC, Riera-Knorrenschild G, Schwertfeger E, et al: Dopaminergic and α-adrenergic control of neurotransmission in human right atrium. J Cardiovasc Pharmacol 1995;26:462-470.

327. Trendelenburg AU, Sutej I, Wahl CA, et al: A re-investigation of questionable subclassifications of presynaptic $α_2$-autoreceptors: Rat vena cava, rat atria, human kidney and guinea-pig urethra. Naunyn-Schmiedeberg's Arch Pharmacol 1997;356:721-737.

328. Parker JD, Newton GE, Landzberg JS, et al: Functional significance of presynaptic α-adrenergic receptors in failing and nonfailing human left ventricle. Circulation 1992;92:1793-1800.

329. Bylund DB, Bond RA, Clarke DE, et al: Adrenoceptors. In: The IUPHAR Compendium of Receptor Characterization and Classification. 1998; pp 58-74.

330. Bristow MR, Minobe WA, Raynolds MV, et al: Reduced $β_1$ receptor messenger RNA abundance in the failing human heart. J Clin Invest 1993;92:2737-2745.

331. Ungerer M, Bohm M, Elce JS, et al: Altered expression of β-adrenergic receptor kinase and $β_1$-adrenergic receptors in the failing human heart. Circulation 1993;87:454-463.

332. Engelhardt S, Bohm M, Erdmann E, et al: Analysis of beta-adrenergic receptor mRNA levels in human ventricular biopsy specimens by quantitative polymerase chain reactions: Progressive reduction of β1-adrenergic receptor mRNA in heart failure. J Am Coll Cardiol 1996;27:146-154.

333. Kreif S, Lonnqvist F, Raimbault S, et al: Tissue distribution of $β_3$-adrenergic receptor mRNA in man. J Clin Invest 1993;91:344-349.

334. Kaumann AJ, Molenaar P: Modulation of human cardiac function through 4 β-adrenoceptor populations. Naunyn-Schmiedeberg's Arch Pharmacol 1997;355:667-681.

335. Bristow MR, Hershberger RE, Port JD, et al: β-Adrenergic pathways in nonfailing and failing human ventricular myocardium. Circulation 1990;82(Suppl D):12-25.

336. Bristow MR, Ginsburg R, Umans V, et al: $β_1$- and $β_2$-Adrenergic receptor subpopulations in nonfailing and failing human ventricular myocardium: Coupling of both receptor subtypes to muscle contraction and selective $β_1$-receptor down-regulation in heart failure. Circ Res 1986;59:297-309.

337. Fowler MB, Laser JA, Hopkins GL, et al: Assessment of β-adrenergic receptor pathway in the intact failing human heart: Progressive receptor down-regulation and subsensitivity to agonist response. Circulation 1986;74:1290-1302.

338. Feldman AM, Cates AK, Vaezev WB, et al: Increase of 40,000 mol wt pertussin toxin substrate (G protein) in the failing human heart. J Clin Invest 1988;82:189-197.

339. Lau CP, Pun KK, Leung WH: Reduced stimulatory guanine nucleotide binding regulatory protein in idiopathic dilated cardiomyopathy. Am Heart J 1991;122:1787-1788.

340. Neumann J, Schmitz W, Scholz H, et al: Increase in myocardial G proteins in heart failure. Lancet 1988;2:936-937.

341. Thomas JA, Marks BH: Plasma norepinephrine in congestive heart failure. Am J Cardiol 1978;41:233-243.

342. Levine TB, Francis GS, Goldsmith SR, et al: Activity of the sympathetic nervous system assessed by plasma hormone levels and their relationship to hemodynamic abnormalities in congestive heart failure. Am J Cardiol 1982;49:1659-1666.

343. Francis GS, Goldsmith SR, Cohn JN, et al: Relationship of exercise capacity to resting left ventricular performance and basal plasma norepinephrine levels in patients with congestive heart failure. Am Heart J 1982;104:725-731.

344. Cohn JN, Levine TB, Olivari MT, et al: Plasma norepinephrine as a guide to prognosis in patients with chronic congestive heart failure. N Engl J Med 1984;311:819-823.

345. Spann JF, Chidsey CA, Poole PE, et al: Mechanism of norepinephrine depletion in experimental heart failure produced by aortic constriction in the guinea pig. Circ Res 1965;17:312.

346. Hasking GJ, Esler MD, Jennings JL, et al: Norepinephrine spillover to plasma in patients with congestive heart failure: Evidence of increased overall and cardiorenal sympathetic nervous activity. Circulation 1986;73:615-621.

347. Eisenhofer G, Friberg P, Rundqvist B, et al: Cardiac sympathetic nerve function in congestive heart failure. Circulation 1996;93: 1667-1676.

348. Davis D, Baily R, Zelis R: Abnormalities in systemic norepinephrine kinetics in human congestive heart failure. Am J Physiol 1988;254:E760-E766.

349. Meredith IT, Eisenhofer G, Lambert GW, et al: Cardiac sympathetic nervous activity in congestive heart failure: Evidence for increased neuronal norepinephrine release and preserved neuronal uptake. Circulation 1993;88:136-145.

350. Leimbach WN, Wallin BG, Victor RG, et al: Direct evidence from intranueral recordings for increased central sympathetic outflow in patients with heart failure. Circulation 1986;73:913-919.

351. Wallin BG, Fagius J: Peripheral sympathetic neural activity in conscious humans. Annu Rev Physiol 1988;50:565-576.

352. Esler M, Jennings G, Korner P, et al: Assessment of human sympathetic nervous system activity from measurements of norepinephrine turnover. Hypertension 1988;11:3-20.

353. Von Lueder TG, Kjekshus H, Edvardsen T, et al: Mechansims of elevated plasma endothelin-1 in CHF: Congestion increases pulmonary synthesis and secretion of endothelin-1. Cardiovasc Res 2004;63:41-50.

354. Kim JK, Augustyniak RA, Sala-Mercado JA, et al: Heart failure alters the strength and mechanisms of arterial baroreflex pressor responses during dynamic exercise. Am J Physiol Heart Circ Physiol 2004;Jun 17 [Epub].

355. Schott P, Singer SS, Kogler H, et al: Pressure overload and neurohumoral activation differentially affect the myocardial proteome. Proteomics 2005 Apr;5(5):1372-1381.

CHAPTER 6

Neurohumoral Axis and Natriuretic Peptides in Heart Failure

John Lynn Jefferies
Anthony C. Chang

Previous chapters have delineated the molecular and cellular alterations and the hemodynamic defense mechanisms that occur in heart failure. This chapter describes the sequential and progressive activation of the sympathetic system and the endocrine cascades with special emphasis on the natriuretic peptides and other relevant biologic markers.

The up-regulation of the renin-angiotensin-aldosterone system (RAS) and increased circulating levels of norepinephrine and endothelin-1 (ET-1) play significant roles in the progression of left ventricular dysfunction in the development of heart failure in the adult population.[1] In a counterregulatory system, the cardiac hormones atrial natriuretic peptide (ANP) and brain natriuretic peptide (also called B-type natriuretic peptide) (BNP) have beneficial actions, such as vasodilation and natriuresis (Fig. 6-1).[2-4] Although there has been an escalation of investigative studies on these cardiac hormones in adults, there is virtually no information in the pediatric population. In addition, the significance of the cytokines and other markers of inflammation are being much more recognized in the pathophysiologic state of heart failure. This chapter reviews the fundamentals of the neurohormonal axis, but focuses on the newer concepts in the use of biochemical markers in the progression, diagnosis, treatment, and prognosis of heart failure.

PATHOPHYSIOLOGY OF HEART FAILURE AND BIOCHEMICAL MARKERS

As discussed in previous chapters, the onset of heart failure with arterial underfilling (manifested by decreased activation of mechanoreceptors in left ventricle, carotid

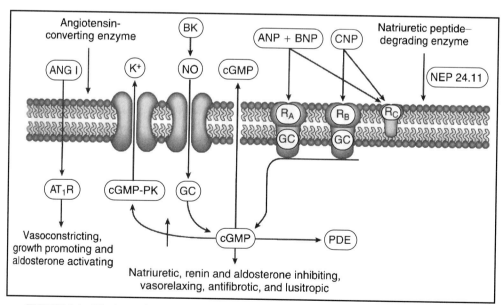

FIGURE 6-1 ■ **The interplay between the renin-angiotensin system and the natriuretic peptides.** The angiotensin system leads to vasoconstriction, fibrosis, decreased diuresis, and sodium retention, whereas the natriuretic system serves as a counterregulatory system with natriuresis, diuresis, vasodilation, antifibrosis, and inhibition of renin and aldosterone. ANG I, angiotensin I; AT₁R, angiotensin type 1 receptor; BK, bradykinin; BNP, brain natriuretic peptide; cGMP, cyclic guanosine-3′, 5′, monophate; CNP, C-type natriuretic peptide; GC, guanylate cyclase; NEP, neutral endopeptidases; PDE, phosphodiesterase; R_A, particulate guanylate cyclase A receptor; R_B, particulate guanylate cyclase B receptor; R_C, particulate guanylate cyclase C receptor. (From Burnett JC, et al: *Alterations in the kidney in heart failure: The cardiorenal axis in the regulation of sodium homeostasis.* In Mann DL [ed]: *Heart Failure: A Companion to Braunwald's Heart Disease,* p. 283, Philadelphia, WB Saunders, 2004.)

sinus, aortic arch, and renal afferent arterioles) leads to a myriad of pathophysiologic adaptations, including stimulation of the adrenergic system, activation of the RAS, and release of substances such as ET and vasopressin. As heart failure progresses, however, the excessive expression of these systems leads to severe vasoconstriction and increases in systemic vascular resistance, sodium and fluid retention, and eventually myocardial fibrosis and apoptosis.

The utility of biochemical markers, such as the natriuretic peptides, in the overall management of heart failure has become progressively more evident in research and clinical medicine. For these biomarkers of heart failure to be useful, a few important caveats should be considered. First, a biomarker assay should be sensitive and specific for heart failure and be able to be performed easily by the facility so that the information is readily available. In addition, these assays should be economically feasible with a favorable ratio relating cost to clinical impact and decision making. The inherent error in the technical measurement performed (coefficient of variation) should be sufficiently low so that any small variation in the biomarker is fairly representative of a clinical change in the spectrum of severity of the disease.[5] This chapter discusses the more commonly used and widely accepted markers and explores the characteristics that make them ideal biologic markers.

SYMPATHETIC NERVOUS SYSTEM

Previous chapters on receptor signaling (in which the adrenergic system and its receptor modifications were detailed) and on the hemodynamic defense system included discussions on the adrenergic system in the presence of heart failure. The discussion in this chapter focuses on the physiologic adaptations and elevation of biologic markers. Heart failure causes a baroreceptor-mediated increase in sympathetic tone that results in several pathophysiologic effects, including tachycardia, increased myocardial contractility, and arterial and venous vasoconstriction. The increase in sympathetic tone is manifested by increased plasma levels of epinephrine and norepinephrine, which mediate the aforementioned pathophysiologic effects.

Norepinephrine is increased in heart failure as a result of increased release and decreased uptake by adrenergic nerve endings, but there also is a concomitant cardiac norepinephrine depletion phenomenon as a result of chronic stimulation. Increased levels of local and circulating norepinephrine as a result of heart failure may lead to myocyte hypertrophy via a dual mechanism of direct stimulation of α-adrenergic and β-adrenergic receptors and indirect activation of the RAS.[6] Norepinephrine also has been shown to be toxic to myocardial cells,[7,8] and the mechanism of this injury is probably via calcium overload or by induction of apoptosis. This cell death can be prevented by concomitant administration of nonselective β-blockade or combined therapy with α-adrenergic and β-adrenergic blockades.[8]

Norepinephrine has been shown to be useful as a heart failure biologic marker. Adult patients with plasma norepinephrine levels greater than 800 pg/mL have a 1-year survival of less than 40%.[9] A multivariate analysis of five significant univariate prognosticators, including heart rate, plasma renin activity, serum sodium, stroke work index, and plasma norepinephrine, found norepinephrine to be the only statistically significant variable.[9] The sympathetic nervous system also exerts renal effects, with stimulation of the RAS, renal vasoconstriction, and direct effects on the proximal convoluted tubule of the kidney. In experimental models of heart failure, renal denervation has been shown to decrease sodium retention.[10] The decreased cardiac adrenergic drive in heart failure is thought to be secondary to increased neuronal release of norepinephrine and decreased neuronal norepinephrine uptake.[11]

The importance of norepinephrine has been delineated further by Anand and colleagues[12] in the Valsartan Heart Failure Trial (Val-HeFT), in which patients with moderate-to-severe heart failure were treated with valsartan, an angiotensin II receptor blocker. In this study, decreases in norepinephrine and BNP were predictors of decreases in morbidity and mortality; to date, this is the largest trial to confirm the prognostic values of these two mediators in patients with moderate-to-severe heart failure. In addition, after heart transplantation, norepinephrine kinetics return to normal, suggesting that these changes in heart failure are functional and reversible.[13] Lastly, a study using the drug moxonidine (a selective imidazoline ligand that acts centrally and directly decreases sympathetic outflow) showed that a decrease in plasma norepinephrine levels was dose related.[14]

RENIN-ANGIOTENSIN-ALDOSTERONE SYSTEM

As discussed previously, the RAS is a regulatory system for blood pressure that acts in concert with the sympathetic nervous system and is activated in heart failure[15,16]; in patients with progressive heart failure, there are marked increases in circulating levels of the RAS components renin, angiotensin II, and aldosterone, all of which can be used as biomarkers for heart failure.[17] The RAS activation and elevation of its biomarkers may not be quite as evident, however, in patients with only mild left ventricular dysfunction.[18] The excessive adrenergic stimulation and activation of the RAS also may play major roles in the progression of cardiac failure to cardiac hypertrophy and fibrosis.

Renin is a key component of the RAS system and is released as a response to sympathetic stimulation of the juxtaglomerular apparatus and to reduction in renal

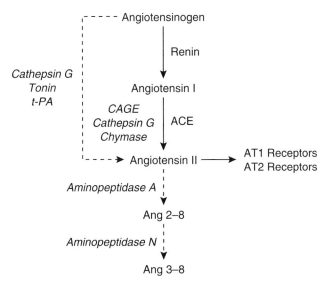

FIGURE 6-2 ■ **The renin-angiotensin cascade.** Angiotensin II is formed by angiotensin I by enzymatic cleavage by the angiotensin-converting enzyme (ACE). Angiotensin II is degraded by aminopeptidases (see text for more details). AT1, angiotensin type 1; AT2, angiotensin type 2; CAGE, chymostatin-sensitive angiotensin II generating enzyme; t-PA, tissue plasminogen activator. (From Lavoie JL, Sigmond CD: *Minireview: Overview of the renin-angiotensin system—an endocrine and paracrine system. Endocrinology* 2003;144: 2179-2183.)

blood flow. Angiotensinogen is first cleaved by renin to form angiotensin I, which subsequently forms angiotensin II via enzymatic action by angiotensin-converting enzyme (ACE) (Fig. 6-2). **Angiotensin II** is a potent peripheral vasoconstrictor and causes vasoconstriction via two mechanisms: by increasing sympathetic tone and arginine vasopressin release and by stimulating angiotensin II type 1 receptors in the vasculature. Angiotensin II also has other influences over release of norepinephrine by the adrenergic nervous system, renal absorption of sodium and water, aldosterone production and release from the adrenal gland, and the sensation of thirst in the central nervous system. Finally, angiotensin II is degraded to angiotensin III and angiotensin IV by aminopeptidases A and N.

The specific receptors angiotensin II type 1 and angiotensin II type 2,[19] which are in the family of G protein–coupled receptors,[20] have different actions and can be found in the heart, kidney, brain, and adrenal gland. Angiotensin II type 1 receptors (which are classified further into angiotensin II type 1a and angiotensin II type 1b subtypes) are found in adult cardiovascular tissue and result in vasoconstrictor effects; angiotensin II type 2 receptors are associated more with fetal tissue and have vasodilatory effects. Both types of receptors can be down-regulated in the presence of severe heart failure. There also is a specific receptor for renin, which can be found in the heart, brain, kidney, placenta, and liver.[21]

Angiotensin II as a biologic marker for heart failure may be theoretically less straightforward compared with norepinephrine. One explanation is that local RAS exist in tissues such as heart, vasculature, adipose tissue, pancreas, gonads, placenta, brain, and vasculature, and there is evidence that the tissue RAS influence vascular and cardiac remodeling.[22-26] In these tissue RAS, conversion of angiotensin I to angiotensin II by enzymes other than ACE (e.g., cathepsin, chymase, and chymostatin-sensitive angiotensin II generating enzyme) has been reported.[27,28] Angiotensin II also can be formed directly from angiotensinogen by cathepsin D or tissue plasminogen activator.[29] The combined central and local RAS create a complex interplay of modulating factors that regulate the cardiovascular system.[30,31]

In addition to its vasoconstrictive effects, angiotensin II may have direct toxic effects on the cardiac myocyte, such as cellular hypertrophy and apoptosis.[32] The degree of activation of angiotensin II as part of the RAS has been shown to be proportional to disease severity of heart failure and seems to correlate with prognosis in adult patients with heart failure.[33] This observation has significant clinical implications because the Val-HeFT and Studies of Left Ventricular Dysfunction (SOLVD) trials reported treatment with ACE inhibitors decreased overall morbidity and mortality in heart failure, and this was concomitantly associated with an attenuation in angiotensin II and other neurohormones.[34]

The adrenal hormone **aldosterone** has potent sodium retention properties and is secreted by the zona glomerulosa in the adrenal gland in response to adrenocorticotropic hormone, angiotensin II, and potassium; it regulates potassium and sodium epithelial cell transport by binding to the inactive cytoplasmic mineralocorticoid receptor.[35-37] Aldosterone can be synthesized in vascular smooth muscle and endothelial cells, brain, blood vessels, and myocardium[38-40]; receptors for aldosterone have been found in the kidney, colon, salivary glands, brain, heart, and blood vessels.[41-43] The distribution of these receptors has been used as a basis for a possible paracrine effect of aldosterone, but this continues to be debated.[44] Aldosterone and its role and manipulation in heart failure are discussed further in Chapter 5.

Elevated levels of aldosterone have been shown to lead to cardiac and vascular fibrosis in animals, but the mechanism is controversial.[45-47] In addition, the interaction of aldosterone with angiotensin II promotes fibrosis by an increase in plasminogen activator inhibitor type 1 expression.[48-52] Elevated levels of aldosterone in humans are associated with endothelial dysfunction, myocardial infarction, left ventricular hypertrophy, and death.[53-55]

NATRIURETIC PEPTIDE HORMONES

A series of past experiments established the endocrinologic properties of the heart.[56] In 1982, de Bold[57] first observed that infusion of atrial tissue extracts resulted in natriuresis in rats. This observation ultimately led to

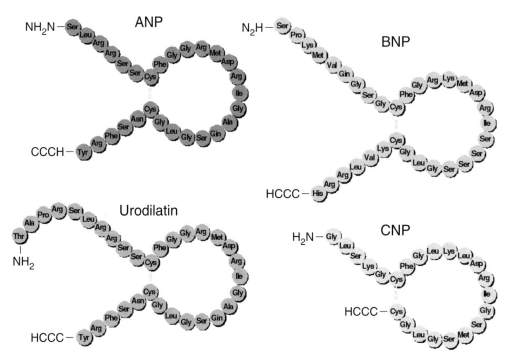

FIGURE 6-3 ■ **Chemical structures of the natriuretic peptides.** The atrial (ANP), B-type (BNP), and C-type (CNP) natriuretic peptides are diagrammatically illustrated. Urodilatin is a synthetic peptide. (Courtesy of *Biosite Diagnostics*, 11030 Roselle Street, San Diego, CA 92121.)

the isolation and reproduction of the hormone ANP. ANP became the first member of a family of peptides that have natriuretic, diuretic, and vasorelaxant properties.[58] These investigations also affirmed the role of these peptides in the endogenous counterregulatory measures against hypertension and volume expansion.[4]

The natriuretic peptides are a group of structurally similar proteins that are genotypically distinct. The three major natriuretic peptides, all of which share a 17-amino acid ring (Fig. 6-3),[59] have a precursor hormone that is encoded by a separate gene with the regulation of each protein being unique. These peptide hormones act on various organs via guanylate cyclase–linked membrane receptors that produce natriuresis, diuresis, and vasodilation of arterial and venous vessels. ANP is released from the atria, whereas BNP is released from the ventricles; a C-type natriuretic peptide (CNP) is derived from the central nervous system and the vascular endothelium. Although myocardial stretch and chamber pressure are the principal mechanisms by which ANP and BNP are activated, additional mediators, such as glucocorticoids, thyroid hormone, ET-1, and angiotensin II (see earlier) also can increase production of these natriuretic peptides.

Natriuretic peptides interact with high-affinity **receptors** on the surface of target cells. Three different receptors (A, B, and C) have been identified in mammalian tissue (Fig. 6-4). Receptors A and B are linked to cascades mediated by the cGMP signaling system, which mediate the vasodilatory and natriuretic effects of these peptides.[60] The A receptor binds ANP and BNP

with a higher affinity for ANP, whereas the B receptor binds CNP. The B receptors predominate in the brain, and the A receptors are more abundant in large blood vessels. A and B receptors are present in the kidney and adrenal glands. The extracellular portion of the receptor is linked to the intracellular portion by a single membrane-spanning section. This intracellular portion contains a guanylyl cyclase catalytic domain that leads to the elevation of cGMP. The C receptor is responsible for

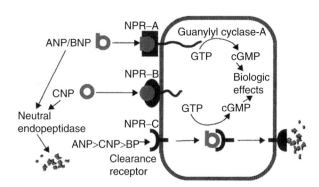

FIGURE 6-4 ■ **Natriuretic peptides and receptors.** The natriuretic peptides, atrial natriuretic peptide (ANP), B-type natriuretic peptide (BNP), and C-type natriuretic peptide (CNP), have different interactions with the receptors for natriuretic peptides. Although ANP and BNP interact mainly with natriuretic peptide receptor A (NPR-A), CNP relates more to natriuretic peptide receptor B (NPR-B). Natriuretic peptide receptor C (NPR-C) (and neutral endopeptidases) is responsible for the degradation of all natriuretic peptides. (From de Lemos JA, McGuire DK, Drazner MH, et al: *B-type natriuretic peptide in cardiovascular disease. Lancet* 2003;362:316-322.)

the clearance of natriuretic peptides: The natriuretic peptides, when bound, are internalized and degraded with subsequent return of the C receptor to the cell surface. ANP, BNP, and CNP bind to this clearance receptor with equal affinity.[61] Natriuretic peptides also can be degraded by cleavage of neutral endopeptidases that are present in renal tubular cells and vascular cells.[62]

Other peptides have been isolated that may be related to the natriuretic peptides. *Dendroaspis* natriuretic peptide, a homologue of ANP, has been reported to be measurable in human plasma and elevated in heart failure. Guanylin and uroguanylin are 15- and 16-amino acid sequences that are produced in the gastrointestinal tract mucosa. They activate guanylyl cyclase, which generates cGMP similar to the natriuretic peptides. It is thought that these hormones may regulate intestinal transport of salt and water, and this may be coordinated with subsequent renal excretion of sodium.[63]

Atrial Natriuretic Peptide

ANP is a cyclic 28-amino acid polypeptide synthesized predominantly from the atria of the normal heart. It is stored in atrial granules as a 126-amino acid prohormone (proANP).[64] After secretion, serine protease corin splits proANP$_{1-126}$ into an N-terminal fragment (consisting of 98 amino acids) and a biologically active ANP in equimolar amounts.[65,66] Both fragments circulate in the plasma. It is suggested that the amino-terminal fragment has biologic actions comparable with the actions of ANP.[67] ANP is removed rapidly from the circulation via hydrolysis and specific receptor activity.[61] N-ANP seems to have a longer half-life and may be more stable for testing, making it a possible biochemical surrogate for the assessment of ANP release from the heart.

Levels of ANP and the prohormone N-ANP in the setting of heart failure and volume overload are elevated because increased tension and resultant stretch on the wall of the atria lead to activation of the cardiac hormonal system.[68] Levels of ANP have been shown to be closely correlated to left atrial pressure.[69] In addition, ANP can be released into the bloodstream after exercise.[70] Although little ANP is produced in the ventricular tissue of normal adults, ANP is present in the ventricular tissue of fetuses and neonates and in hypertrophied ventricles.[71,72] There is even a possible relationship between elevated ANP levels and moderate-to-severe rejection after orthotopic heart transplantation,[73] and levels of ANP and BNP are noted to be elevated by transplanted human hearts.[74] Finally, ANP and BNP levels have been shown to be augmented in the setting of myocarditis.[75]

In animal studies, infusions of low-dose ANP lower blood pressure and reduce peripheral vascular resistance, but at higher doses, infusions result in increases in peripheral vascular resistance, suggesting counterregulatory activation of baroreceptors.[76,77] ANP reduces sympathetic tone in the peripheral vasculature and lowers the threshold of vagal afferent activation, suppressing

reflex vasoconstriction and tachycardia that accompany preload reduction. This effect also helps to maintain a sustained decrease in mean arterial blood pressure. Transgenic mice that overexpress genes encoding for ANP or BNP have levels of natriuretic peptides 10 times higher than normal, and their systolic blood pressures are documented 20 to 30 mm Hg lower than controls.[78]

In the kidney, ANP and BNP increase glomerular filtration and inhibit the reabsorption of sodium, causing natriuresis and diuresis.[79] ANP also causes the vasorelaxation of vascular smooth muscle with resultant reduction in ventricular preload and blood pressure.[80] ANP influences the autonomic nervous system by blocking the sympathetic activity even when cardiac filling pressures are low.[81] ANP causes disruption of the renin-angiotensin-aldosterone axis: An infusion of ANP has been shown not only to decrease the secretion of renin and aldosterone directly, but also seems to attenuate the release of aldosterone indirectly by inhibiting the stimulatory effects of angiotensin II.[82-84] In the renal cortical collecting ducts, ANP inhibits water transport by antagonizing the effects of vasopressin,[85] whereas in the inner medullary collecting duct, ANP blocks the absorption of sodium by stimulating cGMP production.[86-89]

In the brain, ANP is produced within the brain tissue and can act locally. Plasma ANP comes into contact with areas of the brain that are outside the blood-brain barrier. The release of ANP from cultured hypothalamic cells can be provoked by infusions of ET, vasopressin, and norepinephrine, but not angiotensin II.[90-92] ANP inhibits the release of corticotropin and vasopressin through direct effects on the brain. These effects imply extremely well-coordinated central and peripheral actions in controlling fluid and electrolyte balance. Central actions of ANP on the brain even include a decrease in sympathetic tone, perhaps by tonic regulation of baroreceptor signals to the nucleus tractus solitarii.[93,94] Because the A-type natriuretic receptor predominates in areas around the third ventricle, the receptor can bind centrally and peripherally and mediate the effects on thirst and salt ingestion.[95] Transcription of the ANP and BNP genes characterizes cardiac cell growth and has been shown to be directly responsible for proliferation in the fetal heart and trophic growth in the setting of cardiac hypertrophy.[96]

B-Type Natriuretic Peptide

BNP is a cardiac neurohormone produced from the cardiac ventricles in pathophysiologic states, such as systolic or diastolic function, increased left ventricular mass, and low ejection fraction. BNP initially is synthesized as a 134-amino acid peptide named *preproBNP*. PreproBNP is cleaved into ProBNP and a 26-amino acid sequence signal peptide. The 108-amino acid ProBNP sequence is cleaved by furin to form the active BNP$_{77-108}$ and the inactive N-terminal (NT)-proBNP$_{1-76}$ protein.[97] NT-proBNP, which is renally excreted, has a half-life of 120 minutes, whereas the half-life of BNP is 22 minutes. BNP was first identified in porcine brain extract and is present in the human brain, but in much lower concentrations than in the human ventricle. It has been shown that the gene for BNP is located on chromosome 1, organized in tandem with the ANP gene, with these two important genes only 8 kb apart.[98-100]

BNP has cardiovascular and renal effects that are similar to the effects of ANP. BNP causes a decrease in blood pressure by reducing preload secondary to a shift of intravascular fluid into the extravascular compartment, and it increases venous capacitance, which helps to induce a natriuresis that reduces the overall extracellular fluid volume. This latter effect is mediated by direct effects on the renal system and suppression of the renin-angiotensin-aldosterone axis.[101] Similar to ANP, BNP also reduces sympathetic tone in the peripheral vasculature by a myriad of mechanisms, such as suppression of the release of catecholamines, suppression of sympathetic outflow from the central nervous system, inhibition of vasopressin and ET-1, and dampening of baroreceptors.[93,94] The activation threshold of vagal afferents can be reduced by BNP, suppressing reflex tachycardia and vasoconstriction.

BNP infusions in humans at doses sufficient to increase plasma concentrations above normal result in a natriuresis and diuresis that can be independent of blood pressure changes. The infusions result in the reduction of plasma renin and aldosterone concentrations and concomitantly inhibit the aldosterone secretion secondary to angiotensin II stimulation.[102] The drug HS-142-1, which is a competitive antagonist of natriuretic peptide that binds to the A and B receptors,[103] blocks natriuretic-induced diuresis; increases peripheral vascular tone; and increases plasma levels of renin, aldosterone, and catecholamines.[104-107]

Although BNP, ANP, and CNP are produced in the brain, BNP that is produced elsewhere does not cross the blood-brain barrier. The actions of BNP produced locally in the brain reinforce the actions occurring in the other parts of the body; for instance, plasma BNP effects are augmented by the central nervous system inhibition of water ingestion and salt craving.[108,109]

The clinical applications of BNP in adult patients are numerous. The elevation of BNP in the setting of heart failure has been shown to be directly related to morbidity and mortality (Fig. 6-5).[18,110,111] The measurement of BNP also has been shown to be useful in differentiating pulmonary etiologies, such as chronic obstructive pulmonary disease, from cardiac etiologies, such as decompensated heart failure, in patients presenting with dyspnea (Fig. 6-6).[112] BNP can be elevated in systolic and diastolic dysfunction (Fig. 6-7).

Morita and colleagues[113] documented markedly increased levels of BNP in the setting of acute myocardial infarction and postulated that it may reflect the degree

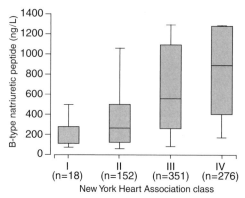

FIGURE 6-5 ■ B-type natriuretic peptide (BNP) concentration in patients with heart failure and New York Heart Association function class. The bars represent the highest and lowest values of BNP measured (ng/L) in patients with New York Heart Association classes I through IV. There appears to be a correlation between BNP level and New York Heart Association classification. (From de Lemos JA, McGuire DK, Drazner MH, et al: *B-type natriuretic peptide in cardiovascular disease. Lancet* 2003;362:316-322.)

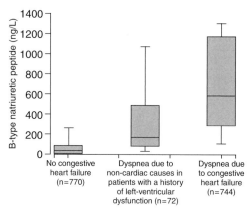

FIGURE 6-6 ■ B-type natriuretic peptide (BNP) concentration in patients with dyspnea. The bars represent the highest and lowest values of BNP measured (ng/L) in patients with no evidence of congestive heart failure versus dyspnea secondary to noncardiac causes (but with history of left ventricular dysfunction) and dyspnea secondary to congestive heart failure. (From de Lemos JA, McGuire DK, Drazner MH, et al: *B-type natriuretic peptide in cardiovascular disease. Lancet* 2003;362:316-322.)

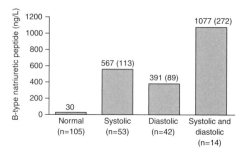

FIGURE 6-7 ■ B-type natriuretic peptide (BNP) concentration in patients with systolic dysfunction, diastolic dysfunction, or both. The bars represent the highest and lowest values of BNP measured (ng/L) in patients with systolic dysfunction, diastolic dysfunction, or both. The values above the bars are the mean values for each group. The patients with systolic and diastolic dysfunction have the highest mean BNP levels. (From de Lemos JA, McGuire DK, Drazner MH, et al: *B-type natriuretic peptide in cardiovascular disease. Lancet* 2003;362:316-322.)

of left ventricular dysfunction, but BNP measured 1 to 4 days after a transmural infarction also can be associated with increased mortality risks independent of left ventricular function.[114-116] Elevated BNP also has been evaluated in the setting of non–ST-segment elevation myocardial infarction and found to be important in identifying patients at higher risks of death and heart failure.[117] Myocardial ischemia[118] and unstable angina[119] can lead to increased BNP levels. BNP levels are increased in many adult patients with essential hypertension and left ventricular hypertrophy.[120] Patients requiring a ventricular assist device have been assessed for changes in BNP levels and have been found to have lower levels after a ventricular assist device was instituted.[121] Elevated levels of BNP also have been noted in patients who have undergone orthotopic heart transplantation. These elevated levels may be evidence of functional adaptation of the transplanted heart.[122] Finally, the measurement of BNP has been proposed as a biochemical screening tool for left ventricular systolic dysfunction in the older adult population,[123] but this has not been widely accepted.

In healthy infants and children, the plasma concentration of BNP increases to a peak immediately after birth, then slowly reaches adult levels by 3 months of age.[124] Shortly after birth, the transitional circulatory changes lead to an increase in left ventricular volume and induce synthesis of BNP. Plasma NT-proBNP has been evaluated in people ranging from neonates to young adults in healthy populations and heart failure patients. In the control population, the normal range of NT-proBNP was 150 to 430 fmol/mL. Measurement of NT-proBNP in children with heart failure revealed elevations above the control levels and reflected the severity of symptoms.[125] In addition, males without cardiac disease have higher serum BNP levels than females.[126] BNP also has been shown to be significantly higher in the elderly population compared with the middle-aged population without heart disease.[127] There does not seem to be circadian rhythm variation of BNP.[126]

BNP has been evaluated in other disease-specific settings. Levels of BNP have been measured in patients with Duchenne muscular dystrophy.[128] In addition, Kawamura and Wago[129] evaluated BNP levels as a useful biochemical marker in the setting of Kawasaki disease and found levels to be elevated in the acute phase and decreased in the convalescent phase. Their results showed that BNP values greater than 50 pg/mL correlated with abnormal ECG changes that are believed to be markers of myocarditis. Lastly, an assessment of ANP and BNP levels before transcatheter closure of atrial septal defects revealed elevated levels before intervention, but a decrease to baseline of control patients was noted after successful closure of the defect.[130]

Plasma BNP also has been used as a prognosticator in the setting of primary pulmonary hypertension and other right ventricular dysfunctional states.[131] BNP levels above normal and, in particular, an increase of levels during follow-up of these patients may be associated with increased mortality. BNP also has been shown to increase in proportion to the degree of right ventricular dysfunction in the setting of pulmonary hypertension[132] and has been used by these same investigators as a marker for the efficacy of vasodilator therapy in patients with primary pulmonary hypertension. Elevation of BNP with right ventricular failure does not seem to be less than that observed with left ventricular systolic or diastolic failure.

In patients with hypertrophic cardiomyopathy, Hasegawa and coworkers[133] showed that there was an elevated serum BNP level compared with normal patients; BNP expression at the level of the ventricular myocyte may be augmented in response to obstruction and diastolic dysfunction. Hayakawa and associates[134] evaluated ANP and BNP levels in pediatric cancer patients undergoing doxorubicin therapy and showed that levels were noted to be significantly elevated in patients with left ventricular dysfunction. It was postulated that serum measurements of ANP and BNP may allow for earlier detection of cardiac damage secondary to chemotherapeutic drugs.

Limited data exist in the setting of surgical intervention in patients with congenital heart disease. There are isolated case reports and small-volume studies that have evaluated BNP values in patients with single-ventricle physiology.[135] These studies suggest that the volume overload to which the heart is subjected with the first palliative operation (i.e., Blalock-Taussig shunt) results in increased production of BNP; the ventricular unloading that occurs with the second palliative procedure (i.e., Glenn anastomosis) results in BNP values in the normal range. Similar results were seen in patients who underwent total cavopulmonary connection (i.e., Fontan operation). Yoshimura and colleagues[136] documented that in the early postoperative period, ANP and BNP levels were significantly lower in the Fontan group, suggesting suppression of the release of these hormones in total cavopulmonary connections. BNP and aldosterone were shown to be increased in the setting of cardiac surgery requiring cardiopulmonary bypass in children and to decrease from preoperative levels[137] after intervention.

The appropriate use of BNP as a valuable diagnostic and clinical tool relies on the rapidity and sensitivity of the bioassay. A bedside assay for the evaluation of BNP levels received approval in 2000 by the U.S. Food and Drug Administration and was shown to be effective in diagnosing heart failure in patients with acute dyspnea in the Breathing Not Properly Multinational Study.[138,139] A fully automated test for quantification of the NT-proBNP received U.S. Food and Drug Administration approval in 2002; its precise roles in assessing and prognosticating heart failure in adults and children with heart failure remain to be elucidated.

C-Type Natriuretic Peptide

The third member of the natriuretic peptide family was first identified in 1990. Similar to BNP, CNP was isolated from pig brain.[140] CNP is structurally different from ANP and BNP and seems to be expressed to a larger extent in the central nervous system and other vascular structures than in the heart; it is more of a local mediator.[141] Two separate CNP molecules have been identified—a 22-amino acid protein and a 53-amino acid protein. Both molecules are derived from the single pro-C-type precursor, but the 22-amino acid CNP is more potent than the 53-amino acid CNP and is present in a higher concentration in the central nervous system, anterior pituitary, kidney, vascular endothelial cells, and plasma.[4]

This B-type receptor is found throughout the central nervous system and interacts with CNP.[142] The receptor predominates in the region of the hypothalamus and other rostral brain regions, where natriuretic peptides inhibit secretion of arginine vasopressin and stimulate sympathetic tone. In contrast with ANP and BNP, CNP does not seem to have significant function as a circulating hormone. It acts locally in the vasculature as a vasodilatory agent and inhibitor of vascular cell proliferation and in the central nervous system, where it has numerous functions.[143,144] The levels of CNP have been measured in the setting of heart failure and found to be no different compared with healthy controls.[145]

INFLAMMATORY CASCADE BIOMARKERS

The inflammatory cascade and its components in heart failure are discussed in more detail in Chapter 3; the various substances in the cascade that are considered potential biomarkers in this milieu are reviewed briefly here. Cytokines that typically are associated with roles in the pathophysiology of heart failure are interleukin (IL)-6 and tumor necrosis factor–α (TNF-α).[146] The implications of other markers, such as ET-1, are becoming more evident, however. Elevated levels of cytokines are associated with a poor prognosis in heart failure[147] and are known to have adverse effects on the myocardial structure and function.[148,149] All of these substances are discussed individually.

Kinins

Kinin peptides are potent vasodilators and have a broad spectrum of activity, including the promotion of diuresis and natriuresis; these agents also protect against ischemia-reperfusion injury by decreasing endothelial adherence of leukocytes. This capability leads to attenuation of disruption of the microvascular barrier, decrease in postischemic leukocyte adherence, and reduction in myocardial injury patterns.[150] In humans, the plasma and tissue kallikrein-kinin system generates **bradykinin** and **kallidin** peptides.[151]

Kinins act via two kinin receptors, type 1 (B1) and type 2 (B2). The B2 receptor typically predominates, whereas B1 receptors are induced by tissue injury.[152] There is even evidence in humans that kinin peptides play a role in the regulation of coronary vascular tone.[153] Kinins also seem to mediate the hypotensive effects of ACE therapy.[154] Kinins play an important role in general biologic processes, such as neutrophil chemotaxis, pain, inflammation, vasodilation, and vascular permeability.[150]

Levels of kinin peptides have been measured in heart failure patients on maximally tolerated ACE therapy who did not have elevated levels of bradykinin or kallidin, although suppression of the kallikrein-kinin system in the face of ACE inhibitor therapy suggests that the activity of the kallikrein-kinin system may be suppressed in heart failure. This suggestion is confirmed further by tissue kallikrein knockout mice, which develop cardiac structural and functional abnormalities.[155]

Endothelin-1

The ETs are peptides released from endothelial cells that possess potent vasoconstrictor properties. The main ET is **ET-1**, which is synthesized via ET-converting enzyme from its precursor, but ET-2 and ET-3 also have roles. ET-1 is a potent cardiac peptide that has been shown to cause sodium retention, vasoconstriction, and mitogenesis. The actions of ET-1 are mediated through receptors ET(A) and ET(B). ET(A) receptors are located on vascular smooth muscles, and ET(B) receptors are located on the endothelium. ET-1 seems to be important in the maintenance of basal vascular tone and blood pressure via the ET(A) receptors, although activation of ET(B) receptors stimulates production of nitric oxide, which may regulate vascular tone by opposing vasoconstriction.[156]

ET-1 is shown to be elevated in the setting of congestive heart failure, especially when the pulmonary vascular resistance is elevated. The main source of ET-1 in heart failure is the pulmonary vascular bed. It is hypothesized to play roles in mediating elevation of cardiac filling pressures and progression of circulatory failure, and high levels of ET-1 are associated with increased mortality in patients with heart failure.[157] In addition, the production of TNF-α can be stimulated by ET-1.[158] ET-1 also may play a role in the progression of pulmonary hypertension in heart failure.[159,160] The severity of pulmonary hypertension is reduced by ET receptor antagonists.[161] These agents also have resulted in improvement in left ventricular performance and a reduction in systemic vascular resistance in patients with heart failure.[162]

It has been postulated that part of the natriuretic effects of the natriuretic peptides (ANP and BNP) as described earlier may be due to the suppression of ET-1 production.[163] The effects of ANP and BNP on ET-1 levels are thought to be mediated through an increase in GMP caused by these cardiac hormones.[4] This postulation was clinically delineated in the Prospective

Randomized Evaluation of Cardiac Ectopy with Dobutamine or Nesiritide Therapy (PRECEDENT) trial substudy group, which showed that short-term infusion of BNP in decompensated heart failure patients caused a reduction in plasma ET-1 levels.[164]

Tumor Necrosis Factor–α

TNF-α (previously known as *cachectin*[165]) was discovered in 1975 and has a central role in the systemic inflammatory response. Plasma concentrations of TNF-α have been documented to be elevated in patients with heart failure.[166] In addition, TNF-α results in depression of myocardial function, and the administration of intravenous TNF-α blockers improved cardiac function in adults with sepsis.[167] TNF-α has been shown to increase nitric oxide synthase activity in vascular smooth muscle.

Serum levels of TNF-α have been shown to be elevated in the patients with heart failure, and the increase in plasma levels has been shown to correlate with the severity of heart failure.[147,166] TNF-α, produced in the failing heart owing to an increase in ventricular wall stress, contributes to the progression of the disease.[168-170] TNF-α has known negative inotropic effects,[171] and in mice with elevated levels of TNF-α, systolic dysfunction develops.[172] TNF-α also has been found to cause changes in the myocardium, including interstitial fibrosis, ventricular remodeling, and apoptosis.[173,174] Patients with high levels of TNF-α are more cachectic and have more advanced heart failure than patients with heart failure and lower TNF-α levels.[175] Patients with heart failure may develop a wasting syndrome known as *cardiac cachexia,* which is associated with a poorer prognosis[176]; TNF-α levels are markedly increased in patients with cardiac cachexia.[177-179] Apoptosis of skeletal muscle frequently is found in patients with heart failure and is associated with decreased exercise capacity.[180]

TNF-α can function as an independent predictor of depressed heart rate variability in patients with heart failure.[181] There are two receptors for TNF-α **(TNFRs 1 and 2)**, and these can be detected as soluble forms. There is a strong correlation between elevated TNFR levels and 30-day mortality in severe heart failure.[182] The levels of TNFR seem to vary over time to a lesser degree than TNF-α or IL-6 levels.[183] Treatment with the TNF-α blocker etanercept has been shown to lead to a dose-dependent improvement in left ventricular ejection fraction and left ventricular remodeling with a possible trend toward improvement in patient functional status.[184] The use of infliximab, a recombinant immunoglobulin human-murine chimeric monoclonal antibody that binds and neutralizes soluble TNF-α, did not improve clinical conditions in patients with moderate-to-severe heart failure.[185]

Arginine Vasopressin

Arginine vasopressin, a hormone secreted by the pituitary gland, is involved in the regulation of plasma osmolality and free water clearance. Similar to the other vasoconstrictors discussed previously, vasopressin levels are elevated in the setting of heart failure.[186,187] There are two types of vasopressin receptors—V1 and V2. In animal studies, the selective blockade of the V1 receptor resulted in an increase in cardiac output without any significant changes in hormone levels or electrolytes; the selective blockade of the V2 receptor resulted, however, in increased plasma vasopressin levels, sodium, and plasma renin activity without changes in cardiac output.[188]

Interleukins

ILs are inflammatory cytokines; they have been studied extensively in adults, and an important role in the pathogenesis of heart failure has been found.[189] **IL-1**, produced by a variety of cells with an important role in the systemic immune response, has been shown to depress myocardial contractility by stimulating nitric oxide synthase.[190] IL-1 also inhibits cardiac myocyte β-adrenergic responsiveness.[191] IL-1 has been shown to regulate growth and expression of certain genes in cardiac myocytes and has been shown to stimulate hypertrophy and re-expression of a fetal gene program[192,193]; these two effects have been linked to apoptosis of myocardial cells. This effect may be mediated through the molecule nitric oxide (see Chapter 3).[194] The mRNA of IL-1 has been shown to be present in the coronaries of patients with dilated cardiomyopathy and in much smaller concentrations in the coronaries of patients with ischemic heart disease.[190]

The levels of the **IL-6** also are increased in the setting of heart failure[166,168] and associated with a worse New York Heart Association class,[195,196] increased lengths of hospital stays for heart failure decompensation, and poorer left ventricular function in the adult population.[147,197-199] The findings of the SOLVD trial[147] were not consistent, however, with these outcomes.

PHARMACOLOGIC THERAPY AND BIOMARKERS

This section briefly reviews the new pharmacologic agents that counter the neurohormonal cascade and their effects on various biomarkers. More detailed discussions occur in other chapters.

Val-HeFT[200] was the largest neurohormone study in patients with symptomatic heart failure. BNP and norepinephrine were measured at baseline and at 4, 12, and 24 months after randomization with either **valsartan** (angiotensin II receptor blocker) or placebo. Valsartan caused sustained reduction in BNP levels and attenuated norepinephrine increase, and this correlated with clinical effects of decreased combined morbidity and mortality, amelioration in symptoms, improvement in left ventricular function and size, and reduced hospitalizations secondary to heart failure. The Val-HeFT II trial showed that **enalapril** treatment resulted in reduced plasma norepinephrine levels compared with an isosorbide dinitrate/hydralazine control group.[33] In Val-HeFT III, the use of **felodipine**, a calcium channel blocker, resulted in a modest reduction in ANP levels compared with therapy with placebo.[201] In the Randomized Evaluation of Strategies for Left Ventricular Dysfunction (RESOLVD) trial, treatment with **candesartan** (angiotensin II receptor blocker) combined with the ACE inhibitor enalapril resulted in a reduction of BNP levels of approximately 30 pg/mL over more than 40 weeks.[202]

Extensive data also exist regarding the use of β blockade in the setting of heart failure. The Cardiac Insufficiency Bisoprolol Study II (CIBIS-II) trial and Metoprolol CR/XL Randomised Intervention Trial in Congestive Heart Failure (MERIT-HF) study group showed favorable long-term effects with the use of **bisoprolol** and **metoprolol**.[203,204] These favorable effects were delineated further by Packer and associates[205] in their evaluation using the β-blocker **carvedilol**. All of these studies documented decreases in markers of activation of the sympathetic nervous system via drug therapy, resulting in improvements in long-term morbidity and mortality (see Chapter 36).

Vasopressin infusions have been used in the setting of heart failure. At our own institution, we have used infusions of calcium and low-dose vasopressin to improve renal perfusion and urine output in patients with medically refractory heart failure. This regimen is controversial, however, because many adult studies show the potential benefits of vasopressin antagonism, as shown in this chapter.

Given the effects of BNP, it has been postulated that the infusion of synthetic BNP may be beneficial in the treatment of decompensated heart failure. **Nesiritide**, an intravenous form of recombinant human BNP from *Escherichia coli* (Natrecor, Scios, Inc, Sunnyvale, Calif), is the first in a new class of drugs for the treatment of decompensated congestive heart failure. Systemic infusion of nesiritide in patients with congestive heart failure results in beneficial hemodynamic actions, including arterial and venous dilation (cGMP mediated) and coronary vasodilation, suppression of the RAS and sympathetic nervous system, and enhanced sodium excretion.[206-208]

The Nesiritide Study Group investigators evaluated the efficacy of synthetic BNP infusion and compared the use of nesiritide with standard intravenous agents in a controlled study design.[209] In the efficacy portion of the trial, patients were randomly assigned to placebo, low-dose nesiritide after bolus infusion (0.3 μg/kg bolus with an infusion of 0.015 μg/kg/min), or high-dose nesiritide after high-dose bolus infusion (0.6 μg/kg bolus with an infusion of 0.03 μg/kg/min). Synthetic BNP infusion resulted in dose-dependent decreases in right atrial pressure, systolic blood pressure, systemic vascular resistance, and pulmonary capillary wedge pressure. There also was an increase in the cardiac

index and no statistically significant change in heart rate. Overall clinical status as assessed by the patient was improved in 60% and 67% of the patients in the low-dose and high-dose groups, respectively, compared with 14% in the placebo group ($P < .001$ for both). Also, there was a statistically significant improvement in the global patient status as per the physician. Patients noted a marked improvement in dyspnea symptoms of 56% and 50% in the low-dose and high-dose groups ($P < .001$ for both groups), respectively. Similarly, fatigue symptoms were markedly decreased in both infusion groups compared with the placebo group. There was a statistically significant decrease in plasma aldosterone levels in both groups, but no significant changes in plasma norepinephrine levels. Urine output also was more improved in the synthetic BNP groups over the duration of the study. Intravenous diuretics were given to fewer patients in the nesiritide groups ($P < .001$ for both).

Nesiritide also has been compared with other pharmacologic therapies. In adults with a history of chronic heart failure and a need for intravenous therapy of decompensated heart failure, nesiritide resulted in a lower 6-month mortality and a trend toward decreased readmissions with low-dose and high-dose infusions.[210] The PRECEDENT trial evaluated nesiritide versus dobutamine in the treatment of acutely decompensated heart failure and found that although dobutamine had substantial chronotropic and proarrhythmic effects, nesiritide reduced ventricular ectopy and did not increase heart rate. In the Vasodilation in the Management of Acute Congestive Heart Failure (VMAC) trial, intravenous synthetic BNP was compared with placebo and intravenous nitroglycerin in the setting of decompensated heart failure. The investigators concluded that nesiritide improved hemodynamics (as measured by pulmonary capillary wedge pressure over 3-hour and 24-hour periods) more effectively than nitroglycerin.[211] Nesiritide also has been studied as a therapy for medically unresponsive pulmonary hypertension. In an isolated case report, nesiritide was given to a patient who was receiving maximal doses of dobutamine, milrinone, and nitroprusside. With the addition of nesiritide, pulmonary artery pressures, transpulmonary gradient, and pulmonary vascular resistance decreased markedly.[212]

Evaluation of the use of aldosterone blockers has been performed in the past, with the most common therapy in use being **spironolactone**. In the Randomized Aldactone Evaluation Study (RALES), the addition of spironolactone reduced mortality by 30% in patients with New York Heart Association class III or IV heart failure who already were being treated with diuretics, digoxin, and ACE inhibitors.[213] The mechanism resulting in these improved outcomes has not been fully elucidated, but one hypothesis is that spironolactone may prevent sudden death by increasing serum potassium or altering uptake of norepinephrine.[214] A substudy of the RALES investigation implicated a connection between the antifibrotic effects of spironolactone and the mortality benefits of therapy.[215] Newer aldosterone blocking agents are being developed. The most notable widely known agent is **eplerenone**. Eplerenone is an aldosterone blocker that selectively blocks the mineralocorticoid receptor, but not the glucocorticoid, progesterone, or androgen receptors. The Eplerenone Post-Acute Myocardial Infarction Heart Failure Efficacy and Survival Study (EPHESUS) evaluated the use of eplerenone versus placebo in patients with heart failure receiving optimal medical therapy.[216] The addition of eplerenone reduced morbidity and mortality among patients with left ventricular dysfunction and heart failure in the setting of myocardial infarction.

Vasopressin antagonism also has been postulated as a possible therapy for chronic heart failure. The ADVANCE trial (A Dose evaluation of a Vasopressin Antagonist in CHF patients undergoing Exercise) evaluated the effect of **conivaptan**, a vasopressin antagonist, on functional capacity in heart failure.[217] Currently other clinical trials are under way that are evaluating the utility of vasopressin antagonist therapy in the treatment of heart failure.[217,218]

Pediatric Data

There are few data on pharmacologic agents and their influence on biomarkers in pediatric patients. We are engaged in a pediatric study at the Texas Children's Hospital in which patients ages 2 to 18 years with New York Heart Association class III or IV heart failure are being treated with nesiritide as first-line therapy, with measurement of biomarkers as part of the protocol. Plasma levels of angiotensin II, renin, aldosterone, vasopressin, ANP, and BNP have been shown to be elevated in patients who had successfully undergone total cavopulmonary connection and bidirectional Glenn procedures. These levels were found to be elevated for years after the surgeries, but lower levels were observed over time.[219] An abnormal exercise capacity and elevated neurohormonal activity have been documented in patients after the Fontan operation.[220,221] A study by Ohuchi and colleagues[222] evaluated cardiac autonomic nervous activity in patients who underwent the Fontan operation. They concluded that in addition to damage secondary to the procedure, the Fontan operation may impair cardiac autonomic activity. ANP and BNP levels also have been measured in patients who have undergone complete surgical repair of tetralogy of Fallot receiving dobutamine. Levels were noted to be elevated before the infusion, but showed a decrease in most patients after infusion, correlating with right-sided pressure and volume overload.[223]

CURRENT STATUS AND FUTURE TRENDS

The implications of biomarker monitoring also must be assessed from the perspective of suppression. If elevated levels of markers such as BNP and norepinephrine have been shown as independent indicators of outcome in adult heart failure patients, perhaps modulation of these markers would have a direct or indirect impact on long-term morbidity and mortality. Additional information is needed in comparative trials of the recombinant BNP versus other cardiotonic medications, such as dobutamine and milrinone, especially in children with decompensated heart failure.

The future of neurohormones as markers and as therapeutic modalities in the pediatric population remains a very early work in progress. More data will be reported in this area of investigation in the near future, but the amount of information currently available is limited. Much of the information presented in this chapter is obtained from the adult literature.[224] Caution must be used in transposing the adult data on to the pediatric heart failure population.

The neurohormonal markers are mere markers, and it is unrealistic to expect any single biomarker to be ideal in the management of heart failure patients, much less serve as a surrogate for clinical treatment efficacy. It is not unreasonable, however, to think that the use of multiple biomarkers could markedly alter current therapeutic strategies. The future of these markers not only may guide initial screening or treatment approaches, but also aid in optimization of therapy in pediatric patients. In addition to the biomarkers discussed in this chapter, there are still new biomarkers being investigated.[225,227]

Key Concepts

■ In a counterregulatory system, the cardiac hormones ANP and BNP have beneficial actions, such as vasodilation and natriuresis.

■ The utility of biochemical markers such as the natriuretic peptides in the overall management of heart failure has become progressively more evident in research and clinical medicine.

■ Heart failure causes a baroreceptor-mediated increase in sympathetic tone that results in several pathophysiologic effects, including tachycardia, increased myocardial contractility, and arterial and venous vasoconstriction. The increase in sympathetic tone is manifested by increased plasma levels of epinephrine and norepinephrine, which mediate the aforementioned pathophysiologic effects.

■ Increased levels of local and circulating norepinephrine as a result of heart failure may lead to myocyte hypertrophy via a dual mechanism of direct stimulation of α-adrenergic and β-adrenergic receptors and indirect activation of the RAS.

■ In patients with progressive heart failure, there are marked increases in circulating levels of the RAS components renin, angiotensin II, and aldosterone, all of which can be used as biomarkers for heart failure.

■ Angiotensin II is a potent peripheral vasoconstrictor and causes vasoconstriction via two mechanisms: by increasing sympathetic tone and arginine vasopressin release and by stimulating angiotensin II type 1 receptors in the vasculature.

- The combined central and local RAS create a complex interplay of modulating factors that regulate the cardiovascular system.
- Elevated levels of aldosterone in humans are associated with endothelial dysfunction, myocardial infarction, left ventricular hypertrophy, and death.
- The three major natriuretic peptides, all of which share a 17-amino acid ring, have a precursor hormone that is encoded by a separate gene with the regulation of each protein being unique. These peptide hormones act on various organs via guanylate cyclase–linked membrane receptors that produce natriuresis, diuresis, and vasodilation of arterial and venous vessels.
- ANP is released from the atria, whereas BNP is released from the ventricles; CNP is derived from the central nervous system and the vascular endothelium.
- Natriuretic peptides interact with high-affinity receptors on the surface of target cells. Three different receptors (A, B, and C) have been identified in mammalian tissue. Receptors A and B are linked to cascades mediated by the cGMP signaling system, which mediate the vasodilatory and natriuretic effects of these peptides. The C receptor is responsible for the clearance of natriuretic peptides.
- Levels of ANP and the prohormone N-ANP in the setting of heart failure and volume overload are elevated because increased tension and resultant stretch on the wall of the atria lead to activation of the cardiac hormonal system.
- BNP is a cardiac neurohormone produced from the cardiac ventricles in pathophysiologic states, such as systolic or diastolic function, increased left ventricular mass, and low ejection fraction.
- In contrast with ANP and BNP, CNP does not seem to have significant function as a circulating hormone. It acts locally in the vasculature as a vasodilatory agent and inhibitor of vascular cell proliferation.
- Cytokines that typically are associated with roles in the pathophysiology of heart failure are IL-6 and TNF-α. The implications of other markers, such as ET-1, are becoming more evident.
- ET-1 is shown to be elevated in the setting of congestive heart failure, especially when the pulmonary vascular resistance is elevated. The main source of ET-1 in heart failure is the pulmonary vascular bed. It has been postulated that part of the natriuretic effects of the natriuretic peptides (ANP and BNP) as described here may be due to the suppression of ET-1 production.
- Serum levels of TNF-α have been shown to be elevated in patients with heart failure. TNF-α has known negative inotropic effects, and TNF-α has been found to cause changes in the myocardium, including interstitial fibrosis, ventricular remodeling, and apoptosis.
- ILs are inflammatory cytokines; they have been studied extensively in adults, and an important role in the pathogenesis of heart failure has been found.
- Systemic infusion of nesiritide in patients with congestive heart failure results in beneficial hemodynamic actions; these include arterial and venous dilation (cGMP mediated) and coronary vasodilation, suppression of the RAS and sympathetic nervous system, and enhanced sodium excretion.

REFERENCES

1. Packer M: The neurohormonal hypothesis: A theory to explain the mechanism of disease progression in heart failure. J Am Coll Cardiol 1992;20:248-254.
2. de Bold AJ: Atrial natriuretic factor: A hormone produced by the heart. Science 1985;230:767-770.
3. Wilkins MR, Redondo J, Brown LA: The natriuretic-peptide family. Lancet 1997;349:1307-1310.
4. Levin ER, Gardner DG, Samson WK: Natriuretic peptides. N Engl J Med 1998;339:321-328.
5. Bozkurt B, Mann DL: Use of biomarkers in the management of heart failure: Are we there yet? Circulation 2003;107:1231-1233.
6. Schrier RW, Abraham WT: Hormones and hemodynamics in heart failure. N Engl J Med 1999;341:577-585.
7. Jiang JP, Downing SE: Catecholamine cardiomyopathy: Review and analysis of pathogenetic mechanisms. Yale J Biol Med 1990; 63:581-591.
8. Mann DL, Kent RL, Parsons B, Cooper GT: Adrenergic effects on the biology of the adult mammalian cardiocyte. Circulation 1992;85: 790-804.
9. Cohn JN, Levine TB, Olivari MT, et al: Plasma norepinephrine as a guide to prognosis in patients with chronic congestive heart failure. N Engl J Med 1984;311:819-823.
10. DiBona GF, Herman PJ, Sawin LL: Neural control of renal function in edema-forming states. Am J Physiol 1988;254:R1017-R1024.
11. Eisenhofer G, Friberg P, Rundqvist B, et al: Cardiac sympathetic nerve function in congestive heart failure. Circulation 1996;93:1667-1676.
12. Anand IS, Fisher LD, Chiang YT, et al: Changes in brain natriuretic peptide and norepinephrine over time and mortality and morbidity in the Valsartan Heart Failure Trial (Val-HeFT). Circulation 2003;107:1278-1283.
13. Rundqvist B, Elam M, Eisenhofer G, Friberg P: Normalization of total body and regional sympathetic hyperactivity in heart failure after heart transplantation. J Heart Lung Transplant 1996;15:516-526.
14. Swedberg K, Bristow MR, Cohn JN, et al: Effects of sustained-release moxonidine, an imidazoline agonist, on plasma norepinephrine in patients with chronic heart failure. Circulation 2002;105:1797-1803.
15. Laragh JH: Hormones and the pathogenesis of congestive heart failure: Vasopressin, aldosterone, and angiotensin II: Further evidence for renal-adrenal interaction from studies in hypertension and in cirrhosis. Circulation 1962;25:1015-1023.
16. Genest J, Granger P, De Champlain J, Boucher R: Endocrine factors in congestive heart failure. Am J Cardiol 1968;22:35-42.
17. Anand IS, Ferrari R, Kalra GS, et al: Edema of cardiac origin: Studies of body water and sodium, renal function, hemodynamic indexes, and plasma hormones in untreated congestive cardiac failure. Circulation 1989;80:299-305.
18. Francis GS, Benedict C, Johnstone DE, et al: Comparison of neuroendocrine activation in patients with left ventricular dysfunction with and without congestive heart failure: A substudy of the Studies of Left Ventricular Dysfunction (SOLVD). Circulation 1990; 82:1724-1729.

19. Timmermans PB, Wong PC, Chiu AT, et al: Angiotensin II receptors and angiotensin II receptor antagonists. Pharmacol Rev 1993; 45:205-251.

20. Sayeski PP, Bernstein KE: Signal transduction mechanisms of the angiotensin II type AT(1)-receptor: Looking beyond the heterotrimeric G protein paradigm. J Renin Angiotensin Aldosterone Syst 2001;2:4-10.

21. Nguyen G, Delarue F, Burckle C, et al: Pivotal role of the renin/prorenin receptor in angiotensin II production and cellular responses to renin. J Clin Invest 2002;109:1417-1427.

22. Lindpaintner K, Ganten D: The cardiac renin-angiotensin system: An appraisal of present experimental and clinical evidence. Circ Res 1991;68:905-921.

23. Grinstead WC, Young JB: The myocardial renin-angiotensin system: Existence, importance, and clinical implications. Am Heart J 1992;123:1039-1045.

24. Bader M, Peters J, Baltatu O, et al: Tissue renin-angiotensin systems: New insights from experimental animal models in hypertension research. J Mol Med 2001;79:76-102.

25. Navar LG, Imig JD, Zou L, Wang CT: Intrarenal production of angiotensin II. Semin Nephrol 1997;17:412-422.

26. Costa M, Majewski H: Facilitation of noradrenaline release from sympathetic nerves through activation of ACTH receptors, beta-adrenoceptors and angiotensin II receptors. Br J Pharmacol 1988;95:993-1001.

27. Liao Y, Husain A: The chymase-angiotensin system in humans: Biochemistry, molecular biology and potential role in cardiovascular diseases. Can J Cardiol 1995;11(Suppl F):13F-19F.

28. Urata H, Ganten D: Cardiac angiotensin II formation: The angiotensin-I converting enzyme and human chymase. Eur Heart J 1993;14(Suppl I):177-182.

29. Grise C, Boucher R, Thibault G, Genest J: Formation of angiotensin II by tonin from partially purified human angiotensinogen. Can J Biochem 1981;59:250-255.

30. Schrier RW: Pathogenesis of sodium and water retention in high-output and low-output cardiac failure, nephrotic syndrome, cirrhosis, and pregnancy (1). N Engl J Med 1988;319:1065-1072.

31. Schrier RW: Body fluid volume regulation in health and disease: A unifying hypothesis. Ann Intern Med 1990;113:155-159.

32. Tan LB, Jalil JE, Pick R, et al: Cardiac myocyte necrosis induced by angiotensin II. Circ Res 1991;69:1185-1195.

33. Francis GS, Cohn JN, Johnson G, et al: Plasma norepinephrine, plasma renin activity, and congestive heart failure: Relations to survival and the effects of therapy in V-HeFT II. The V-HeFT VA Cooperative Studies Group. Circulation 1993;87:VI40-VI48.

34. Benedict CR, Francis GS, Shelton B, et al: Effect of long-term enalapril therapy on neurohormones in patients with left ventricular dysfunction. SOLVD Investigators. Am J Cardiol 1995;75:1151-1157.

35. Arriza JL, Weinberger C, Cerelli G, et al: Cloning of human mineralocorticoid receptor complementary DNA: Structural and functional kinship with the glucocorticoid receptor. Science 1987;237:268-275.

36. Fejes-Toth G, Pearce D, Naray-Fejes-Toth A: Subcellular localization of mineralocorticoid receptors in living cells: Effects of receptor agonists and antagonists. Proc Natl Acad Sci U S A 1998; 95:2973-2978.

37. Bhargava A, Fullerton MJ, Myles K, et al: The serum- and glucocorticoid-induced kinase is a physiological mediator of aldosterone action. Endocrinology 2001;142:1587-1594.

38. Takeda Y, Miyamori I, Yoneda T, et al: Regulation of aldosterone synthase in human vascular endothelial cells by angiotensin II and adrenocorticotropin. J Clin Endocrinol Metab 1996;81: 2797-2800.

39. Hatakeyama H, Miyamori I, Fujita T, et al: Vascular aldosterone: Biosynthesis and a link to angiotensin II-induced hypertrophy of vascular smooth muscle cells. J Biol Chem 1994;269:24316-24320.

40. Gomez-Sanchez CE, Zhou MY, Cozza EN, et al: Aldosterone biosynthesis in the rat brain. Endocrinology 1997;138:3369-3373.

41. Patel PD, Sherman TG, Goldman DJ, Watson SJ: Molecular cloning of a mineralocorticoid (type I) receptor complementary DNA from rat hippocampus. Mol Endocrinol 1989;3:1877-1885.

42. Lombes M, Alfaidy N, Eugene E, et al: Prerequisite for cardiac aldosterone action: Mineralocorticoid receptor and 11 beta-hydroxysteroid dehydrogenase in the human heart. Circulation 1995;92:175-182.

43. Takeda Y, Miyamori I, Inaba S, et al: Vascular aldosterone in genetically hypertensive rats. Hypertension 1997;29:45-48.

44. Mizuno Y, Yoshimura M, Yasue H, et al: Aldosterone production is activated in failing ventricle in humans. Circulation 2001;103:72-77.

45. Brilla CG, Weber KT: Mineralocorticoid excess, dietary sodium, and myocardial fibrosis. J Lab Clin Med 1992;120:893-901.

46. Young M, Head G, Funder J: Determinants of cardiac fibrosis in experimental hypermineralocorticoid states. Am J Physiol 1995; 269:E657-E662.

47. Robert V, Silvestre JS, Charlemagne D, et al: Biological determinants of aldosterone-induced cardiac fibrosis in rats. Hypertension 1995;26:971-978.

48. Brilla CG, Zhou G, Matsubara L, Weber KT: Collagen metabolism in cultured adult rat cardiac fibroblasts: Response to angiotensin II and aldosterone. J Mol Cell Cardiol 1994;26:809-820.

49. Fullerton MJ, Funder JW: Aldosterone and cardiac fibrosis: In vitro studies. Cardiovasc Res 1994;28:1863-1867.

50. Brown NJ, Kim KS, Chen YQ, et al: Synergistic effect of adrenal steroids and angiotensin II on plasminogen activator inhibitor-1 production. J Clin Endocrinol Metab 2000;85:336-344.

51. Loskutoff DJ, Quigley JP: PAI-1, fibrosis, and the elusive provisional fibrin matrix. J Clin Invest 2000;106:1441-1443.

52. Rocha R, Martin-Berger CL, Yang P, et al: Selective aldosterone blockade prevents angiotensin II/salt-induced vascular inflammation in the rat heart. Endocrinology 2002;143:4828-4836.

53. Taddei S, Virdis A, Mattei P, Salvetti A: Vasodilation to acetylcholine in primary and secondary forms of human hypertension. Hypertension 1993;21:929-933.

54. Arora RB: Role of aldosterone in myocardial infarction. Ann N Y Acad Sci 1965;118:539-554.

55. Swedberg K, Eneroth P, Kjekshus J, Wilhelmsen L: Hormones regulating cardiovascular function in patients with severe congestive heart failure and their relation to mortality. CONSENSUS Trial Study Group. Circulation 1990;82:1730-1736.

56. Kisch B: Electron microscopy of the atrium of the heart: I. Guinea pig. Exp Med Surg 1956;14:99-112.

57. de Bold AJ: Atrial natriuretic factor of the rat heart: Studies on isolation and properties. Proc Soc Exp Biol Med 1982;170: 133-138.

58. Kangawa K, Matsuo H: Purification and complete amino acid sequence of alpha-human atrial natriuretic polypeptide (alpha-hANP). Biochem Biophys Res Commun 1984;118:131-139.

59. Cheung BM, Kumana CR: Natriuretic peptides—relevance in cardiovascular disease. JAMA 1998;280:1983-1984.

60. Koller KJ, Goeddel DV: Molecular biology of the natriuretic peptides and their receptors. Circulation 1992;86:1081-1088.

61. Maack T, Suzuki M, Almeida FA, et al: Physiological role of silent receptors of atrial natriuretic factor. Science 1987;238:675-678.

62. Charles CJ, Espiner EA, Nicholls MG, et al: Clearance receptors and endopeptidase 24.11: Equal role in natriuretic peptide metabolism in conscious sheep. Am J Physiol 1996;271:R373-R380.

63. Greenberg RN, Hill M, Crytzer J, et al: Comparison of effects of uroguanylin, guanylin, and Escherichia coli heat-stable enterotoxin STa in mouse intestine and kidney: Evidence that uroguanylin is an intestinal natriuretic hormone. J Invest Med 1997;45:276-282.

64. Ruskoaho H: Cardiac hormones as diagnostic tools in heart failure. Endocr Rev 2003;24:341-356.

65. Wu F, Yan W, Pan J, et al: Processing of pro-atrial natriuretic peptide by corin in cardiac myocytes. J Biol Chem 2002;277: 16900-16905.

66. Yandle TG: Biochemistry of natriuretic peptides. J Intern Med 1994;235:561-576.

67. Vesely DL, Douglass MA, Dietz JR, et al: Three peptides from the atrial natriuretic factor prohormone amino terminus lower blood pressure and produce diuresis, natriuresis, and/or kaliuresis in humans. Circulation 1994;90:1129-1140.

68. Lang RE, Tholken H, Ganten D, et al: Atrial natriuretic factor: A circulating hormone stimulated by volume loading. Nature 1985;314:264-266.

69. Yoshimura M, Yasue H, Okumura K, et al: Different secretion patterns of atrial natriuretic peptide and brain natriuretic peptide in patients with congestive heart failure. Circulation 1993;87:464-469.

70. Yasue H, Yoshimura M, Sumida H, et al: Localization and mechanism of secretion of B-type natriuretic peptide in comparison with those of A-type natriuretic peptide in normal subjects and patients with heart failure. Circulation 1994;90:195-203.

71. Gu J, D'Andrea M, Seethapathy M: Atrial natriuretic peptide and its messenger ribonucleic acid in overloaded and overload-released ventricles of rat. Endocrinology 1989;125:2066-2074.

72. Saito Y, Nakao K, Arai H, et al: Augmented expression of atrial natriuretic polypeptide gene in ventricle of human failing heart. J Clin Invest 1989;83:298-305.

73. Rubin DA, Uretsky BF, Zerbe TR, et al: Increased plasma atrial natriuretic peptide levels after heart transplant: Relation to ventricular expression and severity of rejection. Am Heart J 1994;128:769-773.

74. El Gamel A, Yonan NA, Keevil B, et al: Significance of raised natriuretic peptides after bicaval and standard cardiac transplantation. Ann Thorac Surg 1997;63:1095-1100.

75. Takemura G, Fujiwara H, Takatsu Y, et al: Ventricular expression of atrial and brain natriuretic peptides in patients with myocarditis. Int J Cardiol 1995;52:213-222.

76. Charles CJ, Espiner EA, Richards AM: Cardiovascular actions of ANF: Contributions of renal, neurohumoral, and hemodynamic factors in sheep. Am J Physiol 1993;264:R533-R538.

77. Lappe RW, Smits JF, Todt JA, et al: Failure of atriopeptin II to cause arterial vasodilation in the conscious rat. Circ Res 1985;56:606-612.

78. Ogawa Y, Itoh H, Tamura N, et al: Molecular cloning of the complementary DNA and gene that encode mouse brain natriuretic peptide and generation of transgenic mice that overexpress the brain natriuretic peptide gene. J Clin Invest 1994;93:1911-1921.

79. Marin-Grez M, Fleming JT, Steinhausen M: Atrial natriuretic peptide causes pre-glomerular vasodilatation and post-glomerular vasoconstriction in rat kidney. Nature 1986;324:473-476.

80. Tonolo G, Richards AM, Manunta P, et al: Low-dose infusion of atrial natriuretic factor in mild essential hypertension. Circulation 1989;80:893-902.

81. Floras JS: Sympathoinhibitory effects of atrial natriuretic factor in normal humans. Circulation 1990;81:1860-1873.

82. Richards AM, McDonald D, Fitzpatrick MA, et al: Atrial natriuretic hormone has biological effects in man at physiological plasma concentrations. J Clin Endocrinol Metab 1988;67:1134-1139.

83. Atarashi K, Mulrow PJ, Franco-Saenz R: Effect of atrial peptides on aldosterone production. J Clin Invest 1985;76:1807-1811.

84. Burnett JC Jr, Granger JP, Opgenorth TJ: Effects of synthetic atrial natriuretic factor on renal function and renin release. Am J Physiol 1984;247:F863-F866.

85. Dillingham MA, Anderson RJ: Inhibition of vasopressin action by atrial natriuretic factor. Science 1986;231:1572-1573.

86. Sonnenberg H, Honrath U, Chong CK, Wilson DR: Atrial natriuretic factor inhibits sodium transport in medullary collecting duct. Am J Physiol 1986;250:F963-F966.

87. Zeidel ML, Kikeri D, Silva P, et al: Atrial natriuretic peptides inhibit conductive sodium uptake by rabbit inner medullary collecting duct cells. J Clin Invest 1988;82:1067-1074.

88. Light DB, Schwiebert EM, Karlson KH, Stanton BA: Atrial natriuretic peptide inhibits a cation channel in renal inner medullary collecting duct cells. Science 1989;243:383-385.

89. Zeidel ML: Regulation of collecting duct Na$^+$ reabsorption by ANP 31-67. Clin Exp Pharmacol Physiol 1995;22:121-124.

90. Levin ER, Isackson PJ, Hu RM: Endothelin increases atrial natriuretic peptide production in cultured rat diencephalic neurons. Endocrinology 1991;128:2925-2930.

91. Levin ER, Hu RM, Rossi M, Pickart M: Arginine vasopressin stimulates atrial natriuretic peptide gene expression and secretion from rat diencephalic neurons. Endocrinology 1992;131:1417-1423.

92. Huang W, Lee D, Yang Z, et al: Norepinephrine stimulates immunoreactive (ir) atrial natriuretic peptide (ANP) secretion and pro-ANP mRNA expression from rat hypothalamic neurons in culture: Effects of alpha 2-adrenoceptors. Endocrinology 1992;130:2426-2428.

93. Schultz HD, Gardner DG, Deschepper CF, et al: Vagal C-fiber blockade abolishes sympathetic inhibition by atrial natriuretic factor. Am J Physiol 1988;255:R6-R13.

94. Yang RH, Jin HK, Wyss JM, et al: Pressor effect of blocking atrial natriuretic peptide in nucleus tractus solitarii. Hypertension 1992;19:198-205.

95. Langub MC Jr, Dolgas CM, Watson RE Jr, Herman JP: The C-type natriuretic peptide receptor is the predominant natriuretic peptide receptor mRNA expressed in rat hypothalamus. J Neuroendocrinol 1995;7:305-309.

96. Durocher D, Grepin C, Nemer M: Regulation of gene expression in the endocrine heart. Recent Prog Horm Res 1998;53:7-23.

97. Sawada Y, Suda M, Yokoyama H, et al: Stretch-induced hypertrophic growth of cardiocytes and processing of brain-type natriuretic peptide are controlled by proprotein-processing endoprotease furin. J Biol Chem 1997;272:20545-20554.

98. Tamura N, Ogawa Y, Yasoda A, et al: Two cardiac natriuretic peptide genes (atrial natriuretic peptide and brain natriuretic peptide) are organized in tandem in the mouse and human genomes. J Mol Cell Cardiol 1996;28:1811-1815.

99. Stein BC, Levin RI: Natriuretic peptides: Physiology, therapeutic potential, and risk stratification in ischemic heart disease. Am Heart J 1998;135:914-923.

100. Takeda T, Kohno M: Brain natriuretic peptide in hypertension. Hypertens Res 1995;18:259-266.

101. Hunt PJ, Espiner EA, Nicholls MG, et al: Differing biological effects of equimolar atrial and brain natriuretic peptide infusions in normal man. J Clin Endocrinol Metab 1996;81:3871-3876.

102. Wijeyaratne CN, Moult PJ: The effect of alpha human atrial natriuretic peptide on plasma volume and vascular permeability in normotensive subjects. J Clin Endocrinol Metab 1993;76:343-346.

103. Morishita Y, Sano T, Kase H, et al: HS-142-1, a novel nonpeptide atrial natriuretic peptide (ANP) antagonist, blocks ANP-induced renal responses through a specific interaction with guanylyl cyclase-linked receptors. Eur J Pharmacol 1992;225:203-207.

104. Sano T, Morishita Y, Matsuda Y, Yamada K: Pharmacological profile of HS-142-1, a novel nonpeptide atrial natriuretic peptide antagonist of microbial origin: I. Selective inhibition of the actions of natriuretic peptides in anesthetized rats. J Pharmacol Exp Ther 1992;260:825-831.

105. Honrath U, Matsuda Y, Sonnenberg H: Cardiovascular and renal functional effects of an antagonist of the guanylyl cyclase-linked ANF receptor. Regul Pept 1994;49:211-216.

106. Hirata Y, Matsuoka H, Suzuki E, et al: Role of endogenous atrial natriuretic peptide in DOCA-salt hypertensive rats: Effects of a novel nonpeptide antagonist for atrial natriuretic peptide receptor. Circulation 1993;87:554-561.

107. Wada A, Tsutamoto T, Matsuda Y, Kinoshita M: Cardiorenal and neurohumoral effects of endogenous atrial natriuretic peptide in dogs with severe congestive heart failure using a specific antagonist for guanylate cyclase-coupled receptors. Circulation 1994;89:2232-2240.

108. Blackburn RE, Samson WK, Fulton RJ, et al: Central oxytocin and ANP receptors mediate osmotic inhibition of salt appetite in rats. Am J Physiol 1995;269:R245-R251.

109. Burrell LM, Lambert HJ, Baylis PH: Effect of atrial natriuretic peptide on thirst and arginine vasopressin release in humans. Am J Physiol 1991;260:R475-R479.

110. Koglin J, Pehlivanli S, Schwaiblmair M, et al: Role of brain natriuretic peptide in risk stratification of patients with congestive heart failure. J Am Coll Cardiol 2001;38:1934-1941.

111. Berger R, Huelsman M, Strecker K, et al: B-type natriuretic peptide predicts sudden death in patients with chronic heart failure. Circulation 2002;105:2392-2397.

112. Morrison LK, Harrison A, Krishnaswamy P, et al: Utility of a rapid B-natriuretic peptide assay in differentiating congestive heart failure from lung disease in patients presenting with dyspnea. J Am Coll Cardiol 2002;39:202-209.

113. Morita E, Yasue H, Yoshimura M, et al: Increased plasma levels of brain natriuretic peptide in patients with acute myocardial infarction. Circulation 1993;88:82-91.

114. Omland T, Aakvaag A, Bonarjee VV, et al: Plasma brain natriuretic peptide as an indicator of left ventricular systolic function and long-term survival after acute myocardial infarction: Comparison with plasma atrial natriuretic peptide and N-terminal proatrial natriuretic peptide. Circulation 1996;93:1963-1969.

115. Arakawa N, Nakamura M, Aoki H, Hiramori K: Plasma brain natriuretic peptide concentrations predict survival after acute myocardial infarction. J Am Coll Cardiol 1996;27:1656-1661.

116. Richards AM, Nicholls MG, Yandle TG, et al: Plasma N-terminal pro-brain natriuretic peptide and adrenomedullin: New neurohormonal predictors of left ventricular function and prognosis after myocardial infarction. Circulation 1998;97:1921-1929.

117. Morrow DA, de Lemos JA, Sabatine MS, et al: Evaluation of B-type natriuretic peptide for risk assessment in unstable angina/non-ST-elevation myocardial infarction: B-type natriuretic peptide and prognosis in TACTICS-TIMI 18. J Am Coll Cardiol 2003;41:1264-1272.

118. Tateishi J, Masutani M, Ohyanagi M, Iwasaki T: Transient increase in plasma brain (B-type) natriuretic peptide after percutaneous transluminal coronary angioplasty. Clin Cardiol 2000;23:776-780.

119. Kikuta K, Yasue H, Yoshimura M, et al: Increased plasma levels of B-type natriuretic peptide in patients with unstable angina. Am Heart J 1996;132:101-107.

120. Kohno M, Horio T, Yokokawa K, et al: Brain natriuretic peptide as a cardiac hormone in essential hypertension. Am J Med 1992;92:29-34.

121. Sodian R, Loebe M, Schmitt C, et al: Decreased plasma concentration of brain natriuretic peptide as a potential indicator of cardiac recovery in patients supported by mechanical circulatory assist systems. J Am Coll Cardiol 2001;38:1942-1949.

122. Ationu A, Burch M, Singer D, et al: Cardiac transplantation affects ventricular expression of brain natriuretic peptide. Cardiovasc Res 1993;27:188-191.

123. McDonagh TA, Robb SD, Murdoch DR, et al: Biochemical detection of left-ventricular systolic dysfunction. Lancet 1998;351:9-13.

124. Yoshibayashi M, Kamiya T, Saito Y, et al: Plasma brain natriuretic peptide concentrations in healthy children from birth to adolescence: Marked and rapid increase after birth. Eur J Endocrinol 1995;133:207-209.

125. Mir TS, Marohn S, Laer S, et al: Plasma concentrations of N-terminal pro-brain natriuretic peptide in control children from the neonatal to adolescent period and in children with congestive heart failure. Pediatrics 2002;110:e76.

126. Jensen KT, Carstens J, Ivarsen P, Pedersen EB: A new, fast and reliable radioimmunoassay of brain natriuretic peptide in human plasma: Reference values in healthy subjects and in patients with different diseases. Scand J Clin Lab Invest 1997;57:529-540.

127. Wallen T, Landahl S, Hedner T, et al: Brain natriuretic peptide in an elderly population. J Intern Med 1997;242:307-311.

128. Mori K, Manabe T, Nii M, et al: Plasma levels of natriuretic peptide and echocardiographic parameters in patients with Duchenne's progressive muscular dystrophy. Pediatr Cardiol 2002;23:160-166.

129. Kawamura T, Wago M: Brain natriuretic peptide can be a useful biochemical marker for myocarditis in patients with Kawasaki disease. Cardiol Young 2002;12:153-158.

130. Muta H, Ishii M, Maeno Y, et al: Quantitative evaluation of the changes in plasma concentrations of cardiac natriuretic peptide before and after transcatheter closure of atrial septal defect. Acta Paediatr 2002;91:649-652.

131. Nagaya N, Nishikimi T, Uematsu M, et al: Plasma brain natriuretic peptide as a prognostic indicator in patients with primary pulmonary hypertension. Circulation 2000;102:865-870.

132. Nagaya N, Nishikimi T, Okano Y, et al: Plasma brain natriuretic peptide levels increase in proportion to the extent of right ventricular dysfunction in pulmonary hypertension. J Am Coll Cardiol 1998;31:202-208.

133. Hasegawa K, Fujiwara H, Doyama K, et al: Ventricular expression of brain natriuretic peptide in hypertrophic cardiomyopathy. Circulation 1993;88:372-380.

134. Hayakawa H, Komada Y, Hirayama M, et al: Plasma levels of natriuretic peptides in relation to doxorubicin-induced cardiotoxicity and cardiac function in children with cancer. Med Pediatr Oncol 2001;37:4-9.

135. Wahlander H, Westerlind A, Lindstedt G, et al: Increased levels of brain and atrial natriuretic peptides after the first palliative operation, but not after a bidirectional Glenn anastomosis, in children with functionally univentricular hearts. Cardiol Young 2003;13:268-274.

136. Yoshimura N, Yamaguchi M, Oshima Y, et al: Suppression of the secretion of atrial and brain natriuretic peptide after total cavopulmonary connection. J Thorac Cardiovasc Surg 2000;120:764-769.

137. Ationu A, Singer DR, Smith A, et al: Studies of cardiopulmonary bypass in children: Implications for the regulation of brain natriuretic peptide. Cardiovasc Res 1993;27:1538-1541.

138. Maisel AS, Krishnaswamy P, Nowak RM, et al: Rapid measurement of B-type natriuretic peptide in the emergency diagnosis of heart failure. N Engl J Med 2002;347:161-167.

139. Maisel AS, McCord J, Nowak RM, et al: Bedside B-type natriuretic peptide in the emergency diagnosis of heart failure with reduced or preserved ejection fraction: Results from the Breathing Not Properly Multinational Study. J Am Coll Cardiol 2003;41:2010-2017.

140. Sudoh T, Minamino N, Kangawa K, Matsuo H: C-type natriuretic peptide (CNP): A new member of natriuretic peptide family identified in porcine brain. Biochem Biophys Res Commun 1990;168:863-870.

141. Minamino N, Makino Y, Tateyama H, et al: Characterization of immunoreactive human C-type natriuretic peptide in brain and heart. Biochem Biophys Res Commun 1991;179:535-542.

142. Levin ER, Frank HJ: Natriuretic peptides inhibit rat astroglial proliferation: Mediation by C receptor. Am J Physiol 1991;261:R453-R457.

143. Hunt PJ, Richards AM, Espiner EA, et al: Bioactivity and metabolism of C-type natriuretic peptide in normal man. J Clin Endocrinol Metab 1994;78:1428-1435.

144. Charles CJ, Espiner EA, Richards AM, Donald RA: Central C-type natriuretic peptide augments the hormone response to hemorrhage in conscious sheep. Peptides 1995;16:129-132.

145. Wei CM, Heublein DM, Perrella MA, et al: Natriuretic peptide system in human heart failure. Circulation 1993;88:1004-1009.

146. Shan K, Kurrelmeyer K, Seta Y, et al: The role of cytokines in disease progression in heart failure. Curr Opin Cardiol 1997;12:218-223.

147. Torre-Amione G, Kapadia S, Benedict C, et al: Proinflammatory cytokine levels in patients with depressed left ventricular ejection fraction: A report from the Studies of Left Ventricular Dysfunction (SOLVD). J Am Coll Cardiol 1996;27:1201-1206.

148. Suffredini AF, Fromm RE, Parker MM, et al: The cardiovascular response of normal humans to the administration of endotoxin. N Engl J Med 1989;321:280-287.

149. Torre-Amione G, Kapadia S, Lee J, et al: Expression and functional significance of tumor necrosis factor receptors in human myocardium. Circulation 1995;92:1487-1493.

150. Bhoola KD, Figueroa CD, Worthy K: Bioregulation of kinins: Kallikreins, kininogens, and kininases. Pharmacol Rev 1992;44:1-80.

151. Campbell DJ: The kallikrein-kinin system in humans. Clin Exp Pharmacol Physiol 2001;28:1060-1065.

152. Regoli D, Rhaleb NE, Drapeau G, et al: Basic pharmacology of kinins: Pharmacologic receptors and other mechanisms. Adv Exp Med Biol 1989;247A:399-407.

153. Groves P, Kurz S, Just H, Drexler H: Role of endogenous bradykinin in human coronary vasomotor control. Circulation 1995;92:3424-3430.

154. Gainer JV, Morrow JD, Loveland A, et al: Effect of bradykinin-receptor blockade on the response to angiotensin-converting-enzyme inhibitor in normotensive and hypertensive subjects. N Engl J Med 1998;339:1285-1292.

155. Madeddu P, Varoni MV, Palomba D, et al: Cardiovascular phenotype of a mouse strain with disruption of bradykinin B2-receptor gene. Circulation 1997;96:3570-3578.

156. Haynes WG, Webb DJ: Endothelin as a regulator of cardiovascular function in health and disease. J Hypertens 1998;16:1081-1098.

157. Wei CM, Lerman A, Rodeheffer RJ, et al: Endothelin in human congestive heart failure. Circulation 1994;89:1580-1586.

158. Ruetten H, Thiemermann C: Endothelin-1 stimulates the biosynthesis of tumour necrosis factor in macrophages: ET-receptors, signal transduction and inhibition by dexamethasone. J Physiol Pharmacol 1997;48:675-688.

159. Moraes DL, Colucci WS, Givertz MM: Secondary pulmonary hypertension in chronic heart failure: The role of the endothelium in pathophysiology and management. Circulation 2000; 102:1718-1723.

160. Tsutamoto T, Wada A, Maeda Y, et al: Relation between endothelin-1 spillover in the lungs and pulmonary vascular resistance in patients with chronic heart failure. J Am Coll Cardiol 1994;23:1427-1433.

161. Sakai S, Miyauchi T, Sakurai T, et al: Pulmonary hypertension caused by congestive heart failure is ameliorated by long-term application of an endothelin receptor antagonist: Increased expression of endothelin-1 messenger ribonucleic acid and endothelin-1-like immunoreactivity in the lung in congestive heart failure in rats. J Am Coll Cardiol 1996;28:1580-1588.

162. Kiowski W, Sutsch G, Hunziker P, et al: Evidence for endothelin-1-mediated vasoconstriction in severe chronic heart failure. Lancet 1995;346:732-736.

163. Levin ER: Endothelins. N Engl J Med 1995;333:356-363.

164. Aronson D, Burger AJ: Intravenous nesiritide (human B-type natriuretic peptide) reduces plasma endothelin-1 levels in patients with decompensated congestive heart failure. Am J Cardiol 2002;90:435-438.

165. Carswell EA, Old LJ, Kassel RL, et al: An endotoxin-induced serum factor that causes necrosis of tumors. Proc Natl Acad Sci U S A 1975;72:3666-3670.

166. Levine B, Kalman J, Mayer L, et al: Elevated circulating levels of tumor necrosis factor in severe chronic heart failure. N Engl J Med 1990;323:236-241.

167. Boekstegers P, Weidenhofer S, Zell R, et al: Repeated administration of a F(ab′)2 fragment of an anti-tumor necrosis factor alpha monoclonal antibody in patients with severe sepsis: Effects on the cardiovascular system and cytokine levels. Shock 1994;1:237-245.

168. Torre-Amione G, Vooletich MT, Farmer JA: Role of tumour necrosis factor-alpha in the progression of heart failure: Therapeutic implications. Drugs 2000;59:745-751.

169. Palmieri EA, Benincasa G, Di Rella F, et al: Differential expression of TNF-alpha, IL-6, and IGF-1 by graded mechanical stress in normal rat myocardium. Am J Physiol Heart Circ Physiol 2002;282:H926-H934.

170. Baumgarten G, Knuefermann P, Kalra D, et al: Load-dependent and -independent regulation of proinflammatory cytokine and cytokine receptor gene expression in the adult mammalian heart. Circulation 2002;105:2192-2197.

171. Yokoyama T, Vaca L, Rossen RD, et al: Cellular basis for the negative inotropic effects of tumor necrosis factor-alpha in the adult mammalian heart. J Clin Invest 1993;92:2303-2312.

172. Kubota T, McTiernan CF, Frye CS, et al: Dilated cardiomyopathy in transgenic mice with cardiac-specific overexpression of tumor necrosis factor-alpha. Circ Res 1997;81:627-635.

173. Bradham WS, Bozkurt B, Gunasinghe H, et al: Tumor necrosis factor-alpha and myocardial remodeling in progression of heart failure: A current perspective. Cardiovasc Res 2002;53: 822-830.

174. Aikawa R, Nitta-Komatsubara Y, Kudoh S, et al: Reactive oxygen species induce cardiomyocyte apoptosis partly through TNF-alpha. Cytokine 2002;18:179-183.

175. Torre-Amione G, Kapadia S, Lee J, et al: Tumor necrosis factor-alpha and tumor necrosis factor receptors in the failing human heart. Circulation 1996;93:704-711.

176. Anker SD, Ponikowski P, Varney S, et al: Wasting as independent risk factor for mortality in chronic heart failure. Lancet 1997; 349:1050-1053.

177. Anker SD, Rauchhaus M: Insights into the pathogenesis of chronic heart failure: Immune activation and cachexia. Curr Opin Cardiol 1999;14:211-216.

178. Krown KA, Page MT, Nguyen C, et al: Tumor necrosis factor alpha-induced apoptosis in cardiac myocytes: Involvement of the sphingolipid signaling cascade in cardiac cell death. J Clin Invest 1996;98:2854-2865.

179. Tracey KJ, Morgello S, Koplin B, et al: Metabolic effects of cachectin/tumor necrosis factor are modified by site of production: Cachectin/tumor necrosis factor-secreting tumor in skeletal muscle induces chronic cachexia, while implantation in brain induces predominantly acute anorexia. J Clin Invest 1990; 86:2014-2024.

180. Adams V, Jiang H, Yu J, et al: Apoptosis in skeletal myocytes of patients with chronic heart failure is associated with exercise intolerance. J Am Coll Cardiol 1999;33:959-965.

181. Malave HA, Taylor AA, Nattama J, et al: Circulating levels of tumor necrosis factor correlate with indexes of depressed heart rate variability: A study in patients with mild-to-moderate heart failure. Chest 2003;123:716-724.

182. Ferrari R, Bachetti T, Confortini R, et al: Tumor necrosis factor soluble receptors in patients with various degrees of congestive heart failure. Circulation 1995;92:1479-1486.

183. Dibbs Z, Thornby J, White BG, Mann DL: Natural variability of circulating levels of cytokines and cytokine receptors in patients with heart failure: Implications for clinical trials. J Am Coll Cardiol 1999;33:1935-1942.

184. Bozkurt B, Torre-Amione G, Warren MS, et al: Results of targeted anti-tumor necrosis factor therapy with etanercept (ENBREL) in patients with advanced heart failure. Circulation 2001;103:1044-1047.

185. Chung ES, Packer M, Lo KH, et al: Randomized, double-blind, placebo-controlled, pilot trial of infliximab, a chimeric monoclonal antibody to tumor necrosis factor-alpha, in patients with moderate-to-severe heart failure: Results of the anti-TNF Therapy Against Congestive Heart Failure (ATTACH) trial. Circulation 2003;107:3133-3140.

186. Goldsmith SR, Francis GS, Cowley AW Jr: Arginine vasopressin and the renal response to water loading in congestive heart failure. Am J Cardiol 1986;58:295-299.

187. Goldsmith SR, Dodge D: Response of plasma vasopressin to ethanol in congestive heart failure. Am J Cardiol 1985;55:1354-1357.

188. Naitoh M, Suzuki H, Murakami M, et al: Effects of oral AVP receptor antagonists OPC-21268 and OPC-31260 on congestive heart failure in conscious dogs. Am J Physiol 1994;267:H2245-H2254.

189. Sharma R, Coats AJ, Anker SD: The role of inflammatory mediators in chronic heart failure: Cytokines, nitric oxide, and endothelin-1. Int J Cardiol 2000;72:175-186.

190. Francis SE, Holden H, Holt CM, Duff GW: Interleukin-1 in myocardium and coronary arteries of patients with dilated cardiomyopathy. J Mol Cell Cardiol 1998;30:215-223.

191. Gulick T, Chung MK, Pieper SJ, et al: Interleukin 1 and tumor necrosis factor inhibit cardiac myocyte beta-adrenergic responsiveness. Proc Natl Acad Sci U S A 1989;86:6753-6757.

192. Palmer JN, Hartogensis WE, Patten M, et al: Interleukin-1 beta induces cardiac myocyte growth but inhibits cardiac fibroblast proliferation in culture. J Clin Invest 1995;95:2555-2564.

193. Thaik CM, Calderone A, Takahashi N, Colucci WS: Interleukin-1 beta modulates the growth and phenotype of neonatal rat cardiac myocytes. J Clin Invest 1995;96:1093-1099.

194. de Belder A, Robinson N, Richardson P, et al: Expression of inducible nitric oxide synthase in human heart failure. Circulation 1997;95:1672-1673.

195. Munger MA, Johnson B, Amber IJ, et al: Circulating concentrations of proinflammatory cytokines in mild or moderate heart failure secondary to ischemic or idiopathic dilated cardiomyopathy. Am J Cardiol 1996;77:723-727.

196. Aukrust P, Ueland T, Lien E, et al: Cytokine network in congestive heart failure secondary to ischemic or idiopathic dilated cardiomyopathy. Am J Cardiol 1999;83:376-382.

197. Carlstedt F, Lind L, Lindahl B: Proinflammatory cytokines, measured in a mixed population on arrival in the emergency department, are related to mortality and severity of disease. J Intern Med 1997;242:361-365.

198. Tsutamoto T, Hisanaga T, Wada A, et al: Interleukin-6 spillover in the peripheral circulation increases with the severity of heart failure, and the high plasma level of interleukin-6 is an important prognostic predictor in patients with congestive heart failure. J Am Coll Cardiol 1998;31:391-398.

199. Roig E, Orus J, Pare C, et al: Serum interleukin-6 in congestive heart failure secondary to idiopathic dilated cardiomyopathy. Am J Cardiol 1998;82:688-690, A8.

200. Latini R, Masson S, Anand I, et al: Effects of valsartan on circulating brain natriuretic peptide and norepinephrine in symptomatic chronic heart failure: The Valsartan Heart Failure Trial (Val-HeFT). Circulation 2002;106:2454-2458.

201. McKelvie RS, Yusuf S, Pericak D, et al: Comparison of candesartan, enalapril, and their combination in congestive heart failure: Randomized evaluation of strategies for left ventricular dysfunction (RESOLVD) pilot study. The RESOLVD Pilot Study Investigators. Circulation 1999;100:1056-1064.

202. Cohn JN, Ziesche S, Smith R, et al: Effect of the calcium antagonist felodipine as supplementary vasodilator therapy in patients with chronic heart failure treated with enalapril: V-HeFT III. Vasodilator-Heart Failure Trial (V-HeFT) Study Group. Circulation 1997;96:856-863.

203. The Cardiac Insufficiency Bisoprolol Study II (CIBIS-II): A randomised trial. Lancet 1999;353:9-13.

204. Effect of metoprolol CR/XL in chronic heart failure: Metoprolol CR/XL Randomised Intervention Trial in Congestive Heart Failure (MERIT-HF). Lancet 1999;353:2001-2007.

205. Packer M, Bristow MR, Cohn JN, et al: The effect of carvedilol on morbidity and mortality in patients with chronic heart failure. U.S. Carvedilol Heart Failure Study Group. N Engl J Med 1996;334:1349-1355.

206. Holmes SJ, Espiner EA, Richards AM, et al: Renal, endocrine, and hemodynamic effects of human brain natriuretic peptide in normal man. J Clin Endocrinol Metab 1993;76:91-96.

207. Marcus LS, Hart D, Packer M, et al: Hemodynamic and renal excretory effects of human brain natriuretic peptide infusion in patients with congestive heart failure: A double-blind, placebo-controlled, randomized crossover trial. Circulation 1996;94:3184-3189.

208. Mills RM, LeJemtel TH, Horton DP, et al: Sustained hemodynamic effects of an infusion of nesiritide (human b-type natriuretic peptide) in heart failure: A randomized, double-blind, placebo-controlled clinical trial. Natrecor Study Group. J Am Coll Cardiol 1999;34:155-162.

209. Colucci WS, Elkayam U, Horton DP, et al: Intravenous nesiritide, a natriuretic peptide, in the treatment of decompensated congestive heart failure. Nesiritide Study Group. N Engl J Med 2000;343:246-253.

210. Silver MA, Horton DP, Ghali JK, Elkayam U: Effect of nesiritide versus dobutamine on short-term outcomes in the treatment of patients with acutely decompensated heart failure. J Am Coll Cardiol 2002;39:798-803.

211. Intravenous nesiritide vs nitroglycerin for treatment of decompensated congestive heart failure: A randomized controlled trial. JAMA 2002;287:1531-1540.

212. Bhat G, Costea A: Reversibility of medically unresponsive pulmonary hypertension with nesiritide in a cardiac transplant recipient. ASAIO J 2003;49:608-610.

213. Pitt B, Zannad F, Remme WJ, et al: The effect of spironolactone on morbidity and mortality in patients with severe heart failure. Randomized Aldactone Evaluation Study Investigators. N Engl J Med 1999;341:709-717.

214. Barr CS, Lang CC, Hanson J, et al: Effects of adding spironolactone to an angiotensin-converting enzyme inhibitor in chronic congestive heart failure secondary to coronary artery disease. Am J Cardiol 1995;76:1259-1265.

215. Zannad F, Alla F, Dousset B, et al: Limitation of excessive extracellular matrix turnover may contribute to survival benefit of spironolactone therapy in patients with congestive heart failure: insights from the randomized aldactone evaluation study (RALES). RALES Investigators. Circulation 2000;102:2700-2706.

216. Pitt B, Remme W, Zannad F, et al: Eplerenone: A selective aldosterone blocker, in patients with left ventricular dysfunction after myocardial infarction. N Engl J Med 2003;348:1309-1321.

217. Russell SD, Selaru P, Pyne DA, et al: Rationale for use of an exercise end point and design for the ADVANCE (A Dose evaluation of a Vasopressin ANtagonist in CHF patients undergoing Exercise) trial. Am Heart J 2003;145:179-186.

218. Lee CR, Watkins ML, Patterson JH, et al: Vasopressin: A new target for the treatment of heart failure. Am Heart J 2003;146:9-18.

219. Hjortdal VE, Stenbog EV, Ravn HB, et al: Neurohormonal activation late after cavopulmonary connection. Heart 2000;83:439-443.

220. Driscoll DJ, Danielson GK, Puga FJ, et al: Exercise tolerance and cardiorespiratory response to exercise after the Fontan operation for tricuspid atresia or functional single ventricle. J Am Coll Cardiol 1986;7:1087-1094.

221. Ohuchi H, Yasuda K, Hasegawa S, et al: Influence of ventricular morphology on aerobic exercise capacity in patients after the Fontan operation. J Am Coll Cardiol 2001;37:1967-1974.

222. Ohuchi H, Hasegawa S, Yasuda K, et al: Severely impaired cardiac autonomic nervous activity after the Fontan operation. Circulation 2001;104:1513-1518.

223. Hayabuchi Y, Matsuoka S, Kuroda Y: Plasma concentrations of atrial and brain natriuretic peptides and cyclic guanosine monophosphate in response to dobutamine infusion in patients with surgically repaired tetralogy of Fallot. Pediatr Cardiol 1999;20:343-350.

224. Wang TJ, Larson MG, Levy D, et al: Plasma natriuretic peptide levels and the risk of cardiovascular events and death. N Engl J Med 2004;350:655-663.

225. Han B, Hasin Y: Cardiovascular effects of natriuretic peptides and their interrelation with endothelin-1. Cardiovasc Drugs Ther 2003;17:41-52.

226. Costello JM, Backer CL, Checchia PA, et al: Alterations in the natriuretic hormone system related to cardiopulmonary bypass in infants with congestive heart failure. Pediatr Cardiol 2004; 25:347-353.

227. Jefferies JL and Chang AC: Natriuretic and other biomarkers in heart failure in children and adults. Cardiology in the Young.

CHAPTER 7

The Pressure-Volume Relationship
in Heart Failure

Daniel J. Penny
Jonathan Mynard

Previous chapters have dealt with the molecular and circulatory milieu in heart failure; subsequent chapters focus on the heart itself in its physiologic surroundings. The ability to describe accurately the function of the heart, its metabolic demands, and its interactions with the vasculature is paramount in analyzing the mechanisms of circulatory failure and the effects of interventions in patients with myocardial disease.

In clinical practice, assessment of cardiac function usually is limited to the indirect estimation of ventricular systolic and end-diastolic pressure, estimation of ejection fraction, and, in some echocardiography laboratories, assessment of wall stress. A complete evaluation of cardiac function would extend further, however, ideally to include a relatively load-insensitive indicator of ventricular systolic and diastolic performance, an assessment of the myocardial oxygen consumption and contractile reserve, and an examination of the relationship between ventricular performance and cardiac load.

There has long been an interest in a biomechanical approach to analyzing the performance of the heart, by examining its function in the **pressure-volume relationship.** The examination of cardiac function using a pressure-volume diagram was first described by Frank[1] in 1898 in a theoretical paper, "Die Grundform des arteriellen pulses," which characterized the contractions of the frog ventricle. Over the next 50 years, there was only limited interest in the systematic examination of cardiac function using pressure-volume analysis. In 1955, Katz and coworkers[2] showed that the pressure-volume loop shifted during epinephrine infusion and during asphyxia, and 5 years later Monroe and French[3] showed that the slope of the end-systolic pressure-volume points varied with inotropic stimulation.

Since Suga presented in 1969[4] his analysis of the instantaneous pressure-volume relationship and subsequently developed the concept of "time-varying elastance,"[5,6] there has been heightened interest in the use of the pressure-volume relationship in assessing ventricular performance. This effort has been supported further in recent years with the introduction of the conductance catheter technique, which allows high-fidelity on-line acquisition of pressure-volume data at fast acquisition speeds.[7-9]

PRESSURE-VOLUME RELATIONSHIP OF THE LEFT VENTRICLE

The classic work of Wiggers,[10,11] which described changes in left ventricular pressure and volume during the cardiac cycle, has provided the foundations for current understanding of ventricular function. In Wiggers' schema, the cardiac cycle begins with the onset of depolarization on the ECG, which is soon followed by an increase in pressure within the ventricle. When left ventricular pressure exceeds left atrial pressure, the mitral valve closes. The aortic valve remains closed while aortic pressure still exceeds left ventricular pressure, and ventricular volume remains constant is the so-called **isovolumic contraction.** When left ventricular pressure exceeds aortic diastolic pressure, the aortic valve opens, and the ventricle begins to eject. Consequently the volume of the left ventricle decreases (Fig. 7-1).

Diastole traditionally is assumed to begin with closure of the aortic valve; however, ventricular pressure decay (relaxation) begins before this event. The period of ventricular pressure decay before aortic valve closure was termed *protodiastole* by Wiggers. After aortic valve closure, ventricular pressure continues to decay rapidly. The decay in ventricular pressure results from the energy-requiring calcium uptake to the sarcoplasmic reticulum, together with the passive release of myocardial elastic forces generated during contraction. As the ventricular pressure continues to decay, the mitral valve initially remains closed, and the period of relaxation during which ventricular volume remains constant is termed **isovolumic relaxation.**

When ventricular pressure decreases to less than atrial pressure, the mitral valve opens, and ventricular filling begins; as the ventricle fills, the pressure within initially decreases. This anomalous relationship between pressure and volume is thought to result from "restoring forces," which attempt to restore the shape of the ventricle to that at end diastole. After this time, pressure and volume increase in the ventricle, which exhibits elastic behavior. Later in diastole, the rate of ventricular filling is augmented further by atrial contraction.

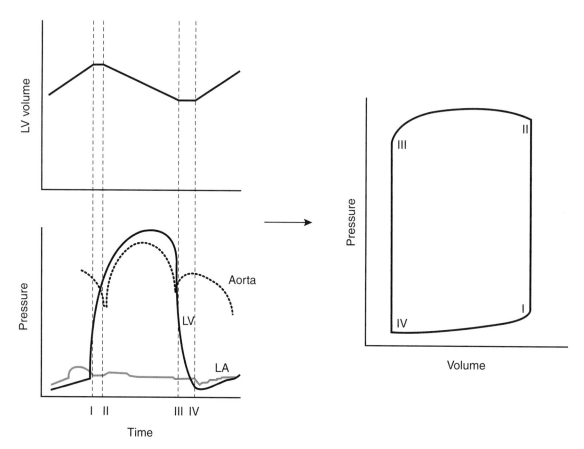

FIGURE 7-1 ■ **Changes in left ventricular (LV) volume and pressures.** *Left panel,* Stylized representation of the changes in LV volume and aortic, LV, and left atrial (LA) pressures during the cardiac cycle. Point I represents the onset of isovolumic contraction, which ends at point II. Isovolumic relaxation begins at point III and continues until point IV. *Right panel,* The same changes in the pressure-volume plane. Beginning at the bottom right-hand corner of the loop, changes in LV pressure and volume during the cardiac cycle can be examined by following the loop in a counter-clockwise direction. Time points I to IV correspond to the same events in the cardiac cycle as those for the left panel.

Although we have considered the changes in left ventricular pressure and volume in the time domain, the essence of the pressure-volume analysis is to consider the time-varying relationship between ventricular pressure and volume, represented by the pressure-volume loop. The pressure-volume loop has four characteristic phases (see Fig. 7-1). Beginning at the bottom right-hand corner of the loop, an initial upstroke (I-II) represents the rapid increase in ventricular pressure, with little volume change—isovolumic contraction. There is then a rapid decrease in ventricular volume, as ventricular ejection proceeds to the end-systolic point (II-III). Ventricular pressure then rapidly falls, with little volume change, as the ventricle enters its isovolumic relaxation phase (III-IV). Finally, ventricular volume increases to its end-diastolic level, reflecting ventricular filling (IV-I).

Looking beyond contractility, the pressure-volume relationship can provide many further insights into cardiovascular function and myocardial failure, and this section focuses on several: the interaction between contractility and load, the coupling between the ventricle and the vascular system, the relationship between ventricular work and oxygen consumption, and the diastolic pressure-volume relationship.

Ventricular Contractility

Suga[12,13] noted that at constant inotropic state, alterations in ventricular load resulted in a population of pressure-volume loops in which, at any time in the cardiac cycle, the pressure-volume points follow a straight line. It was proposed that cardiac contraction could be modeled as a time-varying elastance, with maximal elastance occurring at end systole (**end-systolic elastance [Ees]**), represented by the upper left-hand corner of the pressure-volume loop (Fig. 7-2).[5]

For some, the clinical application of this approach has become narrowly focused on the assessment of maximal elastance as a sole index of ventricular contractility. Although the **end-systolic pressure-volume relationship (ESPVR)** has been considered the "gold standard" measure of ventricular contractility, the importance of other indices should not be underestimated. Kass and coworkers[14] examined the influence of carefully controlled alterations in end-diastolic volume

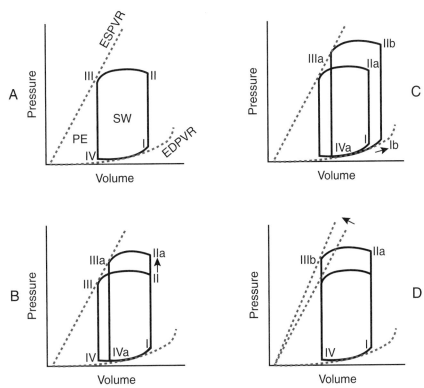

FIGURE 7-2 ■ **Dynamic interactions between ventricular afterload, preload, and contractility.** **A,** The ventricular pressure-volume relationship is bounded by its end-systolic and end-diastolic pressure-volume relationships (ESPVR and EDPVR). **B,** An acute increase in afterload is applied. Pressure at the end of isovolumic contraction is increased (II-IIa), and as ventricular ejection is arrested by the ESPVR (III-IIIa), stroke volume decreases in the absence of any other change. **C** and **D,** The ventricle maintains its stroke volume either by increasing its end-diastolic volume (preload recruitment in **C**) or by increasing its contractility (slope of the ESPVR in **D**) (*see arrows*). When these reserves are exhausted, stroke volume decreases. The changes in pressure-volume relationship observed in left-to-right shunts (e.g., a ventricular septal defect) or insufficiency of the intracardiac valves (e.g., mitral regurgitation or aortic insufficiency) resemble the changes shown in **C** with its increase in end-diastolic volume. The pressure-volume loop area represents the external work of the heart, or stroke work (SW). The potential energy (PE) does not result in SW, but is energy produced during the contraction and comprises the triangular area bounded by the ESPVR and EDPVR lines and the left border of the pressure-volume loop.

and afterload on multiple simultaneously determined ejection and isovolumic phase indices of left ventricular contractility in isolated supported canine ventricles. The influence of load change on each index was compared with its sensitivity to inotropic stimulation, and this sensitivity was contrasted to the response of the ESPVR. There were varying degrees of load sensitivity among the indices, with a generally curvilinear relationship between load and index response for preload and afterload alterations. Nonetheless, over a select range of loading, many indices showed relative load independence, and these often displayed greater sensitivity to inotropic change than to the ESPVR. There is no single gold standard measure that encompasses the complex physiologic processes that determine myocardial contractility; rather, there are numerous measures, each of which provides individual pieces of a complex physiologic jigsaw puzzle.

The use of Ees as a consistent and reproducible index of contractility has been complicated by many factors, including the observation that in the isolated and in vivo heart, there may exist nonlinearity of the ESPVR.[15-18] Although this curvilinearity indicates that in a given situation Ees is a function of vascular loading conditions, under normal conditions a linear relationship, although mathematically convenient, is not essential. Equations for nonlinear ESPVRs have been derived by approximating the relationship using parabolic expressions.[19] Although the relationship may be nonlinear when obtained over a wide range of ventricular load, data obtained in vivo that operate over physiologic ranges of load are usually well represented by a linear model.

Although it is clear that the ESPVR provides a useful measure of ventricular contractility, the pressure-volume approach begins, rather than ends, with an assessment of Ees. The pressure-volume relationship provides a wealth of information about cardiovascular physiology beyond Ees and has proved to be a fertile area of research, which has helped the understanding of cardiovascular hemodynamics.

Contractility and Load

A traditional assessment of ventricular performance would describe ventricular output as a function of four independent determinants: preload, afterload, contractility, and heart rate. It is now clear from several studies[14,20] using the pressure-volume relationship that load and contractility are not independent, but rather interact. Although this view may challenge traditional concepts, it is consistent with some important observations from basic science. The alterations in myocardial cell length (preload), which underpin Starling's law, result from largely length-dependent changes in myocardial activation and excitation-contraction coupling—in other words, alterations in contractility.[21-26] This constant dynamic interplay between ventricular load and contractility may have important homeostatic consequences, allowing stroke volume to be maintained in the face of increased load[20,27] (Fig. 7-3) and potentially providing more favorable energetic efficiency.[20]

Ventriculoarterial Coupling

The intricate coupling between the ventricle and the vasculature is a crucial clinical determinant of cardiovascular function. Although many treatments in a child with heart failure are aimed at augmenting ventricular systolic performance, without the ability of the vasculature to convert within itself the increased pressure work of the ventricle into flow work, these therapeutic strategies would be of little benefit.[28,29] A measure of this interaction between the ventricle and the vasculature would provide a valuable additional tool in the evaluation of cardiovascular performance.

Numerous approaches of varying complexities have been used to quantify the load imposed on the ventricle by the vasculature. Although an overview of the various techniques to characterize vascular load is beyond the scope of this chapter, the use of pressure-volume analysis is considered. This method, initially described by Sunagawa and colleagues,[30] is based on an approximation of mean and end-ejection arterial pressure by the ventricular end-systolic pressure. The model predicts that the ratio of end-systolic pressure to stroke volume remains constant under a steady-state vascular impedance. As a result, the slope of the end-systolic pressure-stroke

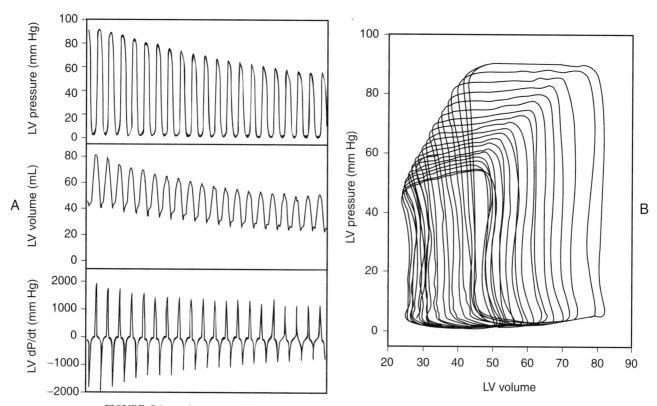

FIGURE 7-3 ■ **Changes in left ventricular (LV) pressure, volume, and rate of change of pressure (dP/dt). A,** Changes in LV pressure, volume, and dP/dt recorded using the conductance catheter technique during caval occlusion. **B,** A series of pressure-volume loops is derived, with a linear end-systolic pressure-volume relationship.

volume relationship equates to the inverse of the effective **arterial elastance (Ea).**[30] The relationship between Ees and effective Ea, as an index of ventriculoarterial coupling, has been used to illustrate how the arterial response determines the physiologic effect of an increase in contractility during inotropic stimulation.[31]

Many studies have used pressure-volume analysis to define the "optimal" relationship between Ea and Ees. Early studies suggested that optimal stroke work would occur when the two elastances were approximately equal.[32,33] These models worked alongside a predicted ejection fraction of only 50%,[19] however, which is considerably lower than that usually observed in normal humans. More recent theoretical studies have predicted that an Ees-to-Ea ratio of 2 is more consistent with an ejection fraction of 60% to 70%,[34] and this has been supported with clinical data from normal subjects.[35] This higher ratio of Ees to Ea would be expected to provide optimal efficiency between ventricular work and oxygen consumption, rather than optimal stroke work. Ventriculoarterial coupling is discussed in more detail in Chapter 8.

Left Ventricular Work and Oxygen Consumption
When an inotrope is administered to increase the work output of the left ventricle, there is usually a concomitant increase in the myocardial demand for metabolic substrates, including oxygen. This increase in oxygen consumption is related at least in part to changes in heart rate, wall tension, and contractility. In addition, inotropic stimulation probably produces intrinsic changes in cardiac oxidative metabolism with increased energy requirements for excitation-contraction coupling—the so-called oxygen-wasting effect.[36-38] As in many critically-ill patients with myocardial disease, the relationship between myocardial oxygen demand and supply is already precarious, and it is imperative that any potentially desirable augmentation of ventricular performance should not be offset by adverse effects on myocardial metabolism and energetics.

Analyses of pressure-volume relationships can provide important information regarding the energetic state of the ventricle. Suga[37] showed that the total energy consumption of the ventricle could be quantified by the specific area in the pressure-volume diagram that is bounded by the ESPVR and EDPVR and the systolic pressure-volume trajectory. In other words, this pressure-volume loop area represents the external work of the heart, or **stroke work**. The **potential energy** does not result in stroke work, but is energy produced during the contraction and comprises the triangular area bounded by the ESPVR and EDPVR lines and the left border of the pressure-volume loop (see Fig. 7-2A). The total pressure-volume area is the combined areas of the stroke work and the potential energy. The scope of the pressure-volume diagram extends beyond cardiac mechanics

to include cardiac energetics and mechanoenergetic coupling under varying contractile conditions.[37,38]

Left Ventricular Diastolic Function
The use of the pressure-volume relationship for the assessment of ventricular diastolic function, the **end-diastolic pressure-volume relationship (EDPVR)**, is based on the assumption that throughout the period during diastole when volume and pressure are increasing, the ventricle exhibits elastic behavior.[39,40] As a result, at any point during this time, the slope of the relationship between pressure and volume represents ventricular compliance. Because the normal pressure-volume relationship at this time is curvilinear, chamber compliance becomes lower as filling proceeds, indicating that the cavity has become stiffer. The pressure-volume curve during this part of diastole usually is assumed to be exponential and to show behavior characteristic of Lagrangian stress so that if pressure is plotted logarithmically and volume linearly, a linear relationship is obtained; it is then possible to calculate its slope and intercept. Ventricular compliance is reduced in patients with ventricular hypertrophy and in patients in whom the cavity is dilated.[41,42]

Analysis along these lines makes many assumptions. The use of the term *compliance* suggests that the walls of the ventricle are passive and that measurements are made under equilibrated conditions. Both of these assumptions can be questioned, even during the period of passive diastole. Equilibrium is not attained because measurements of pressure and volume have to be made as the ventricle fills. As a result, additional dynamic components secondary to the filling process itself must be considered. Of these, the most significant is viscosity. Viscous forces are proportional to the rate of filling and cause the ventricle to appear stiffer than at equilibrium. Viscous forces have been shown experimentally in isolated stretched papillary muscles[43] and may become clinically significant in patients with left ventricular hypertrophy.[44,45] Inertia is another dynamic component of ventricular filling. Inertia results from outward acceleration of the ventricular walls and causes cavity pressure to be lower at the same cavity size compared with the state of equilibrium. Inertial forces are small, however, and even when wall motion is rapid, these seldom result in discrepancies of more than 0.1 mm Hg.

PRESSURE-VOLUME RELATIONSHIP OF THE RIGHT VENTRICLE

The focus so far has been on the use of the pressure-volume relationship in the assessment of left ventricular performance. Similar mathematical formalism has been applied to the right ventricle in terms of its pressure-volume relationship during ejection:[46] the interplay between contractility and load[47] and the close coupling between right ventricular function and the pulmonary vasculature.[48-50] Nonetheless, the normal right ventricular pressure-volume relationship seems to differ from that of the left ventricle. Typically, right ventricular ejection begins early during the pressure increase and continues as ventricular pressure decreases. As a result, phases of isovolumic contraction and relaxation are ill defined or may not exist in the normally loaded right ventricle. Consequently, the form of the pressure-volume loop of the right ventricle differs from the square or rectangle of the normal left ventricular pressure-volume loop and assumes a more triangular shape.[51] When the right ventricle is subjected to a pressure load, ejection during the two "isovolumic" periods ceases, and the overall shape of the pressure-volume loop resembles that of the normal left ventricle.[52,53] Conversely, pressure-volume diagrams obtained from the chronically unloaded left ventricle (e.g., in a patient after the Mustard procedure) may be indistinguishable from the normal right ventricular pattern.[53] These data combined suggest that the normal right ventricular contraction pattern and the pressure-volume relationship reflect loading conditions rather than any intrinsic differences in the properties of the right ventricular myocardium.

Ventricular Interdependence

Having considered the interaction between each ventricle and its respective vascular load, it is timely to consider the interdependence between the ventricles, that is, the effect of volume changes of one ventricle on the other.[54] There are several mechanisms whereby this ventricular interdependence may occur. The heart is enclosed in a noncompliant pericardial sac, with little free space to accommodate acute ventricular dilation. As a result, when right ventricular end-diastolic volume increases, it must do so within the confines of the space allowed for the left

ventricle, limiting left ventricular filling.[55,56] More recent studies using pressure-volume analysis show that in addition to a direct mechanical effect on left ventricular filling, right ventricular dilation may impair left ventricular performance further by reducing its contractility.[57] Another aspect of ventricular interdependence relates to the series relationship between the ventricles, such that the left ventricle requires right ventricular output for its filling.[58] In many situations, the interactions between the two ventricles may have an acute impact on cardiovascular performance in patients with congenital heart disease. In a patient who undergoes banding of the pulmonary artery, distention of the subpulmonary ventricle may alter the performance of the systemic ventricle.[52] During a pulmonary hypertensive crisis, the acute elevation in pulmonary vascular resistance and reduction in pulmonary blood flow result in right ventricular dilation. This dilation may impair left ventricular output, resulting in severe systemic hypotension (Fig. 7-4). In addition, important heart-lung interactions may be present in mechanically ventilated patients, in whom positive end-expiratory pressure, by increasing intrathoracic and pericardial pressures, may accentuate the normal interdependent relationship between the ventricles.[54]

The pressure-volume relationship can provide a detailed assessment of the function of either ventricle or even both simultaneously and is an ideal tool for the assessment of ventricular interdependence. Pinsky and coworkers[59] measured simultaneous right and left ventricular pressures and volumes in anesthetized open-chest, open-pericardium rabbits. Pinsky's group showed that an increase in right ventricular end-diastolic volume resulted in a decrease in left ventricular end-diastolic volume secondary to decreased diastolic compliance, without any change in systolic function. Conversely, increases in left ventricular end-diastolic volume decreased right ventricular end-systolic volume, resulting in an increase in its maximal elastance, but with

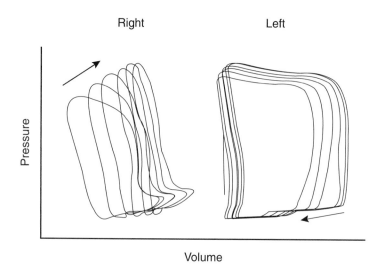

FIGURE 7-4 ■ **The phenomenon of ventricular interdependence.** Simultaneous recordings of pressure-volume loops in the right and left ventricles during occlusion of the main pulmonary artery, showing the phenomenon of ventricular interdependence. As right ventricular pressure and volume increase *(arrow on left)*, left ventricular end-diastolic volume decreases *(arrow on right)*. As left-ventricular end-diastolic volume decreases more than end-systolic volume, left ventricular stroke volume is reduced.

a minimal effect on right ventricular compliance.[60] Santamore and associates[61] showed the effects of intrathoracic pressure on right and left ventricular pressure-volume relationships, suggesting that ventricular interdependence may contribute to the reduction in left ventricular stroke volume during spontaneous inspiration. Santamore and associates[62] also showed that elevations in pericardial (and intrathoracic) pressure, as would exist during positive-pressure ventilation, resulted in further exaggeration of right and left ventricular interdependence. This topic is discussed in more detail in Chapter 8.

PRESSURE-VOLUME RELATIONSHIP IN PRIMARY CARDIAC FAILURE

Heart failure is a term that describes a deterioration of global cardiovascular performance and may incorporate changes in systolic function, diastolic function, and systemic and pulmonary vascular tones. There are few data in the literature that address the changes that occur in the ventricular pressure-volume relationship in children with myocardial failure.[63] Studies in adults have shown, however, that the assessment of the pressure-volume relationship can be used to assess the effects of progressive myocardial failure on integrated cardiovascular performance.

Studies that investigated the matching of ventricular properties to arterial load are particularly important in this respect. As mentioned previously, in normal subjects with an ejection fraction of 60% or more, ventricular elastance is nearly double Ea. This condition affords maximal mechanical efficiency. In patients with moderate heart failure, with ejection fractions of 40% to 59%, ventricular elastance is almost equal to Ea, a condition affording maximal stroke work from a given end-diastolic volume. In patients with severe heart failure, with ejection fractions of less than 40%, ventricular elastance is less than half of Ea, which results in decreased work efficiency. Ventriculoarterial coupling normally is set toward maximizing work efficiency in terms of the relationship between left ventricular work and oxygen consumption. As cardiac function becomes impaired in patients with moderate cardiac dysfunction, ventricular and arterial properties are initially matched to maximize stroke work at the expense of work efficiency. As cardiac dysfunction becomes severe, however, the ventricle and vasculature become uncoupled so that neither the stroke work nor work efficiency is near maximum for patients with severe cardiac dysfunction.[64,65]

The effects of inotropic stimulation also have been assessed in this framework. Studies have shown that the increases in cardiac output during inotropic stimulation depend on vascular characteristics[31]; in depressed hearts, inotropes may modulate ventriculoarterial coupling toward optimization of either stroke work or mechanical efficiency.[65,66] Further studies of children are required to examine whether these mechanisms apply in the immature cardiovascular system.

DEVELOPMENTAL CHANGES IN THE PRESSURE-VOLUME RELATIONSHIP

Considerable changes occur in myocardial structure and function during fetal development.[67] Although it might be expected that developmental changes may alter ventricular performance and inotropic responsiveness during the early neonatal period, data examining these phenomena are inconsistent. The reasons for these inconsistencies are at least partly methodologic. It seems that the conditions under which the assessment is made are crucial in determining the conclusions drawn from neonatal studies. Considerable differences exist between in vivo and in vitro findings and between animal species—the latter probably reflecting species-specific maturational rates in the early postnatal myocardium.

There is some common ground with which one can begin: In intact and isolated cat, rabbit, and rat myocardium, force generation seems to remain below adult levels for many weeks after birth. This situation has been attributed to the reduced numbers of β-adrenoreceptors and altered function of the sarcoplasmic reticulum and organization of myofibrils in the neonate compared with the adult.[68-71] In lambs, the species that has been most studied, some investigators have shown reduced mechanical performance of the left ventricle during the early postnatal period, which seemed to correlate with immaturity of myosin ATPase activity.[72] Other investigators observed an elevated resting left ventricular contractility, however, which decreased as postnatal development progressed.[73]

The effects of postnatal development on the contractile responses to inotropic stimulation also are controversial and seem to be species dependent. The observation of a blunted response of in vitro neonatal rabbit myocardium to β-adrenergic stimulation with isoproterenol, in contrast to a normal response to forskolin (a direct activator of adenylate cyclase), provides an important illustration of maturational differences. These findings suggest that although myocardial adenylate cyclase is well developed in the neonatal heart, its coupling with the β-adrenergic receptor may be functionally incomplete, resulting in reduced responsiveness to adrenergic stimulation.[74] Other studies showed that the inotropic responses to isoproterenol in isolated papillary muscle were fully developed in neonatal rats,[75] but reduced in muscle from neonatal dogs.[76]

In vivo studies also are inconsistent, with one study showing a reduced cardiac output response to isoproterenol in young lambs,[77] but another showing no change in the contractile response (assessed with an isovolumic index) to isoproterenol during postnatal development in piglets.[78] It has been suggested that because resting levels of myocardial contractility measured using an end-systolic index were higher in the younger neonates, the limited reserve seemed to be secondary to a high resting β-adrenergic state.[73,79] The interaction between ventricular load and contractility described in the mature circulation seems to be well developed at birth. In newborn lambs, stepwise increases in afterload increase contractility considerably, which enables the heart to maintain stroke volume at different levels of afterload; this is direct evidence for the existence of homeometric autoregulation in the intact newborn heart.[27] Ea decreases in response to β-adrenergic stimulation in the young neonate, suggesting that the ability to alter ventriculoarterial coupling during inotropic stimulation is well developed even in the early neonatal period.[80]

PRESSURE-VOLUME RELATIONSHIP IN CONGENITAL HEART DISEASE

The pressure-volume relationship might be considered ideal for the assessment of patients with congenital heart disease. In these patients, cardiac load, ventricular interdependence, postoperative bypass-related changes in cardiac function, and inotropic responsiveness all play a crucial role in determining cardiovascular performance. The others (e.g., a ventricular septal defect) and intracardiac valvular insufficiency (e.g., mitral regurgitation or aortic insufficiency) lead to a progressive increase in end-diastolic volume and a shift of the pressure-volume loop to the right on the EDPVR, although no pathophysiologic derangement leads to change in only one parameter without affecting the others (see Fig. 7-2C). More recent investigative studies have provided insight, however, into other, more complex clinical situations in congenital heart diseases and relevant interventions and are discussed in more detail subsequently.

Effects of Cardiac Surgery

Numerous studies of animal models of cardiopulmonary bypass[81] and in adults after cardiac surgery have shown profound perioperative alterations in the pressure-volume relationship. Few studies address, however, the impact of cardiac surgery in the pediatric population. Using the conductance catheter technique during open heart surgery, Chaturvedi and coworkers[82] showed a 40% reduction in left ventricular Ees in infants and children immediately after bypass. The same investigators later showed that these effects could be attenuated by modified ultrafiltration.[83]

Abnormalities of left ventricular diastolic performance are uncommon in infants and children early after biventricular repair of "simple" lesions, as evidenced by a lack of demonstrable deterioration in the EDPVR and time constant of relaxation.[82] These observations contrast considerably, however, with the observations in patients undergoing Fontan operations, in whom pressure decay during isovolumic relaxation is considerably deranged in the early postoperative period, reflecting a dramatic and acute change in ventricular geometry.[84]

Functional Single Ventricle

The sequential palliation of patients with a functionally univentricular circulation imposes rapid and profound alterations in ventricular loading conditions and geometry. The use of pressure-volume analysis in assessing integrated cardiac performance has been explored in this complex group. It was observed in an animal model of the Fontan circulation[85] that the slope of the ESPVR decreased (reduced Ees), and the end-systolic pressure–stroke volume relationship increased (increased Ea). As a result, the Ees-to-Ea ratio decreased, reflecting deterioration in ventriculoarterial coupling, suggesting that stroke work and mechanical efficiency were significantly reduced after Fontan surgery. The Fontan circulation has a contractility-afterload mismatch and an impaired ventriculoarterial coupling, with important negative implications for mechanical efficiency and cardiac functional reserve. Although there are limitations in the development of an acute model in a previously normal animal, these observations show how clinicians can use pressure-volume analysis to study integrated cardiovascular physiology during complex alterations in hemodynamic state.

Tanoue and colleagues[86] brought pressure-volume analysis into the clinical arena, in a detailed comparison of cardiovascular function in patients undergoing Fontan operations with or without a preceding bidirectional cavopulmonary shunt. Tanoue's group showed a more favorable relationship between Ees and Ea in the Fontan circulation of patients who had undergone staged surgery. This finding suggests that correction of afterload mismatch during the interval period between bidirectional cavopulmonary anastomosis and staged Fontan surgery may be important in optimizing the functional outcomes after Fontan operations in high-risk candidates.[87]

Systemic Right Ventricle

In many patients with complex congenital heart disease, staged palliation results in a circulation in which the systemic circulation is supported by a ventricle of right ventricular morphology. There also are many patients who have now reached adulthood after atrial redirection surgery (Mustard or Senning operation) for transposition of the great arteries. Impaired (systemic) right ventricular function has been implicated as a cause of reduced maximal exercise capacity in this group.

Derrick and coworkers[88] used conductance catheters and the pressure-volume relationship to examine the mechanisms of right ventricular impairment in young adults who had undergone Mustard repair. Derrick and coworkers[88] showed that the increases in cardiac index and stroke volume in response to exercise and dobutamine infusion were significantly blunted in Mustard patients compared with controls. This blunting was present despite significantly improved indices of myocardial contraction (ESPVR and preload recruitable stroke work index), enhanced ventriculoarterial coupling, and improved ventricular isovolumic relaxation during dobutamine infusion. No changes were observed in EDPVR, but a key consistent feature in these patients was a failure to augment ventricular filling during tachycardia—manifested by absence of change in peak filling rate.[88]

CURRENT STATUS AND FUTURE TRENDS

This chapter provides an introduction to the present state of the art of pressure-volume analysis in the assessment of global cardiovascular function. We have looked well beyond simple contractility as a marker of cardiac performance and have shown how the pressure-volume relationship can be used to evaluate the metabolic demands of the heart, interactions between the ventricles, and their relationship with the vasculature. The pressure-volume relationship has an important role in the formal assessment of cardiovascular function in the failing heart with or without congenital heart disease. Future research should focus on the use of the pressure-volume relationship as a diagnostic tool and to investigate the global effects of therapeutic interventions in even the immature animal.[89]

Key Concepts

■ The ESPVR provides a useful measure of ventricular contractility, but the pressure-volume approach begins, rather than ends, with an assessment of Ees.

■ Although many treatments in a child with heart failure are aimed at augmenting ventricular systolic performance, without the ability of the vasculature to convert within itself the increased pressure work of the ventricle into flow work, these therapeutic strategies would be of little benefit.

■ The use of the pressure-volume relationship for the assessment of ventricular diastolic function, the EDPVR, is based on the assumption that throughout the period during diastole when volume and pressure are increasing, the ventricle exhibits elastic behavior.

■ Typically, right ventricular ejection begins early during the pressure increase and continues as ventricular pressure decreases. As a result, phases of isovolumic contraction and relaxation are ill defined or may not exist in the normally loaded right ventricle. Consequently, the form of the pressure-volume loop of the right ventricle differs from the square or rectangle of the normal left ventricular pressure-volume loop and assumes a more triangular shape.

■ Ventriculoarterial coupling is normally set toward maximizing work efficiency in terms of the relationship between left ventricular work and oxygen consumption. As cardiac function becomes impaired, in patients with moderate cardiac dysfunction, ventricular and arterial properties are initially matched to maximize stroke work at the expense of work efficiency. As cardiac dysfunction becomes severe, however, the ventricle and vasculature become uncoupled so that neither the stroke work nor work efficiency is near maximum for patients with severe cardiac dysfunction.

■ The others (e.g., a ventricular septal defect) and intracardiac valvular insufficiency (e.g., mitral regurgitation or aortic insufficiency) lead to a progressive increase in end-diastolic volume and a shift of the pressure-volume loop to the right on the EDPVR, although no pathophysiologic derangement leads to change in only one parameter without affecting the others.

■ The Fontan circulation has a contractility-afterload mismatch and an impaired ventriculoarterial coupling, with important negative implications for mechanical efficiency and cardiac functional reserve.

Acknowledgments
We gratefully acknowledge the contribution of Dr. Lara Shekerdemian to this chapter.

REFERENCES

1. Frank O: Die Grundform des arteriellen pulses. Z Biol 1899;37:483-526.
2. Katz AM, Katz LN, Williams FL: Registration of left ventricular volume curves in the dog with the systemic circulation intact. Circ Res 1955;3:588-593.
3. Monroe RG, French GN: Ventricular pressure-volume relationships and oxygen consumption in fibrillation and arrest. Circ Res 1960;8:260-266.
4. Suga H: Time course of pressure-volume relationship of the cardiac ventricle in anesthetized dogs. Nippon Seirigaku Zasshi 1969;31:328-329.
5. Suga H: Left ventricular time-varying pressure-volume ratio in systole as an index of myocardial inotropism. Jpn Heart J 1971;12:153-160.
6. Suga H: Theoretical analysis of a left-ventricular pumping model based on the systolic time-varying pressure-volume ratio. IEEE Trans Biomed Eng 1971;18:47-55.
7. Baan J, Van der Velde ET: Sensitivity of left ventricular end-systolic pressure-volume relation to type of loading intervention in dogs. Circ Res 1988;62:1247-1258.
8. Baan J, Jong TT, Kerkhof PL, et al: Continuous stroke volume and cardiac output from intra-ventricular dimensions obtained with impedance catheter. Cardiovasc Res 1981;15:328-334.
9. Baan J, van der Velde ET, de Bruin HG, et al: Continuous measurement of left ventricular volume in animals and humans by conductance catheter. Circulation 1984;70:812-823.
10. Wiggers CJ: Studies in the consecutive phases of the cardiac cycle. Am J Physiol 1921;56:415-459.
11. Wiggers CJ: Dynamics of ventricular contraction under abnormal conditions (The Henry Jackson Memorial Lecture). Circulation 1952;5:321-348.
12. Suga H: Time course of left ventricular pressure-volume relationship under various end-diastolic volume. Jpn Heart J 1969;10:509-515.

13. Suga H: Time course of left ventricular pressure-volume relationship under various extents of aortic occlusion. Jpn Heart J 1970;11:373-378.

14. Kass DA, Maughan WL, Guo ZM, et al: Comparative influence of load versus inotropic states on indexes of ventricular contractility: Experimental and theoretical analysis based on pressure-volume relationships. Circulation 1987;76:1422-1436.

15. Banerjee A, Brook MM, Klautz RJ, Teitel DF: Nonlinearity of the left ventricular end-systolic wall stress-velocity of fiber shortening relation in young pigs: A potential pitfall in its use as a single-beat index of contractility. J Am Coll Cardiol 1994;23:514-524.

16. Burkhoff D, Sugiura S, Yue DT, Sagawa K: Contractility-dependent curvilinearity of end-systolic pressure-volume relations. Am J Physiol 1987;252:H1218-H1227.

17. Krosl P, Abel FL: Problems with use of the end systolic pressure-volume slope as an indicator of left ventricular contractility: An alternate method. Shock 1998;10:285-291.

18. van der Velde ET, Burkhoff D, Steendijk P, et al: Nonlinearity and load sensitivity of end-systolic pressure-volume relation of canine left ventricle in vivo. Circulation 1991;83:315-327.

19. Kass DA, Kelly RP: Ventriculo-arterial coupling: Concepts, assumptions, and applications. Ann Biomed Eng 1992;20:41-62.

20. Burkhoff D, de Tombe PP, Hunter WC, Kass DA: Contractile strength and mechanical efficiency of left ventricle are enhanced by physiological afterload. Am J Physiol 1991;260:H569-H578.

21. Henderson AH, Cattell MR: Length as a factor in excitation-contraction coupling in heart muscle: An investigation of mechanical transients in strontium-mediated contractions. Eur J Cardiol 1976;4(Suppl):47-51.

22. Henderson AH, Cattell MR: Prolonged biphasic strontium-mediated contractions of cat and frog heart muscle and their response to inotropic influences. J Mol Cell Cardiol 1976;8:299-319.

23. Lakatta EG, Henderson AH: Starling's law reactivated. J Mol Cell Cardiol 1977;9:347-351.

24. Shimizu J, Todaka K, Burkhoff D: Load dependence of ventricular performance explained by model of calcium-myofilament interactions. Am J Physiol Heart Circ Physiol 2002;282:H1081-H1091.

25. Todaka K, Ogino K, Gu A, Burkhoff D: Effect of ventricular stretch on contractile strength, calcium transient, and cAMP in intact canine hearts. Am J Physiol 1998;274:H990-H1000.

26. Stennett R, Ogino K, Morgan JP, Burkhoff D: Length-dependent activation in intact ferret hearts: Study of steady-state $Ca(2^+)$-stress-strain interrelations. Am J Physiol 1996;270:H1940-H1950.

27. Klautz RJ, Teitel DF, Steendijk P, et al: Interaction between afterload and contractility in the newborn heart: Evidence of homeometric autoregulation in the intact circulation. J Am Coll Cardiol 1995;25:1428-1435.

28. Binkley PF, Van Fossen DB, Nunziata E, et al: Influence of positive inotropic therapy on pulsatile hydraulic load and ventricular-vascular coupling in congestive heart failure. J Am Coll Cardiol 1990;15:1127-1135.

29. Binkley PF, Van Fossen DB, Haas GJ, Leier CV: Increased ventricular contractility is not sufficient for effective positive inotropic intervention. Am J Physiol 1996;271:H1635-H1642.

30. Sunagawa K, Sagawa K, Maughan WL: Ventricular interaction with the loading system. Ann Biomed Eng 1984;12:163-189.

31. Freeman GL, Colston JT: Role of ventriculovascular coupling in cardiac response to increased contractility in closed-chest dogs. J Clin Invest 1990;86:1278-1284.

32. Sunagawa K, Maughan WL, Sagawa K: Optimal arterial resistance for the maximal stroke work studied in isolated canine left ventricle. Circ Res 1985;56:586-595.

33. van den Horn GJ, Westerhof N, Elzinga G: Optimal power generation by the left ventricle: A study in the anesthetized open thorax cat. Circ Res 1985;56:252-261.

34. Burkhoff D, Sagawa K: Ventricular efficiency predicted by an analytical model. Am J Physiol 1986;250:R1021-R1027.

35. Starling MR: Left ventricular-arterial coupling relations in the normal human heart. Am Heart J 1993;125:1659-1666.

36. Suga H: Global cardiac function: Mechano-energetico-informatics. J Biomech 2003;36:713-720.

37. Suga H: Ventricular energetics. Physiol Rev 1990;70:247-277.

38. Suga H: Cardiac mechanics and energetics: From Emax to PVA. Front Med Biol Eng 1990;2:3-22.

39. Grossman W, McLaurin LP: Diastolic properties of the left ventricle. Ann Intern Med 1976;84:316-326.

40. Mirsky I: Assessment of passive elastic stiffness of cardiac muscle: Mathematical concepts, physiologic and clinical considerations, directions of future research. Prog Cardiovasc Dis 1976;18:277-308.

41. Peterson KL, Ricci D, Tsuji J, et al: Evaluation of chamber and myocardial compliance in pressure overload hypertrophy. Eur J Cardiol 1978;7(Suppl):195-211.

42. Fester A, Samet P: Passive elasticity of the human left ventricle: The "parallel elastic element." Circulation 1974;50:609-618.

43. Noble MI: The diastolic viscous properties of cat papillary muscle. Circ Res 1977;40:288-292.

44. Gaasch WH, Quinones MA, Waisser E, et al: Diastolic compliance of the left ventricle in man. Am J Cardiol 1975;36:193-201.

45. Gaasch WH, Cole JS, Quinones MA, Alexander JK: Dynamic determinants of left ventricular diastolic pressure-volume relations in man. Circulation 1975;51:317-323.

46. Shoucri RM: Pressure-volume relation in the right ventricle. J Biomed Eng 1993;15:167-169.

47. de Vroomen M, Cardozo RH, Steendijk P, et al: Improved contractile performance of right ventricle in response to increased RV afterload in newborn lamb. Am J Physiol Heart Circ Physiol 2000;278:H100-H105.

48. Lopes Cardozo RH, Steendijk P, Baan J, et al: Right ventricular function in respiratory distress syndrome and subsequent partial liquid ventilation: Homeometric autoregulation in the right ventricle of the newborn animal. Am J Respir Crit Care Med 2000;162:374-379.

49. De Vroomen M, Steendijk P, Lopes Cardozo RH, et al: Enhanced systolic function of the right ventricle during respiratory distress syndrome in newborn lambs. Am J Physiol Heart Circ Physiol 2001;280:H392-H400.

50. D'Orio V, Lambermont B, Detry O, et al: Pulmonary impedance and right ventricular-vascular coupling in endotoxin shock. Cardiovasc Res 1998;38:375-382.

51. Redington AN, Gray HH, Hodson ME, et al: Characterisation of the normal right ventricular pressure-volume relation by biplane angiography and simultaneous micromanometer pressure measurements. Br Heart J 1988;59:23-30.

52. Leeuwenburgh BP, Helbing WA, Steendijk P, et al: Biventricular systolic function in young lambs subject to chronic systemic right ventricular pressure overload. Am J Physiol Heart Circ Physiol 2001;281:H2697-H2704.

53. Redington AN, Rigby ML, Shinebourne EA, Oldershaw PJ: Changes in the pressure-volume relation of the right ventricle when its loading conditions are modified. Br Heart J 1990;63:45-49.

54. Jardin F: Ventricular interdependence: How does it impact on hemodynamic evaluation in clinical practice? Intensive Care Med 2003;29:361-363.

55. Santamore WP, Shaffer T, Papa L: Theoretical model of ventricular interdependence: Pericardial effects. Am J Physiol 1990;259:H181-H189.

56. Santamore WP, Constantinescu M, Shaffer T: Predictive changes in ventricular interdependence. Ann Biomed Eng 1988;16:215-234.

57. Brookes C, Ravn H, White P, et al: Acute right ventricular dilatation in response to ischemia significantly impairs left ventricular systolic performance. Circulation 1999;100:761-767.

58. Robotham JL, Stuart RS, Borkon AM, et al: Effects of changes in left ventricular loading and pleural pressure on mitral flow. J Appl Physiol 1988;65:1662-1675.

59. Pinsky MR, Perlini S, Solda PL, et al: Dynamic right and left ventricular interactions in the rabbit: Simultaneous measurement of ventricular pressure-volume loops. J Crit Care 1996;11:65-76.

60. Janicki JS: Influence of the pericardium and ventricular interdependence on left ventricular diastolic and systolic function in patients with heart failure. Circulation 1990;81:III15-III20.

61. Santamore WP, Heckman JL, Bove AA: Right and left ventricular pressure-volume response to respiratory maneuvers. J Appl Physiol 1984;57:1520-1527.

62. Santamore WP, Heckman JL, Bove AA: Right and left ventricular pressure-volume response to elevated pericardial pressure. Am Rev Respir Dis 1986;134:101-107.

63. Alpert BS, Benson L, Olley PM: Peak left ventricular pressure/volume (Emax) during exercise in control subjects and children with left-sided cardiac disease. Cathet Cardiovasc Diagn 1981;7:145-153.

64. Asanoi H, Sasayama S, Kameyama T: Ventriculoarterial coupling in normal and failing heart in humans. Circ Res 1989;65:483-493.

65. Sasayama S, Asanoi H: Coupling between the heart and arterial system in heart failure. Am J Med 1991;90:14S-18S.

66. Ishizaka S, Asanoi H, Kameyama T, Sasayama S: Ventricular-load optimization by inotropic stimulation in patients with heart failure. Int J Cardiol 1991;31:51-58.

67. Long WH: Autonomic and central neuroregulation of fetal cardiovascular function. In Polin R, Fox, WW (eds): Fetal and Neonatal Physiology. Philadelphia, WB Saunders, 1992, pp 629-645.

68. Maylie JG: Excitation-contraction coupling in neonatal and adult myocardium of cat. Am J Physiol 1982;242:H834-H843.

69. Nakanishi T, Jarmakani JM: Developmental changes in myocardial mechanical function and subcellular organelles. Am J Physiol 1984;246:H615-H625.

70. Anderson PA, Moore GE, Nassar RN: Developmental changes in the expression of rabbit left ventricular troponin T. Circ Res 1988;63:742-747.

71. Nassar R, Reedy MC, Anderson PA: Developmental changes in the ultrastructure and sarcomere shortening of the isolated rabbit ventricular myocyte. Circ Res 1987;61:465-483.

72. Riemenschneider TA, Brenner RA, Wikman-Coffelt J, Mason DT: Maturational changes in cardiac muscle myosin adenosine triphosphatase activity relative to hemodynamic alterations in newborn lambs. Am Heart J 1982;103:834-839.

73. Teitel DF, Sidi D, Chin T, et al: Developmental changes in myocardial contractile reserve in the lamb. Pediatr Res 1985;19:948-955.

74. Artman M, Kithas PA, Wike JS, Strada SJ: Inotropic responses change during postnatal maturation in rabbit. Am J Physiol 1988;255:H335-H342.

75. Mackenzie E, Standen NB: The postnatal development of adrenoceptor responses in isolated papillary muscles from rat. Pflugers Arch 1980;383:185-187.

76. Park IS, Michael LH, Driscoll DJ: Comparative response of the developing canine myocardium to inotropic agents. Am J Physiol 1982;242:H13-H18.

77. Klopfenstein HS, Rudolph AM: Postnatal changes in the circulation and responses to volume loading in sheep. Circ Res 1978;42:839-845.

78. Buckley NM, Gootman PM, Yellin EL, Brazeau P: Age-related cardiovascular effects of catecholamines in anesthetized piglets. Circ Res 1979;45:282-292.

79. Teitel DF, Klautz R, Steendijk P, et al: The end-systolic pressure-volume relationship in the newborn lamb: Effects of loading and inotropic interventions. Pediatr Res 1991;29:473-482.

80. Cassidy SC, Chan DP, Allen HD: Left ventricular systolic function, arterial elastance, and ventricular-vascular coupling: A developmental study in piglets. Pediatr Res 1997;42:273-281.

81. Matsuwaka R, Matsuda H, Shirakura R, et al: Changes in left ventricular performance after global ischemia: Assessing LV pressure-volume relationship. Ann Thorac Surg 1994;57:151-156.

82. Chaturvedi RR, Lincoln C, Gothard JW, et al: Left ventricular dysfunction after open repair of simple congenital heart defects in infants and children: Quantitation with the use of a conductance catheter immediately after bypass. J Thorac Cardiovasc Surg 1998;115:77-83.

83. Chaturvedi RR, Shore DF, White PA, et al: Modified ultrafiltration improves global left ventricular systolic function after open-heart surgery in infants and children. Eur J Cardiothorac Surg 1999;15:742-746.

84. Penny DJ, Lincoln C, Shore D, et al: The early response of the systemic ventricle during transition to the Fontan circulation: An acute hypertrophic cardiomyopathy? Cardiol Young 1992;2:78-84.

85. Szabo G, Buhmann V, Graf A, et al: Ventricular energetics after the Fontan operation: Contractility-afterload mismatch. J Thorac Cardiovasc Surg 2003;125:1061-1069.

86. Tanoue Y, Sese A, Ueno Y, et al: Bidirectional Glenn procedure improves the mechanical efficiency of a total cavopulmonary connection in high-risk Fontan candidates. Circulation 2001;103:2176-2180.

87. Tanoue Y, Sese A, Imoto Y, Joh K: Ventricular mechanics in the bidirectional Glenn procedure and total cavopulmonary connection. Ann Thorac Surg 2003;76:562-566.

88. Derrick GP, Narang I, White PA, et al: Failure of stroke volume augmentation during exercise and dobutamine stress is unrelated to load-independent indexes of right ventricular performance after the Mustard operation. Circulation 2000;102:III154-III159.

89. Stekelenburg-de Vos S, Steendijk P, Ursem NT, et al: Systolic and diastolic ventricular function assessed by pressure-volume loops in the stage 21 venous dipped chick embryo. Pediatr Res 2005;57:16-25.

CHAPTER 8

Systolic and Diastolic Dysfunction

Michael Cheung
Andrew N. Redington

This chapter concentrates on the pathophysiology and clinical manifestations of systolic and diastolic dysfunction in various models of myocardial disease. Fundamental myocardial properties, including the force-velocity relationship and force-frequency relationship (FFR), are discussed first to understand better the changes in ventricular performance associated with disease states. In addition to these intrinsic properties, which are largely derived from in vitro studies of myocardial function, the extrinsic factors affecting systolic performance, such as ventriculovascular coupling and ventricular interaction, are discussed. Mechanisms of diastolic dysfunction are described in terms of phases of diastolic filling and abnormalities of timing. Knowledge of the physiology of muscle shortening and relaxation in vitro is useful in understanding the behavior of the normal heart, the response to disease and therapeutic intervention, and the clinical assessment of myocardial and pump function.

SYSTOLIC FUNCTION AND DYSFUNCTION

Force-Velocity Relationship

Contractile performance of muscle, defined as its ability to do work, can be expressed in different ways, such as by its intrinsic properties and as it is affected by loading conditions. One of the fundamental properties of the myocardium is its **force-velocity relationship**. This relationship defines the ability of the myocyte to shorten more rapidly and to a greater degree when faced with a light load. Conversely, in the face of a heavy load, a muscle shortens more slowly and to a lesser degree. Using in vitro methods of measurement, such as the isovelocity release technique,[1] plots of the load dependence of these shortening velocities yield hyperbolic force-velocity curves (Fig. 8-1). It can be seen that maximal velocity of shortening (V_{max}) occurs at the time of zero load. V_{max} reflects the intrinsic velocity of myosin cross-bridge turnover, which can be measured in vitro as myosin ATPase activity.[2] The x-intercept of this curve where generated force is maximal is designated P_0. For the same contractile state, the changes in performance in the face of changing load are a reflection of the way in which work is performed in the face of a changing hemodynamic environment.

The concept of the maximal velocity of unloaded muscle as being a useful measure of contractility in vivo

was proposed by Sonnenblick.[3,4] Although in vitro studies have increased greatly the understanding of the way in which V_{max}, P_0, and force-velocity relationships may be modulated by alterations in myocardial structure and environment, these measurements in vivo are complicated and flawed. The validity of extrapolating back to zero load for the intact heart continues to be questioned, and the measurement of V_{max} in the in vivo studies has largely fallen out of favor. Some newer tissue Doppler indices have refocused attention on myocardial velocity measurements and may allow clinical and noninvasive insights into this relationship.

Velocity of Circumferential Fiber Shortening

The in vivo measurement of contractility using indices that are independent of load has remained the holy grail of myocardial function assessment (see Chapter 10). The most robust noninvasive index of contractility currently available is the index of **velocity of circumferential fiber shortening** corrected for rate (VCF_C) and indexed to end-systolic wall stress.[5] This index has been used widely in the assessment of acquired and congenital heart disease in children.[6-8]

Since its original description, further assessment of this index has shown that the relationship becomes nonlinear with marked changes in loading conditions.[9] A subsequent study reported the misrepresentation of

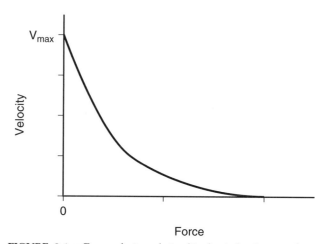

FIGURE 8-1 ■ **Force-velocity relationship for isolated myocardium.** Maximal velocity of shortening (V_{max}) occurs at the time of zero load. The x-intercept of this curve where generated force is maximal is designated P_0.

contractile function when this index is derived from measurements of endocardial dimensions in patients with ventricular hypertrophy.[10] Because subendocardial fibers shorten more than subepicardial fibers, the use of endocardial measurements of fiber shortening overestimates the degree of shortening, with this difference being amplified in the presence of ventricular hypertrophy. Although wall stress in the circumferential direction commonly is used to assess the ventricular afterload, this measurement neglects the effect of radial forces.[11] In this study of patients with a wide range of left ventricular dimensions and mass, the conclusion was that the use of wall stress in the assessment of ventricular afterload may be invalid in patients with abnormal ventricular geometry.

Ventricular Elastance

Although the concept of the time-dependent variation in the slope of the pressure-volume relationship had been stated by earlier investigators, the idea of the time-varying **ventricular elastance** as a measure of contractile function was championed by Suga.[12,13] The acquisition of simultaneous recordings of ventricular pressure and volume data provides important information regarding myocardial function. From the resulting pressure-volume curve, the stiffness of the ventricle can be determined instantaneously for any point in the cardiac cycle. If a family of loops is generated by acute alteration of loading conditions (e.g., preload reduction by transient balloon occlusion of the inferior vena cava), the linear relationship of this time-varying elastance can be plotted with the slope being a relatively load-independent index of ventricular contractility. Analysis of the end-systolic points provides an index of contractility, end-systolic elastance (Ees), which is relatively insensitive to contractile change (e.g., compared with maximal rate of pressure increase [dP/dt$_{max}$]), but is highly resistant to the influence of changes in loading conditions. This resistance makes it a highly desirable index for the experimental assessment of systolic contractile function,[14] particularly when there may be a confounding influence of altered load.

The clinical assessment of ventricular performance using this technique is becoming established because it provides more detailed delineation of the multiple factors involved in determining cardiac function. This concept is exemplified in a study of patients with transposition of the great arteries, in whom a Mustard procedure had been performed. The previously shown failure of stroke volume augmentation had been assumed to be secondary to impaired myocardial responses in the systemic right ventricle. Using pressure-volume analysis during dobutamine stress,[15] right ventricular load–independent contractile indices not only showed an appropriate increase, but also there was a concomitant improvement in indices of myocardial relaxation. There was, however, a failure to increase ventricular filling rate, presumably owing to impaired atrioventricular transport after intra-atrial baffling. By dissecting out the myocardial responses from the load-dependent changes, a more complete and physiologically important description of the circulation was obtained.

Isovolumic Velocity and Acceleration

As mentioned earlier, the ability to assess myocardial velocity using Doppler techniques has refocused attention on the concept of the maximal velocity of unloaded myocardial shortening. The method of tissue Doppler echocardiography is explained in detail elsewhere, but in essence, the Doppler shift principle is applied to the myocardium with exclusion of the blood pool signal through the application of appropriate filters. The principle was first proposed by Isaaz and colleagues[16] and applied to pulse-wave Doppler. Since that time, it has been developed further and applied to M-mode and color Doppler. It is now possible to quantify myocardial movement with high temporal resolution (frame rates >150/sec are routinely achievable using commercially available echocardiographic systems based on digital platforms), and improvements in hardware and software have permitted acquisition of data at frame rates of 500/sec. In addition, the development of on-line analysis software has allowed rapid measurement of acquired data at the bedside.

There has been an interest in myocardial motion during the period of isovolumic contraction as an index of systolic contractile function. From an apical four-chamber transthoracic view, the maximal **isovolumic velocity (IVV)** during this period and first derivative of this with respect to time, **isovolumic acceleration (IVA)**, of the right and left ventricles of the normal heart have been compared with invasive indices of contractility derived from analysis of pressure-volume data.[17,18] Assessment of ventricular long axis function was chosen because longitudinal fibers start to shorten before radial fibers and are the first to be affected by myocardial ischemia[19]; assessment of longitudinal function may have greater potential to detect early changes in global and regional cardiac function.[20]

In an animal model, these isovolumic tissue Doppler indices were challenged by modulation of inotropy with infusions of dobutamine and esmolol, alterations of preload and afterload, and alteration in heart rate by atrial pacing. For the left ventricle, esmolol led to a decrease in IVA and maximal elastance ($P < .03$ and $P < .02$), both of which increased during dobutamine infusion ($P < .02$ and $P < .03$). IVA was unaffected by significant ($P < .001$) acute reduction of ventricular volume and a significantly increased afterload (systolic pressure increase; $P < .001$). With atrial pacing, there was a positive correlation between IVA and dP/dt$_{max}$ ($r^2 = .92$; $P < .05$): As heart rate was increased from 120 to 160 beats/min, there were significant increases in IVA and dP/dt$_{max}$ ($P < .0004$ and $P = .02$). Over the same range of heart rates, there was no significant change in

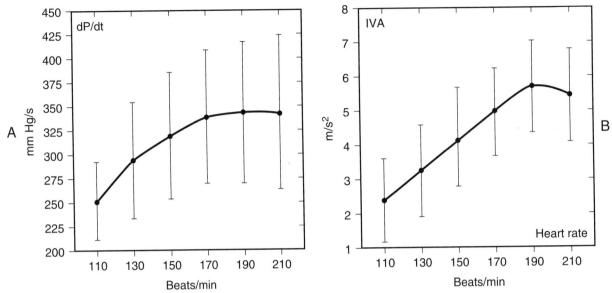

FIGURE 8-2 ■ **Force-frequency relationship.** Simultaneous measurements of the force-frequency relationship by micromanometer derived maximal rate of pressure increase (dP/dt) on the left (**A**) and noninvasive assessment by the novel tissue Doppler-derived index isovolumic acceleration (IVA) on the right (**B**).

maximal elastance ($P = .22$). In contrast, IVV was sensitive to changes in contractility during dobutamine infusion and with changes in heart rate, but it was unable to detect decreased contractility induced by esmolol and, in contrast to IVA, was significantly altered by increased afterload. We found only 9.8% ± 7.8% interobserver and 5.7% ± 4.6% intraobserver variabilities of measurements of IVA. Similar results in terms of resistance to changes in loading conditions and inotropy and ability to measure the FFR were shown for the right ventricle (Fig. 8-2).

As shown in Figure 8-3, IVA starts at the onset of ventricular pressure increase and represents one of the earliest detectable events in systole and reflects the maximal velocity of unloaded shortening. In the systolic phase of the cardiac cycle in vivo, the myocyte is maximally unloaded during the early phase of isovolumic contraction. The changes in myocardial loading conditions within the beating heart modify subsequent myocardial motion. We have shown that in normal hearts, values of IVA for the right ventricle are significantly higher than the values for the left ventricle. In light of the aforementioned load independence, this difference is not purely a reflection of differing loading conditions. Although this observation intuitively may seem incorrect, there are in vitro data to support the findings of superior contractile function of right ventricular compared with left ventricular muscle.

It is beyond the scope of this chapter to discuss the many factors that may modulate the maximal velocity of unloaded shortening.[21] Because this velocity is a reflection of myosin ATPase activity, it is predictably decreased by conditions such as hypothermia,[22]

acidosis,[23] and hypoxia.[24] One of the best-known causes in human disease states are the cardiomyopathies associated with abnormalities of myosin heavy chains (MyHC).[25,26]

Two functionally differing isoforms of MyHC are expressed within mammalian myocardium, α-MyHC and β-MyHC. These isoforms show 93% homology, but α-MyHC shows faster rates of force development,[27]

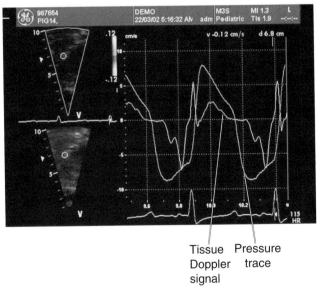

Tissue Doppler signal   Pressure trace

FIGURE 8-3 ■ **Tissue Doppler and isovolumic acceleration (IVA).** This is a tissue Doppler tracing with simultaneous pressure trace showing timing of IVA. IVA occurs at the onset of ventricular pressure increase. Tissue Doppler signal and pressure trace are labeled.

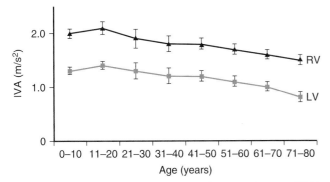

FIGURE 8-4 ■ **Age-related changes in isovolumic acceleration (IVA).** The age-related changes in isovolumic acceleration are shown in 360 normal volunteers. At every age, the right ventricle (RV) has a higher IVA than the left ventricle (LV).

faster myosin ATPase activity,[28] and a greater potential to generate force.[29,30] There is a greater percentage of α-MyHC in the right ventricular myocardium compared with the left ventricle of normal human hearts,[31] and the percentage varies with aging.[32,33] The difference in myocardial performance also has been shown in isolated canine ventricular muscle.[34] Under nearly all loading conditions, right ventricular muscle shortened faster than left ventricular muscle, and time to attain peak total tension of the right ventricle was shorter than that of the left ventricle. Preliminary data obtained in studies of IVA have revealed it to be consistently higher in the right ventricle compared with the left ventricle and to show similar age-related changes (Fig. 8-4).

Isoform switching also has been shown in hypothyroidism[35] and pressure[36] and volume[37] overload. An increase in the proportion of β-MyHC has been described in chronic aortic regurgitation in a rat model,[38] and this is associated with a reduction in the maximum unloaded velocity of shortening of left ventricle papillary muscle in rats with aortic insufficiency relative to controls. Although the general switch in isoforms is similar, there would be subtle differences in this response to pressure compared with volume overload.[39] The overall effect of a switch in MyHC isoform is to contribute toward a reduction in contractility; whether these subtle differences in response to type of load are important clinically is uncertain. If IVA measurement is able to track these changes, its potential as a noninvasive tool to analyze myocardial systolic functional adaptation may be even greater.

Force-Frequency Relationship

First described by Bowditch in 1871,[40] the intrinsic property of the myocardium to alter contractile force with change in rate of stimulation frequency is known as the **force-frequency relationship (FFR)** or the "treppe" effect. Most data support fluctuations in calcium cycling as the underlying mechanism for this phenomenon.[41,42] Because of the complexity of the pathways involved in

this process, there are multiple levels at which the FFR may be modified.

Two major calcium-dependent mechanisms alter the contractile state of the heart. These mechanisms affect either the availability of calcium or the responsiveness of the myofilaments to activation by intracellular calcium. Depolarization of the myocardium permits entry of calcium, leading to the release of a much larger quantity of calcium from intracellular stores within the sarcoplasmic reticulum. Binding of calcium with the myofilament allows actin and myosin to interact and generate force. Relaxation occurs with dissociation of calcium from the myofilament and resequestration into the sarcoplasmic reticulum by an ATPase-dependent calcium pump (SERCA). Modulation of this process can occur by cyclic AMP activation of protein kinases leading to phosphorylation of calcium channels of the sarcolemma or phosphorylation of phospholamban, both of which lead to a greater rate of change of intracellular calcium flux. Other texts[43] and other sections in this book provide a more detailed discussion of the control of calcium cycling and its coupling to contraction.

In vitro studies have shown that the response of the normal myocardium to increasing stimulation rate is to increase force of contractility up to an optimal heart rate at which point force is maximal, after which there is a decline in generated force (Fig. 8-5). The effect of increasing stimulation rate is thought to be an increase in

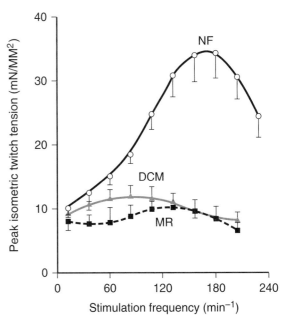

FIGURE 8-5 ■ **Force-frequency relationships in normal and various disease states.** In in vitro studies, the response of the normal myocardium to increasing stimulation rate is to increase force of contractility (up to an optimal heart rate at which point force is maximal). After this point, there is a decline in generated force. These are force-frequency relationships in normal nonfailing (NF) and failing myocardium. Failing myocardium force-frequency relationships are from patients with dilated cardiomyopathy (DCM) and chronic mitral regurgitation (MR). (From Alpert NR, Leavitt BJ, Ittleman FP, et al: *A mechanistic analysis of the force-frequency relation in non-failing and progressively failing human myocardium. Basic Res Cardiol* 1998;93:23-32.)

activity of SERCA through phosphorylation by calcium-dependent calmodulin kinase.[44] The rate-dependent intracellular flux of calcium can be shown through the use of calcium dyes, such as aequorin (Fig. 8-6).[41] Using this approach, dramatically differing responses may be observed in samples of diseased myocardium. In patients with dilated cardiomyopathy, the FFR may become negative; the generated force actually decreases with increasing rate of stimulation (see Fig. 8-5).[45]

Until more recently, in vivo measurements of ventricular FFR have been possible only via cardiac catheterization. The abnormal changes in dP/dt_{max}[46,47] and systolic function[46] have been shown in patients with ventricular hypertrophy versus normal controls.

Abnormal responses in patients with dilated cardiomyopathy also have been shown.[48] Assessment of the FFR using dP/dt_{max} is complicated, however, by the preload dependence of this index (rendering it possible that changes in contractility are underestimated as preload decreases with increasing tachycardia). The use of Ees obviates the confounding variable of changing load. In the original description of maximal elastance as an index of contractility, increases in heart rate through pacing imposed no demonstrable effect on this index.[49]

Previously, we described the derivation of a novel index of ventricular performance, IVA, derived from tissue Doppler echocardiography. IVA is a sensitive index of ventricular contractile function that is relatively independent of changes in loading conditions.[17,18] In these validation studies, we also showed that IVA was able to measure the myocardial FFR, as heart rate was increased by atrial pacing. IVA is a noninvasive technique that can measure the FFR in children with cardiac disease.

The rate-related change in calcium cycling is believed to be the underlying mechanism for the myocardial FFR. It would be expected that the deleterious effects of ischemia-reperfusion on the function of sarcoplasmic reticulum[50] also would affect this relationship. Preliminary studies in neonates undergoing the arterial switch procedure have shown marked postoperative depression of the ventricular FFR compared with preoperative assessment (Fig. 8-7). There is also significantly less depression of the FFR in patients undergoing Fontan completion after previous bidirectional cavopulmonary anastomosis; this is intuitively due to the relatively shorter duration of bypass and aortic cross-clamp, but also may be partly due to the age of the patient at the time of surgery.

Ventricular-Vascular Coupling

As discussed earlier, the myocardial force-velocity relationship dictates that increasing load results in reduced

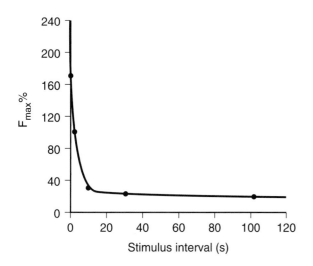

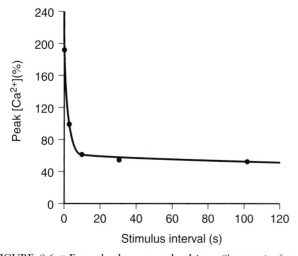

FIGURE 8-6 ■ Force development and calcium. Changes in force development and calcium transients in normal human myocardium using calcium dye. The percent F_{max} and Peak $[Ca^{2+}]_i$ for frequency potential are plotted with values normalized to peak isometric force and calcium at 0.33 Hz, respectively. (From Gwathmey JK, Slawsky MT, Hajjar RJ, et al: *Role of intracellular calcium handling in force-interval relationships of human ventricular myocardium. J Clin Invest* 1990;85:1599-1613.)

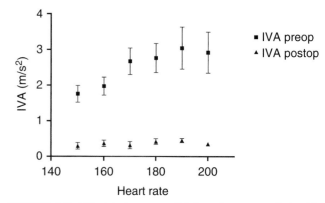

FIGURE 8-7 ■ Ventricular myocardial force-frequency relationship after cardiopulmonary bypass. Disruption of the ventricular myocardial force-frequency relationship in neonates after the arterial switch procedure for transposition of the great arteries. Note the markedly differing force-frequency relationship profile at 6 hours postoperatively *(triangles)* compared with before cardiopulmonary bypass *(squares)*. IVA, isovolumic acceleration.

velocity of contraction and degree of shortening. This is an important factor in determining cardiac performance and output. The systemic vascular bed provides a variable hydraulic load against ejection of blood from the left ventricle. Quantification of vascular load often is represented by the aortic peak systolic or mean pressure; this estimation is an oversimplification, however. Vascular load varies with the cardiac cycle as a result of the combination of the pulsatile nature of blood flow and pressure, elastic properties of blood vessels, and blood inertia and is better represented by **vascular impedance.**

The derivation of the various types of impedance is discussed in detail elsewhere.[51] Fast Fourier transformation of pressure and flow signals to derive an impedance spectrum represents the most complete description that may be obtained clinically and accounts for resistance, compliance, and wave reflection.[52] Input impedance is the ratio of pulsatile pressure and pulsatile flow at a particular arterial site, which depends not only on the local arterial properties, but also on the distal vascular tree.

Another way of considering the effect of vascular load on pump function is by analysis of the ventricular pressure-volume loop. **Effective arterial elastance (Ea)**, which is the ratio of end-systolic pressure and stroke volume, has been proposed as a measure of arterial load.[53,54] From pressure-volume analysis, this is represented by the slope of the line joining the end-diastolic and end-systolic points (Fig. 8-8). If contractility and end-diastolic volume are unchanged, it can be seen that an increase in Ea would result in a smaller stroke volume. Conversely, a reduction in afterload would lead to an increase in stroke volume. The effect of changes in afterload in the setting of reduced contractility may be considered in the same way.

Finally, an alternative approach to the understanding of the effects of afterload is by consideration of the relationship between **power** and **load**. In vitro studies show a bell-shaped curve (Fig. 8-9) representing this relationship, which holds true for the intact heart. Work and power are zero when load is zero and during an isometric contraction when, by definition, the muscle does not shorten. Work and power curves peak at an intermediate load. Chiu and associates[55] showed that in patients with heart failure the curve is shifted to the left, and these patients function on the right-hand descending limb of this relationship. In their study of eight patients with dilated cardiomyopathy, the infusion of sodium nitroprusside initially produced an increase in ventricular power, but a further increase in dosage led to a plateau or decrease in power. Using this form of analysis, the beneficial effects of a decrease in afterload can be seen with a shift along the curve resulting in an increase in the power generated, but that excessive afterload reduction ultimately may be detrimental to pump function and cardiac output.

A similar phenomenon may be seen when abnormal ventricular-vascular coupling is reactive to decreased stroke volume resulting from other hemodynamic problems. Taking the Fontan circulation as an example, the combination of a low stroke volume in the presence of a higher systemic vascular resistance results in demonstrably abnormal ventricular-vascular coupling.[56] Modifying the vascular properties without influencing stroke volume might be expected to be detrimental. Although not addressing ventricular-vascular coupling per se, in a randomized, double-blinded, crossover study of angiotensin-converting enzyme inhibition in a group of Fontan patients, the exercise-induced increase in cardiac index was significantly less in patients while

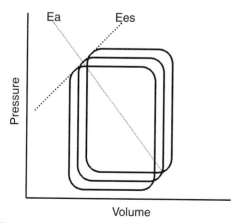

FIGURE 8-8 ■ Concept of arterial elastance (Ea) and ventricular-vascular coupling. The effect of vascular load on pump function is illustrated by analysis of the ventricular pressure-volume loop. Effective Ea, which is the ratio of end-systolic pressure and stroke volume, is a measure of arterial load. From pressure-volume analysis, this is represented by the slope of the line joining the end-diastolic and end-systolic points. Ees, end-systolic elastance.

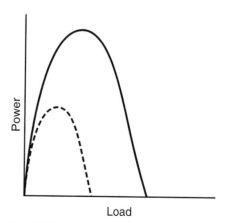

FIGURE 8-9 ■ Relationship of ventricular power and load. The relationship of ventricular power and load in normal hearts (solid line) and in hearts of patients with heart failure (dotted line). A bell-shaped curve represents this relationship. Work and power are 0 when load is 0 and during an isometric contraction when, by definition, the muscle does not shorten. Work and power curves peak at an intermediate load. In patients with heart failure, the curve is shifted to the left.

receiving enalapril compared with placebo.[57] The counter-intuitive acute effects of angiotensin-converting enzyme inhibition in the Fontan circulation emphasize the need to understand all elements of the optimal ventricular-vascular coupling when attempting to modify it to be optimal.

The appropriate afterload for optimal pump function also may be considered in a variety of ways. The definition of optimal function must be determined first: Should it be considered in terms of maximal **efficiency** or rather a measure of maximal stroke volume, power, or cardiac output? The answer depends on prevailing requirements of the body. In most clinical states, we are concerned with performance in terms of cardiac output.

In the normal heart, maximal stroke work and power are generated when the ventricle is subjected to the normal arterial impedance. Theoretically, pressure-volume analysis predicts that loading is optimal in terms of stroke work when the ratio of effective Ea to ventricular elastance is 1 (Ea/Ees = 1).[58] If contractility increases resulting in an increase in Ees, Ea also must increase to maintain maximal stroke work. Because preload changes within a physiologic range do not alter Ees, alterations in ventricular preload do not affect the optimal afterload. Experimental isolated heart studies have shown that maximal stroke work is achieved at a value of Ea/Ees less than 1 and is maintained at near-maximum even at values ranging from 0.3 to 1.3.[59]

Because Ea combines the effects of pulsatile and nonpulsatile loads into a single quantity, a variety of combinations of arterial compliance and systemic resistance values may result in the same measure of Ea. It does not provide information regarding the relative contributions of these factors to total hydraulic load,[60] but it does provide a framework for consideration of the effects of afterload on ventricular performance. Patients with congenital heart disease have primary and secondary problems with ventricular function and the vascular tree. The use of therapies established in the management of adult heart disease may not translate to the care of these children.

DIASTOLIC FUNCTION AND DYSFUNCTION

An understanding of the Wiggers diagram (Fig. 8-10) is helpful in determining the parameters used to assess diastolic function and the factors leading to their derangement. Wiggers divided the cardiac cycle for the left ventricle into eight phases, with three phases during systole and five phases during diastole. Diastolic dysfunction may be described as an abnormality of any of these diastolic phases, but ultimately as abnormal ventricular filling.[61-64] At the start of diastole, myofilaments stop generating tension, and relaxation occurs as an active energy-consuming process. Globally, sufficient

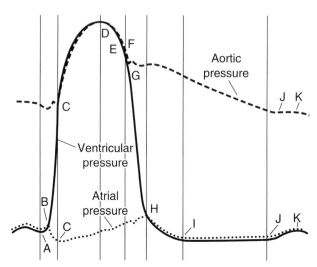

FIGURE 8-10 ■ Wiggers diagram of changes in pressure during the cardiac cycle. Systole begins with isovolumic contraction **(A-C)**, followed by maximum ejection **(C-D)** and ending with a period of reduced ejection **(D-F)**. In the first period of diastole known as *protodiastole* **(F-G)**, the first effects of relaxation are decreases in ventricular and aortic pressures leading to closure of the aortic valve. Ventricular pressure continues to decrease as myocardial relaxation proceeds throughout this period of isovolumic relaxation **(G-H)**. When the ventricular pressure is lower than that of the atrium, the mitral valve opens, and the period of early rapid filling begins **(H-I)**. Ventricular pressure continues to decrease during this phase, albeit at a slower rate. In the normal heart, most ventricular filling (approximately 70%) occurs during this period. A period of diastasis **(I-J)** may be observed when transmitral flow ceases or occurs at a slow rate as pressure in the atrium and ventricle approximate before atrial contraction **(J-K)**.

energy substrates and the mechanisms to regenerate these must be present throughout the myocardium for this process to occur at an appropriate rate and to an adequate extent. Small areas of regional dysfunction may perturb the coordinate mechanisms of relaxation. This regional dysfunction is particularly relevant to the efficiency of active relaxation, whereby ventricular filling depends on elastic recoil or restoring forces after systolic deformation of the myocardium. Additionally, abnormalities of ventricular stiffness or its reciprocal compliance, atrial contraction, and interactions from the adjacent ventricle and pericardium are variably important in different disease states. Fundamentally, however, all of these factors may influence the pressure gradient and blood flow across the atrioventricular valve. Besides these hemodynamic factors, the duration of diastole as a percentage of the total cardiac cycle and the timing of atrial contraction are important determinants of the amount of ventricular filling. The following sections address further the derangements of these different phases of diastole. Clinical examples are used to illustrate diagnosis of these mechanisms of diastolic dysfunction.

Abnormalities of Relaxation and Early Rapid Filling
Assessment of the process of relaxation in vivo is difficult, and although not strictly a reflection of the extent or

timing of this process, attempts have largely centered around measurements of the duration of the isovolumic relaxation period or the rate of pressure decline. None of these methods is able to differentiate between the active relaxation processes and the passive restoring forces of elastic recoil, which act in concert to reduce ventricular pressure during this period.

The **isovolumic relaxation time** (IVRT) can be measured noninvasively using M-mode echocardiographic assessment of the interval from aortic valve closure to mitral valve opening or by Doppler assessment of the period of aortic flow cessation to the onset of mitral valve inflow (see Chapter 10). These two techniques give slightly differing values, but significant changes in IVRT may be indicative of altered relaxation. As can be seen from the Wiggers diagram, for the same rate of relaxation, the higher the pressure at end systole, the longer it will take for the crossover with atrial pressure to occur and result in a longer IVRT. Conversely, higher atrial pressure results in a shortened IVRT. In the absence of altered systolic and diastolic pressures, abnormal myocardial relaxation reduces the rate of pressure decline and causes lengthening of IVRT. IVRT lengthens with normal aging such that values in the elderly are approximately double the values in children. The finding of a significant change in IVRT with aging should be considered in conjunction with other diastolic parameters.

The **time constant of isovolumic relaxation** is measured from invasive recordings of pressure decline. Because it is rare clinically to have simultaneous measurements of atrial and ventricular pressures and aortic flow, exact definition of the period of isovolumic relaxation is difficult. Typically the period is taken to begin with the point of maximal rate of pressure decline (dP/dt_{min}) and to extend to a lower pressure, usually equal to the ventricular end-diastolic pressure. When this curve has been defined, the time for the pressure to decrease by 50%, or pressure half-time, may be measured. For this measurement to be valid, pressure decay during this period should decline as a monoexponential, an assertion that has been questioned.[65] This index is prone to the same limitations as noninvasive measurement of IVRT described earlier.

Early rapid filling begins as ventricular pressure decreases to less than that of atrial pressure. The pressure gradient that develops is the driving force behind blood flow across the atrioventricular valve. If atrial pressure is relatively elevated, peak-filling velocity is increased because of the larger gradient. Conversely, elevation of ventricular pressure causes reduced filling velocity during this phase. When the peak-filling rate is reached, the blood velocity decreases. Because of the rate of pressure increase within the ventricle exceeding the rate of pressure decline secondary to relaxation shortly after mitral valve opening, reversal of the pressure gradient occurs,[66] causing flow deceleration. Blood flow

continues against this pressure gradient because of inertia. Deceleration time, which can be assessed by pulse-wave Doppler, is shorter in hearts with decreased ventricular compliance owing to the more rapid development of this negative pressure gradient.

Abnormal Ventricular Compliance

Ventricular architecture may be altered such that the passive viscoelastic properties of the ventricle become stiffer or less compliant. **Compliance** is the inverse of stiffness and is calculated by the change in volume for a given change in pressure (dV/dP). A structure that is less compliant distends less for a given increase in pressure. Because calculation of compliance requires a measurement of pressure, its quantification requires invasive assessment. A qualitative assessment can be inferred from surrogate measurements (e.g., pulmonary venous Doppler) in the clinical situation.

Invasive assessment of ventricular compliance is possible by analysis of the pressure-volume relationship. It is clear from the pressure-volume loop that compliance is a nonlinear relationship, and that assessment during the period of diastasis, which is the best portion in which to measure passive ventricular properties, is confounded by rapid heart rates. Because the data from a single cardiac cycle are limited, a commonly used approach is to generate a family of loops by alteration of ventricular loading conditions. The diastolic pressure-volume relationship at a particular period of diastole for this series of loops can be analyzed.

Compared with a ventricle of normal compliance, in the presence of decreased compliance, ventricular volume increases relatively less for the same increase in ventricular pressure. Although now rarely used in clinical practice, a noninvasive surrogate of left ventricular pressure can be gained by the use of an apex cardiogram. The basis of this measurement relies on the detection of pressure transmitted to the chest wall at the site of the apex beat as a result of the change in ventricular length during the cardiac cycle. An alternative approach is the assessment of transmitral and pulmonary venous Doppler flow patterns (see Chapter 10).

Abnormal Diastolic Function in Congenital Heart Disease

Important information regarding right ventricular compliance may be gained from the assessment of Doppler flow patterns in the main pulmonary artery. In the absence of significant outflow tract obstruction or elevation of pulmonary artery pressure, decreased right ventricular compliance allows the ventricle to act as a passive conduit to blood flow. This phenomenon of so-called **restrictive right ventricular physiology** was first described in patients with critical pulmonary stenosis after relief of outflow tract obstruction.[67] With the sample volume placed midway between the valve and the bifurcation of the branches of the pulmonary artery,

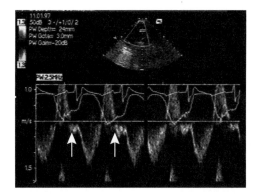

FIGURE 8-11 ■ **Restrictive right ventricular physiology.** Doppler tracing and simultaneous ventricular pressure trace from a patient with restrictive right ventricle physiology after surgical repair of tetralogy of Fallot. The pulse Doppler sample volume is placed in the main pulmonary artery midway between the pulmonary valve and the bifurcation of the branch pulmonary arteries. Note the presence of significant antegrade diastolic flow *(arrows)* coincident with atrial kick on the pressure trace.

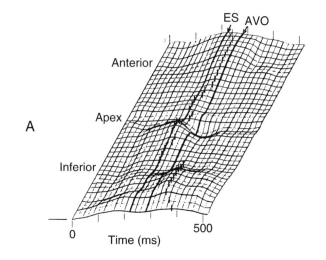

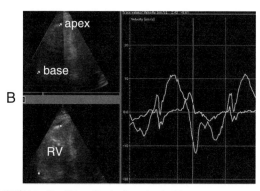

FIGURE 8-12 ■ **Diastolic dysfunction in Fontan patients.** Wall motion abnormalities detected by digitized ventriculograms **(A)** and tissue Doppler echocardiography **(B)** (see text for details). AVO, atrioventricular opening; ES, end systole; RV, right ventricle.

significant antegrade diastolic flow coincident with atrial systole and present throughout the respiratory cycle was detected using pulse-wave Doppler in patients with restriction (Fig. 8-11). This phenomenon subsequently has been most commonly observed after surgical repair of tetralogy of Fallot in the early postoperative period[68] and at late follow-up.[69,70] Clinical signs of right ventricular diastolic dysfunction in the early postoperative period, such as pleural effusions and the requirement for aggressive fluid replacement to maintain cardiac output, are observed frequently in this patient group.

The etiology of this dysfunction has been shown to be myocardial injury at the time of cardiopulmonary bypass.[71] Although problematic in the early postoperative period, the antegrade diastolic flow associated with restriction significantly contributes to forward flow and cardiac output. This finding underscores the importance of maintenance of sinus rhythm and appropriate ventilatory strategy in this group of patients.[72] Although this phenomenon disappears in the midterm postoperative period, it has been shown to recur in some patients at later follow-up.[73] This abnormality has been shown to be beneficial in the long-term by limiting the degree of pulmonary regurgitation and reducing consequent right ventricle dilation and its complications.[69,70]

Abnormalities of systolic[74,75] and diastolic[76-78] systemic ventricular function have been shown after the **Fontan operation**. Although preoperative systolic dysfunction, as measured by the end-systolic wall stress velocity of circumferential fiber shortening corrected for rate, has been shown to normalize at early follow-up,[74,79] the diastolic abnormalities persist and may worsen with time.[80] Incoordinate ventricular wall motion during relaxation and contraction has been shown by angiography. Orthogonal biplane ventricular angiograms were

analyzed in 11 patients before and in 15 patients after the Fontan procedure. Angiograms were recorded at 50 frames/sec, and cavity outlines were manually digitized frame by frame. Regional wall motion was assessed by constructing isometric and contour plots for each beat (Fig. 8-12).[81] Regional abnormalities of relaxation were detected in only 3 of the 11 patients before the Fontan operation, whereas postoperatively (median follow-up 17 months [range 5 to 54 months]) incoordinate diastolic wall motion was detected in 12 of the 15 patients.

Echocardiographic assessment of diastolic filling has revealed multiple abnormalities reflecting deranged ventricular relaxation. In Fontan patients, at a median postoperative interval of 28 months (range 0.03 to 105 months), IVRT was significantly longer than in normal controls and in patients before Fontan surgery.[77] This prolongation of relaxation time is likely a reflection of the nonuniform diastolic wall motion observed in the analysis of ventriculograms causing a reduction in the rate of ventricular pressure decline. In a subsequent follow-up study at a median postoperative interval of

11.4 ± 2 years,[80] IVRT expressed as a Z-score was significantly shorter than at 2.8 ± 2 years postoperatively, and it remained prolonged relative to the normal population. Peak early filling velocities were shown to be significantly lower in the Fontan group, and these changes persisted at late follow-up. Another finding in the Fontan group was the detection of intraventricular flow during the isovolumic relaxation period. Flow from base to apex was detected using pulse-wave Doppler in 80% of the Fontan group compared with 8% of the controls and none of the pre-Fontan group. Flow during this period was not significantly affected by respiration. The presence of intraventricular flow in this period implies the presence of an intracavitary pressure gradient, again most likely caused by incoordinate relaxation. Deceleration time during rapid early filling was significantly shorter in the Fontan group in the early postoperative period and shortened further with increasing follow-up. This short deceleration time indicates more rapid equalization of atrial and ventricular pressures and was attributed to increased ventricular compliance.

Diastolic Abnormalities in Ventricular Hypertrophy

Various structural changes of the myocyte cytoskeleton (e.g., titin isoforms[82]) and density of microtubules[83] and the extracellular matrix (e.g., fibrillar collagen) have been shown to occur with ventricular hypertrophy in response to increased afterload. These patients may show abnormal parameters of relaxation.

In an invasive study of patients with ventricular hypertrophy using conductance catheters, Liu and coworkers[46] showed significantly prolonged relaxation (tau) and decreased compliance (end-diastolic pressure volume relationship). To determine whether decreased compliance in these patients was due to abnormalities of active relaxation or passive structural changes, the same group[84] examined the acute effects of drugs that affect relaxation. In a small study of 14 patients with left ventricular hypertrophy (wall thickness at end diastole 19 ± 4 mm), esmolol infusion caused slowing of relaxation and reduced early rapid filling, and verapamil slowed the time to peak filling. Compliance and end-diastolic pressure relationships were unchanged, however, supporting the hypothesis that decreased compliance in these patients is due to passive structural elements.

A study of children with ventricular hypertrophy secondary to outflow tract obstruction or coarctation showed a different pattern of altered diastolic function.[85] Ten patients ranging from 2.5 to 10.5 years old showed significantly prolonged relaxation compared with controls. There was no significant difference in compliance between patients and controls, however. The method of assessing chamber compliance was slightly different because echocardiography was used to measure changes in volume during acute occlusion of the inferior vena cava. It is interesting to speculate that the early changes in diastolic dysfunction with ventricular hypertrophy are due to relaxation abnormalities, and it is only in the chronic phase that decreased compliance occurs because of structural changes. Our own data in older children after repair of subaortic stenosis showed a more restrictive pattern of filling.[86]

Ventricular Interdependence

Ventricular interdependence describes the way in which changes in performance of a ventricle cause change in the adjacent ventricle via displacement of the ventricular septum. If right ventricular pressure is increased, the septum is displaced leftward, causing compression of the left ventricle and vice versa. The relative degree of change is determined by the relative compliance of the free walls and the septum.[87] If the septum is stiff and the left ventricular free wall is compliant, an increase in right ventricular pressure displaces the septum but causes little change in left ventricular pressure owing to compensation by the compliant left ventricular free wall. Furthermore, since the pericardium surrounds the chambers of the heart, the stiffness of the free wall is significantly influenced by this external constraint.

Volume changes, independent of pressure changes, also may unmask ventricular interdependence. The effect of acute preload reduction by inferior vena cava occlusion is an initial downward parallel shift in the pressure-volume loop, followed by a shift to the left and downward. The slope of the curve is unchanged, implying no change in ventricular compliance. The downward shift is due to removal of the extrinsic effects of ventricular interaction and pericardial constraint. The opposite effect is seen with pericardial effusion. The external compressive effect of an increase in pericardial pressure causes an upward parallel shift in the end-diastolic pressure volume relationship (Fig. 8-13).

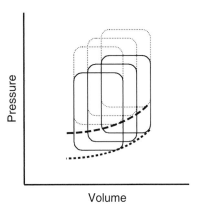

FIGURE 8-13 ■ **Pericardial effusion.** Shift in the end-diastolic pressure-volume relationship secondary to pericardial effusion is seen. Although there is a parallel upward shift in the curve, there is no change in the slope of this relationship, showing no change in ventricular compliance.

The effect of ventricular interaction also has been shown in a small study of patients with atrial septal defects in whom effects of chronic right ventricular volume load on left ventricular diastolic function was investigated.[88] Patients with large shunts (ratio of pulmonary blood flow to systemic blood flow >3:1) were compared with patients with relatively small shunts (pulmonary-to-systemic flow ratio <3:1). The relaxation constant tau for the left ventricle was significantly prolonged in patients with large shunts, indicating impaired left ventricular relaxation. The peak ventricular filling rate normalized because end-diastolic volume was lower. It also was observed that although the left ventricle end-diastolic pressure volume relationship was shifted upward, compliance was unchanged.

Ventricular Cross-Talk

The right ventricle and left ventricle share common myofibers in their superficial layers. It would be surprising if changes in intrinsic myocardial shortening on one side of the heart did not affect its partner on the other side. The magnitude of the change in the right ventricle resulting from a change in the left ventricle is referred to as **cross-talk gain**.[87]

An elegant study of this effect was performed by Damiano and associates[89] using an animal model of electrical isolation of the right ventricle. Onset of left ventricular and right ventricular contraction was varied by sequential pacing of the right atrium and right ventricle. The relative contribution of the left ventricle to right ventricular pressure and output was quantified. When left ventricular contraction occurred before contraction of the right ventricle, distinct double-peaked waveforms were observed in the right ventricular pressure and flow tracings. In this case, the first peak occurred before the onset of left ventricular pressure increase and was attributable to right ventricular contraction. When right ventricular contraction was significantly delayed relative to contraction of the left ventricle, double-peaked waveforms were observed again, but the second peak was due to the right ventricular contraction. Analysis of these data sets allowed calculation of the relative contributions of the left ventricle and right ventricle to these pressure and flow waveforms. Although the right ventricle contributed minimally to the left ventricular pressure, the left ventricle contributed significantly to right ventricular pressure and flow. Approximately 64% of right ventricular pressure was calculated to be due to the left ventricle component. The left ventricle contributed to 68% of the total flow in the pulmonary artery.

A further example of the effect of ventricular cross-talk is provided by the animal study of Hoffman and coworkers,[90] in which the right ventricular free wall was completely excised and replaced by a xenograft pericardial patch. It was noted that the Frank-Starling mechanism for the left ventricle was intact with increasing cardiac output with increasing preload, but output decreased with increasing right ventricle size and during occlusion of right ventricular outflow. Maximal ventricular pressure and stroke work of the left ventricle and right ventricle were linearly related, and both decreased with either increasing right ventricle size or increased right ventricular afterload. It was estimated that the left ventricle contributed 24% of left ventricle stroke work to the generation of right ventricular pressure, and this maintained adequate output, provided that the right ventricle remained small, and afterload was not elevated.

We examined the effect of the pericardium in this relationship in an animal model of normotensive right ventricular dilation by occlusion of the right coronary artery.[91] In the presence of an intact pericardium, right ventricular dilation caused a significant decrease in left ventricular contractility and end-diastolic volume. With the pericardium open, dilation of both ventricles was observed, and there was significantly less impairment of systolic contractile function. Echocardiographic examination during these studies showed that septal shift occurred toward the left ventricle during coronary occlusion, and that the degree of shift was less when the pericardium was open. This study showed for the first time that the reduction in left ventricular systolic function after acute right ventricular dilation was not due purely to changes in diastolic filling, but that the change in left ventricular geometry also was detrimental to left ventricular contraction. It is easy to infer that chronic right ventricular dilation (e.g., after repair of tetralogy of Fallot) may influence left ventricular function. Although far from proving causation, several studies have shown that there is a relationship between impaired right ventricular and left ventricular function in these patients.

Abnormalities of Timing

In the normal heart, early rapid and atrial phases account for approximately 70% and 30% of ventricular filling, respectively. These relative amounts are significantly influenced by changes in relaxation and compliance, and timing of these events has an important role. The time intervals between onset of ventricular relaxation and atrial systole and between atrial systole and ventricular contraction depend on the electrical properties of the sinoatrial and atrioventricular nodes.

Variation in the timing of **atrioventricular delay** has important effects on ventricular filling and cardiac output. The timing of these events and heart rate influence flow patterns as assessed by Doppler echocardiography. With increasing heart rate, the duration of diastole is shortened more significantly than that of ventricular systole. Optimization of atrioventricular delay in patients with dual-chamber pacemakers for complete heart block resulted in a 19% increase in stroke volume.[92] This study and an animal study[93] showed that optimal delay was achieved when ventricular systole began as the mitral valve was moving rapidly toward closure but not yet closed.

Another area of increasing interest, particularly in adult patients, is the beneficial effects of **resynchronization** of ventricular systole.[94,95] Synchrony of ventricular contraction is important in optimizing ventricular efficiency and ejection of blood. Incoordination of relaxation and contraction has important implications for ventricular filling and ejection and energy efficiency.[96] The techniques used to retime the failing heart are discussed in Chapter 39. The results of the Multicenter in Sync Randomized Animal Evaluation (MIRACLE) prospective double-blinded trial[95] have shown significant reductions in left ventricular end-diastolic and end-systolic volumes, reduced left ventricular mass, improved left ventricular ejection fraction, and prolongation of early rapid filling. These improvements were associated with improvements in both symptoms and in New York Heart Association class.

CURRENT STATUS AND FUTURE TRENDS

This chapter has presented some of the fundamental properties of muscle contraction as a basis for understanding the pathologic changes that may occur in disease states. We also have discussed alterations of ventricular and vascular properties that interact to modify blood flow. To optimize ventricular performance, all of these parameters must be considered.

Although the search for an ideal index of contractility continues, there are multiple factors that may affect the eventual ejection of blood from the ventricular cavity. The load dependency of contractile indices must be considered in the assessment of systolic function in these pathologic states. The force-velocity relationship provides the basis of myocardial response to these changes in loading. The index of velocity of circumferential fiber shortening corrected for rate and indexed to end-systolic wall stress or, more accurately, using fiber stress at end systole should be considered for noninvasive assessment. The early studies of myocardial tagging using magnetic resonance imaging have shown some interesting changes in patients with aortic stenosis, and whether these alterations are merely a reflection of changes in load rather than a change in intrinsic contractility is currently unknown. Albeit invasive, the "gold standard" for assessment of contractility is analysis of the pressure-volume loop.

The ventricular force-frequency relationship is an important facet of myocardial function, which is deranged in many forms of cardiac pathology but hitherto largely unexplored in children. The underlying mechanism for this phenomenon seems to be the rate-related changes in calcium cycling within the myocyte. The ability to examine this relationship in vivo has been hampered previously by the lack of a sensitive index of contractile function that is independent of the rate-induced reduction in preload. The novel tissue Doppler index IVA may provide further insights into this mechanism and systolic ventricular contractile properties in various forms of congenital heart disease.

The factors that combine to determine hydraulic load may be targeted in an attempt to improve pump function. Reduction in vascular resistance, delay in wave reflection, and improvement in vascular compliance all contribute to reduce hydraulic load. Strategies employed to bring about these therapeutic changes are essential to ameliorate heart failure in children.

No single index is reflective of diastolic function, and assessment must rely on a combination of measurements. Timing of atrial and ventricular systolic and diastolic events must be considered when data are interpreted. It can be seen, however, that despite the numerous indices of diastolic function that are available and commonly used, the process of ventricular filling is determined by a few basic mechanisms. The final common pathway of these mechanisms is the generation of a pressure gradient across the atrioventricular valve, which provides the energy for blood flow into the ventricular cavity. Future studies of systolic and diastolic function in children with heart failure combining various modalities of investigation will warrant innovative methodologies to assess not only global, but also regional function.[97-99]

Key Concepts

■ One of the fundamental properties of the myocardium is its force-velocity relationship. This relationship defines the ability of the myocyte to shorten more rapidly and to a greater degree when faced with a light load. V_{max} occurs at the time of zero load.

■ The in vivo measurement of contractility using indices that are independent of load has remained the holy grail of myocardial function assessment. The most robust noninvasive index of contractility currently available is the index of velocity of circumferential fiber shortening corrected for rate and indexed to end-systolic wall stress.

■ From the resulting pressure-volume curve, the stiffness of the ventricle can be determined instantaneously for any point in the cardiac cycle. If a family of loops is generated by acute alteration of loading conditions, the linear relationship of this time-varying elastance can be plotted with the slope being a relatively load-independent index of ventricular contractility.

■ There has been an interest in myocardial motion during the period of isovolumic contraction as an index of systolic contractile function. From an apical four-chamber transthoracic view, the maximal isovolumic velocity during this period and first derivative of this with respect to time, isovolumic acceleration, of the right and left ventricles of the normal heart have been compared with invasive indices of contractility derived from analysis of pressure-volume data.

■ The intrinsic property of the myocardium to alter contractile force with change in rate of stimulation frequency is known as the FFR or the "treppe" effect.

■ The rate-related change in calcium cycling is believed to be the underlying mechanism for the myocardial FFR. It would be expected that the deleterious effects of ischemia-reperfusion on the function of sarcoplasmic reticulum also would affect this relationship. Preliminary studies in neonates undergoing the arterial switch procedure have shown marked postoperative depression of the ventricular FFR compared with preoperative assessment.

■ Quantification of vascular load often is represented by the aortic peak systolic or mean pressure; this estimation is an oversimplification, however. Vascular load varies with the cardiac cycle as a result of the combination of the pulsatile nature of blood flow and pressure, elastic properties of blood vessels, and blood inertia and is better represented by vascular impedance.

■ In the normal heart, maximal stroke work and power are generated when the ventricle is subjected to the normal arterial impedance. Theoretically, pressure-volume analysis predicts that loading is optimal in terms of stroke work when the ratio of effective Ea/ventricular elastance is 1 (Ea/Ees = 1).

■ Assessment of the process of relaxation in vivo is difficult, and although not strictly a reflection of the extent or timing of this process, attempts have largely centered around measurements of the duration of the isovolumic relaxation period or the rate of pressure decline.

■ Ventricular architecture may be altered such that the passive viscoelastic properties of the ventricle become stiffer or less compliant. Compliance is the inverse of stiffness and is calculated by dV/dP.

■ The early changes in diastolic dysfunction with ventricular hypertrophy are due to relaxation abnormalities, and it is only in the chronic phase that decreased compliance occurs secondary to structural changes.

REFERENCES

1. Daniels M, Noble MI, ter Keurs HE, Wohlfart B: Velocity of sarcomere shortening in rat cardiac muscle: Relationship to force, sarcomere length, calcium and time. J Physiol 1984;355:367-381.
2. Barany M: ATPase activity of myosin correlated with speed of muscle shortening. J Gen Physiol 1967;50(Suppl):197-218.
3. Sonnenblick EH: Implications of muscle mechanics in the heart. Fed Proc 1962;21:975-990.
4. Brutsaert DL, Sonnenblick EH: Nature of force-velocity relation in heart muscle. Cardiovasc Res 1971;1(Suppl 1):18-33.
5. Colan SD, Borow KM, Neumann A: Left ventricular end-systolic wall stress-velocity of fiber shortening relation: A load-independent index of myocardial contractility. J Am Coll Cardiol 1984;4:715-724.
6. Feltes TF, Pignatelli R, Kleinert S, Mariscalco MM: Quantitated left ventricular systolic mechanics in children with septic shock utilizing noninvasive wall-stress analysis. Crit Care Med 1994;22:1647-1658.
7. Kimball TR, Reynolds JM, Mays WA, et al: Persistent hyperdynamic cardiovascular state at rest and during exercise in children after successful repair of coarctation of the aorta. J Am Coll Cardiol 1994;24:194-200.
8. Leandro J, Dyck J, Poppe D, et al: Cardiac dysfunction late after cardiotoxic therapy for childhood cancer. Am J Cardiol 1994;74:1152-1156.
9. Banerjee A, Brook MM, Klautz RJ, Teitel DF: Nonlinearity of the left ventricular end-systolic wall stress-velocity of fiber shortening relation in young pigs: A potential pitfall in its use as a single-beat index of contractility. J Am Coll Cardiol 1994;23:514-524.
10. Gentles TL, Sanders SP, Colan SD: Misrepresentation of left ventricular contractile function by endocardial indexes: Clinical implications after coarctation repair. Am Heart J 2000;140:585-595.
11. Gentles TL, Colan SD: Wall stress misrepresents afterload in children and young adults with abnormal left ventricular geometry. J Appl Physiol 2002;92:1053-1057.
12. Suga H: Time course of left ventricular pressure-volume relationship under various end-diastolic volume. Jpn Heart J 1969;10: 509-515.
13. Suga H: Time course of left ventricular pressure-volume relationship under various extents of aortic occlusion. Jpn Heart J 1970;11:373-378.
14. Kass DA, Maughan WL, Guo ZM, et al: Comparative influence of load versus inotropic states on indexes of ventricular contractility: Experimental and theoretical analysis based on pressure-volume relationships [erratum appears in Circulation 1988 Mar;77(3):559]. Circulation 1987;76:1422-1436.
15. Derrick GP, Narang I, White PA, et al: Failure of stroke volume augmentation during exercise and dobutamine stress is unrelated to load-independent indexes of right ventricular performance after the Mustard operation. Circulation 2000;102:III154-III159.
16. Isaaz K, Thompson A, Ethevenot G, et al: Doppler echocardiographic measurement of low velocity motion of the left ventricular posterior wall. Am J Cardiol 1989;64:66-75.
17. Vogel M, Schmidt MR, Kristiansen SB, et al: Validation of myocardial acceleration during isovolumic contraction as a novel noninvasive index of right ventricular contractility: Comparison with ventricular pressure-volume relations in an animal model. Circulation 2002;105:1693-1699.
18. Vogel M, Cheung MM, Li J, et al: Noninvasive assessment of left ventricular force-frequency relationships using tissue Doppler-derived isovolumic acceleration: Validation in an animal model. Circulation 2003;107:1647-1652.
19. Jones CJ, Raposo L, Gibson DG: Functional importance of the long axis dynamics of the human left ventricle. Br Heart J 1990;63:215-220.
20. Rushmer RF: Initial phase of ventricular systole: Asynchronous contraction. Am J Physiol 1956;184:H188-H194.
21. ter Keurs HE, de Tombe PP: Determinants of velocity of sarcomere shortening in mammalian myocardium. Adv Exp Med Biol 1993;332:649-665.
22. de Tombe PP, ter Keurs HE: Force and velocity of sarcomere shortening in trabeculae from rat heart: Effects of temperature. Circ Res 1990;66:1239-1254.
23. Ricciardi L, Bottinelli R, Canepari M, Reggiani C: Effects of acidosis on maximum shortening velocity and force-velocity relation of skinned rat cardiac muscle. J Mol Cell Cardiol 1994;26:601-607.
24. Walley KR, Ford LE, Wood LD: Effects of hypoxia and hypercapnia on the force-velocity relation of rabbit myocardium. Circ Res 1991;69:1616-1625.
25. Lowes BD, Gilbert EM, Abraham WT, et al: Myocardial gene expression in dilated cardiomyopathy treated with beta-blocking agents. N Engl J Med 2002;346:1357-1365.

26. Richard P, Charron P, Carrier L, et al: Hypertrophic cardiomyopathy: Distribution of disease genes, spectrum of mutations, and implications for a molecular diagnosis strategy. Circulation 2003; 107:2227-2232.

27. Fitzsimons DP, Patel JR, Moss RL: Role of myosin heavy chain composition in kinetics of force development and relaxation in rat myocardium. J Physiol 1998;513:171-183.

28. Litten RZ 3rd, Martin BJ, Low RB, Alpert NR: Altered myosin isozyme patterns from pressure-overloaded and thyrotoxic hypertrophied rabbit hearts. Circ Res 1982;50:856-864.

29. VanBuren P, Harris DE, Alpert NR, Warshaw DM: Cardiac V1 and V3 myosins differ in their hydrolytic and mechanical activities in vitro. Circ Res 1995;77:439-444.

30. Herron TJ, Korte FS, McDonald KS: Loaded shortening and power output in cardiac myocytes are dependent on myosin heavy chain isoform expression. Am J Physiol Heart Circ Physiol 2001;281:H1217-H1222.

31. Bouvagnet P, Mairhofer H, Leger JO, et al: Distribution pattern of alpha and beta myosin in normal and diseased human ventricular myocardium. Basic Res Cardiol 1989;84:91-102.

32. Boluyt MO, Devor ST, Opiteck JA, White TP: Regional variation in cardiac myosin isoforms of female F344 rats during aging. J Gerontol Ser A Biol Sci Med Sci 1999;54:B313-B317.

33. Lompre AM, Nadal-Ginard B, Mahdavi V: Expression of the cardiac ventricular alpha- and beta-myosin heavy chain genes is developmentally and hormonally regulated. J Biol Chem 1984; 259:6437-6446.

34. Rouleau JL, Paradis P, Shenasa H, Juneau C: Faster time to peak tension and velocity of shortening in right versus left ventricular trabeculae and papillary muscles of dogs. Circ Res 1986;59:556-561.

35. Everett AW, Sinha AM, Umeda PK, et al: Regulation of myosin synthesis by thyroid hormone: Relative change in the alpha- and beta-myosin heavy chain mRNA levels in rabbit heart. Biochemistry 1984;23:1596-1599.

36. Malhotra A, Siri FM, Aronson R: Cardiac contractile proteins in hypertrophied and failing guinea pig heart. Cardiovasc Res 1992;26:153-161.

37. Schwartz K, Apstein C, Mercadier JJ, et al: Left ventricular isomyosins in normal and hypertrophied rat and human hearts. Eur Heart J 1984;5:77-83.

38. Apstein CS, Lecarpentier Y, Mercadier JJ, et al: Changes in LV papillary muscle performance and myosin composition with aortic insufficiency in rats. Am J Physiol 1987;253:H1005-H1011.

39. Dool JS, Mak AS, Friberg P, et al: Regional myosin heavy chain expression in volume and pressure overload induced cardiac hypertrophy. Acta Physiol Scand 1995;155:396-404.

40. Bowditch HP: Uber die Eigentumlichkeiten der Reizbarkeit, welche die Muskelfasern des Herzens zeigen. Ber Konigl Sachs Ges Wissen 1871;23:652.

41. Gwathmey JK, Slawsky MT, Hajjar RJ, et al: Role of intracellular calcium handling in force-interval relationships of human ventricular myocardium. J Clin Invest 1990;85:1599-1613.

42. Alpert NR, Leavitt BJ, Ittleman FP, et al: A mechanistic analysis of the force-frequency relation in non-failing and progressively failing human myocardium. Basic Res Cardiol 1998;93:23-32.

43. Bers D: Excitation-Contraction Coupling and Contractile Force, 2nd ed. Amsterdam. Kluwer Academic Publishers, 2002.

44. Schouten VJ: Interval dependence of force and twitch duration in rat heart explained by Ca^{2+} pump inactivation in sarcoplasmic reticulum. J Physiol 1990;431:427-444.

45. Pieske B, Kretschmann B, Meyer M, et al: Alterations in intracellular calcium handling associated with the inverse force-frequency relation in human dilated cardiomyopathy. Circulation 1995;92: 1169-1178.

46. Liu CP, Ting CT, Lawrence W, et al: Diminished contractile response to increased heart rate in intact human left ventricular hypertrophy: Systolic versus diastolic determinants. Circulation 1993;88:1893-1906.

47. Inagaki M, Yokota M, Izawa H, et al: Impaired force-frequency relations in patients with hypertensive left ventricular hypertrophy: A possible physiological marker of the transition from physiological to pathological hypertrophy. Circulation 1999;99: 1822-1830.

48. Feldman MD, Alderman JD, Aroesty JM, et al: Depression of systolic and diastolic myocardial reserve during atrial pacing tachycardia in patients with dilated cardiomyopathy. J Clin Invest 1988;82:1661-1669.

49. Suga H, Sagawa K, Shoukas AA: Load independence of the instantaneous pressure-volume ratio of the canine left ventricle and effects of epinephrine and heart rate on the ratio. Circ Res 1973;32:314-322.

50. Temsah RM, Netticadan T, Kawabata K, Dhalla NS: Lack of both oxygen and glucose contributes to I/R-induced changes in cardiac SR function. Am J Physiol Cell Physiol 2002;283:C1306-C1312.

51. Nichols WW, O'Rourke MF: McDonald's Blood Flow in Arteries: Theoretical, Experimental and Clinical Principles, 4th ed. London, Arnold, 1998.

52. Nichols WW, Pepine CJ, Geiser EA, Conti CR: Vascular load defined by the aortic input impedance spectrum. Fed Proc 1980;39:196-201.

53. Sunagawa K, Maughan WL, Burkhoff D, Sagawa K: Left ventricular interaction with arterial load studied in isolated canine ventricle. Am J Physiol 1983;245:H773-H780.

54. Kelly RP, Ting CT, Yang TM, et al: Effective arterial elastance | index of arterial vascular load in humans. Circulation 1992; 86:513-521.

55. Chiu YC, Arand PW, Carroll JD: Power-afterload relation in the failing human ventricle. Circ Res 1992;70:530-535.

56. Senzaki H, Masutani S, Kobayashi J, et al: Ventricular afterload and ventricular work in Fontan circulation: Comparison with normal two-ventricle circulation and single-ventricle circulation with Blalock-Taussig shunts. Circulation 2002;105:2885-2892.

57. Kouatli AA, Garcia JA, Zellers TM, et al: Enalapril does not enhance exercise capacity in patients after Fontan procedure. Circulation 1997;96:1507-1512.

58. Sunagawa K, Maughan WL, Sagawa K: Optimal arterial resistance for the maximal stroke work studied in isolated canine left ventricle. Circ Res 1985;56:586-595.

59. De Tombe PP, Jones S, Burkhoff D, et al: Ventricular stroke work and efficiency both remain nearly optimal despite altered vascular loading. Am J Physiol 1993;264:H1817-H1824.

60. Segers P, Stergiopulos N, Westerhof N: Relation of effective arterial elastance to arterial system properties. Am J Physiol Heart Circ Physiol 2002;282:H1041-H1046.

61. Gibson DG, Francis DP: Clinical assessment of left ventricular diastolic function. Heart (British Cardiac Society) 2003;89: 231-238.

62. Zile MR, Brutsaert DL: New concepts in diastolic dysfunction and diastolic heart failure: Part I. Diagnosis, prognosis, and measurements of diastolic function. Circulation 2002;105:1387-1393.

63. Zile MR, Brutsaert DL: New concepts in diastolic dysfunction and diastolic heart failure: Part II. Causal mechanisms and treatment. Circulation 2002;105:1503-1508.

64. Kass DA: Assessment of diastolic dysfunction: Invasive modalities. Cardiol Clin 2000;18:571-586.

65. Frais MA, Bergman DW, Kingma I, et al: The dependence of the time constant of left ventricular isovolumic relaxation (tau) on pericardial pressure. Circulation 1990;81:1071-1080.

66. Van de Werf F, Minten J, Carmeliet P, et al: The genesis of the third and fourth heart sounds: A pressure-flow study in dogs. J Clin Invest 1984;73:1400-1407.

67. Redington AN, Penny DP, Rigby ML, et al: Antegrade diastolic pulmonary arterial flow as a marker right ventricular restriction after complete repair of pulmonary atresia with intact septum and critical pulmonary valve stenosis. Cardiol Young 1992;2: 382-386.

68. Cullen S, Shore D, Redington A: Characterization of right ventricular diastolic performance after complete repair of tetralogy of Fallot: Restrictive physiology predicts slow postoperative recovery. Circulation 1995;91:1782-1789.

69. Gatzoulis MA, Till JA, Somerville J, Redington AN: Mechanoelectrical interaction in tetralogy of Fallot: QRS prolongation relates to right ventricular size and predicts malignant ventricular arrhythmias and sudden death. Circulation 1995;92:231-237.

70. Gatzoulis MA, Clark AL, Cullen S, et al: Right ventricular diastolic function 15 to 35 years after repair of tetralogy of Fallot: Restrictive physiology predicts superior exercise performance. Circulation 1995;91:1775-1781.

71. Chaturvedi RR, Shore DF, Lincoln C, et al: Acute right ventricular restrictive physiology after repair of tetralogy of Fallot: Association with myocardial injury and oxidative stress. Circulation 1999;100:1540-1547.

72. Shekerdemian LS, Bush A, Shore DF, et al: Cardiorespiratory responses to negative pressure ventilation after tetralogy of Fallot repair: A hemodynamic tool for patients with a low-output state. J Am Coll Cardiol 1999;33:549-555.

73. Norgard G, Gatzoulis MA, Josen M, et al: Does restrictive right ventricular physiology in the early postoperative period predict subsequent right ventricular restriction after repair of tetralogy of Fallot? Heart 1998;79:481-484.

74. Sluysmans T, Sanders SP, van der Velde M, et al: Natural history and patterns of recovery of contractile function in single left ventricle after Fontan operation. Circulation 1992;86:1753-1761.

75. Fogel MA, Gupta KB, Weinberg PM, Hoffman EA: Regional wall motion and strain analysis across stages of Fontan reconstruction by magnetic resonance tagging. Am J Physiol 1995;269:H1132-H1152.

76. Penny DJ, Redington AN: Doppler echocardiographic evaluation of pulmonary blood flow after the Fontan operation: The role of the lungs. Br Heart J 1991;66:372-374.

77. Penny DJ, Rigby ML, Redington AN: Abnormal patterns of intraventricular flow and diastolic filling after the Fontan operation: Evidence for incoordinate ventricular wall motion. Br Heart J 1991;66:375-378.

78. Penny DJ, Redington AN: Angiographic demonstration of incoordinate motion of the ventricular wall after the Fontan operation. Br Heart J 1991;66:456-459.

79. Gewillig MH, Lundstrom UR, Deanfield JE, et al: Impact of Fontan operation on left ventricular size and contractility in tricuspid atresia. Circulation 1990;81:118-127.

80. Cheung YF, Penny DJ, Redington AN: Serial assessment of left ventricular diastolic function after Fontan procedure. Heart (British Cardiac Society) 2000;83:420-424.

81. Gibson DG, Prewitt TA, Brown DJ: Analysis of left ventricular wall movement during isovolumic relaxation and its relation to coronary artery disease. Br Heart J 1976;38:1010-1019.

82. Warren CM, Jordan MC, Roos KP, et al: Titin isoform expression in normal and hypertensive myocardium. Cardiovasc Res 2003;59:86-94.

83. Zile MR, Green GR, Schuyler GT, et al: Cardiocyte cytoskeleton in patients with left ventricular pressure overload hypertrophy. J Am Coll Cardiol 2001;37:1080-1084.

84. Kass DA, Wolff MR, Ting CT, et al: Diastolic compliance of hypertrophied ventricle is not acutely altered by pharmacologic agents influencing active processes. Ann Intern Med 1993;119:466-473.

85. Banerjee A, Mendelsohn AM, Knilans TK, et al: Effect of myocardial hypertrophy on systolic and diastolic function in children: Insights from the force-frequency and relaxation-frequency relationships. J Am Coll Cardiol 1998;32:1088-1095.

86. Chan KY, Redington AN, Rigby ML, Gibson DG: Cardiac function after surgery for subaortic stenosis: Non-invasive assessment of left ventricular performance. Br Heart J 1991;66:161-165.

87. Maughan WL, Sunagawa K, Sagawa K: Ventricular systolic interdependence: Volume elastance model in isolated canine hearts. Am J Physiol 1987;253:H1381-H1390.

88. Satoh A, Katayama K, Hiro T, et al: Effect of right ventricular volume overload on left ventricular diastolic function in patients with atrial septal defect. Jpn Circ J 1996;60:758-766.

89. Damiano RJ Jr, La Follette P Jr, Cox JL, et al: Significant left ventricular contribution to right ventricular systolic function. Am J Physiol 1991;261:H1514-H1524.

90. Hoffman D, Sisto D, Frater RW, Nikolic SD: Left-to-right ventricular interaction with a noncontracting right ventricle. J Thorac Cardiovasc Surg 1994;107:1496-1502.

91. Brookes C, Ravn H, White P, et al: Acute right ventricular dilatation in response to ischemia significantly impairs left ventricular systolic performance. Circulation 1999;100:761-767.

92. Leonelli FM, Wang K, Youssef M, et al: Systolic and diastolic effects of variable atrioventricular delay in patients with complete heart block and normal ventricular function. Am J Cardiol 1997;80:294-298.

93. Meisner JS, McQueen DM, Ishida Y, et al: Effects of timing of atrial systole on LV filling and mitral valve closure: Computer and dog studies. Am J Physiol 1985;249:H604-H619.

94. Stellbrink C, Breithardt OA, Franke A, et al: Impact of cardiac resynchronization therapy using hemodynamically optimized pacing on left ventricular remodeling in patients with congestive heart failure and ventricular conduction disturbances. J Am Coll Cardiol 2001;38:1957-1965.

95. St. John Sutton MG, Plappert T, Abraham WT, et al: Effect of cardiac resynchronization therapy on left ventricular size and function in chronic heart failure. Circulation 2003;107:1985-1990.

96. Leclercq C, Kass DA: Retiming the failing heart: Principles and current clinical status of cardiac resynchronization. J Am Coll Cardiol 2002;39:194-201.

97. Eidem BW, McMahon CJ, Cohen RR, et al: Impact of cardiac growth on Doppler tissue imaging velocities: Study in healthy children. J Am Soc Echocardiogr 2004;17:212-221.

98. Hughes ML, Shekerdemian LS, Brizard CP, et al: Improved early ventricular performance with a right ventricle to pulmonary artery conduit in stage I palliation for hypoplastic left heart syndrome: Evidence from strain Doppler echocardiography. Heart 2004;90:191-194.

99. Yu CM, Zhang Q, Fung JW, et al: A novel tool to assess systolic asynchrony and identify responders of cardiac resynchronization imaging. J Am Coll Cardiol 2005;45:677-684.

CHAPTER 9

The Alveolar-Capillary Interface and Pulmonary Edema

Timothy F. Feltes

Previous chapters have focused on cardiovascular adaptations to heart failure; this chapter highlights changes of the alveolar-capillary interface as sequelae of the failing heart. The focus first is on the anatomic features of the alveolar-capillary interface, then the forces involved in normal lung fluid and solute balance with reference to safety factors to prevent fluid accumulation, and finally the pathophysiologic changes observed in pulmonary edema.

ALVEOLAR-CAPILLARY INTERFACE

Assuming satisfactory ventilation and a sufficient volume of mixed venous blood with adequate oxygen carrying capacity, gas exchange becomes a function of the gas transfer characteristics of the alveolar-capillary interface. In heart failure, whether it be high output or low output or acute or chronic, the integrity of the alveolar-capillary interface becomes compromised with unfavorable consequences to gas exchange.

Microvascular Ultrastructure

As described in Fick's law, the rate of gas transfer (Q) is a direct function of a constant reflecting gas solubility (k), gas partial pressure gradient between the alveolus and capillary (ΔP), and alveolar-capillary surface area (A) and is indirectly proportional to the thickness of the alveolar-capillary membrane (T):[1]

$$Q = k\ (\Delta P)\ (A)/T$$

To preserve gas conductance, the integrity of the **alveolar-capillary interface** must be maintained constantly.[2] The alveolar epithelial cells and the capillary endothelial cells with their respective basal laminae constitute the alveolar-capillary membrane, which is involved in alveolar and interstitial clearance of water and solutes. Gas exchange occurs within a segment of lung known as the **acinus.**[3] The airways across which gas exchange occurs include the terminal bronchioles, respiratory bronchioles, alveolar ducts, and alveoli. Coursing with these gas exchange airways are the pulmonary arterioles, which measure less than 100 μm in diameter and which rapidly bifurcate into a mesh of intra-acinar capillaries as these vessels approach the alveoli.[4]

The principal gas and fluid exchange unit of the lung is the **alveolar septum** (Fig. 9-1). In the alveolar septa, capillaries approximately 10 μm in diameter are arranged in an alternating order with adjacent alveoli, which maximizes the air-blood interface and surface area for gas exchange. The capillaries are suspended in interstitium by collagen and elastin cores.[5,6] The capillaries are blanketed by alveolar epithelia composed of type I and type II **pneumocytes.** The type I pneumocytes constitute 95% of the alveolar surface area; these cells are large but thin (<0.1 μm) and offer little resistance to gas transport. The tight junctions that bind alveolar epithelial cells to one another render the cells relatively impervious to solutes and provide a formidable barrier.[7,8] The cuboid type II pneumocytes, outnumbering the type I cells nearly 2:1, are responsible for surfactant production and secretion.

The alveolar septa are asymmetric with thin and thick portions. In the thin portion of the septa, the alveolar epithelium and capillary endothelium have a shared (fused) basement membrane that is ideally designed for gas exchange. This thin alveolar-capillary membrane measures 0.2 to 0.4 mm in diameter.[5] Although the thin portion of the membrane offers little resistance to gas exchange, the fused laminae are highly impervious to solutes, and little fluid filtration can occur across this barrier (keeping the alveoli dry). In contrast, the thick portion of the septum, normally measuring approximately 1 μm in diameter, is where most pulmonary fluid and solute exchange occurs and acts as a fluid sump for the alveolar septum.[9] In contrast to the thin portion of the septum, the alveolar epithelium and capillary endothelium of the thick portion retain their own basal membranes and are separated by interstitium.

The **interstitium** is continuous with intersegmental and interlobal septa of the lung where the pulmonary lymphatics reside. Anatomically the interstitium consists of three connective tissue systems: (1) a sheath of fibers that contains the branching networks of the pulmonary arteries, lymphatic channels, and bronchi; (2) a system that extends from the pleura via intersegmental and interlobular septa and encases the pulmonary veins and other lymphatic communications; and (3) a system of mainly capillaries that connect the former two systems.

Functionally the interstitial pressure in the alveolar septa closely reflects alveolar pressure, whereas the

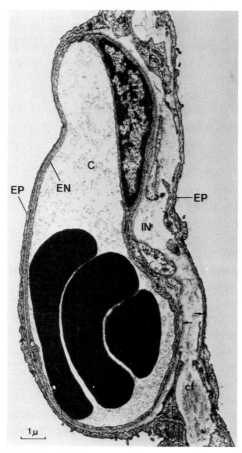

FIGURE 9-1 ■ **The alveolar septum.** The septum is distinguished by a thin portion (left side), composed of a thin alveolar epithelial cell (EP), capillary (C), endothelial cell (EN), and fused basement membranes, and a thick portion (right side), with a basement membrane and interposing interstitium (IN). (From Weibel ER, Bochofen H: *Structural design of the alveolus septum and fluid exchange.* In Fishman AP, Renkin EM [ed]: *Pulmonary Edema.* Baltimore, Williams & Wilkins, 1979, pp 1-20.)

interstitial pressure in the intersegmental and interlobar septa more closely matches that of the pleural space. A pressure gradient is created that favors fluid filtration from the alveolar septa to the interlobar septa of the lung, where the **lymphatic vasculature** is found. From here, fluid and solute filtered at the alveolar-capillary interface make their way into the central venous circulation via pathways of intrapulmonary lymphatics. These lymphatic channels contain a series of vascular valves and smooth muscles by which interstitial fluid (lymph) is actively pumped into the central venous system.

The extracellular matrix not only supports the architecture of the alveolar septa, but also provides strength to the alveolar-capillary barrier. The primary molecule of the **extracellular matrix** is type IV collagen, which seems to be responsible for most of the tensile strength of the extracellular matrix.[10] Other molecules include elastic fibers and proteoglycans. These molecules

connect the extracellular matrix with adjoining cells and account for the sieving properties of the microvascular capillaries and tissue compliance.[9,10]

Forces in Lung Fluid Balance

To maintain fluid balance, fluid in the lung is filtered from the microcirculation into the interstitial space and subsequently returned to the intravascular space via the lymphatic system. **Fluid filtration** (Q_f) in the lung is dictated by the same forces that determine any flow through a system—a balance of driving pressure (ΔP) and conductance (C):

$$Q_f = \Delta P \times C$$

Overall, the driving pressure in lung fluid filtration is a balance of hydrostatic and oncotic forces.[11] The two hydrostatic forces include the **microvascular hydrostatic pressure (P_{mv})**, which tends to push fluid into the interstitium, and the interstitial hydrostatic pressure, called the **perimicrovascular hydrostatic pressure (P_{pmv})**, an opposing force that tends to keep fluid intravascular. P_{mv} is the hydrostatic pressure in the lung capillary bed, or the principal driving force for lung fluid filtration. In addition, P_{mv} is between the mean pulmonary arterial and the left atrial pressures. Although it is controversial whether or not the P_{pmv} is close to alveolar pressure (direct measurement of this pressure is difficult), it seems that P_{pmv} is closer to alveolar pressure than pleural pressure.

Opposing the balance of hydrostatic forces are the two protein-related oncotic forces. **Microvascular oncotic pressure (π_{mv})** acts to keep fluid within the vascular space, and this pressure is probably the same as in large systemic vessels, whereas **perimicrovascular oncotic pressure (π_{pmv})** draws fluid into the interstitium and can be approximated by the lung lymph oncotic pressure and protein concentration.

The oncotic forces influence fluid filtration in the lung as a function of the **reflection coefficient (δ)**, which reflects the permeability property of a barrier or the relative degree of sieving of solutes across the lung microvascular membrane. If the barrier is relatively impervious, δ approximates 1; in contrast, if a barrier offers little resistance to a solute, δ is close to 0. The coefficient δ is a function of the solute's molecular weight; small molecules pass through barriers more easily than larger molecules. For serum proteins, such as albumin and globulin, which make up the primary oncotic forces of the blood, δ is approximately 0.8 (assuming the capillary integrity is maintained). The overall driving pressure equation for fluid filtration in the lung is:

$$\Delta P = (P_{mv} - P_{pmv}) - \delta (\pi_{mv} - \pi_{pmv})$$

One could surmise from the equation that the force that is most influential on lung fluid balance is the P_{mv}.

To complete the equation specific for lung fluid balance, the **filtration coefficient (K_f)**, reflecting the product of hydraulic conductance of the microvascular membrane (or its permeability) and the surface area available for fluid filtration, needs to be considered. When K_f is coupled with the driving pressures in the lung, the forces driving fluid filtration in the lung are finally depicted as the **Starling equation:**[11]

$$Q_f = K_f \left[(P_{mv} - P_{pmv}) - \delta (\pi_{mv} - \pi_{pmv}) \right]$$

Prevention of Pulmonary Edema

Inherent safety factors in the lung suppress interstitial fluid and solute accumulation and airway edema (Table 9-1). Interstitial and alveolar edema is prevented by various factors, such as low filtration coefficient, reflection coefficient that is close to 1, and drainage via lymph and interstitial fluid sumps.

If one were to increase the left atrial pressure in an instrumented dog, one would find no evidence of fluid accumulation in the lung until the left atrial pressure exceeded approximately 23 mm Hg (Fig. 9-2).[12] This observation illustrates that despite incremental increases in P_{mv}, the interstitium stays relatively free of significant fluid accumulation up to significantly elevated pressures.

With an acute increase in pulmonary P_{mv}, **capillary filtration rate** increases immediately but soon tapers (Fig. 9-3). In contrast, **lung lymph flow** slowly increases only after an increase in pulmonary P_{mv}, gradually increasing to a rate equal to the fluid filtration rate.[13] Capillary filtration is initially a function of the hydrostatic gradient between the capillary and interstitium; as increased fluid filtration occurs, however, hydrostatic and oncotic conditions in the interstitium also change. The interstitium is a relatively low-compliant space, so as

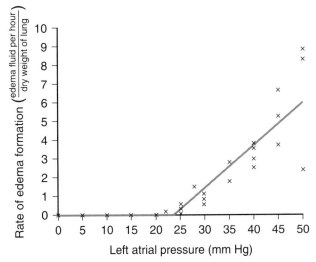

FIGURE 9-2 ■ Left atrial pressure and pulmonary edema. The effects of left atrial pressure on the rate of development of pulmonary edema in an instrumented dog. Pulmonary edema safety factors prevent edema formation until left atrial pressure exceeds 20 mm Hg. (From Guyton AC, Lindsey AE: *Effect of elevated left atrial pressure and decreased plasma protein concentration on the development of pulmonary edema. Circ Res* 7:649, 1959.)

the interstitium fills, the interstitial P_{pmv} begins to increase. This process reduces the transvascular hydrostatic gradient, and filtration begins to decrease. Simultaneously the increased filtration of fluid to the interstitium dilutes out oncotic forces within the interstitium, increasing the transvascular oncotic gradient in favor of intravascular

TABLE 9-1

Safety Factors Protecting Against Pulmonary Edema
Interstitial Edema
Intravascular protein osmotic pressure
K_f relatively low
δ close to 1
Lymphatic drainage
Alveolar Edema
Alveolar gas pressure
K_f extremely low
$\delta = 1$
π_{alv} near 0
Interstitial fluid sumps

From Feltes TF, Hansen TN: Pulmonary edema. In Garson T, Bricker T, Fisher D, et al (eds): The Science and Practice of Pediatric Cardiology. Baltimore, Williams & Wilkins, 1998. δ = reflection coefficient; K_f = filtration coefficient; π_{alv}, microvascular alveolar pressure.

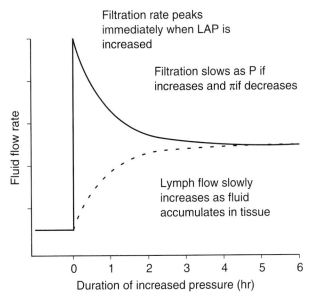

FIGURE 9-3 ■ Left atrial pressure and fluid flow rate. The effect of increase in left atrial pressure (LAP) on pulmonary capillary fluid filtration rate *(solid line)* and lymph flow *(dashed line)*. Pif, pulmonary interstitial fluid pressure; πif, interstitial fluid osmotic pressure. (From Drake RE, Doursout MF: *Pulmonary edema and elevated left atrial pressure: Four hours and beyond. New Physiol Sci* 17:223-226, 2002.)

fluid retention. In this same figure, it is evident that it takes several hours before lung lymph flow matches lymph production. This delay is due in part to the time needed to fill the interstitium with fluid and the transit time for lymph to make its way through the lymphatic drainage system.

The proteoglycans of the **extracellular matrix**, which provide structural support, are highly charged macromolecules; this imparts a marked hydrophilic property to the interstitium.[10] It is speculated that as water filters into the interstitium from the microvasculature, the extracellular matrix holds fluid in a protective semigelatinous state to prevent spillage into the airways until it can be drained via the lymphatic system.[13]

Other mechanisms contribute to the prevention of alveolar and interstitial pulmonary edema. Alveolar edema is inhibited at the level of the alveolar-capillary interface because of tight fusion between alveolar epithelial cells. The microvascular endothelium has a remarkably low filtration coefficient and a reflection coefficient of nearly 1. The alveolar inflation pressure and extremely low alveolar oncotic pressure also help to prevent airway edema. The intravascular oncotic gradient strongly favors intravascular fluid retention.

All of the aforementioned safety factors are only temporarily effective if fluid filtration increases. Eventually the prevention of either alveolar or interstitial edema formation becomes exclusively a function of the pulmonary lymphatic circulation's capacity to drain the interstitium. Normally, lung lymph flow (Q_L) equals lung fluid filtration (Q_f), but has significant reserve capability. As long as Q_L equals or exceeds Q_f, both alveoli and the interstitium remain free of edema fluid. Any impairment of the lymphatic function of the lung can lead, however, to rapid fluid accumulation in the lung regardless of the rate of fluid filtration. A clinical example of this pathophysiology is an infant with congenital pulmonary lymphangiectasis.

The pulmonary lymphatic circulation is composed of a series of vascular channels through which lymph is passively and actively recirculated into the central venous system. The lymphatic vessels contain smooth muscle, which phasically contracts. Little is known about the contractile characteristics of the pulmonary lymphatics and thoracic duct and what influences their ability to drain the pulmonary interstitium. In other tissues, such as the mesenteric lymphatics, nitric oxide decreases the frequency of lymphatic smooth muscle contraction.[14] Likewise, agents such as nitroprusside that increase tissue nitrogen radicals also decrease lymphatic pulsatility.

Finally, the remaining safety factor against development of pulmonary edema is the ability of the pulmonary vascular bed to be recruited. During exercise, cardiac output can increase several times over baseline. Despite such an increase in pulmonary flow, pulmonary edema does not develop. At baseline level of cardiac output in an upright adult, only a portion of the lungs is perfused.[15]

As cardiac output increases, pulmonary vessels are recruited, and pulmonary resistance decreases. Despite an increase in flow, the microvascular hydrostatic pressure remains relatively constant as pulmonary resistance decreases. Lung lymph production increases because more of the microvasculature is engaged in fluid filtration. As the lung develops, lymphatic capillaries develop in parallel with pulmonary arterioles and venules.[3] Vascular recruitment is accompanied by lymphatic channel recruitment that would be capable of maintaining the $Q_L > Q_f$ balance.

Ion Exchange in the Alveolus

Throughout nature, water follows ion transport; this relationship exists in the lung and specifically in the alveolus. **Sodium** is actively pumped from the alveoli, and water follows. In type II alveolar cells, sodium is transported from the alveolar space by differentiated apical sodium channels, then transported into the interstitium via Na+-K+-ATPase pumps along the basolateral surface.[16] In humans, a sodium/glucose cotransport system also has been found to play a role in ion and water transport in the alveolus.[17-20]

Type I cells also may contribute to solute and fluid transport in the alveolus, but these cells have been far less studied than the type II cells. Nonetheless, there is evidence that ion selective pores also may exist near the tight junctions of the type I cells that contribute to the elimination of solute from the airways. Ionic transport from the distal airways is not likely to be limited to the alveoli, but also occurs within the distal airway epithelial cells.[16] Finally, type I epithelial cell aquaporins, or water channels that allow for direct pumping of water from the alveolar space, seem to service a significant role in alveolar-capillary integrity.[21-24]

Extrinsic factors may help to regulate the clearance of fluid from the airways. Catecholamine-dependent transport and cyclic AMP–stimulated **chloride** uptake seem to be important regulators of ion transport from the alveoli and distal airways.[16,25-28] Circulating catecholamines likely contribute to lung fluid clearance in newborns, whereas β2-agonists seem to up-regulate sodium transport from the lung in older mammalian species.[16] Although the mechanism of this increase in solute transport is uncertain, there is evidence to suggest that it is cyclic AMP mediated through an increased transcription of Na+-K+-ATPase, and epithelial sodium channel subunits at the apical and basolateral surfaces.[29-32]

A variety of catecholamine-independent regulators also seem to influence fluid transport from the alveolus. Glucocorticoids have been shown to increase transepithelial sodium uptake in adult and fetal animal lungs.[33,34] Other regulators, such as growth factors, thyroid hormone, and serine protease activity, also have been implicated.[35] Dopamine has been shown to up-regulate Na+-K+-ATPase subunits along the basolateral surface of alveolar epithelial cells.[36]

PULMONARY EDEMA AND HEART FAILURE

Pulmonary edema is simply the accumulation of water and solute in the pulmonary interstitium as a result of perturbations in the equilibrium of the forces discussed earlier (Fig. 9-4). According to the Starling equation, edema can result from increased hydrostatic pressure gradient secondary to increased P_{mv} or decreased P_{pmv}, hypoproteinemia and decreased π_{mv}, or alteration in the lung barrier such that there is an increased K_f or a decreased δ. The various aspects of pulmonary edema are elucidated here.

Cardiogenic Heart Failure

A general schematic of changes that occur in acute and chronically elevated microvascular hydrostatic pressure (e.g., cardiogenic heart failure) is shown in Figure 9-4. The pulmonary microvascular hydrostatic pressure (P_{mv}) can be increased as a result of an increase in left atrial pressure. It is a dynamic number affected by minute-to-minute pulmonary blood flow and resistances proximal and distal to the fluid-filtering sites in the lungs. Gaar and coworkers[37] predicted P_{mv} from attainable hemodynamic measures: mean pulmonary arterial pressure (P_{PA}) and mean left atrial pressure (P_{LA}):

$$P_{mv} = P_{LA} + 0.4 \, (P_{PA} - P_{LA})$$

From this formula, the effects of increasing pulmonary arterial and, even more influential, left atrial pressure on the microvascular hydrostatic pressure are evident.

Whatever the cause, whether an increase in pulmonary blood flow from a left-to-right shunt or increase in left atrial pressure secondary to left ventricular noncompliance or an obstructive lesion, the increased left atrial pressure leads to an obligate increase in P_{mv} and an increase in transmural fluid filtration and lymph production. This flux of fluid and solute to the pulmonary interstitium tests the ability of the pulmonary edema safety factors discussed earlier in preventing pulmonary edema. If lung lymph production exceeds the capacity of the pulmonary lymphatics, interstitial fluid accumulation begins. Eventually, fluid is capable of spilling into the airways, however, and begins to affect gas exchange.

Gas exchange can be affected in the absence of fluid leakage into airspaces in mild interstitial edema. In animal studies of mild hydrostatic pulmonary edema, a significant portion of the interstitial fluid collection occurs within the thick portion of the alveolar septum.[38,39] Because gas exchange between the alveolus and capillary is indirectly proportionate to the thickness of the alveolar capillary membrane, even mild hydrostatic pulmonary edema is significant. Because gas exchange can occur across either side of the alveolar capillary membrane, membrane thickness reflects the harmonic mean thickness (τ_h) of either side of the

membrane. In the lung, a more accurate depiction of Fick's law would be:

$$Q = k(\Delta P) \, (A)/\tau_h$$

Altered Ion Exchange and the Inflammatory Response

The ability to clear fluid from the airways is impaired in patients with hydrostatic pulmonary edema.[40-43] This impairment seems to be unrelated to the pulmonary hemodynamics and suggests down-regulation of alveolar ion and fluid transport. The effect of atrial natriuretic peptide (ANP) has been implicated as one cause of this observation. Increased atrial pressure results in the release of ANP, but this may not be the only source in heart failure. The lungs also may manufacture ANP, particularly in the setting of cardiomyopathy.[44] Although the systemic effects of ANP are to increase sodium and water loss in the urine and systemic vasodilation, ANP seems to have a puzzling effect on the alveolar epithelial cell by directly inhibiting sodium uptake by the alveolar epithelial cell.[16] The clinical impact of this effect has not been established in humans.

The inflammatory responses to heart failure are reviewed thoroughly elsewhere in this book. Nonetheless, some cardiopulmonary interactions that may be mediated by the inflammatory response to heart failure are highlighted here. Work by Yndestad and others[45,46] suggests that up-regulation of **cytokines** is a part of the response to chronic heart failure in adults. T cells from heart failure patients show enhanced gene expression of inflammatory cytokines, which likely have the direct effect of down-regulating sodium transport in the alveoli.[47,48] Specifically, tumor necrosis factor-α, an inhibitor of sodium and water transport in the lung, has been shown to be elevated in patients presenting with acute cardiogenic pulmonary edema who have biologic markers of alveolar-capillary disruption.[49,50] In addition to sodium transport, these proinflammatory agents may alter capillary sieving properties and result in increased spillage of solute and fluid into the interstitium.

Alveolar-Capillary Wall Stress Failure

The need for the alveolar-capillary interface to be thin enough for gas exchange has been emphasized, but it also must be strong enough to withstand the wall stress created by the variations in pulmonary hemodynamics. In certain circumstances, such as in extreme exercise or in pathologic conditions such as cardiogenic pulmonary edema, the stress on the wall of the alveolar-capillary barrier can overcome the strength of the interface.

The stress placed on the wall of capillaries is a function of Laplace's relationship, where wall stress (WS) is directly related to the transmural pressure difference (ΔP), radius of the curve (r), and thickness of the vessel wall (t):[50]

$$WS = (\Delta P) \, (r)/t$$

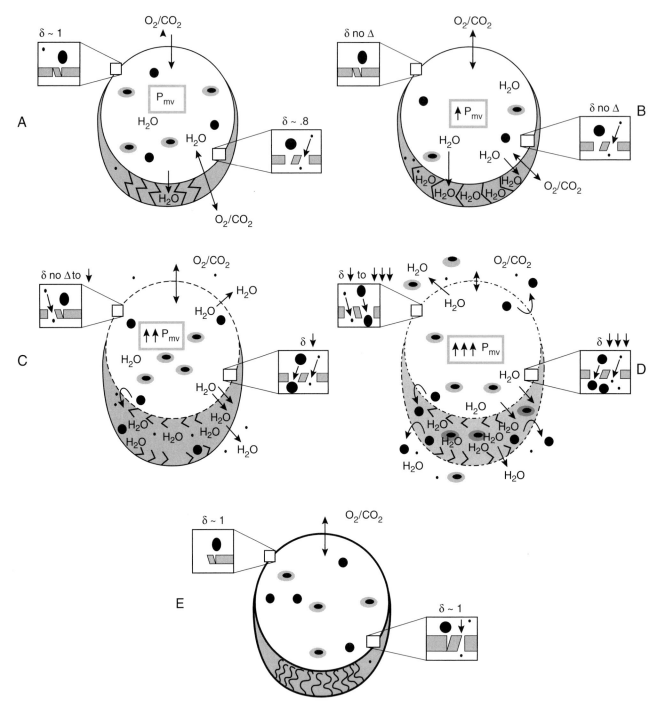

FIGURE 9-4 ■ **Heart failure and pulmonary edema.** Sequencing of acute and chronic cardiogenic heart failure and hydrostatic pulmonary edema. **A,** P_{mv} is the primary Starling force determining fluid filtration in the lung. Colloids *(circles)*, red blood cells *(double circles)*, and water remain largely intravascular. The reflection coefficient (δ) of the alveolar epithelial (~1) and endothelial (~0.8) membranes are high. **B,** When P_{mv} acutely increases with left heart failure, the capillary distends, and filtration of water from the capillary to the interstitial space increases. The edema safety factors are in full force. The interstitial matrix *(jagged lines)* limits the distensibility of the interstitium, causing P_{pmv} to increase and reducing the hydrostatic gradient driving fluid filtration. Water is bound by the hydrophilic glycoproteins in the interstitium, protecting the alveolar space from fluid spillage. The capillary and alveolar membranes maintain a high δ, and little colloid loss to the interstitium or airway occurs. δ does not change significantly for either membrane. **C,** As P_{mv} increases, fluid filtration increases, and the alveolar-capillary membrane stretches. This stretching increases the permeability of the alveolar-capillary membrane (capillary > alveolar), allowing for colloid to enter the interstitium, which reduces the opposing force against hydrostatic pressures driving fluid filtration into the interstitium and alveolar space. The distention of the interstitium results in fragmentation of the extracellular matrix. The leakage of water and colloid into the alveolar space reduces gas exchange.

Continued

FIGURE 9-4 ■ cont'd D, With increasing P_{mv}, structural collapse (stress failure) of the alveolar-capillary membrane occurs, leading to blood, colloid, and fluid spillage into the interstitium and the alveolar space. Limited gas exchange can occur in this setting. **E,** Chronically elevated P_{mv} results in significant pulmonary vascular remodeling along with changes in the extracellular matrix of the alveolar-capillary interface. Although this remodeling may help to reduce fluid and colloid filtration from the microvascular space, it comes at a cost. Hypertrophy of the arterial and venular systems and thickening of the capillary reduce the size of vascular lumens and reduce intrapulmonary blood volume. Thickening of the endothelial and the epithelial basement membranes increases the diffusion barrier for gas exchange.

The thin nature of the capillary accounts for high wall stress that is limited only by the small radius of the capillary. As vessels dilate and hydrostatic pressure increases, as can be seen in heart failure, pulmonary venous hypertension, or left atrial hypertension, loss of structural integrity of the alveolar-capillary membrane may occur.[8,9,51] Borrowing a term from structural engineering, this condition is commonly referred to as *stress failure*. Clinical manifestations of stress failure include hemoptysis, proteinaceous airway fluid, and gas exchange abnormality.[10] In animal studies, disruption of the alveolar-capillary barrier can be seen when P_{mv} exceeds 24 mm Hg.[51]

Studies suggest that stress failure of the alveolar-capillary membrane may be a more common clinical problem than realized. Biologic markers, such as surfactant proteins A and B, are present in the bloodstream of patients with acute cardiogenic pulmonary edema and probably reflect alveolar-capillary disruption.[49,50,52]

Pulmonary Vascular and Extracellular Remodeling

The extracellular matrix resists interstitial edema formation by keeping the interstitial compliance low. In animal studies of acute pulmonary edema, as fluid filters across the microvascular bed of the lung, lymph production exceeds the ability of the lymphatics to drain the interstitium, and interstitial fluid accumulates. As it does so, a critical point is reached when fragmentation of the extracellular matrix can occur. Breakdown of the proteoglycans results in structural failure of these supportive molecules and an increase in interstitial compliance, which results in interstitial fluid accumulation along with the potential for permeability changes in the capillary.[10] Together these changes can contribute to the development of severe pulmonary edema.

Similar to the heart that remodels in response to injury and pressure and volume stresses, the alveolar-capillary barrier also alters its configuration in the presence of chronic hydrostatic stress forces (such as those seen in chronic left heart failure or mitral valve disease). The changes that occur in the pulmonary artery resistance vessels and pulmonary veins in high flow states or in the presence of elevated pulmonary venous pressure have been well described; these changes include peripheralization of vascular smooth muscle, medial hypertrophy of the vessels, and intimal thickening.[53,54] These changes reflect, as West and Mathieu-Costello[8] suggest, the body's attempt to return to a fetal state, when even though pulmonary arterial pressure is high, the microvascular bed is relatively protected from increased pressure because of anatomic (arterial medial hypertrophy) and dynamic (vasoconstriction) factors. Little attention has been paid to the remodeling that occurs in the alveolar-capillary interface under conditions of heart failure, yet such changes have a tremendous impact on gas and solute exchange in these patients.

Several reports in patients with mitral stenosis show that the basement membrane of the capillary and alveolar epithelia is significantly thickened.[55-57] Similar observations can be made in animals exposed to chronic pacing-induced cardiomyopathy.[58] This epithelial thickening is due to increased deposition of type IV collagen. Although this response initially may be protective by decreasing the permeability of the microvascular bed, the increase in thickness of the alveolar-capillary membrane may lead to a more ominous outcome, as in gas diffusion abnormalities.[51,59] This is the likely explanation for the observed reduction in pulmonary transfer factor of carbon monoxide in adult patients with chronic congestive heart failure awaiting cardiac transplantation.[60] In these patients, pulmonary transfer factor of carbon monoxide is decreased as a result of a reduction in pulmonary capillary blood volume and a reduction in the diffusing capacity of the alveolar-capillary membrane in these patients. Data also suggest that remodeling of the pulmonary microvasculature may have a genetic predisposition for abnormal extracellular matrix deposition that can result in gas exchange abnormalities long after correction of the hemodynamic abnormality.[61-63]

The state of health of the vascular endothelium also may contribute to alveolar capillary dysfunction in the heart failure patient. The endothelium plays a crucial role in determining vascular tone in the pulmonary vasculature. A delicate balance between endothelial-derived autocoids, such as vasodilator (nitric oxide) and vasoconstrictor (endothelin), determines pulmonary vascular resistance. In heart failure, in vitro and in vivo studies suggest that nitric oxide–dependent vasodilation of the pulmonary vascular bed is impaired.[53,64,65]

Pulmonary Lymphatic Dysfunction

Maintenance of normal pulmonary lymphatic function is the most effective prevention and management of pulmonary edema formation. Without maintenance of normal pulmonary lymphatic function, the lungs would be rapidly accumulating fluid, flooding the alveoli, and interfering with gas exchange. Little is known about the dynamics of this vascular bed either in its normal state or in pathologic conditions, such as in heart failure. What is known is that lymphatic vessels serve not only as a conduit for lung fluid drainage, but also actively contract to milk lymph toward the central venous system through phasic contraction. The thoracic duct expresses mRNA for smooth muscle actin and myosin and is capable of regulating lung lymph flow, reflecting its ability to adapt to stress conditions similar to vascular structures.[66]

Similar to any vascular system, flow in the lymphatics is a function of resistance. Because the pulmonary lymphatics drain into the central venous system, it stands to reason that increases in central venous pressure can impede pulmonary lymphatic flow. Drainage by the pulmonary lymphatics decreases when the force of contraction of the lymphatic smooth muscle is insufficient to overcome the resistance (Fig. 9-5). This phenomenon is illustrated in a report by Cole and associates.[67] In this series of experiments, the central venous pressure was acutely increased in dogs by creating tricuspid valve

regurgitation and pulmonary stenosis. Abdominal girth was used as an indirect measure of effective lymphatic drainage via the thoracic duct. With right heart failure, there was an associated increase in abdominal girth in the dogs. When the thoracic duct was implanted into the lower pressure pulmonary vein, the ascites and secondary abdominal distention quickly resolved. The effect on outlet pressure lung lymph flow has been shown by other investigators.[68-71] The pulmonary edema seen in patients with cor pulmonale is likely derived from this mechanism.

Maturational Factors

Several cardiac and pulmonary maturational factors likely contribute to cardiopulmonary interaction in heart failure. It is estimated that adults have a complement of about 300×10^6 alveoli with an alveolar surface area of 100 to 140 M^2.[2,3,72] Newborns have nowhere near this surface area partly because of the relative immaturity of the airways. Most infants survive on gas exchange across respiratory bronchioles, and immature alveoli number approximately 20×10^6. During the considerable postnatal growth of the lung, development of the pulmonary capillary bed and intra-acinar vessels closely follows development of the airways.

Similar to the airways, the pulmonary vasculature is immature at birth. There is a theoretical limit as to how much pulmonary vascular recruitment is possible in the very young. Vascular recruitment is an effective safety factor to prevent pulmonary edema when conditions that increase left atrial pressure or increase pulmonary blood flow exist. Animal studies suggest that the degree of recruitment of the pulmonary vascular bed of the newborn is significantly limited.[72] With a lack of vascular recruitment, increases in pulmonary blood flow (e.g., left-to-right shunt) or increases in left atrial pressure (e.g., cardiomyopathy, mitral valve disease) result in a direct increase in microvascular hydrostatic pressure. In addition, the left ventricle of a newborn is less compliant than that of a mature heart because of a high content of noncontractile elements.[73] This situation can lead to much more rapid development of left atrial hypertension under abnormal loading conditions or altered ventricular contractility.

Finally, the tolerance of the pulmonary lymphatics to increases in afterload seems to be age dependent. In a study by Johnson and colleagues,[71] pulmonary lymph flow ceased at much lower outflow pressure in the fetus and young lamb than in the adult sheep (see Fig. 9-5). Pulmonary edema secondary to a reduction in lymphatic drainage would be evident at much lower central venous pressure in an infant than in an older child or adult. This is likely the mechanism for pulmonary edema associated with cor pulmonale or after surgically created cavopulmonary anastomoses (e.g., bidirectional Glenn anastomosis or Fontan procedure).

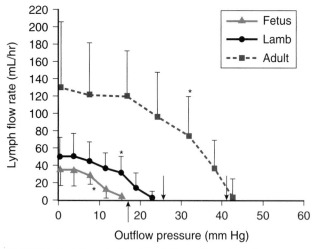

FIGURE 9-5 ■ Thoracic duct lymph flow. Effect of outflow pressure on thoracic duct lymph flow rate in fetuses, lambs, and sheep. In each age group, lymph flow decreases with increasing outflow pressure. Compared with the adult sheep, the fetuses and lambs achieve zero thoracic duct flow at significantly lower outflow pressure. (From Johnson SA, Straten JA, Parellada JA, et al: *Thoracic duct function in fetal, newborn, and adult sheep. Lymphology* 1996;29:50-56.)

CURRENT STATUS AND FUTURE TRENDS

The means by which pneumocytes keep airways dry is only starting to be appreciated. The remodeling of the pulmonary microvasculature, both endothelial and epithelial, in disease states such as heart failure, is poorly understood, and virtually no data exist in regard to understanding of maturational differences to stress factors. Despite its enormous role in the prevention of pulmonary edema, we have almost no knowledge of regulation of the pulmonary lymphatic circulation, especially in pediatric patients. The roles of pulmonary edema safety mechanism and possible therapeutic interventions in heart failure remain to be investigated in children and young adults.[74,75]

Key Concepts

■ The alveolar epithelial cells and the capillary endothelial cells with their respective basal laminae constitute the alveolar capillary membrane, which is involved in alveolar and interstitial clearance of water and solutes.

■ Overall, the driving pressure in lung fluid filtration is a balance of hydrostatic and oncotic forces. The two hydrostatic forces include the P_{mv}, which tends to push fluid into the interstitium, and the P_{pmv}, an opposing force that tends to keep fluid intravascular. P_{mv} is the hydrostatic pressure in the lung capillary bed, or the principal driving force for lung fluid filtration.

■ Opposing the balance of hydrostatic forces are the two protein-related oncotic forces. π_{mv} acts to keep fluid within the vascular space, and this pressure is probably the same as in large systemic vessels, whereas π_{pmv} draws fluid into the interstitium and can be approximated by the lung lymph oncotic pressure and protein concentration.

■ The oncotic forces influence fluid filtration in the lung as a function of δ, which reflects the permeability property of a barrier or the relative degree of sieving of solutes across the lung microvascular membrane.

■ To complete the equation specific for lung fluid balance, the K_f, reflecting the product of hydraulic conductance of the microvascular membrane (or its permeability) and the surface area available for fluid filtration, needs to be considered. When K_f is coupled with the driving pressures in the lung, the forces driving fluid filtration in the lung are finally depicted as the Starling equation: $Q_f = K_f [(P_{mv} - P_{pmv}) - \delta (\pi_{mv} - \pi_{pmv})]$.

■ Pulmonary edema is simply the accumulation of water and solute in the pulmonary interstitium as a result of perturbations in the equilibrium of the forces. According to the Starling equation, edema can result from increased hydrostatic pressure gradient secondary to increased P_{mv} or decreased P_{pmv}, hypoproteinemia and decreased π_{mv}, or alteration in the lung barrier such that there is an increased K_f or a decreased δ.

■ Whatever the cause, whether an increase in pulmonary blood flow from a left-to-right shunt or increase in left atrial pressure from left ventricular noncompliance or an obstructive lesion, the increased left atrial pressure leads to an obligate increase in P_{mv} and an increase in transmural fluid filtration and lymph production.

REFERENCES

1. Weibel ER, Knight BW: A morphogenic study on the thickness of the pulmonary air-blood barrier. J Cell Biol 1964;21:367-384.
2. Weibel ER: Lung morphometry and models in respiratory physiology. In Chang HK, Paiva M (eds): Respiratory Physiology: An Analytical Approach. New York, Marcel Dekker, 1989, pp 1-56.
3. Inselman LS, Mellins RB: Growth and development of the lung. J Pediatr 1981;98:1-15.
4. Staub NC, Albertine KH: The structure of the lungs relative to their principal function. In Murray JF, Nadel JA (eds): Textbook of Respiratory Medicine. Philadelphia, WB Saunders, 1988, pp 12-36.
5. Gehr P, Bachofen M, Weibel ER: The normal lung: Ultrastructure and morphometric estimation of diffusion capacity. Respir Physiol 1978;32:121-140.
6. Weibel ER, Bachofen H: Structural design of the alveolar septum and fluid exchange. In Fishman AP, Renkin EM (eds): Pulmonary Edema. Baltimore, Williams & Wilkins, 1979, pp 1-20.
7. Schneeberger EE, Lynch RD: Structure, function, and regulation of cellular tight junctions. Am J Physiol Lung Cell Mol Physiol 1992;262:L647-L661.
8. West JB, Mathieu-Costello O: Strength of the pulmonary blood-gas barrier. Respir Physiol 1992;88:141-148.
9. West JB, Mathieu-Costello O: Structure of the pulmonary blood-gas barrier. Annu Rev Physiol 1999;61:543-572.
10. Miserocchi G, Negrini D, Passi A, De Luca G: Development of lung edema: Interstitial fluid dynamic and molecular structure. News Physiol Sci 2001;16:66-71.
11. Taylor AE: Capillary fluid filtration: Starling forces and lymph flow. Circ Res 1981;49:557-575.
12. Guyton AC, Lindsey AE: Effect of elevated left atrial pressure and decreased plasma protein concentration on the development of pulmonary edema. Circ Res 1959;7:649.
13. Drake RE, Doursout MF: Pulmonary edema and elevated left atrial pressure: Four hours and beyond. News Physiol Sci 2002; 17:223-226.
14. Von Der Weid P-Y, Zhao J, Van Helden DF: Nitric oxide decreases pacemaker activity in lymphatic vessels of guinea pig mesentery. Am J Physiol Heart Circ Physiol 2001;280:H2707-H2716.
15. Bettinelli D, Kays C, Bailliart O, et al: Effect of gravity and posture on lung mechanics. J Appl Physiol 93:2044-2052, 2002.
16. Matthay MA, Folkesson HG, Clerici C: Lung epithelial fluid transport and the resolution of pulmonary edema. Physiol Rev 2002;82:569-600.
17. Guazzi M: Alveolar-capillary membrane dysfunction in heart failure. Chest 2003;124:1090-1102.
18. Azzam ZS, Vidas D, Saldias FJ, et al: Na, K-ATPase overexpression improves alveolar fluid clearance in a rat model of elevated left atrial pressure. Circulation 2002;105:497-501.
19. Maron MB, Fu Z, Mathieu-Costello O, West JB: Effect of high transcapillary pressures on capillary ultrastructure and permeability coefficients in dog lung. J Appl Physiol 2001;90:638-648.
20. Schneeberger E, McCarthy K: Cytochemical localization of the Na, K-ATPase in rat type II pneumocytes. J Appl Physiol 1986; 20:1584-1589.

21. Maron MB: Dose-response relationship between plasma epinephrine concentration and alveolar liquid clearance. J Appl Physiol 1998;85:1702-1707.

22. Cott GR, Sugahara K, Mason RJ: Stimulation of net active ion transport across alveolar type II cell monolayers. Am J Physiol 1996;250:C222-C227.

23. Goodman BE, Kim KJ, Crandall ED: Evidence for active sodium transport across alveolar epithelium of isolated rat lung. J Appl Physiol 1987;62:2460-2466.

24. Basset G, Crone C, Saumon G: Fluid absorption by rat lung in situ: Pathways for sodium entry in the luminal membrane of alveolar epithelium. J Physiol (Lond) 1987;384:325-345.

25. Fang X, Fukuda N, Barbry P, et al: Novel role for CFTR in fluid absorption from the distal airspaces of the lung. J Gen Physiol 2002;119:199-208.

26. Jiang X, Ingbar DH, O'Grady SM: Adrenergic regulation of ion transport across adult alveolar epithelia cells:effects on Cl- channel activation and transport function in cultures with an apical air interface. J Membr Biol 2001;181:195-204.

27. O'Grady SM, Jiang X, Ingbar DH: Cl- channel activation is necessary for stimulation of Na transport in adult alveolar epithethial cells. Am J Physiol Lung Cell Mol Physiol 2000;278: L239-L244.

28. Walters DV, Olver RE: The role of catecholamines in lung liquid absorption at birth. Pediatr Res 1978;12:239-242.

29. Sakuma T, Folkesson HG, Suzuki S, et al: Beta-adrenergic agonist stimulated alveolar fluid clearance in ex vivo human and rat lungs. Am J Respir Crit Care Med 1997;155:506-512.

30. Sakuma T, Okaniwa G, Nakada T, et al: Alveolar fluid clearance in the resected human lung. Am J Respir Crit Care Med 1994;150:305-310.

31. Dagenais A, Denis C, Vives MF, et al: Modulation of α-Na⁺-K⁺-ATPase by cAMP and dexamethasone in alveolar epithelial cells. Am J Physiol Lung Cell Mol Physiol 2001;281:L217-L230.

32. Minakata Y, Suzuki S, Grygorczyk C, et al: Impact of β-adrenergic agonist on Na⁺ channel and Na⁺-K⁺-ATPase expression in alveolar type II cells. Am J Physiol Lung Cell Mol Physiol 1998;275:L414-L422.

33. Barquin N, Ciccolella DE, Ridge KM, Sznajder JI: Dexamethasone upregulates the Na⁺-K⁺-ATPase in rat alveolar epithelial cells. Am J Physiol Lung Cell Mol Physiol 1997;273:L825-L830.

34. Noda M, Suzuki S, Tsubochi H, et al: Single dexamethasone injection increases alveolar fluid clearance in adult rats. Crit Care Med 2003;31:1183-1189.

35. Lei J, Nowbar S, Mariash CN, Ingbar DH: Thyroid hormone stimulates Na⁺-K⁺-ATPase activity and its plasma membrane insertion in rat alveolar epithelial cells. Am J Physiol Lung Cell Mol Physiol 2003; 285:L762-L772.

36. Barnard ML, Ridge KM, Saldias F, et al: Stimulation of the dopamine 1 receptor increases lung edema clearance. Am J Respir Crit Care Med 1999;160:982-986.

37. Gaar KA, Taylor AE, Owens LJ, Guyton AC: Pulmonary capillary pressure and filtration coefficient in the isolated perfused lung. Am J Physiol 1967;213:910-914.

38. Conforti E, Fenoglio C, Bernocchi G, et al: Morpho-functional analysis of lung tissue in mild interstitial edema. Am J Physiol Lung Cell Mol Physiol 2002;282:L766-L774.

39. Negrini D, Candiani A, Boschetti F, et al: Pulmonary microvascular and perivascular interstitial geometry during development of mild hydraulic edema. Am J Physiol Lung Cell Mol Physiol 2001;281:L1464-L1471.

40. Verghese GM, Ware LB, Matthay BA, Matthay MA: Alveolar epithelial fluid transport and the resolution of clinically severe hydrostatic pulmonary edema. J Appl Physiol 1999;87:1301-1312.

41. Guazzi M, Agostoni P, Bussotti M, Guazzi M: Impeded alveolar-capillary gas transfer with saline infusion in heart failure. Hypertension 1999;34:1202-1207.

42. Guazzi M, Marenzi G, Alimento M, et al: Improvement of alveolar-capillary membrane diffusing capacity with enalapril in chronic heart failure and counteracting effect of aspirin. Circulation 1997;95:1930-1936.

43. Guazzi M, Agostoni P, Guazzi M: Modulation of alveolar-capillary sodium handling as a mechanism of protection of Fas transfer by enalapril, and not by losartan in chronic heart failure. J Am Coll Cardiol 2001;37:398-406.

44. Gutkowska J, Nemer M, Sole MJ, et al: Lung is an important source of atrial natriuretic factor in experimental cardiomyopathy. J Clin Invest 1989;83:1500-1504.

45. Yndestad A, Hom AM, Muller F, et al: Enhanced expression of inflammatory cytokines and activation markers in T-cells from patients with chronic heart failure. Cardiovasc Res 2003;60:141-146.

46. Sharma R, Bolger AP, Li W, et al: Elevated circulating levels of inflammatory cytokines and bacterial endotoxin in adults with congenital heart disease. Am J Cardiol 2003;92:188-193.

47. Dagenais A, Frechette R, Yamagata Y, et al: Down regulation of ENaC activity and expression by TNFα in alveolar epithelial cells. Am J Physiol Lung Cell Mol Physiol 2003;286: L301-L311.

48. Bolger AP, Sharma R, Li W, et al: Neurohormonal activation and the chronic heart failure syndrome in adults with congenital heart disease. Circulation 2002;106:92-99.

49. De Pasquale CG, Arnolda LF, Doyle IR, et al: Prolonged alveolo-capillary barrier damage after acute cardiogenic pulmonary edema. Crit Care Med 2003;31:1060-1067.

50. De Pasquale CG, Bersten AD, Doyle IR, et al: Infarct-induced chronic heart failure increases bidirectional protein movement across the alveolocapillary barrier. Am J Physiol Heart Circ Physiol 2003;284:H2136-H2145.

51. West JB: Cellular responses to mechanical stress: Pulmonary capillary stress failure. J Appl Physiol 2000;89:2483-2489.

52. West JB, Mathieu-Costello O: Structure of the pulmonary blood-gas barrier. Annu Rev Physiol 1999;61:543-572.

53. Driss AB, Devaux MS, Henrion D, et al: Hemodynamic stresses induce endothelial dysfunction and remodeling of pulmonary artery in experimental compensated heart failure. Circulation 2000;101:2764-2770.

54. Stenmark KR: Cellular and molecular mechanisms of pulmonary vascular remodeling. Annu Rev Physiol 1997;59:89-144.

55. Haworth SG, Hall SM, Patel M: Peripheral pulmonary vascular and airway abnormalities in adolescents with rheumatic mitral stenosis. Int J Cardiol 1988;18:405-416.

56. Kay JM, Edwards FR: Ultrastructure of the alveolar-capillary wall in mitral stenosis. J Pathol 1973;111:239-245.

57. Lee YS: Electron microscopic studies of the alveolar-capillary barrier in the patients of chronic pulmonary edema. Jpn Circ J 1979;43:945-954.

58. Townsley MI, Snell KS, Ivey CL, et al: Remodeling of lung interstitium but not resistance vessels in canine pacing-induced heart failure. J Appl Physiol 1999;87:1823-1830.

59. Kingsbury MP, Huang W, Donnelly JL, et al: Structural remodeling of lungs in chronic heart failure. Basic Res Cardiol 2003;98:295-303.

60. Al-Rawas OA, Carter R, Stevenson RD, et al: The alveolar-capillary membrane diffusing capacity and the pulmonary capillary blood volume in heart transplant candidates. Heart 2000;83:156-160.

61. Guazzi M, Pontone G, Brambilla R, et al: Alveolar-capillary membrane conductance: A novel prognostic indicator in heart failure. Eur Heart J 2002;23:467-476.

62. Assayag P, Benamer H, Aubry P, et al: Alteration of the alveolar-capillary membrane diffusing capacity in chronic left heart disease. Am J Cardiol 1998;82:459-464.

63. Guazzi M: Alveolar-capillary membrane dysfunction in heart failure. Chest 2003;124:1090-1102.

64. Ontkean M, Gay R, Greenberg B: Diminished endothelium-derived relaxing factor activity in an experimental model of chronic heart failure. Circ Res 1991;69:1088-1096.

65. Cooper CJ, Jevnikar FW, Walsh T, et al: The influence of basal nitric oxide activity on pulmonary vascular resistance in patients with congestive heart failure. J Am Coll Cardiol 1998;82:609-614.

66. Muthuchamy M, Gashev A, Boswell N, et al: Molecular and functional analyses of the contractile apparatus in lymphatic muscle. FASEB J 2003;17:920-922.

67. Cole WR, Hearst Witte M, Kash SL, et al: Thoracic duct-to-pulmonary vein stent in the treatment of experimental right heart failure. Circulation 1967;36:539-543.

68. Gest AL, Bair DK, Vander Straten MC: Thoracic duct lymph flow in fetal sheep with increased venous pressure from electrically induced tachycardia. Biol Neonate 1993;64:325-330.

69. Drake R, Giesler M, Laine G, et al: Effect of outflow pressure on lung lymph flow in unanesthetized sheep. J Appl Physiol 1985;58:70-76.

70. Drake RE, Gabel JC: Effect of outflow pressure on intestinal lymph flow in unanesthetized sheep. Am J Physiol 1991;260(4 Pt 2): R668-R671.

71. Johnson SA, Straten JA, Parellada JA, et al: Thoracic duct function in fetal, newborn, and adult sheep. Lymphology 1996;29:50-56.

72. Feltes TF, Hansen TN: Effects of an aorticopulmonary shunt on lung fluid balance in the young lamb. Pediatr Res 1989;26:94-97.

73. Friedman WF: The intrinsic physiologic properties of the developing heart. Prog Cardiovasc Dis 1972;15:87-111.

74. L'Her E, Duquesne F, Girou E, et al: Noninvasive continuous positive airway pressure in elderly cardiogenic pulmonary edema patients. Intensive Care Med 2004;30:882-888. Epub 2004 (Feb 28).

75. Wang SM, Lei HY, Huang MC, et al: Therapeutic efficacy of milrinone in the management of enterovirus 71-induced pulmonary edema. Pediatr Pulmonol 2005;39:219-223.

CHAPTER 10

Echocardiographic Quantitation of Ventricular Function

Benjamin W. Eidem

Reliable serial quantitative echocardiographic assessment of ventricular function is an essential tool in the clinician's evaluation and management of adults and children with heart failure. Medical management and timing of surgery often are determined by echocardiographic data to maximize likelihood of recovery. Pediatric patients who require close surveillance of myocardial function can range from an adolescent patient with dilated cardiomyopathy in the outpatient clinic to a neonate after Norwood palliative reconstructive surgery in the immediate postoperative period in the cardiac intensive care setting.

There are critical inherent differences between echocardiographic assessment in adults and children with acquired or congenital heart disease. First, the age and body size spectrum in children is considerably larger, and this creates inherent difficulties in assessing myocardial function as changes occur during maturation of the heart.[1,2] Second, most children with heart failure have congenital heart disease, and palliative or corrective repair of such lesions (e.g., patches for ventricular septal defect) often leads to nongeometric shapes; such alterations render assessments of normal right and left ventricular function more challenging. Third, the pathophysiology of congenital heart disease and its repairs could make the interpretations more difficult because postoperative residua (e.g., chronic pulmonary insufficiency after tetralogy of Fallot repair) are often the etiology of the heart dysfunction. Lastly, many children have only one functional ventricle, and serial assessment of myocardial performance of a single ventricle is a daunting challenge to the echocardiographer.

Although Doppler ultrasound is the mainstay of diagnostic examinations for assessing ventricular function and myocardial performance, a preliminary thorough two-dimensional examination with color Doppler interrogation is essential to assess congenital cardiac anatomy and to evaluate postoperative residua.[3] Failure to perform such a preliminary examination can lead to futile medical therapy or missed opportunities for timely surgical or catheter intervention in the treatment of heart failure. In addition, certain postoperative anatomy and possible residua should be ascertained by other imaging modalities (e.g., angiography, CT, or MRI) in the presence of myocardial dysfunction. For example, a patient with myocardial dysfunction after an arterial switch operation should not be followed by echocardiography as the sole diagnostic methodology without complementary evaluations by

angiography or MRI. Lastly, because systolic dysfunction often is preceded by diastolic dysfunction, quantitative assessment of diastolic function may be predictive of eventual systolic dysfunction in these patients. This chapter discusses in detail current methods of echocardiographic quantitation of systolic and diastolic ventricular performance in children and young adults with heart failure. Echocardiographic findings and noninvasive assessment also are discussed in other chapters addressing specific topics.

ECHOCARDIOGRAPHIC ASSESSMENT OF LEFT VENTRICULAR SYSTOLIC FUNCTION

Left ventricular dimensions often are altered with heart failure with increases in end-diastolic and end-systolic dimensions. It is important to appreciate fully the pathophysiology of various lesions in the interpretation of increased dimensions and shortening fraction. A shortening fraction in the normal range in a patient with aortic regurgitation or mitral regurgitation (MR) would indicate deteriorating function (because one would expect such a patient to possess a supranormal shortening fraction). The progression of findings in regurgitant lesions before heart failure is usually an increase in end-diastolic dimension, followed by an increase in end-systolic dimension, and finally a decrease in shortening fraction as the heart decompensates and fails.

Left ventricular systolic dysfunction has long been recognized to be a powerful predictor of the development of cardiac symptoms and poor long-term outcomes in adults with heart failure.[4-7] In children with congenital heart lesions, the advent of decreased left ventricular systolic function also has been shown to predict poor outcome in many disease states.[8-10] Echocardiographic measures of left ventricular systolic function include M-mode and two-dimensional examinations for dimension and volume changes and Doppler-derived ejection indices of ventricular performance.[11-14] Quantitation of blood flow, such as cardiac output and stroke volume, generally has not been used for assessment of cardiac performance because cardiac output can be preserved until myocardial dysfunction is severe.

Most echocardiographic measures of left ventricular systolic function represent **ejection phase indices,** such as shortening fraction, ejection fraction, velocity of

FIGURE 10-1 ■ **Simpson biplane method of calculating left ventricular ejection fraction. A,** Diagram represents the orthogonal two-chamber and four-chamber views used to calculate systolic and diastolic left ventricular volumes based on the summing of equal sequential slices of left ventricular area. The ventricular volume is calculated by the summation of volumes of ellipsoidal cylinders with radii a_i (apical two-chamber view) and b_i (apical four-chamber view) and the height (L/N), where L is the length of the long axis and N is the number of segments. **B** and **C,** Two-dimensional apical four-chamber view still frames from a patient with dilated cardiomyopathy show the calculation of left ventricular volume using the Simpson method (systole and diastole). LA, left atrium; LV, left ventricle. (**A** from Geva T: *Echocardiography and Doppler ultrasound.* In Garson A, Bricker JT, Fisher DJ, et al [eds]: *Science and Practice of Pediatric Cardiology.* Philadelphia, Williams & Wilkins, 1998, p 819.)

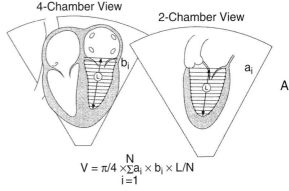

$$V = \pi/4 \times \sum_{i=1}^{N} a_i \times b_i \times L/N$$

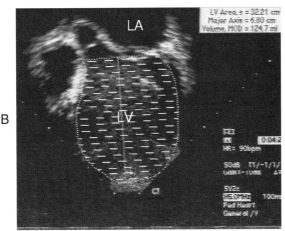

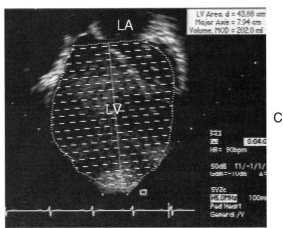

circumferential fiber shortening, changes in peak and mean pressures over time (dP/dt), and systolic time intervals. Some of these rely on geometric assumptions inherent in the elliptical shape of the left ventricle and are influenced significantly by a variety of hemodynamic factors, including altered ventricular preload and afterload, heart rate, left ventricular mass, and myocardial contractility. Unfavorable loading conditions can mimic depressed contractility, and, conversely, contractility can be falsely assessed to be normal in certain situations. The emergence of Doppler-derived measures of ventricular performance has circumvented many of the geometric challenges inherent in the global assessment of ventricular performance, especially in the evaluation of right ventricular performance and quantitative assessment of systolic function in patients with complex ventricular morphologies.[15-20]

Dimension-Derived Indices

One-dimensional wall motion analysis, or M-mode echocardiography, traditionally has been the most common method used to measure left ventricular **shortening fraction**. There are limitations with this relatively crude method of assessing ventricular function. First, contraction of the left ventricle cannot be assumed to be entirely uniform or symmetric. In addition, regional differences in wall motion and wall thickening should be taken into account in the interpretation

of shortening fraction. Finally, a flattened interventricular septum (as observed in patients with right ventricular volume or pressure overload) invalidates such a measurement.

Shortening fraction represents the change in left ventricular short axis diameter (with the cursor between the papillary muscles apical to the mitral valve leaflets):

$$SF\,(\%) = \frac{[LVEDD - LVESD]}{LVEDD} \times 100$$

where *LVEDD* is the left ventricular end-diastolic minor axis dimension, and *LVESD* is the left ventricular end-systolic minor axis dimension. Normal values for shortening fraction range from 28% to 44% with variation for age.

Determination of left ventricular **ejection fraction** (LVEF) is more tedious than calculation of the left ventricular shortening fraction, but more recent improvements in technology (e.g., automated border detection or acoustic quantification) have simplified this procedure. Two-dimensional echocardiography allows measurement of LVEF by quantifying changes in ventricular volume during the cardiac cycle. The geometric model most commonly used to measure LVEF is the modified Simpson biplane method. By using orthogonal apical four-chamber and two-chamber views of the left ventricle, this geometric model calculates left ventricular end-diastolic volume

(LVEDV) and left ventricular end-systolic volume (LVESV) by summing equal sequential slices of left ventricular area from each of these scan planes (Fig. 10-1). LVEF can be calculated as:

$$EF\,(\%) = \frac{[LVEDV - LVESV]}{LVEDV} \times 100$$

More recent studies have validated the ability of three-dimensional echocardiography to obtain accurate and reproducible estimates of left ventricular and right ventricular volumes and ejection fraction.[21] Normal values for LVEF range from 56% to 78%. Similar to shortening fraction, LVEF has been shown to depend on changes in ventricular loading conditions.

Doppler-Derived Indices

Much information can be derived from the **aortic velocity curve**, including peak aortic velocity, acceleration time, ejection time, velocity time integral, peak rate of acceleration, mean acceleration, and acceleration-to-ejection time ratio (Fig. 10-2). Because these indices depend on loading conditions, they have the same limitations as shortening and ejection fraction determinations described previously.

Noninvasive Doppler measurements of peak aortic velocity and peak aortic acceleration time have been

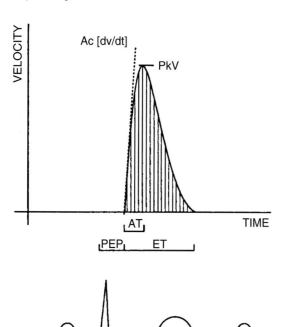

FIGURE 10-2 ■ Aortic velocity curve in assessment of left ventricular systolic function. Graphic representation of aortic velocity curve with peak aortic velocity (PkV), acceleration time (AT), ejection time (ET), and velocity time integral in the shaded area. Additional measurements for left ventricular function assessment include the peak rate of acceleration (Ac[dv/dt]), the mean acceleration (which is PkV/AT), and the AT/ET ratio. PEP, pre-ejection period. (From Silverman NH, Schmidt KG: *The current role of Doppler echocardiography in the diagnosis of congenital heart disease. Cardiol Clin* 1989;7:265-297.)

shown to correlate with other measures of left ventricular systolic function. Previous studies showed that left ventricular ejection force correlated better than peak aortic velocity and peak aortic acceleration time with invasive angiographically-derived LVEF in patients with heart failure.[22,23] Serial changes in peak aortic acceleration time also have shown promise in revealing the extent and rate of recovery of left ventricular systolic function in patients after an acute myocardial infarction and were predictive of the development of congestive heart failure in these patients.[24] In patients with dilated cardiomyopathy, peak aortic Doppler velocity, aortic time velocity integral, and aortic acceleration time all have been shown to be decreased compared with normal controls.[25] Aortic time intervals and Doppler peak velocities are affected, however, by heart rate and loading conditions; studies have documented decreased peak aortic acceleration time and peak aortic velocity with increased heart rate and increased afterload.[26,27]

Mitral regurgitation (MR) is a common finding in patients with heart failure; if MR is present, the peak and mean rate of change in left ventricular systolic pressure can be derived from the ascending portion of the continuous-wave **MR velocity curve** signal (Fig. 10-3).[28] Using the simplified Bernoulli equation, two velocity points along the MR Doppler envelope during the isovolumic contraction period are selected from which a corresponding left ventricular pressure change (rate of pressure rise) can be derived. This change in left ventricular pressure can be divided by the change in time between the two Doppler velocities (1 m/sec and 3 m/sec) to derive the left ventricular dP/dt (so that left ventricular dP/dt = [4 × 3² − 4 × 1²]/time in seconds or 32 mm Hg/time in seconds). Normal mean dP/dt is greater than 1200 mm Hg/sec.

Although more time-consuming to perform, the MR velocity curve and the calculated peak dP/dt correlate accurately with invasive cardiac catheterization measurements.[29] To ascertain peak left ventricular dP/dt noninvasively, the MR signal is digitized to obtain the first derivative of the pressure gradient curve.[30] Similar to other ejection phase indices, left ventricular dP/dt is affected by changes in loading conditions, most notably by increased afterload.

Stress-Velocity Index

There are considerable limitations to the Doppler-derived ejection indices in estimating myocardial performance. Possible sources of error include equating the anatomic area with area of flow, circular or elliptical cross-section models, temporal constancy of the areas and the velocities, and lack of correction for angular deviations.[31]

The rate of left ventricular fiber shortening (average rate of change of the left ventricular circumference in diameters per second) can be assessed noninvasively by M-mode echocardiography. This measurement,

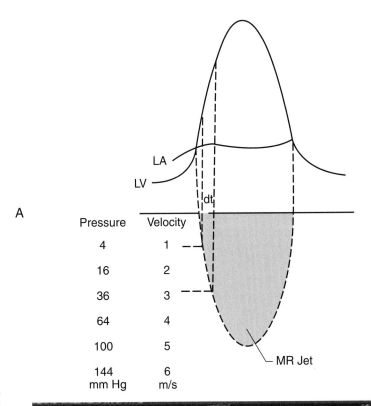

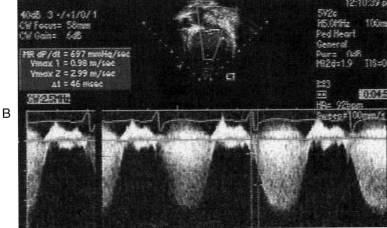

FIGURE 10-3 ■ **Mitral regurgitation curve in assessment of left ventricular systolic function. A,** Calculation of left ventricular pressure over time (dP/dt). The diagram shows the mitral regurgitation (MR) jet and the pressure curves from the left ventricle (LV) and the left atrium (LA) above it. Using the modified Bernoulli equation, the left ventricular dP/dt is the change in left ventricular pressure measured from 1 m/sec to 3 m/sec divided by the change in time between these two left ventricular pressure points: left ventricular dP/dt = (36 mm Hg − 4 mm Hg)/D time in seconds. **B,** Measurement of left ventricular dP/dt in a patient with Duchenne muscular dystrophy. Using the modified Bernoulli equation, the LV dP/dt is the change in left ventricular pressure measured from 1 m/sec to 3 m/sec divided by the change in time between these two left ventricular pressure points: LV dP/dt = (36 mm Hg − 4 mm Hg)/0.046 sec = 697 mm Hg/sec. (**A** from Oh JK, Seward JB, Tajik AJ, et al: *Assessment of ventricular function.* In: *The Echo Manual.* Boston, Little, Brown, 1994, p 63.)

termed the mean **velocity of circumferential fiber shortening (Vcf)**, is normalized for LVEDD and can be obtained from the following equation:

$$Vcf = \frac{[LVEDD - LVESD]}{[LVEDD \times LVET]}$$

where *LVET* is the left ventricular ejection time. It can be simplified to:

$$Vcf = \frac{SF}{LVET}$$

Reported normal values for mean Vcf are 1.5 ± 0.04 circumferences/sec for neonates and 1.3 ± 0.03 circumferences/sec for children 2 to 10 years old.[32,33]

To normalize Vcf for variation in heart rate, LVET is divided by the square root of the R-R interval to derive a rate-corrected mean velocity of circumferential fiber shortening (Vcf$_c$). Normal Vcf$_c$ has been reported to be 1.28 ± 0.22 circumferences/sec in neonates and 1.08 ± 0.14 circumferences/sec in children.[34] Because Vcf$_c$ values are corrected for heart rate, a significant decrease in Vcf$_c$ between neonates and children has been attributed to increased systemic afterload with advancing age. Shortening fraction alone may underestimate ventricular function in newborns. In patients with congenital heart lesions resulting in left ventricular volume overload, mean Vcf$_c$ has been shown to increase, most likely secondary to increased LVEDD and augmented left ventricular contractility with increased left ventricular preload. In contrast, patients with dilated cardiomyopathy with decreased left ventricular systolic function have been reported to have significantly decreased Vcf_c.

Most ejection phase indices, including shortening fraction, ejection fraction, and Vcf_c, depend on the underlying loading state of the left ventricle. Colan and colleagues[35] previously described a **stress-velocity index**, which is an inverse linear relationship between Vcf_c and **end-systolic wall stress** (which most accurately measures left ventricular afterload). The stress-velocity index, in contrast to shortening and ejection fractions or Doppler-derived blood flow velocities, is independent of preload, is normalized for heart rate, and incorporates afterload, resulting in a noninvasive measure of left ventricular contractility that is independent of ventricular loading conditions (Fig. 10-4). Because contractility is the intrinsic ability of the myofibers to generate force, this stress-velocity index can differentiate states of increased ventricular afterload from decreased myocardial contractility. The stress-velocity index has shown significant increases in left ventricular afterload with concomitant decreases in myocardial contractility in patients receiving doxorubicin for treatment of childhood leukemia.[36] More recently, this index has shown improved left ventricular contractility and decreased end-systolic wall stress with amrinone infusion in neonates with postoperative congestive heart failure.[37]

Although this method is theoretically sound and scientifically valid, it is more tedious to perform compared with other methods because the ejection time needs to be obtained from an indirect carotid or brachial artery pulse tracing.[38] In addition, its interpretation needs to take age into account (because the neonatal myocardium exhibits a higher basal contractile state and a greater sensitivity to changes in afterload).[39]

Doppler Tissue Imaging and Strain Rate Imaging

Quantitative assessment of regional left ventricular function has centered on evaluation of segmental endocardial excursion and left ventricular wall thickening.[40] These semiquantitative methods often fail to discriminate between active and passive myocardial motion. Newer echocardiographic modalities, such as Doppler tissue imaging[41-43] and strain rate imaging,[44] offer a potentially more quantitative and accurate approach to the assessment of regional myocardial contraction and relaxation and can correlate with myocardial performance.

Doppler Tissue Imaging (DTI) is a relatively novel method of assessing quantitative longitudinal and radial ventricular function by measuring pulse-wave Doppler velocities directly from underlying myocardium. The systolic velocity (S) is always positive and starts with the first heart sound but ends before the second heart sound. The velocities are heterogeneous depending on ventricular wall and position. The diastolic filling waves consist of the early and late myocardiol motion. Finally, there also are isovolumic Doppler signals that are low velocity biphasic waves during isovolumic contraction and relaxation. Doppler tissue velocities are influenced by sample location because velocities tend to be higher in lateral left ventricular wall and at the base (compared with the apex).

In assessing systolic function, an increase in inotropic state increases DTI velocities, whereas impaired systolic function is manifested by decreased DTI velocities. The rate of annular descent of the atrioventricular valve and the degree of long axis ventricular shortening have been shown to be sensitive echocardiographic indices of ventricular function.[45-49] Studies have shown significant changes in mitral annular DTI velocities in adult patients with left ventricular dysfunction and elevated left ventricular filling pressures.[50-52] Changes in these left ventricular wall motion velocities occur with heart rate and age in the pediatric population.[53]

The deformation or strain of a myocardial tissue segment occurs over the cardiac cycle, and the rate of this deformation is termed the *strain rate*. **Strain rate imaging** is a new echocardiographic technique used to measure regional elongation and shortening of myocardial tissue segments (Fig. 10-5).[54] Preliminary studies have shown regional differences in strain rate in adults after myocardial infarction. Measurements of radial and longitudinal strain rate have been reported in healthy children.[55] In addition, quantification of regional right and left ventricular function by ultrasonic strain rate and strain indices after surgical repair of tetralogy of Fallot in children showed that right ventricular deformation abnormalities are associated with electrical depolarization

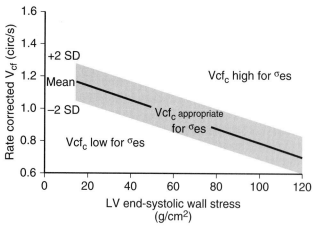

FIGURE 10-4 ■ Stress-velocity index in assessment of left ventricular (LV) systolic function. Graphic representation of the relationship between the mean rate-corrected velocity of circumferential LV fiber shortening (Vcf_c) and the LV end-systolic wall stress (σes). To normalize Vcf for variation in heart rate, it is divided by the square root of the R-R interval to derive a rate-corrected mean velocity of circumferential fiber shortening (Vcf_c). Values above the upper limit of the mean relationship line imply an increased inotropic state, and values below the limit imply a depressed inotropic state. (From Colan SD, Borow KM, Neumann A, et al: *Left ventricular end-systolic wall stress-velocity of fiber shortening relation: A load independent index of myocardial contractility. J Am Coll Cardiol* 1984;4:715-724.)

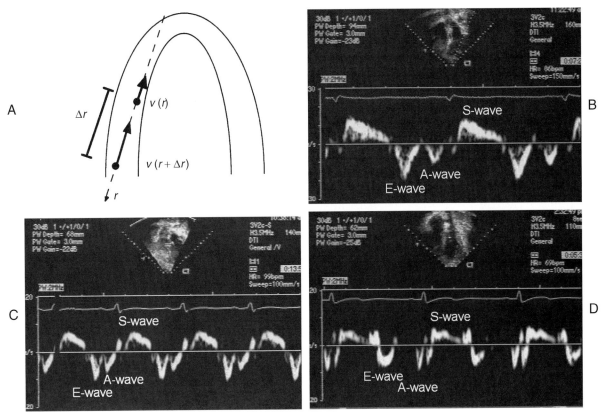

FIGURE 10-5 ■ Doppler tissue imaging for assessment of left ventricular diastolic function. **A,** Diagram depicts estimation of strain rate of tissue segment Δr from tissue velocity. The *r* is the position along the ultrasound beam axis, and the dashed line indicates one of the ultrasound beams. **B** and **C,** Normal mitral annular **(B)** and septal **(C)** Doppler tissue imaging pattern. Note the characteristic normal pattern of a larger early diastolic velocity (E wave) compared with late diastolic velocity (A wave). The S wave is the systolic wave. **D,** Abnormal mitral annular Doppler tissue imaging pattern in a patient with Duchenne muscular dystrophy. Note the reduced early diastolic velocity (E wave) compared with the late diastolic velocity (A wave). (**A** from Heimdal A, Stoylen A, Torp H, et al: *Real-time strain rate imaging of the left ventricle by ultrasound. J Am Soc Echocardiogr* 1998;11:1013-1019.)

abnormalities.[56] Further studies are needed to identify potential applications of strain rate imaging in the regional assessment of myocardial function of right and left ventricles in children with heart failure.

ECHOCARDIOGRAPHIC ASSESSMENT OF LEFT VENTRICULAR DIASTOLIC FUNCTION

Because diastolic dysfunction often precedes systolic dysfunction, careful quantitative assessment of left ventricular diastolic function is mandatory in the noninvasive diagnosis and serial evaluation of patients with heart failure. Left ventricular diastolic dysfunction is associated with abnormalities of ventricular compliance and relaxation and can be shown by characteristic changes in mitral inflow and pulmonary venous Doppler flow patterns and newer modalities, including DTI and color Doppler flow propagation velocity.[57-65]

Inherent limitations exist with these methods, which continue to be refined and studied to yield the most accurate evaluation of diastolic function.

Doppler-Derived Indices
Mitral inflow Doppler, obtained from the apical four-chamber view by positioning a pulsed-wave Doppler sample at the leaflet tips of the mitral valve (to obtain signals for maximal transvalvar velocity), represents the diastolic pressure gradient between the left atrium and left ventricle. Doppler indices include peak filling velocities, acceleration and deceleration rates and times, velocity ratios, and areas under the diastolic filling curve.

The early phase of diastole is based on active **LV** relaxation. The **early diastolic filling wave**, or **E wave**, is the dominant diastolic wave and represents the peak pressure gradient between the left atrium and left ventricle at the onset of diastole. This E wave portion of the diastolic curve is usually 65% ± 4% of the total area of the diastolic curve but is less in disease states that lead to left ventricular noncompliance.[66] The deceleration time of the mitral E wave reflects the time needed for equalization of pressures in the left atrium and left ventricle. The late phase of diastole is the passive **LV** filling phase. The **late diastolic filling wave,** or **A wave**, represents the peak pressure gradient between the left atrium and left ventricle in late diastole at the onset of atrial contraction.

Normal mitral inflow Doppler is characterized by a dominant E wave, a smaller A wave, and a ratio of E and A waves (E:A ratio) between 1 and 3 (Fig. 10-6). Normal duration of mitral deceleration time and isovolumic relaxation time (IVRT) vary with age and have been reported in pediatric and adult populations.[67-69] For assessment of diastolic function, mitral inflow Doppler velocities are affected not only by changes in relaxation

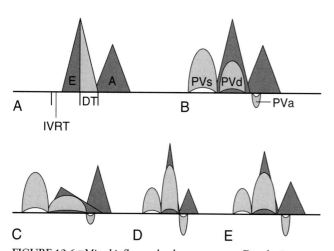

FIGURE 10-6 ■ **Mitral inflow and pulmonary venous Doppler in assessment of left ventricular diastolic function.** Mitral inflow Doppler patterns with pulmonary venous Doppler patterns superimposed. **A,** Mitral inflow pattern alone in a normal subject. E, early flow velocity; A, atrial contraction–related flow velocity; IVRT, isovolumetric relaxation time; DT, deceleration time (peak E wave flow velocity to 0). **B,** The pulmonary venous Doppler flow is now superimposed onto the normal subject's mitral inflow Doppler flow velocities. During atrial contraction, there is retrograde flow. PVs, pulmonary venous flow during systole; PVd, pulmonary venous flow during diastole; PVa, pulmonary venous flow during atrial contraction. **C,** In a subject with an abnormal LV relaxation, there is a diminution of the E/A ratio in the mitral inflow Doppler pattern. The pulmonary venous flow pattern in the same patient exhibits a decrease in the PVd (diastolic) component. **D,** This subject has decreased ventricular compliance and high atrial pressure. There is an exaggerated E/A ratio with a shorter DT than normal as seen in **A**. The pulmonary venous flow pattern is altered with a predominant PVd (diastolic component) and a much smaller PVs (systolic component). The PVa (atrial contraction) component also increases. **E,** "Pseudonormalization" of the mitral inflow Doppler pattern. The mitral inflow pattern is between the situations in **C** and **D** and appears to be normal. The pulmonary venous Doppler pattern remains abnormal, however, with a predominant PVd (diastolic) and a smaller PVs (systolic) component and a relatively larger pulmonary vein retrograde flow in atrial systole (PVa). The mitral inflow Doppler, when used in conjunction with pulmonary venous Doppler, avoids a pseudonormalized mitral inflow pattern being falsely interpreted as "normal." (From Armstrong WF: *Echocardiography.* In Braunwald E, et al: *Heart Disease.* Philadelphia, WB Saunders, 2001, p 175.)

and compliance components of diastolic LV function, but also by a variety of additional anatomic and physiologic factors, including loading conditions, contractility, heart rate, interventricular interaction, valve mobility, respiratory phase, and age.[70] Interpretation of characteristic patterns of mitral inflow must be evaluated carefully with particular attention given to the potential impact of each of these factors on mitral inflow Doppler velocities.

Diastolic dysfunction is manifested by characteristic mitral inflow Doppler patterns. The earliest stage of left ventricular diastolic dysfunction shown by mitral inflow Doppler is **abnormal relaxation** (see Fig. 10-6C). Factors that affect relaxation include loading conditions, contractile state, elastic recoil properties of the ventricle, age, hypertrophied ventricles, myocardial ischemia, and infiltrative cardiomyopathy with normal atrial pressure. Abnormal relaxation is characterized by a reduced E wave velocity, increased A wave velocity, reversed E:A ratio (<1), and a prolonged mitral deceleration time and IVRT.

As diastolic dysfunction progresses, further changes in ventricular relaxation and compliance occur leading to an increase in left atrial pressure. Factors that affect compliance include myocardial properties, interventricular interaction, and ventricular geometry. Increased left atrial pressure normalizes the initial transmitral gradient between the left atrium and left ventricle, producing a transitional **"pseudonormalized" mitral inflow** Doppler pattern with increased E wave velocity and E:A ratio and normalized mitral deceleration and IVRT intervals (see Fig. 10-6E). The pathophysiology is abrupt cessation of early filling as the left ventricular diastolic pressure is increased. This pseudonormal Doppler pattern may be difficult to distinguish from normal mitral inflow Doppler; additional evaluation of pulmonary venous inflow Doppler can be complementary in helping to unmask this advanced degree of left ventricular diastolic dysfunction because the pulmonary venous pattern is abnormal (i.e., forward flow in systole is decreased, forward flow in diastole is increased, and atrial diastolic reversal is more significant and prolonged).

Further deterioration of left ventricular diastolic function results in **restrictive ventricular filling** with an additional increase in left atrial pressure and a concomitant decrease in ventricular compliance. The Doppler pattern of restrictive left ventricular filling is characterized by additional increases in E wave velocity, reduction in A wave velocity, an increased E:A ratio greater than 3, and significant shortening of mitral deceleration time and IVRT (see Fig. 10-6D).

Adult studies have shown that heart failure patients with altered mitral inflow Doppler, and most importantly a restrictive filling pattern, have significantly increased morbidity and mortality.[71,72] Reversal of this restrictive filling pattern with medical therapy to a pattern characteristic of either abnormal relaxation or pseudonormalization has correlated with improved long-term survival in adult heart failure patients.[73]

Pulmonary venous Doppler, combined with mitral inflow Doppler, provides a more comprehensive assessment of left atrial and left ventricular filling pressures.[74-77] Pulmonary venous inflow consists of three distinct Doppler waves: a systolic wave (S wave), a diastolic wave (D wave), and a reversal wave with atrial contraction (Ar wave). In normal adolescents and adults, the characteristic pattern of pulmonary venous inflow consists of a dominant S wave, a smaller D wave, and a small Ar wave of low velocity and brief duration. In neonates and younger children, a dominant D wave is often present with a similar brief low velocity, or even absent, Ar wave.

With worsening left ventricular diastolic dysfunction, left atrial pressure increases, leading to diminished systolic forward flow into the left atrium from the pulmonary veins with relatively increased diastolic forward flow resulting in a diastolic dominance of pulmonary venous inflow. More importantly, the velocity and duration of the pulmonary venous Ar wave are increased. Pediatric and adult studies have shown that an Ar wave duration greater than 30 msec longer than the corresponding mitral A wave duration or a ratio of pulmonary venous Ar wave to mitral A wave duration greater than 1.2 is predictive of elevated left ventricular filling pressure.[78,79] Mitral inflow and pulmonary venous Doppler studies have many pitfalls, and assessment of diastolic function based on this method should be interpreted with caution.

Other methods to evaluate LV diastolic function are being investigated. Studies show that with impaired ventricular relaxation, early diastolic DTI velocity (early filling wave) at the lateral mitral annulus decreases. With increasing diastolic dysfunction, left atrial and left ventricular filling pressures increase, leading to an increased mitral E wave velocity; however, these same changes have been shown to have little impact on DTI E wave velocity at the mitral annulus. DTI velocities also have been shown to be less significantly affected by changes in ventricular filling pressure and loading conditions compared with mitral inflow Doppler velocities.[80-82] Although mitral E wave velocity alone is less reliable as an index of abnormal diastolic function, a ratio of mitral E wave to DTI E wave velocity greater than 15 has been shown to be more predictive of elevated pulmonary capillary wedge pressure. In addition, early diastolic myocardial velocity was found to be the best discriminator between control subjects and patients with diastolic dysfunction.[83] This method to assess diastolic dysfunction needs to take into account that there is substantial heterogeneity in measured velocities within individual myocardial segments consistent with known spatial distribution of myocardial fibers.[84] In addition to DTI, continuous-wave Doppler velocity profile of MR can yield negative left ventricular dP/dt and the time constant of relaxation (τ).[85] Lastly, pulsed Doppler detection of abnormal left ventricular posterior wall diastolic motion dynamics (by placing the sample volume apical to mitral valve sulcus and within the left ventricular endocardium) also can gain insight into global left ventricular diastolic performance.[86]

Color M-Mode Flow Propagation Velocity

Color M-mode Doppler echocardiography has been shown to provide information about diastolic function by measurement of sequential mitral inflow filling waves during propagation from base to apex.[87] Specifically, flow propagation velocity of early transmitral flow from color M-mode recordings inversely correlated with the time constant of relaxation τ (Fig. 10-7).[88] As opposed to mitral inflow Doppler, this propagation velocity has been shown to be significantly less affected by changes in heart rate, left atrial pressure, and loading conditions and may reflect more accurately changes in myocardial relaxation. Numerous studies have shown a significant decrease in flow propagation velocity in patients with diastolic dysfunction of varying etiology. In addition, the ratio of the mitral annular Doppler tissue E-wave velocity to flow propagation velocity has been shown to be a significant predictor of congestive heart failure and outcome in patients after myocardial infarction.[89] This ratio of flow propagation and DTI velocity also may be helpful in distinguishing a normal mitral inflow pattern from one of pseudonormalized mitral inflow.

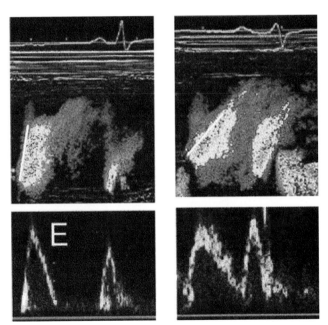

FIGURE 10-7 ■ **Flow propagation velocity (Vp) in assessment of left ventricular diastolic function.** The slope *(yellow line)* of the isovelocity line (from mitral plane to 4 cm apically into the left ventricle) determines Vp. *Top left,* Normal subject. *Top right,* Patient with decreased compliance manifested by decreased slope. *Bottom left and right,* Pulsed-wave Doppler of transmitral flow of these patients. (From Moller JE, Sondergaard E, Seward JB, et al: *Ratio of left ventricular peak E-wave velocity to flow propagation velocity assessed by color M-mode Doppler echocardiography in first myocardial infarction: Prognostic and clinical implications. J Am Coll Cardiol* 2000;35: 363-370.) (See also Color Section.)

ECHOCARDIOGRAPHIC ASSESSMENT OF LEFT VENTRICULAR DYSFUNCTION

Systolic and diastolic dysfunction often can coexist, so a combined measure of left ventricular chamber performance is even more reflective of overall ventricular dysfunction. The **myocardial performance index (MPI)** is a Doppler-derived quantitative measure of global ventricular function that incorporates systolic and diastolic time intervals (Fig. 10-8). This index measures the ratio of total time spent in isovolumic activity divided by the time spent in ventricular ejection. The MPI is defined as the sum of isovolumic contraction time (ICT) and IRT divided by ejection time (ET):

$$MPI = \frac{(ICT + IRT)}{ET}$$

The components of this index are measured from routine pulsed-wave Doppler signals at the atrioventricular valve and ventricular outflow tract of either the left or the right ventricle. To derive the sum of isovolumic contraction time and IRT, the Doppler-derived ejection time for either ventricle is subtracted from the Doppler interval between cessation and onset of the respective atrioventricular valve inflow signal (from the end of the Doppler A wave to the beginning of the Doppler E wave of the next cardiac cycle). The Doppler time intervals should be obtained as close to simultaneous as possible, and consecutive Doppler intervals should not vary by more than 5 to 15 msec. Arrhythmias may render the measurements less accurate.

A recent validation study showed that the MPI (and especially the ratio of shortening fraction to MPI) closely correlate with LV dP/dt over a range of hemodynamic conditions in animal models.[90] Increasing values of the MPI have been shown to correlate with increasing degrees of global ventricular dysfunction. Adult and pediatric studies have established normal values for the MPI. In adults, normal left ventricular and right ventricular MPI values are 0.39 ± 0.05 and 0.28 ± 0.04, whereas in children, similar values for the left ventricle and right ventricle are reported to be 0.35 ± 0.03 and 0.32 ± 0.03.[91] This index is relatively independent of changes in preload and afterload and heart rate, making it particularly appealing in the pediatric population.

Adult studies also have shown the MPI to be a sensitive predictor of outcome in patients with heart failure.[92,93] A simultaneous comparative study showed that correlation between MPI and invasively measured peak +dP/dt during cardiac catheterization was high with $r = 0.82$.[94] The MPI, because it incorporates measures of systolic and diastolic performance, may be a more sensitive early measure of ventricular dysfunction in the absence of other overt changes in isolated systolic or diastolic echocardiographic indices. In addition, because the MPI is a Doppler-derived index, it has been reported to be applied easily to the quantitative assessment of left ventricular and right ventricular function and complex ventricular geometries found in patients with congenital heart disease.

ECHOCARDIOGRAPHIC ASSESSMENT OF RIGHT VENTRICULAR FUNCTION

Echocardiographic functional assessment of a morphologic right ventricle is important for several pediatric patient populations, including patients with (1) transposition of the great arteries who had an atrial switch (Senning or Mustard), (2) tetralogy of Fallot who have pulmonary insufficiency, and (3) single ventricle anatomy of right ventricular morphology. Overall, echocardiographic assessment of right ventricular function has been limited because of the asymmetric and crescentic geometric shape of the right ventricle. Doppler echocardiography historically has been useful in the noninvasive prediction of right ventricular systolic and pulmonary artery pressures.[95] Quantitation of right ventricular systolic function by M-mode or two-dimensional echocardiography has relied, however, on the visual assessment of relative right ventricular wall motion or semiquantitative measurement of fractional area change in right ventricular dimension or volume.[96,97] Newer echocardiographic modalities that have shown promise in quantifying right ventricular function include additional Doppler measures of right ventricular performance (MPI, right ventricular dP/dt, and DTI) and acoustic quantification and three-dimensional echocardiography.

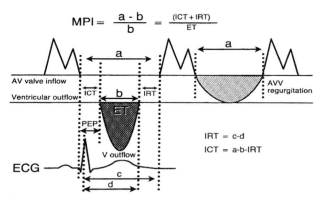

FIGURE 10-8 ■ Myocardial performance index (MPI) for assessment of left ventricular global function. MPI represents the ratio of isovolumic contraction time (ICT) and isovolumic relaxation time (IRT) to ventricular ejection time (ET): MPI = (ICT + IRT)/ET. The duration of ICT + IRT is measured from the cessation of atrioventricular valve (AVV) inflow to the onset of AVV inflow of the next cardiac cycle (interval a). ET is measured from the onset to cessation of ventricular ejection (interval b). MPI = (a − b)/b. Isovolumic time intervals can be measured independently with additional measurements depicted in the diagram. PEP, pre-ejection period. (From Eidem BW, O'Leary PW, Cetta F, et al: *Nongeometric quantitative assessment of right and left ventricular function: Myocardial performance index in normal children and patients with Ebstein anomaly. J Am Soc Echocardiogr* 1998;11:849-856.)

As described previously, the MPI is a Doppler-derived measure of global ventricular function that can be applied to any ventricular geometry. Studies have validated the ability of the **right ventricular MPI** to assess right ventricular function quantitatively in adults and in patients with congenital heart disease. In addition, the MPI has shown prognostic power in discriminating outcome in patients with either right ventricular or left ventricular failure.[98,99] In patients with congenital heart disease with altered right ventricular preload or afterload, the right ventricular MPI has been shown to be relatively independent of changes in loading conditions, making it particularly appealing in this subset of patients.[18] Increasing right ventricular dysfunction is associated with increasing (abnormal) values of right ventricular MPI.

Similar to using MR for calculation of left ventricular dP/dt, the **right ventricular dP/dt**, or the rate of right ventricular pressure change over time, also can be used as a measure of right ventricular systolic function in patients with tricuspid regurgitation. The change in right ventricular pressure can be divided by the change in time between the two Doppler velocities (1 m/sec and 2 m/sec) to derive the right ventricular dP/dt (so that right ventricular dP/dt = $(4 \times 2^2 - 4 \times 1^2)$/time in seconds or 12 mm Hg/time in seconds) (2 m/sec is used as the second Doppler velocity rather than 3 m/sec as with the left ventricular dP/dt). Right ventricular dP/dt has been shown to correlate with invasive measures of right ventricular performance[100] and to be helpful in the serial assessment of right ventricular function in children with hypoplastic left heart syndrome.[101]

A relatively new addition to the quantitative evaluation of right ventricular function is **DTI**. Tricuspid annular motion has been shown to correlate with right ventricular function in previous studies.[102-106] DTI has been shown to be a reproducible noninvasive method of assessing systolic and diastolic annular motion and right ventricular function (Fig. 10-9).[107-110] In contrast to conventional Doppler inflow velocities, preliminary studies in adults and children with DTI have shown these velocities to be relatively independent of loading conditions.[111,112] Comparative measurements of annular versus inflow velocities reveal that the ratio of late-to-early diastolic tricuspid annular velocity showed a higher correlation with right ventricular end-diastolic pressure.[113]

Acoustic quantification uses automated border detection techniques to measure the absolute change and rate of change in right ventricular volume. This modality has been shown to correlate with other invasive methods of right ventricular functional assessment in adults with abnormalities of global right ventricular function.[114,115] Automated border methods also have shown good correlation with MRI in assessing changes in right ventricular volume and systolic function.[116] Feasibility of acoustic quantification in the noninvasive evaluation of right ventricular function in normal children also has been reported.[117] Ongoing investigation is needed to establish the potential of this technique for the identification and serial evaluation of right ventricular dysfunction in children with heart failure.

The advent of **three-dimensional echocardiography** has enabled noninvasive evaluation of right ventricular volume and function. Because three-dimensional echocardiography can evaluate right ventricular geometry in multiple spatial planes, accurate assessment of changes in right ventricular volume during the cardiac cycle are possible.[118-120] Such data collection needs to be rapid, efficient, and automated with minimal motion effects. Application of this new modality to the evaluation of right ventricular systolic failure in adults and children has not yet been reported, but seems to be promising.

ECHOCARDIOGRAPHIC ASSESSMENT OF SINGLE VENTRICULAR FUNCTION

Quantitative measurement of ventricular function in patients with functional single ventricles can be challenging. In most cases, a visual qualitative estimate of systolic function from two-dimensional images is used. Quantitative echocardiographic assessment is limited by complex ventricular geometry often with associated abnormalities of wall motion. Similar to novel techniques used to assess right ventricular function, Doppler echocardiography holds promise in the potential evaluation of global single ventricle function. Only limited studies to date have addressed either dP/dt or the MPI in patients with functional single ventricles.[121] One study showed improved function after cavopulmonary anastomosis in patients with single ventricles when the operation is performed at younger than 1 year of age when using MPI as a measurement of ventricular function.[122] Although there is a paucity of data on these new Doppler indices to predict outcome in patients with complex single ventricle anatomy, early studies show feasibility

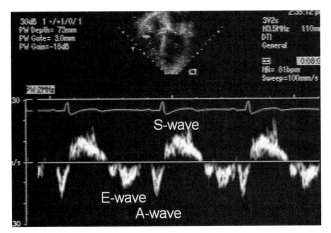

FIGURE 10-9 ■ **Doppler tissue imaging for assessment of right ventricular diastolic function.** Abnormal tricuspid annular Doppler tissue imaging pattern in a patient with Duchenne muscular dystrophy. Note the reduced early diastolic velocity (E wave) compared with the late diastolic velocity (A wave) consistent with abnormal right ventricular function.

of Doppler-derived indices for assessment of single ventricle function (See Chapter 23).

CURRENT STATUS AND FUTURE TRENDS

Assessment of ventricular function using methods of measuring changes in area or volume and Doppler-derived indices have limitations. Although the stress-velocity index is corrected for loading conditions and heart rate, it is cumbersome to perform, especially in the intensive care setting. The Doppler-derived index of combined systolic and diastolic myocardial performance, the MPI, has been shown to be a practical method to assess global ventricular function in children, even with morphologic right ventricles and single ventricles. Additional work using existing technology needs to be completed to validate methods to assess heart failure in children. In addition, few data are available on myocardial function assessment in critically ill children, and more research should be focused on heart failure in the intensive care setting.[123]

Three-dimensional echocardiography holds promise in the nongeometric assessment of ventricular volume and function, but has yet to be evaluated clinically in patients with or without evidence of heart failure. Flow propagation velocity techniques assessed by color M-mode Doppler also can be a strong predictor of heart failure.[124] Finally, it is crucial to use innovative methods, such as tissue velocity imaging, strain rate imaging, and ultrasonic myocardial tissue characterization, to detect myocardial abnormalities before evidence for impaired myocardial contractility and abnormal diastolic function and even early regional myocardial wall motion abnormalities.[125-128]

Key Concepts

■ Although Doppler ultrasound is the mainstay of diagnostic examinations for assessing ventricular function and myocardial performance, a preliminary thorough two-dimensional examination with color Doppler interrogation is essential to assess congenital cardiac anatomy and to evaluate postoperative residua.

■ Because systolic dysfunction is often preceded by diastolic dysfunction, quantitative assessment of diastolic function may be predictive of eventual systolic dysfunction in these patients.

■ The progression of findings in regurgitant lesions before heart failure is usually an increase in end-diastolic dimension, followed by an increase in end-systolic dimension and finally a decrease in shortening fraction as the heart decompensates and fails.

■ Echocardiographic measures of left ventricular systolic function include M-mode and two-dimensional examinations for dimension and volume changes and Doppler-derived ejection indices of ventricular performance. Quantitation of blood flow, such as cardiac output and stroke volume generally has not been used, however, for assessment of cardiac performance because cardiac output can be preserved until myocardial dysfunction is severe.

■ The emergence of Doppler-derived measures of ventricular performance has circumvented many of the geometric challenges inherent in the global assessment of ventricular performance, especially in the evaluation of right ventricular performance and quantitative assessment of systolic function in patients with complex ventricular morphologies.

■ The stress-velocity index, in contrast to shortening/ejection fractions or Doppler-derived blood flow velocities, is independent of preload, is normalized for heart rate, and incorporates afterload, resulting in a noninvasive measure of left ventricular contractility that is independent of ventricular loading conditions.

■ Left ventricular diastolic dysfunction is associated with abnormalities of ventricular compliance and relaxation and can be shown by characteristic changes in mitral inflow and pulmonary venous Doppler flow patterns and newer modalities, including DTI and color Doppler flow propagation velocity.

■ The MPI is a Doppler-derived quantitative measure of global ventricular function that incorporates systolic and diastolic time intervals.

■ The MPI, because it incorporates measures of systolic and diastolic performance, may be a more sensitive early measure of ventricular dysfunction in the absence of other overt changes in isolated systolic or diastolic echocardiographic indices. In addition, because the MPI is a Doppler-derived index, it has been reported to be applied easily to the quantitative assessment of left ventricular and right ventricular function and complex ventricular geometries found in patients with congenital heart disease.

REFERENCES

1. Henry WL, Gardin JM, Ware JH: Echocardiographic measurements in normal subjects from infancy to old age. Circulation 1980;62:1054-1061.

2. De Wolf D, Matthys D, Verhaaren H, et al: Influence of age and low afterload on the stress-velocity relation of the left ventricle. Pediatr Res 1998; 4:600-606.

3. Fraisse A, Colan SD, Jonas RA, et al: Accuracy of echocardiography for detection of aortic arch obstruction after stage I Norwood procedure. Am Heart J 1998;135:230-236.

4. Cintron C, Johnson G, Francis G, et al: Prognostic significance of serial changes in left ventricular ejection fraction in patients with congestive heart failure. Circulation 1993;87:17-23.

5. Cohn JN, Johnson GR, Shabetai R, et al: Ejection fraction, peak exercise oxygen consumption, cardiothoracic ratio, ventricular arrhythmias, and plasma norepinephrine as determinants of prognosis in heart failure. Circulation 1993;87:5-16.

6. Rihal CS, Nishimura RA, Hatle LK, et al: Systolic and diastolic dysfunction in patients with clinical diagnosis of dilated cardiomyopathy: Relation to symptoms and prognosis. Circulation 1994;90:2772-2779.

7. Vasan RS, Larson MG, Benjamin EJ, et al: Congestive heart failure in subjects with normal versus reduced left ventricular ejection fraction: Prevalence and mortality in a population-based cohort. J Am Coll Cardiol 1999;33:1948-1955.

8. Corti R, Binggeli C, Turina M, et al: Predictors of long-term survival after valve replacement for chronic aortic regurgitation: Is M-mode echocardiography sufficient? Eur Heart J 2001;22:866-873.

9. Rubay JE, Shango P, Clement S, et al: Ross procedure in congenital patients: Results and left ventricular function. Eur J Cardiothorac Surg 1997;11:92-99.

10. Jindal RC, Saxena A, Kothari SS, et al: Congenital severe aortic stenosis with congestive heart failure in late childhood and adolescence: Effect on left ventricular function after balloon valvuloplasty. Cathet Cardiovasc Interv 2000;51:168-172.

11. Schiller NB, Shah PM, Crawford M, et al: Recommendation for quantitation of the left ventricle by two-dimensional echocardiography. J Am Soc Echocardiogr 1989;2:358-367.

12. Quinones MA, Waggoner AD, Reduto LA, et al: A new simplified and accurate method for determining ejection fraction with two-dimensional echocardiography. Circulation 1981;64:744-753.

13. Haendchen RV, Wyatt HL, Maurer G, et al: Quantitation of regional cardiac function by two-dimensional echocardiography: I. Patterns of contraction in the normal left ventricle. Circulation 1983;67:1234-1245.

14. Brutsaert DL, Sonnenblick EH: Cardiac muscle mechanics in the evaluation of myocardial contractility and pump function: Problems, concepts, and directions. Prog Cardiovasc Dis 1973;16:337-361.

15. Tei C: New noninvasive index for combined systolic and diastolic ventricular function. J Cardiol 1995;26:135-136.

16. Tei C, Ling LH, Hodge DO, et al: New index of combined systolic and diastolic myocardial performance: A simple and reproducible measure of cardiac function—a study in normals and dilated cardiomyopathy. J Cardiol 1995;26:357-366.

17. Eidem BW, Tei C, O'Leary PW, Seward JB: Nongeometric quantitative assessment of right and left ventricular function: Myocardial performance index in normal children and patients with Ebstein anomaly. J Am Soc Echocardiogr 1998;11:849-856.

18. Eidem BW, O'Leary PW, Tei C, Seward JB: Usefulness of the myocardial performance index for assessing right ventricular function in congenital heart disease. Am J Cardiol 2000;86:654-658.

19. Isaaz K, Munoz del Romeral L, Lee E, Schiller NB: Quantitation of the motion of the cardiac base in normal subjects by Doppler echocardiography. J Am Soc Echocardiogr 1993;6:166-176.

20. Donovan CL, Armstrong WF, Bach DS: Quantitative Doppler tissue imaging of the left ventricular myocardium: Validation in normal subjects. Am Heart J 1995;130:100-104.

21. Jiang L, Siu SC, Handschumacher S, et al: Three-dimensional echocardiography: In vivo validation for right ventricular volume and function. Circulation 1994;89:2342-2350.

22. Stein PD, Sabbah HN: Ventricular performance measured during ejection: Studies in patients of the rate of change ventricular power. Am Heart J 1976;91:599-606.

23. Isaaz K, Ethevenot G, Admant P, et al: A new Doppler method of assessing left ventricular ejection force in chronic congestive heart failure. Am J Cardiol 1989;64:81-87.

24. Sabbah HN, Gheorghiade M, Smith ST, et al: Rate and extent of recovery of left ventricular function in patients following acute myocardial infarction. Am Heart J 1987;114:516-524.

25. Gardin JM, Iseri LT, Elkayam U, et al: Evaluation of dilated cardiomyopathy by pulsed Doppler echocardiography. Am Heart J 1983;106:1057-1065.

26. Harrison MR, Clifton GD, Sublett KL, et al: Effect of heart rate on Doppler indices of systolic function in humans. J Am Coll Cardiol 1989;14:929-935.

27. Harrison MR, Clifton GD, Berk MR, et al: Effect of blood pressure and afterload on Doppler echocardiographic measurements of left ventricular systolic function in normal subjects. Am J Cardiol 1989;64:905-908.

28. Bargiggia GS, Bertucci C, Recusani F, et al: A new method for estimating left ventricular dP/dt by continuous wave Doppler-echocardiography. Circulation 1989;80:1287-1292.

29. Chung N, Nishimura RA, Holmes DR Jr, et al: Measurement of left ventricular dp/dt by simultaneous Doppler echocardiography and cardiac catheterization. J Am Soc Echocardiogr 1992;5:147-152.

30. Chen C, Rodriquez L, Guerrero JL, et al: Noninvasive estimation of the instantaneous first derivative of left ventricular pressure using continuous wave Doppler echocardiography. Circulation 1991;83:2101-2110.

31. Zoghbi WA, Quinones MA: Determination of cardiac output by Doppler echocardiography: A critical appraisal. Herz 1986;11:258-268.

32. Sahn DJ, Deely WJ, Hagan AD, et al: Echocardiographic assessment of left ventricular performance in normal newborns. Circulation 1974;49:232-236.

33. Sahn DJ, Vaucher Y, Williams DE, et al: Echocardiographic detection of large left to right shunts and cardiomyopathies in infants and children. Am J Cardiol 1976;38:73-79.

34. Rowland DG, Gutgesell HP: Noninvasive assessment of myocardial contractility, preload, and afterload in healthy newborn infants. Am J Cardiol 1995;75:18-21.

35. Colan SD, Borow KM, Newmann A: Left ventricular end-systolic wall stress-velocity of fiber shortening relation: A load independent index of myocardial contractility. J Am Coll Cardiol 1984;4:715-724.

36. Lipshultz SE, Colan SD, Gelber RD, et al: Late cardiac effects of doxorubicin therapy for acute lymphoblastic leukemia in childhood. N Engl J Med 1991;324:843-845.

37. Teshima H, Tobita K, Yamamura H, et al: Cardiovascular effects of a phosphodiesterase III inhibitor, amrinone, in infants: Non-invasive echocardiographic evaluation. Pediatr Int 2002;44:259-263.

38. Calabro R, Pisacane C, Pacileo G, et al: Left ventricular midwall mechanics in healthy children and adolescents. J Am Soc Echocardiogr 1999;12:932-940.

39. Crepaz R, Pitscheider W, Radetti G, et al: Age-related variation in left ventricular myocardial contractile state expressed by the stress velocity relation. Pediatr Cardiol 1998;19:463-467.

40. Moynihan PF, Parisi AF, Feldman CL: Quantitative detection of regional left ventricular contraction abnormalities by two-dimensional echocardiography: I. Analysis of methods. Circulation 1981;63:752-760.

41. Garcia MJ, Rodriquez L, Ares M, et al: Differentiation of constrictive pericarditis from restrictive cardiomyopathy: Assessment of left ventricular diastolic velocities in longitudinal axis by Doppler tissue imaging. J Am Coll Cardiol 1996;27:108-114.

42. Garcia MJ, Rodriquez L, Ares M, et al: Myocardial wall velocity assessment by pulsed Doppler tissue imaging: Characteristic findings in normal subjects. Am Heart J 1996;132:648-656.

43. Rychik J, Tian ZY: Quantitative assessment of myocardial tissue velocities in normal children with Doppler tissue imaging. Am J Cardiol 1996;77:1254-1257.

44. Voigt JU, Arnold MF, Karlsson M, et al: Assessment of regional longitudinal myocardial strain rate derived from Doppler myocardial imaging indexes in normal and infarcted myocardium. J Am Soc Echocardiogr 2000;13:588-598.

45. Zaky A, Grabhorn L, Feigenbaum H: Movement of the mitral ring: A study in ultrasound cardiography. Cardiovasc Res 1967;1:121-131.

46. Pai RG, Bodenheimer MM, Pai SM, et al: Usefulness of systolic excursion of the mitral annulus as an index of left ventricular systolic function. Am J Cardiol 1990;67:222-224.

47. Alam M, Hoglund C, Thorstrand C: Longitudinal systolic shortening of the left ventricle: An echocardiographic study in subjects with and without preserved global function. Clin Physiol 1992;12:443-452.

48. Simonson JS, Schiller NB: Descent of the base of the left ventricle: An echocardiographic index of left ventricular function. J Am Soc Echocardiogr 1989;2:25-35.

49. Jones CJ, Raposo L, Gibson DG: Functional importance of the long axis dynamics of the human left ventricle. Br Heart J 1990; 63:215-220.

50. Nagueh SF, Middleton KJ, Kopelen HA, et al: Doppler tissue imaging: A noninvasive technique for evaluation of left ventricular relaxation and estimation of filling pressures. J Am Coll Cardiol 1997;30:1527-1533.

51. Oki T, Tabata T, Yamada H, et al: Clinical application of pulsed Doppler tissue imaging for assessing abnormal left ventricular relaxation. Am J Cardiol 1997;79:921-928.

52. Puleo JA, Aranda JM, Weston MW, et al: Noninvasive detection of allograft rejection in heart transplant recipients by use of Doppler tissue imaging. J Heart Lung Transplant 1998;17:176-184.

53. Mori K, Hayabuchi Y, Kuroda Y, et al: Left ventricular wall motion velocities in healthy children measured by pulsed wave Doppler tissue echocardiography: Normal values and relation to age and heart rate. J Am Soc Echocardiogr 2000;13:1002-1011.

54. Heimdal A, Stoylen A, Torp H, et al: Real-time strain rate imaging of the left ventricle by ultrasound. J Am Soc Echocardiogr 1998;11:1013-1019.

55. Weidemann F, Eyskens B, Jamal F, et al: Quantification of regional left and right ventricular radial and longitudinal function in healthy children using ultrasound-based strain rate and strain imaging. J Am Soc Echocardiogr 2002;15:20-28.

56. Weidemann F, Eyskens B, Mertens L, et al: Quantification of regional right and left ventricular function by ultrasonic strain rate and strain indexes after surgical repair of tetralogy of Fallot. Am J Cardiol 2002;90:133-138.

57. Nishimura RA, Abel MB, Hatle LK, et al: Assessment of diastolic function of the heart: Background and current applications of Doppler echocardiography: Part II. Clinical studies. Mayo Clin Proc 1989;64:181-204.

58. Myreng V, Smiseth OA: Assessment of left ventricular relaxation by Doppler echocardiography. Circulation 1990;81:260-266.

59. Appleton CP, Hatle LK, Popp RL: Relation of transmitral flow velocity patterns to left ventricular diastolic function: New insights from a combined hemodynamic and Doppler echocardiographic study. J Am Coll Cardiol 1988;12:426-440.

60. Thomas JD, Weyman AE: Echo Doppler evaluation of left ventricular diastolic function: Physics and physiology. Circulation 1991;84:977-990.

61. Brun P, Tribouilloy C, Duval AM, et al: Left ventricular flow propagation during early filling is related to wall relaxation: A color M-mode Doppler analysis. J Am Coll Cardiol 1992;20:420-432.

62. Garcia MJ, Ares MA, Asher C, et al: Color M-mode flow velocity propagation: An index of early left ventricular filling that combined with pulse Doppler peak E velocity may predict capillary wedge pressure. J Am Coll Cardiol 1997;29:448-454.

63. Takatsuji H, Mikami T, Urasawa K, et al: A new approach for evaluation of left ventricular diastolic function: Spatial and temporal analysis of left ventricular filling flow propagation by color M-mode Doppler echocardiography. J Am Coll Cardiol 1996;27:365-371.

64. Gonzales-Vilchez F, Ares M, Ayuela J, et al: Combined use of pulsed and color M-mode Doppler echocardiography for the estimation of pulmonary capillary wedge pressure: An empirical approach based on an analytical relation. J Am Coll Cardiol 1999;34:515-523.

65. Stugaard M, Brodahl U, Torp H, et al: Abnormalities of left ventricular filling in patients with coronary artery disease: Assessment by colour Doppler technique. Eur Heart J 1994;15:318-327.

66. Snider AR, Gidding SS, Rocchini AP, et al: Doppler evaluation of left ventricular diastolic filling in children with systemic hypertension. Am J Cardiol 1985;56:921-926.

67. Bryg RJ, Williams GA, Labvitz AJ: Effect of aging on left ventricular diastolic filling in normal subjects. Am J Cardiol 1987;59:971-974.

68. Bessen M, Gardin JM: Evaluation of left ventricular diastolic function. Cardiol Clin 1990;8:315-332.

69. O'Leary PW, Durongpisitkul K, Cordes TM, et al: Diastolic ventricular function in children: A Doppler echocardiographic study establishing normal values and predictors of increased ventricular end diastolic pressure. Mayo Clin Proc 1998;73:616-628.

70. Stoddard MF, Pearson AC, Kern MJ, et al: Influence of alteration in preload on the pattern of left ventricular diastolic filling assessed by Doppler echocardiography in humans. Circulation 1989;79:1226-1236.

71. Xie GY, Berk MR, Smith MD, et al: Prognostic value of Doppler transmitral flow patterns in patients with congestive heart failure. J Am Coll Cardiol 1994;24:132-139.

72. Pinamonti B, DiLenarda A, Sinagra G, et al: Restrictive left ventricular filling pattern in dilated cardiomyopathy assessed by Doppler echocardiography: Clinical, echocardiographic and hemodynamic correlations and prognostic implications. Heart Muscle Disease Study Group. J Am Coll Cardiol 1993;22:808-815.

73. Temporelli PL, Corra U, Imparto A, et al: Reversible restrictive left ventricular diastolic filling with optimized oral therapy predicts a more favorable prognosis in patients with chronic heart failure. J Am Coll Cardiol 1998;31:1591-1597.

74. Klein AL, Takik AJ: Doppler assessment of pulmonary venous flow in healthy subjects and in patients with heart disease. J Am Soc Echocardiogr 1991;4:379-392.

75. Nishimura RA, Abel MD, Hatle LK, et al: Relation of pulmonary vein to mitral flow velocities by transesophageal Doppler echocardiography: Effect of different loading conditions. Circulation 1990;81:1488-1497.

76. Basnight MA, Gonzalez MS, Kershenovich SC, et al: Pulmonary venous flow velocity: Relation to hemodynamics, mitral flow velocity and left atrial volume, and ejection fraction. J Am Soc Echocardiogr 1991;4:547-548.

77. Appleton CP, Gonzalez MS, Basnight MA, et al: Relationship of left atrial pressure and pulmonary venous flow velocities: Importance of baseline mitral and pulmonary venous flow velocity parameters studied in lightly sedated dogs. J Am Soc Echocardiogr 1994;7:264-275.

78. Appleton CP, Galloway JM, Gonzalez MS, et al: Estimation of left ventricular filling pressures using two-dimensional and Doppler echocardiography in adult patients with cardiac disease. J Am Coll Cardiol 1993;22:1972-1982.

79. Yamamoto K, Nishimura RA, Chaliki HP, et al: Determination of left ventricular filling pressure by Doppler echocardiography in patients with coronary artery disease: Critical role of left ventricular systolic function. J Am Coll Cardiol 1997;30:1819-1826.

80. Choong CY, Abascal VM, Thomas JD, et al: Combined influence of ventricular loading and relaxation on the transmitral flow velocity profile in dogs measured by Doppler echocardiography. Circulation 1988;78:672-683.

81. Sohn DW, Chai IH, Lee DJ, et al: Assessment of mitral annulus velocity by Doppler tissue imaging in evaluation of left ventricular diastolic function. J Am Coll Cardiol 1997;30:474-480.

82. Firstenberg MS, Greenberg NL, Main ML, et al: Determinants of diastolic myocardial tissue Doppler velocities: Influences of relaxation and preload. J Appl Physiol 2001;90:299-307.

83. Farias CA, Rodriquez L, Garcia MJ, et al: Assessment of diastolic function by tissue Doppler echocardiography: Comparison with standard transmitral and pulmonary venous flow. J Am Soc Echocardiogr 1999;12:609-617.

84. Galiuto L, Ignone G, DeMaria AN: Contraction and relaxation velocities of the normal left ventricle using pulsed-wave tissue Doppler echocardiography. Am J Cardiol 1998;81:609-614.

85. Chen C, Rodriquez L, Lethor JP, et al: Continuous wave Doppler echocardiography for noninvasive assessment of left ventricular dP/dt and relaxation time constant from mitral regurgitant spectra in patients. J Am Coll Cardiol 1994;23:970-976.

86. Isaaz K, Thompson A, Ethevenot G, et al: Doppler echocardiographic measurement of low velocity motion of the left ventricular posterior wall. Am J Cardiol 1989;64:66-75.

87. Border WL, Michelfelder EC, Glascock BJ, et al: Color M-mode and Doppler tissue evaluation of diastolic function in children: Simultaneous correlation with invasive indices. J Am Soc Echocardiogr 2003;16:988-994.

88. Moller JE, Sondergaard E, Seward JB, et al: Ratio of left ventricular peak E-wave velocity to flow propagation velocity assessed by color M-mode Doppler echocardiography in first myocardial infarction: Prognostic and clinical implications. J Am Coll Cardiol 2000;35:363-370.

89. Moller JE, Sondergaard E, Poulsen SH, et al: Color M-mode and pulsed wave tissue Doppler echocardiography: Powerful predictors of cardiac events after first myocardial infarction. J Am Soc Echocardiogr 2001;14:757-763.

90. Broberg CS, Pantely GA, Barber BJ, et al: Validation of the myocardial performance index by echocardiography in mice: A noninvasive measure of left ventricular function. J Am Soc Echocardiogr 2003;16:814-823.

91. Tei C, Dujardin KS, Hodge DO, et al: Doppler echocardiographic index for assessment of global right ventricular function. J Am Soc Echocardiogr 1996;9:838-847.

92. Tei C, Dujardin KS, Hodge DO, et al: Doppler index combining systolic and diastolic myocardial performance: Clinical value in cardiac amyloidosis. J Am Coll Cardiol 1996;28:658-664.

93. Dujardin KS, Tei C, Yeo TC, et al: Prognostic value of a Doppler index combining systolic and diastolic performance in idiopathic-dilated cardiomyopathy. Am J Cardiol 1998;82:1071-1076.

94. Tei C, Nishimura RA, Seward JB, et al: Noninvasive Doppler-derived myocardial performance index: Correlation with simultaneous measurements of cardiac catheterization measurements. J Am Soc Echocardiogr 1997;10:169-178.

95. Yock PG, Popp RL: Noninvasive estimation of right ventricular systolic pressure by Doppler ultrasound in patients with tricuspid regurgitation. Circulation 1984;70:657-662.

96. Kaul S, Tei C, Hopkins JM, Shah PM: Assessment of right ventricular function using two-dimensional echocardiography. Am Heart J 1984;107:526-531.

97. de Groote P, Millaire A, Foucher-Hossein C, et al: Right ventricular ejection fraction is an independent predictor of survival in patients with moderate heart failure. J Am Coll Cardiol 1998;32:948-954.

98. Yeo TC, Dujardin KS, Tei C, et al: Value of a Doppler-derived index combining systolic and diastolic time intervals in predicting outcome in primary pulmonary hypertension. Am J Cardiol 1998;81:1157-1161.

99. Sebbag I, Rudski LG, Therrien J, et al: Effect of chronic infusion of epoprostenol on echocardiographic right ventricular myocardial performance index and its relation to clinical outcome in patients with primary pulmonary hypertension. Am J Cardiol 2001;88:1060-1063.

100. Anconina J, Danchin N, Selton-Suty C, et al: Noninvasive estimation of right ventricular dP/dt in patients with tricuspid valve regurgitation. Am J Cardiol 1993;71:1495-1497.

101. Michelfelder EC, Vermillion RP, Ludomirsky A, et al: Comparison of simultaneous Doppler and catheter-derived right ventricular dP/dt in hypoplastic left heart syndrome. Am J Cardiol 1996;77:212-214.

102. Frommelt PC, Ballweg JA, Whitstone BN, et al: Usefulness of Doppler tissue imaging analysis of tricuspid annular motion for determination of right ventricular function in normal infants and children. Am J Cardiol 2002;89:610-613.

103. Anzola J: Right ventricular contraction. Am J Physiol 1956;184:567-571.

104. Raines RA, LeWinter MM, Covell JW: Regional shortening patterns in canine right ventricle. Am J Physiol 1976;231:1395-1400.

105. Hammarstrom E, Wranne B, Pinto FJ, et al: Tricuspid annular motion. J Am Soc Echocardiogr 1991;4:331-339.

106. Kukulski T, Hubbert L, Arnold M, et al: Normal regional right ventricular function and its change with age: A Doppler myocardial imaging study. J Am Soc Echocardiogr 2000;13:194-204.

107. Yasuoka K, Harada K, Orino T, Takada G: Right ventricular diastolic filling assessed by conventional Doppler and tissue Doppler imaging in normal children. Tohoku J Exp Med 1999;189:283-294.

108. Vignon P, Spencer K, Mor-Avi V, et al: Quantification of regional systolic and diastolic right ventricular function using color kinesis. Circulation 1996;94(Suppl I) I-668.

109. Arce OX, Knudson OA, Ellison MC, et al: Longitudinal motion of the atrioventricular annuli in children: Reference values, growth related changes, and effects of right ventricular volume and pressure overload. J Am Soc Echocardiogr 2002;15:906-916.

110. Zoghbi WA, Habib JB, Quinones MA: Doppler assessment of right ventricular filling in a normal population: Comparison with left ventricular filling dynamics. Circulation 1990;82:1316-1324.

111. Iwase M, Nagata K, Izawa H, et al: Age-related changes in left and right ventricular filling velocity profiles and their relationship in normal subjects. Am Heart J 1993;126:419-426.

112. Yu CM, Sanderson JE: Right and left ventricular diastolic function in patients with and without heart failure: Effect of age, sex, heart rate, and respiration on Doppler-derived measurements. Am Heart J 1997;34:426-434.

113. Watanabe M, Ono S, Tomomasa T, et al: Measurement of tricuspid annular diastolic velocities by Doppler tissue imaging to assess right ventricular function in patients with congenital heart disease. Pediatr Cardiol 2003;24:463-467.

114. Spencer KT, Garcia MJ, Weinart L, et al: Assessment of right ventricular and right atrial systolic and diastolic performance using automated border detection. Echocardiography 1999;16:643-652.

115. Vignon P, Spencer KT, Mor-Avi V, et al: Evaluation of global and regional right ventricular function using automated border detection techniques. Echocardiography 1999;1:105-116.

116. Geva T, Powell AJ, Crawford EC, et al: Evaluation of regional differences in right ventricular systolic function by acoustic quantification echocardiography and cine magnetic resonance imaging. Circulation 1998;98:339-345.

117. Helbing WA, Bosch HG, Maliepaard C, et al: On-line automated border detection for echocardiographic quantification of right ventricular size and function in children. Pediatr Cardiol 1997;18:261-269.

118. Shiota T, Jones M, Chikada M, et al: Real-time three-dimensional echocardiography for determining right ventricular stroke volume in an animal model of chronic right ventricular volume overload. Circulation 1998;19:1897-1900.

119. Ota T, Fleishman CE, Strub M, et al: Real-time, three-dimensional echocardiography: Feasibility of dynamic right ventricular volume measurement with saline contrast. Am Heart J 1999;137:958-966.

120. Fujimoto S, Mizuno R, Nakagawa Y, et al: Estimation of the right ventricular volume and ejection fraction by transthoracic three-dimensional echocardiography: A validation study using magnetic resonance imaging. Int J Card Imaging 1998;14:385-390.

121. Mahle WT, Coon PD, Wernovsky G, et al: Quantitative echocardiographic assessment of the performance of functionally single right ventricle after the Fontan operation. Cardiol Young 2001;11:399-406.

122. Williams RV, Ritter S, Tani LY, et al: Quantitative assessment of ventricular function in children with single ventricles using the Doppler myocardial performance index. Am J Cardiol 2000;86:1106-1110.

123. Courand JA, Marshall J, Chang Y, et al: Clinical application of wall-stress analysis in the pediatric intensive care unit. Crit Care Med 2001;29:526-533.

124. Moller JE, Sondergaard E, Seward JB, et al: Ratio of left ventricular peak E-wave velocity to flow propagation velocity assessed

by color M-mode Doppler echocardiography in first myocardial infarction. J Am Coll Cardiol 2000;35:363-370.

125. Kiraly P, Kapusta L, Thijssen JM, et al: Left ventricular myocardial function in congenital valvar aortic stenosis assessed by ultrasound tissue-velocity and strain rate techniques. Ultrasound Med Biol 2003;29:615-620.

126. Pacileo G, Calabro P, Limongelli G, et al: Left ventricular remodeling, mechanics, and tissue characterization in congenital aortic stenosis. J Am Soc Echocardiogr 2003;16:214-220.

127. Nii M, Mori K, Kuroda Y: Quantification of the myocardial velocity gradient and myocardial wall thickening velocity in healthy children: A new indicator of regional myocardial wall motion. J Am Soc Echocardiogr 2002;15:624-632.

128. Friedberg MK, Rosenthal DN: New developments in echocardiographic methods to assess right ventricular function in congenital heart disease. Curr Opin Cardiol 2005;20:84-88.

CHAPTER 11

Magnetic Resonance Imaging Assessment in Heart Failure

Tal Geva
Taylor Chung
Andrew J. Powell

Cardiovascular MRI is a noninvasive diagnostic modality that overcomes many of the limitations of echocardiography and cardiac catheterization. Since the 1980s, cardiovascular MRI has evolved from an esoteric test in congenital heart disease imaging into a mainstream diagnostic modality with clinical utility that is rapidly increasing.[1] The validity of cardiovascular MRI in anatomic imaging was recognized in the 1980s,[2,3] but there was no widespread realization of its potential to provide functional information until the late 1990s. In recent years, cardiovascular MRI has been shown to be a useful noninvasive tool in evaluating a variety of congenital and acquired cardiovascular abnormalities that may lead to heart failure in children, including dilated and hypertrophic cardiomyopathies,[4-9] myocarditis,[10-13] transplant rejection,[14-20] cardiac tumors,[21-23] congenital and acquired coronary anomalies,[24-28] myocardial iron load,[29-31] valvular disease,[32-34] constrictive pericardial disease,[11,35,36] and arrhythmogenic right ventricular dysplasia/cardiomyopathy.[37-39] This chapter reviews current applications of cardiovascular MRI in the evaluation of heart failure in patients with congenital and acquired pediatric heart disease.

MRI ACQUISITION

In MRI, magnetic fields and radiofrequency energy are used to stimulate hydrogen nuclei in selected regions of the body to emit radiofrequency waves that are used to construct images. As with other cardiovascular imaging modalities, a thorough understanding of the underlying imaging physics enhances the quality and interpretation of the diagnostic data. A detailed discussion of MRI physics is beyond the scope of this chapter and interested readers are referred to other sources.[40,41]

Cardiac and Respiratory Gating

Magnetic resonance images obtained without synchronization to cardiac and respiratory motions are blurred because the heart and central blood vessels are in relatively rapid motion. A common approach to compensate for cardiac motion is to synchronize image acquisition with the cardiac cycle. Imaging may be synchronized or "gated" with a pulse oximetry trace (so-called peripheral gating) or, more optimally, with a high-quality ECG or vectorcardiogram (VCG) signal. A new technique called *self-gating* has been described that avoids the use of ECG signal altogether.[42]

Because images are constructed over multiple cardiac cycles, respiratory motion can degrade image quality. The most straightforward approach to minimizing respiratory artifacts is to have patients hold their breath during image acquisition. Although this solution is often quite effective, it cannot be used in patients who are too young or too ill to cooperate. In such cases, respiratory motion compensation can be achieved by synchronizing image data acquisition to the respiratory and the cardiac cycles. Respiratory motion can be tracked by a bellows device placed around the torso or by magnetic resonance navigator pulse that concurrently tracks the position of the diaphragm or cardiac border. The principal limitation of respiratory triggering is that it substantially prolongs scan time because image data are accepted only during a portion of the respiratory cycle. Another strategy to minimize respiratory motion artifacts is to acquire multiple images at the same location and average them, minimizing variations caused by respiration. As with respiratory triggering, the disadvantage of this approach is increased scan time.

This discussion highlights the need for faster high-quality MRI techniques that would obviate the needs for cardiac triggering and respiratory motion compensation. Advances in gradient coil performance and parallel acquisition methods have achieved this goal and are becoming widely available.[43,44] Real-time MRI at 30 frames/sec is now possible on commercially available clinical scanners, albeit at the expense of spatial resolution. Given the rapid progress in MRI technology, however, it is conceivable that high quality "real-time" cardiovascular MRI will be available in the near future and that ECG and respiratory triggering may no longer be necessary.

MRI ASSESSMENT OF VENTRICULAR VOLUMES AND MASS

Imaging Techniques

Cardiac-gated gradient echo sequences can be used to produce images at multiple instances over the cardiac cycle in each anatomic location. These images can be displayed in a cine loop format to show the motion of the heart and vasculature over the cardiac cycle. On such cine magnetic resonance images, flowing blood produces a bright signal, and the myocardium and vessel wall are relatively dark ("bright-blood" imaging). ECG-triggered or VCG-triggered **steady-state free precession (SSFP)** is currently the most commonly used cine MRI technique for assessment of ventricular function. The SSFP sequence relies on the ratio of T2-to-T1 relaxations with a resultant high contrast between the blood pool (T2/T1 = 360/1200 = 0.3) and the myocardium (T2/T1 = 75/880 = 0.085), which clearly depicts the boundaries of cardiovascular structures (Fig. 11-1).[45] This sequence is known by several proprietary names, including true fast imaging with steady precession (true FISP), balanced fast field echo (bFFE), and fast imaging employing steady-state acquisition (FIESTA). The acquisition time of SSFP cine MRI is short, typically requiring 4 to 10 seconds for each location depending on heart rate, spatial resolution, and other acquisition parameters. Use of parallel imaging techniques, such as sensitivity encoding (SENSE), allows even shorter acquisition times. The SSFP sequence is highly sensitive to inhomogeneities in the magnetic field, however, such as those induced by implanted metallic devices.

A segmented k-space **fast gradient recalled echo (fast,** also termed "turbo," **GRE)** sequence has been used extensively since the 1990s, and its accuracy and reproducibility in measuring ventricular dimensions and function have been validated.[46-48] Compared with SSFP, the distinction between blood and myocardium on fast GRE images is less sharp, the contrast-to-noise ratio and the temporal resolution are lower, the image acquisition time is longer, and the images are more susceptible to blood flow effects. Fast GRE is less susceptible to inho-

mogeneities in the magnetic field than SSFP. In patients with image artifacts owing to implanted devices, the use of a fast GRE sequence offers an advantage over SSFP.

Image Acquisition

Most modern MRI scanners allow acquisition of ECG-triggered or VCG-triggered SSFP cine MRI during short periods of breath holding. Depending on heart rate and image acquisition parameters (matrix size, number of k-space lines per segment, and the scanner's gradient system capabilities), high-resolution acquisition may last 7 to 10 seconds per slice. A modest decrease in spatial and temporal resolutions lowers the acquisition time to 4 to 5 seconds while producing diagnostically acceptable images. The use of **sensitivity encoding (SENSE)** technology allows a shorter acquisition time by a factor of 2 to 4 (at the expense of reduced signal-to-noise ratio), an increase in spatial resolution while maintaining the same acquisition time, or a combination of the two. Patients are instructed to hold their breath at end expiration to minimize variations in the position of the diaphragm and, consequently, the heart. In patients who are incapable of holding their breath, images are acquired during free breathing with multiple signal averages, with respiratory triggering, or with "real-time" magnetic resonance fluoroscopy.[49,50]

Quantitative evaluation of ventricular function is achieved by obtaining a series of contiguous SSFP cine MRI slices that cover the ventricles in short axis (Fig. 11-2). This imaging involves the following steps:
1. Two-chamber plane (also known as long axial oblique and vertical long axis planes): A slice is

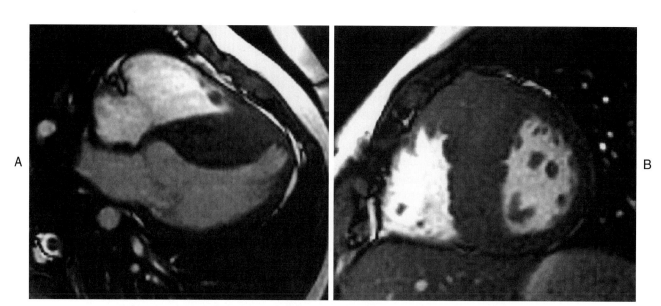

FIGURE 11-1 ■ Steady-state free precession (SSFP) sequence MRI. This is currently the most commonly used cine MRI technique for assessment of ventricular function. This sequence is known by several proprietary names, including true fast imaging with steady precession (true FISP), balanced fast field echo (bFFE), and fast imaging employing steady-state acquisition (FIESTA). The SSFP sequence is highly sensitive to inhomogeneities in the magnetic field, such as those induced by implanted metallic devices. **A,** Four-chamber plane SSFP sequence in a patient with hypertrophic cardiomyopathy. **B,** Short axis plane SSFP sequence in the same patient.

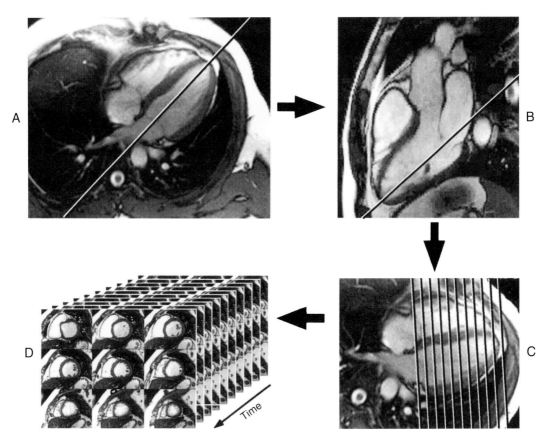

FIGURE 11-2 ■ **Evaluation of ventricular volumes and mass. A,** Using a localizing image obtained in the axial (transverse) plane, a two-chamber (also known as long axial oblique or vertical long axis) plane is prescribed as shown. **B,** Prescription of the four-chamber plane from an end-diastolic image of the previous two-chamber cine sequence. **C,** Prescription of the short axis plane from an end-diastolic image of the previous four-chamber cine sequence extending from the plane of the atrioventricular valves through the cardiac apex. **D,** The short axis stack is viewed in cine mode (see text for details).

prescribed parallel to the plane of the interventricular septum based on previously obtained scout images in the axial (transverse) plane (see Fig. 11-2A). In patients with a biventricular heart and a systemic left ventricle, the slice extends from the center of the mitral valve to the left ventricular apex. In patients with a systemic right ventricle (e.g., atrial switch operation for transposition of the great arteries), it is advantageous to place the slice between the center of the tricuspid valve and the right ventricular apex. In patients with a single ventricle, the slice is placed between the center of the atrioventricular valve to the ventricular apex. This acquisition accounts for the orientation of the ventricles in the transverse plane of the chest.

2. Four-chamber plane (also known as horizontal long axis plane): A slice (or a stack of slices) is prescribed from an end-diastolic image of the previous two-chamber cine sequence, extending between the atrioventricular valve and the ventricular apex (see Fig. 11-2B). This acquisition accounts for the superior-inferior orientation of the ventricles in the chest.

3. Short axis plane: Multiple equidistant slices are prescribed from an end-diastolic image of the previous four-chamber cine sequence covering the ventricles from the plane of the atrioventricular valve to the cardiac apex (see Fig. 11-2C). The first slice is placed at the level of the atrioventricular annuli by connecting the right coronary artery (seen in cross section in the right atrioventricular groove) with the left circumflex coronary artery (seen in the left atrioventricular groove).

4. Subsequent slices are positioned in equidistance through the cardiac apex (see Fig. 11-2D). In most patients, 12 slices cover the ventricles from base to apex with adjustment of slice thickness between 5 and 8 mm and the interslice spacing from 0 to 2 mm. Using these guidelines, the range of ventricular lengths covered is 6 to 12 cm. In some infants, the number of slices can be reduced, whereas in older patients with dilated ventricles, the number of slices may need to be increased. We prefer not to increase the slice thickness greater than 8 mm and interslice spacing greater than 2 mm to avoid partial volume effect and to minimize extrapolation of interslice data.

Image Analysis

Accurate determination of ventricular volume requires clear depiction of the blood-myocardium boundary. Adjustments of the image brightness and contrast on the computer screen can facilitate visualization of that boundary. By tracing the blood-endocardium boundary, the slice's blood pool volume is calculated as the product of its cross-sectional area and thickness (which is prescribed by the operator). The left ventricular papillary muscles and the major trabeculations of the right ventricle are excluded from the blood pool and are considered part of the myocardium. Ventricular volume is determined by summation of the volumes of all slices, and this process can be repeated for each frame in the cardiac cycle to obtain a continuous time-volume loop or may be performed only on end-diastolic (maximal area) and end-systolic (minimal area) frames to calculate diastolic and systolic volumes. From these data, one can calculate left ventricular and right ventricular ejection fractions and stroke volumes. Because the patient's heart rate at the time of image acquisition is known, one can calculate left ventricular and right ventricular outputs. Ventricular mass is calculated by tracing the epicardial borders and calculating the epicardial volume, subtracting the endocardial volume, and multiplying the resultant muscle volume by the specific gravity of the myocardium (1.05 g/mm³).

Most manufacturers of MRI scanners and some third-party companies offer software packages that automatically perform the above-mentioned calculations. Development of algorithms for automatic border detection has facilitated the application of these techniques, but further refinements are required to improve its accuracy.[51-54]

Potential Sources of Errors

Translational motion of the ventricles in the base-to-apex direction is most prominent at the base of the heart. Given that the prescribed short axis slices are fixed in space, there is significant through-plane motion in the basal slices during the cardiac cycle. As a result, the first (and sometimes also the second) most basal slices may contain an atrial blood pool during part of the cardiac cycle because the atrioventricular junction has moved out of the imaging plane during systole. To avoid erroneous inclusion of the atrial blood pool in the calculation of ventricular volume, the image dataset is examined to distinguish between ventricular and atrial structures. In general, when a slice contains a ventricular chamber throughout the cardiac cycle, the chamber's cross-sectional area decreases in systole, and its wall thickness increases. In contrast, in a slice containing ventricular myocardium in diastole and an atrial blood pool in systole, instead of getting smaller and thicker in

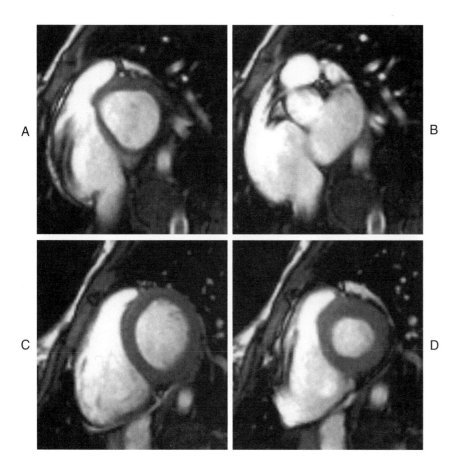

FIGURE 11-3 ■ Selection of basal slices for analysis of ventricular volumes and mass. A and B, Diastolic and systolic frames of the first (most basal) slice. In diastole (A), the presence of left ventricular myocardium and the left anterior descending coronary artery indicates that this frame should be included in the analysis. In systole (B), the left atrium moves into the imaging plane as indicated by the thinning of the wall and the increase in chamber size. C and D, Diastolic and systolic frames of the second slice. In systole (D), the left ventricular wall thickness increases, and chamber size decreases. Diastolic and systolic frames are included in the analysis.

systole, the chamber's cross-sectional area increases, and wall thickness decreases (Fig. 11-3).

Another potential source of error in measurements of ventricular volumes is when the left ventricular papillary muscles and the right ventricular trabeculations are traced in an inconsistent fashion during systole and diastole. Exclusion of the papillary muscles from the blood pool in diastole but not in systole leads to underestimations of end-systolic volume, stroke volume, and ejection fraction. In addition, inconsistent position of the diaphragm during breath holding can lead to spatial variations in the location of the ventricles during acquisition of the short axis images. This source of error in volume calculation can be minimized by instructing the patient to hold his or her breath at end expiration.[55,56]

Accuracy and Reproducibility

The combination of a three-dimensional dataset, clear distinction between the blood pool and the myocardium, and high spatial and temporal resolutions allows for accurate measurements of any cardiac chamber regardless of its morphology and without geometric assumptions. Much research was performed in the late 1980s and early 1990s on in vitro phantoms, animal models, and human subjects to validate the accuracy of cardiovascular MRI measurements of ventricular volumes and mass.[57-63]

More recently, attention has focused on investigating the test characteristics of cardiovascular MRI assessment of chamber dimensions and function (Table 11-1) and on comparison of its accuracy and reproducibility with those of echocardiography and radionuclide techniques.[64-67] Germain and coworkers,[68] in a study of 20 patients with "good echocardiographic windows," found that the mean (±SD) interstudy variability of cardiovascular MRI measurement of left ventricular mass was 6.75% ± 3.8% compared with 11% ± 6.4% for M-mode echocardiography. Bellenger and colleagues[69] calculated that the sample size required to detect changes in left ventricular volumes, ejection fraction, and mass by cardiovascular MRI in patients with heart failure was substantially smaller compared with published values for two-dimensional echocardiography. To detect a 10-mL change in end-diastolic volume (with 90% power and $P < .05$) requires 12 subjects studied by cardiovascular MRI versus 121 patients

TABLE 11-1

Reproducibility of Ventricular Dimensions and Function Measurements by Cardiovascular Magnetic Resonance Imaging

Reference	No. Patients (mean age [yrs])	Diagnoses	Variable	Intraobserver Variability (%)	Interobserver Variability (%)	Interstudy Variability (%)
Semelka et al[64]	11 (44.7)	DCM	LVEDV		4.5±5.3	4.3±3.1
			LVESV		3.3±2.7	4.5±4.6
			LVEF		3.9±1.8	5.8±3.9
			LV mass		3.4±2.9	3.8±3.1
Germain et al[68]	20 (41)	Chest pain, hypertension, cardiomyopathy, valvular heart disease	LV mass	2.0 ± 1.9		6.8±3.8
Bellenger et al[69]	20 (NA)	Heart failure	LVEDV	2.6±1.7	3.3±3.3	2.5±1.3
			LVESV	7.4±4.6	4.2±5.3	3.1±1.9
			LVEF	2.7±0.9	7.3±5.4	4.8±2.9
			LV mass	2.4±2.5	3.1±3	3.0±1.5
Bellenger et al[260]	64 (56±11)	NA	LVEDV	2.8±2.6	5.1±3.7	2.9±1.2
			LVESV	4.6±2.7	5.6±4.9	4.1±2.3
			LVEF	2.1±1.1	9.3±7.8	5.8±2.3
				Within-Subject SD*	95% Range for Change*	
Pattynama et al[261]			RVEDV	13.2 mL	37 mL	
			RVESV	7.8 mL	22 mL	
			RVEF	5.7%	16%	
			RV mass	5.8 g	16 g	

DCM, dilated cardiomyopathy; LV, left ventricle; LVEDV; left ventricular end-diastolic volume; LVEF, left ventricular ejection fraction; LVESV, left ventricular end-systolic volume; LVH, left ventricular hypertrophy; NA, not available; RV, right ventricle; RVEDV; right ventricular end-diastolic volume; RVEF, right ventricular ejection fraction; RVESV, right ventricular end-systolic volume.

TABLE 11-2

Normal Values of Steady-State Free Precession–Based Left Ventricular and Right Ventricular Volumes, Mass, and Ejection Fractions in 60 Subjects*		
	Men (n = 30), Mean ± SD (range[†])	Women (n = 30), Mean ± SD (range[†])
LVEDV index (mL/m²)	82.3 ± 14.7 (53-112)	77.7 ± 10.8 (56-99)
LV ejection fraction (%)	64.2 ± 4.6 (55-73)	64.0 ± 4.9 (54-74)
LV mass index (g/m²)	64.7 ± 9.3 (46-83)	52.0 ± 7.4 (37-67)
RVEDV index (mL/m²)	86.2 ± 14.1 (58-114)	75.2 ± 13.8 (48-103)
RV ejection fraction (%)	55.1 ± 3.7 (48-63)	59.8 ± 5.0 (50-70)

*Age range 20 to 65 years.
† −2 SD to +2 SD
LV, left ventricular; LVEDV, left ventricular end-diastolic volume; RV, right ventricular; RVEDV, right ventricular end-diastolic volume.

examined by two-dimensional echocardiography, a 3% change in ejection fraction requires 15 cardiovascular MRI scans versus 102 echocardiograms, and a 10-g change in mass requires 9 cardiovascular MRI scans versus 273 echocardiograms. Ioannidis and associates[70] compared the accuracy of single-photon emission computed tomography (SPECT) for assessment of left ventricular volumes and ejection fraction with that of cardiovascular MRI. Although the two modalities correlated well, there was a substantial variation in individual measurements by SPECT compared with cardiovascular MRI. One half of the SPECT ejection fraction determinations deviated by at least 5% from cardiovascular MRI–obtained values, and one in four deviated by at least 10%.

Because cardiovascular MRI techniques are evolving rapidly, different sequences may lead to differing measurements of ventricular dimensions and function. Several studies have compared the normal range of left ventricular and right ventricular dimensions and function measured by SSFP cine MRI with values obtained by the fast (turbo) GRE cine technique. Plein and coworkers[71] found that compared with fast GRE, SSFP values of left ventricular end-diastolic and end-systolic volumes were 8.8% and 17.8% higher. Left ventricular mass was 13.8% lower, and ejection fraction was not significantly different between the two techniques. Intraobserver and interobserver variabilities were lower with SSFP measurements compared with fast GRE. In another study, Alfakih and associates[72] showed that right ventricular end-diastolic and end-systolic volumes measured by SSFP are 7.4% and 15.6% higher than by fast GRE. As for the left ventricle, measurements of right ventricular dimension and ejection fraction by SSFP were more reproducible than by fast GRE. The range of SSFP-based left ventricular and right ventricular volumes, mass, and ejection fractions in 60 healthy subjects ranging in age from 20 to 65 years published by Alfakih

and associates[73] is summarized in Table 11-2. SSFP-based normal values of ventricular dimensions in children have not been published.

MRI ASSESSMENT OF MYOCARDIAL FUNCTION

Although ejection fraction and other ejection phase indices, such as shortening fraction and velocity of circumferential fiber shortening, are useful markers of ventricular function and provide valuable prognostic information, they are influenced by preload, afterload, heart rate, and the contractile state of the myocardium. Load-dependent ejection phase indices, such as ejection fraction, can be normal despite depressed contractility, and, conversely, these indices can be depressed despite having normal contractility. Assessment of ventricular function by load-independent indices provides useful information on the contractile state of the myocardium. A detailed discussion of ventricular mechanics is beyond the scope of this chapter and can be found elsewhere in this text.[74,75]

Setser and colleagues,[76] using normalized maximal ventricular power, investigated assessment of the contractile state of the myocardium by cardiovascular MRI. An alternative approach is to adjust ejection phase variables, such as ejection fraction, velocity of fiber shortening, or wall strain to the end-systolic stress. With knowledge of left ventricular end-systolic volume, mass, and pressure (estimated based on mean arterial blood pressure measured by sphygmomanometry), end-systolic stress can be estimated as follows:[75]

$$P = (2/3)\, \sigma_p\, (\ln V_0 - \ln V_c)$$

where V_c is cavity volume, V_0 is chamber volume (cavity volume + myocardial volume), and σ_p is average of orthogonal fiber stresses $(\sigma_{p\phi} + (\sigma_{p\theta})/2$. Experience with this method in cardiovascular MRI is lacking.

Analysis of Regional Wall Motion

A simple qualitative approach is to evaluate visually segmental ventricular wall motion and thickening imaged from long-axis and short-axis gradient echo (SSFP or fast GRE) cine MRI. The left ventricle is divided into 17 segments, as recommended by the American Heart Association,[77] and the right ventricle is divided into 10 segments, as described by Klein and colleagues[78] (Fig. 11-4). Ventricular wall motion is classified as normal (appropriate systolic wall motion toward the center of the ventricle accompanied by myocardial thickening indicative of fiber shortening), hypokinesis (reduced systolic motion and wall thickening), akinesis (no appreciable systolic wall motion and no change in wall thickness), or dyskinesis (outward systolic wall motion without myocardial thickening).

A more objective approach is to define the endocardial and epicardial boundaries of the ventricles throughout the cardiac cycle and, using commercially available software, to analyze quantitatively wall motion and myocardial thickening.[79] The main drawback of this approach is that it is time-consuming, which hinders its acceptance into routine clinical practice. Improvements in automatic border detection can shorten the process, however, and may lead to increased use of this technique.

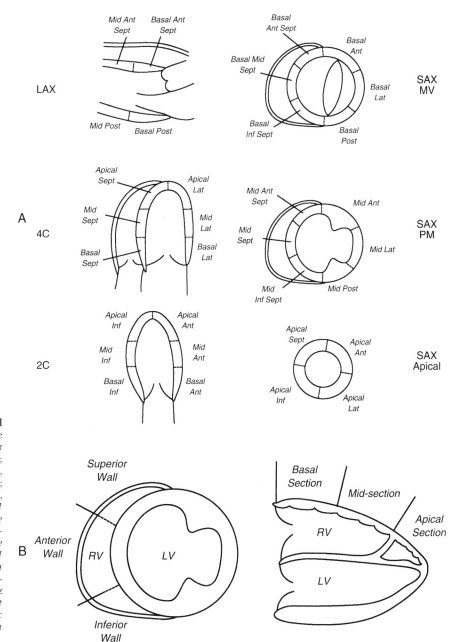

FIGURE 11-4 ■ Regional segmental wall analysis. **A,** Segments of the left ventricle (LV). **B,** Segments of the right ventricular wall. Ant, anterior; Inf, inferior; Lat, lateral; MV, mitral valve; PM, papillary muscles; Post, posterior; RV, right ventricle; SAX, short axis; Sept, septal. (**A** from Cerqueira MD, Weissman NJ, Dilsizian V, et al: *Standardized myocardial segmentation and nomenclature for tomographic imaging of the heart: A statement for healthcare professionals from the Cardiac Imaging Committee of the Council on Clinical Cardiology of the American Heart Association. Circulation* 2002;105:539-542. **B** from Klein SS, Graham TP Jr, Lorenz CH: *Noninvasive delineation of normal right ventricular contractile motion with magnetic resonance imaging myocardial tagging. Ann Biomed Eng* 1998;26:756-763.)

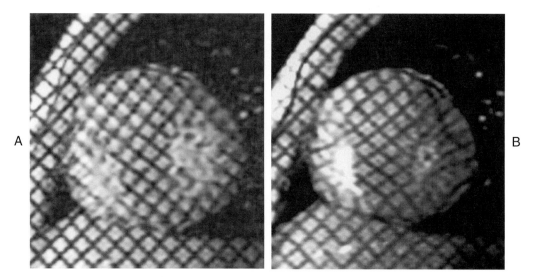

FIGURE 11-5 ■ **Myocardial tagging using spatial modulation of magnetization.** This technique is a modification of cine gradient echo MRI that allows tracking of myocardial motion in two or three spatial dimensions over time. **A,** Diastolic frame shows the undistorted tags before the onset of systole. **B,** Systolic frame shows distortion of the myocardial tags secondary to cardiac motion. Notice the undistorted tags on the chest wall and liver.

Analysis of Myocardial Strain and Stress

Analysis of myocardial strain provides information on regional myocardial function. Although myocardial strain can be calculated from velocity information obtained by phase velocity cine MRI technique (similar to tissue Doppler imaging), most investigators favor a technique called **myocardial tagging using spatial modulation of magnetization (SPAMM)**.[80] This technique is a modification of cine gradient echo MRI that allows tracking of myocardial motion in two or three spatial dimensions over time. Using a preparatory radiofrequency pulse, saturation bands or "tags" that appear as dark lines or stripes are applied across the image at end diastole (Fig. 11-5). On subsequent images, the stripes (tags) remain unchanged on stationary tissue, such as the chest wall and spine, but change their position on moving tissues, such as ventricular myocardium. As the myocardium moves during the cardiac cycle, the tags follow it, and their rotation, translation, and deformation can be tracked, allowing for calculations of myocardial strain and strain rate.[81] This analysis can be done during systole or diastole and in two or three dimensions.[82]

Early studies with myocardial tagging were done mostly by manually tracking the tags, a time-consuming process that hindered the clinical use of this technique. A more recently described technique for the analysis of myocardial tagging data, **harmonic phase imaging (HARP)**, greatly shortens analysis time because it does not require manual tracing of the tags.[83] This technique relies on automatic analysis of the raw MRI data for changes in phase between images (Fig. 11-6). With advances in automatic analysis of the tag data and fast image acquisition and display techniques, it is now possible to evaluate myocardial strain in real time.[84]

Myocardial tagging has been shown to be an important tool in the study of normal left[85-99] and right ventricular mechanics in healthy volunteers.[78] In the clinical arena, analysis of wall strain by myocardial tagging has provided useful information in patients with ischemic and valvular heart disease.[100-111] Kuijpers and colleagues,[112] in a study of 211 patients with chest pain, showed that myocardial tagging detects more segments with regional wall motion abnormalities by dobutamine stress cardiovascular MRI than visual assessment alone. In the field of congenital heart disease, Fogel and colleagues[113-116] used myocardial tagging to characterize patterns of wall motion and strain in patients with functionally single ventricles. As new fast MRI techniques coupled with automatic analysis of myocardial tagging become more widely available, the clinical application of ventricular strain analysis is likely to expand. Further research is required to determine the clinical implications of the strain data and how these data can be used to assess prognosis and guide patient management.

Stress Cardiovascular MRI and Function

There is a growing body of literature on the use of dobutamine stress cardiovascular MRI in the evaluation of myocardial ischemia in adults with coronary artery disease (see discussion in the section on myocardial ischemia later). Several studies have evaluated the use of stress

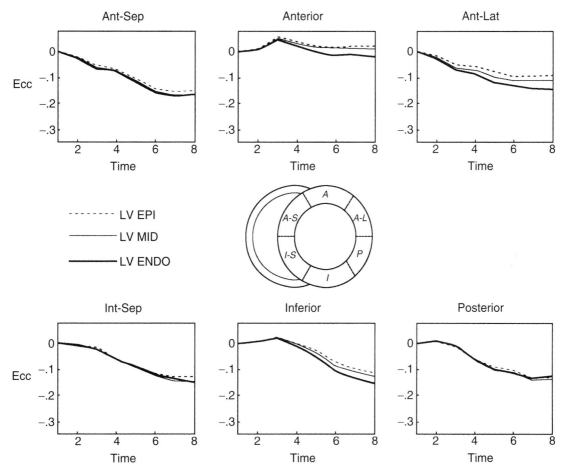

FIGURE 11-6 ■ **Evaluation of regional myocardial strain by tagging analysis.** This technique relies on automatic analysis of the raw MRI data for changes in phase between images. Ant and A, anterior; A-L, anterolateral; A-S, anterior septum; Ecc, strain; ENDO, endocardium; EPI, epicardium; Inf and I, inferior; I-S, inferior-septal; Lat, lateral; LV, left ventricular; MID, midwall; P, posterior; Sep, septal.

cardiovascular MRI in patients with congenital heart disease. First, Tulevski and coworkers[117,118] used a low dose of dobutamine to evaluate the functional reserve of the left and right ventricles in asymptomatic and minimally symptomatic patients with repaired transposition of the great arteries, physiologically corrected transposition of the great arteries, and pulmonary outflow obstruction. Compared with controls, patients with systemic right ventricle had decreased functional reserve. In another study from the same group, Dodge-Khatami and colleagues[119] showed that the functional reserve of the systemic ventricle is comparable in healthy adults and in patients with unoperated, physiologically corrected transposition of the great arteries. Roest and associates[120] showed the feasibility of assessing biventricular dimensions and function by cardiovascular MRI during supine exercise, a method that provides an alternative to pharmacologic stress.

Diastolic Function

Diastole is a complex process during which the force of the myofibers is restored.[121] The diastolic properties of the ventricles are influenced by many factors that are closely interrelated, including heart rate, loading conditions, the contractile state of the myocardium, the material properties of the myocardium (e.g., viscoelastic properties affected by fibrosis, hypertrophy, and other pathologies), ventricular-ventricular interaction, and pericardial constraint. In general, diastole can be divided into early and late phases. The early phase involves active myocardial relaxation and requires active transport of calcium into the sarcoplasmic reticulum. It begins with an isovolumic relaxation period during which the atrioventricular and semilunar valves are closed, followed by an early filling phase. Late diastole is characterized by ventricular filling during atrial contraction, a process that is influenced by ventricular compliance (see Chapters 7 and 8).

As the importance of diastole in many pathologic conditions affecting the cardiovascular system has come into focus, researchers have used various modalities and a wide array of parameters to assess diastolic function. Changes of pressure and chamber dimensions can be assessed invasively by catheterization; nuclear scintigraphy can evaluate ventricular filling; and echocardiography and Doppler ultrasound can measure changes of ventricular dimensions, wall thinning, a wide range of flow-derived variables obtained by Doppler interrogation of the atrioventricular valves and pulmonary veins, myocardial velocities assessed by tissue Doppler imaging, and myocardial strain. With the exception of direct pressure measurements, all of the above-mentioned variables also can be evaluated by MRI.[32,122-135] Helbing and colleagues[32] used cardiovascular MRI to measure blood flow through the tricuspid and pulmonary valves and changes in right ventricular dimensions to assess diastolic function after tetralogy of Fallot repair. Although the data derived from analysis of blood flow and chamber dimensions by MRI are not fundamentally different from similar data obtained by other techniques, MRI offers an advantage in terms of its ability to track tissue motion and deformation during the cardiac cycle using tissue tagging techniques.[131,133-136] Fogel and associates[131] used myocardial tagging to study left ventricular diastolic strain in 11 infants with structurally normal hearts. They showed inhomogeneities in circumferential lengthening (E_2) and radial thinning (E_1). This study characterizes the normal pattern of diastolic myocardial strain in infants, information that can be used to evaluate diastolic function in infants with congenital and acquired heart disease.

One of the challenges of noninvasive assessment of diastolic function is the observation that flow rates are influenced by many variables, and that a normal pattern can be misleading because of "pseudonormalization" related to variations in left atrial pressure and other factors.[137] Investigators have long realized that most of the relaxation process occurs during the isovolumic period of the cardiac cycle, before blood flow or wall motion begins.[121] Early relaxation is best quantified by measuring the rate of left ventricular pressure decay, expressed as the time constant of relaxation, tau (τ).[74,121,138] This variable requires invasive measurement of intracavitary pressure, however, which renders it impractical for longitudinal follow-up. Dong and colleagues[134] showed in a canine model that measurements of the velocity of myocardial untwisting and recoil rate assessed by MRI using tissue tagging correlate closely with τ ($r = -0.86$), and that τ, but not loading conditions, was an independent predictor of the recoil rate. The rate of recoil of torsion derived by tissue tagging may provide a noninvasive, preload-independent isovolumic phase measurement of ventricular relaxation.

MRI ASSESSMENT OF MYOCARDIAL PERFUSION

Compared with the adult population, myocardial ischemia is a rare underlying cause of heart failure in children and young adults. In the pediatric population, ischemia may be associated with congenital coronary abnormalities, such as anomalous origin of a coronary artery from the pulmonary artery or from the opposite sinus of Valsalva,

or acquired conditions, most notably Kawasaki disease. Alternatively the coronary circulation may be compromised in postoperative patients, especially patients whose procedure involved translocation of the coronary arteries (e.g., arterial switch operation). Patients who have undergone heart transplantation also are at risk for the development of accelerated coronary artery disease and abnormalities of the coronary microvasculature.

Most clinicians regard coronary angiography as the gold standard for the diagnosis of ischemia related to coronary artery stenosis. This approach is invasive, carries associated risks, and is expensive, however. A variety of noninvasive modalities are available for the diagnosis of ischemia, including exercise ECG, echocardiography, SPECT, and positron emission tomography (PET). All of these diagnostic tools have drawbacks, as evidenced by the observation that after noninvasive screening, 60% of adult patients undergoing cardiac catheterization do not require revascularization procedures.

Compared with the techniques noted previously, cardiac MRI is a relatively new tool for detection of myocardial ischemia and viability. As a result, the available data on its clinical utility and applicability are considerably more sparse than for the more established techniques. This limitation is perhaps offset by the fact that data specific to children and young adults are scarce for all the noninvasive techniques. The feasibility of assessing myocardial perfusion and viability by cardiovascular MRI in children and patients with congenital heart disease has been shown with encouraging early results.[139]

Myocardial Ischemia

Currently the two most widely used cardiovascular MRI techniques to detect ischemia are dobutamine stress cardiovascular MRI and first-pass myocardial perfusion. **Dobutamine stress cardiovascular MRI** is performed using a protocol similar to dobutamine stress echocardiography with increasing doses of dobutamine up to 40 to 50 µg/kg/min and the addition of atropine if necessary to reach the target heart rate. The goal of the test is to detect ventricular myocardium supplied by a stenotic coronary artery. At rest, the myocardial blood supply-to-demand ratio may be sufficient to allow normal wall motion and thickening. With increasing metabolic demand under pharmacologic stress, however, ischemia may be induced and wall motion becomes impaired. Imaging usually is performed with breath-hold fast cine MRI, providing high-quality images of left ventricular wall motion and thickening. Nagel and coworkers[140] compared the sensitivity and specificity of dobutamine stress cardiovascular MRI with those of dobutamine stress echocardiography in 208 patients for the detection of greater than 50% coronary artery stenosis determined by coronary angiography. Compared with dobutamine stress echocardiography, dobutamine stress cardiovascular MRI was more sensitive (86.2% versus 74.3%), had a higher specificity (85.7% versus 69.8%), and had better accuracy (86% versus 72.7%; $P < .05$ for all). Cardiovascular MRI has a particular advantage over echocardiography in patients who have poor acoustic windows (15% of studies in adults). Hundley and associates[141] reported on 153 patients referred for dobutamine stress cardiovascular MRI after a nondiagnostic dobutamine echocardiogram. The dobutamine stress cardiovascular MRI was completed in an average of 53 minutes and had a sensitivity and specificity of 83% and 83% for detecting coronary artery stenosis greater than 50%. Dobutamine stress cardiovascular MRI can be enhanced further by the use of myocardial tagging, a technique that noninvasively applies grid lines on the myocardium that deform with contraction and facilitate assessment.[112] Using HARP imaging,[84] quantitative assessment of myocardial strain can be calculated rapidly and provide an objective method to diagnosing myocardial ischemia during dobutamine stress testing.[142]

First-pass myocardial perfusion cardiovascular MRI also can be used to diagnose myocardial ischemia. After intravenous injection of a gadolinium-based contrast agent, the enhancement pattern of the myocardium is evaluated during the first transit of the bolus through the heart. The appearance of contrast agent is attenuated in amplitude and rate in regions of compromised coronary blood flow (Fig. 11-7). In practice, the contrast agent (gadopentetate dimeglumine [Magnevist], 0.05 to 0.1 mmol/kg) is infused through a large-bore cannula using a power injector at a rate of 3 to 5 mL/sec. With the patient holding his or her breath, the heart is rapidly imaged in multiple planes for approximately 30 seconds using a cardiac-triggered fast gradient echo hybrid echo-planar pulse sequence. An inversion preparation

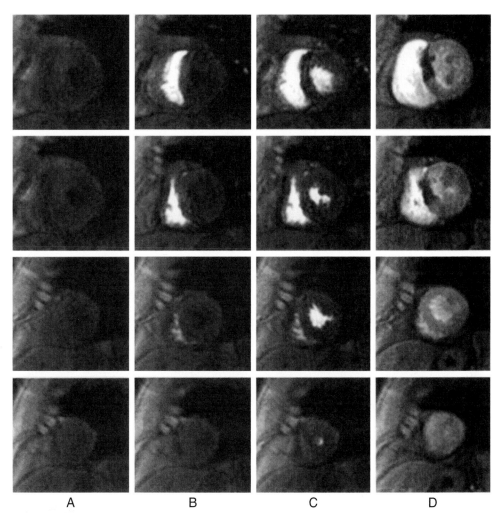

A   B   C   D

FIGURE 11-7 ■ **First-pass myocardial perfusion cardiovascular MRI.** After intravenous injection of a gadolinium-based contrast agent, the enhancement pattern of the myocardium is evaluated during the first transit of the bolus through the heart. First-pass myocardial perfusion is shown in a patient with anterior septal myocardial infarction. **A,** Four short axis slices (*top frame,* basal slice; *bottom frame,* apical slice) before arrival of the contrast agent. **B,** The contrast agent enters the right ventricle. **C,** The contrast agent enters the left ventricle, but not the coronary arteries (note the bright signal from the blood pool but not from the myocardium). **D,** Segments with well-perfused myocardium show bright signal, whereas the hypoperfused anterior septal segment remains dark.

pulse also is used, which minimizes the signal from myocardium and enhances the relative increase in signal intensity produced by the T1-shortening effects of the contrast agent.

Because exercise stress cannot be readily done in the MRI scanner, most perfusion studies are performed with vasodilators such as adenosine or dipyridamole. Qualitative and quantitative analyses have been reported; the latter is done typically by constructing time-intensity curves of myocardial regions and calculating a perfusion reserve index. Nagel and colleagues[143] calculated perfusion reserve by cardiovascular MRI using adenosine in a cohort of 84 patients undergoing diagnostic coronary angiography. They found that MRI had a sensitivity of 88%, a specificity of 90%, and an accuracy of 89% for the detection of coronary artery stenosis greater than 75% by angiography. In another study, 48 patients with suspected coronary artery disease were prospectively studied by MRI, PET, and coronary angiography.[144] Receiver-operator characteristic analysis of the subendocardial upslope data during hyperemia revealed a sensitivity of 87% and specificity of 85% compared with coronary angiography (stenosis >50%) and good agreement with PET.

Myocardial Viability

In addition to detection of ischemia, cardiovascular MRI can be used to differentiate viable from nonviable myocardium (e.g., infarct). This issue is critical because even severely dysfunctional myocardium in patients with coronary artery disease may show functional improvement after revascularization by percutaneous coronary intervention or bypass surgery. **Myocardial delayed enhancement (MDE) imaging** has become the dominant MRI technique to assess viability. It is based on the observation that the "washout" kinetics of standard gadolinium-based intravenous MRI contrast agents is delayed in necrotic myocardium. Consequently, infarcted myocardium appears bright or hyperenhanced compared with viable myocardium when imaged with a segmented inversion recovery fast gradient echo sequence after contrast injection (Fig. 11-8). In practice, MDE imaging is performed 10 to 20 minutes after administration of 0.1 to 0.2 mmol/kg of gadolinium-based contrast agent. MDE is first done using several inversion times to select the one that best nulls the myocardium. Using this inversion time, MDE is performed in short and long axis planes.

Several studies in animals and humans have shown that this technique is effective at identifying the presence, location, and size of acute and chronic myocardial infaction.[145-154] Klein and associates[155] found close agreement between MDE imaging and PET scar size measurements in 31 patients with ischemic heart failure. Because of its superior spatial resolution, MDE is more sensitive than SPECT in patients with small or subendocardial infarctions.[156] Most importantly, the transmural extent of MDE can be used to predict improvement in contractile function after revascularization in patients with acute and chronic coronary artery disease.[157-160] Another promising clinical application of MDE imaging is detection of myocardial fibrosis in patients with

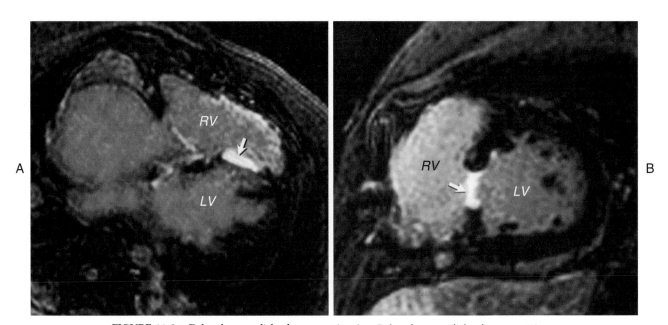

FIGURE 11-8 ■ Delayed myocardial enhancement imaging. Delayed myocardial enhancement imaging in a 7-year-old girl with pulmonary atresia–intact ventricular septum and right ventricle (RV)–dependent coronary arteries who underwent surgical repair with a right ventricular outflow tract patch. **A,** Hyperenhancement and thinning of the mid-septal segment *(arrow),* consistent with nonviable myocardium. **B,** The same segment is seen in the short axis plane *(arrow).* LV, left ventricle.

hypertrophic cardiomyopathy.[7] Kim and Judd[161] showed that the extent of myocardial fibrosis assessed by MDE can be used to stratify risk in these patients. Prakash and associates[139] studied 30 pediatric and congenital heart disease patients with a median age of 13 years (range 0.3 to 40 years) whose diagnoses included repaired congenital heart disease (15), cardiomyopathy (6), cardiac tumor (3), dysplastic left ventricle (2), congenital coronary anomaly (2), and coronary artery aneurysm following Kawasaki disease (2). These investigators found good agreement between MRI evaluation of myocardial perfusion and viability and analysis of segmental wall motion and coronary angiography (n = 10) and SPECT (n = 6). Further studies are needed to validate and expand this initial experience.

MRI ASSESSMENT OF CARDIOMYOPATHY AND MYOCARDITIS

Although echocardiography is the primary diagnostic tool in patients with cardiomyopathy, cardiovascular MRI can provide important information in select patients. As mentioned earlier, cardiovascular MRI is the most reproducible imaging modality for assessment of left ventricular and right ventricular volumes, mass, and ejection fractions. Cardiovascular MRI can assess myocardial morphology, regional function (e.g., wall strain and stress), perfusion, viability, and metabolism.

In dilated cardiomyopathy, the primary goal of the cardiovascular MRI examination is to image the ventricles and quantify their dimensions and function. Cardiovascular MRI also has been used in patients with dilated cardiomyopathy to analyze wall thickening,[162] visualize impaired fiber shortening,[163] and calculate end-systolic stress.[164] Blood flow analysis can be used to quantify valve regurgitation (see discussion in the next section). The presence and extent of myocardial fibrosis can be assessed by myocardial delayed enhancement, which also can be used to detect ventricular thrombi.[165] Several investigators have explored the use of magnetic resonance spectroscopy to evaluate myocardial metabolism in patients with cardiomyopathy.[166-168]

In hypertrophic cardiomyopathy, cardiovascular MRI has been used to study myocardial morphology, mass, function, tissue characteristics, and hemodynamic aspects of the left ventricular outflow tract obstruction and mitral regurgitation. Delayed contrast enhancement can detect scar tissue in the hypertrophied myocardium,[169] a finding that may indicate high risk of adverse outcome.[161]

In patients with myocarditis, cardiovascular MRI can provide information on ventricular dimensions and function, pericardial effusion, valve regurgitation, and, importantly, changes in signal characteristics of the myocardium.[170] Friedrich and associates[12] reported reversible changes in T1-weighted contrast-enhanced myocardial signals in 19 patients during the course of acute myocarditis. They showed focal increases in postcontrast signal intensities early (day 2) in the disease, which subsequently became diffuse, with late resolution by day 84. The authors speculated that the combination of hyperemia secondary to the inflammatory process, slow interstitial wash-in/wash-out kinetics, capillary leakage, and disruption of cell membrane integrity may have led to the accumulation of gadolinium diethylenetriamine penta-acetic acid in the affected myocardium. T2-weighted cardiovascular MRI may detect edema associated with myocardial inflammation.[171] Bellotti and colleagues,[172] in a study of 16 patients with Chagas disease, showed that contrast-enhanced cardiovascular MRI can detect myocardial inflammation and may increase the sensitivity of endomyocardial biopsies. Other investigators reported on the use of cardiovascular MRI in patients with myocarditis secondary to Chagas disease,[13] Lyme disease,[173,174] systemic lupus erythematosus,[175] polymyositis,[176] and eosinophilic myocarditis.[177]

MRI AND BLOOD FLOW ANALYSIS

Quantitative and qualitative assessments of blood flow are used frequently in functional MRI evaluation of congenital and acquired pediatric heart disease.[178] Qualitative evaluation of abnormal flow patterns is used to visualize turbulent flow jets related to stenotic or regurgitant valves or abnormal communications between cardiac chambers or blood vessels (e.g., septal defects, patent ductus arteriosus, systemic-to-pulmonary shunts). Site-specific quantifications of flow rate, flow velocity, stroke volume, and minute flow in principal can be measured across any blood vessel within the central cardiovascular system. Such information provides useful diagnostic information in patients with heart failure.

Imaging Techniques

An ECG-gated **velocity encoded cine MRI (VEC MRI)** sequence, a type of gradient echo sequence, can be used to measure blood flow velocity and quantify blood flow rate.[178,179] The VEC MRI technique is based on the principle that the signal from hydrogen nuclei (such as those in blood) flowing through specially designed magnetic field gradients accumulates a predictable phase shift that is proportional to its velocity. Multiple phase images are constructed across the cardiac cycle in which the signal amplitude (intensity) of each voxel is proportional to mean flow velocity within that voxel. Using specialized software, regions of interest around a vessel are defined, and the flow rate is automatically calculated as the product of the mean velocity and the cross-sectional area (Fig. 11-9).

In practice, an imaging plane is prescribed perpendicular to the vessel of interest, and two sets of multiphase images are reconstructed after a VEC MRI acquisition: a set of magnitude images that provide anatomic information and a set of phase images in

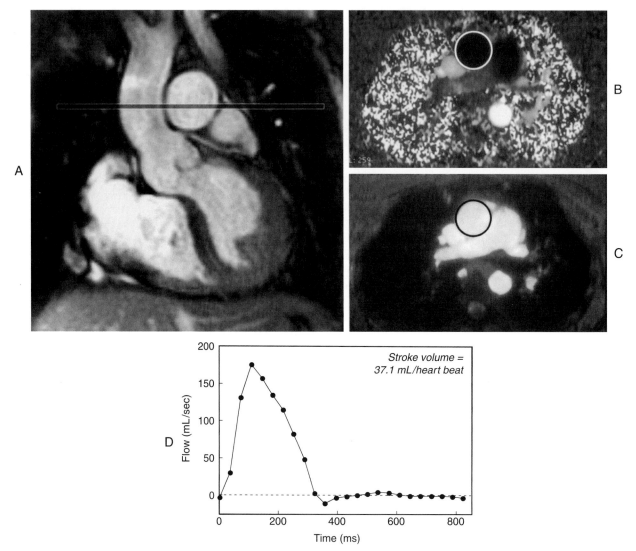

FIGURE 11-9 ■ Phase velocity encoded cine MRI (VEC MRI). An ECG-gated VEC MRI sequence of assessment of blood flow in the ascending aorta. As explained in the text, the VEC MRI technique is based on the principle that the signal from hydrogen nuclei (such as those in blood) flowing through specially designed magnetic field gradients accumulates a predictable phase shift that is proportional to its velocity. Using specialized software, regions of interest around a vessel are defined, and the flow rate is automatically calculated as the product of the mean velocity and the cross-sectional area. **A,** An imaging plane is prescribed perpendicular to the ascending aorta. **B,** Phase image (systolic frame). **C,** Magnitude image. **D,** Flow curve.

which the velocity information is encoded. For each acquisition, the operator prescribes the field of view, matrix size, and slice thickness, which determine spatial resolution. Greil and associates,[180] in an in vitro study using a pulsatile flow model, found that spatial resolution is important for accurate measurements of flow rate by VEC MRI with an optimal number of pixels within the cross section of the vessel of interest of 16 or more. Other variables, such as the angle between the prescribed imaging plane and flow direction, velocity encoding range, flip angle, and slice thickness, also must be considered. Other known caveats of quantitative assessment of blood flow by VEC MRI include flow aliasing and dephasing secondary to turbulent flow.

Aliasing can be avoided by prescribing a velocity encoding range higher than the maximal velocity within the target vessel. Avoiding dephasing secondary to turbulent blood flow can be achieved by shortening the echo time, prescribing a thinner slice thickness, or repositioning the imaging slice proximal or distal to the turbulent jet.

VEC MRI flow calculations have been shown by in vitro and in vivo studies to be accurate and reproducible.[180-189] In vitro studies have shown that measurements of continuous flow are accurate within 5% of reference standard.[190,191] Greil and associates[180] showed that the accuracy and reproducibility of in vitro pulsatile flow measurements by VEC MRI is 0.8% ± 1.5%. Evans and coworkers[187] found a strong correlation ($r^2 = 0.99$) with a 95% confidence interval of ±0.07 L/min over a range of flow rates of 0.125 to 1.9 L/min. Powell and colleagues,[182] in a phantom model that mimics flow condition in the aorta of a child (flow rates 1.25 to 3.5 L/min), found a similarly strong correlation, a close agreement (bias −0.045 L/min), and 95% limits of agreement of −0.19 to 0.1 L/min.

The accuracy of in vivo VEC MRI measurements of blood flow has been shown by numerous studies. Investigators have used ventricular stroke volume, thermodilution, Fick principle, indicator dilution, and flow probe measurements as reference standards, showing strong correlations with VEC MRI.[182,192-200] Hundley and colleagues[198] found that ascending aorta flow in 23 adults was within 4% of flow measurements by the Fick method and within 5% measured by thermodilution. Evans and colleagues,[187] in a study of 10 adult subjects, showed an average difference between pulmonary and systemic flow ratio of 5%. Powell and associates,[182] in a study of 20 volunteers, found that pulmonary-to-systemic flow ratio closely approximated unity (mean ± SD 0.99 ± 0.1; range 0.85 to 1.19). In addition, Beerbaum and coworkers,[181] in a study of 50 children with atrial or ventricular septal defects who underwent concomitant cardiac catheterization, reported a mean difference between VEC MRI and oximetry of 2% (2 SD -20% to +26%). Finally, Powell and colleagues,[201] in a study of 20 patients with atrial septal defect, found a mean difference between VEC MRI and oximetry of 2.3% with a reproducibility of repeat VEC MRI flow measurements of 1.1% ± 4.2% in the main pulmonary artery and 0.7% ± 5.4% in the ascending aorta.

VEC MRI is a useful tool for functional assessment of heart failure in patients with congenital and acquired heart disease. In practice, measurements of blood flow are an integral element of functional assessment by MRI in a wide range of clinical scenarios. Examples include measurements of cardiac output,[198,202] pulmonary-to-systemic flow ratio in patients with intracardiac and extracardiac shunts,[181-183,201,203,204] regional flow to select organs or vascular beds (e.g., patients with vascular malformations),[205-207] valvular regurgitation in patients with native and postoperative lesions (e.g., pulmonary regurgitation after tetralogy of Fallot repair),[208-222] differential lung perfusion (e.g., branch pulmonary artery stenosis),[223-225] atrioventricular valve inflow,[32] estimation of pressure gradient,[221,226,227] and a variety of other clinical scenarios.

Keeping in mind the known limitations of VEC MRI,[178,180,228] site-specific quantifications of flow rate, flow velocity, stroke volume, and minute flow in principle can be measured across any blood vessel within the central cardiovascular system. Pharmacologic stress can be used to provide additional information on functional reserve.[229] Using either dipyridamole or adenosine for vasodilation of the coronary vascular bed, coronary flow reserve can be assessed.[230] An inherent strength of functional assessment by MRI is the ability to measure the same variable by different methods, allowing for internal validation of the functional data. In a patient with an atrial septal defect, the pulmonary-to-systemic flow ratio can be assessed based on (1) flow measurements in the main pulmonary artery and ascending aorta, (2) flow measurements through the tricuspid and mitral valves (typically obtained in a single acquisition perpendicular to plane of the atrioventricular valves), and (3) left ventricular and right ventricular stroke volumes obtained by short axis cine MRI.

Although standard VEC MRI techniques require 2 to 4 minutes of data acquisition in each site, more recent developments of faster imaging strategies (e.g., segmented k-space acquisition and parallel processing) have shortened the acquisition time greatly.[204,231-233] Although these techniques allow for data acquisition during a short period of breath holding (10 to 14 seconds), the physiologic effects of suspended respiration may alter intrathoracic pressure and affect flow measurements. Sakuma and colleagues[234] showed that flow measurements during large lung volume breath holding significantly underestimated cardiac output (4.47 ± 0.63 L/min versus 6.09 ± 0.49 L/min), whereas cardiac output measurements during small lung volume breath holding were similar to those obtained during free breathing. Development of real-time velocity encoded techniques has a potential utility analogous to color Doppler in echocardiography.[217] This technique has proved valuable in providing unique physiologic information in patients with Fontan circulation.[235]

The preceding discussion focused on through-plane flow measurements. When velocity information is measured in the three orthogonal planes (anterior-posterior, superior-inferior, and through-plane), multidimensional flow imaging and shear stress calculation can be accomplished.[236-239] **Three-dimensional flow vector mapping** is a useful adjunct to cine flow imaging because it provides dynamic three-dimensional flow maps that can readily detect abnormal flow patterns (Fig. 11-10).

MRI AND TISSUE CHARACTERIZATION

Assessments of the myocardium, pericardium, blood vessel wall, and extracardiac tissue for pathologic changes can be valuable in patients with heart failure. MRI offers a distinct advantage over other modalities in evaluation of soft tissues because of its ability to discern even minor changes in tissue composition. By manipulations of T1 and T2 weighting and by applying a variety of prepulses or suppression of signals from specific materials (such as fat or water) tissue composition can be evaluated.

Imaging Techniques

Assessments of cardiovascular morphology and tissue characteristics by MRI are based on the use of several

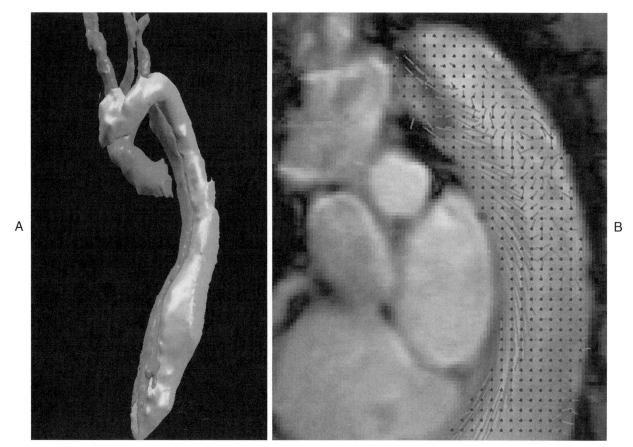

FIGURE 11-10 ■ Three-dimensional flow vector mapping. Aortic dissection in a patient with Marfan syndrome. **A,** Color-coded reconstruction of gadolinium-enhanced three-dimensional magnetic resonance angiography of the aorta. The true aortic lumen is coded in red and the false lumen in yellow. **B,** Systolic frame of three-dimensional flow vector mapping in the descending aorta. Note the streamline flow vectors in the true lumen and the low-velocity (shorter vectors) swirling flow (vectors oriented in different directions) in the false lumen. (See also Color Section)

imaging techniques. A detailed discussion of the technical aspects of these imaging sequences is beyond the scope of this chapter and can be found elsewhere.[40] The following is a brief introduction to some of the commonly used techniques.

Spin echo pulse sequences usually are used to produce images in which flowing blood has low signal intensity and appears dark ("black blood" imaging). Other tissues appear as varying shades of gray. Although cardiac-gated spin echo sequences produce only one image per location and provide only static anatomic information, their advantages include high spatial resolution, excellent blood-myocardium contrast, and decreased artifact from metallic biomedical implants (e.g., sternal wires, stents, prosthetic valves) compared with gradient echo sequences. Spin echo sequences also are modified easily to alter tissue contrast and characterize abnormal structures. When a patient can hold his or her breath, **fast (turbo) spin echo (FSE) with double inversion recovery (DIR) imaging** is a useful pulse sequence.[240,241] This is also a black-blood sequence with the blood signal "nulled" by the inversion pulse rather than relying on blood flow alone. An additional

inversion pulse with short inversion time (150 msec) can be added to null the magnetization from fat (so-called triple inversion recovery) resulting in an image with no signal from blood or fat. In patients who are not able to hold their breath, fast spin echo with double inversion recovery or triple inversion recovery needs to be combined with multiple signal averages to compensate for respiratory motion.

Another method to null the signal from fat or water is based on the difference in their chemical compositions. There is a small difference in the resonant frequency of the signal from protons in H_2O molecules and the CH_2 protons that can be exploited for visualizing water and fat separately.[40]

Clinical Applications

MRI evaluation of tissue characteristics and cardiovascular morphology is a useful tool in patients with heart failure. Examples include assessment of myocardial architecture (e.g., myocardial noncompaction[242,243] and ventricular aneurysm[244]), evaluation of cardiac tumors (Fig. 11-11),[21] vessel wall imaging (e.g., aortic dissection[245,246]), assessment of the myocardium for fatty infiltration or other

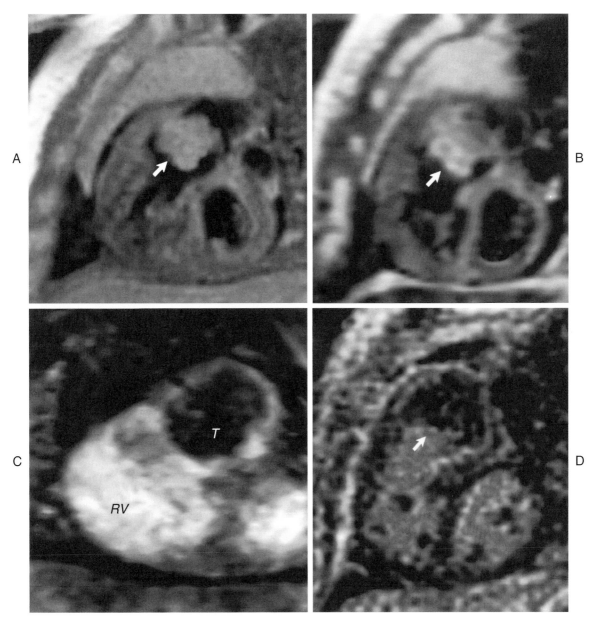

FIGURE 11-11 ■ MRI tissue characterization. Evaluation of tumor characteristics in a newborn with critical subvalvar pulmonary stenosis caused by a large solitary rhabdomyoma attached to the infundibular free wall and the pulmonary valve leaflets. **A,** Proton density–weighted fast spin echo (FSE) with double inversion recovery (DIR) sequence in the short axis plane shows the tumor morphology *(arrow)*. The signal in the tumor is higher (hyperintense) compared with the adjacent myocardium. **B,** T2-weighted FSE-DIR sequence shows moderately high signal intensity from the tumor *(arrow)*. **C,** Gadolinium-enhanced three-dimensional magnetic resonance angiography shows lack of early enhancement of the tumor (T). RV, right ventricle. **D,** Delayed myocardial enhancement sequence shows lack of hyperenhancement of the tumor *(arrow)*, which indicates the tumor is unlikely to be a fibroma.

Continued

pathologic changes (e.g., arrhythmogenic right ventricular cardiomyopathy[37,38]), evaluation of the pericardium (e.g., constrictive pericardium[35,36]) (Fig. 11-12), assessment of myocardial iron load (see discussion in the following section), and imaging of intracardiac thrombus (Fig. 11-13).[165]

In practice, MRI assessment of tissue characteristics is based on the use of several imaging sequences. Standard or fast spin echo is used for morphologic imaging of the myocardium, pericardium, blood vessel walls, and extracardiac structures. Manipulations of image contrast (T1, T2, or proton density-weighted) and the addition of prepulses (e.g., triple inversion recovery, T2 preparation, and fat or water saturation) result in highlighting or suppression of specific tissue characteristics. Gradient echo sequences provide information on signal intensity and, more importantly, on motion of the

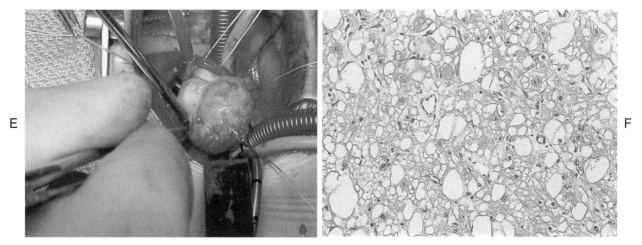

FIGURE 11-11 ■ cont'd. E, Intraoperative photograph of the tumor confirms the MRI characterization of the tumor location, size, and morphology. **F,** Histology of the tumor shows features of rhabdomyoma (hematoxylin-eosin stain). (See also Color Section for Parts E and F)

tissue in question. First-pass myocardial perfusion, early and late enhancement after intravenous administration of gadolinium-based contrast agent, and myocardial tagging can provide additional diagnostic information about tissue characteristics.

Heart failure resulting from iron overload can develop as a result of either excess dietary absorption (hereditary hemochromatosis) or repeated blood transfusions. The most common clinical scenario of cardiac iron overload is seen in patients with thalassemia major, for whom heart failure remains the major cause of death despite the introduction of the iron-chelating agent desferrioxamine.[247] Because of the difficulties in administering desferrioxamine, focusing the most inten-

sive regimens on patients at greatest risk is an important clinical aim. Establishing individual cardiovascular risk is problematic, however, because there is no single parameter able to establish with precision the cardiac iron burden. Although liver biopsy can give a fairly accurate assessment of total body iron burden, there is dissociation between liver and heart iron accumulation. Endomyocardial biopsy has sampling errors, and its invasive nature makes it poorly suited to repeated follow-up assessments. Echocardiography is useful to detect impairment in ventricular systolic function; however, this is a late manifestation of iron overload. Cardiovascular MRI has the potential to quantify the myocardial iron content and help clinicians identify

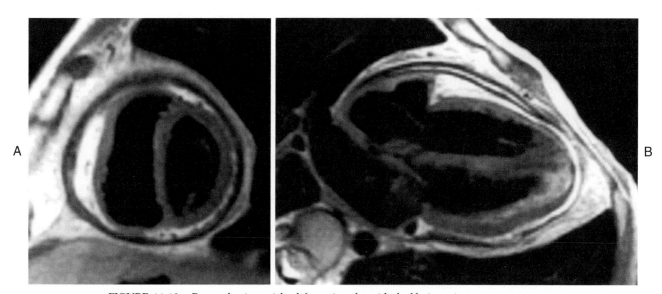

FIGURE 11-12 ■ Proton density–weighted fast spin echo with double inversion recovery sequence. ECG-triggered, breath-hold, proton density–weighted fast spin echo with double inversion recovery images show a markedly thickened pericardium in a 13-year-old girl with constrictive pericarditis. **A,** Short axis plane. **B,** Four-chamber plane.

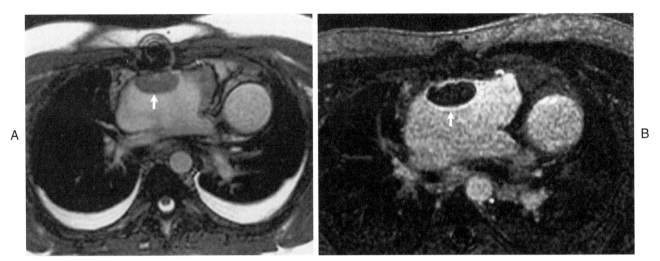

FIGURE 11-13 ■ MRI tissue characterization. MRI evaluation of an intracardiac thrombus in a patient with an atriopulmonary Fontan circulation. **A,** ECG-triggered, breath-hold, steady-state free precession sequence in the axial plane shows a large mobile thrombus *(arrow)* attached to the anterior right atrial wall. Pleural effusion is seen as a bright signal in the posterior aspect of the thorax. **B,** An ECG-triggered, breath-hold gradient echo sequence ordinarily used for assessment of myocardial viability (so-called delayed myocardial enhancement) obtained 2 to 3 minutes after administration of gadopentetate dimeglumine. Note the sharp distinction between the thrombus *(arrow)* and the surrounding blood pool.

patients requiring intensive chelation before they develop systolic dysfunction and the morbidity and mortality associated with overt heart failure. Because iron has strong paramagnetic properties, increasing iron concentration within the liver and myocardium results in a greater signal loss on T1-weighted, T2-weighted, and T2*-weighted imaging (Fig. 11-14). This phenomenon can be exploited to quantify noninvasively the iron load in liver and myocardium and monitor response to chelation therapy. Anderson and colleagues[248,249] developed a gradient echo MRI protocol to measure the T2* parameter of myocardium and liver, with shorter T2* values indicating a higher iron concentration. Using a cardiac-gated fast gradient echo sequence, these investigators imaged the heart at the mid-ventricular level in short axis with varying echo times. The T2* value of a specified region of myocardium was calculated by plotting the signal intensity of that region versus the echo time. In a study of 106 patients with thalassemia major, they showed a progressive decline in ejection fraction as myocardial T2* decreased. There was no significant correlation between myocardial T2* and the conventional parameters of iron status, serum ferritin, and liver iron. Although this approach has promise, larger studies that include longitudinal data are necessary to show whether this cardiovascular MRI technique could truly identify patients at increased risk for heart failure.

MRI SAFETY CONSIDERATIONS

Standard clinical imaging scanners present no known hazards to biologic materials. Guidelines set by the U.S.

Food and Drug Administration keep the strength of the magnetic fields and the deposition of radiofrequency energy well below levels that could cause significant biologic effects. Animal studies evaluating the influence of static magnetic fields have not shown significant biologic effects for fields of 2 Tesla.[250] Millions of patients have undergone MRI studies without any noticeable immediate or long-term sequelae. Pregnancy is presently

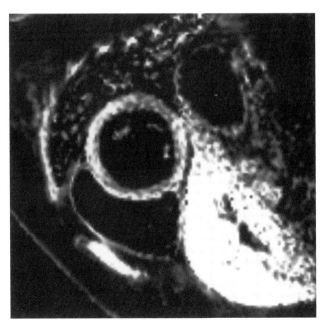

FIGURE 11-14 ■ MRI tissue characterization. Color-coded T2* map of myocardial iron load in a patient with thalassemia. Signal is brighter in the liver compared with the myocardium, indicating higher iron concentration in the liver (see text for discussion). (See also Color Section)

a relative contraindication to MRI, although the magnetic field levels used in clinical imagers have no known effects on the embryo. Many women have undergone MRI during all trimesters of pregnancy without reported ill effect on the mother, fetus, or resultant infant. When maternal and fetal health considerations require diagnostic studies, MRI is preferable to methods that employ x-rays, such as CT or angiography.

Implanted metallic objects are of particular concern in the MRI environment because they potentially could undergo undesirable movements if the magnetic field was sufficiently strong and if they contained sufficient ferromagnetic material. Surgical clips and sternotomy wires implanted in the chest and abdomen are typically only weakly ferromagnetic. These devices quickly become immobilized by surrounding fibrous tissue, and MRI can be used safely to study patients with these implants. The wires and clips may cause image artifact, however. Similarly, MRI can be used to image patients with implanted intravascular coils, stents, and occluding devices when the implants are believed to be immobile. Many centers choose to avoid exposing these patients to MRI for an arbitrarily chosen period of time after implantation (usually for several weeks), but such practice is not supported by conclusive published data. A decision to perform MRI shortly after cardiac surgery or implantation of a biomedical device must weigh the risk-to-benefit ratio for the individual patient.[251]

Numerous devices are considered either a relative or an absolute contraindication to MRI.[251-256] Presence of an intracranial, intraocular, or intracochlear metallic object is considered a contraindication to MRI. The presence of a cardiac pacemaker also is considered a contraindication to MRI,[257] although some reports have suggested that scanning patients who have modern pacemakers may be possible.[258,259]

Because MRI scanners attract ferromagnetic objects, extreme caution should be employed in approaching magnets with objects containing iron or other ferromagnetic materials. Only specially designed MRI-compatible physiologic monitoring equipment should be used in conjunction with MRI studies. There have been several reported cases of patient burns resulting from the use of MRI-incompatible pulse oximeters and ECG monitoring devices.

CURRENT STATUS AND FUTURE TRENDS

Since the mid-1990s, the field of cardiovascular MRI has seen dramatic progress in technical capabilities and clinical applications. Major advances in hardware design, new pulse sequences, and faster image reconstruction techniques allow rapid acquisition of high-resolution images of cardiovascular structures. Current cardio-vascular MRI techniques provide comprehensive assessments of cardiovascular anatomy and function, including quantitative assessments of ventricular dimensions and function, assessments of myocardial function, regurgitation fractions, perfusion and viability, quantification of blood flow rate, and tissue characterization.

As survival for palliative and corrective surgeries continues to improve, serial follow-up with accurate noninvasive imaging, particularly with MRI, becomes even more essential. The future of MRI in assessing a patient with heart failure is virtually unlimited for delineation of anatomy and determination of function and characterization of tissue. The escalation of new technologic advances and innovations in this field of study will continue to improve the capability of MRI to attain important diagnostic information in patients with congenital and acquired pediatric heart disease.[262,263]

Key Concepts

■ ECG-triggered or VCG-triggered SSFP is currently the most commonly used cine MRI technique for assessment of ventricular function. The SSFP sequence relies on the ratio of T2-to-T1 relaxations with a resultant high contrast between the blood pool (T2/T1 = 360/1200 = 0.3) and the myocardium (T2/T1 = 75/880 = 0.085), which clearly depicts the boundaries of cardiovascular structures.

■ Ventricular volume is determined by summation of the volumes of all slices, and this process can be repeated for each frame in the cardiac cycle to obtain a continuous time-volume loop or may be performed only on end-diastolic (maximal area) and end-systolic (minimal area) frames to calculate diastolic and systolic volumes. From these data, one can calculate left and right ventricular ejection fractions and stroke volumes.

■ The combination of a three-dimensional dataset, clear distinction between the blood pool and the myocardium, and high spatial and temporal resolutions allows for accurate measurements of any cardiac chamber regardless of its morphology and without geometric assumptions.

■ A simple qualitative approach is to evaluate visually segmental ventricular wall motion and thickening imaged from long-axis and short-axis gradient echo (SSFP or fast GRE) cine MRI. Ventricular wall motion is classified as normal (appropriate systolic wall motion toward the center of the ventricle accompanied by myocardial thickening indicative of fiber shortening), hypokinesis (reduced systolic motion and wall thickening), akinesis (no appreciable systolic wall motion and no change in wall thickness), or dyskinesis (outward systolic wall motion without myocardial thickening).

■ Analysis of myocardial strain provides information on regional myocardial function. Although myocardial strain can be calculated from velocity information obtained by phase velocity cine MRI technique (similar to tissue Doppler imaging), most investigators favor a technique called myocardial tagging using SPAMM. A more recently described technique for the analysis of myocardial tagging data, HARP, greatly shortens analysis time because it does not require manual tracing of the tags.

■ There is a growing body of literature on the use of dobutamine stress cardiovascular MRI in the evaluation of myocardial ischemia in adults with coronary artery disease. Several studies have evaluated the use of stress cardiovascular MRI in patients with congenital heart disease.

■ As the importance of diastole in many pathologic conditions affecting the cardiovascular system has come into focus, researchers have used various modalities and a wide array of parameters to assess diastolic function. Changes of pressure and chamber dimensions can be assessed invasively by catheterization; nuclear scintigraphy can evaluate ventricular filling; and echocardiography and Doppler ultrasound can measure changes of ventricular dimensions, wall thinning, a wide range of flow-derived variables obtained by Doppler interrogation of the atrioventricular valves and pulmonary veins, myocardial velocities assessed by tissue Doppler imaging, and myocardial strain. With the exception of direct pressure measurements, all of the aforementioned variables also can be evaluated by MRI.

■ Currently the two most widely used cardiovascular MRI techniques to detect ischemia are dobutamine stress cardiovascular MRI and first-pass myocardial perfusion. In addition to detection of ischemia, cardiovascular MRI can be used to differentiate viable from nonviable myocardium (e.g., infarct). MDE imaging has become the dominant MRI technique to assess viability.

■ Cardiovascular MRI is the most reproducible imaging modality for assessment of left ventricular and right ventricular volumes, mass, and ejection fractions. Cardiovascular MRI can assess myocardial morphology, regional function (e.g., wall strain and stress), perfusion, viability, and metabolism.

■ An ECG-gated VEC MRI sequence, a type of gradient echo sequence, can be used to measure blood flow velocity and quantify blood flow rate. Site-specific quantification of flow rate, flow velocity, stroke volume, and minute flow in principle can be measured across any blood vessel within the central cardiovascular system.

■ Assessments of the myocardium, pericardium, blood vessel wall, and extracardiac tissue for pathologic changes can be valuable in patients with heart failure. MRI offers a distinct advantage over other modalities when it comes to evaluation of soft tissues because of its ability to discern even minor changes in tissue composition.

REFERENCES

1. Geva T: Future directions of congenital heart disease imaging. Pediatr Cardiol 2002;23:117-121.
2. Ehman RL, Julsrud PR: Magnetic resonance imaging of the heart: Current status. Mayo Clin Proc 1989;64:1134-1146.
3. Link KM, Formanek AG: MR imaging in congenital heart disease: Where is the leading edge? Ann Radiol (Paris) 1989;32:15-21.
4. Strohm O, Schulz-Menger J, Pilz B, et al: Measurement of left ventricular dimensions and function in patients with dilated cardiomyopathy. J Magn Reson Imaging 2001;13:367-371.
5. Nishimura T, Nagata S, Sakakibara H: Magnetic resonance imaging in familial hypertrophic cardiomyopathy associated with abnormal thallium perfusion and cardiac enzymes. Jpn Circ J 1988;52:395-400.
6. Shiota T, McCarthy PM, White RD, et al: Initial clinical experience of real-time three-dimensional echocardiography in patients with ischemic and idiopathic dilated cardiomyopathy. Am J Cardiol 1999;84:1068-1073.
7. Wilson JM, Villareal RP, Hariharan R, et al: Magnetic resonance imaging of myocardial fibrosis in hypertrophic cardiomyopathy. Tex Heart Inst J 2002;29:176-180.
8. Di Cesare E: MRI of the cardiomyopathies. Eur J Radiol 2001; 38:179-184.
9. Devlin AM, Moore NR, Ostman-Smith I: A comparison of MRI and echocardiography in hypertrophic cardiomyopathy. Br J Radiol 1999;72:258-264.
10. Roditi GH, Hartnell GG, Cohen MC: MRI changes in myocarditis— evaluation with spin echo, cine MR angiography and contrast enhanced spin echo imaging. Clin Radiol 2000;55:752-758.
11. Frank H, Globits S: Magnetic resonance imaging evaluation of myocardial and pericardial disease. J Magn Reson Imaging 1999;10:617-626.
12. Friedrich MG, Strohm O, Schulz-Menger J, et al: Contrast media-enhanced magnetic resonance imaging visualizes myocardial changes in the course of viral myocarditis. Circulation 1998; 97:1802-1809.
13. Bocchi EA, Kalil R, Bacal F, et al: Magnetic resonance imaging in chronic Chagas' disease: Correlation with endomyocardial biopsy findings and gallium-67 cardiac uptake. Echocardiography 1998;15:279-288.
14. Marie PY, Angioi M, Carteaux JP, et al: Detection and prediction of acute heart transplant rejection with the myocardial T2 determination provided by a black-blood magnetic resonance imaging sequence. J Am Coll Cardiol 2001;37:825-831.
15. Lukes DJ, Madhu B, Kjellstrom C, et al: Decreasing ratios of phosphocreatine to beta-ATP correlates to progressive acute rejection in a concordant mouse heart to rat xenotransplantation model. Scand J Immunol 2001;53:171-175.
16. Kanno S, Wu YJ, Lee PC, et al: Macrophage accumulation associated with rat cardiac allograft rejection detected by magnetic resonance imaging with ultrasmall superparamagnetic iron oxide particles. Circulation 2001;104:934-938.
17. Beckmann N, Hof RP, Rudin M: The role of magnetic resonance imaging and spectroscopy in transplantation: From animal models to man. NMR Biomed 2000;13:329-348.
18. Walpoth BH, Muller MF, Celik B, et al: Assessment of cardiac rejection by MR-imaging and MR-spectroscopy. Eur J Cardiothorac Surg 1998;14:426-430.
19. Mousseaux E, Farge D, Guillemain R, et al: Assessing human cardiac allograft rejection using MRI with Gd-DOTA. J Comput Assist Tomogr 1993;17:237-244.
20. Davis SF, Kannam JP, Wielopolski P, et al: Magnetic resonance coronary angiography in heart transplant recipients. J Heart Lung Transplant 1996;15:580-586.
21. Kiaffas MG, Powell AJ, Geva T: Magnetic resonance imaging evaluation of cardiac tumor characteristics in infants and children. Am J Cardiol 2002;89:1229-1233.

22. Villacampa VM, Villarreal M, Ros LH, et al: Cardiac rhabdomyosarcoma: Diagnosis by MR imaging. Eur Radiol 1999;9:634-637.

23. Siripornpitak S, Higgins CB: MRI of primary malignant cardiovascular tumors. J Comput Assist Tomogr 1997;21:462-466.

24. Greil GF, Stuber M, Botnar RM, et al: Coronary magnetic resonance angiography in adolescents and young adults with Kawasaki disease. Circulation 2002;105:908-911.

25. Edelman RR, Manning WJ: Magnetic resonance angiography and flow quantification of coronary arteries. Magn Reson Imaging Clin N Am 1993;1:339-347.

26. Manning WJ, Li W, Cohen SI, et al: Improved definition of anomalous left coronary artery by magnetic resonance coronary angiography. Am Heart J 1995;130:615-617.

27. McConnell MV, Stuber M, Manning WJ: Clinical role of coronary magnetic resonance angiography in the diagnosis of anomalous coronary arteries. J Cardiovasc Magn Reson 2000;2:217-224.

28. Danias PG, Stuber M, McConnell MV, Manning WJ: The diagnosis of congenital coronary anomalies with magnetic resonance imaging. Coron Artery Dis 2001;12:621-626.

29. Jensen PD, Jensen FT, Christensen T, et al: Indirect evidence for the potential ability of magnetic resonance imaging to evaluate the myocardial iron content in patients with transfusional iron overload. Magma 2001;12:153-166.

30. Ooi GC, Chen FE, Chan KN, et al: Qualitative and quantitative magnetic resonance imaging in haemoglobin H disease: Screening for iron overload. Clin Radiol 1999;54:98-102.

31. Mavrogeni SI, Gotsis ED, Markussis V, et al: T2 relaxation time study of iron overload in b-thalassemia. Magma 1998;6:7-12.

32. Helbing WA, Niezen RA, Le Cessie S, et al: Right ventricular diastolic function in children with pulmonary regurgitation after repair of tetralogy of Fallot: Volumetric evaluation by magnetic resonance velocity mapping. J Am Coll Cardiol 1996;28:1827-1835.

33. Vliegen HW, Van Straten A, De Roos A, et al: Magnetic resonance imaging to assess the hemodynamic effects of pulmonary valve replacement in adults late after repair of tetralogy of Fallot. Circulation 2002;106:1703-1707.

34. Colletti PM, DeFrance A, Tak T, et al: Cardiac MRI cine and color Doppler in valvular disease: Correlative imaging. Magn Reson Imaging 1991;9:343-347.

35. Breen JF: Imaging of the pericardium. J Thorac Imaging 2001;16:47-54.

36. White CS: MR evaluation of the pericardium. Top Magn Reson Imaging 1995;7:258-266.

37. Midiri M, Finazzo M: MR imaging of arrhythmogenic right ventricular dysplasia. Int J Cardiovasc Imaging 2001;17:297-304.

38. van der Wall EE, Kayser HW, Bootsma MM, et al: Arrhythmogenic right ventricular dysplasia: MRI findings. Herz 2000;25:356-364.

39. Takahashi N, Ishida Y, Maeno M, et al: Noninvasive identification of left ventricular involvements in arrhythmogenic right ventricular dysplasia: Comparison of 123I-MIBG, 201TlCl, magnetic resonance imaging and ultrafast computed tomography. Ann Nucl Med 1997;11:233-241.

40. Mulkern RV, Chung T: From signal to image: Magnetic resonance imaging physics for cardiac magnetic resonance. Pediatr Cardiol 2000;21:5-17.

41. Sodickson D: Clinical cardiovascular magnetic resonance imaging techniques. In Pennel D (ed): Cardiovascular Magnetic Resonance. New York, Churchill Livingstone, 2002, pp 18-30.

42. Larson AC, White RD, Laub G, et al: Self-gated cardiac cine MRI. Magn Reson Med 2004;51:93-102.

43. Weiger M, Pruessmann KP, Boesiger P: Cardiac real-time imaging using SENSE: SENSitivity Encoding scheme. Magn Reson Med 2000;43:177-184.

44. Setser RM, Fischer SE, Lorenz CH: Quantification of left ventricular function with magnetic resonance images acquired in real time. J Magn Reson Imaging 2000;12:430-438.

45. Carr JC, Simonetti O, Bundy J, et al: Cine MR angiography of the heart with segmented true fast imaging with steady-state precession. Radiology 2001;219:828-834.

46. Bax JJ, Lamb H, Dibbets P, et al: Comparison of gated single-photon emission computed tomography with magnetic resonance imaging for evaluation of left ventricular function in ischemic cardiomyopathy. Am J Cardiol 2000;86:1299-1305.

47. Bellenger NG, Marcus NJ, Davies C, et al: Left ventricular function and mass after orthotopic heart transplantation: A comparison of cardiovascular magnetic resonance with echocardiography. J Heart Lung Transplant 2000;19:444-452.

48. Bellenger NG, Burgess MI, Ray SG, et al: Comparison of left ventricular ejection fraction and volumes in heart failure by echocardiography, radionuclide ventriculography and cardiovascular magnetic resonance: Are they interchangeable? Eur Heart J 2000;21:1387-1396.

49. Kaji S, Yang PC, Kerr AB, et al: Rapid evaluation of left ventricular volume and mass without breath-holding using real-time interactive cardiac magnetic resonance imaging system. J Am Coll Cardiol 2001;38:527-533.

50. Schalla S, Nagel E, Lehmkuhl H, et al: Comparison of magnetic resonance real-time imaging of left ventricular function with conventional magnetic resonance imaging and echocardiography. Am J Cardiol 2001;87:95-99.

51. Fu JC, Chai JW, Wong ST: Wavelet-based enhancement for detection of left ventricular myocardial boundaries in magnetic resonance images. Magn Reson Imaging 2000;18:1135-1141.

52. Makowski P, Sorensen TS, Therkildsen SV, et al: Two-phase active contour method for semiautomatic segmentation of the heart and blood vessels from MRI images for 3D visualization. Comput Med Imaging Graph 2002;26:9-17.

53. Zimmer Y, Akselrod S: An automatic contour extraction algorithm for short-axis cardiac magnetic resonance images. Med Phys 1996;23:1371-1379.

54. Yezzi A Jr, Kichenassamy S, Kumar A, et al: A geometric snake model for segmentation of medical imagery. IEEE Trans Med Imaging 1997;16:199-209.

55. Holland AE, Goldfarb JW, Edelman RR: Diaphragmatic and cardiac motion during suspended breathing: Preliminary experience and implications for breath-hold MR imaging. Radiology 1998;209:483-489.

56. Raichura N, Entwisle J, Leverment J, Beardsmore CS: Breath-hold MRI in evaluating patients with pectus excavatum. Br J Radiol 2001;74:701-708.

57. Ostrzega E, Maddahi J, Honma H, et al: Quantification of left ventricular myocardial mass in humans by nuclear magnetic resonance imaging. Am Heart J 1989;117:444-452.

58. Maddahi J, Crues J, Berman DS, et al: Noninvasive quantification of left ventricular myocardial mass by gated proton nuclear magnetic resonance imaging. J Am Coll Cardiol 1987;10:682-692.

59. Keller AM, Peshock RM, Malloy CR, et al: In vivo measurement of myocardial mass using nuclear magnetic resonance imaging. J Am Coll Cardiol 1986;8:113-117.

60. Katz J, Milliken MC, Stray-Gundersen J, et al: Estimation of human myocardial mass with MR imaging. Radiology 1988;169:495-498.

61. Florentine MS, Grosskreutz CL, Chang W, et al: Measurement of left ventricular mass in vivo using gated nuclear magnetic resonance imaging. J Am Coll Cardiol 1986;8:107-112.

62. Caputo GR, Tscholakoff D, Sechtem U, Higgins CB: Measurement of canine left ventricular mass by using MR imaging. AJR Am J Roentgenol 1987;148:33-38.

63. Koch JA, Poll LW, Godehardt E, et al: In vitro determination of cardiac ventricular volumes using MRI at 1.0 T in a porcine heart model. Int J Cardiovasc Imaging 2001;17:237-242.

64. Semelka RC, Tomei E, Wagner S, et al: Interstudy reproducibility of dimensional and functional measurements between cine

magnetic resonance studies in the morphologically abnormal left ventricle. Am Heart J 1990;119:1367-1373.

65. Semelka RC, Tomei E, Wagner S, et al: Normal left ventricular dimensions and function: Interstudy reproducibility of measurements with cine MR imaging. Radiology 1990;174:763-768.

66. Doherty NE 3rd, Fujita N, Caputo GR, Higgins CB: Measurement of right ventricular mass in normal and dilated cardiomyopathic ventricles using cine magnetic resonance imaging. Am J Cardiol 1992;69:1223-1228.

67. Doherty NE 3rd, Seelos KC, Suzuki J, et al: Application of cine nuclear magnetic resonance imaging for sequential evaluation of response to angiotensin-converting enzyme inhibitor therapy in dilated cardiomyopathy. J Am Coll Cardiol 1992;19:1294-1302.

68. Germain P, Roul G, Kastler B, et al: Inter-study variability in left ventricular mass measurement: Comparison between M-mode echography and MRI. Eur Heart J 1992;13:1011-1019.

69. Bellenger NG, Davies LC, Francis JM, et al: Reduction in sample size for studies of remodeling in heart failure by the use of cardiovascular magnetic resonance. J Cardiovasc Magn Reson 2000;2:271-278.

70. Ioannidis JP, Trikalinos TA, Danias PG: Electrocardiogram-gated single-photon emission computed tomography versus cardiac magnetic resonance imaging for the assessment of left ventricular volumes and ejection fraction: A meta-analysis. J Am Coll Cardiol 2002;39:2059-2068.

71. Plein S, Bloomer TN, Ridgway JP, et al: Steady-state free precession magnetic resonance imaging of the heart: Comparison with segmented k-space gradient-echo imaging. J Magn Reson Imaging 2001;14:230-236.

72. Alfakih K, Thiele H, Plein S, et al: Comparison of right ventricular volume measurement between segmented k-space gradient-echo and steady-state free precession magnetic resonance imaging. J Magn Reson Imaging 2002;16:253-258.

73. Alfakih K, Plein S, Thiele H, et al: Normal human left and right ventricular dimensions for MRI as assessed by turbo gradient echo and steady-state free precession imaging sequences. J Magn Reson Imaging 2003;17:323-329.

74. Colan SD: Assessment of ventricular and myocardial performance. In Fyler DC (ed): Nadas' Pediatric Cardiology. Philadelphia, Hanley & Belfus, 1992, pp 225-248.

75. Regen DM: Calculation of left ventricular wall stress. Circ Res 1990;67:245-252.

76. Setser RM, Sayre K, Flacke S, et al: Assessment of ventricular contractility during cardiac magnetic resonance imaging examinations using normalized maximal ventricular power. Ann Biomed Eng 2001;29:974-982.

77. Cerqueira MD, Weissman NJ, Dilsizian V, et al: Standardized myocardial segmentation and nomenclature for tomographic imaging of the heart: A statement for healthcare professionals from the Cardiac Imaging Committee of the Council on Clinical Cardiology of the American Heart Association. Circulation 2002;105:539-542.

78. Klein SS, Graham TP Jr, Lorenz CH: Noninvasive delineation of normal right ventricular contractile motion with magnetic resonance imaging myocardial tagging. Ann Biomed Eng 1998;26:756-763.

79. Lamb HJ, Singleton RR, van der Geest RJ, et al: MR imaging of regional cardiac function: Low-pass filtering of wall thickness curves. Magn Reson Med 1995;34:498-502.

80. Reichek N: MRI myocardial tagging. J Magn Reson Imaging 1999;10:609-616.

81. Fogel MA: Assessment of cardiac function by magnetic resonance imaging. Pediatr Cardiol 2000;21:59-69.

82. Haber I, Metaxas DN, Axel L: Three-dimensional motion reconstruction and analysis of the right ventricle using tagged MRI. Med Image Anal 2000;4:335-355.

83. Garot J, Bluemke DA, Osman NF, et al: Fast determination of regional myocardial strain fields from tagged cardiac images using harmonic phase MRI. Circulation 2000;101:981-988.

84. Sampath S, Derbyshire JA, Atalar E, et al: Real-time imaging of two-dimensional cardiac strain using a harmonic phase magnetic resonance imaging (HARP-MRI) pulse sequence. Magn Reson Med 2003;50:154-163.

85. Kuijer JP, Marcus JT, Gotte MJ, et al: Simultaneous MRI tagging and through-plane velocity quantification: A three-dimensional myocardial motion tracking algorithm. J Magn Reson Imaging 1999;9:409-419.

86. Fonseca CG, Oxenham HC, Cowan BR, et al: Aging alters patterns of regional nonuniformity in LV strain relaxation: A 3-D MR tissue tagging study. Am J Physiol Heart Circ Physiol 2003;285:H621-H630.

87. Oxenham HC, Young AA, Cowan BR, et al: Age-related changes in myocardial relaxation using three-dimensional tagged magnetic resonance imaging. J Cardiovasc Magn Reson 2003;5:421-430.

88. Tustison NJ, Davila-Roman VG, Amini AA: Myocardial kinematics from tagged MRI based on a 4-D B-spline model. IEEE Trans Biomed Eng 2003;50:1038-1040.

89. McVeigh ER, Atalar E: Cardiac tagging with breath-hold cine MRI. Magn Reson Med 1992;28:318-327.

90. Azhari H, Weiss JL, Shapiro EP: Distribution of myocardial strains: An MRI study. Adv Exp Med Biol 1995;382:319-328.

91. Matter C, Nagel E, Stuber M, et al: Assessment of systolic and diastolic LV function by MR myocardial tagging. Basic Res Cardiol 1996;91(Suppl 2):23-28.

92. Moulton MJ, Creswell LL, Downing SW, et al: Myocardial material property determination in the in vivo heart using magnetic resonance imaging. Int J Card Imaging 1996;12:153-167.

93. Park J, Metaxas D, Axel L: Analysis of left ventricular wall motion based on volumetric deformable models and MRI-SPAMM. Med Image Anal 1996;1:53-71.

94. Dong SJ, Hees PS, Huang WM, et al: Independent effects of preload, afterload, and contractility on left ventricular torsion. Am J Physiol 1999;277:H1053-H1060.

95. Wyman BT, Hunter WC, Prinzen FW, McVeigh ER: Mapping propagation of mechanical activation in the paced heart with MRI tagging. Am J Physiol 1999;276:H881-H891.

96. O'Dell WG, McCulloch AD: Imaging three-dimensional cardiac function. Annu Rev Biomed Eng 2000;2:431-456.

97. Osman NF, Prince JL: Visualizing myocardial function using HARP MRI. Phys Med Biol 2000;45:1665-1682.

98. Ozturk C, McVeigh ER: Four-dimensional B-spline based motion analysis of tagged MR images: Introduction and in vivo validation. Phys Med Biol 2000;45:1683-1702.

99. Power TP, Kramer CM, Shaffer AL, et al: Breath-hold dobutamine magnetic resonance myocardial tagging: Normal left ventricular response. Am J Cardiol 1997;80:1203-1207.

100. Marcus JT, Gotte MJ, Van Rossum AC, et al: Myocardial function in infarcted and remote regions early after infarction in man: Assessment by magnetic resonance tagging and strain analysis. Magn Reson Med 1997;38:803-810.

101. Chin BB, Esposito G, Kraitchman DL: Myocardial contractile reserve and perfusion defect severity with rest and stress dobutamine (99m)Tc-sestamibi SPECT in canine stunning and subendocardial infarction. J Nucl Med 2002;43:540-550.

102. Saito I, Watanabe S, Masuda Y: Detection of viable myocardium by dobutamine stress tagging magnetic resonance imaging with three-dimensional analysis by automatic trace method. Jpn Circ J 2000;64:487-494.

103. Nagel E, Fleck E: Functional MRI in ischemic heart disease based on detection of contraction abnormalities. J Magn Reson Imaging 1999;10:411-417.

104. Mankad R, McCreery CJ, Rogers WJ Jr, et al: Regional myocardial strain before and after mitral valve repair for severe mitral regurgitation. J Cardiovasc Magn Reson 2001;3:257-266.

105. Ungacta FF, Davila-Roman VG, Moulton MJ, et al: MRI-radiofrequency tissue tagging in patients with aortic insufficiency before and after operation. Ann Thorac Surg1998;65:943-950.

106. Geskin G, Kramer CM, Rogers WJ, et al: Quantitative assessment of myocardial viability after infarction by dobutamine magnetic resonance tagging. Circulation 1998;98:217-223.

107. Kramer CM, Rogers WJ, Geskin G, et al: Usefulness of magnetic resonance imaging early after acute myocardial infarction. Am J Cardiol 1997;80:690-695.

108. Kramer CM, Rogers WJ, Theobald TM, et al: Dissociation between changes in intramyocardial function and left ventricular volumes in the eight weeks after first anterior myocardial infarction. J Am Coll Cardiol 1997;30:1625-1632.

109. Kraitchman DL, Wilke N, Hexeberg E, et al: Myocardial perfusion and function in dogs with moderate coronary stenosis. Magn Reson Med 1996;35:771-780.

110. Azhari H, Weiss JL, Rogers WJ, et al: A noninvasive comparative study of myocardial strains in ischemic canine hearts using tagged MRI in 3-D. Am J Physiol 1995;268:H1918-H1926.

111. Setser RM, White RD, Sturm B, et al: Noninvasive assessment of cardiac mechanics and clinical outcome after partial left ventriculectomy. Ann Thorac Surg 2003;76:1576-1586.

112. Kuijpers D, Ho KY, van Dijkman PR, et al: Dobutamine cardiovascular magnetic resonance for the detection of myocardial ischemia with the use of myocardial tagging. Circulation 2003;107:1592-1597.

113. Fogel MA, Weinberg PM, Fellows KE, Hoffman EA: A study in ventricular-ventricular interaction: Single right ventricles compared with systemic right ventricles in a dual-chamber circulation. Circulation 1995;92:219-230.

114. Fogel MA, Gupta KB, Weinberg PM, Hoffman EA: Regional wall motion and strain analysis across stages of Fontan reconstruction by magnetic resonance tagging. Am J Physiol 1995;269:H1132-H1152.

115. Fogel MA, Weinberg PM, Chin AJ, et al: Late ventricular geometry and performance changes of functional single ventricle throughout staged Fontan reconstruction assessed by magnetic resonance imaging. J Am Coll Cardiol 1996;28:212-221.

116. Fogel MA, Weinberg PM, Gupta KB, et al: Mechanics of the single left ventricle: A study in ventricular-ventricular interaction II. Circulation 1998;98:330-338.

117. Tulevski II, van der Wall EE, Groenink M, et al: Usefulness of magnetic resonance imaging dobutamine stress in asymptomatic and minimally symptomatic patients with decreased cardiac reserve from congenital heart disease (complete and corrected transposition of the great arteries and subpulmonic obstruction). Am J Cardiol 2002;89:1077-1081.

118. Tulevski II, Lee PL, Groenink M, et al: Dobutamine-induced increase of right ventricular contractility without increased stroke volume in adolescent patients with transposition of the great arteries: Evaluation with magnetic resonance imaging. Int J Cardiac Imaging 2000;16:471-478.

119. Dodge-Khatami A, Tulevski II, Bennink GB, et al: Comparable systemic ventricular function in healthy adults and patients with unoperated congenitally corrected transposition using MRI dobutamine stress testing. Ann Thorac Surg 2002;73:1759-1764.

120. Roest AA, Kunz P, Lamb HJ, et al: Biventricular response to supine physical exercise in young adults assessed with ultrafast magnetic resonance imaging. Am J Cardiol 2001;87:601-605.

121. Grossman W: Diastolic function and heart failure: An overview. Eur Heart J 1990;11(Suppl C):2-7.

122. Mohiaddin RH, Amanuma M, Kilner PJ, et al: MR phase-shift velocity mapping of mitral and pulmonary venous flow. J Comput Assist Tomogr 1991;15:237-243.

123. Suzuki J, Chang JM, Caputo GR, Higgins CB: Evaluation of right ventricular early diastolic filling by cine nuclear magnetic resonance imaging in patients with hypertrophic cardiomyopathy. J Am Coll Cardiol 1991;18:120-126.

124. Hartiala JJ, Mostbeck GH, Foster E, et al: Velocity-encoded cine MRI in the evaluation of left ventricular diastolic function: Measurement of mitral valve and pulmonary vein flow velocities and flow volume across the mitral valve. Am Heart J 1993;125:1054-1066.

125. Hoff FL, Turner DA, Wang JZ, et al: Semiautomatic evaluation of left ventricular diastolic function with cine magnetic resonance imaging. Acad Radiol 1994;1:237-242.

126. Schwammenthal E, Wichter T, Joachimsen K, et al: Detection of regional left ventricular asynchrony in obstructive hypertrophic cardiomyopathy by magnetic resonance imaging. Am Heart J 1994;127:600-606.

127. Dendale PA, Franken PR, Waldman GJ, et al: Regional diastolic wall motion dynamics in anterior myocardial infarction: Analysis and quantification with magnetic resonance imaging. Coron Artery Dis 1995;6:723-729.

128. Mohiaddin RH, Hasegawa M: Measurement of atrial volumes by magnetic resonance imaging in healthy volunteers and in patients with myocardial infarction. Eur Heart J 1995;16:106-111.

129. Kudelka AM, Turner DA, Liebson PR, et al: Comparison of cine magnetic resonance imaging and Doppler echocardiography for evaluation of left ventricular diastolic function. Am J Cardiol 1997;80:384-386.

130. Eroglu AG, Sarioglu A, Sarioglu T: Right ventricular diastolic function after repair of tetralogy of Fallot: Its relationship to the insertion of a 'transannular' patch. Cardiol Young 1999;9:384-391.

131. Fogel MA, Weinberg PM, Hubbard A, Haselgrove J: Diastolic biomechanics in normal infants utilizing MRI tissue tagging. Circulation 2000;102:218-224.

132. Kroft LJ, Simons P, van Laar JM, de Roos A: Patients with pulmonary fibrosis: Cardiac function assessed with MR imaging. Radiology 2000;216:464-471.

133. Lorenz CH, Flacke S, Fischer SE: Noninvasive modalities: Cardiac MR imaging. Cardiol Clin 2000;18:557-570.

134. Dong SJ, Hees PS, Siu CO, et al: MRI assessment of LV relaxation by untwisting rate: A new isovolumic phase measure of tau. Am J Physiol Heart Circ Physiol 2001;281:H2002-H2009.

135. Paelinck BP, Lamb HJ, Bax JJ, et al: Assessment of diastolic function by cardiovascular magnetic resonance. Am Heart J 2002;144:198-205.

136. Young AA, Cowan BR, Occleshaw CJ, et al: Temporal evolution of left ventricular strain late after repair of coarctation of the aorta using 3D MR tissue tagging. J Cardiovasc Magn Reson 2002;4:233-243.

137. Mandinov L, Eberli FR, Seiler C, Hess OM: Diastolic heart failure. Cardiovasc Res 2000;45:813-825.

138. Taylor AJ, Bergin JD: Noninvasive assessment of systolic and diastolic function: Important clues to differentiating types of congestive heart failure. Postgrad Med 1993;94:55-70.

139. Prakash A, Powell AJ, Krishnamurthy R, Geva T: Magnetic resonance imaging evaluation of myocardial perfusion and viability in congenital and acquired pediatric heart disease. Am J Cardiol 2004;93:657-661.

140. Nagel E, Lehmkuhl HB, Bocksch W, et al: Noninvasive diagnosis of ischemia-induced wall motion abnormalities with the use of high-dose dobutamine stress MRI: Comparison with dobutamine stress echocardiography. Circulation 1999;99:763-770.

141. Hundley WG, Hamilton CA, Thomas MS, et al: Utility of fast cine magnetic resonance imaging and display for the detection of myocardial ischemia in patients not well suited for second harmonic stress echocardiography. Circulation 1999;100:1697-1702.

142. Kraitchman DL, Sampath S, Castillo E, et al: Quantitative ischemia detection during cardiac magnetic resonance stress testing by use of FastHARP. Circulation 2003;107:2025-2030.

143. Nagel E, Klein C, Paetsch I, et al: Magnetic resonance perfusion measurements for the noninvasive detection of coronary artery disease. Circulation 2003;108:432-437.

144. Schwitter J, Nanz D, Kneifel S, et al: Assessment of myocardial perfusion in coronary artery disease by magnetic resonance: A

comparison with positron emission tomography and coronary angiography. Circulation 2001;103:2230-2235.

145. Dendale P, Franken PR, Block P, et al: Contrast enhanced and functional magnetic resonance imaging for the detection of viable myocardium after infarction. Am Heart J 1998;135: 875-880.

146. Kim RJ, Fieno DS, Parrish TB, et al: Relationship of MRI delayed contrast enhancement to irreversible injury, infarct age, and contractile function. Circulation 1999;100:1992-2002.

147. Gerber BL, Garot J, Bluemke DA, et al: Accuracy of contrast-enhanced magnetic resonance imaging in predicting improvement of regional myocardial function in patients after acute myocardial infarction. Circulation 2002;106:1083-1089.

148. Perin EC, Silva GV, Sarmento-Leite R, et al: Assessing myocardial viability and infarct transmurality with left ventricular electromechanical mapping in patients with stable coronary artery disease: Validation by delayed-enhancement magnetic resonance imaging. Circulation 2002;106:957-961.

149. Motoyama S, Kondo T, Anno H, et al: Relationship between thrombolytic therapy and perfusion defect detected by Gd-DTPA-enhanced fast magnetic resonance imaging in acute myocardial infarction. J Cardiovasc Magn Reson 2001;3:237-245.

150. Sandstede JJ, Lipke C, Beer M, et al: Analysis of first-pass and delayed contrast-enhancement patterns of dysfunctional myocardium on MR imaging: Use in the prediction of myocardial viability. AJR Am J Roentgenol 2000;174:1737-1740.

151. Lauerma K, Niemi P, Hanninen H, et al: Multimodality MR imaging assessment of myocardial viability: Combination of first-pass and late contrast enhancement to wall motion dynamics and comparison with FDG PET-initial experience. Radiology 2000;217:729-736.

152. Kim RJ, Hillenbrand HB, Judd RM: Evaluation of myocardial viability by MRI. Herz 2000;25:417-430.

153. Bax JJ, de Roos A, van Der Wall EE: Assessment of myocardial viability by MRI. J Magn Reson Imaging 1999;10:418-422.

154. Kim RJ, Chen EL, Lima JA, Judd RM: Myocardial Gd-DTPA kinetics determine MRI contrast enhancement and reflect the extent and severity of myocardial injury after acute reperfused infarction. Circulation 1996;94:3318-3326.

155. Klein C, Nekolla SG, Bengel FM, et al: Assessment of myocardial viability with contrast-enhanced magnetic resonance imaging: Comparison with positron emission tomography. Circulation 2002;105:162-167.

156. Wagner A, Mahrholdt H, Holly TA, et al: Contrast-enhanced MRI and routine single photon emission computed tomography (SPECT) perfusion imaging for detection of subendocardial myocardial infarcts: An imaging study. Lancet 2003;361:374-379.

157. Kim RJ, Wu E, Rafael A, et al: The use of contrast-enhanced magnetic resonance imaging to identify reversible myocardial dysfunction. N Engl J Med 2000;343:1445-1453.

158. Choi KM, Kim RJ, Gubernikoff G, et al: Transmural extent of acute myocardial infarction predicts long-term improvement in contractile function. Circulation 2001;104:1101-1107.

159. Knuesel PR, Nanz D, Wyss C, et al: Characterization of dysfunctional myocardium by positron emission tomography and magnetic resonance: Relation to functional outcome after revascularization. Circulation 2003;108:1095-1100.

160. Beek AM, Kuhl HP, Bondarenko O, et al: Delayed contrast-enhanced magnetic resonance imaging for the prediction of regional functional improvement after acute myocardial infarction. J Am Coll Cardiol 2003;42:895-901.

161. Kim RJ, Judd RM: Gadolinium-enhanced magnetic resonance imaging in hypertrophic cardiomyopathy: In vivo imaging of the pathologic substrate for premature cardiac death? J Am Coll Cardiol 2003;41:1568-1572.

162. Buser PT, Auffermann W, Holt WW, et al: Noninvasive evaluation of global left ventricular function with use of cine nuclear magnetic resonance. J Am Coll Cardiol 1989;13:1294-1300.

163. MacGowan GA, Shapiro EP, Azhari H, et al: Noninvasive measurement of shortening in the fiber and cross-fiber directions in

the normal human left ventricle and in idiopathic dilated cardiomyopathy. Circulation 1997;96:535-541.

164. Fujita N, Duerinekx AJ, Higgins CB: Variation in left ventricular regional wall stress with cine magnetic resonance imaging: Normal subjects versus dilated cardiomyopathy. Am Heart J 1993;125:1337-1345.

165. Mollet NR, Dymarkowski S, Volders W, et al: Visualization of ventricular thrombi with contrast-enhanced magnetic resonance imaging in patients with ischemic heart disease. Circulation 2002;106:2873-2876.

166. von Kienlin M, Beer M, Greiser A, et al: Advances in human cardiac 31P-MR spectroscopy: SLOOP and clinical applications. J Magn Reson Imaging 2001;13:521-527.

167. Skrabek RQ, Anderson JE: Metabolic shifts and myocyte hypertrophy in deflazacort treatment of mdx mouse cardiomyopathy. Muscle Nerve 2001;24:192-202.

168. Pohost GM, Meduri A, Razmi RM, et al: Cardiac MR spectroscopy in the new millennium. Rays 2001;26:93-107.

169. Bogaert J, Goldstein M, Tannouri F, et al: Original report: Late myocardial enhancement in hypertrophic cardiomyopathy with contrast-enhanced MR imaging. AJR Am J Roentgenol 2003;180:981-985.

170. Gagliardi MG, Bevilacqua M, Di Renzi P, et al: Usefulness of magnetic resonance imaging for diagnosis of acute myocarditis in infants and children, and comparison with endomyocardial biopsy. Am J Cardiol 1991;68:1089-1091.

171. Gagliardi MG, Polletta B, Di Renzi P: MRI for the diagnosis and follow-up of myocarditis. Circulation 1999;99:458-459.

172. Bellotti G, Bocchi EA, de Moraes AV, et al: In vivo detection of Trypanosoma cruzi antigens in hearts of patients with chronic Chagas' heart disease. Am Heart J 1996;131:301-307.

173. Veluvolu P, Balian AA, Goldsmith R, et al: Lyme carditis: Evaluation by Ga-67 and MRI. Clin Nucl Med 1992;17:823.

174. Globits S, Bergler-Klein J, Stanek G, et al: Magnetic resonance imaging in the diagnosis of acute Lyme carditis. Cardiology 1994;85:415-417.

175. Been M, Thomson BJ, Smith MA, et al: Myocardial involvement in systemic lupus erythematosus detected by magnetic resonance imaging. Eur Heart J 1988;9:1250-1256.

176. Ohata S, Shimada T, Shimizu H, et al: Myocarditis associated with polymyositis diagnosed by gadolinium-DTPA enhanced magnetic resonance imaging. J Rheumatol 2002;29:861-862.

177. Takahashi N, Murakami Y, Shimada T, et al: Detection of eosinophilic myocarditis using contrast-enhanced magnetic resonance imaging: Case report. Can Assoc Radiol J 2001;52:20-22.

178. Powell AJ, Geva T: Blood flow measurement by magnetic resonance imaging in congenital heart disease. Pediatr Cardiol 2000;21:47-58.

179. Pelc NJ, Herfkens RJ, Shimakawa A, Enzmann DR: Phase contrast cine magnetic resonance imaging. Magn Reson Q 1991;7:229-254.

180. Greil G, Geva T, Maier SE, Powell AJ: Effect of acquisition parameters on the accuracy of velocity encoded cine magnetic resonance imaging blood flow measurements. J Magn Reson Imaging 2002;15:47-54.

181. Beerbaum P, Korperich H, Barth P, et al: Noninvasive quantification of left-to-right shunt in pediatric patients: Phase-contrast cine magnetic resonance imaging compared with invasive oximetry. Circulation 2001;103:2476-2482.

182. Powell AJ, Maier SE, Chung T, Geva T: Phase-velocity cine magnetic resonance imaging measurement of pulsatile blood flow in children and young adults: In vitro and in vivo validation. Pediatr Cardiol 2000;21:104-110.

183. Hundley WG, Li HF, Lange RA, et al: Assessment of left-to-right intracardiac shunting by velocity-encoded, phase-difference magnetic resonance imaging: A comparison with oximetric and indicator dilution techniques. Circulation 1995;91:2955-2960.

184. Papaharilaou Y, Doorly DJ, Sherwin SJ: Assessing the accuracy of two-dimensional phase-contrast MRI measurements of complex unsteady flows. J Magn Reson Imaging 2001;14:714-723.

185. Robertson MB, Kohler U, Hoskins PR, Marshall I: Quantitative analysis of PC MRI velocity maps: Pulsatile flow in cylindrical vessels. Magn Reson Imaging 2001;19:685-695.

186. Wise RG, Newling B, Gates AR, et al: Measurement of pulsatile flow using MRI and a Bayesian technique of probability analysis. Magn Reson Imaging 1996;14:173-185.

187. Evans AJ, Iwai F, Grist TA, et al: Magnetic resonance imaging of blood flow with a phase subtraction technique: In vitro and in vivo validation. Invest Radiol 1993;28:109-115.

188. Zananiri FV, Jackson PC, Goddard PR, et al: An evaluation of the accuracy of flow measurements using magnetic resonance imaging (MRI). J Med Eng Technol 1991;15:170-176.

189. Steinman DA, Frayne R, Zhang XD, et al: MR measurement and numerical simulation of steady flow in an end-to-side anastomosis model. J Biomech 1996;29:537-542.

190. Firmin DN, Nayler GL, Kilner PJ, Longmore DB: The application of phase shifts in NMR for flow measurement. Magn Reson Med 1990;14:230-241.

191. Ku DN, Biancheri CL, Pettigrew RI, et al: Evaluation of magnetic resonance velocimetry for steady flow. J Biomech Eng 1990;112:464-472.

192. Sondergaard L, Thomsen C, Stahlberg F, et al: Mitral and aortic valvular flow: Quantification with MR phase mapping. J Magn Reson Imaging 1992;2:295-302.

193. Firmin DN, Nayler GL, Klipstein RH, et al: In vivo validation of MR velocity imaging. J Comput Assist Tomogr 1987;11:751-756.

194. Kondo C, Caputo GR, Semelka R, et al: Right and left ventricular stroke volume measurements with velocity-encoded cine MR imaging: In vitro and in vivo validation. AJR Am J Roentgenol 1991;157:9-16.

195. Rebergen SA, van der Wall EE, Doornbos J, de Roos A: Magnetic resonance measurement of velocity and flow: Technique, validation, and cardiovascular applications. Am Heart J 1993;126:1439-1456.

196. Rebergen SA, Chin JG, Ottenkamp J, et al: Pulmonary regurgitation in the late postoperative follow-up of tetralogy of Fallot: Volumetric quantitation by nuclear magnetic resonance velocity mapping. Circulation 1993;88:2257-2266.

197. Rebergen SA, Ottenkamp J, Doornbos J, et al: Postoperative pulmonary flow dynamics after Fontan surgery: Assessment with nuclear magnetic resonance velocity mapping. J Am Coll Cardiol 1993;21:123-131.

198. Hundley WG, Li HF, Hillis LD, et al: Quantitation of cardiac output with velocity-encoded, phase-difference magnetic resonance imaging. Am J Cardiol 1995;75:1250-1255.

199. Matsumura K, Nakase E, Haiyama T, et al: Determination of cardiac ejection fraction and left ventricular volume: Contrast-enhanced ultrafast cine MR imaging vs IV digital subtraction ventriculography. AJR Am J Roentgenol 1993;160:979-985.

200. Pelc LR, Pelc NJ, Rayhill SC, et al: Arterial and venous blood flow: Noninvasive quantitation with MR imaging. Radiology 1992;185:809-812.

201. Powell AJ, Tsai-Goodman B, Prakash A, et al: Comparison between phase-velocity cine magnetic resonance imaging and invasive oximetry for quantification of atrial shunts. Am J Cardiol 2003;91:1523-1525, A9.

202. Hundley WG, Meshack BM, Willett DL, et al: Comparison of quantitation of left ventricular volume, ejection fraction, and cardiac output in patients with atrial fibrillation by cine magnetic resonance imaging versus invasive measurements. Am J Cardiol 1996;78:1119-1123.

203. Brenner LD, Caputo GR, Mostbeck G, et al: Quantification of left to right atrial shunts with velocity-encoded cine nuclear magnetic resonance imaging. J Am Coll Cardiol 1992;20:1246-1250.

204. Beerbaum P, Korperich H, Gieseke J, et al: Rapid left-to-right shunt quantification in children by phase-contrast magnetic resonance imaging combined with sensitivity encoding (SENSE). Circulation 2003;108:1355-1361.

205. Buonocore MH: Estimation of total coronary artery flow using measurements of flow in the ascending aorta. Magn Reson Med 1994;32:602-611.

206. Kolbitsch C, Lorenz IH, Hormann C, et al: The impact of increased mean airway pressure on contrast-enhanced MRI measurement of regional cerebral blood flow (rCBF), regional cerebral blood volume (rCBV), regional mean transit time (rMTT), and regional cerebrovascular resistance (rCVR) in human volunteers. Hum Brain Mapp 2000;11:214-222.

207. Sommer G, Noorbehesht B, Pelc N, et al: Normal renal blood flow measurement using phase-contrast cine magnetic resonance imaging. Invest Radiol 1992;27:465-470.

208. Geva T, Sahn, DJ, Powell AJ: Magnetic resonance imaging of congenital heart disease in adults. Prog Pediatr Cardiol 2003;17:21-39.

209. Holmqvist C, Oskarsson G, Stahlberg F, et al: Functional evaluation of extracardiac ventriculopulmonary conduits and of the right ventricle with magnetic resonance imaging and velocity mapping. Am J Cardiol 1999;83:926-932.

210. Walker PG, Houlind K, Djurhuus C, et al: Motion correction for the quantification of mitral regurgitation using the control volume method. Magn Reson Med 2000;43:726-733.

211. Walker PG, Oyre S, Pedersen EM, et al: A new control volume method for calculating valvular regurgitation. Circulation 1995;92:579-586.

212. Globits S, Higgins CB: Assessment of valvular heart disease by magnetic resonance imaging. Am Heart J 1995;129:369-381.

213. Reid SA, Walker PG, Fisher J, et al: The quantification of pulmonary valve haemodynamics using MRI. Int J Cardiovasc Imaging 2002;18:217-225.

214. Dohmen PM, Hotz H, Lembcke A, et al: Magnetic resonance imaging of stentless xenografts for reconstruction of right ventricular outflow tract. Semin Thorac Cardiovasc Surg 2001;13:24-27.

215. Kuehne T, Saeed M, Reddy G, et al: Sequential magnetic resonance monitoring of pulmonary flow with endovascular stents placed across the pulmonary valve in growing swine. Circulation 2001;104:2363-2368.

216. Helbing WA, de Roos A: Clinical applications of cardiac magnetic resonance imaging after repair of tetralogy of Fallot. Pediatr Cardiol 2000;21:70-79.

217. Nayak KS, Pauly JM, Kerr AB, et al: Real-time color flow MRI. Magn Reson Med 2000;43:251-258.

218. Arrive L, Najmark D, Albert F, et al: Cine MRI of mitral regurgitation in planes angled along the intrinsic cardiac axes. J Comput Assist Tomogr 1994;18:569-575.

219. Ohnishi S, Fukui S, Kusuoka H, et al: Assessment of valvular regurgitation using cine magnetic resonance imaging coupled with phase compensation technique: Comparison with Doppler color flow mapping. Angiology 1992;43:913-924.

220. Nishimura F: Oblique cine MRI for the evaluation of aortic regurgitation: Comparison with cineangiography. Clin Cardiol 1992;15:73-78.

221. Mitchell L, Jenkins JP, Watson Y, et al: Diagnosis and assessment of mitral and aortic valve disease by cine-flow magnetic resonance imaging. Magn Reson Med 1989;12:181-197.

222. Metcalfe MJ, Jones RA, Redpath TW, et al: Low-field cine magnetic resonance imaging in aortic valve disease. Br J Radiol 1989;62:1063-1066.

223. Fogel MA, Weinberg PM, Rychik J, et al: Caval contribution to flow in the branch pulmonary arteries of Fontan patients with a novel application of magnetic resonance presaturation pulse. Circulation 1999;99:1215-1221.

224. Fratz S, Hess J, Schwaiger M, et al: More accurate quantification of pulmonary blood flow by magnetic resonance imaging than by lung perfusion scintigraphy in patients with Fontan circulation. Circulation 2002;106:1510-1513.

225. Henk CB, Schlechta B, Grampp S, et al: Pulmonary and aortic blood flow measurements in normal subjects and patients after

single lung transplantation at 0.5 T using velocity encoded cine MRI. Chest 1998;114:771-779.

226. Rupprecht T, Nitz W, Wagner M, et al: Determination of the pressure gradient in children with coarctation of the aorta by low-field magnetic resonance imaging. Pediatr Cardiol 2002; 23:127-131.

227. Ebbers T, Wigstrom L, Bolger AF, et al: Estimation of relative cardiovascular pressures using time-resolved three-dimensional phase contrast MRI. Magn Reson Med 2001;45:872-879.

228. van der Geest RJ, Reiber JH: Quantification in cardiac MRI. J Magn Reson Imaging 1999;10:602-608.

229. Pennell DJ, Firmin DN, Burger P, et al: Assessment of magnetic resonance velocity mapping of global ventricular function during dobutamine infusion in coronary artery disease. Br Heart J 1995;74:163-170.

230. Schwitter J, DeMarco T, Kneifel S, et al: Magnetic resonance-based assessment of global coronary flow and flow reserve and its relation to left ventricular functional parameters: A comparison with positron emission tomography. Circulation 2000;101: 2696-2702.

231. Shibata M, Sakuma H, Isaka N, et al: Assessment of coronary flow reserve with fast cine phase contrast magnetic resonance imaging: Comparison with measurement by Doppler guide wire. J Magn Reson Imaging 1999;10:563-568.

232. Rodriguez-Gonzalez AO: Arterial flow determined with half Fourier echo-planar imaging. Arch Med Res 2000;31:470-485.

233. Thompson RB, McVeigh ER: Fast measurement of intracardiac pressure differences with 2D breath-hold phase-contrast MRI. Magn Reson Med 2003;49:1056-1066.

234. Sakuma H, Kawada N, Kubo H, et al: Effect of breath holding on blood flow measurement using fast velocity encoded cine MRI. Magn Reson Med 2001;45:346-348.

235. Hjortdal VE, Emmertsen K, Stenbog E, et al: Effects of exercise and respiration on blood flow in total cavopulmonary connection: A real-time magnetic resonance flow study. Circulation 2003;108:1227-1231.

236. Be'eri E, Maier SE, Landzberg MJ, et al: In vivo evaluation of Fontan pathway flow dynamics by multidimensional phase-velocity magnetic resonance imaging. Circulation 1998; 98:2873-2882.

237. Kohler U, Marshall I, Robertson MB, et al: MRI measurement of wall shear stress vectors in bifurcation models and comparison with CFD predictions. J Magn Reson Imaging 2001;14:563-573.

238. Oyre S, Ringgaard S, Kozerke S, et al: Accurate noninvasive quantitation of blood flow, cross-sectional lumen vessel area and wall shear stress by three-dimensional paraboloid modeling of magnetic resonance imaging velocity data. J Am Coll Cardiol 1998;32:128-134.

239. Morgan VL, Roselli RJ, Lorenz CH: Normal three-dimensional pulmonary artery flow determined by phase contrast magnetic resonance imaging. Ann Biomed Eng 1998;26:557-566.

240. Edelman RR, Chien D, Kim D: Fast selective black blood MR imaging. Radiology 1991;181:655-660.

241. Simonetti OP, Finn JP, White RD, et al: "Black blood" T2-weighted inversion-recovery MR imaging of the heart. Radiology 1996;199:49-57.

242. Bax JJ, Atsma DE, Lamb HJ, et al: Noninvasive and invasive evaluation of noncompaction cardiomyopathy. J Cardiovasc Magn Reson 2002;4:353-357.

243. Hamamichi Y, Ichida F, Hashimoto I, et al: Isolated noncompaction of the ventricular myocardium: Ultrafast computed tomography and magnetic resonance imaging. Int J Cardiovasc Imaging 2001;17:305-314.

244. Frances CD, Shlipak MG, Grady D: Left ventricular pseudoaneurysm: Diagnosis by cine magnetic resonance imaging. Cardiology 1999;92:217-219.

245. Sakuma H, Bourne MW, O'Sullivan M, et al: Evaluation of thoracic aortic dissection using breath-holding cine MRI. J Comput Assist Tomogr 1996;20:45-50.

246. Moore NR, Parry AJ, Trottman-Dickenson B, et al: Fate of the native aorta after repair of acute type A dissection: A magnetic resonance imaging study. Heart 1996;75:62-66.

247. Olivieri NF, Nathan DG, MacMillan JH, et al: Survival in medically treated patients with homozygous beta-thalassemia. N Engl J Med 1994;331:574-578.

248. Anderson LJ, Wonke B, Prescott E, et al: Comparison of effects of oral deferiprone and subcutaneous desferrioxamine on myocardial iron concentrations and ventricular function in beta-thalassaemia. Lancet 2002;360:516-520.

249. Anderson LJ, Holden S, Davis B, et al: Cardiovascular T2-star (T2*) magnetic resonance for the early diagnosis of myocardial iron overload. Eur Heart J 2001;22:2171-2179.

250. Wolff S, James TL, Young GB, et al: Magnetic resonance imaging: Absence of in vitro cytogenetic damage. Radiology 1985;155: 163-165.

251. Shellock FG: Metallic surgical instruments for interventional MRI procedures: Evaluation of MR safety. J Magn Reson Imaging 2001;13:152-157.

252. Shellock FG, Shellock VJ: Cardiovascular catheters and accessories: Ex vivo testing of ferromagnetism, heating, and artifacts associated with MRI. J Magn Reson Imaging 1998;8:1338-1342.

253. Sawyer-Glover AM, Shellock FG: Pre-MRI procedure screening: Recommendations and safety considerations for biomedical implants and devices. J Magn Reson Imaging 2000;12:92-106.

254. Rutledge JM, Vick GW 3rd, Mullins CE, Grifka RG: Safety of magnetic resonance imaging immediately following Palmaz stent implant: A report of three cases. Cathet Cardiovasc Interv 2001;53:519-523.

255. Jagannathan NR: Magnetic resonance imaging: Bioeffects and safety concerns. Indian J Biochem Biophys 1999;36:341-347.

256. Edwards MB, Taylor KM, Shellock FG: Prosthetic heart valves: Evaluation of magnetic field interactions, heating, and artifacts at 1.5 T. J Magn Reson Imaging 2000;12:363-369.

257. Ordidge RJ, Shellock FG, Kanal E: A Y2000 update of current safety issues related to MRI. J Magn Reson Imaging 2000;12:1.

258. Hofman MB, de Cock CC, van der Linden JC, et al: Transesophageal cardiac pacing during magnetic resonance imaging: Feasibility and safety considerations. Magn Reson Med 1996;35:413-422.

259. Gimbel JR, Johnson D, Levine PA, Wilkoff BL: Safe performance of magnetic resonance imaging on five patients with permanent cardiac pacemakers. Pacing Clin Electrophysiol 1996;19:913-919.

260. Bellenger NG, Francis JM, Davies CL, et al: Establishment and performance of a magnetic resonance cardiac function clinic. J Cardiovasc Magn Reson 2000;2:15-22.

261. Pattynama PM, Lamb HJ, Van der Velde EA, et al: Reproducibility of MRI-derived measurements of right ventricular volumes and myocardial mass. Magn Reson Imaging 1995;13:53-63.

262. Aladl UE, Hurwitz GA, Dey D, et al: Automated image registration of gated cardiac single-photon emission computed tomography and magnetic resonance imaging. J Magn Reson Imaging 2004;19:283-290.

263. Kunz RP, Oellig F, Krummenauer F, et al: Assessment of left ventricular function by breath-hold cine MR imaging: Comparison of different steady-state free precession sequences. J Magn Reson Imaging 2005;21(2):140-148.

CHAPTER 12

Assessment of Heart Failure by Cardiac Catheterization

Glenn Leonard, Jr.
Henri Justino
Ronald Grifka

The quest for understanding the functioning of the heart and the vascular system has existed for centuries. Although necropsy studies provided excellent opportunities to study cardiac anatomy in tremendous detail, cardiac catheterization emerged as a means of obtaining information about the cardiovascular system in the living organism. In 1711, Hales experimented with biventricular catheterization in horses, but the first human cardiac catheterization is attributed to Forssmann in 1929, when he passed a catheter through his own antecubital vein and advanced it into the right atrium. Forssmann paved the way for the rapid explosion of knowledge that has occurred, beginning with diagnostic catheterization and leading up to the current era of advanced therapeutic catheterization for a wide variety of congenital and acquired cardiovascular diseases.

The advent of ultrasound and MRI as noninvasive means of studying the cardiovascular system has led to the reappraisal of the role of invasive catheterization. This chapter describes some of the methods for assessment of ventricular performance in the cardiac catheterization laboratory. Some of the methods described have been relegated to the status of historic importance, having been supplanted by noninvasive methods of obtaining the same information. Nonetheless, despite the increasingly important roles of noninvasive imaging modalities, some of the most robust indices of ventricular systolic and diastolic function, as discussed in this chapter, are still obtainable only by direct catheterization. This chapter reviews the available methods for assessing cardiac function in the cardiac catheterization laboratory, then explores their clinical usefulness in pediatric heart disease (see also Chapters 7 and 8).

EVALUATION OF CARDIOVASCULAR FUNCTION

Cardiovascular function is the result of the interaction of a variety of complex factors, including preload, afterload, intrinsic myocardial systolic function (contractility), diastolic function, valvular function, atrioventricular and ventriculovascular coupling, and cardiac rhythm.

Cardiac Output Determination

The main role of the heart is as a pump, and assessment of pump function in terms of its output should be an important factor in the overall assessment of cardiac function. A general nonspecific assessment of cardiac function can be ascertained from determination of cardiac output, as measured by an indicator dilution method (e.g., thermodilution) or calculated by the Fick method. Cardiac output is extremely load dependent, however, and heart failure does not imply pump failure. A patient may have a low cardiac output despite grossly normal myocardial contractility (e.g., pericardial tamponade, severe mitral stenosis, or massive systemic arteriovenous malformation). Pump function as determined by the cardiac output is relatively insensitive in detection of heart failure, unless it is interpreted in the context of the accompanying loading conditions. Assessment of preload and afterload is paramount in assessment of cardiac function.

Pressure Measurement

Pressure measurement in various cardiac chambers and vessels aids in creating the context in which the cardiac output may be interpreted. Assessment of preload requires the measurement of the filling pressures (left ventricular end-diastolic pressure [LVEDP], pulmonary capillary wedge pressure, or left atrial pressure for the left side of the heart and right atrial pressure or right ventricular end-diastolic pressure [RVEDP] for the right side). The filling pressures are easy to measure, can be assessed continuously by indwelling catheters, and are useful in the serial assessment of circulatory function in the cardiac catheterization laboratory and in the intensive care unit. Filling pressures are poor surrogates of preload when abnormal chamber filling characteristics exist because the filling pressure depends in large part on the compliance of the atrium and ventricle.

Application of the length-tension relationship (derived from the isolated muscle preparation) to the analysis of ventricular function requires expressing length in the context of a three-dimensional ventricle (i.e., volume). A more accurate estimate of preload is the ventricular end-diastolic volume (EDV), which is not as readily measured as end-diastolic pressure and is not as practical to follow on a minute-to-minute basis. The most accurate translation of preload is a more difficult entity to calculate still and involves correction of the EDV for the wall thickness (i.e., the end-diastolic wall stress). Because of the complexity involved in measuring end-diastolic wall stress or ventricular EDV, the filling pressures are used as surrogates for these parameters.

Similarly, although aortic pressure is used as a simple surrogate for afterload because it is easy to measure and easy to track closely, a more accurate representation of left ventricular afterload is the systemic vascular resistance (SVR). The measurement of SVR is superior because it incorporates not only the aortic pressure, but also the central venous pressure and the cardiac output, providing a more accurate measurement of the physiologic milieu. An even more accurate assessment of the left ventricular afterload is the aortic impedance, which incorporates even more factors, including aortic compliance and blood viscosity. In drawing comparisons again to the isolated muscle preparation, the idealized measure of left ventricular afterload would be the systolic wall stress. This value is extremely complex to calculate, however, because none of its components (pressure, wall thickness, and left ventricular volume) is constant during systole; wall stress ideally would need to be integrated over the duration of systole.

Ventricular Volume Determination

Cardiac angiography can provide qualitative information regarding anatomic and functional abnormalities and quantitative information about chamber size and various ejection phase indices of ventricular performance. Ventricular systolic and diastolic dimensions, area, and wall thickness may be measured directly, and volume, ejection fraction, mass, and wall stress may be calculated.

Techniques for calculating left and right ventricular volumes by angiography require algorithms with numerous geometric assumptions and a large margin of error, especially for the right ventricle. Nevertheless, quantitative analysis of ventricular volume from contrast ventriculograms has been the gold standard against which all other imaging modalities have been compared. Algorithms for calculation of ventricular volumes are based on studies of anatomically normal left ventricles. When studying ventricular volumes in the setting of congenital heart disease, various assumptions may not hold true, owing to developmental abnormalities in ventricular size, geometry, and position within the thorax. In the setting of congenitally malformed hearts, ventricular volume is obtained more easily by echocardiography or MRI; ventricular volumes now are rarely calculated from contrast ventriculograms in most pediatric cardiac catheterization laboratories.

The most common method used for measuring left ventricular volume is the **area-length method**, introduced by Dodge and colleagues.[1] This method requires an excellent-quality left ventriculogram without ectopic beats. The first step in determining left ventricular volume

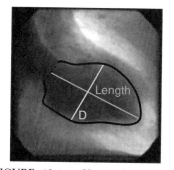
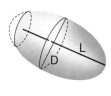

$$V = \pi/6 \; LD^2$$

FIGURE 12-1 ■ **Ventricular volume determination: area-length method.** On the left, a right anterior oblique view of the left ventriculogram at end diastole, with manually traced endocardial outline and calculated axial length and diameter (D). On the right, left ventricular volume represented as an ellipsoid with major diameter (L) and minor diameter (D). In this example, only one plane is used. (From Sheehan FH: http:/www.avnrt.com/docs/arealen.jpg.) (See also Color Section)

is to trace the left ventricle silhouette at the outermost margin of the radiographic contrast area, including trabeculations and papillary muscles within the perimeter. The left ventricular contour is compared with an ellipsoid of revolution. The diameter (D) of the ellipse is computed from the area (A) enclosed by the contour and its longest length (L). The volume is calculated using the mean of areas computed from single or biplane techniques (Fig. 12-1).[2]

A more accurate volume calculation results from using the biplane method, right anterior oblique (RAO) and left anterior oblique (LAO) views, and the resultant ellipsoid of minor diameters, D_{rao} and D_{lao}. The corresponding volume equation is used:[2]

$$V = (4/3) \; \pi([L/2] \; [M/2] \; [N/2]) = (\pi/6) \; LMN$$

where V is volume, L is long axis, and M and N are short axes of the ellipsoid. M and N are calculated by using the area-length method:

$$A_{rao} = \pi(L_{rao}/2)(M/2); \; M = 4A_{rao}/\pi L_{rao}$$

$$A_{lao} = \pi(L_{lao}/2)(N/2); \; N = 4A_{lao}/\pi L_{lao}$$

Combining the equations yields:

$$V = 8/3\pi(A_{rao} \times A_{lao}/L_{min})$$

The measured volume is corrected for the space occupied by trabeculae and papillary muscles, using a regression equation. Dodge and colleagues,[1] using the area-length method, were the first to develop values for corrected left ventricular volume. Graham and coworkers[3] later refined this technique to make it more applicable to children. This refinement was achieved by re-evaluating Dodge's regression equation. The regression equation used by Dodge and colleagues[1] would yield a negative result for corrected volume when the calculated volume was less than 2.1 cm³. Graham and coworkers[3] proposed two separate regression equations: one table for calculated volumes less than 15 cm³ and another table for calculated volumes greater than 15 cm³. Normal values were defined for patients younger than and older than 2 years of age:[3]

$$V' = 0.733 \ (V) \text{ for volumes} <15 \text{ cm}^3$$

$$V' = 0.974 \ (V) - 3.1 \text{ cm}^3 \text{ for volumes} >15 \text{ cm}^3$$

The area-length method has been validated extensively in vitro and in vivo. Measured volumes agree closely with known values ($r = .995$; standard error of the estimate = 8.2 mL). Accuracy and variability in the application of this method in the clinical setting have been well characterized.[4]

In adults, the normal left ventricular EDV is 70 ± 20 (SD) mL/m². Graham and coworkers[3] found normal left ventricular volumes of 42 ± 10 cm³/m² for children younger than 2 years old and 73 ± 11 cm³/m² for children older than 2 years. The abrupt increase in the range of normal values for children older than 2 years is problematic, reflecting some of the inherent inaccuracies in the regression equations that have been developed.

The applicability of the area-length method, which compares the left ventricle with an ellipsoid, is questionable when applied to the right ventricle or a geometrically distorted left ventricle caused by a disease state (e.g., the left ventricle is known to change from an ellipsoid shape to a much more spherical shape in severe dilated cardiomyopathy).

The **Simpson rule** is independent of assumptions regarding ventricular shape. Biplane cineangiography can be performed in the straight posteroanterior and lateral views, or in 30 degrees RAO and 60 degrees LAO, or other angulated projections (e.g., 45 degrees RAO, and 60 degrees LAO with 25 degrees cranial).[2] The ventricular chamber is divided into a series of discs that are added to the total volume. The details of derivation of the Simpson rule are beyond the scope of this chapter, but for illustrative purposes, Figure 12-2 shows the Simpson rule applied to the left ventricle.

The right ventricle, in part because of its more complex internal geometry, has not been studied as extensively as the left ventricle. Because of its complex geometry, the prolate ellipsoid model is not appropriate for calculating right ventricular volume. The most widely used method employed for volume determination of the right ventricle is the Simpson rule[5,6]; normal values for right ventricular volumes in children have been proposed using the Simpson rule.[5]

ASSESSMENT OF VENTRICULAR PERFORMANCE

Conductance Catheter Technique

The calculation of a time-varying ventricular volume (i.e., frame-by-frame analysis of volume) from an angiogram can be arduous and time-consuming, despite the availability of software programs that can aid in the calculation of the ventricular volume from any of the methods discussed. The emergence of conductance catheters, integrated with high-fidelity pressure sensors, has permitted the generation of real-time pressure-volume loops (Fig. 12-3). The analysis of pressure-volume loops in the cardiac catheterization laboratory provides a powerful method of assessing myocardial performance. Different loading conditions, infusion of vasoactive drugs, and acute interventional procedures may be performed to generate variably loaded pressure-volume loops.[7]

Baan and associates[8] were the first to develop the conductance volumetric method. Briefly, a conductance catheter typically contains 8 to 12 electrodes spaced 7 to 15 mm apart. An electrical field is generated between the electrodes, and the potential produced by the current is measured. The conductances from the electrode pairs are summed and converted to volume using a signal conditioner, assuming that the current flows through all the blood in the ventricular chamber. The catheter also contains a high-fidelity pressure transducer at its tip to allow for simultaneous pressure recording. Real-time pressure-volume loops can be generated and analyzed. As a result, numerous indices of ventricular systolic and diastolic performance can be derived. Additionally, transient changes in loading conditions can be imposed

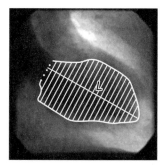
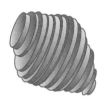

$$V = \Sigma_{i=1}^{n} \ \pi/4 \ D_i^2 \ \Delta L$$

FIGURE 12-2 ■ Simpson rule method for left ventricular volume. On the left, a right anterior oblique view of the left ventriculogram at end diastole, with manually traced endocardial outline and calculated axial length (L) subdivided into segments. On the right, representation of left ventricular volume as the summed volumes of graduated discs with diameter (D_i) and thickness ΔL_i. The Riemann sum of the disc volumes is processed according to the Simpson rule, allowing for a smooth (not stepped) endocardial curvature. (From Sheehan FH: http://www.avnrt.com/docs/arealen.jpg.) (See also Color Section)

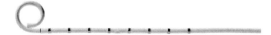

FIGURE 12-3 ■ Conductance catheter. The outermost electrodes of this conductance catheter generate an intracavitary electrical field, and the remaining electrodes measure the potential difference and derive the time-varying conduction for each of the five ventricular segments. The total ventricular volume is derived from the sum of the five segmental conductances. (Used by permission from Millar Instruments, Inc.)

(e.g., pharmacologic manipulation, volume infusion, inferior vena cava or pulmonary artery occlusion), allowing the generation of a family of pressure-volume loops. Because the conductance catheter method is relatively independent of ventricular geometry, it lends itself well to the study of ventricular function in the realm of congenital heart disease, especially when assessing abnormal right ventricles.[9-15]

A potential drawback of this technique is that other structures, such as the myocardium and surrounding tissue, also conduct current, so-called parallel conductance.[14-19] If the parallel conductance is not taken into consideration, significant errors may be introduced in determining volume measurement. Parallel conductance can be estimated typically by injecting a small volume of hypertonic saline into the pulmonary artery for the left ventricle or into the femoral vein for the right ventricle, which transiently augments the ventricular conductance signal.[8,14,18] Several studies have found a negligible impact of parallel conductance on volume measurements.[14,18] Conductance catheters have given cardiologists the ability to generate real-time pressure-volume loops for a wide variety of indices of systolic and diastolic function, allowing for the discrimination of ventricular chamber function with respect to primary systolic, diastolic, and vascular loading factors.[19]

Basic Cardiac Parameters

Before discussing the advantages of pressure-volume loop analysis, we should define some basic parameters of ventricular performance that can be obtained in the cardiac catheterization laboratory. **Stroke volume**, the amount of blood ejected with each heartbeat, is the difference between EDV and end-systolic volume. **Ejection fraction** is the ratio of the ventricular stroke volume to the EDV. **Cardiac output** is the product of stroke volume and heart rate. In the absence of intracardiac shunts or valvular regurgitation, angiographic measurement of stroke volume should correlate with other independent measures of stroke volume, such as the Fick calculation or thermodilution method. If an intracardiac shunt or valvular regurgitation is present, angiographic measurement of stroke volume exceeds that determined by the Fick and thermodilution methods. The difference between the two yields the **regurgitant fraction**.

Preload represents all the factors that contribute to passive ventricular wall stress (or tension) at the end of diastole.[21] Changing compliance of the ventricles makes end-diastolic pressure less reliable than the EDV as a measure of preload. Because the right ventricular and left ventricular EDVs are difficult to measure, however, preload often is estimated by using the end-diastolic pressure (RVEDP and LVEDP). Preload is determined by the law of LaPlace and defined by the equation:

$$\text{wall stress } \sigma = PR/2h$$

where P is chamber pressure, R is chamber radius, and h is wall thickness.[22,23] This equation can be applied to the left and right ventricles. Patients with compensated dilated cardiomyopathy have an increase in wall stress as a result of an increase in radius of the ventricular chamber, but cardiac muscle compensates with hypertrophy (an increase in thickness) to restore the wall stress to normal. In the cardiac catheterization laboratory, the preload, or ventricular end-diastolic pressure, is taken at the nadir after the transmitted atrial A wave, usually at the point on the ventricular pressure tracing that coincides with the onset of the q wave of the ECG tracing.

Afterload is similarly described as interaction of the factors that contribute to total myocardial wall stress (or tension) during systolic ejection.[21] Afterload is the force that resists myofibril shortening and varies throughout systole. Acutely increasing afterload results in decreases in stroke volume and ejection fraction. The effect of afterload also can be illustrated using the law of LaPlace. A child with aortic stenosis has increased afterload secondary to the increased pressure needed to eject blood through the stenotic orifice. When compensated, the left ventricle hypertrophies (wall thickness increases) to restore wall stress to normal.[23,24] Indices of afterload include aortic pressure, total peripheral resistance, arterial impedance (arterial elastance [Ea]), and myocardial peak wall stress.

Pressure-Volume Analysis

It is best to understand the interaction between pressure, volume, and contractility by analyzing pressure-volume loops (Fig. 12-4). Using the left ventricle as a model, myocardial contraction begins at end diastole (the point marked *EDV*). This starts the period of **isovolumic contraction**, when there is an increase in left ventricular pressure without change in left ventricular volume. When the pressure in the left ventricular chamber exceeds aortic pressure, the aortic valve opens, and left ventricular volume decreases as blood is ejected. When contraction reaches its peak at end systole, the myocardial fibers begin to relax. The left ventricular pressure decreases to less than aortic pressure, and the aortic valve closes. This starts the period of **isovolumic relaxation**, when there is a rapid decrease in left ventricular pressure without a change in volume. The mitral valve opens, and ventricular filling begins. The EDV is reached at the point marked *EDV,* starting the curve over again.

The upper left hand corner of any given pressure-volume loop represents end systole, the point of **maximal elastance (E max)**. A group of pressure-volume loops can be obtained by applying a brief alteration of preload or afterload (the most commonly used method of altering preload is a transient balloon occlusion of the inferior vena cava). The upper left hand corners of each pressure-volume loop within this series of loops can be

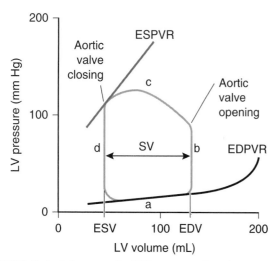

FIGURE 12-4 ■ Left ventricular (LV) pressure-volume loop. The various phases of the LV pressure-volume loop are depicted in the diagram. Line *a* denotes ventricular filling; *b,* isovolumetric contraction; *c,* ventricular ejection; and *d,* isovolumetric relaxation. EDPVR, end-diastolic pressure-volume relationship; EDV, end-diastolic volume; ESPVR, end-systolic pressure-volume relationship; ESV, end-diastolic volume. (From Klabunde RE: Textbook of Cardiovascular Physiology Concepts. Lippincott, Williams and Wilkins, 2004, Figure 4-4, p. 67)

FIGURE 12-5 ■ Left ventricular (LV) volume pressure relationship and inotropic state. Diagram shows the end-systolic pressure-volume relationship (ESPVR) line with positive inotropic agent (line shifted to the left) and negative inotropic agent (line shifted to the right). EDPVR, end-diastolic pressure-volume relationship. (From Burkhoff D: Mechanical properties of the heart and its interaction with the vascular system. http:/www.columbia.edu/itc/hs/medical/heartsim.)

connected to each other, and define the **end-systolic pressure-volume relationship (ESPVR).** The ESPVR intercepts the *x*-axis at a volume defined as Vo (the volume at which the ventricle cannot develop any pressure in systole). ESPVR, over physiologic ranges, is relatively linear. The slope of the ESPVR, **end-systolic elastance (Ees)** in units of elastance, mm Hg/mL, is a relatively load-independent index of ventricular contractility.[25-27] An increase in contractility is reflected in a leftward shift of the ESPVR (i.e., steeper line), whereas a rightward shift indicates decreased contractility (Fig. 12-5).

Because in the physiologic range ESPVR can be approximated as a straight line, it can be described by an equation relating its slope (Ees) and volume axis intercept (Vo):

$$Pes = Ees\ (Ves - Vo)$$

where Pes and Ves refer to the pressure and volume at end systole, respectively.

The volume axis intercept is extrapolated from the ESPVR line and subject to large errors. Also, Ees depends on ventricular size, which has hindered attempts at defining normal values for Ees despite correcting for ventricular size. There are some limitations when using the ESPVR as a clinical measure of left ventricular contractility. Despite the various inherent limitations, left ventricular pressure-volume analysis provides a powerful tool to aid in understanding the interaction of contractile state and load to produce ventricular performance.[28-33]

The **left ventricular end-diastolic pressure-volume relationship (EDPVR)**, in contrast to the left ventricular ESPVR, is nonlinear and represents the relationship

between pressure and volume during ventricular diastole. The slope (dP/dV) of the EDPVR is the ventricular elastance or stiffness. The chamber stiffness depends on where along the curve it is measured. Its reciprocal (dV/dP), or inverse of the slope, is compliance or distensibility.[9,34-36] The early part of the EDPVR curve is relatively linear, but the slope increases as the ventricle continues to fill. A shift of the curve leftward indicates an increase in stiffness, and a shift rightward indicates an increase in compliance (Fig. 12-6). (See other chapters for more in-depth discussion.)

Ventricular energetics can be understood in the pressure-volume plane (Fig. 12-7). The area contained within the left ventricular pressure-volume loop is the **stroke work**, or the external work performed by the ventricle. The remaining area under the ESPVR is the **potential energy** produced by the ventricular contraction but not resulting in external work. The sum of the two is equal to the total **pressure-volume area (PVA)**. Suga and colleagues[58] compared this estimate of mechanical energy expenditure with the myocardial oxygen consumption (MVO_2), and it was determined that MVO_2 was linearly related to the PVA. Most positive inotropic interventions shift the MVO_2-PVA relation upward, indicating an increase in energy demands.

Further understanding of ventricular energetics can be obtained through analysis of ventriculoarterial coupling (see other chapters). Optimal transfer of energy from the ventricles to their respective arterial circulations requires appropriate matching of these mechanical systems. How the ventricles adapt to their respective afterloads defines maximal external work output. **Afterload**, or total peripheral resistance, is represented

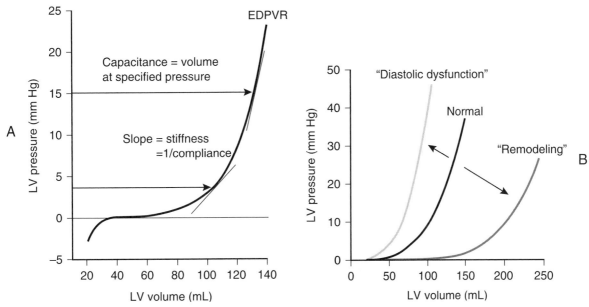

FIGURE 12-6 ■ **End-diastolic pressure-volume relationship. A,** Nonlinearity of end-diastolic pressure-volume relationship (EDPVR). Terms used are depicted, including ventricular stiffness (slope of EDPVR at a given volume), compliance (mathematical reciprocal of stiffness), and chamber capacitance (volume at a specific filling pressure). **B,** Changes in the passive component of diastole (i.e., shift of end-diastolic pressure-volume relationship [EDPVR]). A leftward/upward–shifted EDPVR (decreased ventricular capacitance) results in a need for increased filling pressure to achieve filling volumes necessary for the heart to generate a normal stroke volume and blood pressure. Conversely a rightward/downward–shifted EDPVR (increased ventricular capacitance) occurs in all forms of dilated cardiomyopathy and is commonly referred to as "ventricular remodeling." LV, left ventricular. (From Burkhoff D: *Diastolic heart failure. J Am Coll Cardiol* 2004;44:1543-1549).

on the pressure-volume diagrams as the **arterial elastance (Ea)** (Fig. 12-8). It is the ratio of end-systolic pressure to end-systolic volume:

$$Ea = Pes/ESV$$

Ventriculoarterial coupling is described as the relationship between the Ea and Ees: Ea/Ees. The ratio of these elastances defines the efficiency of the myocardium. In a failing ventricle, it is implied that there is less than maximal work output, which creates a ventriculoarterial mismatch. This type of analysis has been employed to evaluate ventricular energetics in the Fontan circulation.[37] Szabo and associates[37] showed a decrease in contractility in the Fontan circulation by way of a decrease in Ees

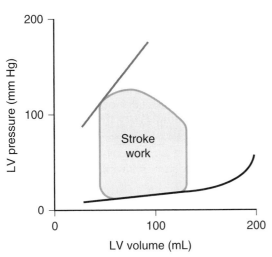

FIGURE 12-7 ■ **Stroke work.** The ventricular stroke work is the area bounded within the ventricular pressure-volume loop. The remaining area under the end-systolic pressure-volume relationship is the potential energy produced by the ventricular contraction but not resulting in external work. The sum of the two is equal to the total pressure-volume area, which correlates with myocardial oxygen consumption. LV, left ventricular. (From Klabunde RE: Textbook of Cardiovascular Physiology Concepts. Lippincott, Williams and Wilkins, 2004, Figure 1, p. 17)

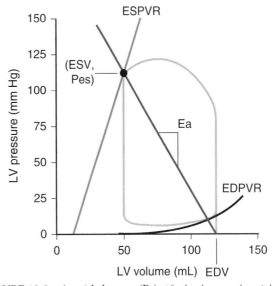

FIGURE 12-8 ■ **Arterial elastance (Ea).** Afterload, or total peripheral resistance, is represented on pressure-volume diagrams as the effective Ea. It is the ratio of end-systolic pressure to stroke volume: Ea = Pes/ESV. EDPVR, end-diastolic pressure-volume relationship; ESPVR, end-systolic pressure-volume relationship; ESV, end-systolic volume; LV, left ventricular; Pes, end-systolic pressure. (From Burkhoff D: http://www.columbia.edu/itc/hs/medical/heartsim. Mechanical properties of the heart and its interaction with the vascular system.

(i.e., a decrease in the slope of the ESPVR); accompanied by an increase in Ea; this results in an increased Ea/Ees. The implication was that the Fontan circulation created a ventriculoarterial mismatch by increased impedance (caused by the additional connection of the pulmonary vascular bed to the systemic vasculature) and decreased contractility, predicting limited functional reserve.

Information that can be obtained from analyses of pressure-volume loops thus includes (1) end-systolic and end-diastolic pressures and volumes, (2) stroke volume and cardiac output, (3) left ventricular filling dynamics by the slope of the EDPVR, (4) stroke work (area within the pressure-volume loops; i.e., external work) and potential energy (residual area under the ESPVR slope), (5) contractile state of the ventricle by the slope of the ESPVR, and (6) ventriculovascular coupling.[20]

Evaluation of Systolic Function and Contractility

Systolic function should be viewed as a composite interaction between preload, afterload, and contractility. The concepts of preload, afterload, and contractility were developed from isolated muscle experiments. When analyzed individually, each of these concepts was easily defined. Converting the concepts to a composite interaction relevant to the intact cardiovascular system has been challenging, however. When analyzing ventricular performance, it is best not to separate changes in ventricular performance from changes in contractility, but rather to describe how the heart functions either as a pump (considering variables that represent output) or as a contracting muscle (considering variables of pressure, force, or stress).

The heart is a complex organ with many contributing factors that help define its overall function. In simple terms, when describing the heart as a pump, we are interested in input and output. The relationship between the two is illustrated by the well-known Frank-Starling relationship (Fig. 12-9). When preload (EDV) is increased, the normal heart is capable of increasing its force of contraction and as a result increases stroke volume; this also depends on the state of inotropy and the imposed afterload. Changes in venous return cause a ventricle to move along a single Frank-Starling curve that is defined by the existing conditions of afterload and inotropy. An upward shift of the curve represents an increase in contractility or a decrease in afterload, and a downward shift of the curve represents a depression of contractility or an augmentation of afterload.

In general, left ventricular performance is considered impaired if there is an increase in ventricular EDV, while stroke volume (or cardiac index or both) and work are within normal limits or reduced. Afterload and preload are more descriptive of the heart as a pump, whereas **contractility** is more of an attribute of the heart as a muscle. Contractility is influenced primarily by biochemical and hormonal changes and classically

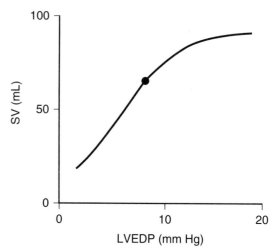

FIGURE 12-9 ■ **Frank-Starling mechanism.** Increasing venous return to the left ventricle increases the left ventricular end-diastolic pressure (LVEDP) and volume, which increases ventricular preload. The end result is an increase in stroke volume (SV). The normal operating point in adult subjects is an LVEDP of about 8 mm Hg and a stroke volume of 70 mL per beat. (From Klabunde RE: Textbook of Cardiovascular Physiology Concepts. Lippincott, Williams and Wilkins, 2004, Figure 4-8, p. 73.)

has been regarded as independent of preload or afterload.[22] Contractility is not synonymous with systolic function. Rather, systolic function is a factor of contractility, afterload, and preload and can be impaired while contractility is normal.

The maximum rate of increase of **ventricular pressure dP/dt_{max}** is one of the most extensively studied parameters of myocardial contractility.[22,24,38] It is highly sensitive to acute changes in contractility. A reduced slope of the ventricular pressure curve signifies impaired contractility. Under normal circumstances, dP/dt is believed to be independent of changes in afterload, but sensitive to changes in preload. The effect is enhanced in ventricles with increased contractility, but reduced in ventricles with depressed contractility. Several attempts have been made to desensitize dP/dt to the effect of changing preload.

In the early 1960s, Gleason and Braunwald were the first to report dP/dt in patients. They studied 40 healthy adult patients with micromanometer-tipped catheters and obtained a dP/dt_{max} in the range of 841 to 1696 mm Hg/sec in the left ventricle and 223 to 296 mm Hg/sec in the right ventricle. By altering myocardial contractility with maneuvers such as exercise and infusion of norepinephrine or isoproterenol, they showed a significant increase in dP/dt.[22] Numerous studies followed to assess dP/dt, each with a different method of altering contractility. These studies showed that isometric and dynamic exercise, tachycardia by atrial pacing or atropine, β-agonists, and digitalis glycosides all produced increases in dP/dt_{max}.

Few studies have been done in humans to assess the changes in dP/dt induced by alterations in afterload and preload. The studies seem to indicate that dP/dt_{max} tends to increase slightly with moderate increases in left ventricular preload and shows little change with alterations in afterload. Although changes in dP/dt reflect acute changes in inotropy in a given individual, dP/dt is less useful in comparisons between individuals, especially when there has been chronic left ventricular pressure or volume overload. Peak dP/dt generally is increased in patients with chronic aortic stenosis, although contractility is normal or decreased in most of these patients. Accurate measurement of dP/dt requires a pressure measurement system with excellent frequency-response characteristics. Because this level of high-fidelity recording is not possible using fluid-filled catheters, micromanometer-tipped catheters usually are required to achieve this frequency-response range.

Evaluation of Diastolic Function and Relaxation/Stiffness

Diastole is characterized by a set of separate but interrelated phases, defined as relaxation, filling, and end diastole. The most common parameters used to assess diastolic function can be measured in the cardiac catheterization laboratory. The diastolic function measurements can be divided into measurements that reflect the process of active relaxation and measurements that reflect passive stiffness. These measurements are the time constant of relaxation, or tau (τ), which is representative of active relaxation; passive relaxation (dP/dV), which is subcategorized into chamber stiffness (Kc), and myocardial stiffness (Km); its inverse, compliance (dV/dP); and the ventricular end-diastolic pressure.[9,34,35,39-41] Other parameters, such as isovolumic relaxation time and peak negative dP/dt, are not true representations of ventricular relaxation, but depend on such things as heart rate and peak systolic pressure. The above-mentioned parameters have been used predominantly for the left ventricle, but also have been derived for the right ventricle.[20]

When the aortic and pulmonary valves close, the ventricular pressures decline in an exponential fashion during isovolumic relaxation. Isovolumic relaxation can be studied using a high-fidelity, micromanometer-tipped catheter, and the peak rate of ventricular pressure decline (peak negative dP/dt) and the time constant of isovolumic ventricular pressure decline, τ, can be calculated.[43,53]

The maximum rate of ventricular pressure decline, **peak negative dP/dt**, is one of the simplest ways of quantifying the time course of left ventricular pressure decline. Peak negative dP/dt is altered, however, by changes in loading conditions and by conditions that change myocardial relaxation.[43] Because of the load dependency of peak negative dP/dt and the fact that it uses information from only one point on the left ventricular pressure-time plot, other indices have been introduced that analyze the time course of left ventricular isovolumic pressure more completely.[40]

The **relaxation constant** τ was first introduced by Weiss and coworkers[52] in 1976 and was derived from micromanometric recordings of left ventricular pressure. It is the inverse slope of the linear relationship between the natural log of ventricular diastolic pressure plotted against time, $\ln P = \ln p_0 - t/\tau$, or more simply, the time it takes for ventricular pressure to decline by approximately two thirds of its initial value.[28,40,53] It also has been shown that τ is only minimally affected by loading conditions and is a more reliable parameter to evaluate early diastolic relaxation than peak negative dP/dt.[28,40] It increases with slower ventricular relaxation and decreases with faster relaxation (e.g., sympathetic stimulation) and can be used for the left and right ventricles. Leeuwenburgh and colleagues[43] showed that isovolumetric relaxation time during early diastole is shorter in the right ventricle than in the left ventricle, but it occurs within the period of left ventricular isovolumetric relaxation. Normal adult values of τ have been derived,[24] but it has been more difficult to obtain normal values of τ in children because of the lack of controls. Krogmann and associates[56] were first to evaluate τ in children.

In addition to active relaxation, passive viscoelastic properties contribute to the process that returns the myocardium to its resting force and length. The properties typically are regarded as ventricular (chamber stiffness) and myocardial properties (muscle stiffness). Ventricular (passive) elastic properties are related directly to the symptoms experienced by patients, whereas the myocardial properties reflect the functional status of the heart muscle itself and may or may not be influenced by the organ as a whole.

Chamber stiffness (Kc) assesses the ability of the ventricle to distend under pressure and can be derived from the EDPVR. Ideally the passive EDPVR should be constructed from points that are obtained after relaxation is complete and at slow filling rates so that viscous effects are not present. This is during the period of mid-to late diastole when the influence of active ventricular relaxation and atrial related filling rates are minimal. When the EDPVR is obtained, the chamber stiffness generally is defined as a change in pressure relative to a change in volume (dP/dV). Because the pressure-volume relationship is nonlinear, the chamber stiffness depends on the point on the curve at which it is measured. Most indices of chamber stiffness change with changing ventricular volumes. The most commonly used equation for assessing chamber stiffness is:

$$P = ae^{KcV}$$

where P is the LVEDP, a is the y intercept constant, e is the base of the natural logarithm, Kc is the chamber stiffness constant or slope, and V is left ventricular EDV.[28,40] When chamber stiffness increases, the pressure-volume curve shifts to the left, and the chamber stiffness constant is increased.[54]

Studies that have defined the chamber stiffness constant are based on earlier work done by Mirsky.[57] Only a few pediatric studies have been performed that examined the passive properties of the ventricle. Banerjee and coworkers[28] analyzed the effect of hypertrophy on diastolic function in children using the common exponential curve equation. The chamber stiffness constant was calculated as the slope of the linear regression between left ventricular EDV (dP/dV) versus LVEDP. In addition, Sandor and Olley[34] studied 13 pediatric patients, 10 of whom had congenital heart disease, and determined values for chamber and myocardial stiffness.

Myocardial stiffness (Km) can be quantified using the myocardial stress-strain relationship and represents the resistance of the myocardium to stretching when it is subjected to a stress. The calculation of stress is difficult and involves a geometric model of the left ventricle, whereas the calculation of strain requires some assumption of the unstressed left ventricular volume. Muscle stiffness is the slope of the myocardial stress-strain relationship. Calculation of myocardial stiffness is achieved by plotting instantaneous left ventricular diastolic wall stress against left ventricular mid-wall strain from the lowest diastolic to end-diastolic pressure or from the end of the rapid filling phase to the peak a wave:

$$\sigma = ae^{k\varepsilon}$$

where σ is the left ventricular end-diastolic stress, a is the y intercept constant, e is the base of the natural logarithm, k is the myocardial stiffness constant or slope, and ε is left ventricular end-diastolic strain. At any given strain, myocardial stiffness is equal to the slope $(d\sigma/d\varepsilon)$ of a tangent drawn to the stress-strain relationship at that strain. When myocardial stiffness is increased, the stress-strain relationship shifts to the left so that for any given change in myocardial length (strain), there is greater increase in force (wall stress) that develops to resist this deformation. In addition, the slope of the $d\sigma/d\varepsilon$-versus-stress relationship becomes steeper, and the myocardial stiffness constant increases when myocardial stiffness is increased.[54] Theoretical and technical difficulties in determining these indices have limited their clinical usefulness.

CURRENT STATUS AND FUTURE TRENDS

Most of the aforementioned parameters also have been applied to the right ventricle. Because of the complexity of the right ventricle in shape, location, and geometry, however, there continues to be a paucity of studies regarding its function compared with the left ventricle. Redington[42] pointed out the fact that since the 1970s, the number of publications concerning the left ventricle outnumbered publications for the right ventricle by 10 to 1. Since the 1990s, there has been an increase in interest in the study of the right ventricle. This increased research is expected to have the greatest impact on pediatric cardiology and on adults with congenital heart disease.

Further understanding of the physiology of the right ventricle will lead to better interpretation of the aforementioned techniques when assessing systolic and diastolic performance. The right ventricle and left ventricle pump against different vascular beds, and the right ventricle expends only about one quarter of the external work expended by the left ventricle. The pressure-volume tracing of the right ventricle is different (more triangular in shape than that of the left ventricle) but can resemble the left ventricular pressure-volume loop when faced with an increased afterload, such as in pulmonary stenosis or single right ventricle. Right ventricular and left ventricular diastolic properties also are different. Nevertheless, despite the inherent differences in left ventricular and right ventricular properties, they remain inextricably linked.[42-46]

Despite important advances in noninvasive imaging techniques, some of the most robust parameters important to the understanding of cardiac function still can be obtained only by invasive assessment in the cardiac catheterization laboratory. Although some of the concepts discussed in this chapter have direct clinical applicability, others are used predominantly for research purposes.[59] Human studies involving pediatric subjects are lacking, especially studies of right ventricular performance and diastolic function in the setting of congenital heart disease.[60]

Key Concepts

■ Filling pressures are poor surrogates of preload when abnormal chamber filling characteristics exist because the filling pressure depends in large part on the compliance of the atrium and ventricle.

■ The idealized measure of left ventricular afterload is the systolic wall stress. This value is extremely complex to calculate, however, because none of its components (pressure, wall thickness, and left ventricular volume) is constant during systole; wall stress ideally would need to be integrated over the duration of systole.

■ The applicability of the area-length method, which compares the left ventricle with an ellipsoid, is questionable when applied to the right ventricle or a geometrically distorted left ventricle caused by a disease state (e.g., the left ventricle is known to change from an ellipsoid shape to a much more spherical shape in severe dilated cardiomyopathy).

■ Because the conductance catheter method is relatively independent of ventricular geometry, it lends itself well to the study of ventricular function in congenital heart disease, especially when assessing abnormal right ventricles.

■ Conductance catheters have enabled cardiologists to generate real-time pressure-volume loops for a wide variety of indices of systolic and diastolic function, allowing for the discrimination of ventricular chamber function with respect to primary systolic, diastolic, and vascular loading factors.

■ Preload represents all the factors that contribute to passive ventricular wall stress (or tension) at the end of diastole. Changing compliance of the ventricles makes end-diastolic pressure less reliable than EDV as a measure of preload. Because the right ventricular and left ventricular EDVs are difficult to measure, however, preload is often estimated by using the end-diastolic pressure (RVEDP, LVEDP).

■ Afterload is similarly described as all the factors that contribute to total myocardial wall stress (or tension) during systolic ejection. It is the force that resists myofibril shortening and varies throughout systole. Indices of afterload include aortic pressure, total peripheral resistance, Ea, and myocardial peak wall stress.

■ The left ventricular EDPVR, in contrast to the left ventricular ESPVR, is nonlinear and represents the relationship between pressure and volume at the time of complete ventricular relaxation (end-diastole). The slope (dP/dV) of the EDPVR is the ventricular elastance or stiffness. The early part of the curve is relatively linear, but the slope increases as the ventricle continues to fill. A shift of the curve leftward indicates an increase in stiffness, and a shift rightward indicates an increase in compliance.

■ The area contained within the left ventricular pressure-volume loop is the stroke work, or the external work performed by the ventricle. The remaining area under the ESPVR is the potential energy produced by the ventricular contraction but not resulting in external work. The sum of the two is equal to the PVA. MVO_2 was linearly related to the PVA.

■ Afterload, or total peripheral resistance, is represented on the pressure-volume diagrams as the effective Ea. It is the ratio of end-systolic pressure to stroke volume: Ea = Pes/SV.

■ Ventriculoarterial coupling is described as the relationship between the Ea and Ees: Ea/Ees. The ratio of these elastances defines the efficiency of the myocardium.

■ When analyzing ventricular performance, it is best not to separate changes in ventricular performance from changes in contractility, but rather to describe how the heart functions either as a pump (considering variables that represent output) or as a contracting muscle (considering variables of pressure, force, or stress).

■ Contractility is not synonymous with systolic function. Rather, systolic function is a factor of contractility, afterload, and preload and can be impaired while contractility is normal.

■ The diastolic function measurements can be divided into measurements that reflect the process of active relaxation and measurements that reflect passive stiffness, including the time constant of relaxation, or τ, which is representative of active relaxation; passive relaxation (dP/dV), which is subcategorized into chamber stiffness and myocardial stiffness; its inverse,

compliance (dV/dP); and the ventricular end-diastolic pressure.

■ It also has been shown that τ is only minimally affected by loading conditions and is a more reliable parameter to evaluate early diastolic relaxation than negative dP/dt.

■ In addition to active relaxation, passive viscoelastic properties contribute to the process that returns the myocardium to its resting force and length. The properties typically are regarded as ventricular (chamber stiffness) and myocardial properties (muscle stiffness).

■ Chamber stiffness assesses the ability of the ventricle to distend under pressure and can be derived from the EDPVR. When the EDPVR is obtained, the chamber stiffness generally is defined as a change in pressure relative to a change in volume (dP/dV).

■ Myocardial stiffness can be quantified using the myocardial stress-strain relationship and represents the resistance of the myocardium to stretching when it is subjected to a stress. Calculation of myocardial stiffness is achieved by plotting instantaneous left ventricular diastolic wall stress against left ventricular midwall strain from the lowest diastolic to end-diastolic pressure or from the end of the rapid filling phase to the peak a wave.

REFERENCES

1. Dodge HT, Sandler H, Ballew DW: The use of biplane angiocardiography for the measurement of left ventricular volume in man. Am Heart J 1960;60:762-776.

2. Fifer MA, Grossman W: Measurement of ventricular volumes, ejection fraction, mass, wall mass, and regional wall motion. In Baim DS, Grossman W (eds): Grossman's Cardiac Catheterization, Angiography and Intervention, 6th ed. Philadelphia. Lippincott, Williams and Wilkins. 2000, pp. 353-366.

3. Graham TP, Jarmakani JM, Canent RV: Left heart volume estimation in infancy and childhood. Circulation 1971;43:895-904.

4. McKay RG, Spears JR, Aroesty JM: Instantaneous measurement of left and right ventricular stroke volume and pressure-volume relationship with an impedence catheter. Circulation 1984;69:703-710.

5. Graham TP, Jarmakani JM, Atwood GF: Right ventricular volume determinations in children. Circulation 1972;47:144-153.

6. Gentzler H, Briselli MF, Gault JH: Angiographic estimation of right ventricular volume in man. Circulation 1974;50:324-330.

7. Witsenburg M, van der Velde E, Klautz R: Acute effects of balloon valvuloplasty and pacing on left ventricular performance in children with moderate pulmonary valve stenosis, analysed by systolic and diastolic pressure-volume relationships. Eur Heart J 1994; 15:83-88.

8. Baan J, Van Der Velde E, De Bruin H: Continuous measurement of left ventricular volume in animals and humans by conductance catheter. Circulation 1984;70:812-823.

9. Sandor GS, Patterson M, Tipple M: Left ventricular systolic and diastolic function after total correction of tetralogy of Fallot. Am J Cardiol 1987;60:1148-1151.

10. Senzaki H, Masutani S, Kobyashi J: Ventricular afterload and ventricular work in Fontan circulation. Circulation 2002;105: 2885-2892.

11. Chaturvedi R, Kilner P, White P: Increased airway pressure and simulated branch pulmonary artery stenosis increase pulmonary regurgitation after repair of tetralogy of Fallot. Circulation 1997;95:643-649.

12. Chaturvedi R, Lincoln C, Gothard J: Left ventricular dysfunction after open repair of simple congenital heart defects in infants and children: Quantitation with the use of a conductance catheter immediately after bypass. J Thorac Cardiovasc Surg 1998;115:77-83.

13. Redington A, Oldershaw P, Shinebourne E: A new technique for the assessment of pulmonary regurgitation and its application to the assessment of right ventricular function before and after repair of tetralogy of Fallot. Br Heart J 1988;60:57-65.

14. White P, Redington A: Right ventricular volume measurement: Can conductance do it better? Physiol Meas 2000;21:R23-R41.

15. White P, Bishop A, Conroy B: The determination of volume of right ventricular casts using a conductance catheter. Eur Heart J 1995;16:1425-1429.

16. White PA, Chaturvedi RR, Shore D: Left ventricular parallel conductance during cardiac cycle in children with congenital heart disease. Am J Physiol 1997;42:H295-H302.

17. Szwarc R, Ball H: Simultaneous LV and RV volumes by conductance catheter: Effects of lung insufflation on parallel conductance. Am J Physiol 1998;275:H653-H661.

18. White PA, Chaturvedi RR, Bishop AJ: Does parallel conductance vary during systole in the human right ventricle? Cardiovasc Res 1996;32:901-908.

19. White P, Brookes C, Ravn H: Validation and utility of novel reduction technique for determination of parallel conductance. Am J Physiol Heart Circ Physiol 2001;280:H475-H482.

20. Piper C, Horstkotte D, Wiemer M: Real-time pressure-volume measurements: A new diagnostic tool for the assessment of valvar heart disease. J Heart Valve Dis 2003;12:420-422.

21. Norton J: Toward consistent definitions for preload and afterload. Adv Physiol Educ 2001;25:53-61.

22. Fifer MA, Grossman W: Mesurement of ventricular volumes, ejection fraction, mass, wall mass, and regional wall motion. In Baim DS, Grossman W (eds): Grossman's Cardiac Catheterization, Angiography and Intervention, 6th ed. Philadelphia. Lippincott, Williams and Wilkins, 2000, pp. 353-366.

23. Dorn GW, Donner R, Assey ME: Alterations in left ventricular geometry, wall stress, and ejection performance after correction of congenital aortic stenosis. Circulation 1998;78:1358-1364.

24. Little WC: Assessment of normal and abnormal cardiac function. In Braunwald E, Zipes DP, Libby P, Bonou R (eds.): Heart Disease: A Textbook of Cardiovascular Medicine, 6th ed. Philadelphia. WB Saunders. 2001, pp. 479-502.

25. Sagawa K: The end-systolic pressure-volume relation of the ventricle: Definition, modifications and clinical use. Circulation 1981; 63:1223-1227.

26. Suga H, Sagawa K: Instantaneous pressure-volume relationship and their ratio in the excised, supported canine left ventricle. Circ Res 1974;35:117-126.

27. McKay R, Aroesty J, Heller G: Left ventricular pressure-volume diagrams and end-systolic pressure-volume relations in human beings. J Am Coll Cardiol 1984;3:301-312.

28. Banerjee A, Mendelsohn AM, Knilans TK: Effect of myocardial hypertrophy on systolic and diastolic function in children: Insights from the force frequency and relaxation-frequency relationship. J Am Coll Cardiol 1998;32:1088-1095.

29. Schreuder J, Steendijk P, Van der Veen F: Acute and short-term effects of partial left ventriculectomy in dilated cardiomyopathy: Assessment by pressure-volume loops. J Am Coll Cardiol 2000;36: 2104-2114.

30. Peterson K, Tsuji J, Johnson A: Diastolic left ventricular pressure-volume and stress-strain relation in patients with valvular aortic stenosis and left ventricular hypertrophy. Circulation 1978;58: 77-89.

31. Dekker A, Barenbrug P, van der Veen F: Pressure-volume loops in patients with aortic stenosis. J Heart Valve Dis 2003;12:325-332.

32. Hon J, Steendijk P, Petrou M: Influence of clenbuterol treatment during six weeks of chronic right ventricular pressure overload as studied with pressure-volume analysis. J Thorac Cardiovasc Surg 2001;122:767-774.

33. Caputo M, Schreuder J, Fino C: Assessment of myocardial performance with ventricular pressure-volume relations: Clinical application in cardiac surgery. Ital Heart J 2000;1:269-274.

34. Sandor GS, Olley PM: Determination of left ventricular diastolic chamber stiffness and myocardial stiffness in patients with congenital heart disease. Am J Cardiol 1982;49:771-779.

35. Sandor GS, Puterman ML, Patterson M: Effect of pressure loading, volume loading and surgery on left ventricular chamber and myocardial stiffness in congenital heart disease, with a reevaluation of normal pediatric values. J Am Coll Cardiol 1986;8:371-378.

36. Gaasch WH, Levine HJ, Quinines MA: Left ventricular compliance: Mechanisms and clinical implications. Am J Cardiol 1976;38: 645-653.

37. Szabo G, Buhmann V, Graf A: Ventricular energetics after the Fontan operation: Contractility-afterload mismatch. J Thorac Cardiovasc Surg 2003;125:1061-1069.

38. Penny D: The basics of ventricular function. Cardiol Young 1999; 9:210-223.

39. Brutsaert DL, Sys SU, Gillebert TC: Diastolic failure: Pathophysiology and therapeutic implications. J Am Coll Cardiol 1993; 22:318-325.

40. Mandinov L, Eberli FR, Seiler C: Diastolic heart failure. Cardiovasc Res 2000;45:813-825.

41. Kass DA: Assessement of diastolic dysfunction: Invasive modalities. Cardiol Clin 2000;18:571-586.

42. Redington AN: Right ventricular function. Cardiol Clin 2002;20: 341-349.

43. Leeuwenburgh B, Steendijk P, Helbing WA: Indexes of diastolic RV function: Load dependence and changes after chronic RV pressure overload in lambs. Am J Physiol Heart Circ Physiol 2002;282:H1350-H1358.

44. Brookes C, Ravn H, White P: Acute right ventricular dilatation in response to ischemia significantly impairs left ventricular systolic performance. Circulation 1999;100:761-767.

45. Brookes C, White P, Bishop A: Validation of a new intraoperative technique to evaluate load-independent indices of right ventricular performance in patients undergoing cardiac operations. J Thorac Cardiol Surg 1998;116:468-476.

46. Redington A, Gray H, Hodson M: Characterization of the normal right ventricular pressure-volume relation by biplane angiography and simultaneous micomanometer pressure measurements. Br Heart J 1988;59:23-30.

47. Eichhorn EJ, Willard JE, Alvarez L: Are contraction and relaxation coupled in patients with and without congestive heart failure? Circulation 1992;85:2132-2139.

48. Derrick GP, Narang I, White PA: Failure of stroke volume augmentation during exercise and dobutamine stress is unrelated to load-independent indexes of right ventricular performance after the mustard operation. Circulation 2000;102(Suppl III):III-154-III-159.

49. Shishido T, Sugimachi M, Kawaguchi O: Novel method to estimate ventricular contractility using interventricular pulse wave velocity. Am J Physiol 1999;277:H2409-H2415.

50. Amirhamzeh M, Dean D, Jia C: Validation of right and left ventricular conductance and echocardiography for cardiac function studies. Ann Thorac Surg 1996;62:1104-1109.

51. Moss R, Fitzsimons D: Frank-Starling relationship: Long on importance, short on mechanism. Circ Res 2002;90:11-13.

52. Weiss JL, Fredericksen JW, Weisfeldt ML: Hemodynamic determinants of the time course of fall in canine left ventricular pressure. J Clin Invest 1976;58:751-756.

53. Zile MR, Brutsaert DL: New concepts in diastolic dysfunction and diastolic heart failure: I. Diagnosis, prognosis, measurements of diastolic function. Circulation 2002;105:1387-1393.

54. Zile MR, Catalin BF, Gaasch WH: Diastolic heart failure-abnormalities in active relaxation and passive stiffness of the left ventricle. N Engl J Med 2004;350:1953-1959.

55. Amoore JN, Santamore WP, Bove AA: The influence of ventricular interdependence on indices of left ventricular function. In Ingels NB, Daughters GT, Baan J, et al (eds): Systolic and

Diastolic Function of the Heart. Amsterdam, the Netherlands, IOS Press, 1996, p 123.

56. Krogmann ON, Rammos S, Jakob M: Left ventricular diastolic dysfunction late after coarctation repair in childhood: Influence of left ventricular hypertrophy. J Am Coll Cardiol 1993;21:1454-1460.

57. Mirsky I: Assessment of passive elastic stiffness of cardiac muscle: Mathematical concepts, physiologic and clinical considerations, directions of future research. Prog Cardiovasc Dis 1976;28: 277-308.

58. Suga H, Hayashi T, Shirahata M: Regression of cardiac oxygen consumption on ventricular pressure-volume area in dog. Am J Physiol 1981;240:H320-H325.

59. Ishida M, Tomita S, Nakatani T, et al: Acute effects of direct cell implantation into the heart: A pressure-volume study to analyze cardiac function. J Heart Lung Transplant 2004;23:881-888.

60. Kanter JP, Hellebrand WE: Recent advances in non-interventional pediatric cardiac catheterization. Curr Opin Cardiol 2005; 20:75-79.

CHAPTER 13

The Economic Aspects of Heart Failure

Anthony C. Chang

Health care spending varies widely from country to country, with many countries spending less than 5% of the gross domestic product (GDP) and other countries spending significantly more. The health care expenditure for the United States, the world's largest health care market, exceeds $1 trillion per annum and 15% of the GDP (increasing from $10 billion and 3.8% of the GDP in 1950) with per capita spending for health care presently the highest in the world ($5440 in 2002).[1] The United States consumes about 40% of all health care expenditures, while comprising only 5% of the world population. Germany and Japan, with comparable GDPs per capita as the United States, spend about half as much per capita on health care expenditure per person (Fig. 13-1).

In the United States, most health care costs are due to increased service intensity—more health care workers per patient to provide more technologically advanced care. Although the United States spends more money per capita on health care than other countries, universal health care economic questions inevitably arise in all countries in dealing with heart failure: Who gets a heart transplant when there is a shortage of donors? Who will pay for state-of-the-art implantable ventricular assist devices? What medications can decrease hospital usage? Can specialized outpatient heart failure clinics decrease

hospital admission rates? Will children all over the world have equal access to medical and surgical therapies for heart failure?

Overall, governments around the world attempt to maximize market efficiency, while distributing health care resources and services. All countries must decide on three basic health economic decisions: (1) how much to allocate to health care services, (2) the methods to pay for those services, and (3) the means to distribute those services to the population.

PRIMER OF HEALTH CARE ECONOMICS

Supply and demand for health care services are discussed briefly here. Physicians tend to consider medical decisions in terms of need, whereas medical economists attempt to focus more on demand. Although the law of **demand** states that as one lowers the price, the greater the quantity demanded, the law of **supply** states that the higher the price, the greater is the quantity firms are willing to produce. As the demand increases, the price and the output correspondingly increase, and the size of the price and output increase depends on the amount of the demand increase and the supply responsiveness, called **elasticity**. If the supply is elastic, an

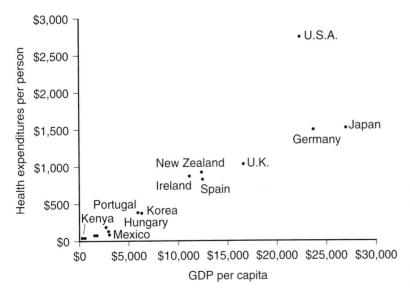

FIGURE 13-1 ■ **Health expenditures versus income.** The health expenditure per person (in U.S. dollars) is plotted against gross domestic product (GDP) per capita (in U.S. dollars). As shown, the United States is alone in its relatively high health expenditure per person for its GDP. (From Getzen TE: *Health Economics: Fundamentals and Flow of Funds.* New York, John Wiley & Sons, 1997, p. 419.)

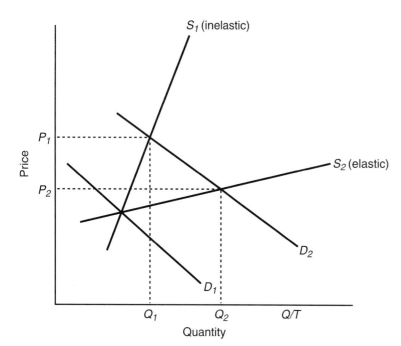

FIGURE 13-2 ■ **Different supply elasticities with increased demand.** The graph shows demand (D) and supply (S) curves with price (P) on the vertical axis and quantity (Q) of medical services on the horizontal axis. With the demand increase from D_1 to D_2, an elastic supply results in a larger increase in quantity of medical services (Q_2 versus Q_1), but an inelastic supply has a higher price increase (P_1 versus P_2). (From Feldstein PJ: *Health Care Economics.* Albany, NY, Delmar Publishers, 1999, p 47.)

increase in demand leads to increases in price and output; if the supply is relatively inelastic, however, a large price increase results in only a small increase in output (Fig. 13-2).

Two fundamental concepts are involved in demand: opportunity cost and marginal return. **Opportunity cost** is what must be given up to do or obtain something; in other words, the highest valued alternative that must be foregone. The opportunity cost of a medical education would include the foregone income one could have earned had one not gone to school. **Marginal return** is another analytic concept for health care. As a health program increases in size or in expenditure, the health output initially increases, but eventually increases at a more gradual rate (Fig. 13-3). The relationship between input and output in health care is not linear. A strategy in allocating resources to maximize the return from each of the programs (e.g., heart transplantation,

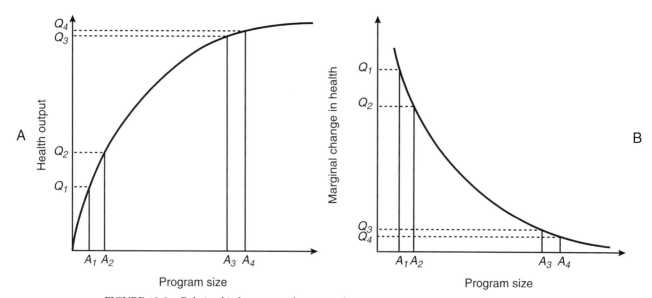

FIGURE 13-3 ■ **Relationship between total output and program size. A,** An increase in program size (on the horizontal axis) from A_1 to A_2 yields a larger increase in health output (on the vertical axis; Q_1 to Q_2) compared with a similar size increase from A_3 to A_4 (Q_3 to Q_4). **B,** This nonlinear relationship is depicted as program size on the horizontal axis and marginal change in health on the vertical axis. (From Feldstein PJ: *Health Care Economics.* Albany, NY, Delmar Publishers, 1999, p 22.)

mechanical assist devices, and outpatient management team) in decreasing mortality and morbidity of heart failure should include determination of marginal returns on each program.

Health care use and funding differ from country to country. In the United States, about 50% or more of the spending is to compensate for the hospital (≥35%) and the physician (about 20%).[2] The remainder is spent on drugs, nursing homes/home health, and other (including administration, public health, and research). The sources of funds include the government (almost 50%) and employer insurance (about 33%) with a fraction from self-pay (about 15% to 20%).

There are several economic analytic methods to determine clinical outcome for the resource expended. **Cost-benefit analysis** is an analytic technique that balances pros and cons of cost of health care and lives saved as part of public decision making; it provides a common ground for physicians and economists. The physician strives to use medical and surgical means to ameliorate the health of each individual patient, whereas the health care economist has to consider societal burden and budget constraints. Cost-benefit analysis compares different therapies in different areas of medicine, but measures cost and clinical outcomes in monetary terms. An example of cost-benefit analysis is whether coronary artery surgery or ventricular assist device implantation adds a sufficient number of years to life expectancy to justify the cost.[3]

Cost-effective analysis, an abbreviated form of the cost-benefit analysis, analyzes and compares the cost of several alternatives without directly translating the benefit (e.g., lives saved or cases prevented) into dollars. This type of analysis can determine which programs or inputs are least costly for achieving a given objective and can be used to compare several methods of intervention. A cost-effectiveness ratio can be determined, and the ratio typically provides a quantitative relationship between resources expended and health care outcomes. Cost per life saved among three programs to reduce neonatal mortality can be used as a case example (Table 13-1). The data show that the cost per life saved is much less with prenatal care compared with neonatal

intensive care units. A threshold for cost-effective care of $50,000 per quality-adjusted life-year gained is suggested.[4] The high prevalence of heart failure and its substantial economic burden render heart failure a good study model for cost-effectiveness analyses.

A specific type of cost-effectiveness analysis is **cost utility analysis**, which incorporates morbidity and quality-of-life measures (quality-adjusted life-years) into the clinical outcomes.[5] Such analyses in heart failure studies are lacking because there is an absence of quality-of-life weights.[6] Lastly, another type of economic cost analysis is **cost minimization analysis**. This analysis gathers solely information about the resources expended without taking into consideration clinical outcomes; the outcomes are presumed to be equivalent.

ECONOMIC BURDEN OF HEART FAILURE IN ADULTS

Mortality from coronary artery disease decreased by 50% between 1970 and 1990, and the two main contributing factors were changes in lifestyle (cessation of smoking, attention to hypertension, and reduction of cholesterol) and advent of coronary care units. Lifestyle changes not only are relatively inexpensive compared with state-of-the-art coronary care units in the effort to reduce mortality from coronary heart disease, but also were shown to be more effective.[7] Survivors of coronary heart disease now die from ischemic cardiomyopathy and heart failure, however, as the population ages and deaths from myocardial infarction diminishes. Epidemiologic studies of the increasing prevalence of heart failure reaching epidemic proportions showed that it is a consequence of improved survival coupled with minimal changes in disease prevention.[8] Heart failure is now one of the most prevalent and chronic diseases worldwide, with the prevalence about 20 million worldwide and expected to reach 10 million in the United States alone by 2007 with more than 500,000 new cases per annum.[9]

Data are limited on direct costs in heart failure. Health care use in heart failure encompasses not only

TABLE 13-1

Cost-Effectiveness Analysis: Cost per Lives Saved Among Three Programs to Reduce Neonatal Mortality		
	No. Lives Saved per 1000 Additional Participants	Cost of Each Program per 1000 Additional Participants	Cost per Life Saved
Prenatal care	4.5	$176,000	$39
Teenage family planning	0.6	$122,000	$203
Neonatal intensive care unit	2.8	$13,616,000	$4778

From Joyce T, Corman H, Grossman M: A cost-effective analysis of strategies to reduce infant mortality. Med Care 1988;26:348-360.

hospital admissions and stay, but also other items, such as rate of rehospitalization, inpatient and outpatient physician services, ambulance transportation, concomitant drugs administered, therapy for comorbidities, and laboratory and diagnostic tests performed. In addition, approximately 50,000 of heart failure patients in the United States potentially could benefit from some form of permanent cardiac replacement or assistance.[10] The research on new pharmacologic agents or new surgical technology is usually overhead cost in the production of drugs of new technology. The economic burden does not take into account work lost by patients and care provided by nonpaid caretakers. Lastly, there is no price valuation for human suffering from heart failure. One Italian study showed that among patients admitted for heart failure, 82% had difficulty with mobility, and 88% had limitations with everyday activities.[11]

Heart failure is the leading cause of hospitalization in the United States in adults older than age 65 and results in more than 3 million hospitalizations annually, with 50% of these patients readmitted within 6 months of initial discharge. Heart failure now accounts for more than 5% of total health care expenditures in the United States with an estimated cost of $21 to $40 billion.[12,13] Hospitalizations for heart failure are proportionally the greatest expenditure and account for 60% to 75% of overall cost of heart failure (with an average of $7000 to $10,000 per admission). Approximately 90% of resources are used by patients in New York Heart Association classes III and IV.[14] The associated morbidity and mortality with heart failure and its resource use are staggering worldwide.[15,16] Interventional measures to reduce disease severity and hospitalizations would reduce the economic burden of heart failure effectively.

One strategy to reduce resource use and improve clinical outcome is to provide early diagnosis and institute early vasoactive therapy for acute decompensated heart failure.[17] New diagnostic modalities, such as the biomarker B-type natriuretic peptide, can be useful to diagnose and monitor heart failure serially (see Chapter 6). In addition, nesiritide therapy has been shown to reduce health care use in patients with acute decompensated heart failure.[18] In chronic heart failure therapy, many drug studies have concomitant cost-effectiveness analyses that accompanied the efficacy assessments. Drugs such as valsartan, enalapril, bisoprolol, and carvedilol all have been shown to reduce cost per patient in chronic heart failure resource use.[19-23] Studies also compared drugs in the same class in cost-effectiveness. One study showed that patients treated with carvedilol experienced fewer total hospitalizations and emergency department visits compared with patients treated with metoprolol, despite a higher pharmacy cost.[24] Evidence exists that varying drug dosages used for heart failure can lead to different cost-effectiveness.[25] As the number of patients with ventricular assist device and cardiac resynchronization therapy increases,

cost-effectiveness of these types of therapy will be necessary to conform with cost-containment measures in the current economic milieu.[26,27]

An additional strategy to minimize health care costs in heart failure patients is to provide an inpatient and outpatient health care setting in which there is a focused effort in caring for these patients to reduce overall hospital usage.[28] The concept of **disease management** is defined as a population-based system in which there is recognition that patients at risk for adverse events are identified, subjected to a continuous intervention, and monitored for changes in outcome. A heart failure disease management program can be associated with decreased hospital use and cost at a single center or in a multicenter venue,[29,30] especially if a multidisciplinary approach to include nurse specialists is used.[31,32] There is also evidence for lower mortality and lower resource use when heart failure patients are followed by specialists and family practitioners (versus family practitioners alone or with no cardiovascular follow-up).[33] In addition, an outpatient heart failure clinic was shown to reduce hospital resources (admissions and length of stay).[34] Practice guidelines that include identification of risk factors for development of heart failure, serial assessment of guideline goals and risk for progression of disease, and promotion of evidence-based management of heart failure have been shown to be useful.[35] Even home monitoring in the form of electronic devices can reduce medical resource use.[36] Lastly, one study proposed that the heart failure disease management programs should be evaluated in the context of a retail pricing strategy known as leader pricing, the practice of pricing certain popular items at below cost (called loss-leader) to bring more customers into the store.[37]

ECONOMIC LESSONS FOR HEART FAILURE IN CHILDREN

There are major differences between adults and children with heart failure from the economic perspective. First, although more improvement in heart health resulted from public health awareness rather than expensive application of new medical technology, this concept is not applicable to pediatric patients with heart failure. In children, heart failure is due to ventricular dysfunction from prior palliative or corrective surgeries or from dilated cardiomyopathy.[38] Second, the pediatric heart failure population is relatively small compared with the adult heart failure population, and this has an impact on research and development in certain medical or surgical therapies (particularly advances in surgical devices, such as smaller ventricular assist devices). Third, clinicians who care for pediatric heart failure patients need to collaborate to delineate not only drug profiles, but also cost-effectiveness of the various therapies because the number of available pediatric patients for clinical trials is limited. Important lessons can be gleaned, however, from experience in adult heart failure and the economic burden it imposes on health care. Lastly, as children with congenital heart disease survive into adulthood, these adults with congenital heart disease who may have heart failure are steadily increasing in number and can benefit from the adult heart failure experience.[39] Overall, there are few data on cost per life saved among children with heart failure, but information will be forthcoming as this population increases in volume.

CURRENT STATUS AND FUTURE TRENDS

All health care systems strive for lower cost, higher quality, greater efficiency, and equal access. As the intensity of services increases as a result of new technology, it will be a continual challenge to maintain cost, while improving quality. In the future, care of heart failure patients will include use of frequent electronic communications between the patient and the primary care team.[40] Patients will have access to higher quality heart failure programs, but will have to be willing to have ownership in their health care and to pay for the quality. High-quality, high-efficiency care is necessary to care for pediatric heart failure patients. Economic analyses, including methods of evaluating cost-effectiveness of therapies in heart failure in children, will be essential to enable society to make better and more informed decisions.

Key Concepts

■ In the United States, most health care costs are due to increased service intensity—more health care workers per patient to provide more technologically advanced care.

■ Overall, governments around the world attempt to maximize market efficiency, while distributing health care resources and services. All countries must decide on three basic health economic decisions: (1) how much to allocate to health care services, (2) the methods to pay for those services, and (3) the means to distribute those services to the population.

■ Physicians tend to consider medical decisions in terms of need, whereas medical economists attempt to focus more on demand.

■ As the demand increases, the price and the output will correspondingly increase, and the size of the price and output increase depends on the amount of the demand increase and the supply responsiveness, called elasticity.

■ Opportunity cost is what must be given up to do or obtain something; in other words, the highest valued alternative that must be foregone. Marginal return is another analytic concept for health care. As a health program increases in size or in expenditure, the health output initially increases, but eventually increases at a more gradual rate.

■ Cost-benefit analysis is an analytic technique that attempts to balance pros and cons of cost of health care and lives saved as part of public decision making; it provides a common ground for physicians and economists.

■ Cost-effective analysis, an abbreviated form of the cost-benefit analysis, analyzes and compares the cost of several alternatives without directly translating the benefit (e.g., lives saved or cases prevented) into dollars.

■ A specific type of cost-effectiveness analysis is cost utility analysis, which incorporates morbidity and quality-of-life measures (quality-adjusted life-years) into clinical outcomes.

■ Epidemiologic studies of the increasing prevalence of heart failure reaching epidemic proportions showed that it is a consequence of improved survival coupled with minimal changes in disease prevention.

■ Heart failure is the leading cause of hospitalization in the United States in adults older than age 65 and results in more than 3 million hospitalizations annually, with 50% of these patients readmitted within 6 months of initial discharge.

■ One strategy to reduce resource usage and improve clinical outcome is to provide early diagnosis and institute early vasoactive therapy for acute decompensated heart failure.

■ An additional strategy to minimize health care costs in heart failure patients is to provide an inpatient and outpatient health care setting in which there is a focused effort in caring for these patients to reduce overall hospital usage.

■ The concept of disease management is defined as a population-based system in which there is recognition that patients at risk for adverse events are identified, subjected to a continuous intervention, and monitored for changes in outcome.

REFERENCES

1. Barlett DL, Steele JB: Critical Condition. New York, Doubleday, 2004.
2. U.S. Office of the Actuary, Health Care Financing Administration, 1995-2000.
3. Getzen ET: Economic evaluation of health services. In: Health Economics: Fundamentals and Flow of Funds. New York, John Wiley & Sons, 1997, pp. 24-57.
4. Bozzette SA: Routine screening for HIV infection: Timely and cost-effective. N Engl J Med 2005;352:620-622.
5. Schleinitz MD, Heidenreich PA: A cost-effectiveness analysis of combination antiplatelet therapy for high-risk acute coronary syndromes: Clopidogrel plus aspirin versus aspirin alone. Ann Intern Med 2005;142:251-259.
6. Lee WC, Chavez YE, Baker T, et al: Economic burden of heart failure: A summary of recent literature. Heart Lung 2004;33: 362-371.

7. Goldman L, Cook F: The decline in ischemic heart disease mortality rates: An analysis of the comparative effects of medical interventions and changes in lifestyle. Ann Intern Med 1984;101: 825-836.

8. McCullough PA, Philbin EF, Spertus JA, et al: Confirmation of a heart failure epidemic: Findings from the Resource Utilization Among Congestive Heart Failure (REACH) study. J Am Coll Cardiol 2002;39:60-69.

9. Galbreath AD, Krasuski RA, Smith B, et al: Long term healthcare and cost outcomes of disease management in a large, randomized community-based population with heart failure. Circulation 2004;110:3518-3526.

10. Evans RW: Costs and insurance coverage associated with permanent mechanical cardiac assist/replacement devices in the United States. J Card Surg 2001;16:280-293.

11. Albanese MC, Plewka M, Gregori D, et al: Use of medical resources and quality of life of patients with chronic heart failure: A prospective survey in a large Italian community hospital. Eur J Heart Fail 1999;1:411-417.

12. Gilbert EM: Cost-effectiveness of beta-blocker treatment in heart failure. Rev Cardiovasc Med 2002;3(Suppl 3):S42-S47.

13. Abraham WT, Scarpinato L: Higher expectations for management of heart failure: Current recommendations. J Am Board Fam Pract 2002;15:39-49.

14. Szucs TD: The growing healthcare burden of CHF. J Renin Angiotensin Aldosterone Syst 2000;1(Suppl 1):2-6.

15. Ryden-Bergsten T, Anderson F: The health care costs of heart failure in Sweden. J Intern Med 1999;246:275-284.

16. Selke B, Brunot A, Lebrun T: Economic repercussions of cardiac insufficiency in France. Arch Mal Coeur Vaiss 2003;96:191-196.

17. Saltzberg MT: Beneficial effects of early initiation of vasoactive agents in patients with acute decompensated heart failure. Rev Cardiovasc Med 2004;5(Suppl 4):S17-S27.

18. Lenz TL, Foral PA, Malesker MA, et al: Impact of nesiritide on health care resource utilization and complications in patients with decompensated heart failure. Pharmacotherapy 2004;24: 1137-1146.

19. Reed SD, Friedman JY, Velazquez EJ, et al: Multinational economic evaluation of valsartan in patients with chronic heart failure: Results from the Valsartan Heart Failure Trial (Val-HeFT). Am Heart J 2004;148:122-128.

20. Abarca J, Malone DC, Armstrong EP, et al: Angiotensin-converting enzyme inhibitor therapy in patients with heart failure enrolled in a managed care organization: Effect on costs and probability of hospitalization. Pharmacotherapy 2004;24:351-357.

21. Glick H, Cook J, Kinosian B, et al: Costs and effects of enalapril therapy in patients with symptomatic heart failure: An economic analysis of the Studies of Left Ventricular Dysfunction (SOLVD) Treatment Trial. J Card Fail 1995;1:371-380.

22. CIBIS-II Investigator: Reduced costs with bisoprolol treatment for heart failure: An economic analysis of the second Cardiac Insufficiency Bisoprolol Study (CIBIS-II). Eur Heart J 2001;22: 1021-1031.

23. Fowler MB, Vera-Llonch M, Oster G, et al: Influence of carvedilol on hospitalizations in heart failure: Incidence, resource utilization, and costs. U.S. Carvedilol Heart Failure Study Group. J Am Coll Cardiol 2001;37:1692-1699.

24. Luzier AB, Antell LA, Chang LL, et al: Reimbursement claims analysis of outcomes with carvedilol and metoprolol. Ann Pharmacother 2002;36:386-391.

25. Sculpher MJ, Poole L, Cleland J, et al: Low dose vs high doses of angiotensin converting enzyme inhibitor lisinopril in chronic heart failure: A cost effectiveness analysis based on the Assessment of Treatment with Lisinopril and Survival (ATLAS) study. The ATLAS Study Group. Eur J Heart Fail 2000;2:447-454.

26. Morales DL, Argenziano M, Oz MC: Outpatient left ventricular assist device support: A safe and economical therapeutic option for heart failure. Prog Cardiovasc Dis 2000;43:55-66.

27. Nichol G, Kaul P, Huszti E, et al: Cost-effectiveness of cardiac resynchronization therapy in patients with symptomatic heart failure. Ann Intern Med 2004;141:343-351.

28. Stewart S: Financial aspect of heart failure programs of care. Eur J Heart Fail 2005;7:423-428.

29. Whellan DJ, Gaulden L, Gattis WA, et al: The benefit of implementing a heart failure disease management program. Arch Intern Med 2001;161:2223-2228.

30. Tsuyuki RT, Fradette M, Johnson JA, et al: A multicenter disease management program for hospitalized patients with heart failure. J Card Fail 2004;10:473-480.

31. McAlister FA, Stewart S, Ferrua S, et al: Multidisciplinary strategies for the management of heart failure patients at high risk for admission: A systematic review of randomized trials. J Am Coll Cardiol 2004;44:810-819.

32. Stewart S, Horowitz JD: Specialist nurse management programmes: Economic benefits in the management of heart failure. Pharmacoeconomics 2003;21:225-240.

33. Ezekowitz JA, van Walraven C, McAllister FA, et al: Impact of specialist followup in outpatients with congestive heart failure. Can Med Assoc J 2005;172:189-194.

34. Gregoroff SJ, McKelvie RS, Szabo S: The impact of an outpatient heart failure clinic on hospital costs and admissions. Int J Health Care Qual Assur Inc Leadership Health Serv 2004;17:i-xi.

35. Desai S, Jessup M: Practice guidelines: Role of internists and primary care physicians. Med Clin North Am 2004;88: 1369-1380.

36. Mehra MR, Uber PA, Choomsky DB, et al: Emergence of electronic home monitoring in chronic heart failure rationale, feasibility, and early results with the HomMed Sentry Observer System. Congest Heart Fail 2000;6:137-139.

37. Hauptman PJ, Bednarek HL: The business concept of leader pricing as applied to heart failure disease management. Dis Manage 2004;7:226-234.

38. Kay JD, Colan SD, Graham TP: Congestive heart failure in pediatric patients. Am Heart J 2001;142:923-928.

39. Somerville J: Grown up congenital heart disease: Medical demands look back look forward 2000. Thorac Cardiovasc Surg 2001;49:21-26.

40. Frist WH: Health care in the 21st century. N Engl J Med 2005;352: 267-272.

CHAPTER 14

Clinical Recognition of Congestive Heart Failure in Children

Carolyn A. Altman
Grace Kung

Heart failure is the inability of the heart and neuro-hormonal systems to supply sufficient cardiac output to keep up with metabolic demands. Perturbation of one or more of the determinants of cardiac output (heart rate, contractility, preload, and afterload) can result in heart failure. Clinical recognition of heart failure relies on knowledge of the mechanisms that result in the mismatch between cardiac capability and systemic demands and the differential diagnoses for heart failure depending on age, history, physical examination, and laboratory evaluation.

In pediatric patients, typical clinical scenarios of congestive heart failure include volume overload from intracardiac or extracardiac shunts, pressure overload from outflow obstruction, intrinsic cardiac muscle contractility disorder, persistent tachycardia or bradycardia, and lack of atrioventricular synchrony. Cardiac output also may be insufficient because of increased metabolic demands, such as severe anemia, sepsis, or hyperthyroidism. The time of heart failure onset, especially in the first year of life, can be useful to determine the etiology. This chapter focuses on the specific clinical presentation and potential differential causative diagnoses of heart failure by age group: the fetus, the neonate during the first few days of life, the neonate during the first week of life, the neonate from 2 to 6 weeks of life, infancy, and childhood/adolescence. The reader is referred to chapters in other general pediatric cardiology textbooks for a generalized discussion of history and physical examination.

CLINICAL MANIFESTATIONS AND DIFFERENTIAL DIAGNOSES OF HEART FAILURE BY AGE

The Fetus

Fetal congestive heart failure may result from congenital heart defects with outflow obstruction, inflow obstruction, or severe atrioventricular valvar insufficiency. Other causes include premature closure of the patent foramen ovale or patent ductus arteriosus, bradyarrhythmias such as complete atrioventricular block, tachyarrhythmias such as atrial flutter or supraventricular tachycardia, fetal infections including myocarditis, dilated cardiomyopathies, cardiac tumors, and twin-to-twin transfusion syndrome. High output failure in fetuses may stem from severe anemia (Rh isoimmune disease, α-thalassemia), extracardiac shunts (vein of Galen or other arteriovenous malformations, teratomas), or hyperthyroidism. Shunts at the ventricular level do not manifest themselves yet as heart failure in the setting of high fetal pulmonary vascular resistance. Many cardiomyopathies may not present until later in infancy or childhood.

Important components of the maternal **history** include any chronic medical or psychiatric diseases, infections during pregnancy, or medication use during pregnancy. A family history of congenital heart disease or prior fetal demise is also important. The perception of decreased fetal movement can occur in fetuses with heart failure. Severe fetal congestive heart failure also can manifest as hydrops fetalis (excess fetal water with pleural effusions, pericardial effusions, and ascites).

Fetal echocardiography is the main diagnostic tool of fetal cardiac assessment. Echocardiographic investigation includes careful assessment for congenital heart disease, ventricular function, ventricular size discrepancy, semilunar or atrioventricular valvar insufficiency, flow across the patent foramen ovale and patent ductus arteriosus, intracardiac masses, heart rate and rhythm, umbilical arterial and venous flow patterns, and ductus venosus flow (see Chapter 25).

The Neonate

First Few Days of Life The neonatal period is a time of transition away from the fetal circulation and metabolism and recovery from the birth process. Removal of the placenta increases systemic vascular resistance, and oxygen consumption doubles ex utero.[1-3] Neonatal myocardium is less compliant than adult myocardium, and the filling of one ventricle more significantly decreases the distensibility of the other.[4,5] Although contractility increases postnatally, neonatal myocardium operates near the upper limits of the Frank-Starling curve with little reserve.[6-9]

Neonates are unable to tolerate significant changes in loading conditions or heart rate and are more vulnerable to the development of heart failure. This vulnerability may be particularly true for neonates who are small for gestational age or premature, who may have relatively hypoplastic myocardial fibers or limited cardiac energy stores (see Chapter 26).[10,11]

Etiologies for congestive heart failure most commonly manifesting in the first day of life include birth asphyxia, fetal distress, toxemia of pregnancy, fetal or neonatal myocarditis, sepsis, bradyarrhythmias or tachyarrhythmias, structural anomalies associated with marked pulmonary or tricuspid regurgitation, hypocalcemia, hypoglycemia, severe anemia, or hyperviscosity syndrome.[12] Congenital heart defects associated with marked hypoxia and poor cardiac output (obstructed total anomalous pulmonary venous return, transposition with an intact ventricular septum and severely restrictive atrial septum, hypoplastic left heart syndrome with a severely restrictive atrial septum) manifest soon after birth as well, but usually not as isolated heart failure. Although intracardiac shunt lesions are unlikely to cause symptoms during the early neonatal period because pulmonary vascular resistance is still likely to be high, obligatory extracardiac shunts from systemic arteriovenous malformations can cause symptoms during this period.

A careful **history** should be obtained concerning the prenatal course for maternal medical (connective tissue diseases, diabetes, congenital heart disease, cardiomyopathy) or psychiatric conditions; medications; infections (TORCH and human immunodeficiency virus); and results of prenatal echocardiograms, ultrasounds, amniocentesis, or other laboratory data. Family history for congenital heart disease, cardiomyopathy, unexplained deaths, or spontaneous abortions should be documented. Birth history is important with regard to prolonged rupture of membranes, maternal infection, presence of meconium, Apgar scores, or other evidence for fetal distress. Family history for congenital or acquired heart disease should be ascertained.

Physical examination includes signs of heart failure that are related to the etiology of failure and involvement of the left or right heart (or both). Left-sided heart failure with elevated left ventricular end-diastolic pressure causes pulmonary venous congestion. This condition results in rapid shallow breathing or tachypnea (>60 breaths/min in the neonate or >40 breaths/min in the older infant), dyspnea, and increased work of breathing evidenced by retractions (subcostal, intercostal, or suprasternal), grunting, and nasal flaring. Wheezes are more likely than rales as the pulmonary auscultatory finding in infants with heart failure. Pulmonary or bronchial compression by enlarged pulmonary arteries or other cardiac structures (i.e., the massively enlarged right atrium in Ebstein anomaly or dilated left atrium in large left-to-right shunts) also can result in early respiratory distress and even respiratory failure. Right-sided heart failure manifests with systemic congestion. If fetal hydrops was present, persistent ascites, pleural effusions, pericardial effusions, and skin edema persist. Enlargement and firmness of the liver is more common than peripheral edema or jugular venous distention as a sign of systemic venous congestion in the neonate and infant, although puffy eyelids can be present.

A consistent resting sinus tachycardia greater than 150 beats/min compensates for decreased stroke volume and is a cardinal sign of cardiac compromise; hypotension may result with failure of this compensatory mechanism. Resting heart rates greater than 220 to 230 beats/min are more likely to reflect a primary tachyarrhythmia than sinus tachycardia.[13,14] Complete heart block with escape rhythm of less than 55 beats/min are more likely to be associated with symptoms of heart failure and cardiomyopathy.[15,16] Severely asphyxiated neonates can have a relative bradycardia with resting heart rates of 90 to 110 beats/min.[12] In addition to resting heart rate, four extremity blood pressure measurements are necessary.

The precordial activity may be normal, excessive (in high output failure), or quiet (with depressed myocardial contractility). A single second heart sound may reflect pulmonary hypertension or congenital heart disease. An audible gallop in a neonate is concerning because innocent third heart sounds are unlikely to be appreciated on auscultation in this age group. With fast heart rates, it may be difficult to distinguish third from fourth heart sounds: S_3 is a low-frequency sound best appreciated at the apex or left sternal border and can be heard in normal children, whereas S_4 is associated with rapid filling of the ventricle during atrial contraction (secondary to decreased compliance) and usually is considered abnormal.

A heart murmur early in the neonatal period is commonly atrioventricular valve regurgitation. High-velocity tricuspid regurgitation in the setting of pulmonary hypertension or right ventricular outflow tract obstruction generates a holosystolic murmur at the lower left and right sternal borders. A prominent to-and-fro murmur along the left sternal border is a classic finding for tetralogy of Fallot with absent pulmonary valve. Continuous murmurs or bruits are heard over systemic or cerebral arteriovenous malformations, so auscultation should include over the cranium and the liver areas. Cyanosis may result from congenital heart disease, pulmonary disease, sepsis, hypoglycemia, polycythemia, or low cardiac output. Marked pallor raises concern for anemia. Cool, pale or mottled extremities with diminished pulse volume and capillary refill are universal signs of poor cardiac output. Neonates with high output failure have bounding central pulses. Jitteriness and possible seizures suggest hypocalcemia or hypoglycemia.

Initial **laboratory evaluation** includes chest radiography to evaluate for cardiomegaly, pulmonary edema, regional atelectasis, and possible contributing processes such as pneumonia. ECG distinguishes the sinus tachycardia of heart failure from other tachyarrhythmias or bradyarrhythmias. Low-voltage (<5 mm) QRS complexes in the limb leads, low-amplitude or inverted T waves, and small or absent Q waves in V5 and V6 are the classically described findings in myocarditis.[17] Findings such as ischemia-related ST-T wave changes, ventricular hypertrophy, and atrial enlargement are not specific for a single diagnosis. Examination of blood gases may reveal a metabolic acidosis with elevated lactate from the inability of output to match metabolic demand. A mixed respiratory and metabolic acidosis with hypercarbia may be present in asphyxia or pneumonia/sepsis, whereas hypoxemia may be related to structural heart disease or pulmonary disease. Hemoglobin as well as glucose and calcium levels should be checked. Clinical suspicion for infection guides the necessity for obtaining viral and bacterial cultures. Echocardiography shows cardiac structure, pressure data, and functional status. Further laboratory evaluations of cardiomyopathies are described in detail in Chapters 18, 19, and 20.

First Week of Life Beyond the first day of life, causes of congestive heart failure in neonates can be broadly categorized as causes more likely to occur within the first week of life and causes more likely to present between 1 and 6 weeks of life.[12] During the first week of life, defects dependent on a patent ductus arteriosus for systemic circulation (e.g., hypoplastic left heart syndrome, critical aortic stenosis, or interrupted aortic arch) often present with increasing tachypnea, tachycardia, diminished pulses, and worsening perfusion with evidence of heart failure. The rapid development of cardiogenic shock is a common presentation and can be confused with neonatal sepsis.[18]

In the **physical examination** of a neonate and of any child, it is essential simply to observe (e.g., level of comfort, general appearance, breathing pattern, mental alertness, nutritional status, color and perfusion, and genetic abnormalities) to appreciate a basal undisturbed state. In hypoplastic left heart syndrome and critical aortic stenosis, upper and lower extremity pulses are equally poor with symmetric pulse oximetry readings. The upper extremity pulses usually are preserved in interrupted aortic arch and coarctation, whereas pedal pulses and perfusion deteriorate. Pedal pulse oximetry is useful in identifying right-to-left ductal shunting. Murmurs are often absent, particularly in the setting of depressed ventricular function. A single second heart sound may reflect a single semilunar valve or pulmonary hypertension. In laboratory evaluation, cardiomegaly on chest radiograph had 85% sensitivity and 95% specificity for congenital heart disease in the study by Pickert and colleagues[18] reviewing critically ill infants with sepsis/meningitis or left heart obstructive lesions presenting to a pediatric emergency department in the first month of life.

Lesions dependent on the ductus for pulmonary blood flow (critical pulmonary stenosis, pulmonary atresia/intact ventricular septum) also present at this time, with signs of progressive cyanosis and right heart failure. A right ventricular impulse is present near the lower left sternal border or over the xiphoid. An impulse that is localized and sharp is a tap, whereas an impulse that is diffuse and slower rising is termed a heave. The second heart sound may be single. These patients may have a systolic murmur at the lower left sternal border from tricuspid regurgitation or at the upper left sternal border from right ventricular outflow tract obstruction. Chest radiograph shows decreased pulmonary perfusion and the upturned apex associated with right ventricular hypertrophy. ECG shows right ventricular hypertrophy except in the setting of right ventricular hypoplasia.

Although patency of the ductus is life preserving in patients with otherwise no systemic or pulmonary blood flow, persistent patency of the ductus arteriosus may result in congestive heart failure in premature neonates, particularly infants weighing less than 1500 g.[19,20] Classic signs of ductal patency include a long systolic or continuous murmur, bounding pulses, cardiomegaly, and increased pulse pressure with signs of heart failure.

Although infants with severe perinatal asphyxia present acutely at birth with cardiogenic shock and myocardial dysfunction, some infants with a relatively uneventful perinatal and postpartum course develop progressive respiratory distress, cardiomegaly, hepatomegaly, oxygen requirement, diminished pulses, atrioventricular valve regurgitation, and ventricular dysfunction with clinical findings of heart failure in the first days of life.[5,21] A pulmonary vascular bed with persistent pulmonary vasoconstriction may be the primary etiology, or this could result from hypoglycemia, sepsis, or pneumonia.[5,22] Pre- and post-simultaneous pulse oximetry can suggest this entity with right-to-left ductal shunting by the lower postductal saturations.

Other systemic diseases can affect cardiac output in this age group. Neonatal hyperthyroidism is a rare cause of high output heart failure.[12] Cardiovascular collapse also can result from adrenal insufficiency.[23] Laboratory data classically show hypoglycemia, hyponatremia, and hyperkalemia.[12]

From 2 to 6 Weeks of Life Lesions most typically manifesting with failure beyond the first week of life include lesions with increasing left-to-right shunts as pulmonary vascular resistance decreases. These shunt lesions include ventricular septal defects, complete atrioventricular canal defects, aortopulmonary windows, truncus arteriosus, unobstructed total anomalous pulmonary venous return, and persistent patent ductus arteriosus.[12] Patients with shunts at multiple levels present earlier than patients with a single lesion. Isolated atrial septal defects are unlikely to generate symptoms during this period.

Other important lesions that may present with failure during the first 6 weeks of life include coarctation of the aorta, heart muscle abnormalities such as those resulting from myocarditis or Pompe disease, endocardial fibroelastosis, and anomalous left coronary artery from the pulmonary artery (ALCAPA).[12] Infants with ALCAPA present with failure secondary to left ventricular ischemia or infarction as flow in the left coronary becomes retrograde from the right with decreasing pulmonary vascular resistance, bypassing the microcoronary circulation to flow into the pulmonary artery. These infants may exhibit periods of intense irritability or infantile angina, particularly with feeding.[27] The physical examination may reveal the holosystolic murmur of mitral regurgitation from infarcted mitral papillary muscles, in addition to the previously described signs of failure. The ECG can raise the index of suspicion for this lesion, with the pattern of deep (≥ 3 mm) or wide (≥ 30 msec) Q waves or a QR pattern in I, AVL, or left chest leads and the absence of Q waves in the inferior leads II,II, and AVF.[28] These findings are not totally specific because dilated cardiomyopathy and myocarditis may have similar findings (see Chapters 17 and 18).[28]

In addition to the questions outlined in the prior sections, it is important to obtain an accurate feeding history, including whether breastfeeding or bottle feeding, length of time for feeding to be completed (most infants should complete a feeding in ≤ 30 minutes), number of ounces fed, alertness during feeding, and increased respiratory rate or sweating with feeding. Choking, gagging, or coughing with feeds can occur in an infant attempting to suck while breathing rapidly. Increasing circulating catecholamines result in resting tachycardia, pallor, and diaphoresis, especially with feeds.[24-26] In addition, irritability and fussiness with feeding can be secondary to myocardial ischemia. Systemic venous congestion involving the gastrointestinal tract can cause gut wall edema, hypomotility, and abnormal absorption, resulting in abdominal discomfort, feeding intolerance, or emesis. Poor weight gain results from the inability to eat sufficient calories to supply the increased metabolic demands.[25-26]

On **physical examination**, the infant may appear cachectic and tachypneic with sweat on the forehead. Precordial activity is increased. Harrison's groove, a line of depression near the diaphragm attachment of the rib cage, can be observed. A right ventricular impulse is palpable in the setting of right ventricular volume/pressure overload. The presence of a holosystolic murmur suggests a ventricular septal defect or atrioventricular valvar regurgitation. Patent ductus arteriosus, aortopulmonary window, and truncus arteriosus usually generate continuous murmurs with continued flow or runoff into the pulmonary arteries in diastole. Diastolic rumbles are mid-diastolic filling turbulence generally associated with a pulmonary-to-systemic flow ratio of at least 2:1. A gallop and a hyperdynamic precordium can be present with volume overload lesions.

Hypothyroidism has been reported to cause signs and symptoms of low cardiac output in this age group.[12] Infants may exhibit lethargy, constipation, cool and dry skin, hypothermia, resting bradycardia, and cardiomegaly. Endocarditis in neonates can present with heart failure, feeding difficulties, tachycardia, respiratory distress, changing murmurs, and hypotension.[29,30]

Although it is helpful to categorize the most likely etiology of heart failure based on a neonate's age, overlap occurs within these and the other groups. Neonates with hypoplastic left heart syndrome most typically present with ductal closure at 2 to 3 days of age, but can present on the first day of life. Myocarditis, dilated cardiomyopathies, and functional cardiomyopathies secondary to sustained arrhythmias, renal failure, or hypertension can manifest anytime.[12]

Infants After 6 Weeks to 1 Year Old

Infants may present in heart failure or with lesions that can precipitate heart failure beyond the neonatal period with any of the lesions described previously as typically presenting beyond the first week of life. Coarctation of the aorta is well known to present late. In the study by Wren and coworkers[31] of 1590 infants diagnosed with congenital heart disease by 1 year of age, 27% of infants with coarctation were undiagnosed by 6 weeks of age, and 20% were still undiagnosed by 3 months. In the same study, two thirds of infants with aortic valve stenosis were undiagnosed at 6 weeks of age, and 45% were undiagnosed by 12 weeks of age.[31]

Kawasaki disease may cause heart failure secondary to myocarditis or myocardial infarction, with the risk for coronary arteritis greatest in infants younger than 1 year of age.[32-34] Impaired ventricular contractility can occur in septic shock in infants and young children and contributes significantly to mortality.[35-37] Myocardial dysfunction is particularly a characteristic component of meningococcal septic shock and has been associated with elevated serum cardiac troponin I.[36,37]

Older Children and Adolescents

Older children and adolescents are more likely to have symptomatic heart failure from acquired or operated cardiac conditions, rather than newly recognized or unoperated congenital heart disease.[38] There are exceptions to this generalization, however. Large left-to-right shunts from large atrial septal defects, intractable arrhythmias or severe tricuspid regurgitation in Ebstein anomaly of the tricuspid valve, tricuspid regurgitation and right ventricular dysfunction in ventricular inversion with L-transposed great arteries, and aortic valve prolapse and regurgitation with ventricular septal defects all may result in heart failure in children beyond infancy. Right heart failure can occur in older patients with Eisenmenger syndrome.

Patients with repaired or palliated congenital heart disease may develop heart failure with chronic or progressive volume or pressure overload. Such patients include those with single ventricle physiology and atrioventricular regurgitation, pulmonary vein obstruction, aortic arch obstruction, Fontan baffle obstruction, bradyarrhythmias or tachyarrhythmias, or ventricular dysfunction. The development of severe mitral regurgitation after atrioventricular canal repair or aortic regurgitation after aortic valvotomy/valvuloplasty, truncus repair, or Ross procedure can result in left heart failure. Prosthetic valve dysfunction can cause acute failure. Progressive pulmonary insufficiency after tetralogy of Fallot can result in progressive right ventricular dysfunction. Progressive right ventricular dysfunction may elicit symptoms of "left heart" failure in patients status post atrial switch operation or palliated ventricular inversion with L-transposed great arteries (see Chapter 27).

Acquired disease resulting in heart failure in children and teenagers includes acute rheumatic fever with aortic, mitral, or tricuspid insufficiency. Dilated cardiomyopathy in children results from a large array of diseases, including genetically acquired primary muscular or metabolic disorders, infectious diseases (e.g., myocarditis or secondary to systemic disease), arrhythmias, toxins or drugs, Kawasaki disease, or myocardial dysfunction after congenital heart surgery.[39] Hypothyroidism or hyperthyroidism may be associated with low output or high output heart failure.[38] Renal disease or hypertension or both may result in left heart failure, and pulmonary hypertension or cystic fibrosis can result in cor pulmonale with right heart failure.[38] Restrictive, constrictive, and hypertrophic cardiomyopathies all can elicit signs and symptoms of heart failure in this age group.

Endocarditis can complicate the course of otherwise asymptomatic congenital heart defects (such as simple bicuspid aortic valve or small ventricular septal defect), and more complex operated disease. Endocarditis with abrupt structural change (acute mitral or aortic insufficiency, rupture of aortic sinus into left or right atrium, dehisced mechanical valve) can cause the rapid development of severe heart failure from the sudden volume overload.[30] Heart failure may develop more insidiously in slowly progressive valvar insufficiency in subacute endocarditis.

As with other age groups, the **history** can provide valuable clues to the presence of symptomatic heart failure. A decrease in exercise capacity may be shown by decreased stamina compared with peers. In patients who are limited in their exercise capacity by underlying structural heart disease, it is important to investigate changes in exercise tolerance compared with their own baseline over time. Children may not admit to easy fatigability while playing, but may increase or add nap times and duration of sleeping at night. They simply may avoid any strenuous physical activity altogether.

Weight loss or weight gain must be questioned. Weight gain may arise from rapid collection of edema; this may be accompanied by complaints of abdominal pain and distention from hepatic congestion, gut edema, or ascites. Teenagers may complain of ill-fitting clothes. Weight loss results from the chronic anorexia and nausea from gut edema. Older children may experience paroxysmal nocturnal dyspnea.[38] Excessive sweating is a nonspecific symptom of failure. Although pediatric patients do not usually complain of pedal edema, their parents may note periorbital edema, particularly on awakening in the morning. Patients with established heart failure who are well controlled medically may exhibit more symptoms if "tipped over" by intercurrent infection, arrhythmia, anemia, metabolic disorder, or dietary/fluid indiscretion. An admission of chest pain, especially associated with exercise, can indicate ischemia.

On **physical examination**, tachycardia, tachypnea, hepatomegaly, cool extremities, and diminished perfusion are classic findings of heart failure. Rales are less common than wheezes in younger children. Jugular venous distention may be present in older children. Ascites is more common than peripheral pedal edema in most children and adolescents. In older children, a lateral and downward displaced apical impulse from the normal location of the midclavicular line at the fifth intercostal space indicates cardiac enlargement. A hyperactive precordium can be present. Auscultatory findings depend on the underlying etiology of heart failure, but an S3 gallop, S4 gallop, or both often can be heard. In older children with heart failure, pulsus paradoxus (exaggeration of the normal inspiratory and expiratory variation in blood pressure) and pulsus alternans (alternating strong and weak pulse) may be palpated.

The starting **laboratory examination** in older patients is similar to infants, with close evaluations of the chest radiograph, ECG, and echocardiogram. B-type natriuretic peptide is a neurohormone synthesized in the cardiac ventricles, and levels are increased in decompensated congestive heart failure.[40,41] Measuring B-type natriuretic peptide levels has been found to be useful in helping to differentiate dyspnea from heart failure versus other causes in adults.[42] In addition, N-terminal pro–B-type natriuretic peptide levels in children positively correlated with a clinical heart failure score and negatively correlated with ejection fraction.[43] Measurement of these peptides may be useful in pediatric patients in trying to distinguish increased respiratory distress from a large left-to-right shunt, mitral regurgitation, or left ventricular dysfunction from an intercurrent pneumonia or other lung disease (see Chapter 6).

A valuable adjunct in older children with symptoms primarily related to exertion or exercise intolerance is formal exercise testing. Symptoms during exertion and exercise capacity often do not correlate well with the routine cardiopulmonary assessment at rest.[44] Exercise testing can quantitate functional capacity, measuring respiratory, cardiac, and metabolic responses to exercise.[45] Peak oxygen consumption provides an objective measure of cardiopulmonary reserve.[45] The degree of exercise intolerance in adults with heart failure correlates with prognosis.[46,47] Adults with heart failure have exaggerated metabolic and respiratory responses to exercise compared with normals.[45] In a study of children with dilated cardiomyopathy, at the anaerobic threshold and at peak exercise, the systolic blood pressure, oxygen consumption, oxygen consumption for heart rate, tidal volume, exercise duration, carbon dioxide production, and minute ventilation were lower than in controls.[45] Ventilatory equivalents for oxygen and carbon dioxide were higher in the cardiomyopathy group at anaerobic threshold and peak exercise. These measures provided at exercise testing may prove valuable in guiding changes in medications and other management decisions in the future.

CURRENT STATUS AND FUTURE TRENDS

Four parameters of heart failure that could be used in classifying heart failure have been described: myocardial function, functional capacity (ability to maintain daily activities and achieve maximal exercise capacity), functional outcomes (mortality, need for transplant), and degree of activation of compensatory mechanisms (e.g., neurohumoral responses).[48] The most well-recognized and widely used classification is the **New York Heart Association classification** for adults (Table 14-1). This functional capacity classification system assigns patients to one of four classes

TABLE 14-1

New York Heart Association Classification	
Class I	No limitations to normal exertion
Class II	Symptoms on ordinary exertion
Class III	Symptoms with less than ordinary exertion
Class IV	Symptoms at rest

depending on the degree of effort needed to elicit symptoms of angina, fatigue, dyspnea, or palpitations.[49] More quantitative assessments of left ventricular systolic function can be obtained with echocardiography (ejection fraction, shortening fraction), but these lack the sensitivity of symptoms and correlate poorly with exercise capacity on formal exercise testing.[48]

In an effort to capture the evolution and progression of heart failure in adult patients, which would be even more useful in evaluating and managing heart failure, the **American Heart Association and the American College of Cardiology** devised a new classification system (Table 14-2).[50] This staging system acknowledges the patient's course is a continuum, advancing from one stage to the next. Therapeutic interventions before the development of structural or functional heart disease in patients at risk (stage A) or the development of symptoms in patients with structural or functional abnormalities (stage B) may improve outcome. These guidelines do not include assessment of heart failure in children, however.

TABLE 14-2

American Heart Association and American College of Cardiology Classification of Heart Failure		
Stage	Description	Examples
A	Patients at high risk of developing HF because of the presence ofconditions that are strongly associated with the developmentof HF. Such patients have no identified structural or functional abnormalities of the pericardium, myocardium, or cardiac valves and have never shown signs or symptoms of HF	Systemic hypertension, coronary artery disease, diabetes mellitus, history of cardiotoxic drug therapy or alcohol abuse, personal history of rheumatic fever, family history of cardiomyopathy
B	Patients who have developed structural heart disease that is strongly associated with the development of HF, but who have never shown signs or symptoms of HF	Left ventricular hypertrophy or fibrosis, left ventricular dilation or hypocontractility, asymptomatic valvular heart disease, previous myocardial infarction
C	Patients who have current or prior symptoms of HF associated with underlying structural heart disease	Dyspnea or fatigue due to left ventricular systolic dysfunction; asymptomatic patients who are undergoing treatment for prior symptoms of HF
D	Patients with advanced structural heart disease and marked symptoms of HF at rest despite maximal medical therapy and who require specialized interventions	Patients who are frequently hospitalized for HF and cannot be safely discharged from the hospital; patients in the hospital awaiting heart transplantation; patients at home receiving continuous intravenous support for symptom relief or being supported with a mechanical circulatory assist device; patients in a hospice setting for the management of HF

HF, heart failure.

Classification of heart failure in pediatric patients is difficult to establish because of the wide strata of ages yielding different normative respiratory and heart rates, the range of different developmental stages allowing widely different exercise capabilities (e.g., feeding versus riding a bike), and the variety of different etiologies for heart failure (e.g., pump dysfunction, large

TABLE 14-3

Ross Scoring System of Heart Failure in Infants			
	0 points	1 point	2 points
Volume per feed (oz)	>3.5	2.5-3.5	<2.5
Time per feed (min)	<40 min	>40 min	
Respiratory rate	<50/min	50-60/min	>60/min
Respiratory pattern	Normal	Abnormal	
Peripheral perfusion	Normal	Decreased	
S$_3$ or diastolic rumble	Absent	Present	
Liver edge from costal margin	<2 cm	2-3 cm	>3 cm
Totals			
No CHF:	0-2 points		
Mild CHF:	3-6 points		
Moderate CHF:	7-9 points		
Severe CHF:	10-12 points		

CHF, congestive heart failure.

TABLE 14-4

Ross Classification of Heart Failure in Infants	
Class I	No limitations or symptoms
Class II	Mild tachypnea or diaphoresis with feeding in infants
	Dyspnea on exertion in older children
	No growth failure
Class III	Marked tachypnea or diaphoresis with feeds or exertion
	Prolonged feeding times
	Growth failure from CHF
Class IV	Symptoms at rest with tachypnea, retractions, grunting, or diaphoresis

CHF, congestive heart failure.

shunts, metabolic disorders).[48] In 1992, Ross and colleagues[51] published a scoring system for infants based on volume consumed per feeding, time taken per feeding, respiratory rate, heart rate, respiratory pattern, peripheral perfusion, presence of a diastolic rumble or S$_3$, and hepatomegaly (Table 14-3).

The Ross classification, paralleling the New York Heart Association classification scheme, evolved into a more sophisticated classification (Table 14-4).[48,52] The class of heart failure using this classification system was shown to have a corresponding incremental increase in

TABLE 14-5

Pediatric Clinical Heart Failure Score			
	SCORE (POINTS)		
	0	1	2
History			
Diaphoresis	Head only	Head and body During exercise	Head and body At rest
Tachypnea	Rare	Several times	Frequent
Physical Examination			
Breathing	Normal	Retractions	Dyspnea
Respiratory rate/min			
0-1 yr	<50	50-60	>60
1-6 yr	<35	35-45	>45
7-10 yr	<25	25-35	>35
11-14 yr	<18	18-28	>28
Heart rate			
0-1 yr	<160	160-170	>170
1-6 yr	<105	105-115	>115
7-10 yr	<90	90-100	>100
11-14 yr	<80	80-90	>90
Liver edge from costal margin	<2 cm	2-3 cm	>3 cm

Modified from Ross and Reithmann.

plasma norepinephrine levels, which decreased on resolution of heart failure by surgical or medical management.[52-54] Lymphocyte β-adrenergic receptor density was shown to decrease incrementally with higher classes of failure.[54] For children from infancy through adolescence, Reithmann and associates[55] devised another heart failure scoring system including clinical values and showed significantly decreased post-receptor adenylate cyclase activity in children with scores greater than 6. The scoring system represents the merging of the Ross and Reithmann classifications (Table 14-5), and has been used in several clinical failure investigations.[43,56] Carvedilol use correlated with lower failure score and increased ejection fraction.[56]

Finally, the New York University Pediatric Heart Failure Index is a scoring system for children of all ages that incorporates signs and symptoms of heart failure, but also awards points for medications, the presence of single ventricle physiology, and radiographic and echocardiographic data (Table 14-6).[57] Higher scores represent increased failure. Patients undergoing surgery for large left-to-right shunts were shown to decrease their heart failure scores.[57] Given the variability in prescribing different failure medications and the fact the medications already are included in the scoring system, analyzing the benefits of medications would be difficult

TABLE 14-6

Score	Signs and Symptoms
+2	Abnormal ventricular function by echo or gallop
+2	Dependent edema
+2	Failure to thrive or cachexia
+1	Marked cardiomegaly by x-ray or by physical examination
+1	Reported physical activity intolerance or prolonged feeding
+2	Poor perfusion by physical examination
+1	Pulmonary edema by x-ray or auscultation
+2	Resting sinus tachycardia
+2	Retractions
+1	Liver <4 cm below costal margin
+2	Liver >4 cm below costal margin
+1	Mild-to-moderate observed tachypnea or dyspnea
+2	Moderate-to-severe observed tachypnea or dyspnea
+1	Digoxin
+1	Low-to-moderate diuretic use
+2	High diuretic dose or >1 diuretic
+1	ACE inhibitors or non–ACE inhibitor vasodilator or angiotensin receptor blockers
+	β-Blockers
+2	Anticoagulants not related to prosthetic valve
+2	Antiarrhythmic agents or AICDs
+2	Single ventricle

New York University Pediatric Heart Failure Index

ACE, angiotensin-converting enzyme; AICDs, automatic implantable cardioverter defibrillators.

with this system. Data evaluating correlation between morbidity and mortality and the degree of heart failure based on any of these scoring systems are lacking. Eventual future classifications most likely would involve objective data, such as biomarkers.[58,59]

Key Concepts

■ Etiologies for congestive heart failure most commonly manifesting in the first day of life include birth asphyxia, fetal distress, toxemia of pregnancy, fetal or neonatal myocarditis, sepsis, bradyarrhythmias or tachyarrhythmias, structural anomalies associated with marked pulmonary or tricuspid regurgitation, hypocalcemia, hypoglycemia, severe anemia, or hyperviscosity syndrome.

■ Wheezes are more likely than rales as the pulmonary auscultatory finding in infants with heart failure. Pulmonary or bronchial compression by enlarged pulmonary arteries or other cardiac structures (i.e., the massively enlarged right atrium in Ebstein anomaly or dilated left atrium in large left-to-right shunts) also can result in early respiratory distress and even respiratory failure.

■ Enlargement and firmness of the liver are more common than peripheral edema or jugular venous distention as a sign of systemic venous congestion in neonates and infants, although puffy eyelids can be present.

■ With fast heart rates, it may be difficult to distinguish third from fourth heart sounds: S_3 is a low-frequency sound best appreciated at the apex or left sternal border and can be heard in normal children, whereas S_4 is associated with rapid filling of the ventricle during atrial contraction (secondary to decreased compliance) and usually is considered abnormal.

■ In the physical examination of a neonate and of any child, it is essential simply to observe (e.g., level of comfort, general appearance, breathing pattern, mental alertness, nutritional status, color and perfusion, and genetic abnormalities) to appreciate a basal undisturbed state.

■ Lesions most typically presenting with failure beyond the first week of life include lesions with increasing left-to-right shunts as pulmonary vascular resistance decreases. These shunt lesions include ventricular septal defects, complete atrioventricular canal defects, aortopulmonary windows, truncus arteriosus, unobstructed total anomalous pulmonary venous return, and persistent patent ductus arteriosus. Other important lesions that may present with failure during the first 6 weeks of life include coarctation of the aorta, heart muscle abnormalities such as those resulting from myocarditis or Pompe disease, endocardial fibroelastosis, and ALCAPA.

■ Large left-to-right shunts from large atrial septal defects, intractable arrhythmias or severe tricuspid regurgitation in Ebstein anomaly of the tricuspid valve, tricuspid regurgitation and right ventricular dysfunction in ventricular inversion with L-transposed great arteries, and aortic valve prolapse and regurgitation with ventricular septal defect all may result in heart failure in children beyond infancy.

■ Four parameters of heart failure that could be used in classifying heart failure have been described: myocardial function, functional capacity (ability to maintain daily activities and achieve maximal exercise capacity), functional outcomes (mortality, need for transplant), and degree of activation of compensatory mechanisms (e.g., neurohumoral responses).

REFERENCES

1. Stopfkuchen H: Changes of the cardiovascular system during the perinatal period. Eur J Pediatr 1987;146:545.
2. Lister G, Walter TK, Versmold HT, et al: Oxygen delivery in lambs: Cardiovascular and hematologic development. Am J Physiol 1979;237:H668.
3. Lister G, Moreau G, Moss M, Talner NS: Effects of alterations of oxygen transport on the neonate. Semin Perinatol 1984;8:192.
4. Romero T, Covell J, Friedman WF: A comparison of pressure-volume relations of the fetal, newborn, and adult hearts. Am J Physiol 1972;222:1285.
5. Adams JM: Neonatology. In Garson AJ, Bricker JT, Fisher DJ, Neish SR (eds): The Science and Practice of Pediatric Cardiology. Philadelphia, Williams & Wilkins, 1998, pp 2835-2836.
6. Riemenshchneider TA, Breener RA, Mason DT: Maturational changes in myocardial contractile state of newborn lambs. Pediatr Res 1981;15:349.
7. Berman W Jr, Musselman J: Myocardial performance in the newborn lamb. Am J Physiol 1979;237:H66.
8. Teitel DF, Sidi D, Chin T, et al: Developmental changes in the myocardial contractile reserve in the lamb. Pediatr Res 1985;19:948.
9. Emmanoulides GC, Moss AJ, Monset-Couchard M, et al: Cardiac output in newborn infants. Biol Neonate 1970;15:186.
10. Takahashi N, Nishida H, Arai T, Kaneda Y: Abnormal cardiac histology in severe intrauterine growth retardation infants. Acta Paediatr Jpn 1995;37:341.
11. Schultz K, Weisenbach J: Cardiomegaly in hypoglycaemic small-for-gestational-age infant. 1982;23:69.
12. Artman M, Graham TP Jr: Congestive heart failure in infancy: Recognition and management. Am Heart J 1982;103:1040.
13. Fisher DJ, Gross DM, Garson A: Rapid sinus tachycardia—differentiation from supraventricular tachycardia. Am J Dis Child 1983;137:164.
14. Garson A: Arrhythmias. In Garson A (ed): The Electrocardiogram in Infants and Children: A Systematic Approach. Philadelphia, Lea & Febiger, 1983, p 231.
15. Eronen M, Siren MK, Ekblad H, et al: Short and long-term outcome of children with congenital complete heart block diagnosed in utero or as a newborn. Pediatrics 2000;106:86.
16. Groves AM, Allen LD, Rosenthal E: Outcome of isolated congenital complete heart block diagnosed in utero. Heart 1997;78:95.
17. Friedman RA, Schowengerdt KO, Towbin JA: Myocarditis. In Garson AJ, Bricker JT, Fisher DJ, Neish SR (eds): The Science and Practice of Pediatric Cardiology. Philadelphia, Williams & Wilkins, 1998, p 1785.
18. Pickert CB, Moss MM, Fiser DH: Neonatal infection versus congenital obstructive left heart disease. Pediatr Emerg Care 1998;14:263.
19. Mikhail M, Lee W, Toews W, et al: Surgical and medical experience with 734 premature infants with patent ductus arteriosus. J Thorac Cardiovasc Surg 1982;83:349.
20. Ghosh PK, Lubliner J, Mogilnar M, et al: Ligation of patent ductus arteriosus in very low birthweight premature neonates. Thorax 1985;40:533.
21. Cabal LE, Udayakumar D, Siassi B, et al: Cardiogenic schock associated with perinatal asphyxia in term infants. J Pediatr 1980;96:705.
22. Rowe RD, Hoffman T: Transient myocardial ischemia of the newborn infant: A form of severe cardiorespiratory distress in full-term infants. J Pediatr 1972;81:243.
23. Sommerville RJ, Nora JJ, Clayton GW, McNamara DG: Adrenal insufficiency mimicking heart disease in infancy. Pediatrics 1968;42:691.
24. Dzimiri N, Galal O, Moorji A, et al: Regulation of sympathetic activity in children with various congenital heart diseases. Pediatr Res 1995;38:55.
25. Buchhorn R, Hammersen A, Bartmus D, Bursch J: The pathogenesis of heart failure in infants with congenital heart disease. Cardiol Young 2001;11:498.
26. Farrell AG, Schamberger MS, Olson IL, Leitch CA: Large left-to-right shunts and congestive heart failure increase total energy expenditure in infants with ventricular septal defect. Am J Cardiol 2001;87:1128.
27. Bland EF, White PD, Garland J: Congenital anomalies of the coronary arteries: Report of an unusual case associated with cardiac hypertrophy. Am Heart J 1933;8:787.
28. Johnsrude CL, Perry JC, Cecchin F, et al: Differentiating anomalous left main coronary artery originating from the pulmonary artery in infants from myocarditis and dilated cardiomyopathy by electrocardiogram. Am J Cardiol 1995;75:71.
29. Millard DD, Shulman ST: The changing spectrum of neonatal endocarditis. Clin Perinatol 1983;15:587.
30. Ferrieri P, Gewitz MH, Gerber MA, et al: Unique features of infective endocarditis in childhood. Pediatrics 2002;109:931.
31. Wren C, Richmond R, Donaldson L: Presentation of congenital heart disease in infancy: Implications for routine examination. Arch Dis Child Fetal Neonatal Educ 1999;80:F49.
32. Gersony WM: Diagnosis and management of Kawasaki disease. JAMA 1991;265:2699.
33. Dajani AS, Taubert KA, Gerber MA, et al: Diagnosis and therapy of Kawasaki disease in children. Circulation 1993;87:1776.
34. Honkanen VE, Mc Crindle BW, Laxer RM, et al: Clinical relevance of the risk factors for coronary artery inflammation in Kawasaki disease. Pediatr Cardiol 2003;24:122.
35. Feltes TF, Pignatelli R, Kleinert S, Mariscalco MM: Quantitated left ventricular systolic mechanics in children with septic shock utilizing noninvasive wall-stress analysis. Crit Care Med 1994;22:1647.
36. Thiru Y, Pathan N, Bignall S, et al: A myocardial cytotoxic process is involved in the cardiac dysfunction of meningococcal septic shock. Crit Care Med 2000;28:2979.
37. Hagmolen H, Wiegman A, van den Hoek GJ, et al: Life-threatening heart failure in meningococcal septic shock in children: Non-invasive measurement of cardiac parameters is of important prognostic value. Eur J Pediatr 2000;159:277.
38. Artman M, Parrish MD, Graham TP: Congestive heart failure in childhood and adolescence: Recognition and management. Am Heart J 1983;105:471.
39. Kay JD, Colan SD, Graham TP: Congestive heart failure in pediatric patients. Am Heart J 2001;142:923.
40. Maeda K, Takayoshi T, Wada A, et al: Plasma brain natriuretic peptide as a biochemical marker of high left ventricular end-diastolic pressure in patients with symptomatic left ventricular dysfunction. Am Heart J 1998;135:825.
41. Muders F, Kromer EP, Griese DP, et al: Evaluation of plasma natriuretic peptides as markers for left ventricular dysfunction. Am Heart J 1997;134:442.

42. McCullough PA, Nowak RM, McCord J, et al: B-type natriuretic peptide and clinical judgement in emergency diagnosis of heart failure. Circulation 2002;106:416.

43. Mir TS, Marohn S, Laer S, et al: Plasma concentration of N-terminal and Pro-brain natriuretic peptide in control children from the neonatal to adolescent period and in children with congestive heart failure. Pediatrics 2002;110:e76.

44. Carell ES, Murali S, Schulman D, et al: Maximal exercise tolerance in chronic congestive heart failure: Relationship to resting ventricular function. Chest 1994;106:1746.

45. Guimaraes GV, Bellotti G, Mocelin AO, et al: Cardiopulmonary exercise testing in children with heart failure secondary to idiopathic dilated cardiomyopathy. Chest 2001;120:816.

46. Sullivan MJ, Hawthorne MH: Exercise intolerance in patients with chronic heart failure. Prog Cardiovasc Dis 1995;38:1.

47. Mancini DM, Eisen H, Kussmaul W, et al: Value of peak exercise VO$_2$ for optimal cardiac transplantation in ambulatory patients with failure. Circulation 1991;83:778.

48. Ross RD: Grading the graders of congestive heart failure in children. J Pediatr 2001;138:618.

49. The Criteria Committee of the New York Heart Association: Diseases of the Heart and Blood Vessels: Nomenclature and Criteria for Diagnosis, 6th ed. Boston, Little, Brown, 1964, p 112.

50. Hunt SA, Baker DW, Chin MH, et al: ACC/AHA guidelines for the evaluation and management of chronic heart failure in the adult: Executive summary: A report of the American College of Cardiology/American Heart Association Task Force on Practice Guidelines (Committee to Revise the 1995 Guidelines for the Evaluation and Management of Heart Failure). J Am Coll Cardiol 2001;38:2101.

51. Ross RD, Bollinger RO, Pinsky WW: Grading the severity of congestive heart failure in infants. Pediatr Cardiol 1992;13:72.

52. Ross RD, Daniels SR, Schwartz DC, et al: Plasma norepinephrine levels in infants and children with congestive heart failure. Am J Cardiol 1987;59:911.

53. Ross RD, Daniels SR, Schwartz DC, et al: Return of plasma norepinephrine to normal after resolution of congestive heart failure in congenital heart disease. Am J Cardiol 1987;60:1411.

54. Wu JR, Chang HR, Huang TY, et al: Reduction in lymphocyte B-adrenergic receptor density in infants and children with heart failure secondary to congenital heart disease. Am J Cardiol 1996;77:170.

55. Reithmann C, Reber D, Kozlik-Feldmann R, et al: Post-receptor defect of adenyl cyclase in severely failing myocardium from children with congenital heart disease. Eur J Pharmacol 1997;330:79.

56. Laer S, Mir TS, Behn F, et al: Carvedilol therapy in pediatric patients with congestive heart failure: A study investigating clinical and pharmacokinetic parameters. Am Heart J 2002;143:916.

57. Connolly D, Rutkowski M, Auslender M, Artman M: The New York University Pediatric Heart Failure Index: A new method of quantifying chronic heart failure severity in children. J Pediatr 2001;138:644.

58. Westerlind A, Wahlander H, Lindstedt G, et al: Clinical signs of heart failure are associated with increased level of natriuretic peptide types B and A in children with congenital heart defects or cardiomyopathy. Acta Paediatr 2004;93:340.

59. Jefferies JL, Chang AC: Natriuretic peptides and other biomarkers in heart failure in children and adults. Cardiology in the Young (in press).

CHAPTER 15

Classification of Types of Heart Failure

Antonio R. Mott
John P. Breinholt

In the traditional physiology paradigm, the heart serves as a pump that provides the energy to facilitate blood flow through the blood vessels—arteries and veins. In the current era, the paradigm is revised such that the heart is regarded as a muscle that can be conditioned and is susceptible to a deconditioned state. Additionally, the blood vessels are dynamic, prone to react to changes in blood pressure.[1] The circulatory system is a dynamic system with complex interactions with other organ systems. In a consensus statement, the National Heart, Lung, and Blood Institute defines cardiac failure as occurring when:[2]

> … [A]n abnormality of cardiac function causes a heart to fail to pump blood at a rate required by the metabolizing tissues or when the heart can do so only with an elevated filling pressure. The heart's inability to pump a sufficient amount of blood to meet the needs of the body tissues may be due to insufficient or defective cardiac filling and/or impaired contraction and emptying. Compensatory mechanisms increase blood volume and raise cardiac filling pressures, heart rate, and cardiac muscle mass to maintain the heart's pumping function and cause redistribution of blood flow. Eventually, however, despite these compensatory mechanisms, the ability of the heart to contract and relax progressively declines, and the heart failure worsens.

Heart failure is common in adults. Approximately 5 million people in the United States are treated for heart failure at an annual cost of $25.8 billion.[3,4] Although the incidence of heart failure in children has yet to be defined, cardiac failure is commonly due to systemic diseases, congenital heart disease, cardiomyopathy, tachyarrhythmia, and post cardiac surgery. Regardless of the etiology, timely diagnosis and effective treatment of cardiac failure are important in preventing short-term and long-term sequelae. This chapter provides an overview of the traditional classification scheme for the different types of cardiac failure.

Cardiac failure in children, similar to that in adults, can be classified into different types. As with any descriptive classification system, there are inherent overlap and a tendency to oversimplify the complex interactions and pathophysiology of the circulatory system. The following subclassifications of cardiac failure are described:

1. Acute heart failure versus chronic heart failure
2. High cardiac output syndrome versus low cardiac output syndrome
3. Right heart failure versus left heart failure
4. Forward cardiac failure versus backward cardiac failure
5. Systolic cardiac failure versus diastolic cardiac failure

ACUTE VERSUS CHRONIC HEART FAILURE

The rate at which the onset of heart failure symptoms occurs has an impact on the clinical manifestations and distinguishes acute from chronic heart failure. Time permits compensatory mechanisms to be activated to preserve adequate oxygen delivery to the tissues. This time line is a continuum, however, and the boundaries of acute and compensated or decompensated chronic heart failure are often blurred.

Acute heart failure occurs when the body's compensatory mechanisms do not have the time to become effective, and there is inadequate oxygen delivery to the tissues followed by the onset of symptoms of heart failure. In pediatric patients, **fulminant myocarditis** is a classic example of acute decompensated heart failure resulting in a sudden reduction in cardiac output and inadequate organ perfusion. Another example is sudden hemodynamic deterioration resulting from severe **valvular insufficiency** secondary to endocarditis,[5] trauma,[6] or rupture of sinus of Valsalva aneurysm.[7]

Chronic heart failure can occur with the slow and insidious onset of impaired cardiac output, allowing the body's compensatory mechanisms to become activated, preserving organ perfusion.[8] Nevertheless, patients with chronic failure can have an exacerbation of heart failure and present with signs and symptoms consistent with acute heart failure.

HIGH VERSUS LOW CARDIAC OUTPUT FAILURE

High Cardiac Output Failure

In high cardiac output failure, cardiac output is increased to provide for the needs of the tissues. These patients may appear relatively asymptomatic, and on physical examination, there is usually tachycardia, warm skin, and a widened pulse pressure. Possible etiologies for high output cardiac failure include anemia, congenital or acquired arteriovenous malformations, hyperthyroidism, vitamin deficiencies, and pregnancy.

In children, **anemia** can occur in various scenarios, such as iron deficiency anemia resulting from malnutrition and hemoglobinopathies such as sickle cell disease. Chronic anemia in the absence of underlying cardiac disease is not likely to cause significant cardiac symptoms.[9,10] **Congenital arteriovenous malformations** occur embryologically as a result of delayed development and maturation of the vascular supply to an organ and appear as embryonic capillary networks. These entities manifest as small hemangiomas or as large clusters of blood vessels, commonly in the lower extremities. Osler-Weber-Rendu disease, or hereditary hemorrhagic telangiectasia, is a condition associated with arteriovenous malformations in the lungs and liver. Vein of Galen aneurysms are large cerebral arteriovenous malformations that manifest in the newborn period with cardiomegaly and early hemodynamic compromise.[11] Acquired arteriovenous malformations are commonly due to penetrating trauma or procedures such as central line placement. **Hyperthyroidism** also can lead to high output heart failure with symptoms likely to be amplified in the presence of coexisting heart disease, whether congenital or acquired.[12] Nevertheless, neonatal thyrotoxicosis is likely to cause cardiac embarrassment even in the absence of congenital heart disease. Common physical examination findings are tachycardia and a widened pulse pressure. **Beriberi**, caused by thiamine deficiency usually of greater than 3 months' duration, can cause high output heart failure. This deficiency is rare in industrialized nations, but is endemic in parts of the undeveloped world. The main affected populations are infants age 1 to 4 months and adults with illnesses such as gastrointestinal disorders, alcoholism, and human immunodeficiency virus. In affected individuals, thiamine treatment yields improvement within 24 hours.[13]

Lastly, a high cardiac output state can occur in the first trimester of pregnancy. This risk is of particular importance to women with congenital heart disease; there are now approximately 1 million adults with either palliated or repaired congenital heart defects.[14] As women contemplate the risks of pregnancy with coexisting heart disease, this particular risk must be weighed carefully with regard to its risk to the mother and fetus.[15]

Low Cardiac Output Failure

Low cardiac output failure is more common than high output failure in pediatric patients. Primary pump or primary cardiac muscle dysfunction, in addition to changes in systemic or pulmonary vascular resistance, are at the core of this form of cardiac failure. Common causes of low cardiac output include acute myocarditis, dilated cardiomyopathy, chronic tachyarrhythmia, coronary anomalies, and cardiac postoperative sequelae.[16]

In contrast to high output heart failure, patients with low output heart failure appear ill or toxic. Prominent signs of low cardiac output include resting tachycardia, cool extremities, pallor, oliguria, and systemic vasoconstriction. Intracardiac monitoring reveals increased central venous and left atrial pressures. Systemic blood pressure and mixed venous saturation also are decreased. The pulse pressure is usually narrowed. Tachycardia (particularly resting tachycardia) and increased systemic vascular resistance are compensatory mechanisms that promote improved oxygen delivery to the organs. Tachycardia and increased systemic resistance also increase the energy demands on the cardiac muscle. Similar to in high output heart failure, identification and treatment of the underlying etiology are vital to proper management.

RIGHT VERSUS LEFT HEART FAILURE

In pediatric patients, the preponderance of congenital heart defects provides a unique opportunity for the clinician to diagnose and manage predominant right or left heart failure (see Chapter 16). As in other types of heart failure, right and left heart failure can coexist in the same patient because the pulmonary and systemic circulations are in series. These categories and the possible permutations between categories (e.g., left systolic dysfunction observed with myocarditis versus right diastolic dysfunction seen after repair of tetralogy of Fallot) can lead to further confusion, but create interesting clinical scenarios.

Each ventricle has a unique anatomic and compensatory profile that warrants review. The right ventricle is the predominant ventricle in utero, responsible for providing 65% of the combined cardiac output to the fetus.[17] During postnatal transitioning, pulmonary vascular resistance decreases. As a result, afterload decreases, and the right ventricular wall becomes thin and compliant with a contractile profile that adapts to the decreased resistance of the pulmonary vascular bed.[18] The right ventricular contractile sequence consists of contraction of the spinal muscles, movement of the right ventricular free wall toward the interventricular septum, and assistance from the "wringing" nature of left ventricular contraction that aids in right ventricular cavity emptying (see Chapter 16). Other factors affecting right ventricular systolic and diastolic function include preload, afterload, and intrathoracic pressure.[19] Overall the right ventricle is less able to adapt to the wide range of afterload conditions.

Although the right ventricle is the predominant ventricle in utero, the left ventricle becomes thick walled, highly contractile, and more adaptive to provide constant output over a varied range of afterload conditions after birth. The interventricular septum most closely emulates the anatomic and physiologic characteristics of the left ventricle. Its specific role continues to be defined. Abnormalities of the interventricular septum can impede systolic and diastolic properties of the right ventricle and left ventricle. Left ventricular systolic and diastolic function also is affected by preload, afterload, and intrathoracic pressure.

Right Heart Failure

Right ventricular failure is common in pediatric patients and often is due to right-sided obstructive or regurgitant lesions, pulmonary hypertension, cor pulmonale, and acute graft rejection after orthotopic cardiac transplantation. Although the work profile of the right ventricle is quite different from the left ventricle, the right ventricle performs an important role in providing cardiac output (preload to the left atrium). Right ventricular output abruptly decreases with minimal alterations in afterload, and systolic dysfunction ensues. Diastolic dysfunction also can cause right heart failure. In the presence of diastolic dysfunction, the ventricle does not relax, and ventricular filling is compromised. Diastolic dysfunction is more common than previously believed. Common clinical findings of right heart failure include hepatomegaly with or without pulsatility, abdominal ascites, and lower extremity edema. Jugular venous distention is noted more commonly in older patients because jugular veins are difficult to assess in infants. Infants may present with difficulty feeding or diaphoresis while feeding, possibly associated with a catecholamine surge that occurs when they are confronted with eating while in respiratory distress.[20,21]

Right ventricular outflow tract obstruction can lead to right heart failure. A neonate with a left-sided obstructive lesion, such as critical coarctation of the aorta, also can present with right heart failure. This phenomenon is due to the dominance of the right ventricle in utero. In addition, **tricuspid or pulmonary insufficiency**, especially when both are present concomitantly, can lead to right ventricular failure.[22] Pathologic states, such as **elevated pulmonary vascular resistance** caused by primary or secondary pulmonary hypertension, can result in right heart failure. These patients also can present with cyanosis secondary to shunting at the atrial level. Cor pulmonale also is common in pediatric patients, especially former premature infants with residual chronic lung disease (see Chapter 28). Other causes of cor pulmonale include advanced obstructive sleep apnea from tonsillar hypertrophy with or without obesity.[23] Volume overload lesions, such as atrial septal defect or partial anomalous pulmonary venous connection, usually do not lead to overt right ventricular failure.

Left Heart Failure

Left heart failure is common in pediatric patients. Although the left ventricle is capable of responding to various changes in afterload, different pathologic states can compromise left ventricular function and lead to left ventricular failure. In the presence of left heart failure, there usually is increased systemic vascular resistance. Common clinical findings of left heart failure include tachycardia and decreased skin perfusion; left heart failure also can produce symptoms and signs of right heart failure when biventricular failure occurs.

Myocarditis is a common etiology of left heart failure.[24] Other etiologies include **coronary artery anomalies** (i.e., anomalous origin of the left coronary artery from the pulmonary artery), **left ventricular outflow tract obstruction** (including valvar and subvalvar aortic stenosis and aortic arch obstruction), **aortic or mitral regurgitation**, and **acute rejection** after orthotopic cardiac transplantation. In addition, systemic ventricular failure can occur in morphologic right ventricles in patients who had an atrial switch operation.[25,26] In the absence of confounding conditions, left-to-right shunt lesions, such as ventricular septal defect or patent ductus arteriosus, usually do not lead to left ventricular failure. Left heart failure can be systolic, which presents as an abnormality in the contractile properties of the ventricle. Likewise, left heart failure also can present as diastolic dysfunction (see later). In the presence of diastolic dysfunction, the ventricle does not relax, and ventricular filling is compromised (see Chapter 8). The primary etiology determines the extent and onset of left heart failure. As such, elucidating the cause of left heart failure is as important as its recognition and treatment.

FORWARD VERSUS BACKWARD HEART FAILURE

Heart failure can develop in two circulatory directions.[27] In forward failure, there is inadequate delivery of blood to the arterial system; this pathophysiologic state can occur via the pulmonary artery or the aorta, affecting end-organ perfusion in either vascular bed. In backward failure, incomplete return of blood to the ventricle results in increased pressure directed toward the source of filling for the ventricle in accordance with Starling's law (Fig. 15-1). The concept of backward heart failure was first introduced by Hope in 1932.[28] He hypothesized

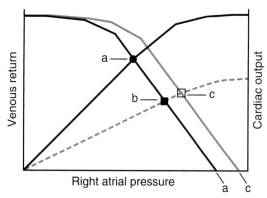

FIGURE 15-1 ■ Forward and backward heart failure via "Guyton diagrams." The venous return is seen on the y-axis, and right pressure is plotted on the x-axis. With decrease in contractility and forward heart failure, the circulating blood volume is increased *(dashed line)*. Darkened box *b* shows decrease in cardiac output and venous return with an increase in right atrial pressure. The increase in mean circulatory filling pressure shifts the relationship between venous return and right atrial pressure upward and to the right toward a steady state *(open box c)*. Venous return, cardiac output, and right atrial pressure are increased. (From Katz AM: Organ physiology: *The failing heart as a weakened pump*. In Katz A [ed]: *Heart Failure Pathophysiology, Molecular Biology and Clinical Management*. Philadelphia, Lippincott Williams & Wilkins, 2000, pp 35-69.)

that when the ventricle fails to eject its contents, blood pools and pressure increases in the atrium and the venous system emptying into that ventricle.

Right-sided forward failure occurs most commonly in the presence of a right ventricle with **decreased systolic function** or **right ventricular outflow tract obstruction**. The right ventricle cannot empty adequately, resulting in decreased blood flow to the pulmonary vasculature. Initially the right ventricle hypertrophies and later dilates with resulting decreased output. Right-sided backward failure also can result from significant **tricuspid stenosis and regurgitation**[29] or **severe pulmonary hypertension**. There is progressive right atrial enlargement and elevated central venous pressure and impedance to blood inflow to the right ventricle. Severe forward failure can lead to backward failure, especially in the presence of increased right ventricular end-diastolic and systolic pressures.

Because the heart is a bipartite structure, the left ventricle and right ventricle have an innate interdependence. **Mitral valve stenosis** with resulting left atrial hypertension and left ventricular backward failure also causes increased impedance to pulmonary artery flow and emptying of the right ventricle. In patients with **hypertrophic cardiomyopathy**, the limited left ventricular cavity reduces filling and leads to backward failure. In the presence of **myocarditis** or **dilated cardiomyopathy**, there is an increase in ventricular wall tension (fulfilling the law of LaPlace) and decreased forward flow from the left ventricle. In patients with severe **left ventricular outflow tract obstruction**, there also

is decreased forward flow from the left ventricle to the aorta. As a result, the left ventricle develops inappropriate concentric hypertrophy, diastolic dysfunction, and left atrial hypertension. This sequela results in impaired filling, increased pulmonary capillary wedge pressure, and ultimately left-sided backward heart failure and right-sided forward heart failure from elevated right-sided pressures.

Backward and forward failure can often coexist in the same patient because the circulatory system is in continuum. Although vasodilators are the mainstay of therapy for forward heart failure, diuretics remain popular pharmacologic agents for backward failure (see Chapter 32). Overaggressive use of diuretic agents could reduce preload and worsen forward failure.

SYSTOLIC VERSUS DIASTOLIC HEART FAILURE

Systolic cardiac failure and diastolic cardiac failure are differentiated by failure of ventricular ejection with decreased inotropy (systolic failure) and abnormal ventricular filling with decreased lusitropy (diastolic failure). Although both types of heart failure can occur together, each has distinct characteristics when they occur alone (Table 15-1 and Fig. 15-2).[30]

Systolic Heart Failure

Systolic heart failure is closely associated with such conditions as **myocardial infarction** and **pulmonary embolus**, two conditions that are relatively rare in children. Conditions leading to global systolic dysfunction

TABLE 15-1

Systolic Versus Diastolic Heart Failure		
Characteristic	Systolic Heart Failure	Diastolic Heart Failure
Clinical Features		
Symptoms (e.g., dyspnea)	Yes	Yes
Congestive state (e.g., hepatomegaly)	Yes	Yes
Exercise capacity	Decreased	Decreased
Cardiac output augmentation	Decreased	Decreased
Left Ventricular Structure and Function		
Ejection fraction	Decreased	Normal
Left ventricular mass	Increased	Increased
Relative wall thickness	Decreased	Increased
End-diastolic volume	Increased	Normal
End-diastolic pressure	Increased	Increased
Left atrial size	Increased	Increased

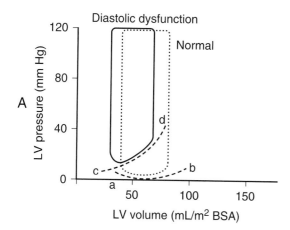

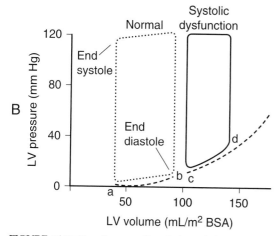

FIGURE 15-2 ■ **Systolic versus diastolic heart failure.** Schematic diagrams of diastolic (**A**) and systolic (**B**) dysfunction. **A,** The pressure volume curve depicts diastolic dysfunction with elevated end-diastolic pressure volume relationship curve (up and to the left as seen in *cd*). Normal pressure volume curve is depicted with a dotted line. **B,** The solid line depicts systolic dysfunction with the pressure volume curve displaced to the right. There is compensatory volume increase. BSA, body surface area; LV, left ventricular. (From Zile MR: *Diastolic dysfunction: Detection, consequences, and treatment: II. Diagnosis and treatment of diastolic dysfunction. Mod Concepts Cardiovasc* 1990;59:1-14.)

that are more likely to occur in children include **myocarditis** and **dilated cardiomyopathy**; pathologic states resulting in regional systolic dysfunction usually involve coronary ischemia or infarction (**coronary anomalies** or **Kawasaki disease**).[31] Anatomic lesions that also can result in systolic failure include coarctation of the aorta, which causes increased afterload that often leads to ventricular dysfunction. Systolic dysfunction manifests as forward failure because the impaired ventricle is unable to deliver blood adequately to its end organs. In left ventricular systolic failure, the kidneys are poorly perfused, leading to water and salt retention.

Diastolic Heart Failure

Diastolic heart failure largely comprises two abnormalities: decreased diastolic compliance and slowed or impaired ventricular relaxation (as seen in hypertrophic

cardiomyopathy or restrictive cardiomyopathy). True diagnostic criteria have not been established, however, despite continued efforts by the American Heart Association, American College of Cardiology, and the European Study Group on Diastolic Heart Failure. The American Heart Association and American College of Cardiology indicate that "the diagnosis of diastolic heart failure is generally based on the finding of typical symptoms and signs of heart failure in a patient who is shown to have a normal left ventricular ejection fraction and no valvular abnormalities on echocardiogram."[32] The European Study Group also adds "evidence of abnormal left ventricular relaxation, filling, diastolic distensibility or diastolic stiffness."[33] A more recent proposal has been made to establish a classification system for diastolic failure: This proposal includes clinical signs and symptoms of congestive heart failure, echocardiographic evidence of normal systolic function, and evidence of diastolic dysfunction.[34]

Etiologies of diastolic dysfunction include **anatomic obstruction** that prevents normal ventricular filling (i.e., pulmonary venous obstruction or mitral stenosis[35]), **reduction in ventricular compliance** (i.e., heart transplant rejection), **external forces** (i.e., pericardial effusion), and **suboptimal hemodynamics** (i.e., elevated pulmonary vascular resistance after the Fontan procedure). Diastolic heart failure also is present frequently in **cardiomyopathy** patients, particularly hypertrophic (concentric) and restrictive types,[36] and patients with systemic hypertension with resultant hypertrophy. It often manifests clinically as dyspnea and exercise intolerance. This manifestation is likely due to an increased ventricular filling pressure that translates to increased upstream venous pressure leading to pulmonary or systemic congestion. This is a form of backward heart failure.

Although similar in clinical presentation, there are differences between patients with systolic or diastolic heart failure. The mortality rate for diastolic heart failure is less (5% to 8%) relative to systolic heart failure (10% to 15%).[37] Although additional evidence is needed to elucidate the significance, studies have shown that brain natriuretic peptide levels are higher in systolic heart failure patients than diastolic heart failure patients.

CURRENT STATUS AND FUTURE TRENDS

Heart failure is a clinical entity that occurs when there is an inability of the heart and its compensatory mechanisms to deliver adequate oxygen to the tissues. Heart failure has been classified into several broad categories, but as with any descriptive classification system, there is overlap and a tendency to oversimplify the complex interactions and pathophysiologic states. Despite the subclasses, timely recognition and treatment of heart failure are important in the prevention of long-term sequelae.[38,39] Much insight into these various subclasses of heart failure has been gained in adults with heart failure but remains to be gained in children.[40,41]

Key Concepts

■ The rate at which the onset of heart failure symptoms occurs affects the clinical manifestations and distinguishes acute from chronic heart failure. Time permits compensatory mechanisms to be activated to preserve adequate oxygen delivery to the tissues. This time line is a continuum, however, and the boundaries of acute and compensated or decompensated chronic heart failure are often blurred.

■ In pediatric patients, fulminant myocarditis is a classic example of acute decompensated heart failure resulting in a sudden reduction in cardiac output and inadequate organ perfusion. Another example is sudden hemodynamic deterioration resulting from severe valvular insufficiency secondary to endocarditis, trauma, or rupture of sinus of Valsalva aneurysm.

■ Possible etiologies for high output cardiac failure include anemia, congenital or acquired arteriovenous malformations, hyperthyroidism, vitamin deficiencies, and pregnancy.

■ Common causes of low cardiac output include acute myocarditis, dilated cardiomyopathy, chronic tachyarrhythmia, coronary anomalies, and cardiac postoperative sequelae.

■ Right ventricular failure is common in pediatric patients and often is due to right-sided obstructive or regurgitant lesions, pulmonary hypertension, cor pulmonale, and acute graft rejection after orthotopic cardiac transplantation.

■ In forward failure, there is inadequate delivery of blood to the arterial system; this pathophysiologic state can occur via the pulmonary artery or the aorta, affecting end-organ perfusion in either vascular bed. In backward failure, incomplete return of blood to the ventricle results in increased pressure directed toward the source of filling for the ventricle in accordance with Starling's law.

■ Diastolic heart failure largely comprises two abnormalities: decreased diastolic compliance and slowed or impaired ventricular relaxation (as seen in hypertrophic cardiomyopathy or restrictive cardiomyopathy).

■ Etiologies of diastolic dysfunction include anatomic obstruction that prevents normal ventricular filling (i.e., pulmonary venous obstruction or mitral stenosis), reduction in ventricular compliance (i.e., heart transplant rejection), external forces (i.e., pericardial effusion), and suboptimal hemodynamics (i.e., elevated pulmonary vascular resistance after Fontan procedure). Diastolic heart failure also is present frequently in cardiomyopathy patients, particularly hypertrophic (concentric) and restrictive types, and patients with systemic hypertension with resultant hypertrophy.

REFERENCES

1. Katz AM: Organ physiology: The failing heart as a weakened pump. In Katz A (ed): Heart Failure Pathophysiology, Molecular Biology and Clinical Management. Philadelphia, Lippincott Williams & Wilkins, 2000, pp 35-69.
2. Lenfant C: Report of the Task Force on Research in Heart Failure. Circulation 1994;90:1118-1123.
3. American Heart Association: Heart Disease and Stroke Statistics—2004 Update. Dallas, American Heart Association, 2003.
4. Massie BM, Shah NB: Evolving trends in the epidemiologic factors of heart failure: Rationale for preventive strategies and comprehensive disease management. Am Heart J 1997;133:703-712.
5. Lechner E, Dickerson HA, Fraser CD, et al: Vasodilatory shock after surgery for aortic valve endocarditis treated with low dose vasopressin. Pediatr Cardiol 2004;25(5):558-561.
6. Onorati F, DeSanto LS, Carozza A, et al: Marfan syndrome as a predisposing factor for traumatic aortic insufficiency. Ann Thorac Surg 2004;77:2192-2194.
7. Arora R, Trehan V, Rangasetty UM, et al: Transcatheter closure of ruptured sinus of Valsalva aneurysm. J Interv Cardiol 2004;17:53-58.
8. Givertz MM, Colucci WS, Braunwald E: Clinical aspects of heart failure: High-output failure; pulmonary edema. In Braunwald E, (ed): Heart Disease: A Textbook of Cardiovascular Medicine. Philadelphia, WB Saunders, 2001, pp 531-561.
9. Francis GS, Gassler JP, Sonneblick EH: Pathophysiology and diagnosis of heart failure. In Fuster V, Alexander RW, O'Rourke RA, et al (eds): Hurst's the Heart. New York, McGraw-Hill, 2001, pp 655-685.
10. Hebert PC, Van der Linden P, Biro G, et al: Physiologic aspects of anemia. Crit Care Med 2004;20:187-212.
11. Brunelle F: Arteriovenous malformations of the vein of Galen in children. Pediatr Radiol 1997;27:501-513.
12. Cavallo A, Joseph CJ, Casta A: Cardiac complications in juvenile hyperthyroidism. Am J Dis Child 1984;138:479-482.
13. Curran JS, Lewis AB: Vitamin deficiencies and excesses. In Behrman RE, Kliegman R, Jenson HB (eds): Nelson Textbook of Pediatrics. Philadelphia, WB Saunders, 2000, p 179.
14. Brickner ME, Hillis LD, Lange RA: Congenital heart disease in adults: First of two parts. N Engl J Med 2000;342:256-263.
15. Veldtman GR, Connolly HM, Grogan M, et al: Outcomes of pregnancy in women with tetralogy of Fallot. J Am Coll Cardiol 2004;44:181-183.
16. Wessel DL: Managing low cardiac output syndrome after congenital heart surgery. Crit Care Med 2001;29:S220-S230.
17. Fineman JR, Soifer SJ: The fetal and neonatal circulations. In Chang AC, Hanley FL, Wernovsky G, Wessel D (eds): Pediatric Cardiac Intensive Care. Baltimore, Williams & Wilkins, 1998, pp 17-24.
18. Hines R: Right ventricular function and failure: A review. Yale J Biol Med 1991;64:295-307.
19. Rushmer RF, Thal N: The mechanics of ventricular contraction: A cinefluorographic study. Circulation 1951;4:219-228.
20. Freed MD: Congestive heart failure. In Fyler DC, Nadas AS (eds): Nadas' Pediatric Cardiology. Philadelphia, Hanley & Belfus, 1992, pp 63-72.
21. Talner N: Heart failure. In Emmanouilides GC, Adams FH, Moss AJ (eds): Moss and Adams' Heart Disease in Infants, Children, and Adolescents: Including the Fetus and Young Adult, vol 2. Baltimore, Williams & Wilkins, 1995, pp 1746-1773.
22. Pflamer A, Eicken A, Angustin N, et al: Symptomatic neonates with Ebstein anomaly. J Thorac Cardiovasc Surg 2004;127:1208-1209.
23. Zohar Y, Talmi YP, Frenkel H, et al: Cardiac function in obstructive sleep apnea patients following uvulopalatopharyngoplasty. Otolaryngol Head Neck Surg 1992;107:390-394.
24. Gagliardi MG, Bevilacqua M, Bassano C, et al: Long term follow up of children with myocarditis treated by immunosuppression

and of children with dilated cardiomyopathy. Heart 2004;90:1167-1171.

25. Chang AC, Wernovsky G, Wessel DL, et al: Surgical management of late right ventricular failure after Mustard or Senning repair. Circulation 1992;86:II-140-II-149.

26. Benzaquen BS, Webb GD, Colman JM, et al: Arterial switch operation after Mustard procedures in adult patients with transposition of the great arteries: Is it time to revise our strategy? Am Heart J 2004;147:E8.

27. Stevenson LW: Clinical use of inotropic therapy for heart failure: Looking backward or forward? Circulation 2003;108:492-497.

28. Hope JA: A Treatise on the Diseases of the Heart and Great Vessels, and on the Affections Which May Be Mistaken for Them. Philadelphia, Lea & Blanchard, 1842.

29. Messika-Zeitoun D, Thomson H, Bellamy M, et al: Medical and surgical outcome of tricuspid regurgitation caused by flail leaflets. J Thorac Cardiovasc Surg 2004;128:296-302.

30. Aurigemma GP, Gaasch WH: Clinical practice: Diastolic heart failure. N Engl J Med 2004;351:1097-1105.

31. DeWolf D, Vercruysse T, Suys B, et al: Major coronary anomalies in childhood. Eur J Pediatr 2002;161:637-642.

32. Hunt SA, Baker DW, Chin MH, et al: ACC/AHA Guidelines for the evaluation and management of chronic heart failure in the adult: Executive summary: A report of the American College of Cardiology/American Heart Association Task Force on Practice Guidelines (Committee to Revise the 1995 Guidelines for the Evaluation and Management of Heart Failure). Circulation 2001; 104:2996-3007.

33. How to diagnose diastolic heart failure. European Study Group on Diastolic Heart Failure. Eur Heart J 1998;19:990-1003.

34. van Kraaij DJ, van Pol PE, Ruiters AW, et al: Diagnosing diastolic heart failure. Eur J Heart Fail 2002;4:419-430.

35. Schaverien MV, Freedom RM, McCrindle BW: Independent factors associated with outcomes of parachute mitral valve in 84 patients. Circulation 2004;109:2309-2313.

36. Chinnaiyan KM, Leff CB, Marsalese DL: Constrictive pericarditis versus restrictive cardiomyopathy: Challenges in diagnosis and management. Cardiol Rev 2004;12:314-320.

37. Zile MR, Baicu CF: Alterations in ventricular function: Diastolic heart failure. In Mann DL (ed): Heart Failure. Philadelphia, WB Saunders, 2003, pp 209-227.

38. McElhinney DB, Colan SD, Moran AM, et al: Recombinant human growth hormone treatment for dilated cardiomyopathy in children. Pediatrics 2004;114:e452-e458.

39. Zareba KM, Lavigne JE, Lispshultz SE: Cardiovascular effects of HAART in infants and children of HIV infected mothers. Cardiovasc Toxicol 2004;4:271-280.

40. Zile MR, Baicu CF, Gaasch WH: Diastolic heart failure—abnormalities in active relaxation and passive stiffness of the left ventricle. N Engl J Med 2004;350:1953-1959.

41. Egan JR, Festa M, Cole AD, et al: Clinical assessment of cardiac performance in infants and children following cardiac surgery. Intensive Care Medicine 2005;31:568-573.

CHAPTER 16

Right Ventricular Dysfunction in Congenital Heart Disease

Timothy C. Slesnick
Anthony C. Chang

The right ventricle has been perceived as a relatively passive conduit between the two circulations, but is in fact a complex pump with its unique physiology of ejection, interaction with its adjacent left ventricle, influence by respirations, and myriad of congenital anomalies. Since the 1970s, there have been increasing investigations into the role of the right ventricle in healthy and diseased states. Early studies indicated that even complete destruction of the right ventricular free wall in dogs resulted in no overall impairment of cardiac function and only minimal increase in venous pressures.[1] Since then, many groups have shown that in the presence of stressors, such as increased preload or afterload,[2,3] impaired coronary perfusion,[4] or systemic disease such as septic shock,[5-10] the function of the right ventricle can be affected with clinical and hemodynamic consequences.

In adults, the frequency of right heart failure has been estimated to be equal to that of left heart failure.[11] In children, the etiologies of right ventricular failure often differ from etiologies seen in adults, and the percentage of right heart failure is relatively high with clinicians often underestimating its early stages. Patients with tetralogy of Fallot can experience isolated right ventricular failure if they are subjected to prolonged periods of pulmonary valve insufficiency (see Chapter 21). In addition, other patients (e.g., patients with congenitally corrected transposition of the great arteries) have a morphologic right ventricle as their systemic ventricle and are subject to potential deterioration of its function. Finally, some patients have single right ventricle anatomy (e.g., patients with hypoplastic left heart syndrome), and the right ventricle is subjected to increased pressure and volume workload (see Chapter 23). As in adults, the prognosis and therapies available in right heart failure are often determined largely by the etiology, and similar to the adult experience, biventricular failure usually carries a worse prognosis than right ventricular dysfunction alone.

Little is known about the right ventricle and its long-term fate in a variety of congenital heart defects. This chapter delineates the role of the right ventricle in children and young adults with heart failure and discusses the diagnosis and management of right ventricular dysfunction and failure in the context of congenital heart disease. Right ventricular failure in the clinical contexts of elevated pulmonary vascular resistance, acute respiratory distress syndrome, and sepsis is discussed elsewhere in this text (see Chapters 28 and 29).

DIFFERENCES BETWEEN THE RIGHT AND LEFT VENTRICLES

Embryology and Morphology

From an embryologic standpoint, the developments of the right ventricle and left ventricle are distinct and intricately interdependent. The embryonic heart is composed of mesodermal tissue that begins formation in week 3 of gestation. Around day 22 of gestation, the primary heart tube lengthens and begins to bend to the right, a process called *looping*; the ventricular loop forms with inlet and outlet portions.[12,13] The inlet portion eventually gives rise to the left ventricle; the right ventricle and outflow tracts are derived from the outlet portion. As the primary tube loops, it also forms inner and outer curvatures. Distinct portions of the outer curvature balloon out, forming the apical portions of both ventricles.[12] The trabeculations of these apical segments possess characteristic morphologies that allow the two developing ventricles to be identified as left or right by day 24 of gestation.[13]

At the same time that the apical segments of the future ventricles are ballooning out from the outer curvature, changes in the inner curvature facilitate the establishment of an inlet and outlet segment for each ventricle. The tricuspid valve and inlet portion of the right ventricle arise from the ventricular loop in an area called the *primary ring*.[14] The right ventricular outflow tract arises from the outlet portion of the primary heart tube, termed the *bulbus cordis*, after separating from the primitive aorta (division complete by 9 weeks gestation).[15-17] The muscular interventricular septum forms at the same time between the two ballooning apical segments.[12,14]

In utero, the right ventricle is the dominant ventricle and produces 66% of the cardiac output as a result of shunting across the foramen ovale and ductus arteriosus.[2] After birth, the pulmonary vascular resistance (PVR) decreases, and the foramen ovale and ductus arteriosus close. These changes equalize right-sided and left-sided cardiac outputs, and the low afterload against which the right ventricle pumps allows it to become a thin-walled, highly compliant structure.

Geometry and Shape

The left ventricle has a well-defined "prolate ellipsoid"[3,18] structure, which can readily be studied for precise calculations of volume and function, but the right ventricular geometry is not as easily characterized. Although its highly compliant nature is designed for sustained low-pressure perfusion, the right ventricular structure does change readily based on its loading conditions.[19] Even in the healthy heart, deriving a geometric formula for right ventricular volumetric calculations is difficult and imprecise. Also, there is greater variation in regional wall thickness in the right ventricle than the left ventricle,[20] further complicating mathematical evaluation. Various models have been used in the past, including tetrahedron[2] as well as hemielliptical[21,22] and ellipsoidal shell subtraction techniques (Fig. 16-1).[23-25] None of these geometric shapes yields as precise a correlation with autopsy specimens, however, as those performed on the left ventricle.

The right ventricle is composed of primarily two components: the sinus, which generates pressure during systole, and the conus, or infundibulum, which regulates this pressure.[11,18] The crista supraventricularis separates these two portions and is in continuity with the tricuspid valve, the right ventricular free wall, and intraventricular septum (IVS).[17] It is controversial whether the inlet portion of the right ventricle is separate from the sinus and should be considered a third

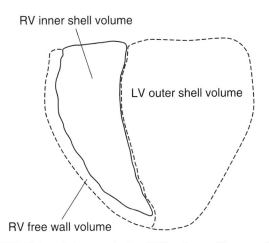

FIGURE 16-1 ■ Right ventricular (RV) volume. Diagram of the ellipsoidal shell subtraction technique of calculating RV volume. RV volume is represented by subtracting the left ventricular (LV) outer shell volume and the RV free wall volume from the total biventricular volume. (From Feneley MP, Elbeery JR, Gaynor JW, et al: Ellipsoidal shell subtraction model of right ventricular volume: Comparison with regional free wall dimensions as indexes of right ventricular function. Circ Res 1990;67:1427-1436.)

portion of the ventricle,[18] similar to the three regions seen in the left ventricle. The character of the apical trabeculations in the right ventricle morphologically distinguishes it from the left ventricle in that the trabeculations in the right ventricle are much more coarse. In patients with abnormal anatomy or single ventricles, the specific characteristics of the trabeculations, rather than spatial relationships, allow definitive identification of a right ventricle versus a left ventricle.[12]

Coronary Artery Perfusion

The coronary blood supply of the right ventricle also differs from that of the left ventricle. The right coronary artery (RCA) provides perfusion to the right ventricular free wall and the inferior one third of the IVS, and the left anterior descending branch of the left coronary artery provides flow to the superior two thirds of the IVS. Although the left coronary artery and its branches fill during diastole only, the RCA fills during systole and diastole under normal conditions. When afterload is increased, however, the RCA fills primarily during diastole in a manner similar to the left-sided coronary circulation. This "dual filling" of the RCA and continuous perfusion of the right ventricle is believed to account for the relatively minimal depression in right ventricular function observed with near-occlusion of the RCA in the absence of other hemodynamic disease.[2,4,11]

In animal models, near-total occlusion of the RCA in the absence of other stressors shows only minimal changes in overall systemic hemodynamics.[4] When stressors, such as increased afterload, are applied, however, increasing degrees of RCA obstruction cause an exaggerated response compared with that seen with isolated elevation of afterload.[4,26] In diseased states, RCA perfusion occurs predominantly during diastole. When right ventricular dysfunction reaches a level where systemic hemodynamics become altered and diastolic blood pressure begins to decrease, RCA perfusion decreases, leading to further deterioration of right ventricular function.[26,27] Figure 16-2 illustrates the effects on cardiac output, systemic pressures, and left and right ventricular diastolic pressures caused by changing right ventricular peak systolic pressures (with and without occluding the RCA). Further studies have shown that as RCA perfusion decreases, and dysfunction occurs, the heart's ability to compensate, even with assistance from inotropic agents to increase contractility, is impaired.[28,29]

Contraction and Myocardial Performance

The mechanism of contraction and function is complex in the right ventricle. Systole starts earlier and ends later than in the left ventricle, allowing a longer period for ventricular emptying.[25] The cardiac contraction mechanism for the right ventricle itself consists of three distinct phases that proceed from apex to cone in peristaltic waves. First, the spiral muscles contract; second, the right ventricular free wall moves inward toward the IVS;

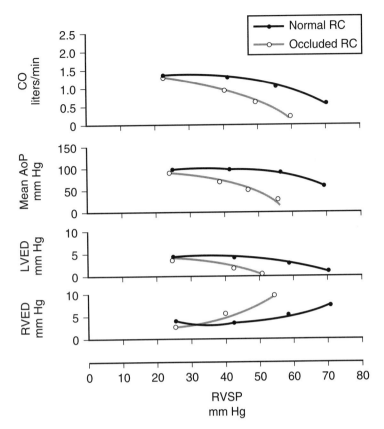

FIGURE 16-2 ■ Right ventricular hemodynamic profile in failure. Composite graphs of data on canine models relating cardiac output (CO), mean aortic pressure (AoP), left ventricular end-diastolic pressure (LVED), and right ventricular end-diastolic pressure (RVED) to right ventricular systolic pressure (RVSP) from states of control to just before total decompensation. (From Brooks H, Kirk ES, Vokonas PS, et al: Performance of the right ventricle under stress: Relation to right coronary flow. J Clin Invest 1971;50:2176-2183.)

and third, the left ventricle contracts, producing a "wringer"-type action that further aids in emptying the right ventricle.[2,11,30] Although these three phases exist universally in the contraction of the right ventricle, performance and efficiency of the right ventricle are influenced further by other factors.

Right ventricular performance is determined by intrinsic and extrinsic factors. The myocytes and the length of their stretch affect the contractility of the ventricle. The myofibrils in the right ventricle are histologically identical to the myofibrils in the left ventricle, indicating that the contractile differences between the two ventricles are influenced more by the different loading conditions, geometry, and outflow impedance than the intrinsic histology.

Among the extrinsic factors influencing right ventricular performance, changes in **afterload** have a major effect on short-term and long-term right ventricular function. As a thin-walled structure, the right ventricle is poorly able to compensate for increased pulmonary pressures and undergoes progressive dilation with increased myofibril stretch using the Frank-Starling mechanism to restore cardiac output. This dilation is in contrast to the left ventricle, where an increased afterload generally causes hypertrophy to maintain cardiac output. It has been shown that the right ventricular ejection fraction (RVEF) is at least twice as sensitive as the left ventricular ejection fraction (LVEF) to changes in afterload. Processes that increase pulmonary vascular

tone and pressure also lead to an increase in shearing stress on the endothelium of the pulmonary vasculature, leading to an imbalance of vasoactive mediators. Levels of nitric oxide (NO) and prostaglandin I_2 decrease with an increase in thromboxane A_2, leading to an increased contractile tone and an increased propensity for thrombus formation.[31] Overall, an acute increase in right-sided afterload typically is met with a dramatic decrease in RVEF.[32]

Preload, as determined by ventricular compliance and venous return, establishes myofiber length before contraction and plays an important role in right ventricular performance. Increased preload leads to increased myofibril stretch and increased contractility,[8] but chronic increase in preload also leads to dilation. The effect of changing preloads on right ventricular function is shown when examining normal respiratory variation in the right ventricle. With inspiration, there is decreased intrathoracic pressure leading to increased venous return and increased preload.[33] The increased preload causes an increased stroke volume, a prolonged ejection time, and an increase in contractility shown by increased peak E and A wave velocities and integrals. These changes in right heart physiology with respiration are more pronounced in diseased states. Patients who have undergone a Fontan-type operation no longer have a right ventricle in series with their circulation and have pulmonary blood flow via passive venous return so that they are extremely sensitive to respiratory effects.

Patients in whom the right ventricle is still in series, but in whom diastolic function is impaired, as seen in restrictive disease processes, also show exaggerated responses to changes in respiratory motions.[19] Finally, patients placed on mechanical ventilation exhibit abnormal right ventricular function caused by altered preload, afterload, and IVS motion.[2]

The geometry of the right ventricle affects contractility and efficacy. A higher percentage of segmental shortening occurs in the myocytes in the conus than in the midventricular area, influencing contractility.[34] The constraint from the pericardium and the function and position of the IVS modify the limits of right ventricular function. The pericardium is much less compliant than the myocardium, and even in healthy states, the pericardium limits cardiac dilation. In disease states, the constraints of the pericardium are more pronounced, and the combination of the pericardium and the IVS can effectively cause tamponade physiology on the right ventricle.

Although the RVEF is less than that of the LVEF, its end-diastolic volume is larger. The influence that the function and geometry of the left ventricle has on the performance of the right ventricle, termed **ventricular interdependence**, cannot be overstated. Under controlled states, the IVS bows into the right ventricular cavity, causing a cross section of the left ventricle to resemble a circle, while that of the right ventricle is crescentic in form. When right-sided pressures increase, the IVS shifts first to the midline, then bows into the left ventricle, causing an internal tamponade on the left ventricle with impairment of its function and systemic hemodynamic alterations.[2] The degree of distention of either ventricle affects the compliance and distensibility

of the other ventricle through the motion and position of the IVS.[33,35,36] All of these effects are more significant when the pericardium is intact.[2,11,19,33,37] Although the most obvious source of this ventricular interdependence is the shared septum, other factors, such as the pericardium and shared external muscle bundles, contribute to this interventricular cross-talk. In addition, the contraction of the right ventricle has little to no direct effect on the left ventricle, but contraction of the left ventricle generates a pressure waveform in the right ventricle that is nearly identical to the normal right ventricular systolic pressure waveform. It is believed that a part of the external mechanical work done on the right ventricle is derived from the contraction of shared muscle fibers.[19,35]

After examining the ranges of intrinsic and extrinsic factors that alter right ventricular function, clearly it is the summation of these factors that predicts how an individual would respond to acute and chronic changes. A decrease in myocyte contractility may be well compensated by altered loading conditions and not produce measurable changes in right ventricular function. Conversely, a patient with preserved myocardial contractility may fail under unfavorable loading conditions.

Pressure-Volume Flow Loop

Construction of pressure volume curves allows further understanding of right ventricular function (see Chapter 7). The left ventricle produces a square- or rectangular-shaped pressure-volume loop[38] designed to maximize work and cycle efficiency, whereas the right ventricular pressure-volume loop is triangular in shape (Fig. 16-3).[3,20,38] In the healthy right ventricle, there is little to no period of either isovolumic contraction

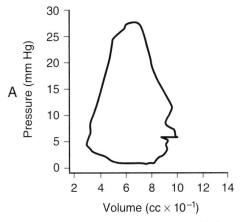
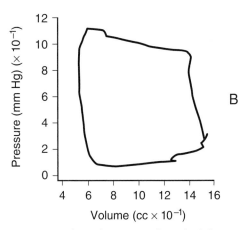

FIGURE 16-3 ■ **Normal right and left ventricular pressure volume loops. A** and **B,** The left ventricle **(B)** has a pressure volume loop that resembles a square with clear isovolumic contraction and relaxation phases, whereas the right ventricle **(A)** has a pressure volume loop that resembles a triangle without a distinct isovolumic contraction or relaxation phase. In processes of increased right ventricular afterload, however, the right ventricular pressure volume loop starts to resemble the left ventricular pressure volume loop. (From Redington AN, Gray HH, Hudson ME, et al: Characterisation of the normal right ventricular pressure-volume relation by biplane angiography and simultaneous micromanometer pressure measurements. Br Heart J 1988;59:23-30.)

or relaxation. Ejection from the ventricle begins during the pressure upstroke in the right ventricle, minimizing isovolumic contraction. Similarly, ejection continues after the ventricular pressure peaks and has begun to decline, with 60% of the stroke volume ejected after the peak systolic pressure.[38] This distinctive ventricular ejection, which continues with decline in right ventricular pressure and even after a negative pressure gradient exists between the right ventricle and the main pulmonary artery, is primarily due to inertia and the low impedance in the pulmonary vascular bed.[28]

The time between peak systolic pressure and the closure of the semilunar valve has been termed the **hangout interval**, and it has been the focus of considerable investigation. Although the hangout interval does not represent a precise physiologic event, it is a helpful concept to assess the opposition to flow or impedance in the pulmonary circulation. Its duration in the systemic circulation is generally less than 15 msec, but in the pulmonary circulation it can last 80 msec.[38,39] Clinically, this phenomenon can be observed by the delayed closure of the pulmonic valve (P_2) compared with the aortic valve (A_2) and the physiologic splitting of S_2. Any process that increases pulmonary resistance decreases this interval, and factors that decrease resistance (inspiration) increase the interval.[38-40] Pulmonary hypertension markedly decreases the interval, whereas pulmonary valve stenosis with post-stenotic dilation increases it, and S_2 is more widely split.[39]

Cycle efficiency relates the mechanical work done by a ventricle to the maximal work possible for a given change in pressure and volume. Because a square loop yields the maximal efficiency, the left ventricle is more mechanically efficient, but the right ventricle is more energy efficient. For a given stroke volume, the external mechanical stroke work done by the right ventricle can be 20% required by the left ventricle.[38] Because the myofibrils in the two ventricles are histologically similar, primarily the loading conditions determine the pressure and volume curves and their composite loop. As illustrated later, disease processes that alter normal right heart hemodynamics shift and distort the pressure volume loops.

EVALUATIONS OF STRUCTURE AND FUNCTION IN THE RIGHT VENTRICLE

Right ventricular failure can be detected on **clinical examination** via its cardiac and systemic manifestations. There may be a palpable heave felt best at the lower left sternal border secondary to right ventricular dilation. The underlying cardiac disease determines the presence and qualities of cardiac murmurs, and the intensity and split of S_2 help distinguish pulmonary hypertension (decreased split, loud P_2) from pulmonic stenosis with post-stenotic dilation (increased split,

softer P_2). Occasionally a dilated main pulmonary artery is palpable as a pulsatile structure during systole in the second right intercostal space. Systemically the most common signs of right heart failure in children are tachypnea and hepatomegaly, while altered laboratory values include elevated lactate (secondary to liver dysfunction). Increased right-sided pressures may be visible in the neck veins, and dependent peripheral edema occurs.

Aside from physical examination, accurate evaluation of the right ventricle is more difficult than evaluation of the left ventricle for several reasons, but it is crucial in the diagnosis and treatment of many types of cardiovascular diseases. Pressure measurements using direct access to pulmonary arteries and veins are more difficult and invasive than those for systemic arteries and veins. As mentioned earlier, the right ventricular geometry is far more complex than the left ventricular geometry, so right ventricular volumes are difficult to calculate via mathematical models. Finally, conventional thinking that the role of the right heart was believed to be less important than is realized today promulgated fewer studies of normal and abnormal values for pressures and volumes in the right heart compared with those of the left heart. Despite these barriers, accurate evaluation of the right ventricle can be accomplished via a variety of methods.

Right atrial, right ventricular, and pulmonary artery **pressure measurements** typically are performed using invasive monitoring catheters, such as central venous lines, Swan-Ganz catheters, and right heart cardiac catheterization lines. In a healthy patient, normal pressure measurements include mean right atrial pressures of 1 to 4 mm Hg, right ventricular pressures of 24 to 29/3 to 5 mm Hg, and pulmonary artery pressures of 20 to 22/7 to 10 mm Hg with mean pulmonary artery pressures of 11 to 12 mm Hg.[41] A diagnostic fluid challenge can increase right atrial pressure dramatically in the face of significant right ventricular dysfunction. Most authorities consider a right ventricular systolic pressure greater than 35 mm Hg pressure overload.[3] If the left atrial pressure also is measured, either directly or via a pulmonary artery wedge pressure, the PVR can be calculated and is typically 100 to 250 dynes/sec/cm[5] or 1.2 to 3 Wood units.[11,41] Mathematical models, such as Fourier transformations, can help evaluate pulmonary vascular mechanics, impedance, and right ventricular energetics and have been shown to be valid for evaluation of cardiopulmonary systems.[24,42]

Volumetric measurements of the right heart are accomplished by invasive and noninvasive methods. Besides its irregular geometry, the right ventricle is located retrosternally, making it difficult to image with modalities such as echocardiography (see Chapter 10).[43] Other methods, such as cardiac catheterization and radionuclide studies, are invasive so that establishing normal values on healthy individuals is difficult.

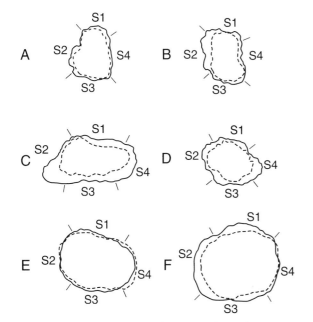

FIGURE 16-4 ■ **Evaluation of right ventricular indices.** Diagrams illustrate right ventricular end-diastolic and end-systolic sizes in normal and various disease states (long and short axis). **A** and **B,** Normal subjects. **C** and **D,** Patients with transposition of the great arteries after atrial switch operation, but no overt heart failure. **E** and **F,** Patients with transposition of the great arteries after atrial switch operation and with clinical heart failure. (From Trowitzsch E, Colan SD, Sanders SP: Global and regional right ventricular function in normal infants and infants with transposition of the great arteries after Senning operation. Circulation 1985;72:1008-1014.)

Over time, several well-accepted imaging and mathematical methods have been derived to evaluate right ventricular volumes and function (Fig. 16-4). Most frequently, Simpson's rule is used to calculate volume by dividing a structure (the right ventricle) into a series of slices, each of which is measured for cross-sectional area. This method has been shown to have good correlation among various imaging modalities and postmortem specimens in animals and humans.[38,44] Right ventricular end-diastolic volumes (RVEDV) in healthy individuals are 62 to 78 mL/m², and right ventricular end-systolic volumes (RVESV) are 21 to 30 mL/m², yielding stroke volumes of 39 to 48 mL/m² and RVEF 51% to 70% (typically slightly lower than the LVEF owing to the larger RVEDV).[28,38,44,45] RVEF is highly influenced by loading conditions and its dynamic surroundings (respiratory variations) so that an individual value of RVEF can be difficult to interpret.

Chest radiographs tend to be of minimal diagnostic value at discerning specifics about the right heart other than gross dilation and presence of normal, increased, or decreased pulmonary vasculature. **ECG** yields slightly more information by showing the conducting axis of the heart and evidence of right atrial or right ventricular dilation and hypertrophy. The duration and dispersion of the QRS complex have been shown to correlate with RVEDV and right ventricular mass in

some disease processes (e.g., tetralogy of Fallot). In these patients, prolonged QRS duration (>180 msec) or increased dispersion also has been shown to correlate with an increased risk of malignant tachyarrhythmias.[46-50] Overall, plain film radiographs and ECGs are used as screening rather than diagnostic tools for right heart disease.

Echocardiography can provide noninvasive, highly accurate information on the right heart. Two-dimensional echocardiography allows visualization of the right atrium, right ventricle, and main and segmental pulmonary arteries. Doppler echocardiography further allows quantification of flow velocities through vessels and valves, and calculations of pressures can be made.[11,48,51,52] As a result of the RVEF characteristics and influence by the respiratory cycle, Doppler investigations of the tricuspid valve (specifically the transtricuspid flow for early-to-late diastolic filling ratio) to assess right ventricular diastolic function is tedious at best and may be inaccurate. Subsegmental analysis of wall motion helps assess global and regional functions.[43] New techniques, such as integrated backscatter analysis, help evaluate structural composition (collagen content and myofiber disarray) and intrinsic contractility of the right ventricular myocardium.[53] Three-dimensional echocardiography may improve diagnostic capabilities because it does not require geometric assumptions for volume calculations and can provide real-time evaluation of the right heart.[54] Real-time three-dimensional stress echocardiography has been used in adults to evaluate left ventricular function and volumes, but so far few, if any, studies have examined its role in pediatrics.[55]

MRI and **high-resolution CT** are emerging rapidly as superior diagnostic options for evaluation of the right ventricle (see Chapter 11). MRI currently offers superior anatomic and functional details without exposure to radiation, but the speed and availability of CT render it a promising alternative modality in the future. MRI has become the noninvasive diagnostic method of choice for defining right ventricular anatomy and function parameters, such as right ventricular mass, wall thickness, and ejection fraction.[52] Similar to three-dimensional echocardiography, MRI provides information without making geometric assumptions so that volume, cardiac output, ejection fraction, and wall thickness all can be calculated.[34,44,56,57] Spatial relationships also can be precisely defined, including intracardiac and vascular stenoses or dilations, regional wall motion, and soft tissue composition. Evaluation of MRI data can be time-consuming and often involves the operator tracing the exact endocardial borders so as not to include trabeculae or papillary muscles, but the results have proved to be accurate and reproducible over multiple studies.[34,44,48,52,57]

Nuclear scans, including the first-pass technique and equilibrium gated pool scans, have been used since the 1920s[58]; with the increasing quality of echocardiography and growing use of MRI, however, nuclear studies now

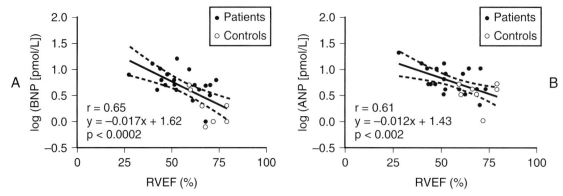

FIGURE 16-5 ■ **Natriuretic peptides as biomarkers for right ventricular failure.** Levels of B-type natriuretic peptide (BNP) and atrial natriuretic peptide (ANP) correlate with right ventricular ejection fraction (RVEF). The solid lines delineate the linear regression, and the dotted lines are 95% confidence intervals of the regression line. (From Tulevski I, Dodge-Khatami A, Groenink M, et al: Right ventricular function in congenital cardiac disease: Noninvasive quantitative parameters for clinical follow-up. Cardiol Young 2003;13:397-403.)

are used less frequently. The scans can be used to define anatomy and function and are not dependent on geometric assumptions for calculations.[44,58] All nuclear medicine studies involve exposure to radioactive agents, however. In pediatrics, the lower blood volumes produce lower count rates, and adjacent structures frequently overlap, making interpretation more difficult. Because the data are averaged over multiple cardiac cycles, simultaneous pressure measurements are not possible,[38] limiting the applications of the information.

Cardiac catheterization is the gold standard for evaluation of pressure and volume measurements of the right ventricle, but its invasive nature and exposure to radiation and contrast agents limit the frequency with which it can be performed. In general, angiography tends to overestimate right ventricular volumes compared with cadaver specimens because of the inclusion of trabeculae and papillary muscles, but good correlation has been shown.[38,44] Thermodilution catheters also have been shown to measure rates of flow accurately, but they tend to be inaccurate at measuring volumes in pressure overloaded right ventricles.[59] Angiographic pressure and volumetric data allow generation of pressure-volume loops for the right ventricle, as discussed earlier, which has aided greatly in understanding of the function of the right ventricle in healthy and diseased states.

In addition to imaging modalities, several **biochemical markers** have been found to correlate with cardiac function and failure, specifically atrial and brain natriuretic peptides (see Chapter 6). Atrial natriuretic peptide has strong diuretic and systemic vasorelaxant effects, in addition to inhibiting the renin-angiotensin-aldosterone system and the sympathetic nervous system. Secretion occurs primarily in the atria under physiologic conditions, but occurs in the atria and ventricles at significantly higher levels in congestive heart failure.[60] Atrial natriuretic peptide secretion begins

in utero when the apical left ventricle balloons out from the outer curvature, allowing the cells to be distinguished from primary myocardium.[12] B-type natriuretic peptide is secreted primarily from the ventricles in physiologic and diseased states, but at much higher levels when the heart is failing. RVEF has been shown to correlate inversely with serum levels of both natriuretic peptides, which can be measured using monoclonal antibodies and radioimmunoassays.[48,60,61] Following of biochemical markers such as atrial and B-type natriuretic peptides serially may allow clinicians to monitor therapy and recovery from heart failure accurately, but further studies establishing criteria still are needed (Fig. 16-5).

MECHANISMS OF RIGHT VENTRICULAR FAILURE

Failure of the right ventricle occurs secondary to volume or pressure overload. In pediatric patients, these conditions occur most commonly as a result of congenital heart disease.

Volume Overload Lesions

Volume overload is caused most often by either uncorrected congenital heart disease, such as an **atrial septal defect** or **tricuspid regurgitation** (often occurring with Ebstein anomaly), or after corrective surgery for congenital heart disease, as in the case of a child with **repaired tetralogy of Fallot** and **pulmonary insufficiency**.[62-64] The common underlying element among these lesions is the presence of increased blood flow into the right ventricle, leading to progressive dilation of the right ventricle. Although dilation improves cardiac output by shifting the right ventricular function along a Starling curve, there are limitations to this compensatory mechanism. Additionally, many of these conditions lead to arrhythmias, from dilation of the right atrium with atrial arrhythmias (atrial septal defect), accessory pathways with supraventricular tachyarrhythmias (Ebstein anomaly),[65] or malignant ventricular tachyarrhythmias (repaired tetralogy of Fallot).[46-50]

Pressure Overload Lesions

Many congenital heart lesions also may lead to pressure overload on the right ventricle before and after surgical correction. As mentioned before, the thin-walled, highly compliant right ventricle is extremely sensitive to changes in afterload, and the pressure-overloaded ventricle dramatically changes its hemodynamics in the acute and chronic settings. The two most common scenarios in which pressure overload occurs are right ventricular outflow tract obstruction, such as that seen in tetralogy of Fallot, or lesions that leave the right ventricle as the systemic ventricle, such as transposition of the great arteries after an atrial switch operation or congenitally corrected transposition of the great arteries (see Chapter 27). The single right ventricle as seen in hypoplastic left heart syndrome is discussed in Chapter 23.

In **tetralogy of Fallot**, the right ventricle is subjected to pressure overload and hypoxia from birth, which leads to progressive hypertrophy, fibrosis, and myofibrillar disorganization. Even after surgical correction, a degree of right ventricular outflow obstruction often is encountered, sometimes with concomitant pulmonary insufficiency, leading to volume overload as well.[48,62,63,66] In patients with repaired tetralogy of Fallot, right ventricular systolic function can be abnormal, with decreased right ventricular stroke volumes, RVEF, and right ventricular filling during exercise or dobutamine stress.[48,67] Many patients develop aneurysms or akinetic areas in the right ventricular outflow tract, which have been shown to be independent risk factors for right ventricular dilation and hypertrophy, with a negative effect on RVEF.[63] Surgical scarring and fibrosis add to the inherently abnormal myocardium, leading to impaired diastolic function and an increased incidence of arrhythmias.[64,66]

Patients with transposition of the great arteries who have undergone an **atrial switch operation** (Senning or Mustard) have a right ventricle that is subjected to a different type of pressure overload. In these children, the right ventricle has become the systemic ventricle and now is pumping against systemic arterial pressures. Although fractional shortening can be preserved or slightly decreased, RVEDV and RVESV are greater than in controls.[43,68] The right ventricular geometry becomes round, and the IVS bows toward the left ventricle.[68] Function is impaired at times by frequent arrhythmias (reports range from 13% to 100% of patients with rhythm disturbances after an atrial switch operation) secondary to chamber dilation, suture lines, and occasional direct damage to the sinoatrial node intraoperatively.[48,51,69,70] Over time, the tricuspid valve becomes incompetent when subjected to systemic pressures,

leading to volume overload in addition to the preexisting pressure overload.

Similarly, patients who have **congenitally corrected transposition of the great arteries** (atrioventricular and ventriculoarterial discordance) have a systemic right ventricle, with similar problems as patients with transposition of the great arteries after an atrial switch operation. Congenitally corrected transposition of the great arteries rarely occurs without other hemodynamically significant anomalies, and these other cardiac abnormalities are believed to contribute to the long-term morbidity and mortality.[45] Late mortality after classic repairs for congenitally corrected transposition of the great arteries is high in most studies because of the inferior capacity of the right ventricle and the tricuspid valve to function as the systemic ventricle.[71,72] Other groups have shown adequate function of the right ventricle, however, as a systemic ventricle in long-term studies.[45] The double-switch procedure allows the left ventricle to be brought into series as the systemic ventricle, but long-term follow-up is not yet available for this repair. Regardless of the type of surgery, the risk for arrhythmias is high in these patients, with many developing complete heart block secondary to abnormal position and fibrosis through the atrioventricular node (2% per year) and 48% requiring pacemaker placement.[48,51,72,73]

A large body of literature indicates that a left ventricle is superior to a right ventricle as the systemic ventricle, particularly when atrioventricular valve incompetence develops.[73-75] The results of stress testing on the right ventricle as a systemic ventricle are mixed. Patients with transposition of the great arteries tend to have decreased exercise tolerance with impaired diastolic filling, heart rate response, and systolic function.[76] Tulevski and colleagues found that patients with transposition of the great arteries who had undergone an atrial switch procedure had decreased right ventricular filling, decreased RVESV and RVEDV, and decreased right ventricular stroke volume in response to dobutamine stress.[77] Patients with congenitally corrected transposition of the great arteries exhibited more normal responses and augmentation of volumes when stressed with dobutamine, but still exhibited decreased maximal heart rates.[48,73,76,77]

One final mechanism of altered right ventricular function occurs in patients placed on a **left ventricular assist device**. In adult studies, 20% of patients placed on a left ventricular assist device have right ventricular failure, and the mechanism for depressed right ventricular function is multifactorial. When a patient is placed on a left ventricular assist device, the left heart is unloaded, causing a shift of blood volume from the pulmonary to the systemic circulation, increasing the right ventricular preload. Unloading the left ventricle causes a decrease in the afterload against which the right ventricular contracts, which increases right ventricular function.

With an unloaded left ventricle, however, the IVS shifts to the left, altering the volume and geometry of the right ventricle. This shift of the IVS causes decreased compliance and contraction of the right ventricle. In healthy hearts, this decreased contractility is generally well tolerated with maintenance of the cardiac output. Patients with underlying right ventricular dysfunction may experience right-sided failure, however, as a result of these changes. Placing a patient on a left ventricular assist device for left heart failure may unmask biventricular failure. Right heart function always must be followed closely in these patients, particularly during the initial time on mechanical support.[11,78]

Regardless of whether volume, pressure, or combined overload is the cause of right ventricular failure, decreased coronary perfusion diminishes the compensatory mechanisms of the ventricle.[4,26] Animal studies have shown that occlusion of the RCA with normal pulmonary vasculature caused a decrease in contractility, but no change in cardiac output. Occlusion of the RCA in the presence of progressive pulmonary artery obstruction caused a greater increase in right-sided pressures and a decrease in cardiac output than a similar increase in pulmonary pressure with intact coronary perfusion. As obstruction increased, systemic decompensation occurred, and this threshold was lower in animals with impaired coronary perfusion. Additionally, in the presence of above-normal levels of RCA perfusion, this threshold was higher than in controls, indicating that hyperperfusion helps to improve right ventricular function and cardiac performance.[4] A vicious cycle can occur as right ventricular failure begins, wherein decreasing right ventricular function causes a decrease in systemic arterial pressure. Because the perfusion of the RCA occurs primarily during diastole in diseased states, this decreased systemic pressure leads to decreased perfusion, which causes worsening right heart failure.[26,27]

Pressure-Volume Relationship in Right Ventricular Dysfunction

When subjected to volume overload, the RVESV and RVEDV increase, preserving cardiac output with a decrease in RVEF.[44,62,63] Right ventricular mass also tends to increase over time, which may help to maintain low wall stress.[50] The pressure-volume loop for the right ventricle maintains its geometric configuration, but shifts to the right along the volumetric axis (Fig. 16-6, left column). Different congenital heart disease lesions produce small differences in the pressure volume loops, but the relative lack of isovolumic contraction and relaxation remain.[3,37] Chronic changes in right ventricular volume overload are tolerated better than acute alterations, and the surrounding structures (pericardium and left ventricle) along with intrinsic factors, such as myocardial disease, play important roles in how quickly a change in preload would alter function.[19] In chronic

right ventricular volume overload, the right ventricular end-diastolic pressure may not be elevated despite a relatively large increase in RVEDV.

Patients with congenital heart disease causing pressure overload on the right ventricle show several important changes in their pressure volume relationships. In the acute setting, RVESV is increased, while RVEDV remains the same, decreasing stroke volume and cardiac output.[26,32] Over time, the right ventricle undergoes hypertrophy and dilation to increase RVEDV and restore cardiac output. Although the exact nature of the pressure overload does affect the relationships, the periods of isovolumic contraction and relaxation become more prominent regardless of whether the obstruction is subpulmonic, valvar, or supravalvar (pulmonary vascular bed) in origin.[3,32] Ejection still may occur during pressure increase in the ventricle, but reduces to less than 5% of total stroke volume during the pressure decline, essentially eliminating the hangout interval. In these right ventricular pressure overload lesions, the overall geometry of the pressure volume loop of the right ventricle resembles that of the normal left ventricle (Fig. 16-6, middle column), and cycle efficiency is higher than in the normal right ventricle.[3] In the face of increased afterload, the right ventricular stroke work can increase dramatically for extended periods (years), showing a contractile reserve not possible in the normal left ventricle.[19]

Patients with transposition of the great arteries who have undergone an atrial switch operation have a morphologic left ventricle ejecting against the pulmonary circulation. It also has been shown that the pressure-volume loop for the left ventricle in this lesion closely resembles a normal right ventricular pressure-volume relationship (Fig. 16-6, right column).[3] These loops provide further proof that the intrinsic properties of the two ventricles are nearly identical, but the loading conditions and outflow impedance largely determine their function and efficiency.

ACUTE AND LONG-TERM TREATMENT OF RIGHT VENTRICULAR FAILURE

Therapeutic modalities for right heart failure include volume management, pharmacologic agents, mechanical support, and palliative and corrective surgeries. Most studies have focused on short-term or intermediate-term results, so the long-term efficacy of some agents discussed here are still unknown. In addition, some of the mechanisms used in treating left heart failure may or may not pertain to right heart disease because there are distinct differences between the two ventricles and the relevant vascular systems. The right heart and its failure in pulmonary hypertension and its effects secondary to mechanical ventilation are discussed further in Chapter 28.

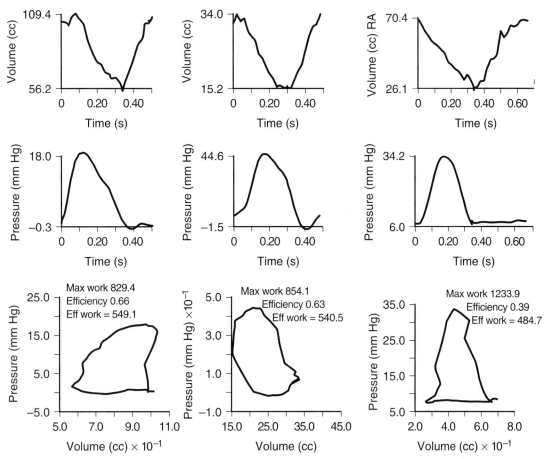

FIGURE 16-6 ■ **Ventricular pressure-volume loops in congenital heart disease.** In the left column, right ventricular volume, pressure, and pressure-volume loop from a patient with a large atrial septal defect are shown. Although the morphology of the curve remains similar to a normal right ventricle, the volumes are increased. In the middle column, the right ventricular pressure-volume loop in a patient with tetralogy of Fallot is shown. There is a period of isovolumic contraction, causing the loop to resemble more closely that of the normal left ventricle. In the column on the right, a left ventricular pressure volume loop in a patient with transposition of the great arteries after a Mustard procedure is shown. The loop shows similar morphology to that of a normal right ventricular pressure-volume relationship. Max, maximum; Eff, effective. (From Redington AN, Rigby ML, Shinebourne EA, et al: Changes in the pressure-volume relation of the right ventricle when its loading conditions are modified. Br Heart J 1990;63:45-49.)

Preload and Volume

Volume status, along with ventricular compliance, determines preload and can be manipulated to augment right ventricular function. In patients with normal PVR, volume expansion can increase preload to maximize stretch and contractility, increasing cardiac output.[9] If PVR is increased, volume expansion may result in an increase in pulmonary pressure, afterload, wall stress, myocardial oxygen requirement, and tricuspid regurgitation, all of which are detrimental to right ventricular function. Although children with volume overload can be treated judiciously with diuretics to improve the above-mentioned factors, this volume contraction may result in a shift to a lower contractile state along the Starling curve.

Inotropic Agents

Inotropic agents help to increase myocardial contractility and are used in short-term therapy. These agents often are given with diuretics to allow relief of congestion and decrease wall stress and oxygen demand, but maintain contractility.[2,8,11] β-**Adrenergic agonists** (e.g., dopamine, dobutamine, epinephrine) increase production of cyclic AMP (cAMP), whereas **phosphodiesterase inhibitors** (e.g., milrinone, amrinone) inhibit breakdown of cAMP; both lead to increased calcium concentrations in the myocardial cells (see Chapters 33 and 34).[11,79] Various agents have been shown to improve preload recruitable stroke work, decrease PVR, and improve active relaxation of the right ventricle in animal models.[24,80] The increased contractility increases myocardial oxygen demand[17,81] and anaerobic metabolism, however, leading to lactic acidosis. Over time, the myocardium becomes desensitized to the elevated calcium levels, and contractility again decreases. Increasing intracellular calcium stores also predispose the myocardium to arrhythmias secondary to calcium release.[80] Lastly, the beneficial effects of inotropic agents on contractility are blunted in diseased or damaged hearts, further limiting the number of patients who benefit from inotropic therapy.[29] Some of the inotropes also function as vasoconstrictors by stimulating α-receptors in the systemic and pulmonary arterial systems, which results in mixed effects on right ventricular function. Vasoconstriction causes an increase in afterload, but helps improve coronary perfusion by increasing aortic diastolic pressures. The balance of these two factors determines whether right ventricular function would be helped or hindered by vasoconstrictors.[2,11]

Thyroxine and **glucagon** have been shown to increase right ventricular function via their positive inotropic and chronotropic effects.[17] Both compounds cause an increase in cAMP levels leading to increased contractility, and triiodothyronine actively binds to myocyte nuclei and improves relaxation via Na+,K+-ATPase channels.[17,82,83] Although experience with these medications is small, one randomized adult study found improved exercise tolerance and hemodynamics on levothyroxine compared with placebo in patients with dilated cardiomyopathy.[84]

One alternative to inotropic agents is levosimendan, a **calcium-sensitizing agent**. Levosimendan binds to troponin C and increases myocardial calcium sensitivity during systole (without effects on relaxation kinetics), increasing contractility without increasing cAMP or calcium concentrations (see Chapter 38). Additionally, it opens potassium-dependent ATP channels and decreases sensitivity to calcium in the pulmonary vasculature, leading to pulmonary vasodilation.[80] Levosimendan also has been shown to have beneficial short-term effects in patients with decompensated left ventricular failure[79] and has been shown to increase right ventricular contractility and possibly to decrease PVR in animal models.[80,85] Human trials evaluating levosimendan and its effects on right heart function are still lacking, however.

Vasodilating Agents

When PVR is elevated, vasodilator therapy helps the failing right ventricle by decreasing afterload. A reduced afterload also allows a decline in RVEDV, producing decreased wall tension and myocardial oxygen requirement. The dilated pulmonary vasculature also increases left ventricular preload, which increases mean arterial pressure and RCA perfusion pressure. Systemic and selective pulmonary vasodilators are available in the treatment of right ventricular failure.

Systemic vasodilators (e.g., nitroglycerin, nitroprusside, hydralazine) effectively decrease pulmonary vascular tone, but have several detrimental side effects (see Chapter 35). Systemic vasodilation occurs with decreased aortic diastolic pressures, leading to decreased RCA perfusion, worsening ischemia, and inhibited compensatory mechanisms. Pulmonary vasodilation also counteracts hypoxic vasoconstriction in the lungs, worsening ventilation-perfusion mismatch, and leads to systemic desaturation.

Calcium channel blockers have been shown to lower pulmonary arterial pressures and PVR effectively in short-term and long-term studies of patients with pulmonary hypertension. There is a significant reduction in mortality rate and improvement in symptoms in patients who respond to calcium channel blockers.[86] Similar to other nonspecific vasodilators, systemic hypotension often limits use of calcium channel blockers.

Selective pulmonary vasodilators are advantageous in that they decrease right ventricular afterload without causing systemic hypotension. At present, a variety of agents are approved for use in the United States, including inhaled NO, various forms of prostacyclin (intravenous, inhaled, and subcutaneous), and oral endothelin-1 blockers.[87]

Inhaled NO was the first approved selective pulmonary vasodilator and was formerly known as endothelium-derived relaxing factor. In a healthy person, NO is released continuously from the pulmonary endothelium and mediates vasodilation through increasing cyclic GMP levels[88] and interactions with acetylcholine and substance P. Basal endothelial release of NO is believed to vary in the different vascular systems (much lower in the coronary bed), contributing to the low resting pulmonary vascular tone. Injury to the endothelium interrupts the continual release and contributes to the development of increasing PVR.[89] Inhaled NO has been shown to cause pulmonary vasodilation,[88] and because it binds quickly to plasma proteins and hemoglobin to form methemoglobin, it does not result in systemic vasodilation.[90-92] Inhaled NO has been shown to be effective at decreasing pulmonary artery pressures in adult and pediatric patients,[88,90,92] with an increased cardiac output also observed in some studies.[90] Therapy can be monitored using exhaled levels of NO and nitric dioxide (should be <5 ppm) and methemoglobin levels (should be <5%).[91] There has been no proven survival benefit to inhaled NO, and rebound hypertension can occur, so patients must be weaned off of therapy in a judicious fashion.[88,90]

Prostacyclin, also known as prostaglandin I_2, has beneficial effects on PVR in intravenous, inhaled, and subcutaneous forms. It is synthesized in pulmonary endothelial cells, acting as a pulmonary smooth muscle vasorelaxant and stimulating release of NO.[93-95] Additionally, prostacyclin is a potent platelet aggregation inhibitor,[94-97] and it serves as a physiologic antagonist to thromboxane A_2, known to play an important proaggregatory role in pulmonary vascular damage.[31,98] One disadvantage of prostacyclin therapy is that its short half-life makes it difficult to monitor levels, and its stable carbacyclin derivative must be followed. Additionally, the most reliable method of monitoring therapy is through urinary excretion of its metabolites (not widely available).[31]

Intravenous prostacyclin (epoprostenol) has been used for long-term therapy in pulmonary hypertension since 1984.[99] In many patients, epoprostenol reduces pulmonary artery pressures and PVR, improves exercise capacity and quality of life, and in some series showed a survival benefit as well.[94,95,100] Additionally, long-term studies show benefit beyond that produced through isolated pulmonary vasodilation, indicating that part of epoprostenol's benefit also is derived from the antithrombotic and antiproliferative effects of prostacyclin and may reverse some of the underlying disease process.[87,97] Most studies have examined epoprostenol's role in treating patients with primary pulmonary hypertension, but several groups have examined its role in treating patients with congenital heart disease leading to pulmonary hypertension, with similar results.[101] Side effects result from systemic vasodilation and may include headache, facial flushing, abdominal cramping, diarrhea, nausea, jaw pain, and thrombocytopenia.[87,96,100,102] Epoprostenol requires an indwelling catheter, with risks of line infections and sepsis. Tolerance has been reported, and rebound pulmonary hypertension occurs quickly because of the short half-life (1 to 2 minutes) if the continuous infusion is interrupted.[87]

Iloprost, a stable prostacyclin analogue that can be administered in inhaled form, has several advantages over epoprostenol. Thus far, neither tolerance nor rebound pulmonary hypertension has been reported.[93,103,104] The compound undergoes rapid spontaneous hydrolysis, so systemic side effects are less common, but may include headache, flushing, jaw pain, and cough.[98,104] Inhaled prostacyclin is less expensive, more potent, and easier to administer than inhaled NO.[103,105] Results of clinical trials with iloprost have been mixed, however. Hoeper and coworkers[104] showed improvements in symptoms, cardiopulmonary hemodynamics, and exercise capacity, but Machherndl and colleagues[98] found no hemodynamic or symptomatic improvements. No survival benefits have been shown so far.[104,105] Because some of epoprostenol's efficacy is derived from its antithrombotic and antiproliferative effects, it is not known if iloprost achieves sufficient plasma levels to have similar effects.[104] Studies on its effects in children with right heart failure resulting from congenital heart disease are still needed.

Treprostinil is another prostacyclin analogue that has a longer half-life than the other preparations (3 hours),[87] allowing administration via a continuous subcutaneous infusion. Studies have shown improvements in exercise capacity, symptoms, and cardiopulmonary hemodynamics

in adult patients.[106] Side effects are similar to other prostacyclin medications, with the addition of gastrointestinal hemorrhages and pain at the infusion site, prompting many patients to discontinue therapy.[87,96,106] At present, there have been no studies showing improved survival with treprostinil.

Endothelin has been shown to be a potent pulmonary vasoconstrictor, it enhances smooth muscle cell proliferation, and plasma levels correlate with pulmonary arterial pressures and PVR.[107-113] High concentrations of endothelin have been measured in serum and in the lungs of adult and pediatric patients with elevated pulmonary pressures.[113] Blockade of endothelin receptors with the oral medication bosentan, a **nonselective ET$_{A/B}$ blocker**, has been shown to decrease inflammation, prevent pulmonary fibrosis, and decrease pulmonary arterial pressures in animal models.[111,114] Several short-term studies involving pediatric[108,115] and adult[107,110,116] patients with severe pulmonary hypertension (caused by primary pulmonary hypertension, scleroderma, or congenital heart disease) have shown beneficial effects on cardiopulmonary hemodynamics (increased cardiac output, stroke volume, and cardiac index with decreased PVR and pulmonary artery pressures). Adult studies also have shown improvement in exercise capacity and a delay in time to clinical worsening, which have not been shown in pediatric patients.[107,110]

A comparison study reviewed several studies on epoprostenol, treprostinil, and bosentan and concluded that treatment with bosentan was more cost-effective than the other medications.[117] Because ET$_B$ receptors are believed to mediate pulmonary vasodilation, sitaxsentan (a selective ET$_A$ blocker) may exert beneficial effects without hindering vasodilation and has been shown to improve several hemodynamic parameters in short-term studies.[109] Side effects from endothelin blockers are rare, but include flushing, headaches, and increases in hepatic transaminases, which are dose dependent and reversible on discontinuation of the medications.[87,102,107,108,110,115]

Invasive Therapies

Besides optimizing pressure and volume relationships in the right heart, therapy for right ventricular failure also should focus on maintenance of normal conduction. The sinus node artery is a branch off the RCA before the ventricular branches,[4] so any process impairing RCA filling may lead to arrhythmias. Atrial and ventricular dysrhythmias lead to decreased function, and several causes of right ventricular pressure and volume overload (such as those seen with tetralogy of Fallot) have been associated with increased incidences of malignant tachyarrhythmias and sudden cardiac death.[47] All arrhythmias should be treated aggressively to optimize function. Additionally, **electrical resynchronization** via atrioventricular pacing in right heart failure has been shown to increase cardiac output and pressure over time in the acute setting and may represent a novel therapy in the chronic setting as well.[118]

For some patients, pharmacologic therapy is insufficient to maintain adequate right ventricular function, and more invasive treatment is necessary. In patients with acute right heart failure, **mechanical circulatory support** can allow the right ventricle to rest and recover from the insult or alternatively provide a bridge to transplantation, especially if biventricular dysfunction is present (see Chapters 45-47). Extracorporeal membrane oxygenation can be used for full cardiopulmonary support in infants and children.[119,120] Mechanical assist devices, such as pulmonary artery balloon counterpulsation[121] and right ventricular assist devices, have been used in adults. Thus far, experience in pediatric patients involves primarily short-term devices and either biventricular[122] or left ventricular support.[119,120] As technology advances, the size and availability of these devices are becoming less prohibitive to pediatric use, and experience with right heart mechanical assistance is forthcoming.

Surgical strategies, such as correction of underlying anatomic abnormalities, through either surgery or interventional cardiac catheterization, also are necessary in many patients with right heart failure when the initial hemodynamic abnormalities have been stabilized. The timing of these interventions is paramount in caring for children with congenital heart disease. Relief of pressure obstruction or sources of volume overload can lead to significant improvements in pressure volume relationships, symptoms, and pulmonary disease. In some patients, the underlying anatomy may not be amenable to complete correction, and palliative surgical measures can be an alternative strategy. Establishing a bidirectional cavopulmonary anastomosis from the superior vena cava to the right pulmonary artery allows partial volume decompression of the right heart and often significant improvement of right ventricular hemodynamics; this can be an element of a surgical strategy for right ventricular failure. In addition, banding of the pulmonary artery in certain patients with a failing systemic right ventricle after the atrial switch operation for transposition of the great arteries can improve left ventricular function and tricuspid valve incompetence.

CURRENT STATUS AND FUTURE TRENDS

As increasing numbers of children survive cardiac surgeries, the fate of the right ventricle in certain patient subpopulations becomes more important. Although its complex geometry and physiology render the right ventricle more difficult to study than the left ventricle, cardiologists need to continue to be vigilant of right ventricular dysfunction during its early decompensation. Noninvasive modalities, such as three-dimensional echocardiography and MRI, can be useful in serial evaluations of right ventricular function, especially if complemented by biomarkers, such as B-type natriuretic peptide. In addition, innovative technology still needs to be explored for long-term continual surveillance of right ventricular function.[123]

Although selective pulmonary vasodilators have allowed some improvements in the care of pediatric patients with right ventricular dysfunction, long-term studies of pharmacologic agents that would improve right ventricular function on a sustained basis are still needed. Surgery to overcome right ventricular failure in older children and young adolescents with previously palliative or repaired congenital heart disease is still a challenge.[124] Finally, as mechanical circulatory support devices become smaller and more commercially available, their use to support the right ventricle can allow a bridge to transplantation or recovery.[125]

Key Concepts

■ The right ventricle has been perceived as a relatively passive conduit between the two circulations, but is in fact a complex pump with its unique physiology of ejection, interaction with its adjacent left ventricle, influence by respirations, and myriad of congenital anomalies.

■ The left ventricle has a well-defined "prolate ellipsoid" structure, which can readily be studied for precise calculations of volume and function, but the right ventricular geometry is not as easily characterized. Although its highly compliant nature is designed for sustained low-pressure perfusion, the right ventricular structure does change readily based on its loading conditions.

■ Although the left coronary artery and its branches fill during diastole only, the RCA fills during systole and diastole under normal conditions. When afterload is increased, however, the RCA fills primarily during diastole in a manner similar to the left-sided coronary circulation.

■ The cardiac contraction mechanism for the right ventricle itself consists of three distinct phases that proceed from apex to cone in peristaltic waves. First, the spiral muscles contract; second, the right ventricular free wall moves inward toward the IVS; and third, the left ventricle contracts, producing a "wringer"-type action that further aids in emptying the right ventricle.

■ The myofibrils in the right ventricle are histologically identical to the myofibrils in the left ventricle, indicating that the contractile differences between the two ventricles are influenced more by the different loading conditions, geometry, and outflow impedance than the intrinsic histology.

■ Among the extrinsic factors influencing right ventricular performance, changes in afterload have a major effect on short-term and long-term right ventricular function.

As a thin-walled structure, the right ventricle is poorly able to compensate for increased pulmonary pressures and undergoes progressive dilation with increased myofibril stretch using the Frank-Starling mechanism to restore cardiac output. This dilation is in contrast to the left ventricle, where an increased afterload generally causes hypertrophy to maintain cardiac output.

■ Under controlled states, the IVS bows into the right ventricular cavity, causing a cross section of the left ventricle to resemble a circle, whereas that of the right ventricle is crescentic in form. When right-sided pressures increase, the IVS shifts first to the midline, then bows into the left ventricle, causing an internal tamponade on the left ventricle with impairment of its function and systemic hemodynamic alterations.

■ Although the most obvious source of this ventricular interdependence is the shared septum, other factors, such as the pericardium and shared external muscle bundles, contribute to this interventricular cross-talk.

■ The left ventricle produces a square- or rectangular-shaped pressure volume loop designed to maximize work and cycle efficiency, whereas the right ventricular pressure volume loop is triangular in shape. In the healthy right ventricle, there is little to no period of either isovolumic contraction or relaxation.

■ This distinctive ventricular ejection, which continues with decline in right ventricular pressure and even after a negative pressure gradient exists between the right ventricle and the main pulmonary artery, is primarily due to inertia and the low impedance in the pulmonary vascular bed.

■ Cycle efficiency relates the mechanical work done by a ventricle to the maximal work possible for given changes in pressure and volume. Because a square loop yields the maximal efficiency, the left ventricle is more mechanically efficient, but the right ventricle is more energy efficient. For a given stroke volume, the external mechanical stroke work done by the right ventricle can be 20% required by the left ventricle.

■ MRI has become the noninvasive diagnostic method of choice for defining right ventricular anatomy and function parameters, such as right ventricular mass, right ventricular wall thickness, and RVEF. Similar to three-dimensional echocardiography, MRI provides information without making geometric assumptions, so volumes, cardiac outputs, ejection fractions, and wall thicknesses all can be calculated.

■ RVEF has been shown to correlate inversely with serum levels of both natriuretic peptides, which can readily be measured using monoclonal antibodies and radioimmunoassays.

■ A large body of literature indicates that a left ventricle is superior to a right ventricle as the systemic ventricle, particularly when atrioventricular valve incompetence develops.

■ Chronic changes in right ventricular volume overload are far better tolerated than acute alterations, and the surrounding structures (pericardium and left ventricle) along with intrinsic factors, such as myocardial disease, play an important role in how quickly a change in preload would alter function. In chronic right ventricular volume overload, the right ventricular end-diastolic pressure may not be elevated despite a relatively large increase in RVEDV.

■ In these right ventricular pressure overload lesions, the overall geometry of the pressure volume loop of the right ventricle resembles that of the normal left ventricle, and cycle efficiency is higher than in the normal right ventricle. In the face of increased afterload, the right ventricular stroke work can increase dramatically for extended periods (years), showing a contractile reserve not possible in the normal left ventricle.

■ In patients with normal PVR, volume expansion can increase preload to maximize stretch and contractility, increasing cardiac output. If PVR is increased, volume expansion may result in an increase in pulmonary pressure, afterload, wall stress, myocardial oxygen requirement, and tricuspid regurgitation, all of which are detrimental to right ventricular function.

■ When PVR is elevated, vasodilator therapy helps the failing right ventricle by decreasing afterload. A reduced afterload also allows a decline in RVEDV, producing decreased wall tension and myocardial oxygen requirement. The dilated pulmonary vasculature also increases left ventricle preload, which increases mean arterial pressure and RCA perfusion pressure.

■ In some patients, the underlying anatomy may not be amenable to complete correction, and palliative surgical measures can be an alternative strategy. Establishing a bidirectional cavopulmonary anastomosis from the superior vena cava to the right pulmonary artery allows partial volume decompression of the right heart and often significant improvement of right ventricular hemodynamics; this can be an element of a surgical strategy for right ventricular failure. In addition, banding of the pulmonary artery in certain patients with a failing systemic right ventricle after the atrial switch operation for transposition of the great arteries can improve right ventricular function and tricuspid valve incompetence.

REFERENCES

1. Starr I, Jeffers WA, Meade RH: The absence of conspicuous increments of venous pressure after severe damage to the right ventricle of the dog, with a discussion of the relation between clinical congestive failure and heart disease. Am Heart J 1943;26:291-301.

2. Hines R: Right ventricular function and failure: A review. Yale J Biol Med 1991;64:295-307.

3. Redington AN, Rigby ML, Shinebourne EA, Oldershaw PJ: Changes in the pressure-volume relation of the right ventricle when its loading conditions are modified. Br Heart J 1990;63:45-49.

4. Brooks H, Kirk ES, Vokonas PS, et al: Performance of the right ventricle under stress: Relation to right coronary flow. J Clin Invest 1971;50:2176-2183.

5. Reuse C, Frank B, Contempre B, Vincent JL: Right ventricular function in septic shock. Intensive Care Med 1988;14:486-487.

6. D'Orio V, Lambermont B, Detry D, et al: Pulmonary impedance and right ventricular-vascular coupling in endotoxin shock. Cardiovasc Res 1998; 38:375-382.

7. Dhainaut JF, Lanore JJ, de Gournay JM, et al: Right ventricular dysfunction in patients with septic shock. Intensive Care Med 1988;14(Suppl 2):488-491.

8. Schneider AJ, Teule GJ, Groeneveld AB, et al: Biventricular performance during volume loading in patients with early septic shock, with emphasis on the right ventricle: A combined hemodynamic and radionuclide study. Am Heart J 1988;116:103-112.

9. Hoffman MJ, Greenfield LJ, Sugarman HJ, Tatum JL: Unsuspected right ventricular dysfunction in shock and sepsis. Ann Surg 1983;198:307-319.

10. Kimchi A, Ellrodt AC, Berman DS, et al: Right ventricular performance in septic shock: A combined radionuclide and hemodynamic study. J Am Coll Cardiol 1984;4:945-951.

11. Mebazaa A, Karpati P, Renaud E, Algotsson L: Acute right ventricular failure-from pathophysiology to new treatments. Intensive Care Med 2003;30:185-196.

12. Moorman A, Webb S, Brown NA, et al: Development of the heart: (1) Formation of the cardiac chambers and arterial trunks. Heart 2003;89:806-814.

13. O'Rahilly R: The timing and sequence of events in human cardiogenesis. Acta Anat 1971;79:70-75.

14. Anderson RH, Webb S, Brown NA, et al: Development of the heart: (2) Septation of the atriums and ventricles. Heart 2003;89:949-958.

15. Licata RH: The human embryonic heart in the ninth week. Am J Anat 1954;94:73-125.

16. Heerdt PM, Pleimann BE: The dose-dependent effects of halothane on right ventricular contraction pattern and regional inotropy in swine. Anesth Analg 1996;82:1152-1158.

17. Stobierska-Dzierzek B, Awad H, Michler RE: The evolving management of acute right-sided heart failure in cardiac transplant recipients. J Am Coll Cardiol 2001;38:923-931.

18. Anderson RH, Ho SY: The anatomy of the morphologically right ventricle. In Redington AN, et al (eds): The Right Heart in Congenital Heart Disease. London, Greenwich Medical Media LTD, 1998, pp 1-8.

19. Redington AN: Right ventricular function. In Redington AN, et al (eds): The Right Heart in Congenital Heart Disease. London, Greenwich Medical Media LTD, 1998, pp 17-24.

20. Maughan WL, Shoukas AA, Sagawa K, Weisfeldt ML: Instantaneous pressure-volume relationship of the canine right ventricle. Circ Rese 1979;44:309-315.

21. Boak, JG, Bove AA, Kreulen J, Spann JF: A geometric basis for calculation of right ventricular volume in man. Cathet Cardiovasc Diag 1977;3:217-230.

22. Hebert FL, Chemla D, Gerard O, et al: Angiographic right and left ventricular function in arrhythmogenic right ventricular dysplasia. Am J Cardiol 2004; 93:728-733.

23. Feneley MP, Elbeery JR, Gaynor JW, et al: Ellipsoidal shell subtraction model of right ventricular volume: Comparison with regional free wall dimensions as indexes of right ventricular function. Circ Res 1990;67:1427-1436.

24. McGovern JJ, Cheifetz IM, Craig DM, et al: Right ventricular injury in young swine: Effects of catecholamines on right ventricular function and pulmonary vascular mechanics. Pediatr Res 2000;48:763-769.

25. Reedy T, Chapman CB: Measurement of right ventricular volume by cineangiofluorography. Am Heart J 1963;66:221-225.

26. Guyton AC, Lindsey AW, Gilluly JJ: The limits of right ventricular compensation following acute increase in pulmonary circulatory resistance. Circ Res 1954;2:326-332.

27. Fineberg MH, Wiggers CJ: Compensation and failure of the right ventricle. Am Heart J 1936;11:255-263.

28. Friedman BJ, Lozner EC, Curfman GD, et al: Characterization of the human right ventricular pressure-volume relation: Effect of dobutamine and right coronary artery stenosis. J Am Coll Cardiol 1984;4:999-1005.

29. Greyson C, Garcia J, Mayr M, Schwartz GG: Effects of inotropic stimulation on energy metabolism and systolic function of ischemic right ventricle. Am J Physiol 1995;268:H1821-H1828.

30. Rushmer R, Thal N: The mechanics of ventricular contraction: A cinefluorographic study. Circulation 1951;4:219-228.

31. Adatia I, Barrow SE, Stratton PD, et al: Thromboxane A2 and prostacyclin biosynthesis in children and adolescents with pulmonary vascular disease. Circulation 1993;88:2117-2122.

32. Ghignone M, Girling L, Prewitt RM: Effect of increased pulmonary vascular resistance on right ventricular systolic performance in dogs. Am J Physiol 1984;246:339-343.

33. Weber KT, Janicki JS, Schroff S, Fishman AP: Contractile mechanics and interaction of the right and left ventricles. Am J Cardiol 1981;47:686-695.

34. Klein SS, Graham Jr TP, Lorenz CH: Noninvasive delineation of normal right ventricular contractile motion with magnetic resonance imaging myocardial tagging. Ann Biomed Eng 1998;26:756-763.

35. Taylor RR, Covell JW, Sonnenblick EH, Ross J: Dependence of ventricular distensibility on filling of the opposite ventricle. Am J Physiol 1967;213:711-718.

36. Lazar JM, Flores AR, Grandis DJ, et al: Effects of chronic right ventricular pressure overload on left ventricular diastolic function. Am J Cardiol 1993;72:1179-1182.

37. Dell'Italia LJ, Walsh RA: Right ventricular diastolic pressure-volume relations and regional dimensions during acute alterations in loading conditions. Circulation 1988;77:1276-1282.

38. Redington AN, Gray HH, Hodson ME, et al: Characterisation of the normal right ventricular pressure-volume relation by biplane angiography and simultaneous micromanometer pressure measurements. Br Heart J 1988;59:23-30.

39. Shaver JA: Clinical implications of the hangout interval. Int J Cardiol 1984;5:391-398.

40. Dell'Italia LJ, Walsh RA: Acute determinants of the hangout interval in the pulmonary circulation. Am Heart J 1988;116:1289-1297.

41. Vargo TA: Cardiac catheterization: Hemodynamic measurements. In Garson AJ, et al (eds): The Science and Practice of Pediatric Cardiology. Baltimore, Williams & Wilkins, 1998, pp 961-993.

42. Attinger EO, Anne A, McDonald DA: Use of Fourier series for the analysis of biological systems. Biophys J 1966;6:291-304.

43. Trowitzsch E, Colan SD, Sanders SP: Global and regional right ventricular function in normal infants and infants with transposition of the great arteries after Senning operation. Circulation 1985;72:1008-1014.

44. Helbing WA, Rebergan SA, Maliepaard C, et al: Quantification of right ventricular function with magnetic resonance imaging in children with normal hearts and with congenital heart disease. Am Heart J 1995;130:828-837.

45. Dimas AP, Moodie DS, Sterba R, Gill CG, et al: Long-term function of the morphologic right ventricle in adult patients with corrected transposition of the great arteries. Am Heart J 1989; 118:526-530.

46. Gatzoulis MA, Till JA, Somerville J, Redington AN: Mechano-electrical interaction in tetralogy of Fallot: QRS prolongation relates to right ventricular size and predicts malignant ventricular arrhythmias and sudden death. Circulation 1995; 92:231-237.

47. Neffke JG, Tulevski II, van der Wall EE, et al: ECG determinants in adult patients with chronic right ventricular pressure overload caused by congenital heart disease: Relation with plasma neurohormones and MRI parameters. Heart 2002;88:266-270.

48. Tulevski II, Dodge-Khatami A, Groenink M, et al: Right ventricular function in congenital cardiac disease: Noninvasive quantitative

parameters for clinical follow-up. Cardiol Young 2003;13: 397-403.

49. Therrien J, Siu SC, Harris L, et al: Impact of pulmonary valve replacement on arrhythmia propensity late after repair of tetralogy of Fallot. Circulation 2001;103:2489-2494.

50. Gray R, Greve G, Chen R, et al: Right ventricular myocardial response to chronic pulmonary regurgitation in lambs: Disturbances of activation and conduction. Pediatr Res 2003;54:529-535.

51. Hijazi ZM, Hellenbrand WE: The right ventricle in congenital heart disease. Cardiol Clin 1992;10:91-110.

52. Wei L, Davlouros PA, Kilner PJ, et al: Doppler-echocardiographic assessment of pulmonary regurgitation in adults with repaired tetralogy of Fallot: Comparison with cardiovascular magnetic resonance imaging. Am Heart J 2004;147:165-172.

53. Pacileo G, Limongelli G, Verrengia M, et al: Backscatter evaluation of myocardial functional and textural findings in children with right ventricular pressure and/or volume overload. Am J Cardiol 2004;93:594-597.

54. Mizelle KM, Rice MJ, Sahn DJ: Clinical use of real-time three-dimensional echocardiography in pediatric cardiology. Echocardiography 2000;17:787-790.

55. Takuma S, Cardinale C, Homma S: Real-time three-dimensional stress echocardiography. Echocardiography 2000;17:791-794.

56. Doherty 3rd NE, et al: Measurement of right ventricular mass in normal and dilated cardiomyopathic ventricles using cine magnetic resonance imaging. Am J Cardiol 1992;69:1223-1228.

57. Pattynama PM, Lamb HJ, Van der Velde EA, et al: Reproducibility of MRI-derived measurements of right ventricular volumes and myocardial mass. Magn Reson Imaging 1995;13:53-63.

58. Berger HJ, Matthay RA, Pytlik LM, et al: First-pass radionuclide assessment of right and left ventricular performance in patients with cardiac and pulmonary disease. Semin Nucl Med 1979;9:275-295.

59. Hoeper MM, Tongers J, Leppert A, et al: Evaluation of right ventricular performance with a right ventricular ejection fraction thermodilution catheter and MRI in patients with pulmonary hypertension. Chest 2001;120:502-507.

60. Tulevski II, Groenink M, van der Wall EE, et al: Increased brain and atrial natriuretic peptides in patients with chronic right ventricular pressure overload: Correlation between plasma neurohormones and right ventricular dysfunction. Heart 2001;86:27-30.

61. Yasue H, Yoshimura M, Sumida H, et al: Localization and mechanism of secretion of B-type natriuretic peptide in comparison with those of A-type natriuretic peptide in normal subjects and patients with heart failure. Circulation 1994;90:195-203.

62. Geva T, Sandweiss BM, Gauvreau K, et al: Factors associated with impaired clinical status in long-term survivors of tetralogy of Fallot repair evaluated by magnetic resonance imaging. J Am Coll Cardiol 2004;43:1068-1074.

63. Davlouros PA, Kilner PJ, Hornung TS, et al: Right ventricular function in adults with repaired tetralogy of Fallot assessed with cardiovascular magnetic resonance imaging: Detrimental role of right ventricular outflow aneurysms or akinesia and adverse right-to-left ventricular interaction. J Am Coll Cardiol 2002; 40:2044-2052.

64. Helbing WA, Niezen RA, Le Cessie S, et al: Right ventricular diastolic function in children with pulmonary regurgitation after repair of tetralogy of Fallot: Volumetric evaluation by magnetic resonance velocity mapping. J Am Coll Cardiol 1996;28:1827-1835.

65. Ahel V, Kilvain S, Rozmanic V, et al: Right atrial reduction for tachyarrhythmias in Ebstein's anomaly in infancy. Tex Heart Inst J 2001;28:297-300.

66. Gatzoulis MA, Clark AL, Cullen S, et al: Right ventricular diastolic function 15 to 35 years after repair of tetralogy of Fallot: Restrictive physiology predicts superior exercise performance. Circulation 1995;91:1775-1781.

67. Gatzoulis MA, Elliott JT, Guru V, et al: Right and left ventricular systolic function late after repair of tetralogy of Fallot. Am J Cardiol 2000; 86:1352-1357.

68. Redington AN, Rigby ML, Oldershaw B, et al: Right ventricular function 10 years after the Mustard operation for transposition of the great arteries: Analysis of size, shape, and wall motion. Br Heart J 1989; 62:455-461.

69. Beerman LB, Neches WH, Fricker FJ, et al: Arrhythmias in transposition of the great arteries after the Mustard operation. Am J Cardiol 1983;51:1530-1534.

70. Duster MC, Bink-Boelkens MTE, Wampler D, et al: Long-term follow-up of dysrhythmias following the Mustard procedure. Am Heart J 1985;109:1323-1326.

71. Devaney EJ, Charpie JR, Ohye RG, and Bove EL: Combined arterial switch and Senning operation for congenitally corrected transposition of the great arteries: Patient selection and intermediate results. J Thorac Cardiovasc Surg 2003;125:500-507.

72. Lundstrom U, Bull C, Wyse RK, Somerville J: The natural and "unnatural" history of congenitally corrected transposition. Am J Cardiol 1990;65:1222-1229.

73. Connelly MS, Liu PP, Williams WG, et al: Congenitally corrected transposition of the great arteries in the adult: Functional status and complications. J Am Coll Cardiol 1996;27:1238-1243.

74. Ohuchi H, Hiraumi Y, Tasato H, et al: Comparison of the right and left ventricle as a systemic ventricle during exercise in patients with congenital heart disease. Am Heart J 1999;137:1185-1194.

75. Paul MH, Wessel HU: Exercise studies in patients with transposition of the great arteries after atrial repair operations (Mustard/Senning): A review. Pediatr Cardiol 1999;20:49-55.

76. Tulevski II, Lee PL, Groenink M, et al: Dobutamine-induced increases of right ventricular contractility without increased stroke volume in adolescent patients with transposition of the great arteries: Evaluation with magnetic resonance imaging. Int J Card Imaging 2000;16:471-478.

77. Tulevski II, van der Wall EE, Groenink M, et al: Usefulness of magnetic resonance imaging dobutamine stress in asymptomatic and minimally symptomatic patients with decreased cardiac reserve from congenital heart disease (complete and corrected transposition of the great arteries and subpulmonic obstruction). Am J Cardiol 2002;89:1077-1081.

78. Farrar DJ, Compton PG, Hershon JJ, Hill JD: Right ventricular function in an operating room model of mechanical left ventricular assistance and its effects in patients with depressed left ventricular function. Circulation 1985;72:1279-1285.

79. Slawsky MT, Colucci WS, Gottlieb SS, et al: Acute hemodynamic and clinical effects of levosimendan in patients with severe heart failure. Study investigators. Circulation 2000;102:2222-2227.

80. De Witt BJ, Ibrahim IN, Bayer E, et al: An analysis of responses to levosimendan in the pulmonary vascular bed of the cat. Anesth Analg 2002;94:1427-1433.

81. Yamada O, Kamiya T, Suga H: Right ventricular mechanical and energetic properties. Jpn Circ J 1989;53:1260-1268.

82. Tidholm A, Falk T, Gundler S, et al: Effect of thyroid hormone supplementation on survival of euthyroid dogs with congestive heart failure due to systolic myocardial dysfunction: A double-blind, placebo-controlled trial. Res Vet Sci 2003;75:195-201.

83. Ascheim DD, Hryniewicz K: Thyroid hormone metabolism in patients with congestive heart failure: The low triiodothyronine state. Thyroid 2002;12:511-515.

84. Moruzzi P, Doria E, Agostini PG, et al: Usefulness of L-thyroxine to improve cardiac and exercise performance in idiopathic dilated cardiomyopathy. Am J Cardiol 1994;73:374-378.

85. Leather HA, Ver Eycken K, Segers P, et al: Effects of levosimendan on right ventricular function and ventriculovascular coupling in open chest pigs. Crit Care Med 2003;31:2339-2343.

86. Rich S, Kaufmann E, Levy PS: The effect of high doses of calcium-channel blockers on survival in primary pulmonary hypertension. N Engl J Med 1992;327:76-81.

87. Sulica R, Poon M: Current medical treatment of pulmonary arterial hypertension. Mt Sinai J Med 2004;71:103-114.

88. Roberts Jr JD, et al: Inhaled nitric oxide in congenital heart disease. Circulation 1993;87:447-453.

89. Celermajer DS, et al: Role of endothelium in the maintenance of low pulmonary vascular tone in normal children. Circulation 1994;89:2041-2044.

90. Bhorade S, Christenson J, O'Connor M, et al: Response to inhaled nitric oxide in patients with acute right heart syndrome. Am J Respir Crit Care Med 1999;159:571-579.

91. Ware LE: Inhaled nitric oxide in infants and children. Crit Care Nurs Clin North Am 2002;14:1-6.

92. Pepke-Zaba J, Higenbottam T, Dinh-Xuan AT, et al: Inhaled nitric oxide as a cause of selective pulmonary vasodilation in pulmonary hypertension. Lancet 1991;338:1173-1174.

93. Kelly LK, Porta NF, Goodman DM, et al: Inhaled prostacyclin for term infants with persistent pulmonary hypertension refractory to inhaled nitric oxide. J Pediatr 2002;141:830-832.

94. Barst RJ, Rubin LJ, Long WA, et al: A comparison of continuous intravenous epoprostenol (prostacyclin) with conventional therapy for primary pulmonary hypertension. The Primary Pulmonary Hypertension Study Group. N Engl J Med 1996;334:296-302.

95. Hinderliter AL, Willis PW 4th, Barst RJ, et al: Effects of long-term infusion of prostacyclin (epoprostenol) on echocardiographic measures of right ventricular structure and function in primary pulmonary hypertension. Primary Pulmonary Hypertension Study Group. Circulation 1997;95:1479-1486.

96. Gildea TR, Arroliga AC, Minai OA: Treatments and strategies to optimize the comprehensive management of patients with pulmonary arterial hypertension. Cleve Clin J Med 2003;70 (Suppl 1):S18-S27.

97. McLaughlin VV, Genthner DE, Panella MM, Rich S: Reduction in pulmonary vascular resistance with long-term epoprostenol (prostacyclin) therapy in primary pulmonary hypertension. N Engl J Med 1998;338:273-277.

98. Machherndl S, Kneussl M, Baumgartner H, et al: Long-term treatment of pulmonary hypertension with aerosolized iloprost. Eur Respir J 2001;17:8-13.

99. Higenbottam T, Wheeldon D, Wells F, Wallwork J: Long-term treatment of primary pulmonary hypertension with continuous intravenous epoprostenol (prostacyclin). Lancet 1984;1: 1046-1047.

100. Badesh DB, Tapson VF, McGoon MD, et al: Continuous intravenous epoprostenol for pulmonary hypertension due to the scleroderma spectrum of disease: A randomized, controlled trial. Ann Intern Med 2000;132:425-434.

101. Rosenzweig EB, Kerstein D, Barst RJ: Long-term prostacyclin for pulmonary hypertension with associated congenital heart defects. Circulation 1998;99:1858-1865.

102. Mehta S: Drug therapy for pulmonary arterial hypertension: What's on the menu today? Chest 2003;124:2045-2049.

103. Lowson SM, Doctor A, Walsh BK, Doorley PA: Inhaled prostacyclin for the treatment of pulmonary hypertension after cardiac surgery. Crit Care Med 2002;30:2762-2764.

104. Hoeper MM, Schwarze M, Ehlerding S, et al: Long-term treatment of primary pulmonary hypertension with aerosolized iloprost, a prostacyclin analogue. N Engl J Med 2000;342:1866-1870.

105. Olschewski H, Simonneau G, Galie N, et al: Inhaled iloprost for severe pulmonary hypertension. N Engl J Med 2002;347: 322-329.

106. Simonneau G, Barst RJ, Galie N, et al: Continuous subcutaneous infusion of treprostinil, a prostacyclin analogue, in patients with pulmonary arterial hypertension: A double-blind, randomized, placebo-controlled trial. Am J Respir Crit Care Med 2002; 165:800-804.

107. Channick RN, Simonneau G, Sitbon O, et al: Effects of the dual endothelin-receptor antagonist bosentan in patients with pulmonary hypertension: A randomised placebo-controlled study. Lancet 2001;358:1119-1123.

108. Barst RJ, Ivy D, Dingemanse J, et al: Pharmacokinetics, safety, and efficacy of bosentan in pediatric patients with pulmonary arterial hypertension. Clin Pharmacol Ther 2003;73:372-382.

109. Givertz MM, Colucci WS, LeJemtel TH, et al: Acute endothelin A receptor blockade causes selective pulmonary vasodilation in patients with chronic heart failure. Circulation 2000;101:2922-2927.

110. Rubin LJ, Badesh DB, Barst RJ, et al: Bosentan therapy for pulmonary arterial hypertension. N Engl J Med 2002;346:896-903.

111. Filep JP, Fournier A, Foldes-Filep E: Acute pro-inflammatory actions of endothelin-1 in the guinea-pig lung: Involvement of ETA and ETB receptors. Br J Pharmacol 1995;115:227-236.

112. Allen SW, Chatfield BA, Koppenhafer SA, et al: Circulating immunoreactive endothelin-1 in children with pulmonary hypertension: Association with acute hypoxic pulmonary vasoreactivity. Am Rev Respir Dis 1993;148:519-522.

113. Jia B, Zhang S, Chen Z, et al: Plasma endothelin 1 concentrations in children with congenital heart defects. Min Pediatr 1998; 50:99-103.

114. Pearl JM, Wellmann SA, McNamara JL, et al: Bosentan prevents hypoxia-reoxygenation-induced pulmonary hypertension and improves pulmonary function. Ann Thorac Surg 1999;68: 1714-1722.

115. Ivy D, Doran A, Claussen L, et al: Weaning and discontinuation of epoprostenol in children with idiopathic pulmonary arterial hypertension receiving concomitant bosentan. Am J Cardiol 2004;93:943-946.

116. Galie N, Hinderliter AL, Torbicki A, et al: Effects of the oral endothelin-receptor antagonist bosentan on echocardiographic and doppler measures in patients with pulmonary arterial hypertension. J Am Coll Cardiol 2003;41:1380-1386.

117. Highland KB, Strange C, Mazur J, Simpson KN: Treatment of pulmonary arterial hypertension: A preliminary decision analysis. Chest 2003;124:2087-2092.

118. Dubin AM, Feinstein JA, Reddy M, et al: Electrical resynchronization: A novel therapy for the failing right ventricle. Circulation 2003;107:2287-2289.

119. Beghetti M, Rimensberger PC: Mechanical circulatory support in pediatric patients. Intensive Care Med 2000;26:350-352.

120. Duncan BW: Mechanical circulatory support for infants and children with cardiac disease. Ann Thorac Surg 2002;73:1670-1677.

121. Miller DC, Moreno-Cabral RJ, Stinson EB, et al: Pulmonary artery balloon counterpulsation for acute right ventricular failure. J Thorac Cardiovasc Surg 1980;80:760-763.

122. Williams MR, Quaegebeur JM, Hsu DT, et al: Biventricular assist device as a bridge to transplantation in a pediatric patient. Ann Thorac Surg 1996;62:578-580.

123. Kjellstrom B, Linde C, Bennett T, et al: Six years followup of an implanted SvO2 sensor in the right ventricle. Eur J Heart Failure 2004;6:627-634.

124. Poirier NC, Yu JH, Brizard CP, et al: Long term results of left ventricular reconditioning and anatomic correction for systemic right ventricular dysfunction after atrial switch procedures. J Thorac Cardiovasc Surg 2004;127:975-981.

125. Furukawa K, Motomura T, Nose Y: Right ventricular failure after left ventricular assist device implantation: The need for an implantable right ventricular assist device. Artif Organs 2005; 29:369-377.

CHAPTER 17

Acute Myocarditis

Alan B. Lewis

A conceptual framework for myocarditis as a triphasic process has emerged in recent years, with each phase having unique pathogenetic and clinical features.[1] Myocarditis is initiated by viral infection and is characterized by inflammation of the myocardium accompanied by myocellular necrosis. Enteroviruses, particularly coxsackievirus B (CVB), and adenoviruses are the predominant viral agents associated with acute myocarditis, although numerous other viral agents also have been implicated. Viral proliferation triggers a host immunologic response usually resulting in viral clearance. In a subset of individuals, however, a secondary phase evolves in which an autoimmune response is initiated by ongoing T cell proliferation, cytokine activation, and cross-reacting antibodies.[2] This phase is followed by a chronic phase in which immune-mediated changes and dilated cardiomyopathy predominate.

Overall, the effector mechanisms of immune-mediated myocardial injury in myocarditis are more cellular based than humoral in origin. Eventually, progressive adverse remodeling results in the development of dilated cardiomyopathy (see Chapter 18). Management decisions must take into account the particular phase of this disease continuum and be targeted to the underlying pathogenesis. This chapter highlights advances in the understanding of the complex pathogenetic and clinical continuum that constitutes the wide spectrum of myocarditis and addresses current and future therapeutic modalities.

EPIDEMIOLOGY AND PATHOGENESIS

Myocarditis is defined as inflammation of the myocardium in association with nonischemic myocellular necrosis.[3] The incidence of myocarditis is difficult to ascertain because of the varied clinical expression, ranging from absent or minimal symptoms to cardiogenic shock and death. Population estimates of prevalence frequently range from 1 to 10 per 100,000 persons. The incidence in young, male military recruits in Finland over a 20-year period was nearly 15 per 100,000 (0.015%).[4] In contrast, a large autopsy series in Japan found myocarditis in 0.11% of more than 370,000 autopsies.[5] The prevalence of acute myocarditis may have declined in recent years in the United States. The percentage of patients with biopsy-proven myocarditis at a single large referral center declined from 20% in

1985 to less than 2% in 1996.[6] Infants and young children may be more prone to the development of myocarditis because of a higher overall rate of enteroviral and adenoviral infections.[7] Epidemics, particularly of CVB, have been observed in neonates.

Viruses are the most common etiology of myocarditis, but other infectious agents or noninfectious causes are numerous (Table 17-1). The enteroviruses, particularly CVB3 and CVB4, have long been recognized as common etiologic agents. With the advent of molecular techniques, initially using in situ hybridization and more recently polymerase chain reaction (PCR) to detect viral genomes, the importance of coxsackievirus has been confirmed and additional viruses have emerged as major agents.[8] Adenovirus type C (types 2 and 5) was the most commonly detected viral pathogen in recent series, with enteroviruses second.[9,10] Other viruses causing myocarditis are considerably less common and include cytomegalovirus, influenza A, hepatitis C,[11] parvovirus,[12] Epstein-Barr virus, herpes simplex virus, respiratory syncytial virus, and human immunodeficiency virus.[13] A bacteria that causes myocarditis that deserves mention is diphtheria, which can lead to arrhythmias and conduction defects. In addition, hematogenously acquired bacterial myocarditis can be associated with bacterial endocarditis. *Trypanosoma cruzi* can cause myocarditis and results in Chagas' disease, which is endemic in South America.

Giant cell myocarditis is uncommon in children, but is characterized by giant cell inflammatory infiltrate in the myocardium with prominent myocyte necrosis and has a high mortality rate compared with lymphocytic myocarditis. Rarely, autoimmune diseases, such as lupus, rheumatoid arthritis, and ulcerative colitis, may be complicated by myocarditis. Among noninfectious toxins, cocaine abuse has been associated with acute onset of severe left ventricular dysfunction.[14]

IMMUNOLOGIC PHASES OF MYOCARDITIS

Three interrelated mechanisms result in myocardial injury from the aforementioned infectious agents, including direct invasion of the myocardial cells, production of a myocardial toxin, and immune-mediated myocardial damage.[15] That the immunologically mediated changes led by T lymphocytes and macrophages

TABLE 17-1

Etiologic Agents of Myocarditis					
Viral	**Rickettsial**	**Bacterial**	**Fungal**	**Spirochetal**	**Protozoal**
Coxsackievirus	Scrub typhus	Diphtheria	Candidiasis	Syphilis	Chagas
Adenovirus	Rocky mountain spotted	Tuberculosis	Aspergillosis	Lyme disease	*Toxoplasma*
	fever (*Rickettsia rickettsii*)	*Streptococcus*	Cryptococcosis	(*Borrelia burgdorferi*)	
Cytomegalovirus	Q fever (*Coxiella burnetii*)	*Staphylococcus*	Histoplasmosis	Leptospirosis	Malaria
Echovirus		Meningococcus	Coccidioidomycosis		
Epstein-Barr virus		*Mycoplasma*	Blastomycosis		
Herpes simplex virus		Brucellosis			
Influenza A virus					
Respiratory syncytial					
virus					
HIV					
Hepatitis C virus					
Parvovirus B19					
Mumps					
Rubeola					
Varicella					

are the predominant mechanisms that result in myocardial injury (Fig. 17-1).[16] The infectious process and sequelae of the cellular immune-mediated myocarditis can be delineated in three phases.

Phase 1: Viral Infection and Proliferation

Phase 1 is an induction phase during which the virus itself plays a major role. The predominance of coxsackievirus and adenoviruses as causative agents of myocarditis may be explained by the discovery of a specific common receptor for both viruses.[17] The **coxsackie-adenoviral receptor** (CAR) is a transmembrane protein with immunoglobulin-like domains that binds CVB and adenovirus type C and allows internalization of viral genome (Fig. 17-2). The coxsackie-adenoviral receptor also serves as an internalizing receptor for many other enteroviruses.[18] The receptor gene has been cloned and mapped to chromosome 2q11.2.[19] Bowles and Towbin[20] speculated that polymorphisms in the coxsackie-adenoviral receptor gene or mutations in specific binding regions, along with variations in the virus itself, may account for the cardiotropic virulence of CVB and adenoviruses. An additional factor that may influence cardiovirulence is the role of coxsackie-adenoviral receptor coreceptors in increasing the binding efficiency of coxsackie-adenoviral receptor. CVB uses a complement **deflecting protein decay accelerating factor** (DAF), whereas adenovirus uses integrins $\alpha_{v\beta3}$ and $\alpha_{v\beta5}$.[1] Acting collaboratively, the receptor-coreceptor complex facilitates binding, uncoating of the virus, and internalization of viral genome.

Interesting histopathologic differences have been identified between enterovirus-induced myocarditis and myocarditis caused by adenovirus.[16] Coxsackievirus myocarditis is associated with typical lymphocytic infiltrate, edema, and myocyte necrosis (Fig. 17-3),

whereas the inflammatory infiltrate is less extensive in adenoviral disease, but fibrosis tends to predominate. T cell activation by adenoviruses seems to be less robust, although the mechanism for this response is not understood.

Much of the understanding of the pathophysiology of myocarditis comes from murine models of CVB myocarditis. During the initial viral phase, lasting approximately 4 days, CVB enters the body through the gastrointestinal tract (or, in the case of adenovirus, through the respiratory tract) and migrates to lymphoid tissue, where it is harbored in immune cells and evades immune clearance. The virus may be transported to the myocardium or other target organs. Proliferating virus also produces focal myocyte necrosis from a direct cytopathic effect. A polymorphonuclear and mononuclear cell response is triggered, accompanied by antibody production that results in viral clearance.

At this point, the immune system should down-regulate and return to baseline. In susceptible individuals, these viral **neoantigens**, acting through MHC class I and II molecules on cell membranes, may promote ongoing activation of the immune system. Changes of the myocardial cell as a result of the viral infection induce a neoantigen that is recognized by the cytotoxic T lymphocytes. Even an endogenous cardiac antigen such as myosin can be a substrate to lead to this immune activation.[21] Further T cell–mediated myocyte destruction may be initiated by exposure of myocardial antigens that cross-react with viral antigens. Antibodies that cross-react with the viral particles and the myocardial proteins further the damage (this phenomenon is called *myocardial mimicry*). Finally, antibodies are produced against the β-adrenergic receptors and the mitochondrial ADP-ATP translocator.[22]

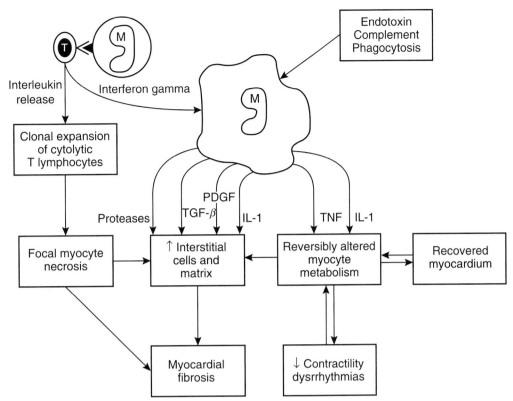

FIGURE 17-1 ■ Cellular pathways mediating reversible and irreversible immune injury to the heart. The heart and its immunomodulatory response to an insult such as myocarditis is illustrated. The myocardial antigen is presented to T lymphocytes (*T*) by macrophages (*M*). This leads to differentiation of T cells with stimulation by release of cytokines. In addition, factors that can stimulate myocardial fibrosis, such as transforming growth factor (TGF)-β, platelet-derived growth factor (PDGF), interleukin (IL)-1, and tumor necrosis factor (TNF) are released and lead to increased interstitial cells and matrix and reversibly altered myocyte metabolism. All of these changes potentially can lead to myocardial fibrosis that is irreversible. (From Lange LG and Schreiner, GF: Immune mechanisms of cardiac disease. N Engl J Med 1994;330:1129-1135.)

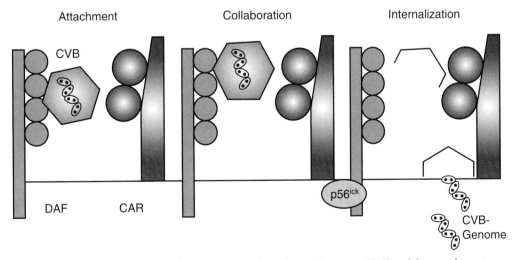

FIGURE 17-2 ■ Collaboration of receptors. Coxsackie-adenoviral receptor (CAR) and the complement deflecting protein accelerating factor (DAF) act as coreceptors to enhance the binding efficiency of coxsackievirus B (CVB) onto the DAF-CAR complex, permit uncoating of the viral genome, and facilitate internalization. CAR is a transmembrane protein with immunoglobulin-like domains that binds CVB and adenovirus type C and allows internalization of viral genome. CAR also serves as an internalizing receptor for many other enteroviruses. Coxsackievirus B uses a DAF. Acting collaboratively, the receptor-coreceptor complex facilitates binding, uncoating of the virus, and internalization of viral genome. (From Liu PP and Mason, JW: Advances in the understanding of myocarditis. Circulation 2001;104:1076-1082.)

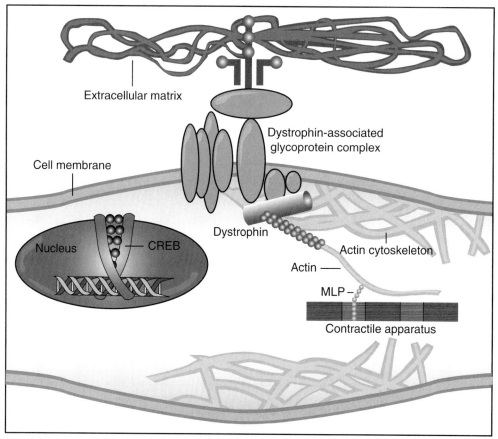

FIGURE 17-3 ■ Dystrophin cleavage by enteroviral protease 2A. This diagram shows the cardiac myocyte and the role of dystrophin. Dystrophin and the dystrophin-associated glycoprotein complex is an essential intracellular cytoskeletal protein that links the contractile system via actin to the sarcolemma and extracellular matrix. This protein is directly cleaved by enteroviral protease 2A, leading to dysfunction of this protein. CREB, cyclic AMP response-element binding protein; MLP, muscle LIM (Lin-11, Isl-1, Mec-3) protein. (From Leiden JM: The genetics of dilated cardiomyopathy: Emerging clues to the puzzle. N Engl J Med 1997;337:1081.)

Phase 2: Autoimmunity

During phase 2 of the disease process, lymphocytes and macrophages predominate, but the proliferating virus is generally absent from the myocardium, although viral RNA may be detected by PCR.[23] Myocardial inflammation and injury are perpetuated, however, as the activated immune system continues to target the host myocardium to result in a chronic autoimmune myocarditis. The mechanisms by which **T lymphocytes** can effect injury during myocarditis to infected and uninfected cells include accumulation of activated macrophages, production of antibody and antibody-dependent cell-mediated cytotoxicity, direct lysis by antibody and complement, cytolysis via perforin (a protein that induces increased membrane permeability), and direct action of cytotoxic T cells.[24] The delicate balance of all of these mechanisms determines the degree of myocardial injury.

The MHC presenting cells (e.g., macrophages) stimulate the production of **CD4 T helper cells** and **CD8** **cytotoxic T cells** to result in a cellular amplification of the immune response. The activation of these helper T cells leads to formation and differentiation of other effector T cells, which lead to cytokine production. **Natural killer cells**, activated by interferon, can offer some protection against the virus by increasing its clearance.

The T cells target infected myocytes and destroy them by direct T cell–mediated cytolysis or via proinflammatory **cytokines**. These cytokines provide a molecular infrastructure for immune modulation of cardiac function. Patients with acute myocarditis have marked expression of interferon-γ; interleukins (IL)-1, IL-6, IL-8, and IL-10[25]; and tumor necrosis factor (TNF)-α.[26] These cytokines not only enhance further the immune reaction and T cell proliferation, but also induce apoptosis and cause ventricular dysfunction.[27] In addition, the cytokine macrophage chemotactic factor recruits monocytes that later become **macrophages**, which release cytotoxic factors such as proteases and cytokines (such as transforming growth factor-β, platelet-derived growth factor, TNF-α, and IL-1). These soluble factors can cause reversible myocardial dysfunction by interfering with function of the myocardial adrenergic β-receptor and G_i, the inhibitory protein that regulates adrenergic-receptor function.[28] Conversely, IL-12 has been shown to be protective by reducing viral replication, inflammation, and myocyte necrosis and improving survival.[29] **Cell adhesion molecules** also may contribute to the pathogenesis of myocarditis.[30] Intercellular adhesion molecule I has been discovered to promote leukocyte adherence and transendothelial migration, and its expression is up-regulated by the cytokines IL-1 and TNF-α.

Cytokine activation induces expression of **nitric oxide synthase**. In the murine CVB3 myocarditis model, nitric oxide synthase activity appears by day 4 and peaks by day 8 after virus inoculation.[31] Nitric oxide production is part of the host protective response against the virus, but also may be toxic to the myocardium by inhibiting adrenergic stimulation. The net effect of T cell amplification, cytokine activation, and nitric oxide synthase induction destroys infected and noninfected myocytes, reducing the total number of contractile units and establishing the substrate for ventricular remodeling and progression to dilated cardiomyopathy.

Phase 3: Progression to Dilated Cardiomyopathy

There is increasing evidence that viral myocarditis is the substrate for the development of many cases of dilated cardiomyopathy. Coxsackieviral protease can cleave **dystrophin**, a major component of the myocardial cytoskeleton[32] and the sarcoglycan complex in myocytes.[16,33] In CVB3 myocarditis in the mouse, viral protease 2A has been shown to cleave dystrophin, and this leads to chronic dilated cardiomyopathy (see Fig. 17-3). Defects in the dystrophin gene also have been associated with X-linked dilated cardiomyopathy.[34,35] The disruption of the dystrophin and other components of the cytoskeleton leads to ventricular dilation and remodeling and may explain partially the development of marked ventricular dilatation and dilated cardiomyopathy after viral myocarditis. It remains unclear, however, why this progression develops in some individuals and not others.

Additional factors for a prolonged state of auto-immunity may include persistence of nonreplicating coxsackievirus genome. Enteroviral RNA can be detected in 35% of patients with dilated cardiomyopathy[36] and may promote continued protease-mediated disruption of the cytoskeleton. In addition, enteroviral proteins may contribute directly to myocardial injury. Persistent interstitial inflammation leads to continual fibrosis secondary to growth factor–induced fibroblast proliferation and abnormal extracellular matrix with collagen formation.

Chronic activation of adrenergic and renin-angiotensin systems results in defective excitation-contraction coupling caused by diastolic Ca^{2+} channel leak that depletes sarcoplasmic reticulum Ca^{2+} and reduced sarcoplasmic reticulum Ca^{2+} reuptake.[37] Continued cytokine production leads to myocardial dysfunction secondary to mechanisms described previously. Lastly, the process of **apoptosis**, with its characteristic features such as chromatin aggregation, nuclear and cytoplasmic aggregation, and formation of apoptotic bodies, also is part of progression to dilated cardiomyopathy. A sustained complex interplay between the viral genome and the heart leads to ongoing changes months and years after the initial infection.

CLINICOPATHOLOGIC SUBTYPES OF MYOCARDITIS

Lieberman and colleagues[38] have proposed a clinico-pathologic classification of viral myocarditis that divides patients into four distinct subtypes based on their presenting symptoms, clinical courses, outcomes, and histologies. **Fulminant myocarditis** is characterized by a distinct, sudden onset of cardiac failure, severe left ventricular dysfunction, and cardiogenic shock. Endomyocardial biopsy reveals extensive inflammation and numerous foci of myocyte necrosis. Immunosuppression does not seem to influence the clinical outcome. Intensive cardiovascular support usually includes intravenous inotropic agents, and mechanical assist devices may be required. If patients survive the acute insult, there is a high likelihood of complete recovery. In a multi-institutional review, 3 out of 4 fulminant myocarditis patients[28] and 7 out of 15 pediatric patients who required mechanical circulatory support[39] survived with recovery of normal ventricular function.

Acute myocarditis constitutes the largest group of patients. An interstitial aggregation of mononuclear cells, including lymphocytes, plasma cells, and eosinophils, is seen frequently in early myocarditis. Necrosis of the myocardium with loss of cross-striations of the muscle fibers also can be seen, particularly with coxsackievirus. The onset of cardiac symptoms is often indistinct, and patients seem to develop a more gradual deterioration in ventricular function. Early right ventricular endomyocardial biopsy reveals active or borderline myocarditis, but inflammation is absent on subsequent biopsy specimens. Patients may undergo spontaneous recovery or may respond to immunosuppression. Alternatively, patients may develop progressive left ventricular dysfunction and dilation typical of dilated cardiomyopathy. Acute lymphocytic myocarditis without cardiac failure is an uncommon cause of sudden, nontraumatic death in young individuals. Of 1961 cases of sudden death reported in 13 published series, 5% had lymphocytic myocarditis at necropsy.[40]

Two additional infrequent chronic categories have been recognized. **Chronic active myocarditis** is characterized by indistinct onset of congestive heart failure with left ventricular dysfunction. Endomyocardial biopsy reveals active or borderline myocarditis with persistence of inflammation and occasional giant cells with extensive fibrosis on subsequent biopsy specimens. There is a slowly progressive deterioration in ventricular function. Immunosuppression does not seem to alter the overall course, although brief, unsustained improvement may be observed. **Chronic persistent myocarditis** is the final and least common category. Patients present with atypical chest pain, palpitations, and ventricular arrhythmias, but symptoms of congestive heart failure are absent. Ventricular function is generally normal. Endomyocardial biopsy reveals a lymphocytic infiltrate that persists on subsequent biopsy specimens. Patients with acute myocarditis may present with similar atypical chest pain and ventricular arrhythmias without congestive heart failure. Immunosuppressive therapy has not been shown to be useful in the management of chronic persistent myocarditis.

PATHOPHYSIOLOGY OF VENTRICULAR DYSFUNCTION IN MYOCARDITIS

The murine model of viral myocarditis caused by the encephalomyocarditis virus has allowed detailed hemodynamic measurements during the first 2 weeks after virus inoculation.[41] Three distinct clinical stages have been identified. During the first stage (days 1 to 3), systolic ventricular performance was hyperdynamic and characterized by increases in contractility, cardiac output, and end-systolic pressure. Diastolic function decreased slightly, however. The increase in ventricular function may be mediated by sympathetic activation. The most dramatic changes were observed during the second stage (days 4 to 7) and consisted of progressive,

severe depression of contractility, stroke volume, cardiac output, and chamber compliance, while marked left ventricular dilation developed, and end-diastolic pressure increased. The last stage of recovery (days 8 to 14) was characterized by significant improvements in ventricular compliance and stroke volume, but only slight recovery of contractility. The left ventricle remained markedly dilated with increased end-diastolic volume. The detailed time course provided by the murine model may serve to aid understanding of the hemodynamic alterations in human acute myocarditis in which the initial hyperdynamic phase is unlikely to be appreciated.

The myriad pathophysiologic changes observed with myocarditis can be summarized as follows: (1) Increase in sympathetic nervous system input leads to vasoconstriction and increased afterload; (2) Congestive heart failure with increased end-diastolic pressure and volume leads to pulmonary venous congestion and pulmonary edema; (3) Ventricular dilation leads to mitral annular dilation and regurgitation, which exacerbates the increased left atrial volume and pressure; and (4) Eventual fibrosis leads to scar formation and ventricular ectopy and overall decreased ventricular compliance.

CLINICAL ASPECTS OF MYOCARDITIS

Establishment of the diagnosis of myocarditis requires a broad complement of noninvasive and invasive modalities (Table 17-2).[42] The clinical history and presentation may be highly varied depending on age and subtype of myocarditis (see earlier), so a high index of suspicion is needed, especially in subclinical cases. In many patients, symptom onset may be indistinct and progress slowly over days to weeks. In others, a fulminant, rapidly progressive deterioration in cardiac output results in cardiovascular collapse and shock. Resting tachycardia is invariably present in children who are more critically ill with myocarditis. Neonates and infants may

TABLE 17-2

Diagnostic Modalities for Evaluation of Suspected Myocarditis		
Noninvasive	Serologic	Invasive
Chest radiograph	CPK-MB	Cardiac catheterization
ECG	Troponin I, T	Right ventricular endomyocardial biopsy for histology (Dallas criteria) and PCR
Echocardiogram	C-reactive protein	
MRI	BNP	
Antimyosin scintigraphy MRI	Erythrocyte sedimentation rate	
Endotracheal aspirate PCR	Tracheal aspirate for PCR	
	Viral cultures	
	Viral antibodies	
	Autoantibodies (antimyosin)	
	TNF-α	

BNP, B-type natriuretic peptide; CPK-MB, creatine phosphokinase MB fraction; PCR, polymerase chain reaction; TNF, tumor necrosis factor.

TABLE 17-3

Differential Diagnosis of Myocarditis by Age
Newborn and Infant
Sepsis
Hypoxia
Hypoglycemia
Hypocalcemia
Structural heart disease
Idiopathic dilated cardiomyopathy
Barth syndrome
Endocardial fibroelastosis
Anomalous left coronary artery from the pulmonary artery
Cerebral arteriovenous malformation
Child
Idiopathic dilated cardiomyopathy
X-linked dilated cardiomyopathy
Autosomal-dominant dilated cardiomyopathy
Anomalous left coronary artery from the pulmonary artery
Endocardial fibroelastosis
Chronic tachyarrhythmia
Pericarditis

From Towbin JA: Myocarditis. In Allen HD, Gutgesell HP, Clark EB, and Driscoll D (eds): Moss and Adams' Heart Disease in Infants, Children, and Adolescents. Philadelphia, Lippincott Williams & Wilkins, 2001.

present with fever, poor appetite, diaphoresis, lethargy, irritability, or respiratory distress, whereas older children and adolescents present with symptoms of lethargy, low-grade fever, decreased appetite, respiratory distress, syncope, or abdominal pain. A few patients may present with substernal chest pain mimicking myocardial infarction[43] or with ventricular arrhythmias. Other conditions can mimic myocarditis. Table 17-3 lists the differential diagnosis of myocarditis by age.

Clinical Evaluation

The physical examination may show a gallop rhythm with a quiet precordium. The skin often feels cool to the touch, and the pulses are thready in quality. In addition, the pansystolic murmur of mitral regurgitation often can be auscultated toward the apex. Hepatomegaly also is palpated frequently in these children.

The ECG typically shows a common constellation of findings in myocarditis with resting sinus tachycardia, low QRS voltages, and T wave flattening or inversion (Fig. 17-4). A pattern of myocardial infarction (wide Q waves and ST-segment changes) also can be observed. Bundle branch block–induced prolongation of the QRS may be evident. A widening of the QRS duration may indicate global myocardial ischemia and warrants heightened vigilance. The atrioventricular node may be involved, resulting in prolongation of atrioventricular conduction and leading to heart block varying from first degree to third degree in 20% of patients, with return of atrioventricular conduction within 7 days in 67% of patients who had advanced atrioventricular block.[44] Supraventricular tachycardia, including atrial ectopic tachycardia and atrial fibrillation/flutter,[45] can occur, so special attention to P waves and the axis should be made. Ventricular ectopy, including bigeminy, trigeminy, nonsustained ventricular tachycardia, or sustained ventricular tachycardia, may be an ominous warning for sudden death.[40] Any sudden onset of arrhythmias in a child with no prior history of dysrhythmias, especially

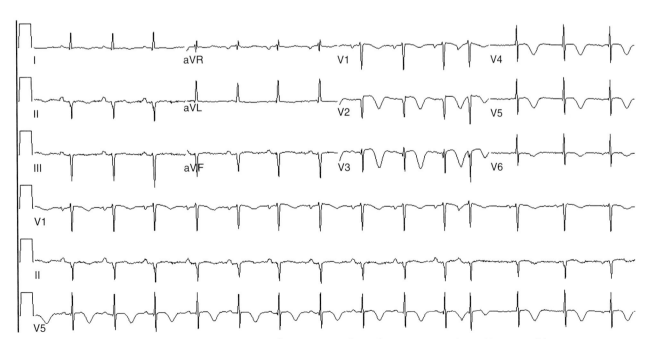

FIGURE 17-4 ■ ECG in a patient with acute myocarditis. The ECG in a patient with myocarditis shows resting tachycardia with low QRS voltages and T wave flattening/inversions. In some cases, ST-segment changes also can be seen.

ventricular in nature, should raise suspicion for myocarditis.[46]

The chest radiograph may show cardiomegaly, pulmonary venous engorgement, and pulmonary edema in patients with acute myocarditis. Increased heart size may not be present, however, particularly in patients with a fulminant onset or with only ventricular arrhythmias.

Echocardiography is the most useful noninvasive diagnostic modality. Evidence of severe left ventricular dysfunction and decreased shortening and ejection fractions is present in most patients, even patients in whom the left ventricle is not dilated and the heart size is not enlarged on chest radiography. Left ventricular function may be normal, however, in patients presenting only with ventricular ectopy. Segmental dyskinesis is common. As a result of the left ventricular and annular dilation, mitral regurgitation is frequently noted. Pericardial effusion also can be seen in some patients with myocarditis. If left ventricular dilation and dysfunction are present, careful examination of the entire endocardial surface of the left ventricle should be performed to search for mural thrombus. Finally, it is important to identify the origins of the right and left coronary arteries, particularly in infants and young children, to exclude the diagnosis of anomalous origin of the left coronary artery from the pulmonary artery. There also is some evidence that noninvasive screening with MRI may help to select a group of patients with myocarditis.[47]

Blood tests (e.g., complete blood count, erythrocyte sedimentation rate, and other chemistry profiles) usually are not helpful to confirm the diagnosis of myocarditis, but the presence of a low serum bicarbonate and an elevated serum creatinine can be ominous predictors for impending cardiovascular collapse. Serologic markers of myocardial injury frequently are elevated, including creatinine phosphokinase MB fraction, troponin I,[48] and C-reactive protein,[49] and may be followed serially to assess ongoing inflammation and injury. Increased levels of autoantibodies against myosin and the adenine nucleotide translocator protein have been reported in myocarditis and correlate with progressive worsening of ventricular function.[50,51]

Cardiac catheterization often shows diminished cardiac output with elevated end-diastolic pressures and pulmonary artery pressures. Right ventricular endomyocardial biopsy using the Dallas criteria for histologic classification continues to be the "gold standard" for the diagnosis of myocarditis, although there are limitations to this as a diagnostic criterion for myocarditis.[52] The Dallas criteria emphasize the significance of myocyte necrosis or vacuolization that is manifested by histologic findings of cellular disintegration with lymphocytes and sarcolemma with the presence of macrophages (Fig. 17-5).[53] First biopsy samples are classified as (1) myocarditis with or without fibrosis, (2) borderline myocarditis, and (3) no myocarditis.

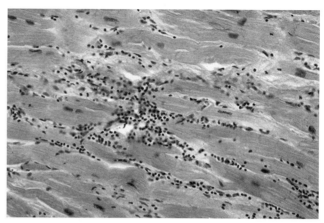

FIGURE 17-5 ■ **Histology of acute myocarditis from right ventricular endomyocardial biopsy.** There is an extensive lymphocytic interstitial infiltrate in association with injured and necrotic myocytes. (From Webpath, with the permission of Edward C. Klatt, MD, Florida State University College of Medicine, Tallahassee, Fla.)

Subsequent biopsy samples have a different classification scheme (ongoing, resolving, and resolved myocarditis with or without fibrosis). Biopsy is valuable in differentiating acute myocarditis from dilated cardiomyopathy for treatment and prognosis. Confirmation of myocarditis permits immunosuppressive therapy to be used appropriately. The chance of complete recovery of ventricular function is much greater for acute myocarditis than dilated cardiomyopathy; this is particularly important for patients with a fulminant presentation in whom continued inotropic or mechanical support is warranted, rather than premature listing for cardiac transplantation. Meticulous attention to technique is essential, however, particularly in young myocarditis patients receiving inotropic support in which the risk of biopsy-related perforation may be increased.[54] Some cardiologists also advocate the use of biopsy samples from other sites in the heart, such as the left ventricle. Lastly, the use of immunocytochemical techniques employing monoclonal antibodies may be valuable in differentiating the different types of lymphocytes found in the myocardium (the suppressor/cytotoxic lymphocyte is more predominant in active myocarditis). Expression of TNF-α in the myocardium may be prognostic in patients with myocarditis.[55]

Improvement in diagnostic accuracy can be achieved by using immunohistochemical markers for lymphocytes and applying PCR techniques (Fig. 17-6) to detect the presence of a viral genome (e.g., enteroviruses, adenovirus, cytomegalovirus, parvovirus, respiratory syncytial virus, Epstein-Barr virus, herpes simplex virus, and influenza A virus) in the biopsy specimen.[56-58] In view of the inherent risks of endomyocardial biopsy, PCR has been applied to other, more readily obtained specimens. Although blood PCR rarely has been useful in identifying viral RNA, endotracheal aspirates obtained in intubated patients have correlated highly

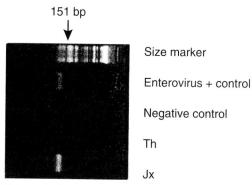

151 bp

Size marker

Enterovirus + control

Negative control

Th

Jx

FIGURE 17-6 ■ Polymerase chain reaction (PCR) for enterovirus. This PCR amplification process identifies specific portions of a viral genome and is a sensitive and specific test. The 151-bp band on the agarose gel shown here is a PCR-positive band for the enterovirus + control and for patient Jx. The negative control and patient Th are devoid of any band. (From Towbin JA: Myocarditis. In Allen HD, Gutgesell HP, Clark EB, and Driscoll D: [eds]: Moss and Adams' Heart Disease in Infants, Children, and Adolescents. Philadelphia, Lippincott Williams & Wilkins, 2001.)

with PCR analysis of endomyocardial biopsy specimens.[59] PCR of tracheal aspirates in intubated patients should be considered strongly in the diagnostic evaluation of myocarditis.

Using immunohistochemistry and PCR as adjuncts to the standard Dallas criteria, the European Study of Epidemiology and Treatment of Inflammatory Heart Disease reported a 17% prevalence of inflammation, whereas virus was detected in only 11% of adults with clinically suspected myocarditis.[60] Endomyocardial biopsy in children with suspected myocarditis showed histology compatible with myocarditis in 20% (8 of 41).[61] Viral genomes in another series were found by PCR in 46% (12 of 26) of children with a clinical diagnosis of myocarditis.[62] Antimyosin scintigraphy can identify myocardial inflammation with high sensitivity, but has low specificity; it may be useful in selecting individuals more likely to have a positive endomyocardial biopsy.

Therapeutic Strategies

The first line of treatment of myocarditis is the management of heart failure and hemodynamic instability. Patients with mild-to-moderate cardiac failure should be treated with conventional pharmacologic agents, including diuretics, angiotensin-converting enzyme inhibitors, and digoxin. Captopril may have a selective advantage over other angiotensin-converting enzyme inhibitors because of its ability to act as an oxygen-free radical scavenger and lessen ongoing myocardial injury.[63] Digoxin should be used with caution and in low dosage and without a loading dose in view of increased expression of inflammatory cytokines and mortality in murine myocarditis treated with high-dose digitalis.[64] Anticoagulation with aspirin, warfarin, or intravenous heparin may be used to prevent mural thrombus formation when the left ventricle is markedly dilated, and contractile function is severely depressed.

After stabilization, β-adrenergic antagonists, such as carvedilol may be introduced cautiously and titrated up over 6 to 8 weeks (see Chapter 36). β Blockade in general, and carvedilol in particular, reduces mortality and improves left ventricular ejection fraction in chronic heart failure. β-Antagonists are contraindicated, however, in patients with acute, severe cardiac failure, particularly if inotropic agents are required. Circulating catecholamines influence the production of cytokines through β-receptor stimulation. Carvedilol has been shown to reduce myocardial injury and mortality in murine myocarditis possibly by increasing the production of IL-12 and interferon,[65] allowing the activated immune system to return to the resting state.

Ventricular ectopy is common and should be treated aggressively with intravenous lidocaine. Intravenous amiodarone also may be used to treat high-grade ventricular ectopy, although it has potential for drug-related hypotension. Patients with ventricular arrhythmias often need longer term therapy and require close surveillance indefinitely.[66] Temporary transvenous pacing may be initiated for patients with complete heart block; great care must be exercised, however, because of the increased risk of electrode perforation of inflamed myocardium.

Extracardiac issues are important to manage in patients with myocarditis. Assisted ventilation along with continuous positive airway pressure relieves the excess work of breathing, improves pulmonary edema and oxygenation, and may exert a beneficial effect on left ventricular afterload.[67] In the setting of low cardiac output, severe ventricular dysfunction, and absence of cardiac reserve, the sedation needed for endotracheal intubation may precipitate further decompensation, however, and lead to cardiac arrest. Additional extracardiac issues involve central nervous system conditions, such as cerebral thromboemboli or encephalitis, and other organ system conditions, such as acute renal failure or hepatitis.

Patients with fulminant myocarditis and cardiogenic shock require aggressive intervention to support circulation (see Chapter 37). Filling pressure should be adequate to maintain cardiac output and may need to be at a level greater than 10 mm Hg. Intravenous inotropic agents should be initiated as soon as possible, but excessively high doses are to be avoided given the propensity of an inflamed myocardium to have arrhythmias. When low cardiac output and elevated systemic vascular resistance are present, a phosphodiesterase inhibitor, such as milrinone, should be considered. Milrinone has the advantages that it does not increase myocardial oxygen consumption (as it does not increase heart rate) and improves diastolic properties of the heart (lusitropy).

Mechanical circulatory support with extracorporeal membrane oxygenation or ventricular assist devices may be lifesaving in patients with fulminant myocarditis in whom inotropic agents are ineffective in maintaining adequate cardiac output. Diagnostic catheterization can be performed while on mechanical support in these children.[68] In a retrospective, multicenter review, Duncan and associates[39] reported 80% survival (12 of 15) in children receiving mechanical support. Of these patients, 60% (9 of 15) were weaned successfully from mechanical support with 7 long-term survivors; all 7 ultimately recovered normal ventricular function. The remaining six patients were bridged to transplantation. Circulatory support with mechanical assist devices is justified for acute, fulminant myocarditis with excellent prospects for recovery of ventricular function; it is underused as a therapy in these children (see Chapters 45-47).

Immunosuppression for the treatment of acute myocarditis is controversial. Immunosuppressive agents, administered early in the course of murine myocarditis, increase viral replication, myocellular necrosis, and mortality.[69,70] If there is a role for immunosuppression, it should be initiated only during the autoimmune phase of the disease process. In contrast, intravenous immunoglobulin (IVIG) improves the outcome of murine myocarditis by reducing myocellular necrosis, plasma catecholamines, and interferon-γ. It also may contain neutralizing antibodies to the causative virus.[71,72] The utility of IVIG may be limited in the clinical setting, however, because few patients present during the initial viral phase when IVIG may be most useful. In a retrospective, case-controlled study of children with recent-onset cardiac failure from left ventricular dysfunction, IVIG seemed to increase the probability of return to normal ventricular function, but had no improvement in survival.[73] More recently, a prospective, randomized, placebo-controlled trial was conducted to evaluate whether IVIG improves left ventricular ejection fraction in adults with recent-onset dilated cardiomyopathy and myocarditis.[74] Significant improvement in left ventricular ejection fraction was noted at 1 year, but there was no difference between the placebo- and IVIG-treated patients.

There have been numerous, small, nonrandomized studies of immunosuppression for myocarditis that have reported conflicting positive and negative results. Agents used have included prednisone, cyclophosphamide, cyclosporine, azathioprine, and OKT3. The U.S. Myocarditis Treatment Trial randomized adults with biopsy-proven myocarditis to conventional therapy alone or an immunosuppression regimen of steroids with azathioprine or cyclosporine.[75] Control and immunosuppressed patients had similar recovery of left ventricular function with no difference in overall mortality. A retrospective review of biopsy-proven myocarditis in children treated by steroids with or without IVIG or conventional therapy alone showed no significant difference in recovery of ventricular function or survival.[76] In addition, immunosuppressive therapy with azathioprine or cyclosporine associated with prednisone improved the prognosis of children with active myocarditis.[77,78] Steroid treatment seems to benefit a subset of children with ventricular ectopic rhythm and myocarditis.[79] Immunosuppression with OKT3 has been reported to improve ventricular function in pediatric myocarditis.[80] As in most of the other reported series, the findings are limited by the lack of randomized controls and the small cohort.

Despite the absence of valid outcome data, most pediatric cardiologists report using some form of immunomodulation in the management of myocarditis patients. In a survey of pediatric cardiologists in North America in 2000, 92% of respondents used immunomodulatory agents. Of these, 43% used IVIG alone (2 g/kg), 13% used steroids only (for 1 to 6 months), and 44% combined IVIG with steroids. In the absence of large, randomized, placebo-controlled trials of biopsy-proven (or other PCR-positive evidence) acute viral myocarditis, the potential for benefits from IVIG and immunosuppression remains uncertain.

OUTCOME IN PATIENTS WITH MYOCARDITIS

The outcome for all forms of myocarditis is difficult to discern because it is likely that a significant number of cases are subclinical and never come to medical attention, whereas others are identified at necropsy as the cause of sudden unexpected death. Conventional estimates are that one third of patients with acute myocarditis undergo complete recovery; one third improve clinically, but have persistent ventricular dysfunction; and one third develop chronic cardiac failure, leading to death or transplantation. Outcomes may be better estimated, however, according to the clinicopathologic group. More recent data suggest better outcomes with freedom from death or cardiac transplantation of 79% after 2 years.[81]

Survival of 132 adults with biopsy-proven acute myocarditis was 45% at 11 years, but was 93% in 15 patients with fulminant myocarditis.[82] Encouraging results also were noted in children undergoing mechanical support for fulminant myocarditis.[39] Overall survival in this critically ill population was 80%. Conversely the prognosis in giant cell myocarditis is especially poor, with a 70% 1-year mortality or need for transplantation.[83] Survival of acute myocarditis in neonates also remains poor.

CURRENT STATUS AND FUTURE TRENDS

The focus for the future needs to be on improved diagnostic capabilities and strategies to prevent and treat myocarditis better. The low yield of positive results from current endomyocardial biopsy methods mandates that new noninvasive imaging and molecular diagnostic techniques, such as reverse transcription PCR,[84] are developed to reduce reliance on tissue diagnosis using endomyocardial biopsy. Increasing availability of DNA microarrays is helpful in the understanding of the complex host-viral interactions.[85] Preventive strategies incorporating immunization against CVB3 and cardiotropic strains of adenovirus should be explored. Mumps virus, eradicated with vaccines, was proved to be the etiologic agent in 90% of myocardial specimens from endocardial fibroelastosis patients.[86]

The coxsackie-adenovirus receptor, so vital for myocyte attachment and internalization of virus, is a potential target for therapeutic intervention. Antiviral therapy in general is unlikely to be useful, however, because most acute myocarditis patients present after the viral replication phase has passed. Persistence of the viral genome into the dilated cardiomyopathy phase may allow for strategies to target selectively noninfectious transcriptional expression.[1,87] Modulation of inflammatory cytokines may mitigate the deleterious effects of inflammation on the myocardium after the initial phase. Interferon-γ and IL-12 have been shown to suppress inflammation without altering viral replication in murine myocarditis.[88] At present, no anticytokine regimens have been reported in human myocarditis, but future therapy could include a molecular cocktail or gene therapy to modulate the inflammatory cascade.[89]

Key Concepts

■ Myocarditis is defined as inflammation of the myocardium in association with nonischemic myocellular necrosis. The incidence of myocarditis is difficult to ascertain because of the varied clinical expression, ranging from absent or minimal symptoms to cardiogenic shock and death.

■ Three interrelated mechanisms result in myocardial injury from the aforementioned infectious agents, including direct invasion of the myocardial cells, production of a myocardial toxin, and immune-mediated myocardial damage. The immunologically mediated changes led by T lymphocytes and macrophages are the predominant mechanisms that result in myocardial injury.

■ The net effect of T cell amplification, cytokine activation, and nitric oxide synthase induction destroys infected and noninfected myocytes, reducing the total number of contractile units and establishing the substrate for ventricular remodeling and progression to dilated cardiomyopathy.

■ The disruption of the dystrophin and other components of the cytoskeleton leads to ventricular dilation and remodeling and may explain partially the development of marked ventricular dilatation and dilated cardiomyopathy after viral myocarditis.

■ The myriad pathophysiologic changes observed with myocarditis can be summarized as follows: (1) Increase in sympathetic nervous system input leads to vaso-constriction and increased afterload; (2) Congestive heart failure with increased end-diastolic pressure and volume leads to pulmonary venous congestion and pulmonary edema; (3) Ventricular dilation leads to mitral annular dilation and regurgitation, which exacerbates the increased left atrial volume and pressure; and (4) Eventual fibrosis leads to scar formation and ventricular ectopy and overall decreased ventricular compliance.

■ Circulatory support with mechanical assist devices is justified for acute, fulminant myocarditis with excellent prospects for recovery of ventricular function; it is underused as a therapy in these children.

■ In the absence of large, randomized, placebo-controlled trials of biopsy-proven (or other PCR-positive evidence) acute viral myocarditis, the potential for benefits from IVIG and immunosuppression is uncertain.

REFERENCES

1. Liu PP, Mason JW: Advances in the understanding of myocarditis. Circulation 2001;104:1076-1082.
2. Bowles NE, Towbin JA: Molecular aspects of myocarditis. Curr Opin Cardiol 1998;13:179-184.
3. Aretz HT: Myocarditis: The Dallas criteria. Hum Pathol 1987;18:619-624.
4. Karjalainen J, Heikkila J: Incidence of three presentations of acute myocarditis in young men in military service: A 20-year experience. Eur Heart J 1999;20:1120-1125.
5. Wakafuji S, Okada R: Twenty year autopsy statistics of myocarditis incidence in Japan. Jpn Circ J 1986;50:1288-1293.
6. McCarthy RE, Boehmer JP, Hruban RH, et al: Long term outcome of fulminant myocarditis as compared with acute (nonfulminant) myocarditis. N Engl J Med 2000;342:690-695.
7. Kaplan MH: Coxsackievirus infection in children under three months of age. In Bendinelli M, Friedman H (eds): Coxsackieviruses: A General Update. New York, Plenum Press, 1988, pp 221-240.
8. Kandolf R, Ameis D, Kirschener P, et al: In situ detection of enteroviral genomes in myocardial cells by nucleic acid hybridization: An approach to the diagnosis of viral heart disease. Proc Natl Acad Sci U S A 1987;84:6272-6276.
9. Martin AB, Webber S, Fricker FJ, et al: Acute myocarditis: Rapid diagnosis by PCR in children. Circulation 1994;90:330-339.
10. Bowles NE, Jiyuan N, Kearney DL, et al: Detection of viruses in myocardial tissues by polymerase chain reaction: Evidence of adenovirus as a common cause of myocarditis in children and adults. J Am Coll Cardiol 2003;42:466-472.
11. Matsumori A, Yutani C, Ikeda Y, et al: Hepatitis C virus from the hearts of patients with myocarditis and cardiomyopathy. Lab Invest 2000;80:1137-1142.
12. Schowengerdt KO, Ni J, Denfield SW, et al: Association of parvovirus B19 genome in children with myocarditis and cardiac allograft rejection: Diagnosis using the polymerase chain reaction. Circulation 1997;96:3549-3554.
13. Barbaro G, Di Lorenzo G, Grisorio B, et al: Incidence of dilated cardiomyopathy and detection of HIV in myocardial cells of HIV-positive patients. N Engl J Med 1998;330:1093-1099.
14. Saltzberg MT: Secondary and infiltrative cardiomyopathies. Curr Treat Options Cardiovasc Med 2000;2:373-384.
15. Virmani R, Burke AP: Infective disease of the myocardium. In Narula J, Virmani R, Ballester M, et al (eds): Heart Failure: Pathogenesis and Treatment. London, Martin Dunitz, 2002, pp. 403-422.

16. Lange LG, Schreiner GF: Immune mechanisms of cardiac disease. N Engl J Med 1994;330:1129-1135.

17. Bergelson JM, Cunningham JA, Droguett G, et al: Isolation of a common receptor for coxsackie B viruses and adenoviruses 2 and 5. Science 1997;275:1320-1323.

18. Martino T, Petric M, Weingart H, et al: The coxsackie-adenovirus receptor (CAR) is used by reference strains and clinical isolates representing all 6 serotypes of coxsackievirus group B, and by swine vesicular disease virus. J Virol 2000;271:99-108.

19. Bowles KR, Gibson J, Wu J, et al: Genomic organization and chromosomal localization of the human coxsackievirus B-adenovirus receptor gene. Hum Genet 1999;105:354-359.

20. Bowles N, Towbin J: Molecular aspects of myocarditis. Curr Infect Dis Rep 2000;2:308-314.

21. Caforia ALP, Grazzini M, Mann JM, et al: Identification of alpha and beta-cardiac myosin heavy chain isoforms as major autoantigens in dilated cardiomyopathy. Circulation 1992;85:1734-1742.

22. Schulze K, Becker BF, Schauer R, et al: Antibodies to ADP-ATP carrier—an autoantigen in myocarditis and dilated cardiomyopathy—impair cardiac function. Circulation 1990;81:959-969.

23. Reeto KN, Osman SA, Illavia SJ, et al: Quantitative analysis of viral RNA kinetics in coxsackievirus B induced murine myocarditis: Biphasic pattern of clearance following acute infection, with persistence of residual viral RNA throughout and beyond the inflammatory phase of disease. J Gen Virol 2000;81:2755-2762.

24. Woodruff JF: Viral myocarditis: A review. Am J Pathol 1980;101:427-484.

25. Satoh M, Tamura G, Segawa I, et al: Expression of cytokine genes and presence of enteroviral genomic RNA in endomyocardial biopsy tissues of myocarditis and dilated cardiomyopathy. Virchows Arch 1996;427:503-509.

26. Matsumori A, Yamada T, Suzuki H, et al: Increased circulating cytokines in patients with myocarditis and cardiomyopathy. Br Heart J 1994;72:561-566.

27. Bryant D, Becker L, Richardson J, et al: Cardiac failure in transgenic mice with myocardial expression of tumor necrosis factor-alpha. Circulation 1998;97:1375-1381.

28. Wiechmann RJ, Wollmering M, Bristow MR: IL-1 Inhibits β-adrenergic responsiveness in intact human ventricular myocardium (abstract). J Am Coll Cardiol 1991;17(Suppl A):57A.

29. Shoi T, Matsumori A, Nishio R, et al: Protective role of interleukin-12 on viral myocarditis. J Med Cell Cardiol 1997;29:2327-2334.

30. Springer TA: Adhesion receptors of the immune system. Nature 1990;346:425-434.

31. Mikami S, Kawashima S, Kanazawa K, et al: Expression of nitric oxide synthase in a murine model of viral myocarditis induced by coxsackievirus B3. Biochem Biophys Res Commun 1996;220:983-989.

32. Badorff C, Lee GH, Lamphear BJ, et al: Enteroviral protease 2A cleaves dystrophin: evidence of cytoskeletal disruption in acquired cardiomyopathy. Nat Med 1999;5:320-326.

33. Lee GH, Badorff C, Knowlton K: Dissociation of sarcoglycans and the dystrophin carboxyl terminus from the sarcolemma in enteroviral cardiomyopathy. Circ Res 2000;87:489-495.

34. Towbin JA, Hejtmancik JF, Brink P, et al: X-linked dilated cardiomyopathy (XLCM): Molecular genetic evidence of linkage to the Duchenne muscular dystrophy gene at the Xp21 locus. Circulation 1993;87:1854-1865.

35. Xiong D, Lee GH, Badorff C, et al: Dystrophin deficiency markedly increases enterovirus-induced cardiomyopathy: A genetic predisposition to viral heart disease. Nat Med 2002;8:872-877.

36. Fujioka S, Kitaura Y, Ukimura A, et al: Evaluation of viral infection in the myocardium of patients with idiopathic dilated cardiomyopathy. J Am Coll Cardiol 2000;36:1920-1926.

37. Marks AR: A guide for the perplexed: Towards an understanding of the molecular basis of heart failure. Circulation 2003;107:1456-1459.

38. Lieberman EB, Grover HM, Herskowitz A, et al: Clinicopathologic description of myocarditis. J Am Coll Cardiol 1991;18:1617-1626.

39. Duncan BW, Bohn DJ, Atz AM, et al: Mechanical circulatory support for the treatment of children with acute fulminant myocarditis. J Thorac Cardiovasc Surg 2001;122:440-448.

40. Theleman KP, Kuiper JJ, Roberts WC: Acute myocarditis (predominantly lymphocytic) causing sudden death without heart failure. Am J Cardiol 2001;88:1078-1083.

41. Nishio R, Sasayama S, Matsumori A: Left ventricular pressure-volume relationship in a murine model of congestive heart failure due to acute viral myocarditis. J Am Coll Cardiol 2002;40:1506-1514.

42. Batra AJ, Lewis AB: Acute myocarditis. Curr Opin Pediatr 2001;13:234-239.

43. Angelini A, Calzolari V, Calabrese F, et al: Myocarditis mimicking acute myocardial infarction: Role of endomyocardial biopsy in the differential diagnosis. Heart 2000;84:245-250.

44. Batra AS, Epstein D, Silka MJ: The clinical course of acquired complete heart block in children with acute myocarditis. Pediatr Cardiol 2002;24:495-497.

45. Shah SS, Hellenbrand WE, Gallagher PG: Atrial flutter complicating neonatal coxsackie B2 myocarditis. Pediatr Cardiol 1998;19:185-186.

46. Ino T, Okubo M, Akimoto K, et al: Corticosteroid therapy for ventricular tachycardia in children with silent lymphocytic myocarditis. J Pediatr 1995;126:304-308.

47. Gagliardi MG, Bevilacqua M, DiRenzi P, et al: Usefulness of magnetic resonance imaging for diagnosis of acute myocarditis in infants and children, and comparison with endomyocardial biopsy. Am J Cardiol 1991;68:1089-1091.

48. Briassoulis G, Papadopoulos G, Zavras N, et al: Cardiac troponin I in fulminant adenovirus myocarditis treated with a 24-hour infusion of high-dose intravenous immunoglobulin. Pediatr Cardiol 2000;21:391-394.

49. Kaneko K, Kanda T, Hasegawa A, et al: C-reactive protein as a prognostic marker in lymphocytic myocarditis. Jpn Heart J 2000;41:41-47.

50. Lauer B, Schannwell M, Kuhl U, et al: Antimyosin autoantibodies are associated with deterioration of systolic and diastolic left ventricular function in patients with chronic myocarditis. J Am Coll Cardiol 2000;35:11-18.

51. Schultheiss HP, Schulze K, Domer A: Significance of the adenine nucleotide translocator in the pathogenesis of viral heart disease. Mol Cell Biochem 1996;163/164:319-327.

52. Webber SA, Boyle GJ, Jaffe R, et al: Role of right ventricular endomyocardial biopsy in infants and children with suspected or possible myocarditis. Br Heart J 1994;72:360-363.

53. Aretz H, Billingham M, Edwards W, et al: Myocarditis: A histologic definition and classification. Am J Cardiovasc Pathol 1987;1:3-14.

54. Pophal SG, Sigfusson G, Booth KL, et al: Complications of endomyocardial biopsy in children. J Am Coll Cardiol 1999;34:2105-2110.

55. Jibiki T, Terai M, Tateno S, et al: Expression of tumor necrosis factor-alpha protein in the myocardium in fatal myocarditis. Pediatr Int 2000;42:43-47.

56. Martin AB, Webber S, Fricker FJ, et al: Acute myocarditis: Rapid diagnosis by PCR in children. Circulation 1994;90:330-333.

57. Bowles NF, Richardson PJ, Olsen EGJ, Archard LC: Detection of coxsackie-B-virus specific RNA sequences in myocardial biopsy samples from patients with myocarditis and dilated cardiomyopathy. Lancet 1986;1:1120-1122.

58. Bowles NE, Ni J, Kearney DL, et al: Detection of viruses in myocardial tissues by polymerase chain reaction: Evidence of adenovirus as a common cause of myocarditis in children and adults. J Am Coll Cardiol 2003;42:466-472.

59. Akhtar N, Ni J, Stromberg D, et al: Tracheal aspirate as a substrate for polymerase chain reaction of viral genome in childhood pneumonia and myocarditis. Circulation 1999;99:2011-2018.

60. Hufnagal G, Pankuweit S, Richter A, et al: The European Study of Epidemiology and Treatment of Cardiac Inflammatory Diseases (ESETCID): First epidemiological result. Herz 2000;25: 279-285.

61. Webber SA, Boyle GJ, Jaffe R, et al: Role of right ventricular endomyocardial biopsy in infants and children with suspected or possible myocarditis. Br Heart J 1994;72:360-363.

62. Calabrese F, Rigo E, Milanesi O, et al: Molecular diagnosis of myocarditis and dilated cardiomyopathy in children: Clinicopathologic features and prognostic implications. Diagn Mol Pathol 2002;11:212-221.

63. Rezkalla S, Kloner RA, Khatib G, Khatib R: Beneficial effects of captopril in acute coxsackievirus B3 murine myocarditis. Circulation 1990;81:1039-1046.

64. Matsumori A, Igata H, Ono K, et al: High doses of digitalis increase the myocardial production of proinflammatory cytokines and worsen myocardial injury in viral myocarditis: A possible mechanism of digitalis toxicity. Jpn Circ 1999;63:934-940.

65. Nishio R, Shioi T, Sasayama S, Matsumori A: Carvedilol increases the production of interleukin-12 and interferon-gamma and improves the survival of mice infected with encephalomyocarditis virus. J Am Coll Cardiol 2003;41:340-345.

66. Friedman RA, Kearney DL, Moak JP, et al: Persistence of ventricular arrhythmias after resolution of occult myocarditis in children and young adults. J Am Coll Cardiol 1994;24:780-783.

67. Shekerdemian L, Bohn D: Cardiovascular effects of mechanical ventilation. Arch Dis Child 1999;80:475-480.

68. Booth KL, Roth SJ, Perry SB, et al: Cardiac catheterization of patients supported by extracorporeal membrane oxygenation. J Am Coll Cardiol 2002;40:1681-1686.

69. Estrin M, Herzum M, Buie C, Huber SA: Immunosuppressives in murine myocarditis. Eur Heart J 1987;8(Suppl J):259-262.

70. Tomioka N, Kishimoto C, Matsumori A, Kawai C: Effects of prednisolone on acute viral myocarditis in mice. J Am Coll Cardiol 1986;7:868-872.

71. Kishimoto C, Takamatsu N, Kawamata H, et al: Immunoglobulin treatment ameliorates murine myocarditis associated with reduction of neurohumoral activity and improvement of extracellular matrix change. J Am Coll Cardiol 2000;36:1979-1984.

72. Weller AH, Hall M, Huber SA: Polyclonal immunoglobulin therapy protects against cardiac damage in experimental coxsackievirus-induced myocarditis. Eur Heart J 1992;13:115-119.

73. Drucker N, Colan S, Lewis AB, et al: Gamma globulin treatment of acute myocarditis in the pediatric population. Circulation 1994;89:252-257.

74. McNamara DM, Holubkov R, Starling RC, et al: Controlled trial of intravenous immune globulin in recent-onset dilated cardiomyopathy. Circulation 2001;103:2254-2259.

75. Mason JW, O'Connell JB, Herskowitz A, et al: A clinical trial of immunosuppressive therapy for myocarditis. N Engl J Med 1995;333:269-275.

76. English RF, Webber SA: Outcomes of pediatric acute myocarditis. J Am Coll Cardiol 2003;41(Suppl A):491A.

77. Kleinert S, Weintraub RG, Wilkinson JL, et al: Myocarditis in children with dilated cardiomyopathy: Incidence and outcome after dual therapy immunosuppression. J Heart Lung Transplant 1997;16:1248-1252.

78. Camargo PR, Snitcowsky R, da Luz PL, et al: Favorable effects of immunosuppressive therapy in children with dilated cardiomyopathy and active myocarditis. Pediatr Cardiol 1995;16:61-68.

79. Balaji S, Wiles HB, Sens MA, et al: Immunosuppressive treatment for myocarditis and borderline myocarditis in children with ventricular ectopic rhythm. Br Heart J 1994;72:354-359.

80. Ahdoot J, Galindo A, Alejos JC, et al: Use of OKT3 for acute myocarditis in infants and children. J Heart Lung Transplant 2000;19:1118-1121.

81. Lee KJ, McCrindle BW, Bohn DJ, et al: Clinical outcomes of acute myocarditis in childhood. Heart 1999;82:226-233.

82. McCarthy RE, Boehmer JP, Hruban RH, et al: Long term outcome of fulminant myocarditis as compared with acute (nonfulminant) myocarditis. N Engl J Med 2000;342:690-695.

83. Cooper LT Jr: Giant cell myocarditis: Diagnosis and treatment. Herz 2000;25:291-298.

84. Bendig JW, Franklin OM, Hebden AK, et al: Coxsackie B3 sequences in the blood of a neonate with congenital myocarditis, plus serological evidence of maternal infection. J Med Virol 2003;70:606-609.

85. Taylor LA, Carthy CM, Yang D: Host gene regulation during coxsackievirus B3 infection in mice: Assessment by microarrays. Circ Res 2000;87:328-334.

86. Ni J, Bowles NE, Kim Y-H, et al: Viral infection of the myocardium in endocardial fibroelastosis: Molecular evidence for the role of mumps virus as an etiological agent. Circulation 1997;95:133-139.

87. Wessely R, Klingel K, Santana LF, et al: Transgenic expression of replication-restricted enteroviral genomes in heart muscle induces defective excitation-contraction coupling and dilated cardiomyopathy. J Clin Invest 1998;102:1444-1453.

88. Nishio R, Matsumori A, Shioi T, et al: Treatment of experimental viral myocarditis with interleukin-10. Circulation 1999;100:1102-1108.

89. Liu H, Hanawa H, Yoshida T, et al: Effect of hydrodynamics-based gene delivery of plasmid DNA encoding interleukin-1 receptor antagonist-Ig for treatment of rat autoimmune myocarditis: Possible mechanism for lymphocytes and noncardiac cells. Circulation 2005;111:1593-1600.

CHAPTER 18

Dilated Cardiomyopathy

Gul H. Dadlani
William G. Harmon
Steven E. Lipshultz

The epidemiology of pediatric cardiomyopathy was investigated in two large, multicenter studies in the United States and Australia.[1,2] These studies reported an annual incidence of all cases of pediatric cardiomyopathy to be between 1.13 and 1.24 cases per 100,000 children. Dilated cardiomyopathy (DCM) accounted for most cases (51% to 58%), and hypertrophic cardiomyopathy (HCM) was identified in 25% to 42% of patients, with the remaining cases classified as restrictive or unspecified disease.[1-3] Risk factors for the development of pediatric cardiomyopathy included age, gender, race, ethnic background, and the presence of an affected family member.[3]

More than 50% of pediatric cardiomyopathy cases are children younger than 1 year old.[1-3] This early incidence may represent the effects of genetic defects on critical intracellular pathways. The incidence peaks again in adolescence. Lower socioeconomic status is associated with a higher incidence of cardiomyopathy. These data suggest that genetic and environmental factors increase the risk of cardiomyopathy. Boys have a higher incidence as a result of an X-linked expression of cardiomyopathy, as seen with mutations in the dystrophin and taffazin genes in Duchenne and Becker muscular dystrophies. In addition, the presence of a family member with a cardiomyopathy increases the incidence for all first-degree relatives: 9% to 20% of cardiomyopathies are inherited.[3]

DCM is a heterogeneous group of myocardial disorders that results in ventricular dilation and impaired systolic contractile function. Myocardial function requires a delicate intracellular and extracellular balance to maintain optimal cardiac output. Clinical manifestations in children vary from asymptomatic left ventricular dysfunction to florid congestive heart failure (CHF). Dysfunction of the myocyte may occur at many levels and can be attributed to primary genetically transmitted disorders that intrinsically affect the myocyte or to secondary extracellular injuries from myriad sources. Hypoxic events, infections, environmental or toxin exposures, autoimmune reactions, arrhythmias, nutritional deficiencies, and abnormal autonomic responses are only a few examples of disease processes implicated in the development of DCM. Regardless of the exact mechanism, myocardial injury and myocyte loss beyond a critical

point result in varying degrees of ventricular dysfunction. This chapter focuses on the pathophysiology, evaluation, and management of DCM.

MOLECULAR AND PATHOPHYSIOLOGIC BASIS OF DILATED CARDIOMYOPATHY

DCM is a complex disorder that requires an understanding of myocyte biology, macroscopic myocardial structure and function, and the neurohumoral compensatory mechanisms seen in heart failure. These topics are discussed in other chapters and are not addressed in detail in this chapter. Briefly, cardiac myocytes are composed of myofibrils containing contractile proteins longitudinally arranged into units called **sarcomeres**. Each sarcomere is composed of specialized contractile (myosin, actin, troponin, and tropomyosin) and other cytoskeletal proteins (dystrophin, desmin, taffazin, lamin A/C, titin) that interact to produce myocyte contraction. The myocyte cell membrane, or **sarcolemma**, has deep invaginations (T tubules), which allow for the rapid spread of action potentials and the inflow of extracellular calcium into the intracellular space. Extracellular calcium inflow stimulates the release of intracellular calcium from the sarcoplasmic reticulum. The **sarcoplasmic reticulum** is an intracellular network of fine tubules that surrounds the myofibrils and regulates intracellular calcium concentrations.

Release of intracellular calcium causes an elevation in calcium concentrations that subsequently triggers sarcomere contraction. Intracellular calcium is actively resequestered back into the sarcoplasmic reticulum by a calcium-ATPase ion channel. This calcium-ATPase channel is regulated by phospholamban, a protein on the membrane of the sarcoplasmic reticulum.[4,5] The generation of contractile force depends on normal electrical conduction for cell depolarization, intercellular and intracellular calcium signaling, adequate force generation, and appropriate transmission of force through the intracellular cytoskeleton.

From a macroscopic level, contractile function in the myocardium requires a critical mass of myocytes to maintain adequate cardiac output in a growing child. Ongoing somatic and cardiac growth occurs during childhood.

Newborns have a finite number of myocytes, and the overall number of these myocytes decreases with age, as some are normally lost by apoptosis. The remaining myocytes support the increasing metabolic demands of growing children.

Because **myocytes** are terminally differentiated cells, they usually do not undergo cell division. Somatic growth of the heart muscle occurs mainly by hypertrophy of the remaining myocytes. Myocyte injury (from either a genetic or an exogenous cause) may initiate cellular necrosis, regional fibrosis with collagen deposition surrounding the affected region, and hypertrophy of the adjacent viable cells. Myocyte loss leads to impaired contractile function, decreased cardiac output, increased myocardial oxygen consumption, increased end-systolic and end-diastolic volumes, increased peripheral resistance, and activation of compensatory mechanisms that attempt to maintain cardiac output. The loss of even a few myocytes during childhood may have much larger ramifications as the individual grows and remains dependent on a reduced number of cardiac myocytes over subsequent decades of life.

Myocyte injury and reduction in cardiac output trigger many compensatory responses. The Frank-Starling relationship is one of the mechanisms at work in the failing heart. In early heart failure, increased preload (increased end-diastolic volume) increases diastolic stretch, enlarging stroke volume and cardiac output. Other mechanisms include activation of the neurohumoral axis through the renin-angiotensin-aldosterone system, sympathetic nervous system, vasopressin, and natriuretic peptides, all of which increase systemic vascular resistance and intravascular volume. These mechanisms maintain blood pressure and improve cardiac output in the short-term, but they may have detrimental long-term effects on ventricular remodeling and function. Additionally, long-term heart failure may be associated with the reinitiation of fetal genetic programming and the differential expression of alternative contractile protein isoforms. This modified gene expression is the myocyte's attempt to improve mechanical efficiency.[6-8] As mentioned, these compensatory mechanisms may be useful to maintain cardiac output in the short-term, but often become maladaptive over time.

PRIMARY DILATED CARDIOMYOPATHIES

Primary cardiomyopathies are disorders intrinsic to the myocardium that occur without a secondary cause (i.e., exposure to toxins, ischemia, infections, or other systemic diseases).[4] These disorders may present as any one of the three pathologic forms (dilated, hypertrophic, or restrictive) of myocardial disease. A single disease process may display phenotypic features of multiple pathologic types or progress from one type to another over time. An estimated 10% of HCMs have features of a DCM.[10]

Although cardiomyopathies previously were believed to be idiopathic, many forms of DCM and HCM now have been linked to genetic defects in structural and functional proteins in the cardiac myocyte. Although the precise cause is unclear in many cases, 30% of patients with idiopathic cardiomyopathies have a genetic abnormality to explain the heart failure.[4,8,9] As the genetic code continues to unravel, more genetic causes will become evident. Of idiopathic DCMs, 9% to 20% have a familial component and probably a genetic cause.[1-3]

DCM is defined by impaired contractile function that culminates with chamber enlargement. The generation of contractile force sufficient to maintain cardiac output is a complex process requiring normal electrical conduction, normal intercellular and intracellular calcium signaling, appropriate energy production, sufficient force generation from the sarcomere proteins, and adequate force transmission from the sarcomere through to the extracellular matrix via cytoskeletal proteins. A defect in any of the critical proteins that regulate or are actively involved in this pathway theoretically can lead to DCM.

Primary cardiomyopathies commonly are found in association with **neuromuscular disorders** because myocytes and skeletal muscles share many of the same contractile proteins (Table 18-1). Although the exact mechanisms of heart failure progression remain undetermined, there are unique mechanisms of myocyte dysfunction in DCM and HCM. Genetic disorders display variable modes of inheritance, often showing a variable degree of penetrance. Such factors may complicate the clinical recognition of these complex disorders.

Inherited DCMs are distinguished by a diverse heterogeneity in the number of possible loci affected in the genome and by a wide spectrum of clinical phenotypes that are associated with this disease process. Several genetic loci have been attributed to DCM (Table 18-2). Examples include conduction abnormalities seen in

TABLE 18-1

Common Neuromuscular Disorders Associated with Cardiomyopathies
Friedreich ataxia
Becker muscular dystrophy
Myotonic dystrophy
Barth syndrome
Nemaline myopathy
Multiple lentiginosis
Duchenne muscular dystrophy
Emery-Dreifuss muscular dystrophy
Limb-girdle muscular dystrophy
Juvenile progressive spinal muscular atrophy
Myotubular myopathy

From Denfield SW, Gajarski RJ, Towbin JA: Cardiomyopathies. In Garson A, Bricker JT, Fisher DJ, et al (eds): The Science and Practice of Pediatric Cardiology, 2nd ed. Baltimore, Williams & Wilkins, 1998.

TABLE 18-2

Genetic Aspects of Primary Dilated Cardiomyopathies

Defective Gene Product	Gene Function	Genetic Mapping	Inheritance	Associated Symptoms
Sarcomere Proteins				
Cardiac troponin T	Forms part of the tropomyosin complex that regulates contraction of actin and myosin in the sarcomere	1q32	Familial	DCM, HCM
Actin	Thin filaments in sarcomere	15q14	Familial	DCM, HCM
Myosin-binding protein C	Binds myosin heavy chains and titin in elastic filaments. Located in sarcomere A bands	11p11.2	Familial	DCM, HCM
Myosin (beta heavy chain)	Thick filament contractile protein	14q12	Familial	DCM, HCM
Titin	Large sarcomere-cytoskeletal protein that contributes to sarcomere organization	2q24	Familial, autosomal dominant	DCM/HCM, tibial MD
Tropomyosin (alpha)	Sarcomere protein that regulates thin filament activation	15q22	Familial	DCM, HCM
Cytoskeletal Proteins				
Desmin	Cytoskeletal intermediate filament involved in force transmission	2p35	Autosomal dominant, familial	DCM
Sarcoglycan (alpha)	Transmembrane protein that associates with dystrophin and links cytoskeleton to the extracellular matrix	17q12-21	Familial, autosomal recessive	DCM/HCM, limb-girdle MD
Metavinculin	Cytoskeletal microfilaments	10q22	Familial	DCM
Dystrophin	Large cytoskeletal protein involved in force transduction and membrane stabilization	Xp21	X-linked recessive	DCM, Duchenne MD, Becker MD
Tafazzin	Unknown function	Xq28	X-linked recessive	Infantile DCM, Barth syndrome, LV non-compaction
Dystrobrevin (alpha)	Sarcolemma protein complex	18q12.1	Autosomal dominant	DCM, LV noncompaction
Lamin A + C	Nuclear envelope proteins forming intermediate filaments	1q21	Autosomal dominant, autosomal recessive, X-linked recessive	Emery-Dreifuss MD, limb-girdle MD, conduction defects, partial lipodystrophy
Telethonin	Z-disc complex	17q12	Familial	DCM
Channelopathies				
Phospholamban	Inhibitor of the SR calcium-ATPase, regulating relaxation of cardiac muscle	6q22	Familial, autosomal dominant	DCM
Cardiac ryanodine receptor	Calcium channel in the SR	1q42	Autosomal dominant	AVRD
Cell Membrane Proteins				
Desmoplakin	Cell adhesion molecule forming desmosomes	6p24	Autosomal dominant, autosomal recessive	AVRD
Plakoglobin	Cell adhesion molecule forming desmosomes	17q21	Autosomal recessive, familial	AVRD, Naxos disease

AVRD, arrhythmogenic right ventricular dysplasia; DCM, dilated cardiomyopathy; HCM, hypertrophic cardiomyopathy; MD, muscular dystrophy; LV, left ventricular; SR, sarcoplasmic reticulum.
Data summarized from OMIM (Online Mendelian Inheritance In Man) website, May, 2003.

association defects in lamin A + C, which are intermediate filaments that form nuclear envelope proteins.[4,11] Intracellular calcium kinetics are regulated by the protein phospholamban, defects of which have been identified in patients with dilated disease.[4,5] Mitochondrial defects lead to abnormalities in energy generation. Defects in sarcomere proteins (myosin, actin, and troponin T) can decrease force generation, and abnormalities in cytoskeletal proteins (dystrophin, sarcoglycan alpha, titin, desmin, and taffazin) can decrease transmission of the contractile force.[4] Ongoing molecular analysis of these critical pathways no doubt will lead to the further identification of loci central to the development of various cardiomyopathies.

HCM has been linked to specific defects in sarcomere proteins (beta cardiac myosin heavy chain, troponin T, myosin binding protein C, myosin light chains, actin, troponin I, alpha tropomyosin, and titin) and nonsarcomeric proteins that potentially are involved in energy use.[4,12,13] HCM is characterized histologically by myocyte disarray, misalignment of the myocardial cells, myocyte hypertrophy, and interstitial fibrosis.[4,11,12] Many defects leading to the hypertrophic phenotypic have been hypothesized to cause inefficient use of ATP.[12] Defects in the same sarcomere proteins, but located at different gene loci, may result in a dilated phenotype. It seems that sarcomere proteins have multiple binding regions, and that defects in the regions that function in force generation or transmission lead to a dilated phenotype, whereas mutations affecting energy use may lead to a hypertrophic phenotype.[4] HCM is discussed in more detail in Chapter 20.

Primary cardiomyopathies occur in one of four inheritance patterns (Fig. 18-1): autosomal dominant, autosomal recessive, X-linked, or mitochondrial. **Autosomal dominant** inheritance is the most common pattern and usually has a varying degree of phenotypic expression.[4,20] Affected individuals have a 50% chance of passing the gene onto their offspring. Phenotypic expression may vary and ranges from asymptomatic left ventricular dysfunction to rapidly progressing heart failure. In contrast, **autosomal recessive** inheritance requires that an affected individual receive two copies of a defective gene (one from each parent), with affected homozygous individuals tending to have a more uniform phenotypic expression. **X-linked disorders** affect only male offspring because they have only one copy of an X chromosome; asymptomatic females carry the affected gene to the next generation. **Mitochondrial disorders** show maternal inheritance because abnormal mitochondria are passed from the mother to all of the offspring. Phenotypic expression may vary depending on the percentage of abnormal mitochondria inherited.

Left ventricular noncompaction is a rare form of a primary cardiomyopathy.[14] This disorder is characterized by a developmental arrest in the normal compaction of the ventricular endocardium resulting in prominent trabeculations with deep recesses within the myocardium. The left ventricle is more commonly affected, although abnormalities can exist in both ventricles. The spectrum of clinical features consists of ventricular hypertrophy and dilation, systolic and diastolic ventricular dysfunction, ECG abnormalities, systemic thromboemboli, supraventricular and ventricular arrhythmias, CHF, and sudden death. Congenital heart defects, mitochondrial myopathies, Barth syndrome, and dysmorphic features may be present. Phenotypic expression varies, and age at presentation may range from infancy to early adulthood. Many infants have recovery of some degree of systolic function for a period (years) before eventual deterioration.[14]

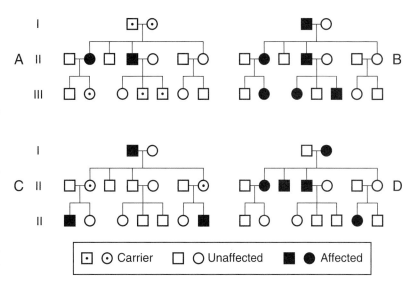

FIGURE 18-1 ■ Inheritance patterns in dilated cardiomyopathy. Autosomal recessive **(A)**, autosomal dominant **(B)**, X-linked **(C)**, and mitochondrial **(D)** inheritance are shown. In autosomal recessive traits, gene carrier parents (heterozygotes) have a 25% chance of having homozygous children with the disease, and the disease skips generations because of the production of heterozygous offspring who become carriers of the defective gene. The autosomal dominant diseases show a 50% likelihood of offspring receiving a copy of the abnormal gene, and these heterozygotes become affected. No skipping of generations occurs. In X-linked disorders, only males are affected, females are gene carriers, and no male-to-male transmission occurs. In mitochondrial diseases, maternal inheritance occurs. With all offspring receiving abnormal mitochondria (heteroplasmy), the offspring may or may not develop disease. (From Towbin JA: Pediatric myocardial disease. Pediatr Clin North Am 1999;46:289-308.)

Endocardial fibroelastosis is a cardiomyopathy that is characterized by excessive endocardial thickening secondary to proliferation of fibrous and elastic fibers.[15,16] Primary or secondary causes may lead to a common pathologic end point. Thickening of the endocardium leads to decreased compliance, dilation or contraction of the ventricular chamber, diastolic dysfunction, atrial enlargement, progressive CHF, arrhythmias, thromboemboli, and sudden death. Primary forms have been described in mucopolysaccharidosis I, carnitine deficiency, Barth syndrome, and idiopathic familial disorders.[16] Secondary forms of endocardial fibroelastosis have been attributed to viral infections and congenital heart defects, such as aortic stenosis, hypoplastic left heart syndrome, and complete heart block. Polymerase chain reaction analyses of postmortem specimens with endocardial fibroelastosis showed the presence of mumps viral RNA.[15] Fetal echocardiogram can detect endocardial fibroelastosis in utero. Age at presentation ranges from infancy (<1 year old) to occasionally later childhood or early adulthood. After diagnosis, the prognosis is poor, with most patients developing progressive CHF.

Arrhythmogenic right ventricular dysplasia is a genetic disorder involving atrophy of the myocardium, followed by fibrosis and fatty infiltrates, usually in the region of the right ventricular free wall.[17-19] Patients with this condition typically present with recurrent, sustained episodes of ventricular tachycardia or fibrillation that originate from the right ventricle. A left bundle branch block pattern on the surface ECG is characteristic. The resting ECG may show a wide QRS interval in the right precordial leads (V_1 to V_3), T wave inversion in the right precordial leads, and a normal QTc interval. Patients have varying degrees of right ventricular dysfunction and may experience palpitations, dizziness, syncope, or sudden death as a result of ventricular ectopy.

Although no infectious agents have been consistently identified, viral genomes have been isolated by polymerase chain reaction in some patients with arrhythmogenic right ventricular dysplasia.[17] Ventricular fibrillation secondary to arrhythmogenic right ventricular dysplasia is a significant cause of sudden cardiac death, especially with exercise in teenagers and young adults.[17-19] About one third of patients have a familial form with autosomal dominant inheritance; there may be incomplete penetrance and variable phenotypic expression.[19] Autosomal recessive forms also have been documented.[19] Genetic mutations have been found in cardiac ryanodine receptors and in desmosomes, which are protein complexes that form the major cell adhesion junctions in cardiac and epidermal tissues.[19] Abnormal strength of the affected myocardial tissue may lead to early apoptosis and the characteristic pathologic features because the cardiac tissue is under such high mechanical stress.

SECONDARY CAUSES OF DILATED CARDIOMYOPATHY

DCM may develop secondary to many possible alterations in the delicate extracellular environment of the cardiac myocyte (Table 18-3). Myocytes require a constant supply of oxygen and nutrients, which are closely regulated by neurohumoral, endocrine, immunologic, and inflammatory stimuli. Myocyte injury may occur via hypoxia, nutritional deficiency, infection, inflammation, toxin exposure, or arrhythmia. Regardless of the specific cause, myocyte loss or injury beyond a critical point leads to the development of varying degrees of ventricular dysfunction. The more common etiologies for DCM in children are discussed subsequently.

Myocarditis is a major contributor to the development of ventricular dysfunction and DCM in children and adults. Although myocarditis can occur as a result of bacterial, fungal, or protozoan infections, viral myocarditis predominates. Adenovirus and enterovirus are two of the most common viruses isolated from patients with DCM; however, many other viruses have been implicated as causal agents.[21,22] Viral infection may lead to direct myocardial injury or induce a harmful immunoinflammatory response. This response may involve complement activation and may lead to varying degrees of cytokine expression, which promotes progressive myocyte loss.

More recent reports have identified a specific coxsackievirus-adenovirus receptor on the myocardial cell membrane, which may explain the apparent susceptibility of the heart to this infection (see Chapter 17). Viral infections also have been found to disrupt cytoskeletal architecture, decreasing myocardial efficiency. This disruption has been associated with viral protease 2A expression. This viral protein cleaves dystrophin and is at least partially responsible for the loss of cardiac function seen with some forms of viral myocarditis.[22]

The increased prevalence and improved survival of children with **human immunodeficiency virus (HIV)** infection mandate an increased awareness of its cardiovascular complications. HIV-related cardiac complications include focal myocarditis, pericarditis, pericardial effusions, endocarditis, idiopathic left ventricular dysfunction, systemic hypertension, pulmonary hypertension, arrhythmias, premature coronary artery disease, acquired immunodeficiency syndrome (AIDS)– related cardiac tumors, and autonomic dysfunction.[23] DCM may occur in the setting of HIV through damage to the cardiac myocyte from direct HIV infection; coinfection with other viruses, bacteria, or parasites; autoimmune reactions; drug-related cardiotoxicities; nutritional deficiencies; endocrine abnormalities; inflammatory mediators; or autonomic dysregulation.[23]

The incidence of DCM is estimated to be 8% to 15% in HIV-infected children and adults.[23] Cardiovascular complications have surpassed pulmonary complications

TABLE 18-3

Secondary Causes of Dilated Cardiomyopathies	
Infections	*Ischemia*
Viral	Hypoxia
Bacterial	Birth asphyxia
Fungal	Drowning
Protozoan (Chagas/toxoplasmosis)	Kawasaki disease
Rickettsial (Rocky Mountain spotted fever)	Coronary artery malformation
Spirochetal (Lyme disease)	Premature coronary artery disease
Arrhythmias	*Toxins*
Supraventricular tachycardia	Anthracyclines
Atrial flutter	Radiation
Ectopic atrial tachycardia	Other chemotherapeutic agents
Ventricular tachycardia	Sulfonamide sensitivity
Bradycardia	Penicillin sensitivity
	Iron (hemachromatosis)
	Copper
Endocrine	
Hyperthyroidism/hypothyroidism	*Systemic Disorders*
Diabetes mellitus (infant of a diabetic mother)	Systemic lupus erythematosus
Excess catecholamines (pheochromocytoma or neuroblastoma)	Juvenile rheumatoid arthritis
Congenital adrenal hyperplasia	Polyarteritis nodosa
	Kawasaki disease
Storage Diseases	Osteogenesis imperfecta
Glycogen storage diseases	Noonan syndrome
Mucopolysaccharidoses	Peripartum cardiomyopathy
Sphingolipidoses	Hemolytic uremic syndrome
	Leukemia
Nutritional Deficiencies	Amyloidosis
Protein: kwashiorkor	Sarcoidosis
Thiamine: beriberi	Reye syndrome
Vitamin E	
Selenium	
Carnitine	
Phosphate	

From Denfield SW, Gajarski RJ, Towbin JA: Cardiomyopathies. In Garson A, Bricker JT, Fisher DJ, et al (eds): The Science and Practice of Pediatric Cardiology, 2nd ed. Baltimore, Williams & Wilkins, 1998.

as the leading causes of morbidity and mortality for HIV infection in children.[24] The early recognition of ventricular dysfunction and other cardiovascular complications through routine screening, combined with aggressive medical therapy, may improve the morbidity and mortality rates for this subgroup of patients (Table 18-4). As therapy for HIV improves and children live longer, the prevalence of DCM is likely to continue to increase.

Another secondary cause of DCM is **chemotherapy** and other cancer treatments, such as radiation. Pediatric cancer survival has improved markedly with the use of anthracyclines, radiation, and other chemotherapy agents. It is estimated that 1 of every 250 adults in the United States will be a survivor of childhood cancer by the end of 2010.[25] Although survival is improved, the morbidity from the cardiovascular complication of these agents is substantial. Long-term survivors of childhood cancer are a growing population of young adults at risk for premature cardiovascular disease. Children differ from adult cancer survivors in that they undergo somatic and myocardial growth and have a longer potential life span after chemotherapy. Loss of myocytes from cancer therapy during childhood may predispose pediatric cancer patients to progressive ventricular dysfunction and cardiomyopathy in later life. Direct chemotherapy-associated myocardial damage may occur by free radical damage, mitochondrial injury, apoptosis, or inflammatory or autoimmune responses. Indirect mechanisms of myocardial damage seen after successful treatment of childhood cancer include growth hormone deficiency, endothelial (vascular) injury, and autonomic dysfunction.

TABLE 18-4

Recommended Screening for Children with HIV Infection
Perform a baseline echocardiogram at the time of HIV diagnosis
Follow-up echocardiograms are recommended every 1-2 yr in asymptomatic children with HIV
Annual echocardiograms are recommended in children with HIV-related symptoms
Any child with a cardiovascular abnormality or abnormal ventricular function should receive care guided by a pediatric cardiologist
Echocardiograms also may be warranted in children with unexplained persistent pulmonary symptoms to exclude cardiac disease and in patients with viral coinfections who are at risk for myocarditis
Prevention of modifiable cardiovascular risk factors and routine cardiovascular risk assessments with lipid profiles, ECGs, exercise stress tests, Holter monitors, and serum biomarkers such as: C-reactive protein and B-type natriuretic peptides also may be beneficial

HIV, human immunodeficiency virus.

Anthracycline agents commonly are used to treat many types of childhood cancers. They cause varying degrees of ventricular dysfunction in the acute and chronic phases (>1 year) after administration (Table 18-5). About 65% of cancer survivors have some degree of ventricular dysfunction detectable 6 years after anthracycline exposure.[26] Risk factors for the development of anthracycline-related cardiac dysfunction include higher cumulative doses (generally ≤550 mg/m^2), rapid administration, younger age, increased duration (years) of survival, female gender, African-American race, and concomitant use of some specific chemotherapeutic agents (i.e., amsacrine, which is no longer used in the United States).[25] In addition to systolic ventricular dysfunction,

TABLE 18-5

Recommended Screening for Children After Anthracycline Exposure
Perform a baseline echocardiogram before anticancer therapy
Serial echocardiograms during anticancer therapy based on treatment protocols are of unproved efficacy
Serial echocardiograms after anticancer therapy (every 1-2 yr) are recommended, depending on the relative risk of cardiotoxicity
Any child with a cardiovascular abnormality or abnormal ventricular function should receive care guided by a pediatric cardiologist
Prevention of modifiable cardiovascular risk factors and routine cardiovascular risk assessments should be encouraged

long-term survivors may show evidence of a restrictive cardiomyopathy after anthracycline therapy. Mediastinal radiation causes inflammation in the coronary arteries and diffuse interstitial fibrosis in the myocardium, which may lead to premature coronary artery disease or to a restrictive cardiomyopathy.[27]

Hypoxic-ischemic injury may occur in children secondary to a specific systemic illness, secondary to injury, or during the birth process, which can cause global hypoxia in the infant and lead to acute myocyte injury or loss. Elevations in cardiac troponin T have been identified in otherwise healthy full-term infants and correlate with low Apgar scores.[28] Birth-associated hypoxia has been attributed to compression of the umbilical cord, placental compromise, and maternal disorders. Children also may be at risk for myocardial injury from hypoxia after drowning, acute life-threatening events, or severe systemic illnesses.

Insufficient coronary artery perfusion may occur secondary to congenital anomalies of the coronary arteries, palliated congenital heart disease, acquired coronary artery abnormalities, or premature coronary artery disease. An **anomalous left coronary artery from the pulmonary artery** is a congenital abnormality that commonly presents with severe heart failure in infancy. As the pulmonary artery resistance decreases, the perfusion pressure across the distribution of the left coronary artery decreases, and hypoperfusion of the myocardium ensues. Echocardiograms may reveal regional wall motion abnormalities or global hypokinesis. Infants with complex congenital heart disease palliated with systemic-to-pulmonary artery shunts may be at risk for myocardial ischemia. The continuous arterial supply of blood into the pulmonary arteries may lower aortic diastolic pressure, reducing coronary artery perfusion pressure and opening the possibility of myocardial ischemia. See Chapter 47 for further discussion.

Kawasaki disease is a pediatric vasculitis that may damage the coronary arteries permanently. It is the most common cause of acquired heart disease in children in the United States. Coronary artery aneurysms occur in about 25% of untreated patients and in less than 5% of patients treated with intravenous gamma globulins during the acute and convalescent stages of the disease.[29] Although most aneurysms regress, patients with residual coronary disease remain at risk for myocardial ischemia and sudden death secondary to latent coronary artery stenosis and thrombosis. The sites of regressed aneurysms also may remain abnormal, with evidence of excessive intimal hypertrophy and endothelial dysfunction.[30] The long-term ramifications of Kawasaki disease are unknown.[30-32] Identifying and quantifying coronary artery calcifications may be useful in the risk stratification of this population.[32] Research needs to define which patients are at risk for subsequent coronary artery disease as teenagers or young adults. Patients with Kawasaki disease with residual coronary artery abnormalities should be followed continually because of their risk of myocardial ischemia.

Atherosclerotic disease with ischemic cardiomyopathy is a major public health concern. Atherosclerosis starts in childhood; prevention should be focused on reduction of modifiable risk factors in children. Obesity is an increasing health problem for children in the United States, with a prevalence of 12% to 21%.[33] Obesity, type 2 diabetes, insulin insensitivity, hypertension, dyslipidemias, and systemic inflammation may predispose children to the early development of atherosclerosis.[33,34] Coronary artery perfusion also can be affected by illicit drug use (cocaine) and other stimulant medications.

DCM may present after sustained **rhythm disturbances,** such as supraventricular tachycardias (especially ectopic atrial tachycardias), ventricular tachycardias, or marked bradycardia from congenital or acquired conduction abnormalities. Tachycardias can cause decreased diastolic filling times, decreased myocardial perfusion, and atrioventricular dyssynchrony that may lower cardiac output and ventricular function, if sustained. Bradycardia may elevate end-diastolic volumes, leading to chamber enlargement and ventricular dysfunction (see Chapter 24).

Nutritional disorders also can be a secondary cause of DCM. Myocytes require a constant supply of glucose, free fatty acids, amino acids, vitamins, and other micronutrients to meet their energy requirements. Conversely, an excess of certain vitamins, minerals, electrolytes, or other essential nutrients can lead to progressive ventricular dysfunction and a cardiomyopathy. Protein wasting from eating disorders, HIV infection, or other chronic illnesses may cause ventricular dysfunction. Calcium and magnesium deficiencies can impair inotropy and predispose patients to arrhythmias. Micronutrients, such as copper, selenium, thiamine, and carnitine, are vital coenzymes that maintain the energy production for the myocyte; deficiencies can lead to the development of cardiomyopathy. Anemia (from iron deficiency, sickle cell disease, renal failure, or other chronic illnesses) causes a high-output state as increased cardiac output is used to compensate for the decrease in oxygen-carrying capacity. High output causes increased myocardial demand and can progress to DCM. Excess amounts of iron (in hemochromatosis and in patients requiring long-term packed red blood cell transfusions) may lead to iron overload, and iron deposition in the myocardium may cause secondary myocardial damage. Wilson disease is associated with myocardial copper deposits and has been associated with progressive ventricular dysfunction.

Additional miscellaneous conditions warrant mention. Cocaine use can lead to DCM; the etiology is believed to be secondary to cocaine's ability to block norepinephrine reuptake and release of dopamine and its coronary vasospastic effects. Several systemic diseases, such as systemic lupus erythematosus and rheumatoid arthritis, rarely can be associated with DCM. Lastly, endocrine and metabolic causes of DCM include obesity and diabetes (both diseases escalating in frequency among children and adolescents) and thyroid disorders (hyperthyroidism and hypothyroidism occasionally can result in ventricular dysfunction).

DIAGNOSTIC METHODOLOGY FOR DILATED CARDIOMYOPATHY

The gross **pathologic appearance** of DCM is a globular heart with severe biventricular dilation. Ventricular dysfunction leads to accumulation of blood within the ventricles and subsequently elevates end-diastolic pressures, leading to atrial enlargement. Intramural thrombi also may be present, caused by the stasis of blood in the dilated ventricles. On gross pathologic inspection, the myocardium may be pale, with a thin, translucent endocardium, which may or may not be accompanied by focal sclerosis (i.e., endocardial fibroelastosis).[20] Scarring and fibrosis of the myocardium may form irritable foci and a substrate for malignant ventricular arrhythmias. The overall weight of the heart is increased proportionately to the degree of compensatory myocardial hypertrophy. The right ventricular free wall may appear parchment-like and have fibrous or fatty infiltrates in arrhythmogenic right ventricular dysplasia. In left ventricular noncompaction, the left ventricular myocardium has deep recesses and characteristic trabeculations.

Microscopic evaluation of the heart typically reveals histologic features of myocyte hypertrophy, myocyte degeneration, and varying amounts of interstitial fibrosis.[20] In addition, the myocytes are often elongated. Depending on the cause of DCM, other unique histologic findings also may be present, including lymphocyte or giant cell infiltrates in myocarditis or myocyte disarray in primary cardiomyopathies. Electron microscopy also may be useful to identify ultrastructural abnormalities in mitochondria, T tubules, and Z bands.[20]

The **signs and symptoms** of a patient with DCM depend on age and the degree of ventricular dysfunction; they range from asymptomatic ventricular dysfunction to overt CHF. As compensatory responses fail, cardiac output decreases, and symptoms of CHF appear. The rate of symptom progression varies and depends on the nature of the underlying disease. Infants in CHF usually present with feeding intolerance because this activity represents most of their daily work. These symptoms consist of tachypnea, increased respiratory effort with retractions, feeding intolerance, diaphoresis with feeding, prolong periods of irritability, and failure to thrive.

Children and adults initially may present with exercise intolerance or dyspnea with exertion because they are unable to increase cardiac output to meet increased systemic demands. As ventricular dysfunction worsens, they may display symptoms of left-sided and right-sided heart failure, including fatigue, orthopnea, tachypnea, dyspnea, and edema. Mesenteric ischemic symptoms also may appear if cardiac output is unable to perfuse the gastrointestinal tract adequately. Resulting gastrointestinal symptoms may include nausea, anorexia, vomiting, and prolonged abdominal pain after meals. Children of any age may present with palpitations, dizziness, presyncope, or syncope if supraventricular or ventricular arrhythmias are present. Unexplained palpitations of new onset, syncope, respiratory distress, or gastrointestinal symptoms should alert clinicians to screen for a cardiac cause.

The **physical examination** findings of CHF also vary with the degree of ventricular dysfunction and the age of the patient. Vital signs may provide crucial evidence to the diagnosis of DCM. The most striking feature is an elevated heart rate (for age) with decreased heart rate variability. Tachycardia initially compensates for the decreased stroke volume. Pulses may be weak with a narrow pulse pressure, as the systemic vascular resistance increases and cardiac output decreases. The blood pressure is low to normal and may be maintained until just before cardiovascular collapse. The respiratory rate may be elevated. Cyanosis is uncommon.

Physical examination may reveal jugular venous distention in older children; however, this distention is uncommon in infants. Chest examination can reveal increased work of breathing, intercostal retractions, and nasal flaring in infants with pulmonary edema. Bronchial edema may lead to airway obstruction and "cardiac wheezing" in infants. Auscultation of the chest may reveal rales in older children. Cardiomegaly can compress the left main stem bronchus, with subsequent atelectasis and decreased left-sided aeration.

Cardiac examination may reveal cardiomegaly, increased precordial impulse, or lateral displacement of the apical impulse. The heart sounds are usually distant or muffled. Murmurs may not be present, although mitral regurgitation may be audible if the enlarged left ventricle is causing dilation of the mitral valve annulus and incompetency of the valve. An extra heart sound may be audible as a gallop rhythm, secondary to elevated ventricular filling pressures. Abdominal examination can reveal hepatomegaly and ascites. Nonspecific generalized abdominal pain also may be present from mesenteric ischemia. Dependent edema is common and can be seen in the eyelids and scrotum of infants or in the legs of children and adults.

Coexisting symptoms also may suggest the cause of cardiomyopathy. Hypoglycemia, a primary metabolic acidosis with an anion gap, or hyperammonemia may suggest a metabolic disorder. Encephalopathy with progressive neurodevelopmental decline could be consistent with a metabolic disorder, mitochondrial disease,

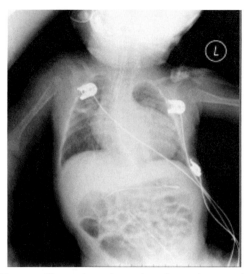

FIGURE 18-2 ■ **Chest radiography in idiopathic cardiomyopathy.** Chest radiograph of a 3-month-old infant with idiopathic dilated cardiomyopathy shows cardiomegaly with a cardiothoracic diameter of greater than 0.5.

or storage disease. Neuromuscular symptoms, such as weakness, hypotonia, myotonia, or ataxia, may suggest an inborn error of metabolism or congenital myopathy.[35]

Chest radiography classically reveals cardiomegaly with a cardiac-to-thoracic diameter ratio of greater than 0.5 to 1 (Fig. 18-2). Cardiomegaly typically results from left atrial and left ventricular enlargement. The left atrial enlargement may elevate the left main stem bronchus and cause airway obstruction or atelectasis in the left lung field. In younger children, lung fields often appear hyperexpanded, with flattening of the diaphragm. Elevated pulmonary venous pressures lead to pulmonary congestion and resultant small airway edema. Infants and small children, as a result of the small caliber of their airways, may have obstructive airway symptoms consistent with this characteristic radiographic finding. Varying degrees of pulmonary venous congestion with progression to overt pulmonary edema may occur over time. Pleural effusions may be present.

ECG usually reveals sinus tachycardia with an elevated heart rate for age and decreased heart rate variability (Fig. 18-3). Nonspecific ST-T segment and T wave changes are seen in the left precordial and inferior leads. T wave inversion in the left precordial leads suggests repolarization abnormalities. Atrial enlargement and ventricular hypertrophy also may be seen. Arrhythmias are common in DCM patients and may consist of atrial arrhythmias (supraventricular tachycardia, atrial flutter, and atrial fibrillation) or ventricular tachycardias.[36] Overall, ECGs have considerable variability. A study reported that resting ECG findings correlated poorly with myocyte histologic findings from endomyocardial biopsy specimens.[37]

Two-dimensional transthoracic **echocardiography** is a relatively simple, noninvasive procedure useful for identifying, quantifying, and assessing the degree of

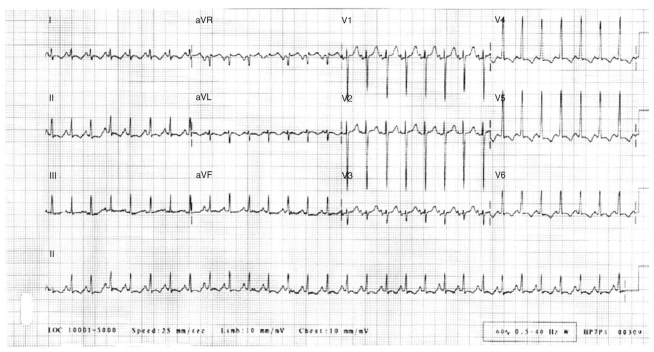

FIGURE 18-3 ■ ECG in idiopathic dilated cardiomyopathy. ECG of a 3-month-old infant with idiopathic dilated cardiomyopathy shows diffuse ST-segment abnormalities.

ventricular dysfunction over time in DCM patients. Characteristic findings include ventricular enlargement and globally decreased contractile function, without regional wall motion abnormalities (Fig. 18-4). Indices of left ventricular function that may be measured by echocardiography include shortening fraction, ejection fraction, mean circumferential fiber shortening, ratio of the left ventricular pre-ejection period to ejection time, myocardial performance index, ventricular wall thickness or mass, and wall stress analyses.[20,38,39] Load-independent assessment of left ventricular contractility can

be measured by the stress velocity index.[40] These echocardiographic measurements have been useful predictors of outcomes in certain subgroups of DCM patients. In children with HIV infection, abnormalities in contractility, fractional shortening, and increased wall thickness independently predict mortality. Childhood cancer survivors with ventricular dysfunction have decreased wall thickness and elevated systemic afterload after anthracycline exposure.[38]

Routine echocardiography also should be performed to rule out congenital heart disease, regional wall

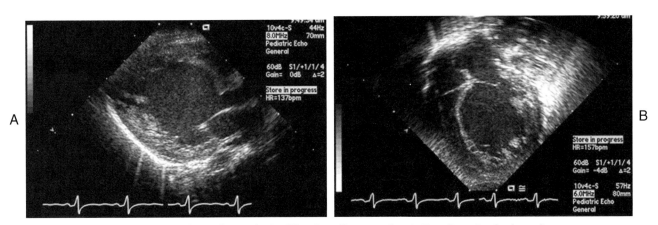

FIGURE 18-4 ■ Echocardiography in dilated cardiomyopathy. A, Two-dimensional echocardiogram (parasternal long axis) of a 3-month-old infant with idiopathic dilated cardiomyopathy shows severe left ventricular enlargement. **B,** Two-dimensional echocardiogram (apical four-chamber view) of a 3-month-old infant with idiopathic dilated cardiomyopathy shows severe left ventricular and left atrial enlargement.

motion abnormalities, anomalous origins of the coronary arteries (especially an anomalous left coronary artery from the pulmonary artery), endocardial fibroelastosis, abnormal papillary muscle function, and intramural thrombi. Color and pulse-wave Doppler echocardiography can determine the presence and degree of mitral regurgitation, assess cardiac output by aortic flow velocities, assess the degree of diastolic dysfunction by atrioventricular valve inflow patterns, and estimate pulmonary artery and right ventricular pressures. Echocardiography also is useful for evaluating cardiomyopathy patients longitudinally. Changes in ventricular function, intramural thrombi, wall stress, and valvar regurgitation can be followed over time and used to guide medical therapy.

Cardiac catheterization with endomyocardial biopsy can obtain useful diagnostic and prognostic information in patients with DCM. This invasive procedure is limited, however, by its inherent risks and limited sensitivity. Potential complications of cardiac catheterization and endomyocardial biopsy include hemorrhage, vascular injury, thromboemboli, transient conduction abnormalities, arrhythmias, cardiac perforation with tamponade, and death. The overall incidence of complications ranges from 1% to 6% with a mortality rate of less than 1% in adults.[41]

Catheterization can assess the hemodynamics of left ventricular end-diastolic, pulmonary capillary wedge, pulmonary artery, and central venous pressures, which may help direct therapy. Endomyocardial biopsy remains the gold standard to exclude myocarditis and may be useful in the diagnosis of metabolic abnormalities, mitochondrial defects, and infiltrative disease (hemochromatosis, amyloidosis, and sarcoidosis). Biopsy results are often nonspecific, showing myocyte hypertrophy and fibrosis.[20] Polymerase chain reaction analysis and electron microscopy may provide more definitive diagnoses, which may affect prognosis and treatment greatly. Polymerase chain reaction analysis is available for many of the common causes of viral myocarditis, including enteroviruses, adenovirus, cytomegalovirus, herpes simplex virus, Epstein-Barr virus, respiratory syncytial virus, influenza virus, and HIV.

The definitive indications for cardiac catheterization with endomyocardial biopsy are unclear. In patients with a high likelihood of infectious, infiltrative, or metabolic diseases, an endomyocardial biopsy may be diagnostic. Biopsies also may be useful in rapidly deteriorating diseases, when transplantation may be needed. A cardiac catheterization with coronary artery angiography also may be needed if the coronary artery origins cannot be delineated by echocardiography. Randomized trials are necessary to determine the exact indications for endomyocardial biopsy.

Myocardial perfusion scans are useful for differentiating ischemic DCM from idiopathic DCM in patients at high risk for coronary artery disease. In children, the routine use of radionucleotide studies is not indicated, unless regional wall motion abnormalities exist.

Acute myocardial injury or inflammation can be detected with **biomarkers,** such as cardiac troponins I and T. These biomarkers are intracellular cytoskeletal proteins that are sensitive and specific for acute myocyte injury. Serum elevation of cardiac troponin T or I at the onset of DCM should alert clinicians to look for ischemia, myocarditis, or an acute inflammatory process as the cause of the cardiomyopathy. Patients with infectious causes for cardiomyopathy may have an elevated white blood cell count with a lymphocytosis. Blood and nasopharyngeal cultures for viruses are usually nondiagnostic. Patients presenting with CHF can have heart failure progression monitored with B-type natriuretic peptide levels. These hormones are secreted from the ventricular myocardium in response to chamber dilation.[42] B-type natriuretic peptide levels may be useful in evaluating transplantation rejection and potentially in managing DCM in children (see Chapter 6).[42] Depending on the age and presentation of the DCM patient, a metabolic evaluation with blood and urine analysis should be considered.[35] In the future, molecular testing will be commercially available to screen for heritable genetic defects that lead to DCM.

TREATMENT STRATEGY FOR DILATED CARDIOMYOPATHY

The short-term and long-term management of a patient with DCM should incorporate preventive health measures that include identification and risk stratification of high-risk patients and the institution of primary and secondary prevention protocols. Short-term and long-term management is based on each patient's degree of ventricular dysfunction.

Short-Term Management
The acute management of a child newly diagnosed with DCM should include the following:
1. Rule out treatable or correctable causes of DCM, such as myocarditis or ischemia (usually from an anomalous left coronary artery).
2. Minimize the risk of complications from DCM, especially the risks of thromboembolic events and supraventricular and ventricular arrhythmias.
3. Provide supportive care for CHF symptoms.

All patients with newly diagnosed and unexplained ventricular dysfunction should be screened for active myocardial injury with cardiac troponin T or I analysis. Ongoing injury from treatable causes, such as myocarditis, ischemia from an anomalous left coronary artery or other coronary artery abnormality, hypoxia, or exposure to a cardiotoxin, should be evaluated and treated. Antiretroviral therapy should be considered for HIV infection. Limited evidence indicates that intravenous immunoglobulin has been beneficial for treating children with acute viral myocarditis.[43,44] The discovery of an anomalous left coronary artery from the pulmonary artery requires prompt surgical correction.

Intramural thrombi form as a result of stasis in cardiac chambers during times of low cardiac output. The risks of intramural thrombi and systemic thromboemboli in children are unknown, but they are estimated to range from 3% to 50% in adults with DCM.[45] If an intramural thrombus is detected by echocardiography, systemic anticoagulation is indicated, unless contraindications exist. When the thrombus has stabilized, the patient may be converted to oral anticoagulation with warfarin. The value of preventive anticoagulation alone or in combination with aspirin for antiplatelet therapy is unclear, but anticoagulation may be useful.

Arrhythmias are a potential cause of sudden death in these patients. Newly diagnosed patients may benefit from Holter monitoring or inpatient telemetry if ventricular function is severely depressed. Electrolyte imbalances (calcium, magnesium, and potassium) should be corrected. If supraventricular or ventricular arrhythmias persist, they should be treated to improve an already diminished cardiac output. The choice of an antiarrhythmic drug should be balanced against its potential to depress ventricular function further or cause proarrhythmic side effects. Temporary or permanent pacing may be needed for marked bradyarrhythmias. Biventricular pacing may improve atrioventricular synchrony and has improved symptoms in adults with CHF secondary to ischemia, but its usefulness in children with nonischemic DCM is unknown.

The short-term management of patients with heart failure arising from DCM should consist of the same supportive care as used in the management of CHF stemming from other conditions. Acute symptoms can be controlled with intravenous inotropes, such as dopamine and dobutamine, and with a diuretic for volume reduction. Phosphodiesterase inhibitors (milrinone) or nitroprusside for afterload reduction may have additive benefits. When the acute decompensation has been controlled, patients are converted to an oral regimen of afterload reduction with angiotensin-converting enzyme inhibitors and diuretics. Digoxin and β-blockers also may be beneficial. Spironolactone and angiotensin receptor blocking agents can modify further the renin-angiotensin-aldosterone axis, although their usefulness is undetermined in children. Lastly, novel agents such as B-type natriuretic peptide analogue can be initiated.

Compared with adults, children and young adults rarely have ischemic cardiomyopathies. The diverse heterogeneity of primary and secondary cardiomyopathies in this population creates a therapeutic dilemma because many disease processes are unique and may not conform to standard heart failure management strategies. This difference was evident in a report of long-term survivors of childhood cancer after anthracycline therapy. In these patients, ventricular function initially improved with afterload reduction by angiotensin-converting enzyme inhibitors, but progressive ventricular dysfunction subsequently developed during intermediate follow-up at 8 years.[46] Randomized trials are needed to determine the best therapeutic regimen for each disease process.

Long-Term Management

The natural history of DCM depends on the cause (primary versus secondary) and on any coexisting risk factors. Primary cardiomyopathies are usually progressive, despite aggressive anticongestive medical therapy, whereas secondary causes may or may not be progressive. Although many children with secondary cardiomyopathies recover ventricular function, children with marked myocardial injury in early childhood (anthracycline exposure, viral myocarditis) probably should be followed continually.

Patients who progress to intractable CHF may benefit from surgical palliative therapies before heart transplantation is considered. Surgical palliation with bridging techniques, such as ventricular assist devices, intra-aortic balloon pumps, and extracorporeal membrane oxygenation, has allowed some patients who normally would not have survived to live long enough to receive a heart transplantation.

Partial left ventriculectomy (Batista procedure) is another form of surgical palliation that involves reducing left ventricular mass by surgical resection.[47] This procedure theoretically alters the geometry of the left ventricle to improve contractility. It has been used as a bridge to transplantation or as an alternative to transplantation if contraindications exist. Its usefulness, especially in pediatric patients, is limited.[47-49]

Figure 18-5 summarizes a preventive health strategy for patients with various forms of pediatric ventricular dysfunction. Primary prevention avoids myocyte injury altogether and is the best strategy, when possible. Primary preventive techniques have been applied successfully to prevent HIV and some chemotherapy-related disease. Infants with vertically transmitted HIV infection have benefited from prenatal and postnatal administration of zidovudine.[43,50] Children receiving anthracycline therapy can be pretreated with dexrazoxane, a potent iron chelator that functions as a free radical scavenger, to prevent anthracycline-related cardiotoxicity.[51] Children with ventricular dysfunction also are likely to benefit from reducing modifiable cardiovascular risk factors, such as hypertension, diabetes, hypercholesterolemia, smoking, and obesity. Secondary prevention strategies prevent ongoing myocardial injury from occurring after the initial insult. Many of the acute and chronic measures discussed previously are included in this category. Children should be encouraged to eat a well-balanced diet and to participate in regular physical activity or a cardiac rehabilitation program whenever possible.

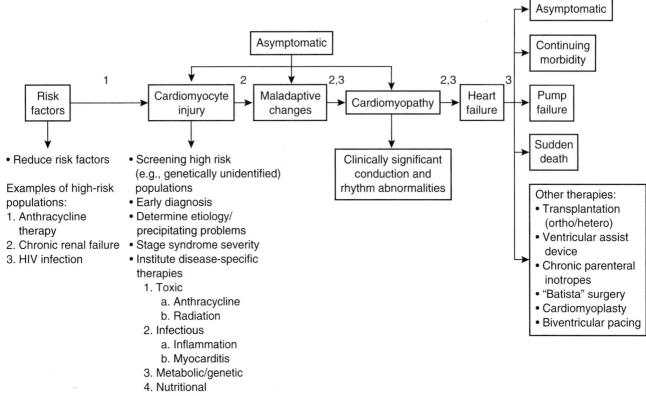

FIGURE 18-5 ■ **Preventive strategy for ventricular dysfunction.** A preventive health strategy for patients with various forms of pediatric ventricular dysfunction. (1) Primary prevention—prevents myocyte injury by decreasing the risk of exposure to causative agents. (2) Secondary prevention— prevents further myocardial injury by screening high-risk populations, modifying reducible risk factors, identifying myocyte injury, and instituting disease-specific therapies early. (3) Potential sites of benefit from neurohormonal regulation to slow the progression of ventricular dysfunction. (From Dadlani GH, Harmon WG, Simbre II VC, et al: *Cardiomyocyte injury to transplant: Pediatric management. Curr Opin Cardiol* 2003;18:91-97.)

In addition, routine screening for some high-risk groups is recommended.

The outcome of children with DCM depends on the cause of the disease and age at presentation. Four outcomes are possible after the initial recognition of ventricular dysfunction: (1) resolution of the ventricular dysfunction, (2) improvement in the degree of dysfunction without complete resolution, (3) progressive deterioration in ventricular dysfunction leading to the need for cardiac transplantation, or (4) death (see Fig. 18-5). Traditionally, approximately one third of children presenting with DCM stemming from myocarditis recover completely, another one third improve but with some residual dysfunction, and the remaining one third die or require transplantation.[20] In 2003, the Pediatric Cardiomyopathy Registry estimated the median age of diagnosis to be 1.8 years for children with DCM in the United States.[1] Of these children, 12.7% required heart transplantation, and 13.6% died within 2 years of the initial diagnosis.[1] Other reports have estimated the 1-year survival rate to be 63% to 70%, the 5-year survival rate to be 34% to 66%, and the 10-year survival rate 3% to be 50%.[20] Sudden death may occur at any stage regardless

of ventricular function and may be precipitated by comorbidities, such as progressive ventricular dysfunction, CHF, arrhythmias, conduction disturbances, or thromboembolic events.

CURRENT STATUS AND FUTURE DIRECTIONS

DCM can be a devastating disease for infants and children that may lead to heart transplantation or death. Most cases are idiopathic; however, myocarditis and neuromuscular disorders account for many cases. Males are at increased risk as a result of gender-linked inheritance patterns, and many children present with the disease before 1 year of age. Progression of heart failure and mortality are highest in the first 2 years after the diagnosis. Multicenter randomized studies are needed to guide medical therapy and screening protocols for high-risk groups. In addition, gene-based therapy and myocyte progenitor cell transplantation hold great promise as therapeutic alternatives. Lastly, surgical options such as mitral valve surgery and new miniaturized ventricular assist devices and their influences on molecular remodeling of the failed ventricle can be considered in the near future.[54,55] In the future, genetic screening[56] also may identify individuals predisposed for myocardial risk, such as individuals with immunologic defects that predispose them to myocarditis or defects in DNA repair mechanisms that may predispose them to free radical injury from anthracycline. Identifying these high-risk groups may allow physicians to tailor medical therapy to prevent subsequent myocardial injury.

Key Concepts

■ More than 50% of pediatric cardiomyopathy cases occur in children younger than 1 year old. This early incidence may represent the effects of genetic defects on critical intracellular pathways.

■ Myocyte injury (from either a genetic or an exogenous cause) may initiate cellular necrosis, regional fibrosis with collagen deposition surrounding the affected region, and hypertrophy of the adjacent viable cells. Myocyte loss leads to impaired contractile function, decreased cardiac output, increased myocardial oxygen consumption, increased end-systolic and end-diastolic volumes, increased peripheral resistance, and activation of compensatory mechanisms that attempt to maintain cardiac output.

■ Although cardiomyopathies previously were believed to be idiopathic, many forms of DCM and HCM now have been linked to genetic defects in structural and functional proteins in the cardiac myocyte. Of idiopathic DCMs, 9% to 20% have a familial component and probably a genetic cause.

■ The generation of contractile force sufficient to maintain cardiac output is a complex process requiring normal electrical conduction, normal intercellular and intracellular calcium signaling, appropriate energy production, sufficient force generation from the sarcomere proteins, and adequate force transmission from the sarcomere through to the extracellular matrix via cytoskeletal proteins. A defect in any of the critical proteins that regulate or are actively involved in this pathway theoretically can lead to DCM.

■ Primary cardiomyopathies commonly are found in association with neuromuscular disorders because myocytes and skeletal muscles share many of the same contractile proteins.

■ It seems that sarcomere proteins have multiple binding regions, and that defects in the regions that function in force generation or transmission lead to a dilated phenotype, whereas mutations affecting energy use may lead to a hypertrophic phenotype.

■ Primary cardiomyopathies occur in one of four inheritance patterns: autosomal dominant, autosomal recessive, X-linked, or mitochondrial. Autosomal dominant inheritance is the most common pattern and usually has a varying degree of phenotypic expression.

■ Left ventricular noncompaction is a rare form of a primary cardiomyopathy. This disorder is characterized by a developmental arrest in the normal compaction of the ventricular endocardium resulting in prominent trabeculations with deep recesses within the myocardium.

■ Endocardial fibroelastosis is a cardiomyopathy that is characterized by excessive endocardial thickening secondary to proliferation of fibrous and elastic fibers. Primary or secondary causes may lead to a common pathologic end point.

■ Arrhythmogenic right ventricular dysplasia is a genetic disorder involving atrophy of the myocardium, followed by fibrosis and fatty infiltrates, usually in the region of the right ventricular free wall. Patients with this condition typically present with recurrent, sustained episodes of ventricular tachycardia or fibrillation that originate from the right ventricle.

■ HIV-related cardiac complications include focal myocarditis, pericarditis, pericardial effusions, endocarditis, idiopathic left ventricular dysfunction, systemic hypertension, pulmonary hypertension, arrhythmias, premature coronary artery disease, AIDS-related cardiac tumors, and autonomic dysfunction. DCM may occur in the setting of HIV through damage to the cardiac myocyte from direct HIV infection; coinfection with other viruses, bacteria, or parasites; autoimmune reactions; drug-related cardiotoxicities; nutritional deficiencies; endocrine abnormalities; inflammatory mediators; or autonomic dysregulation.

■ Direct chemotherapy-associated myocardial damage may occur by free radical damage, mitochondrial injury, apoptosis, or inflammatory or autoimmune responses. Indirect mechanisms of myocardial damage seen after successful treatment of childhood cancer include growth hormone deficiency, endothelial (vascular) injury, and autonomic dysfunction.

■ In addition to systolic ventricular dysfunction, long-term survivors may show evidence of a restrictive cardiomyopathy after anthracycline therapy. Mediastinal radiation causes inflammation in the coronary arteries and diffuse interstitial fibrosis in the myocardium, which may lead to premature coronary artery disease or to a restrictive cardiomyopathy.

■ Compared with adults, children and young adults rarely have ischemic cardiomyopathies. The diverse heterogeneity of primary and secondary cardiomyopathies in this population creates a therapeutic dilemma because many disease processes are unique and may not conform to standard heart failure management strategies.

Acknowledgments

The authors thank Svjetlana Tisma-Dupanovic, MD, Peter Chang, DO, and Sarah Duffy, BS, for their contributions to this chapter.

REFERENCES

1. Lipshultz SE, Sleeper LA, Towbin JA, et al: The incidence of pediatric cardiomyopathies in two regions of the United States. N Engl J Med 2003;348:1647-1655.

2. Nugent AW, Daubeney PE, Chondros P, et al: The epidemiology of childhood cardiomyopathy in Australia. N Engl J Med 2003; 348:1639-1646.

3. Strauss A, Lock JE: Pediatric cardiomyopathy—a long way to go. N Engl J Med 2003;348:1703-1705.

4. Seidman JG, Seidman C: The genetic basis for cardiomyopathy: From mutation identification to mechanistic paradigms. Cell 2001; 104:557-567.

5. Schmitt JP, Kamisago M, Asahi M, et al: Dilated cardiomyopathy and heart failure caused by a mutation in phospholamban. Science 2003;299:1410-1413.

6. Kajstura J, Leri A, Finato N, et al: Myocyte proliferation in end-stage cardiac failure in humans. Proc Natl Sci U S A 1998;95: 8801-8805.

7. Quaini F, Cigola E, Lagrasta C, et al: End-stage cardiac failure in humans is coupled with the induction of proliferating nuclear antigen and nuclear mitotic division in ventricular myocytes. Circ Res1994;75:1050-1063.

8. Francis GS, Wilson-Tang WH: Pathophysiology of congestive heart failure. Rev Cardiovasc Med 2003;4(Suppl 2):S14-S20.

9. Kamran Baig MK, Goldman JH, Caforio AL, et al: Familial dilated cardiomyopathy: Cardiac abnormalities are common in asymptomatic relatives and may represent early disease. J Am Coll Cardiol 1998;31:195-201.

10. Shimizu M, Ino H, Yamaguchi M, et al: Autopsy findings in siblings with hypertrophic cardiomyopathy caused by Arg92Trp mutation in the cardiac troponin T gene showing dilated cardiomyopathy like features. Clin Cardiol 2003;26:536-539.

11. Brodsky GL, Muntoni F, Miocic S, et al: Lamin A/C gene mutation associated with dilated cardiomyopathy with variable skeletal muscle involvement. Circulation 2000;101:473-476.

12. Crilley JG, Boehm EA, Blair E, et al: Hypertrophic cardiomyopathy due to sarcomeric gene mutations is characterized by impaired energy metabolism irrespective of the degree of hypertrophy. J Am Coll Cardiol 2003;41:1776-1782.

13. Braunwald E, Seidman CE, Siwart U: Contemporary evaluation and management of hypertrophic cardiomyopathy. Circulation 2002;106:1312-1316.

14. Pignatelli RH, McMahon CJ, Dreyer WJ, et al: Clinical characterization of left ventricular noncompaction in children: A relatively common form of cardiomyopathy. Circulation 2003;108: 2672-2678.

15. Ni J, Bowles NE, Kim YH, et al: Viral infection of the myocardium in endocardial fibroelastosis: Molecular evidence for the role of mumps virus as an etiological agent. Circulation 1997;95:133-139.

16. De Letter EA, Piette MH: Endocardial fibroelastosis as a cause of sudden unexpected death. Am J Forensic Med Pathol 1999; 20:357-363.

17. Bowles NE, Ni J, Marcus F, Towbin JA: The detection of cardiotropic viruses in the myocardium of patients with arrhythmogenic right ventricular dysplasia/cardiomyopathy. J Am Coll Cardiol 2002;39:892-895.

18. Marcus F, Towbin J, Zareba W, et al: Arrhythmogenic right ventricular dysplasia/cardiomyopathy (ARVD/C): A multidisciplinary study: Design and protocol. Circulation 2003;107:2975-2978.

19. Alcalai R, Metzger S, Rosenheck S, et al: A recessive mutation in desmoplakin causes arrhythmogenic right ventricular dysplasia, skin disorder, and wholly hair. J Am Coll Cardiol 2003;42:319-327.

20. Towbin JA: Pediatric myocardial disease. Pediatr Clin North Am 1999;46:289-308.

21. Bowles NE, Kearney DL, Pauschinger M, et al: Detection of viruses in myocardial tissues by polymerase chain reaction: Evidence of adenovirus as a common cause of myocarditis in children and adults. J Am Coll Cardiol 2003;42:466-472.

22. Calabrese F, Rigo E, Milanesi O, et al: Molecular diagnosis of myocarditis and dilated cardiomyopathy in children: Clinicopathologic features and prognostic implications. Diagn Mol Pathol 2002;11:212-221.

23. Harmon WG, Dadlani G, Fisher S, Lipshultz SE: Myocardial and pericardial disease in HIV. Curr Treat Options Cardiovasc Med 2002;4:497-509.

24. Langston C, Cooper ER, Goldfarb J, et al: HIV-related mortality in infants and children: Data from the pediatric pulmonary and cardiovascular complications of vertically transmitted HIV study. Pediatrics 2001;107:328-336.

25. Grenier MA, Lipshultz SE: Epidemiology of anthracycline cardiotoxicity in children and adults. Semin Oncol 1998;(Suppl 10): 25:72-85.

26. Simbre VC, Adams MJ, Deshpande SS, et al: Cardiomyopathy caused by antineoplastic therapies. Curr Treat Options Cardiovasc Med 2001;3:493-505.

27. Adams MJ, Hardenbergh P, Constine LS, Lipshultz SE: Radiation-associated cardiovascular disease. Crit Rev Oncol Hematol 2003;45:55-75.

28. Simbre II VC, Sinkin R, Hart S, et al: Unsuspected myocardial injury in otherwise healthy newborns (abstract). Pediatr Res 2002;51:37A

29. Harmon WG, Lipshultz SE: Kawasaki syndrome. In Burg FD, Ingelfinger JR, Polin RA, Gershon AA (eds): Gellis and Kagan's Current Pediatric Therapy, 17th ed. Philadelphia, WB Saunders, 2001, pp 550-553.

30. Furuyama H, Odagawa Y, Katoh C, et al: Assessment of coronary function in children with a history of Kawasaki disease using 15 O-water positron emission tomography. Circulation 2002; 105:2878-2884.

31. Kahwaji IY, Connuck DM, Tafari N, Dahdah NS: A national survey on the pediatric cardiologist's clinical approach for patients with Kawasaki disease. Pediatr Cardiol 2002;23:639-646.

32. Dadlani GH, Gingell RL, Orie JD, et al: Kawasaki patients with coronary artery calcifications detected by ultrafast CT scan: A pediatric population that may be at risk for early atherosclerosis (abstract). Circulation 2001;104:2439.

33. Bacha F, Saad R, Gungor N, et al: Obesity, regional fat distribution, and syndrome X in obese black versus white adolescents: Race differential in diabetogenic and atherogenic risk factors. J Clin Endocrinol Metab 2003;88:2534-2540.

34. Ford E: C-reactive protein concentration and cardiovascular disease risk factors in children: Findings from the national health and nutrition examination survey 1999-2000. Circulation 2003;108:1053-1058.

35. Schwartz ML, Cox GF, Lin AE, et al: Clinical approach to genetic cardiomyopathy in children. Circulation 1996;94:2021-2038.

36. Friedman RA, Moak JP, Garson Jr A: Clinical cause of idiopathic dilated cardiomyopathy in children. J Am Coll Cardiol 1991; 18:152.

37. Nugent AW, Davis AM, Kleinert S, et al: Clinical, electrocardiographic, and histologic correlations in children with dilated cardiomyopathy. J Heart Lung Transplant 2001;20:1152-1157.

38. Lipshultz SE: Ventricular dysfunction clinical research in infants, children and adolescents. Prog Pediatr Cardiol 2000;12:1-28.

39. Ocal B, Oguz D, Karademir S, et al: Myocardial performance index combining systolic and diastolic myocardial performance in doxirubicin treated patients and its correlation to conventional echo/Doppler indices. Pediatr Cardiol 2002;23:522-527.

40. Colan SD, Parness IA, Spevak PJ, Sanders SP: Developmental modulation of myocardial mechanics: Age- and growth-related alterations in afterload and contractility. J Am Coll Cardiol 1992;19:619-629.

41. Wu LA, Lapeyre AC, Cooper LT: Current role of endomyocardial biopsy in the management of dilated cardiomyopathy and myocarditis. Mayo Clin Proc 2001;76:1030-1038.

42. Claudius I, Yueh-Tze L, Ruey-Kang C, et al: Usefulness of B-type natriuretic peptide as a noninvasive screening tool for cardiac allograft pathology in pediatric heart transplant recipients. Am J Cardiol 2003;92:1368-1370.

43. Lipshultz SE, Fisher SD, Lai WW, Miller TL: Cardiovascular monitoring and therapy for HIV-infected patients. Ann N Y Acad Sci 2001;946:236-273.

44. Lipshultz SE, Orav EJ, Sanders SP, Colan SD: Immunoglobulins and left ventricular structure and function in pediatric HIV infection. Circulation 1995;92:2220-2225.

45. Sirajuddin RA, Miller AB, Geraci SA: Anticoagulation in patients with dilated cardiomyopathy and sinus rhythm: A critical literature review. J Card Fail 2002;8:48-53.

46. Lipshultz SE, Lipsitz SR, Sallen SE, et al: Long-term enalapril therapy for left ventricular dysfunction in doxorubicin-treated survivors of childhood cancer. J Clin Oncol 2002;20:4517-4522.

47. Chiu SN, Wu MH, Wang JK, et al: Heart transplantation and the Batista operation for children with refractory heart failure. Jpn Circ J 2001;65:289-293.

48. Nakamoto S, Oku H, Fukuhara H, et al: Partial left ventriculotomy in association with dilated cardiomyopathy: Echocardiographic folllow-up. Jpn Circ J 2002;66:104-106.

49. Claus M, Beling M, Grohmann A, et al: Long-term results after partial left ventriculectomy. Int J Cardiol 2003;89:223-230.

50. Lipshultz SE, Easley KA, Orav EJ, et al: Absence of cardiac toxicity of zidovudine in infants. Pediatric Pulmonary and Cardiac Complications in Vertically Transmitted HIV Infection Study Group. N Engl J Med 2000;343:759-766.

51. Lipshultz SE: Dextrazone for protection against cardiotoxic effects of anthracyclines in children. J Clin Oncol 1996;14:328-331.

52. Lipshultz SE, Fisher SD, Lai WW, Miller TL: Cardiovascular risk factors, monitoring and therapy for HIV-infected patients. AIDS 2003;17:S96-S122.

53. Dadlani GH, Harmon WG, Simbre VC II, et al: Cardiomyocyte injury to transplant: Pediatric management. Curr Opin Cardiol 2003;18:91-97.

54. Geha AS, El-Zein C, Massad MG: Mitral valve surgery in patients with ischemic and nonischemic dilated cardiomyopathy. Cardiology 2004;101:15-20.

55. Vatta M, Stetson SJ, Jimenez S, et al: Molecular normalization of dystrophin in the failing left and right ventricle of patients treated with either pulsatile or continuous flow-type ventricular assist devices. J Am Coll Cardiol 2004;43:811-817.

56. Burkett EL, Hershberger RE: Clinical and genetic issues in familial dilated cardiomyopathy. J Am Coll Cardiol 2005;45:969-981.

CHAPTER 19

Restrictive Cardiomyopathy and Constrictive Pericarditis

Susan W. Denfield

Cardiomyopathies are defined as diseases of the myocardium associated with cardiac dysfunction.[1] According to the World Health Organization (WHO) definition, restrictive cardiomyopathy (RCM) is characterized by restrictive filling and reduced diastolic volume of either or both ventricles with normal or near-normal systolic function and wall thicknesses; increased interstitial fibrosis may be present. RCM may be idiopathic or associated with another disease. Pericarditis is an inflammation of the pericardium that may be idiopathic or associated with another disease. Constrictive pericarditis is a form of cardiac compression resulting from a diseased, usually scarred, pericardium that restricts cardiac filling.[2]

Although RCM is a disease of the myocardium, and constrictive pericarditis is a disease of the pericardium, their clinical presentations can be similar. Both diseases can result in heart failure as defined by a panel of the National Heart, Lung and Blood Institute:[3] Heart failure occurs when an abnormality of cardiac function causes the heart to fail to pump blood at a rate required by the metabolizing tissues or when the heart can do so only with elevated filling pressure. The heart's inability to pump a sufficient amount of blood to meet the needs of the body tissues may be due to insufficient or defective cardiac filling or impaired contraction and emptying or both.[3]

Differentiating RCM from constrictive pericarditis is important because the approaches to treatment are distinctly different. This chapter reviews the epidemiology, etiologies, pathology, pathophysiology, clinical presentation, diagnostic evaluation, outcome, and management of pediatric patients with RCM and those with constrictive pericarditis. In total, 26 case reports and series consisting of 129 pediatric patients with RCM and 21 case reports and series of pediatric patients with constrictive pericarditis from 1957 to the present are reviewed.[4-50]

RESTRICTIVE CARDIOMYOPATHY

Of the four types of cardiomyopathy categorized by the WHO (dilated, hypertrophic, restrictive, and arrhythmogenic right ventricular cardiomyopathy), RCM is the least common.[1] In children, RCM accounts for only 2.5% to 5% of the diagnosed cardiomyopathies.[4,5,51,52] In the Australian study by Nugent and colleagues,[51] RCM accounted for 2.5% of the cardiomyopathies diagnosed in children younger than 10 years of age. This finding is similar to the two-region U.S. study by Lipshultz and associates,[52] who reported that RCM or other specified types (not dilated or hypertrophic) accounted for only 3% of the cardiomyopathies in children younger than 18 years old. The higher 5% reported by Denfield and Lewis[5] were from single institutions and may have been due to referral bias.

The incidence of cardiomyopathies is higher in children younger than 1 year of age when all types of cardiomyopathy are considered.[51,52] RCM may be an exception, however. In the Nugent study,[52] the incidence of all types of cardiomyopathy except RCM declined rapidly after infancy to their maximum study age of 10 years. In the studies of RCM in children, the average age at the time of diagnosis was 6 years (range 0.1 to 19 years) (Table 19-1).[4-29] Only two of the patients were 19 years old at the time of diagnosis, with the remaining patients younger than 18 years. At the time of diagnosis, 7% were 1 year old or younger, 81% were between 2 and 11 years old, and 12% were between 12 and 19 years old. Whether this apparent difference

TABLE 19-1

Demographics and Clinical Features of Children with Restrictive Cardiomyopathy	
Percent of cardiomyopathies	2.5-5%
Mean/median age at presentation (range)	5.8/4.7 yr (0.1-19 yr)
Female-to-male ratio %	57%:43%
Positive family history	30%
Presenting complaints:	
Respiratory—DOE, "asthma," cough/pneumonia	47%
Abnormal PE—ascites, hepatomegaly, edema, gallop, loud P_2, murmur	21%
Congestive heart failure (not otherwise defined)	10%
Syncope	10%
Other*	≤10%

*Includes sudden death, palpitations, fatigue, embolic events, incidental cardiomegaly on chest x-ray, and positive family history.
 DOE, dyspnea on exertion; PE, physical examination
 (Data compiled from references 4-29.)

in usual age of onset is due to case ascertainment or true differences in the disease onset is unknown.

Gender differences also have been reported in cardiomyopathies. Beyond infancy, boys had a higher incidence of cardiomyopathy than girls in the Lipshultz study.[52] Only hypertrophic and unspecified cardiomyopathies occurred with higher frequency in boys in the Nugent study, with RCM occurring with equal frequency in boys and girls.[51] In contrast, of the 113 subjects in whom gender was reported in the RCM studies reviewed, 57% were female (16 subjects were not specified by gender). If all 16 were males, the male-to-female ratio would be 50:50, suggesting there is not a male predominance in RCM and raising the possibility that there is actually a female predominance (see Table 19-1). Sporadic and familial cases of RCM are reported. Of the published cases, 30% of patients in whom family history was reported had a positive family history.

Genetic Aspects

Mutations in three genes (transthyretin, desmin, and troponin I) have been identified to date that may result in a RCM phenotype.[53-56] Transthyretin mutations result in RCM with amyloidosis and have been reported only in adults.[54] Desmin is a myofibrillar protein that is the chief intermediate filament of skeletal and cardiac muscle.[55] It maintains the structural and functional integrity of the myofibrils and functions as a cytoskeletal protein, linking Z bands to the plasma membrane. Mutations in the desmin gene may cause RCM with or without skeletal myopathy and with or without conduction system disease. The inheritance pattern usually is autosomal dominant, but sporadic mutations have been identified.[55]

Troponin I mutations have been identified in patients with RCM and hypertrophic cardiomyopathy.[53] The RCM and the hypertrophic cardiomyopathy phenotypes can be expressed in the same family; this indicates that idiopathic RCM can be part of the clinical expression of sarcomeric contractile protein disease. The diversity of the phenotypic expression of troponin mutations in families suggests that additional genetic factors or environmental factors or both play a role in disease expression. De novo mutations and autosomal dominant transmission have been documented in RCM patients and their families.[53]

Clinical Features

RCM has multiple causes and may result from myocardial diseases including infiltrative or noninfiltrative processes, storage diseases, endomyocardial diseases, myocarditis, and after cardiac transplantation (Table 19-2).[57] The pathology and histology vary with the underlying disease process. In adults, endomyocardial fibrosis (EMF) in the tropics and amyloidosis outside the tropics are the most common causes of RCM.[58] Cardiac amyloidosis is virtually unheard of in children. In pediatric patients, EMF may be the most common cause of RCM in

TABLE 19-2

Causes of Restrictive Cardiomyopathies in Children and Adults	
Myocardial	Glycogen storage diseases
Idiopathic	Endomyocardial
Familial	Endomyocardial fibrosis
Scleroderma	Hypereosinophilia syndrome
Myocarditis	(Löffler endocarditis)
Cardiac transplantation	Endocardial fibroelastosis
Pseudoxanthoma	Carcinoid
elasticum	Metastatic cancers
Diabetic cardiomyopathy	Radiation
Amyloidosis	Drugs
Sarcoidosis	Anthracyclines
Gaucher disease	Serotonin
Hurler disease	Methysergide
Fatty infiltration	Ergotamine
Hemochromatosis	Mercurials
Fabry disease	Busulfan

the tropics. Outside the tropics, idiopathic RCM is probably most common in children based on reported cases in the literature.[4-29]

Endomyocardial fibrosis (EMF) was first described by Davies in 1948.[59] It occurs most frequently in tropical and subtropical Africa (particularly Uganda and Nigeria), but is found in tropical and subtropical regions throughout the world. It is seen occasionally in temperate climates, usually in individuals who previously lived in tropical areas. The disease affects both genders equally and occurs most often in adolescents and young adults[60]; it is also more common in blacks.[61]

The disease is most commonly biventricular, followed by purely left ventricular involvement in approximately 40% of the cases and purely right ventricular involvement in 10%.[61] The symptom complex varies with the sites of involvement. Symptoms of pulmonary venous congestion result from left-sided disease, whereas signs and symptoms of systemic venous congestion result from right-sided disease. Involvement of the mitral or tricuspid valve apparatus can result in significant valvular regurgitation. Medical and surgical therapies are palliative.

The histology of EMF is characterized by fibrosis of the endocardium of varying thickness. Histologic changes occur in predominantly three areas: the left ventricular apex, the mitral valve apparatus, and the right ventricular apex, which may extend to the supporting structures of the tricuspid valve. In severe cases, the process may extend to the outflow tracts. Small patches of fibroelastosis may occur in the outflow tracts, but the elastin component is believed to be secondary and not a primary part of the process. Cellular infiltrates are not prominent. Although EMF occurs in areas where parasitic diseases that result in eosinophilia are common, the cause of the process is still unknown. Eosinophilia is not typically a prominent feature, in contrast to Löffler endocarditis.

Hypereosinophilic syndrome (HES), or **Löffler endocarditis**, is similar to EMF in many respects. It is debated whether these diseases are variants of the same disease. Although there are pathologic and clinical similarities, there are important contrasts as well. HES typically is seen in temperate climates and is more common in men. Hypereosinophilia is present. HES includes persistent eosinophilia with 1500 eosinophils/mm³ for at least 6 months or until death with evidence of organ involvement. Usually a variety of organs besides the heart are involved, including the lungs, bone marrow, and brain.[62] The cause of the eosinophilia is usually unknown, but may be leukemic or secondary to parasitic, allergic, granulomatous, hypersensitivity, or neoplastic disorders.[63] Cardiac histologic findings include varying degrees of eosinophilic myocarditis (not characteristically seen in EMF), inflammatory reaction in the small intramural coronary vessels with thrombosis and fibrinoid changes, and endocardial mural thrombosis and fibrotic thickening.[61]

The clinical picture in HES may include weight loss, fever, cough, rash, and heart failure. Systemic embolism is frequent, and death is usually secondary to the cardiac manifestations of the disease. Therapy for hypereosinophilia includes corticosteroids, hydroxyurea, or vincristine, but this therapy usually is not directed by the cardiologist. Cardiac therapy includes digoxin, diuretics, afterload reduction, and anticoagulation. Surgical approaches include mitral and tricuspid valve repair or replacement; excision of the fibrotic endocardium may be useful for symptom palliation of intractable heart failure. Pediatric case reports and case series of HES and EMF patients report a relatively high reoperation rate secondary to dysfunction of mechanical or bioprosthetic valves with recurrent thrombosis, fibrosis, or tearing despite anticoagulation.[64,65] Significant cardiac symptoms may persist despite all modalities of therapy.[65]

Many **metabolic disorders** including infiltrative and storage diseases and specific enzyme deficiencies can result in RCM. These diseases include lysosomal disorders, such as Hurler syndrome, Gaucher disease, and Fabry disease, and glycogen storage diseases, which can be lysosomal disorders or result from cytoplasmic enzyme deficiencies. **Hemochromatosis** may be a primary or secondary disease resulting from iron overload with subsequent dysfunction of multiple organs, including the heart. Either RCM or more commonly dilated cardiomyopathy may result from hemochromatosis. **Sarcoidosis** is a noncaseating granulomatous disorder that is more common in adults than in children. The granulomatous inflammatory process can affect the heart and result in RCM. Systolic dysfunction, pericarditis, conduction system disease, and sudden death also may occur. Although a common cause of RCM in adults,

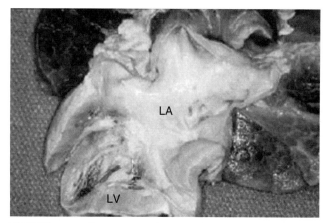

FIGURE 19-1 ■ Restrictive cardiomyopathy. The left atrium (LA) is massively dilated, dwarfing the size of the left ventricle (LV), in this autopsy specimen from a patient with restrictive cardiomyopathy. (See also Color Section)

cardiac **amyloidosis** as a cause for RCM in pediatric patients was not found in the literature search. **Drugs** and therapeutic agents, such as anthracyclines, serotonin, methysergide, ergotamine, mercurial agents, and busulfan, have been reported to cause RCM.[66-69] Mediastinal **radiation** also has resulted in RCM.[70] Outside the tropics, the **idiopathic form** of RCM is probably the most common form in children. Although the family history is positive in only approximately 30% of this population, a genetic basis or predisposition for the development of the disease is likely.

Figure 19-1 shows the pathology of this disease and the typical appearance of a heart from a patient with idiopathic RCM. The left atrium dwarfs the left ventricle, and the left ventricular cavity size is normal with no appreciable left ventricular hypertrophy. In most cases, the heart is otherwise structurally normal, although there have been rare reports of patients who also have atrial septal defects or small, hemodynamically insignificant ventricular septal defects.[9,28] The histology in idiopathic RCM is nonspecific, revealing varying degrees of fibrosis and myocyte hypertrophy.

The pathophysiology of RCM is as follows: Diastolic function is affected primarily by ventricular compliance, stiffness, and relaxation. In the normal heart, the phase of rapid or early filling occurs as the left ventricular pressure declines to less than the pressure in the left atrium, just after the mitral valve opens, and accounts for most ventricular filling.[71,72] The duration of the next phase, called *diastasis,* varies and is heart rate dependent, permitting less than 5% of filling. The last phase of diastole is atrial systole and accounts for approximately 15% of normal ventricular filling. In the classic description of RCM, ventricular filling is completed in early diastole with little or no filling in late diastole. In this model, restrictive physiology results from increased myocardial stiffness with decreased compliance causing a marked ventricular pressure increase with small changes in volume.

The earliest phase of clinical diastole is isovolumic relaxation, which is an active energy-requiring process for the uptake of calcium ions into the sarcoplasmic reticulum. Ischemia and hypertrophy can result in abnormal relaxation secondary to changes in calcium uptake. Gewillig and coworkers[10] reported on six children with RCM who by catheterization and echocardiography had parameters suggesting delayed relaxation and restrictive filling as the mechanisms for RCM. In their patients, early filling contributed approximately 56%; mid-diastolic filling, 28%; and atrial filling, 16% to total ventricular filling. These investigators suggested that the restrictive hemodynamics were caused by dysfunction and delay of active relaxation of the ventricle rather than increased intrinsic stiffness of the ventricular wall.[10] It is likely that as diastolic diseases become better understood that RCM is likely to result from abnormal stiffness or abnormal relaxation or both depending on the underlying cause of the disease and disease progression.

The clinical presentation is summarized in Table 19-1 as the presenting complaints of pediatric patients reported in the English literature. In children, RCM frequently masquerades as other diseases. The most common presenting symptoms initially may appear to be pulmonary related. Children with RCM frequently have a history of recurrent lower respiratory tract infections or asthma. Referral to a cardiologist eventually occurs when cardiomegaly is noted on chest x-ray.

The second most common reason for referral is abnormal physical examination findings. Patients who have ascites, hepatomegaly, and edema frequently are referred to a gastroenterologist first. Referral to a cardiologist occurs when additional cardiac signs or symptoms occur, a chest x-ray is noted to be abnormal, or no specific gastrointestinal etiology is found for the edema and hepatomegaly. Earlier referral to a cardiologist occurs when the presenting sign is an abnormal heart sound, such as a murmur, gallop, or loud P_2.

Congestive heart failure and syncope each account for approximately 10% of the presenting complaints. Syncope in these patients may be related to ischemia, arrhythmias, or thromboembolism.[9,10] Ischemia and arrhythmias may be the most common causes of syncope and sudden death in this patient population.[9] In one case, no definitive mechanism for syncopal episodes was found, but an arrhythmia was ruled out, and there were no ischemic changes on treadmill.[5] Two children had sudden cardiac death as their presentation at ages 6 and 16 years, presumably secondary to familial RCM because there were 13 other affected family members in five generations.[12] A positive family history was an infrequent reason for referral in the published reports; however, 30% of patients in whom a family history was reported had a positive family history.

Clinical Evaluation

The physical examination commonly reveals a gallop rhythm and a loud P_2. Hepatomegaly, ascites, and edema

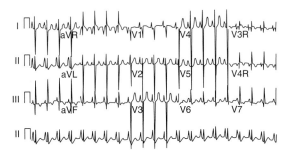

FIGURE 19-2 ■ ECG in a patient with restrictive cardiomyopathy. ECG from a 2-year-old child with restrictive cardiomyopathy shows sinus rhythm with right atrial enlargement, right-axis deviation, a QS pattern in V1, ST-segment depression in the inferolateral leads, and T wave inversion in III.

also commonly are found. The ECG is extremely useful in screening for RCM because approximately 98% of ECGs are abnormal (Fig. 19-2).[4-10,12-25,28] The most common abnormalities are right or left atrial (or both) enlargement; ST-segment depression and ST-T wave abnormalities are also frequently present. Right and left ventricular hypertrophy and conduction abnormalities also can be seen.

A Holter evaluation can be useful not only for rhythm evaluation, but also for ST-segment analysis. Rivenes and associates[9] reported Holter results in 12 patients, 8 of whom had ischemic changes with ST-segment depression of 3 to 12.7 mm, most evident at higher heart rates. In one patient, ventricular tachycardia was preceded by chest pain and ST-segment depression of 8.2 mm, but she was successfully resuscitated (Fig. 19-3). Three case reports also showed ischemic or infarct patterns on ECG and autopsy, and in some children, chest pain related to the ischemia was identified, suggesting this is an important cause of morbidity and mortality in these patients.[6,15,16]

Of the pediatric studies reporting arrhythmias, approximately 15% of the patients had arrhythmias or conduction disturbances or both.[4,5,7-9,19,23,25,28] Atrial flutter was the most commonly reported arrhythmia. High-grade second-degree and third-degree heart block were the next most commonly reported disturbances. Atrial fibrillation and atrial tachycardias, Wolff-Parkinson-White syndrome with supraventricular tachycardia, symptomatic sinus bradycardia requiring pacing, and ventricular tachycardia and torsades de pointes also were reported.

The chest x-ray seems to be a useful screening test because it is abnormal in approximately 90% of cases.[4-10,13-22,28] Cardiomegaly and pulmonary venous congestion are the most common abnormalities. The echocardiogram is usually diagnostic (Fig. 19-4). On two-dimensional imaging, classic cases show markedly dilated atria, often dwarfing the size of the ventricles. Typically there is normal or near-normal left ventricular systolic function and absence of significant hypertrophy or dilation. Based on studies reporting systolic functional parameters, 30% may present with or develop a depressed shortening or ejection fraction.[4,8,10,28]

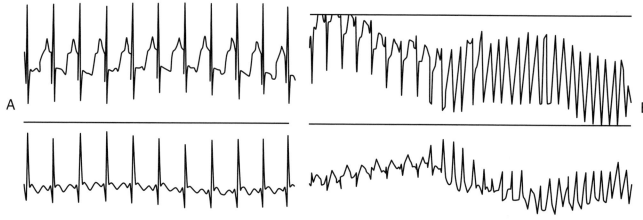

FIGURE 19-3 ■ Holter monitoring in a patient with restrictive cardiomyopathy. A, Holter monitor tracing from a 10-year-old outpatient shows 8-mm ST-segment depression at a heart rate of 135 beats/min.
B, Holter monitor tracing from the same patient when she was admitted to the hospital with chest
pain. During an episode of chest pain, she developed sinus tachycardia, ST-segment depression, and
ventricular tachycardia from which she was successfully cardioverted.

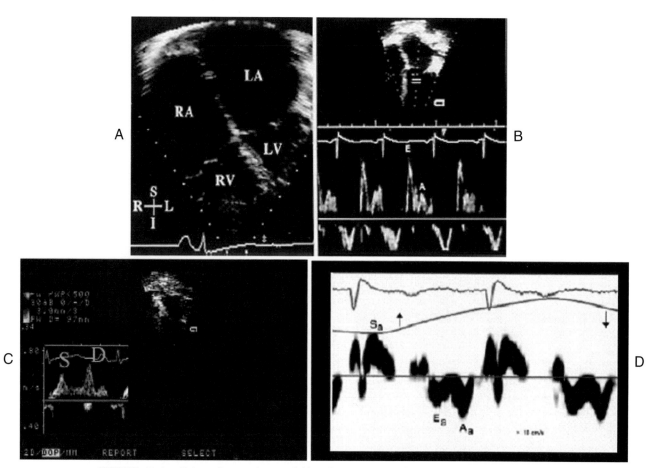

FIGURE 19-4 ■ Echocardiogram from a child with restrictive cardiomyopathy. A, Severe biatrial
enlargement, dwarfing the size of the ventricles. B, Mitral inflow with an increased E/A ratio and a
shortened deceleration time. C, Doppler tracing from the right upper pulmonary vein shows
increased diastolic flow velocity compared with systolic flow with a shortened deceleration time.
D, Tissue Doppler imaging reveals a pseudonormal Ea Aa pattern and an increased E/Ea ratio. Aa, atrial
contraction; D, diastole; Ea, early diastolic velocity; E/A ratio, early-to-late diastolic filling ratio; LA,
left atrium; LV, left ventricle; RA, right atrium; RV, right ventricle; S, systole; Sa, systolic wave at annulus.

Reported shortening fractions have been as low as the low 20% range with ejection fractions as low as the upper 30% range. In addition, 40% have or develop mild, sometimes progressive, left ventricular hypertrophy.[4,5,8,10,28] Varying patterns of hypertrophy have been reported, including, concentric, mid-septal bulge, apical hypertrophy, and atypical hypertrophy. The subset of patients with hypertrophy may have a troponin I mutation. The mixed restrictive/hypertrophic phenotype can result in a confusing clinical picture in terms of diagnosis and optimal therapeutic approaches.

During two-dimensional imaging, the presence of thrombi should be addressed. Thrombotic and embolic events have been described in approximately 21% of pediatric patients with idiopathic RCM reported in seven studies.[4,5,7,8,10,24,28] In HES and EMF, there may be obliteration of the apex by thrombus, and the atrioventricular valve apparatus frequently is involved in the pathologic process with thickening of valve leaflets and decreased excursion, particularly of the mitral valve. In idiopathic RCM, the valves are typically normal in appearance. Pericardial thickening on two-dimensional evaluation suggests constrictive pericarditis and not RCM.

Doppler patterns of diastolic dysfunction have been well characterized in adults, and pediatric data have been reported. Typical findings in adults with RCM include an increased early-to-late diastolic filling ratio (E/A ratio). Although numerous studies have characterized Doppler findings in adults with RCM, only a few pediatric studies have described Doppler findings in children with RCM.[7,8,10,25] Some children in some of these studies did not have complete Doppler data because all the pediatric studies were retrospective. In the patients described, the findings consistent with restrictive filling and increased left ventricular end-diastolic pressure included elevated E/A ratios, short mitral deceleration times, increased pulmonary vein atrial reversal velocity and duration, and pulmonary vein atrial reversal duration greater than mitral A duration.[7,8,25] Restrictive hemodynamics typically are believed to be caused by increased ventricular wall stiffness; however, idiopathic RCM also may result from disorders of delayed active relaxation. The Gewillig study[10] described six children with idiopathic RCM whose Doppler profiles were consistent with restrictive filling with elevated E/A ratios and shortened deceleration times, but who also had parameters suggesting dysfunction and delay of active relaxation of the ventricle. In their patients, mitral inflow patterns revealed a prominent mitral L wave with mid-diastolic filling accounting for approximately 28% of total ventricular filling. The left ventricular pressure curve showed a small, but steady decline during mid-diastolic filling on cardiac catheterization, implying the driving force for filling was ventricular suction and not increased left atrial pressure. In adults, Doppler tissue imaging has been used to help differentiate between RCM and

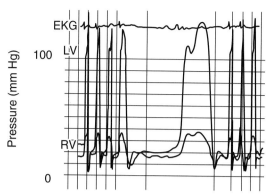

FIGURE 19-5 ■ Cardiac catheterization. Pressure tracing during cardiac catheterization shows the dip and plateau or square root sign, which may be seen in either restrictive cardiomyopathy or constrictive pericarditis.

constrictive pericarditis, but this modality needs further evaluation in children.[73,74]

Cardiac catheterization is an important part of the evaluation in patients with RCM and may be performed at the time of diagnosis. Catheterization can help differentiate between RCM and constrictive pericarditis, although virtually all hemodynamic features can overlap.[75] Both diseases typically have an early diastolic dip and subsequent plateau pattern, also called the *square root sign* (Fig. 19-5).[61,75] In classic RCM, the left ventricular end-diastolic pressure, left atrial pressure, and pulmonary capillary wedge pressure are markedly elevated and at least 4 to 5 mm Hg (preferably 10 mm Hg) greater than the right atrial pressure and right ventricular end diastolic pressure. In cases in which the pressures are essentially equal, volume loading may bring out the differences in pressure between the right and left sides.

Pulmonary hypertension is frequently present at the time of initial catheterization in addition to elevated left or right ventricular end-diastolic pressures in RCM.[4,8,25,27-29] The initial pulmonary vascular resistance index may range from normal to 13.6 U:m[2].[4,8,25,27-29] In studies providing follow-up data 0.3 to 8 years after presentation, the pulmonary vascular resistance index ranged from normal to 30 U:m[2].[4,28,29] The pulmonary vasculature frequently remains reactive with some studies suggesting response to inhaled nitric oxide.[27] In the study by Weller and associates,[28] 40% were precluded from orthotopic heart transplantation, however, due to an elevated and nonreactive pulmonary vascular resistance at the time they were evaluated for cardiac transplantation.[28] None of the studies predicted when or in whom fixed pulmonary vascular resistance would develop.

In patients who undergo endomyocardial biopsy, most specimens are nondiagnostic, revealing varying degrees of fibrosis and hypertrophy. Increased numbers of mitochondria are seen in some patients, as is an increase in glycogen, but endomyocardial biopsy is rarely diagnostic of a specific etiology and is not without risk.[4,8,10] Desmin myopathy has been seen in skeletal muscle biopsy and cardiac tissue, however, leading to an etiologic diagnosis.[24,55] Desmin myopathy can signify impending skeletal myopathy or conduction system disease and should be evaluated for in any biopsy tissue obtained.

Children with RCM are hemodynamically fragile; case series and reports in children with RCM have reported deterioration and death during or shortly after catheterization and biopsy.[4,17] Although cardiac catheterization is useful, careful consideration of the risk-to-benefit ratio of the information that is likely to be obtained by the biopsy should be undertaken before catheterization.

The prognosis in children with RCM is poor[4,5,7,8,25,28]; one half of the children die within 2 years of diagnosis. The prognosis in RCM seems to be significantly worse than in patients with hypertrophic cardiomyopathy or dilated cardiomyopathy, in which the 2-year mortality rates are reported to be 12.7% and 13.6%.[52] In RCM, heart failure–related deaths are the most common, but sudden cardiac death also has been reported to be a common cause of death in children with RCM.[9] In the study by Rivenes and associates,[9] sudden cardiac death occurred in 28% of children with an annual mortality rate of 7%; this is comparable to a 31% incidence of sudden death in children with hypertrophic cardiomyopathy reported by Maron and colleagues.[76] In review of the literature reports in which data on sudden death were available, approximately 12% of children died suddenly.[6,9,12,17,28] Patients who seem to be at greater risk for sudden death include patients who present with signs and symptoms of ischemia, such as syncope and chest pain.[9]

Poor prognostic factors for death from heart failure include cardiomegaly and pulmonary venous congestion on chest x-ray, age younger than 5 years, thromboembolism, and elevated pulmonary vascular resistance index.[7,8,28] Children with heart failure also are at risk from ischemic complications.[9] In the studies reviewed, approximately 50% of patients died, 30% were alive receiving a variety of medical therapies, and 20% had undergone cardiac transplantation. Of patients undergoing cardiac transplantation, 80% were alive.

Therapeutic Strategies

There was no consistent approach to therapy in the studies reviewed. At present, medical therapy remains supportive. Any therapy with potential for hemodynamic effects should be started with the patient hospitalized because of the fragile nature of these patients. Diuretics are useful in patients with signs and symptoms of systemic or pulmonary venous congestion, but overdiuresis should be avoided because these patients are sensitive to alterations in preload. Due to the 21% incidence of thromboembolic events, antiplatelet therapy or anticoagulants should be administered.

Medications were given in a variety of combinations, including digoxin, afterload-reducing agents, calcium channel blockers, and β-blockers. Because of the small number of patients in each study, and the lack of uniformity of treatment even within studies, the benefits or risks of these therapies could not be determined accurately. Bengur and coworkers [77] reported that captopril lowered the aortic pressure by 24% without an increase in cardiac output when administered during cardiac catheterization to four pediatric patients with RCM. These authors suggested that captopril should not be used in patients with RCM. In the studies that reported the use of angiotensin-converting enzyme inhibitors in some patients, acute decompensation was not reported, but no therapeutic or symptomatic benefit was noted.[4,5,8,25,28,29] In adults with diastolic heart failure, the use of angiotensin-converting enzyme inhibitors has been suggested, but data are limited in adults as well.[78] Modulation of the neurohumoral activation may affect fibroblast activity, interstitial fibrosis, intracellular calcium handling, and myocardial stiffness. The risks and benefits of angiotensin-converting enzyme inhibitors in pediatric RCM remain to be determined.

In adults with diastolic dysfunction, tachycardia is poorly tolerated, so β-blockers or some calcium channel blockers have been suggested as part of the treatment regimen.[78] In the pediatric study by Rivenes and associates,[9] β-blocker therapy was suggested to blunt rapid heart rates, given the apparent ischemia risk in their patient population in whom significant ST-segment depression was noted at higher heart rates. Subsequently, three children younger than 5 years old were reported who were begun on propranolol (n = 2) or metoprolol (n = 1) but who did not tolerate β-blocker therapy.[79] In the first patient, episodes of pallor, weakness, and listlessness occurred; this patient was on telemetry, and no arrhythmias were documented. These episodes stopped when propranolol was discontinued. The second patient developed staring spells and profound diaphoresis; one episode occurred while the patient was in the hospital and terminated with the administration of a high dextrose infusion (50% dextrose) before a blood glucose value was obtained. Propranolol was discontinued, and the episodes ceased. The patient who received metoprolol became irritable and restless after 2 to 3 days on the medication with some improvement initially after stopping the drug. Further studies are needed to determine the role of β-blocker therapy in this disease.

Because current medical therapy seems to be ineffective, and the development of pulmonary hypertension is common, and mortality is high, cardiac transplantation should be the therapy of choice. When comparing survival with RCM with survival after cardiac transplantation, it is evident that cardiac transplantation results in longer survival.[28] Most patients should be evaluated and placed on the transplantation waiting list at the time of presentation. While waiting for transplantation, patients should have Holter monitoring performed every 6 months or as symptoms dictate to evaluate for signs of ischemia, ventricular arrhythmias, or developing conduction disturbances. Implantable defibrillators should be considered for patients with evidence of ischemia and ventricular arrhythmias, and strenuous physical activity should be avoided.

CONSTRICTIVE PERICARDITIS

The clinical presentation of patients with RCM and constrictive pericarditis can be similar, as can results of diagnostic tests used to try to differentiate between these two clinical entities. If isolated bands of constriction occur, constrictive pericarditis can present similarly to tricuspid or mitral stenosis or subpulmonary or pulmonary stenosis.[80-84] The differentiation of constrictive pericarditis from other pathologic processes is important because of the differences in outcome and treatment of the various disease states.

Clinical Features

In children, constrictive pericarditis has been reported to account for 0.7% to 13% of all cases of pericarditis.[33,37] Although it has been reported in children younger than 10 years old, it is uncommon.[31,33,36] A male predominance has been reported in children.[31,36]

Two **syndromes** have been described in children that are associated with the development of constrictive pericarditis. Mulibrey nanism is a rare autosomal recessive disorder that also has been called *Perheentupa syndrome* or *constrictive pericarditis with dwarfism.*[46]

It is characterized by short stature; triangular face; yellowish dots on ocular fundi; long, shallow, J-shaped sella turcica; and constrictive pericarditis. Another autosomal recessive disorder has been described that includes pericarditis (constrictive), arthritis, and camptodactyly.[45,48] The locus responsible for this syndrome has been assigned by homozygosity mapping to a 1.9 cM interval on chromosome 1q25-31.[85] This syndrome also has been termed *familial fibrosing serositis.*[45] The common feature seems to be fibrosis of serous membranes. DeLine and Cable[50] also reported a cluster of cases that occurred in two generations of a family. The pericarditis phenotype in this family included effusive and constrictive pericarditis. Familial clustering of common etiologies for pericarditis was not present in their patient cohort, leading the investigators to postulate possible autosomal dominant inheritance with incomplete penetrance based on the family pedigree. Lastly, although a specific syndrome has not been identified, there has been an unusually frequent association of atrial septal defects with constrictive pericarditis.[40] Ascertainment bias has not been completely excluded as a cause for this association.

There are multiple causes of constrictive pericarditis (Table 19-3). Tuberculosis historically has been the leading cause of constrictive pericarditis throughout the world and remains a dominant cause in developing countries. Idiopathic and a combination of other infectious agents are the most common etiologies in developed nations. Connective tissue diseases and vasculitis, malignancies, therapeutic irradiation, and cardiopericardial

TABLE 19-3

Reported Associations or Causes of Constrictive Pericarditis in Children and Adults	
Idiopathic	Uremia (on dialysis)
Infectious	Hemorrhagic disorders (resulting in hemopericardium)
Tuberculosis	Atrial septal defect (unrepaired)
Viral	Drugs
Bacterial	Procainamide
Fungal	Methysergide
Parasitic	Practolol
Connective tissue diseases	Hydralazine
Rheumatoid arthritis	Cromolyn sodium
Systemic lupus erythematosus	Penicillins
Dermatomyositis	Isoniazid
Scleroderma (includes CREST syndrome)	Minoxidil
Sarcoidosis	Phenylbutazone
Familial/syndrome/genetic	Porphyria cutanea tarda
Family cluster	Asbestosis
Mulibrey nanism	Whipple syndrome
Pericarditis (constrictive), arthritis, and camptodactyly	Chylopericardium
Radiation	Cholesterol pericarditis
Cardiac surgery	ICD patches
Chest trauma (blunt or penetrating)	Epicardial pacemaker
Malignancy	Chemical trauma—sclerotherapy of esophageal varices
Myocardial infarction	

CREST, calcinosis, Raynaud phenomenon, esophageal involvement, sclerodactyly, and telangiectasia; ICD, implantable cardioverter defibrillator.

surgery may result in constrictive pericarditis. The incidence after cardiac surgery is low (<0.2%).[86]

The pathology of constrictive pericarditis involves inflammation of the pericardium with subsequent healing that results in a thick or thin scar that restricts cardiac filling.[2] The thickened pericardium consists of an increased number of fibrous strands with foci of inflammation.[87] In some cases, calcification may ensue. The development of an underlying atrophic myocarditis also has been suggested as a cause of myocardial dysfunction. There is usually total or near-total obliteration of the pericardial space. Localized bands of constriction can occur, however, that can mimic stenosis of any of the cardiac valves.[2,80-84,87]

The pathophysiology of constrictive pericarditis is mainly due to loss of pericardial compliance.[86] This loss results in three major effects: (1) dissociation of intrathoracic and intracardiac pressures with respiration; (2) increased right and left ventricular interdependence; and (3) impaired diastolic filling with increased dependence on heart rate. In constrictive pericarditis, the total amount of blood entering the heart does not vary much with the respiratory cycle.[86] As a result of the constriction from the pericardium, the cardiac chambers are isolated from the changes in intrathoracic pressure. The pulmonary veins are intrathoracic and are not isolated from the changes in intrathoracic pressure. Vena cava flow continues to be affected by changes in intrathoracic pressure as well. During inspiration, there is a reduction in the velocity of diastolic flow in the pulmonary veins and a subsequent reduction in left-sided filling. The ventricles in constrictive pericarditis are pathologically coupled (increased right and left ventricular interdependence). The inspiratory reduction in left ventricular filling is associated with an increase in diastolic filling in the right ventricle, and the ventricular septum shifts to the left. The opposite effects are seen on exhalation, and the septum shifts to the right. This shifting results in the septal bounce seen on echocardiography. These changes also result in an expiratory reduction of flow in the vena cava, increased hepatic flow reversal, and decreased tricuspid flow velocity.

Diastolic filling of all cardiac chambers is impaired by the fibrotic pericardium. Ventricular filling is initially rapid due to elevated atrial pressures with 75% of filling occurring in the first 25% of diastole.[86] By mid-diastole, the rapid filling abruptly declines because of the noncompliant pericardium. An increase in heart rate is an effective means of maintaining cardiac output in constrictive pericarditis because filling is severely limited in late diastole. The cardiac output depends more on heart rate in this condition than in normal states.

Patients with constrictive pericarditis can have myriad clinical presentations. In the chronic form of constrictive pericarditis, symptoms are typically present for years before the diagnosis is made because a specific cause is rarely determined. Pediatric patients come to attention most frequently because of ascites and hepatomegaly, but dyspnea and failure to thrive also are common.[30,31,33-35,42,47,49] Protein-losing enteropathy also may occur.[32,35] Constrictive pericarditis also may have a more acute (days to months) or subacute (arbitrarily defined as 3 to 12 months) presentation, following an infectious illness or a primary purulent pericarditis. In some cases, a sterile pericardial effusion associated with meningitis or sepsis may occur, but during the recovery phase of these illnesses, constrictive pericarditis can develop.[37] In these cases, signs and symptoms of constrictive pericarditis occur within days to months of the inciting illness. This form of the disease may be transient.[43]

Clinical Evaluation

In children, the most common physical findings in the chronic and more acute forms include hepatomegaly and ascites. Peripheral edema usually is less marked than the ascites and hepatomegaly. There is often prominent jugular venous distention. Kussmaul sign (inspiratory jugular venous distention) may be present. Muffled heart sounds are more frequent in children with this disease than diastolic filling sounds.

The ECG is usually abnormal, but nonspecific. Frequent findings include relatively low-voltage QRS complexes and nonspecific ST-T wave abnormalities. Notched P waves and right atrial enlargement were reported in some patients and less commonly findings of ventricular hypertrophy and conduction delays.[30,31,33,34,47,49] Arrhythmias were uncommon, with atrial flutter reported in one.[35] Chest x-rays are usually abnormal in children, but nonspecific. Some degree of cardiomegaly, venous congestion, and pleural effusions were commonly reported.[31,34,42,49,47] Pericardial calcification has been reported in approximately 21% of children with constrictive pericarditis.[41]

A thickened pericardium may be present on transthoracic echocardiogram (Fig. 19-6); the absence of a thickened pericardium does not exclude constrictive pericarditis. In other cases, a thick pericardium may be present, but the signs and symptoms of constrictive pericarditis may be absent. A thick pericardium alone does not warrant the diagnosis of constrictive pericarditis. Transesophageal echocardiography may show the thickened pericardium better in some views. On two-dimensional imaging, a septal bounce may be present. Changes in the transseptal gradient during diastole may account for the septal displacement.[86] Dilation of the atria and inferior vena cava also may be present.

Doppler flow patterns also are useful in diagnosing constrictive pericarditis and differentiating it from RCM. The effects of the respiratory cycle on venous flow patterns and atrioventricular valve inflow patterns can be helpful. Superior vena cava flow is normally biphasic with peak systolic flow greater than diastolic.[86] During inspiration in constrictive pericarditis, the following may be seen: a decrease in systolic or diastolic flow or an increase in reversal of flow.[86] In the hepatic veins,

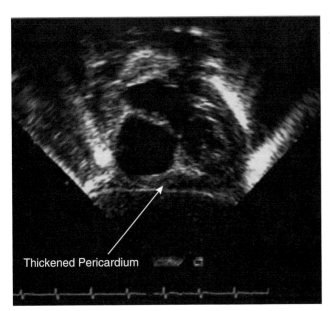

FIGURE 19-6 ■ Echocardiography in a patient with constrictive pericarditis. Subcostal image shows a thickened pericardium in a child with constrictive pericarditis.

there is decreased overall flow with decreased flow reversal and increased diastolic forward flow. During inspiration, there is increased right ventricular filling, but a decreased rapid filling period. The peak E and A waves are increased, but E deceleration time is decreased. During expiration, the opposite changes occur. Pulmonary venous flow reflects diastolic function and left atrial and ventricular filling. In constrictive pericarditis, the intrathoracic pulmonary vein flow is dissociated from the encased intracardiac structures and pressure. Peak systolic and diastolic velocities decrease with inspiration and increase with expiration. Diastolic flow remains greater than systolic flow throughout respiration, however. Left ventricular filling (flow integrals) decreases with inspiration, as does the rapid filling period. Isovolumic relaxation time increases. Mitral valve flow velocities decrease with decline in peak E and A waves and duration. Reciprocal changes occur with expiration. Doppler tissue imaging and strain rate also have been used to differentiate RCM from constrictive pericarditis in adults, in whom impaired diastolic function distinguishes patients with intrinsic myocardial disease from patients with pericardial disease.[73,74]

CT also may detect pericardial thickening. In children, the pericardium is normally less than 2 mm thick.[47] Secondary associated findings include a dilated inferior vena cava, acute angulation of the interventricular septum, a deformed ventricular contour, and pericardial calcification. The inferior vena cava-to-aorta ratio should be less than 3. MRI is an additional technique for identifying a thickened pericardium; however, calcification may not be well seen with MRI. Atrial and inferior vena cava enlargement, abnormal septal configuration, and narrowed tubular-appearing ventricles also may be seen with MRI.[2,88]

Cardiac catheterization may be useful in this disease. Constrictive hemodynamics closely resemble that of RCM. In constrictive pericarditis, right atrial pressure tracings reveal a prominent early diastolic y descent.[87] The a and v waves have a similar peak pressure, resulting in the M configuration. The right and left ventricular diastolic pressure tracings show an early dip and plateau pattern (the square root sign). This pattern reflects the early rapid filling in the first third of diastole. The elevated pressure resulting in the plateau causes an elevation in mean venous pressure. In classic constrictive pericarditis, there is elevation and equalization of the right atrial, right ventricular, left atrial, and left ventricular end-diastolic pressures to within 4 to 5 mm Hg.[87] Pulmonary hypertension usually is less marked than in RCM. It is unusual for the right ventricular and pulmonary artery systolic pressures to exceed 50 mm Hg.

In limited cases, **endomyocardial biopsy** may be necessary to help distinguish constrictive pericarditis from RCM. The findings in constrictive pericarditis are nonspecific. The absence of myopathic findings lends support to the diagnosis of constrictive pericarditis, whereas the presence of myopathic changes suggests RCM.

Rarely, exploratory thoracotomy is necessary to differentiate constrictive pericarditis from RCM. If constrictive pericarditis is identified, pericardiectomy at the time also may be curative and is the treatment of choice. In patients with RCM, exploratory thoracotomy is not a benign procedure, however, and may result in death.[28] Every effort should be made to establish the diagnosis of RCM without exploratory thoracotomy.

Therapeutic Strategies

In the acute to subacute forms of constrictive pericarditis, the constrictive process may be transient. Medical therapy may result in resolution of the disease process. In these forms, a preceding infectious illness or pericarditis typically can be identified weeks to several months before symptom onset.[2,43] The chronic form of constrictive pericarditis requires surgical intervention; 70% to 80% of patients are improved or cured.[31,39] In adults, predictors of poor prognosis in constrictive pericarditis include underlying malignancy, previous pericardial surgery, New York Heart Association class IV at presentation, myocardial atrophy, and myocardial inflammation and scarring.[86] Predictors of outcome are less well defined in children.

In the acute to subacute forms, immediate surgical intervention may not be necessary. Any underlying infectious cause should be treated if identified. Diuretics are used for the management of fluid retention. Several case reports and case series have suggested the use of anti-inflammatory doses of aspirin or steroids with close observation and follow-up.[44,89] If symptoms and follow-up evaluation reveal resolution of the findings of constrictive pericarditis, surgery may be avoided. If symptoms do not resolve or chronic constrictive pericarditis is diagnosed, pericardiectomy is the treatment of choice, with as complete resection as possible.

CURRENT STATUS AND FUTURE DIRECTIONS

In most patients, it is possible to distinguish between RCM and constrictive pericarditis without an exploratory thoracotomy (Table 19-4). There continue to be cases, however, in which the hemodynamic profile has so much overlap that thoracotomy is required for diagnosis. Henein and coworkers[90] have suggested that in overlap cases in which pericardial disease is found the term *restrictive pericarditis* should be applied. Because of the significant morbidity and mortality associated with thoracotomy in patients with RCM, less invasive means of confirming the diagnosis need to continue to be developed. In children, ongoing assessment and validation of noninvasive techniques, such as Doppler tissue imaging and evaluation of pericardial slippage by MRI, are needed to help differentiate constrictive pericarditis from RCM.

Because the only definitive therapy for RCM at present is cardiac transplantation, better medical therapies are needed for the treatment of RCM. Improved methods of risk stratification are needed for RCM patients to identify the patients at greatest risk for thromboembolism, rapid progression of elevated pulmonary vascular resistance, and sudden death. In addition, a more in-depth understanding of the molecular mechanisms of these diseases[91] and innovations in diagnostic imaging (e.g., cardiac phosphorus-31 two-dimensional chemical shift imaging)[92,93] may elucidate these diseases in the near future.

Key Concepts

■ According to the WHO definition, RCM is characterized by restrictive filling and reduced diastolic volume of either or both ventricles with normal or near-normal systolic function and wall thicknesses; increased interstitial fibrosis may be present. RCM may be idiopathic or associated with another disease.

■ Pericarditis is an inflammation of the pericardium that may be idiopathic or associated with another disease. Constrictive pericarditis is a form of cardiac compression resulting from a diseased, usually scarred, pericardium that restricts cardiac filling.

■ Of the four types of cardiomyopathy categorized by the WHO (dilated, hypertrophic, restrictive, and arrhythmogenic right ventricular cardiomyopathy), RCM is the least common.

■ Mutations in three genes (transthyretin, desmin, and troponin I) have been identified to date that may result in a RCM phenotype.

TABLE 19-4

Restrictive Cardiomyopathy versus Constrictive Pericarditis		
	Restrictive Cardiomyopathy	Constrictive Pericarditis
ECG		
Atrial enlargement	Nearly universal	May be present
LVH or RVH or both	Common	Usually absent
Low-voltage QRS	Unusual	Common
ST-T wave abnormality	Common	Common
Chest x-ray		
Calcification	Absent	≤21%
Echocardiogram		
Pericardial thickening	Absent	May be thickened
Atrial dilation	Marked	May be enlarged
Wall thicknesses	Normal to mild hypertrophy	Usually normal
Systolic function	Normal to depressed	Normal
Septal bounce	Absent	Usually present
Doppler: respiratory flow changes	Occasional	Usually marked
Gated MRI/CT	Normal pericardium	Usually thickened
Cardiac catheterization	PWP and LVEDP may exceed RAP and RVEDP by >4 mm Hg	RAP = PWP, RVEDP = LVEDP (usually within 4 mm Hg)
	RSVP often >50 mm Hg	RVSP usually <50 mm Hg
RV endomyocardial biopsy	Usually abnormal (frequently nonspecific)	Usually normal

LVEDP, left ventricular end-diastolic pressure; LVH, left ventricular hypertrophy; PWP, pulmonary wedge pressure; RAP, right atrial pressure; RV, right ventricular; RVEDP, right ventricular end-diastolic pressure; RVH, right ventricular hypertrophy; RVSP, right ventricular systolic pressure

- RCM has multiple causes and may result from myocardial diseases including infiltrative or noninfiltrative processes, storage diseases, endomyocardial diseases, myocarditis, and after cardiac transplantation.
- The pathophysiology of RCM is as follows: Diastolic function is affected primarily by ventricular compliance, stiffness, and relaxation. In the classic description of RCM, ventricular filling is completed in early diastole with little or no filling in late diastole. In this model, restrictive physiology results from increased myocardial stiffness with decreased compliance causing a marked ventricular pressure increase with small changes in volume.
- The ECG is extremely useful in screening for RCM because approximately 98% of ECGs are abnormal. The most common abnormalities are right or left atrial (or both) enlargement; ST-segment depression and ST-T wave abnormalities are also frequently present.
- In classic RCM, the left ventricular end-diastolic pressure, left atrial pressure, and pulmonary capillary wedge pressure are markedly elevated and at least 4 to 5 mm Hg (preferably 10 mm Hg) greater than the right atrial pressure and right ventricular end-diastolic pressure.
- The prognosis in children with RCM is poor; one half of the children die within 2 years of diagnosis. The prognosis in RCM seems to be significantly worse than in patients with hypertrophic cardiomyopathy or dilated cardiomyopathy, in which the 2-year mortality rates are reported to be 12.7% and 13.6%.
- At present, medical therapy remains supportive. Any therapy with potential for hemodynamic effects should be started with the patient hospitalized because of the fragile nature of these patients. Diuretics are useful in patients with signs and symptoms of systemic or pulmonary venous congestion, but overdiuresis should be avoided because these patients are sensitive to alterations in preload. Due to the 21% incidence of thromboembolic events, antiplatelet therapy or anticoagulants should be administered.
- Because current medical therapy seems to be ineffective, and the development of pulmonary hypertension is common, and mortality is high, cardiac transplantation should be the therapy of choice.
- The clinical presentation of patients with RCM and constrictive pericarditis can be similar, as can results of diagnostic tests used to try to differentiate between these two clinical entities.
- The pathophysiology of constrictive pericarditis is mainly due to loss of pericardial compliance. This loss results in three major effects: (1) dissociation of intrathoracic and intracardiac pressures with respiration, (2) increased right and left ventricular interdependence, and (3) impaired diastolic filling with increased dependence on heart rate.
- An increase in heart rate is an effective means of maintaining cardiac output in constrictive pericarditis because filling is severely limited in late diastole. The cardiac output depends more on heart rate in this condition than in normal states.
- If symptoms and follow-up evaluation reveal resolution of the findings of constrictive pericarditis, surgery may be avoided. If symptoms do not resolve or chronic constrictive pericarditis is diagnosed, pericardiectomy is the treatment of choice, with as complete resection as possible.

REFERENCES

1. Richardson P, McKenna W, Bristow M, et al: Report of the 1995 World Health Organization/International Society and Federation of Cardiology Task Force on the Definition and Classification of Cardiomyopathies. Circulation 1996;93:841-842.
2. Spodick DH: Constrictive pericarditis. In Spodick DH (ed): The Pericardium: A Comprehensive Textbook. New York, Marcel Dekker, 1997, pp 214-259.
3. Braunwald E (chair): Report of the Task Force on Research in Heart Failure. Bethesda, Md, National Heart, Lung and Blood Institute, 1994.
4. Denfield SW, Rosenthal G, Gajarski RJ, et al: Restrictive cardiomyopathies in childhood etiologies and natural history. Tex Heart Inst J 1997;24:38-44.
5. Lewis AB: Clinical profile and outcome of restrictive cardiomyopathy in children. Am Heart J 1992;123:1589-1593.
6. Harris LC, Rodin AE, Nghiem QX: Idiopathic, nonobstructive cardiomyopathy in children. Am J Cardiol 1968;21:153-165.
7. Cetta F, O'Leary PW, Seward JB, et al: Idiopathic restrictive cardiomyopathy in childhood: Diagnostic features and clinical course. Mayo Clin Proc 1995;70:634-640.
8. Chen S, Balfour IC, Jureidini S: Clinical spectrum of restrictive cardiomyopathy in children. J Heart Lung Transplant 2001;20:90-92.
9. Rivenes SM, Kearney DL, Smith EO, et al: Sudden death and cardiovascular collapse in children with restrictive cardiomyopathy. Circulation 2000;102:876-882.
10. Gewillig M, Mertens L, Moerman P, et al: Idiopathic restrictive cardiomyopathy in childhood: A diastolic disorder characterized by delayed relaxation. Eur Heart J 1996;17:1413-1420.
11. Mehta AV, Ferrer PL, Pickoff AS, et al: M-mode echocardiographic findings in children with idiopathic restrictive cardiomyopathy. Pediatr Cardiol 1984;5:273-280.
12. Fitzpatrick AP, Shapiro LM, Rickards AF, et al: Familial restrictive cardiomyopathy with atrioventricular block and skeletal myopathy. Br Heart J 1990;63:114-118.
13. Toussaint M, Planche C, Villain E, et al: Restrictive cardiomyopathy in children: Ultrastructural findings. Virchows Arch A 1987;412:27-29.
14. Sapire DW, Casta A, Swischuk LE, et al: Massive dilatation of the atria and coronary sinus in a child with restrictive cardiomyopathy and persistence of the left superior vena cava. Cathet Cardiovasc Diagn 1983;9:47-53.
15. Erath GH, Graham TP, Smith CW, et al: Restrictive cardiomyopathy in an infant with massive biatrial enlargement and normal ventricular size and pump function. Cathet Cardiovasc Diagn 1978;4:289-296.
16. Ishijima M, Kawai S, Okada R, et al: An autopsy case of cardiomyopathy with restrictive physiology in a child. Heart Vessels 1990;5:70-73.

17. Maki T, Niimura I, Nishikawa T, et al: An atypical case of cardiomyopathy in a child: Hypertrophic or restrictive. Heart Vessels 1990;5:84-87.

18. Schieber RA, Lurie PR, Neustein HB: Restrictive cardiomyopathy with pseudotumor formation of the left ventricle. Pediatr Cardiol 1982;3:153-159.

19. Miyazaki A, Ichida F, Suzuki Y, et al: Long-term follow-up of a child with idiopathic restrictive cardiomyopathy. Heart Vessels 1990;(Suppl 5):74-76.

20. Nishikawa T, Tanaka Y, Sasaki Y, et al: A case of pediatric cardiomyopathy with severely restrictive physiology. Heart Vessels 1992;7:206-210.

21. Aroney C, Bett N, Radford D: Familial restrictive cardiomyopathy. Aust N Z J Med 1988;18:877-878.

22. Izumi T, Masani F, Mitsuma S, et al: Juvenile cases of restrictive cardiomyopathy without eosinophilia. Heart Vessels 1990; 5:77-79.

23. Rapezzi C, Ortolani P, Binetti G, et al: Idiopathic restrictive cardiomyopathy in the young: Report of two cases. Int J Cardiol 1990;29:121-126.

24. Bertini E, Bosman C, Bevilacqua M, et al: Cardiomyopathy and multicore myopathy with accumulation of intermediate filaments. Eur J Pediatr 1990;149:856-858.

25. Neudorf U, Bolte A, Lang D, et al: Diagnostic findings and outcome in children with primary restrictive cardiomyopathy. Cardiol Young 1996;6:44-47.

26. Angelini A, Calzolari V, Thiene G, et al: Morphologic spectrum of primary restrictive cardiomyopathy. Am J Cardiol 1997; 80:1046-1050.

27. Hughes ML, Kleinert S, Keogh A, et al: Pulmonary vascular resistance and reactivity in children with end-stage cardiomyopathy. J Heart Lung Transplant 2000;19:701-794.

28. Weller RJ, Weintraub R, Addonizio LJ, et al: Outcome of idiopathic restrictive cardiomyopathy in children. Am J Cardiol 2002;90: 501-506.

29. Kimberling MT, Balzer DT, Hirsch R, et al: Cardiac transplantation for pediatric restrictive cardiomyopathy: Presentation, evaluation and short term outcome. J Heart Lung Transplant 2002;21: 455-459.

30. Shea DW, Kirklin JW, Dushane JW: Chronic constrictive pericarditis in children. Am J Dis Child 1957;93:430-435.

31. Roshe J, Shumacker HB: Pericardiectomy for chronic cardiac tamponade in children. Surgery 1959;46:1152-1161.

32. Plauth WH, Waldmann TA, Wochner DR, et al: Protein-losing enteropathy secondary to constrictive pericarditis in childhood. Pediatrics 1964;34:636-648.

33. Simcha A, Taylor JFN: Constrictive pericarditis in childhood. Arch Dis Child 1971;46:515-519.

34. Idriss FS, Nikaidoh H, Muster A: Constrictive pericarditis simulating liver disease in children. Arch Surg 1974;109:223-226.

35. Greenwood RD, Rosenthal A, Cassady R, et al: Constrictive pericarditis in childhood due to mediastinal irradiation. Circulation 1974;50:1033-1039.

36. Griese GG: Chronic pericarditis in children. Wisc Med J 1975;74: S21-S24.

37. Strauss AW, Santa-Maria M, Goldring D: Constrictive pericarditis in children. Am J Dis Child 1975;129:822-826.

38. Cumming GR, Kerr D, Ferguson CC: Constrictive pericarditis with dwarfism in two siblings (mulibrey nanism). J Pediatr 1976; 88:569-572.

39. Van der Horst RL, Le Roux BT: Pericardiectomy in children. Thorax 1976;31:391-393.

40. Harada K, Seki I, Okuni M: Constrictive pericarditis with atrial septal defect in children. Jpn Heart J 1978;19:531-543.

41. Van der Horst RL: Pericardial calcification in childhood. Cardiovasc Radiol 1978;1:265-267.

42. Haycock GB, Jordan SC: Chronic pericardial constriction with effusion in childhood. Arch Dis Child 1979;54:890-895.

43. Allaria A, Michelli D, Capelli H, et al: Transient cardiac constriction following purulent pericarditis. Eur J Pediatr 1992;151:250-251.

44. Hugo-Hamman CT, Scher H, De Moor MMA: Tuberculous pericarditis in children: A review of 44 cases. Pediatr Infect Dis J 1994;13:13-18.

45. Verma UN, Misra R, Radhakrisnan S, et al: A syndrome of fibrosing pleuritis, and synovitis with infantile contractures of fingers and toes in 2 sisters: "Familial fibrosing serositis." J Rheumatol 1995;22:2349-2355.

46. Lapunzina P, Rodriguez I, de Matteo E, et al: Mulibrey nanism: Three additional patients and a review of 39 patients. Am J Med Genet 1995;55:349-355.

47. Chen S-J, Li Y-W, Wu M-H, et al: CT and MRI findings in a child with constrictive pericarditis. Pediatr Cardiol 1998; 19:259-262.

48. Buendia A, Attie F, Martinez-Lavin M: The syndrome of pericarditis, arthritis, and camptodactyly: An under-recognized cause of pericardial constriction in children? Cardiol Young 1999; 9:526-528.

49. Gomes Ferreira SMA, Gomes Ferreira A, do Nascimento Morais A, et al: Constrictive chronic pericarditis in children. Cardiol Young 2001;11:210-213.

50. DeLine JM, Cable DG: Clustering of recurrent pericarditis with effusion and constriction in a family. Mayo Clin Proc 2002;77: 39-43.

51. Nugent AW, Daubeney PEF, Chondros P, et al: The epidemiology of childhood cardiomyopathy in Australia. N Engl J Med 2003;348:1639-1646.

52. Lipshultz SE, Sleeper CA, Towbin JA, et al: The incidence of pediatric cardiomyopathy in two regions of the United States. N Engl J Med 2003;348:1647-1655.

53. Morgensen J, Kubo T, Duque M, et al: Idiopathic restrictive cardiomyopathy is part of the clinical expression of cardiac troponin I mutations. J Clin Invest 2003;111:209-216.

54. Jacobson R, Ittmann M, Buxbaum JN, et al: Transthyretin IIe 122 and cardiac amyloidosis in African-Americans: 2 case reports. Tex Heart Inst J 1997;24:45-52.

55. Dalakas MC, Park K-Y, Semino-Mora C, et al: Desmin myopathy: A skeletal myopathy with cardiomyopathy caused by mutations in the desmin gene. N Engl J Med 2000;342:770-780.

56. Goldfarb LG, Park K-Y, CerveneKova L, et al: Missense mutations in desmin associated with familial cardiac and skeletal myopathy. Nat Genet 1998;19:402-403.

57. Pahl E, Miller SA, Griffith BP, et al: Occult restrictive hemodynamics after pediatric heart transplantation. J Heart Lung Transplant 1995;14:1109-1115.

58. Kushwaha SS, Fallon JT, Fuster V: Restrictive cardiomyopathy. N Engl J Med 1997;336:267-276.

59. Davies JNP: Endocardial fibrosis in Africans. East Afr Med J 1948;25:10.

60. Johnson RA, Palacios I: Nondilated cardiomyopathies. Adv Intern Med 1984;30:243-274.

61. Wynne J, Braunwald E: The cardiomyopathies and myocarditides. In Braunwald E, Zipes DP, Libby P (eds): Heart Disease: A Textbook of Cardiovascular Medicine, 6th ed. Philadelphia, WB Saunders, 2001, pp 1774-1782.

62. Weller PF, Bubley GJ: The idiopathic hypereosinophilia syndrome. Blood 1994;83:2759.

63. Felice PV, Sawicki J, Anto J: Endomyocardial disease and eosinophilia. Angiology 1993;44:869.

64. Radford DJ, Garlick RB, Pohlner PG: Multiple valvar replacements for hypereosinophilia syndrome. Cardiol Young 2002;12:67-70.

65. Santos CL, Moraes CR, Santos FL, et al: Endomyocardial fibrosis in children. Cardiol Young 2001;11:205-209.

66. Mortensen SA, Olsen HS, Baandrup U: Chronic anthracycline cardiotoxicity: Haemodynamic and histopathological manifestations suggesting a restrictive endomyocardial disease. Br Heart J 1986;55:274-282.

67. Bu'Lock FA, Mott MG, Oakhill A, et al: Left ventricular diastolic function after anthracycline chemotherapy in childhood: Relation with systolic function, symptoms and pathophysiology. Br Heart J 1995;73:340-350.

68. Mason JW, Billingham ME, Friedman JP: Methysergide-induced heart disease: A case of multivalvular and myocardial fibrosis. Circulation 1977;56:889-890.

69. Billingham ME: Pharmacotoxic myocardial disease: An endomyocardial study. Heart Vessels 1985;(Suppl 1):278-282.

70. Gottdiener JS, Katin MJ, Borer JS, et al: Late cardiac effects of therapeutic mediastinal irradiation: Assessment by echocardiography and radionuclide angiography. N Engl J Med 1983;308:569-572.

71. Opie LH: Normal and abnormal cardiac function. In Braunwald E, Zipes DP, Libby P (eds): Heart Disease: A Textbook of Cardiovascular Medicine, 6th ed. Philadelphia, WB Saunders, 2001, pp 463-464.

72. Child JS, Perloff JK: The restrictive cardiomyopathies. Cardiol Clin 1988;6:289-316.

73. Palka P, Lange A, Donnelly JE, et al: Differentiation between restrictive cardiomyopathy and constrictive pericarditis by early diastolic Doppler myocardial velocity gradient at the posterior wall. Circulation 2000;102:655-662.

74. Rajagopalan N, Garcia MJ, Rodriguez L, et al: Comparison of new Doppler echocardiographic methods to differentiate constrictive pericardial heart disease and restrictive cardiomyopathy. Am J Cardiol 2001;87:86-94.

75. Schoenfeld MH: The differentiation of restrictive cardiomyopathy from constrictive pericarditis. Cardiol Clin 1990;8:663-671.

76. Maron BJ, Henry WL, Clark CE, et al: Asymmetric septal hypertrophy in childhood. Circulation 1976;53:9-19.

77. Bengur AR, Beekman RH, Rocchini AP, et al: Acute hemodynamic effects of captopril in children with a congestive or restrictive cardiomyopathy. Circulation 1991;83:523-527.

78. Zile MR, Brutsaert DL: New concepts in diastolic dysfunction and diastolic heart failure: Part II. Circulation 2002;105:1503-1508.

79. Denfield SW: Sudden death in children with restrictive cardiomyopathy. Cardiac Electrophysiol Rev 2002;6:163-167.

80. Barros JL, Perez Gomez F: Pulmonary stenosis due to external compression by a pericardial band. Br Heart J 1967;29:947-949.

81. Chesler E, Mitha AS, Matisson RE, et al: Subpulmonic stenosis as a result of noncalcific constrictive pericarditis. Chest 1976;69:425-427.

82. Nishimura RA, Kazmier FJ, Smith HC, et al: Right ventricular outflow obstruction caused by constrictive pericardial disease. Am J Cardiol 1985;55:1447-1448.

83. Ramdas GP, Ryad T, Sammy W: Constrictive pericarditis causing extrinsic mitral stenosis and a left heart mass. Clin Cardiol 1996;19:517-519.

84. McGinn JS, Zipes DP: Constrictive pericarditis causing tricuspid stenosis. Arch Intern Med 1972;129:487-490.

85. Bahabri SA, Suwairi WM, Laxer RM, et al: The camptodactyly-arthropathy-coxa vara-pericarditis syndrome. Arthritis Rheum 1998;41:730-735.

86. Myres RBH, Spodick DH: Constrictive pericarditis: Clinical and pathophysiologic characteristics. Am Heart J 1999;138:219-232.

87. Brockington GM, Zebede J, Pandian NG: Constrictive pericarditis. Cardiol Clin 1990;8:645-661.

88. Vick WG, Rokey R: Cardiovascular magnetic resonance evaluation of the pericardium in health and disease. In Manning W, Pennell DJ (eds): Cardiovascular Magnetic Resonance. Philadelphia, Churchill Livingstone, 2002, pp 355-363.

89. Sagrista-Sauleda J, Angel J, Sanchez A, et al: Effusive-constrictive pericarditis. N Engl J Med 2004;350:469-475.

90. Henein MY, Rakhit RD, Sheppard MN, et al: Restrictive pericarditis. Heart 1999;82:389-392.

91. Petrich BG, Eloff BC, Lerner DL, et al: Targeted activation of c-Jun N-terminal kinase in vivo induces restrictive cardiomyopathy and conduction defects. J Biol Chem 2004;279:15330-15338.

92. Schocke MF, Zoller H, Vogel W, et al: Cardiac phosphorus-31 two-dimensional chemical shift imaging in patients with hereditary hemochromatosis. Magn Reson Imaging 2004;22:515-521.

93. Francone M, Dymarkowski S, Kalantzi M, et al: Real-time cine MRI of ventricular septal motion: A novel approach to assess ventricular coupling. J Magn Reson Imaging 2005;21:305-309.

CHAPTER 20
Hypertrophic Cardiomyopathy

Jeffrey A. Towbin

Hypertrophic cardiomyopathy (HCM) is defined by its wall thickening—hence the term *hypertrophic heart disease*.[1-3] The major impact of this disorder on human health is based on its predilection to be inherited; its reputation as the most common cause of sudden death in young, healthy, athletic individuals[4-7]; and its potential to develop heart failure.[8-10] Heart failure can occur secondary to diastolic factors or secondary to the development of systolic dysfunction, so-called burned-out HCM.[8-10] No matter what the cause of untoward clinical features, HCM is a significant burden on health care finances, not to mention the untold price of the tragedies in affected families.

In the pediatric age range, the underlying etiologies responsible for HCM and the variable age range of onset differentiates the childhood form of the disease from the adult form.[11] In infants, ventricular hypertrophy associated with systolic dysfunction is more the rule than the exception. In addition, overlap disorders, in which HCM coexists with other atypical features, are more common during childhood, further confounding the presentations, treatments, and outcomes compared with adult disease. This chapter describes the similarities and differences.

NORMAL CARDIAC STRUCTURE

A brief review of the normal cardiac molecular structure is presented here; more details can be found in earlier chapters. Cardiac muscle fibers comprise separate cellular units (myocytes) connected in series.[12] In contrast to skeletal muscle fibers, cardiac fibers do not assemble in parallel arrays, but bifurcate and recombine to form a complex three-dimensional network. Cardiac myocytes are joined at each end to adjacent myocytes at the **intercalated disc**, the specialized area of interdigitating cell membrane (Fig. 20-1). The intercalated disc contains **gap junctions** (containing connexins) and **mechanical junctions**, composed of **adherens junctions** (containing N-cadherin, catenins, and vinculin) and **desmosomes** (containing desmin, desmoplakin, desmocollin, and desmoglein). Cardiac myocytes are surrounded by a thin membrane (sarcolemma), and the interior of each myocyte contains bundles of longitudinally arranged myofibrils. The myofibrils are formed by repeating sarcomeres, the basic contractile units of cardiac muscle composed of interdigitating thin (actin) and thick (myosin) filaments that give the muscle its characteristic striated appearance.[13,14]

The **thick filaments** are composed primarily of myosin, but additionally contain myosin-binding proteins C, H, and X. The **thin filaments** are composed of cardiac actin; α-tropomyosin (α-TM); and cardiac troponins T, I, and C (cTnT, cTnI, cTnC). In addition, myofibrils contain a third filament formed by the giant filamentous protein, **titin**, which extends from the Z-disc to the M line and acts as a molecular template for the layout of the sarcomere. The Z-disc at the borders of the sarcomere is formed by a lattice of interdigitating proteins that maintain myofilament organization by cross-linking antiparallel titin and thin filaments from adjacent sarcomeres (Fig. 20-2). Other proteins in the Z-disc include α-actinin, nebulette, telethonin/T-cap, capZ, MLP, myopalladin, myotilin, Cypher/ZASP, filamin, and FATZ.[13-16]

Finally, the **extrasarcomeric cytoskeleton**, a complex network of proteins linking the sarcomere with the sarcolemma and the **extracellular matrix**, provides structural support for subcellular structures and transmits mechanical and chemical signals within and between cells. The extrasarcomeric cytoskeleton has intermyofibrillar and subsarcolemmal components, with the intermyofibrillar cytoskeleton composed of intermediate filaments, microfilaments, and microtubules.[15-20] **Desmin** intermediate filaments form a three-dimensional scaffold throughout the extrasarcomeric cytoskeleton with desmin filaments surrounding the Z-disc, allowing for longitudinal connections to adjacent Z-discs and lateral connections to subsarcolemmal costameres.[19,20]

Microfilaments composed of nonsarcomeric actin (mainly γ-actin) also form complex networks linking the sarcomere (via α-actinin) to various components of the costameres. **Costameres** are subsarcolemmal domains located in a periodic, gridlike pattern, flanking the Z-discs and overlying the I bands, along the cytoplasmic side of the sarcolemma. These costameres are sites of interconnection between various cytoskeletal networks linking sarcomere and sarcolemma and are believed to function as anchor sites for stabilization of the sarcolemma and for integration of pathways involved in mechanical force transduction. Costameres contain three principal components: the focal adhesion-type complex, the spectrin-based complex, and the

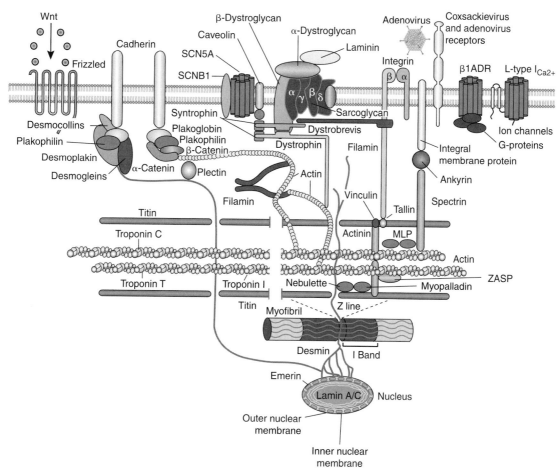

FIGURE 20-1 ■ Cardiac myocyte cytoarchitecture. Schematic of the interactions between dystrophin and the dystrophin-associated proteins in the sarcolemma and intracellular cytoplasm (dystroglycans, sarcoglycans, syntrophins, dystrobrevin, sarcospan) at the carboxy-terminal end of the dystrophin. The integral membrane proteins interact with the extracellular matrix via α-dystroglycan-laminin α2 connections. The amino-terminus of dystrophin binds actin and connects dystrophin with the sarcomere intracellularly, the sarcolemma, and the extracellular matrix. Additional sarcolemmal proteins include ion channels, adrenergic receptors, integrins, and the coxsackie and adenoviral receptors. Cell-cell junctions, including cadherins and the plakin and other desmosomal family proteins, also are notable. Also shown is the interaction between intermediate filament proteins (i.e., desmin) with the nucleus. MLP, muscle LIM protein. (See also Color Section)

Sarcomeric Assembly

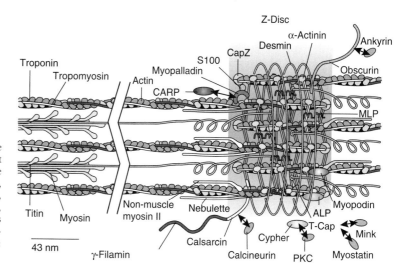

FIGURE 20-2 ■ Z-disc architecture. The Z-disc of the sarcomere comprises multiple interacting proteins that anchor the sarcomere. The proteins involved in the Z-disc structure include α-actinin, MLP, Cypher (ZASP), and others. ALP, actinin-associated LIM protein; CapZ, actin capping protein; MLP, muscle LIM protein; T-Cap, telethonin. (From Pyle WG, Solaro RJ: At the crossroads of myocardial signaling: The role of Z-discs in intracellular signaling and cardiac function. Circ Res 2004;94: 296-305.) (See also Color Section)

dystrophin/dystrophin-associated protein complex.[21,22] The focal adhesion-type complex, composed of cytoplasmic proteins (i.e., vinculin, talin, tensin, paxillin, zyxin), connect with cytoskeletal actin filaments and with the transmembrane proteins α-dystroglycan, β-dystroglycan, α-sarcoglycan, β-sarcoglycan, γ-sarcoglycan, δ-sarcoglycan, dystrobrevin, and syntrophin.[17,18] Several actin-associated proteins are located at sites of attachment of cytoskeletal actin filaments with costameric complexes, including α-actinin and the muscle LIM protein, MLP.

The C-terminus of **dystrophin** binds β-dystroglycan (see Fig. 20-1), which interacts with α-dystroglycan to link to the extracellular matrix (via α-2-laminin). The N-terminus of dystrophin interacts with actin. Also notable, voltage-gated sodium channels colocalize with dystrophin, β-spectrin, ankyrin, and syntrophins, whereas potassium channels interact with the sarcomeric Z-disc and intercalated discs.[23-25] Because arrhythmias and conduction system diseases are common in children and adults with all forms of cardiomyopathy, this interaction could play an important role. Disruption of the links from the sarcolemma to the extracellular matrix at the dystrophin C-terminus and to the sarcomere and nucleus via N-terminal dystrophin interactions could lead to a "domino effect" disruption of systolic function, diastolic dysfunction, and development of arrhythmias.

HYPERTROPHIC CARDIOMYOPATHY

HCM is a complex cardiac disease with unique pathophysiologic characteristics and a great diversity of morphologic, functional, and clinical features.[1-3] Although HCM has been regarded largely as a relatively uncommon cardiac disease, the prevalence of echocardiographically defined HCM in a large cohort of apparently healthy young adults selected from a community-based general population was reported to be 0.2%.[26] HCM is considered to occur secondary to diastolic dysfunction, a disease of relaxation of the ventricular myocardium.[27,28] Systolic function is preserved or hypercontractile, and left ventricular outflow tract obstruction may occur.

Clinical Features
HCM is a primary myocardial disorder with an autosomal dominant pattern of inheritance that is characterized by hypertrophy of the left ventricle (with or without right ventricle) with histologic features of myocyte hypertrophy, myofibrillar disarray, and interstitial fibrosis.[1-3] HCM is one of the most common inherited cardiac disorders, with a prevalence in young adults of 1 in 500.[3] Various names have been given to this disorder, including hypertrophic obstructive cardiomyopathy and idiopathic subaortic stenosis. These names reflect textbook features of asymmetric septal hypertrophy and left ventricular outflow tract obstruction. This description of the disease

is based primarily on patients with severe symptoms seen in tertiary hospital referral centers. Epidemiologic studies suggest that a wide spectrum of clinical manifestations of varying severity and prognosis is present in community populations.

The first clinical description of HCM was reported in 1869[29] in France, and it was recognized to be a genetic disorder in the late 1950s. Since then, numerous clinical and pathologic studies of HCM have been performed. Since the 1990s, molecular genetic studies have provided important insights into the pathogenesis of HCM and have provided a new perspective for the diagnosis and management of patients with this disorder.[30]

Clinical Evaluation
The classic features of HCM include myocyte hypertrophy, myofiber disarray, and patchy fibrosis.[1-3] In some patients, mitochondrial proliferation or morphologic abnormalities with or without inclusion material, glycogen stores, vacuolization, or desmin deposits may be seen.[11,46,47] Similar to dilated cardiomyopathy (DCM), metabolic and mitochondrial abnormalities may be causative, and the same blood, urine, and muscle studies should be obtained. In addition, fibroblasts for α-1,4-glycosidase (acid maltase) deficiency to diagnose Pompe disease should be considered.[11]

Affected individuals with HCM exhibit significant variability in their clinical presentation. They may be asymptomatic or present with symptoms ranging from palpitations and dizziness to syncope and sudden death. The age of onset of symptoms varies, with some patients presenting at birth or during childhood and others presenting in their 40s or 50s. Most commonly, patients present before age 20.[11]

The physical examination in subjects with HCM may or may not be fruitful. Because of the ventricular relaxation disorder, the ventricular stiffness may result in an S_4 gallop. In patients with left ventricular outflow tract obstruction, an outflow murmur may be heard. Otherwise, the examination is typically normal unless a restrictive component or heart failure exists, in which case jugular venous distention, hepatomegaly, and other signs of heart failure may be evident.

The diagnosis of HCM relies on echocardiography, Holter monitoring, and exercise testing; histopathology also may be useful. In addition, in small children, metabolic studies may be useful in determining the etiology of disease.[11] The primary modality for the diagnosis of HCM is transthoracic echocardiography. The hallmark diagnostic feature of HCM is asymmetric hypertrophy of the interventricular septum, with or without systolic anterior motion of the mitral valve and hypercontractile systolic function as seen by M-mode (Fig. 20-3). Doppler and color Doppler interrogation identifies outflow tract obstruction when it occurs. It is now recognized that the obstructive form of HCM occurs in less than 25% of affected individuals. Studies of kindreds with HCM have

Hypertrophic Cardiomyopathy

1 month old   8 month old

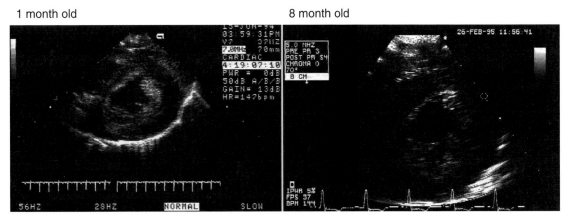

FIGURE 20-3 ■ **Echocardiography in dilated cardiomyopathy.** *Left panel,* Parasternal short-axis echocardiogram. Concentric hypertrophy in a 1-month-old infant. Note the small left ventricular chamber. *Right panel,* Similar view shows worsening left ventricular hypertrophy, and a smaller chamber size at 8 months of age in the same infant.

shown that the distribution and severity of left ventricular hypertrophy may vary considerably, that asymmetric hypertrophy is no longer an essential requirement for the diagnosis of this disorder, and that even within the same family the features may differ.

The diagnosis of HCM generally requires exclusion of secondary causes of hypertrophy, such as hypertension or aortic stenosis; however, in some individuals, particularly in older age groups, these conditions may coexist. The differentiation of HCM from physiologic left ventricular hypertrophy may be difficult, particularly in competitive athletes. The extent of left ventricular hypertrophy also may vary among different mutant genes. Individuals with β-MHC gene mutations usually develop moderate or severe hypertrophy with a high disease penetrance, whereas individuals with cTnT gene mutations reportedly have only mild or clinically undetectable hypertrophy.[31,32] Unusual forms of hypertrophy have been reported, localized to the left ventricular apex (cTnI mutations)[33] or midcavity (cardiac actin and MLC gene mutations).[34,35] The extent of left ventricular hypertrophy also may vary between members of a single family with the same gene mutation, as previously noted. These observations may be explained by a modifying role of additional genetic and environmental factors, such as blood pressure, exercise, diet, and body mass. More recently, tissue Doppler imaging and strain rate echocardiography, real-time methods that measure wall motion and thickening, have been used to detect subclinical systolic and diastolic dysfunction.[36-38]

The ECG may be normal in HCM or have associated left ventricular hypertrophy or biventricular hypertrophy. Giant QRS complexes are common in patients with Pompe disease or left ventricular noncompaction.[11,39] Pre-excitation also may be noted in patients with

HCM.[11,40,41] Ventricular, atrial, or supraventricular arrhythmias may be seen on surface ECG as well. Patients with restrictive physiology may show atrial enlargement. Holter monitoring also may show arrhythmias.[42-45]

Risk stratification has been reported with the use of exercise testing, with blunting or reduction of blood pressure or blunting of heart rate response to exercise being associated with increased risk.[4] In particular, blood pressure reduction by more than 15 mm Hg or failure to increase blood pressure by more than 25 mm Hg is associated with increased risk. Other associated risk factors include syncope, nonsustained ventricular tachycardia, severe left ventricular hypertrophy on echocardiography (>3 cm in adults), and family history of premature death.[5]

Natural History

The natural history of HCM varies; some individuals remain asymptomatic throughout life, and others may develop progressive symptoms with or without heart failure or experience sudden death.[1-3] Longitudinal echocardiographic studies have documented left ventricular remodeling with age. Progressive increases in left ventricular wall thickness have been reported in individuals during adolescence and early adult life. In some individuals, left ventricular wall thickness may increase in later life.[48] Age-related reductions in left ventricular wall thickness, associated with myocyte loss and fibrosis, also have been described in individuals with long-standing disease ("burnt-out" HCM).[8-10] Ten percent to 20% of individuals with HCM may develop DCM, whereas 10% to 16% of affected adults develop atrial fibrillation. This risk of atrial fibrillation is increased in individuals with left atrial enlargement.[2,3]

HCM is a frequent cause of sudden death, particularly in young individuals and competitive athletes.[4-7]

Estimates of the prevalence of sudden death vary according to the population studied, ranging from less than 1% in the general community to 3% to 6% in tertiary care hospital referral centers. Various mechanisms for sudden death have been proposed, including ventricular bradyarrhythmias secondary to sinus node and atrioventricular conduction abnormalities and tachyarrhythmias triggered by reentrant depolarization pathways related to myofibrillar disarray and fibrosis, abnormal Ca^{2+} homeostasis, myocardial ischemia, left ventricular diastolic dysfunction, and left ventricular outflow tract obstruction.

Various risk stratification algorithms based on clinical parameters have been proposed to identify individuals with an increased propensity for sudden death. Given the complexity of mechanisms that may precipitate sudden death, it is not surprising that no single risk factor has been identified. Conflicting results have been found for the positive predictive value of young age at diagnosis, history of syncope, severity of symptoms, left ventricular wall thickness, left ventricular outflow tract gradient, left atrial size, atrial fibrillation, and exercise response of blood pressure and heart rate. Genotype also has been suggested to predict outcome. The mechanisms whereby HCM gene mutations influence prognosis are unknown. Although some HCM mutations that alter the charge of the encoded amino acid have been associated with a poor outcome, other mutations that alter charge have a good prognosis.[49,50] Genetic studies and animal model studies, including electrophysiologic studies in mouse models, may provide important insights into the differential propensity for sudden death between different HCM gene mutations. These genotype-phenotype correlations have come into question, however.[51]

Diastolic heart failure refers to individuals with effort intolerance, dyspnea, venous congestion, and pulmonary edema in the face of diastolic dysfunction. Also known as heart failure with preserved systolic function, this form of heart failure typically occurs in individuals with HCM or restrictive cardiomyopathy (RCM).[9,10,27,28,42-45,52] Diastolic dysfunction, which is necessary in this disorder, refers to abnormal diastolic distensibility, filling, or left ventricular relaxation.

Pathophysiologically, diastolic function is determined by the passive elastic properties of the left ventricle and by the process of active relaxation. Combinations of increased myocardial mass and altered extramyocardial collagen lead to abnormal passive elastic properties, and the effects of impaired myocardial relaxation stiffen the left ventricle further.[27] Analysis of pressure volume loops shows that the diastolic pressure volume line is displaced upward and leftward (Fig. 20-4), with reduced capacity to fill at low left atrial pressures. The ejection fraction is normal, and end-diastolic pressure is elevated. Relatively small increases in central blood volume or venous tone elevation increase in arterial stiffness or both can lead to significant increases in left atrial and pulmonary venous pressures, resulting in acute pulmonary edema (see Chapters 7 and 8 for more detailed discussions).[9]

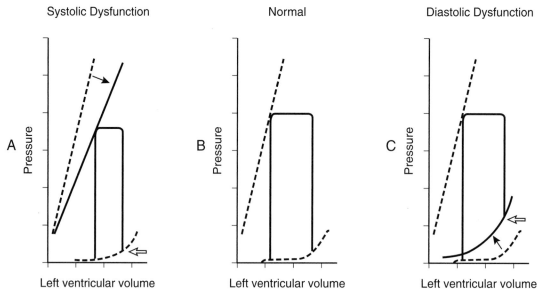

FIGURE 20-4 ■ Left ventricular pressure volume loops in systolic and diastolic dysfunction. In systolic dysfunction, left ventricular contractility is depressed, and the end-systolic pressure volume line is displaced downward and to the right (*black arrow* in **A**); as a result, there is a diminished capacity to eject blood into the high-pressure aorta. **B** is the pressure-volume loop in normal hearts. In diastolic dysfunction, the diastolic pressure volume line is displaced upward and to the left (*black arrow* in **C**), and the end-diastolic pressure is normal (*open arrow* in **A**); in diastolic dysfunction, the ejection fraction is normal, and the end-diastolic pressure is elevated (*open arrow* in **C**). (See also Color Section)

Hypertrophic Cardiomyopathy:
A Disease of the Sarcomere

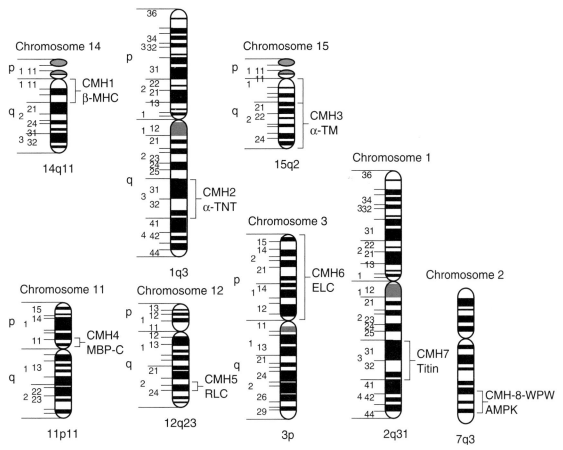

FIGURE 20-5 ■ Genetic location of hypertrophic cardiomyopathy–causing genes. (See also Color Section)

Genetics Aspects

The first gene for familial HCM was mapped to chromosome 14q11.2-q12 using genome-wide linkage analysis in a large Canadian family.[53] Soon afterward, familial HCM locus heterogeneity was reported[54] and subsequently confirmed by the mapping of the second familial HCM locus to chromosome 1q3 and of the third locus to chromosome 15q2.[55,56] Carrier and associates[57] mapped the fourth familial HCM locus to chromosome 11p11.2. Multiple other loci subsequently were reported, including loci on chromosomes 7q3,[58] 3p21.2-3p21.3,[59] 12q23-q24.3,[59] 19p13.2-q13.2,[60] and 15q14 (Fig. 20-5).[61] More recently, new loci on chromosomes 2q31,[62] 11p15.1,[63] 6q13,[64] and 3p25[65] were identified. Several other families are not linked to any known familial HCM loci, indicating the existence of additional familial HCM–causing genes (Table 20-1).

Most of the disease-causing genes identified to date code for proteins that are part of the sarcomere, which is a complex structure with an exact stoichiometry and multiple sites of protein-protein interactions.[30,66,67] These include three **myofilament proteins**, the β-myosin heavy chain (β-MyHC), the ventricular myosin essential

TABLE 20-1

Hypertrophic Cardiomyopathy Genetics		
CHR Locus	**Gene**	**Protein**
Xq22	α-Gal	α-Galactosidase
Xq24	LAMP-2	Lysomal-associated membrane protein 2
Xq28	G4.5	Tafazzin
1q32	TNNT2	Cardiac troponin T
2q31	TTN	Titin
3p21.2	MELC	Myosin essential light chain
3p25	CAV3	Caveolin-3
6q13	MYO6	Unconventional myosin VI
7q31	AMPK	AMP-kinase
11p11	MYBPC3	Myosin binding protein C
11p15.1	MLP	Muscle LIM protein
12q23	MRLC	Myosin regulatory light chain
14q12	MYH7	β-Myosin heavy chain
15q14	ACTC	Cardiac actin
15q22	TPM1	α-Tropomyosin
19p13.2	CTNNI	Cardiac troponin I

light chain 1 (MLC-1s/v), and the ventricular myosin regulatory light chain 2 (MLC-2s/v); four thin filament proteins, cardiac actin, cTnT, cTnI, and α-TM; and one myosin-binding protein, cardiac myosin binding protein C (cMyBP-C) (see Table 20-1).

Each of these proteins is encoded by multigene families that exhibit tissue-specific, developmental, and physiologically regulated patterns of expression.[68] The giant protein titin[62] and its interactive Z-disc protein, MLP, also have been identified.[63] In addition, the gene located on chromosome 7q3 associated with HCM and Wolff-Parkinson-White syndrome was identified as AMP kinase, which has been suggested to play a role in energy metabolism and cause infiltration of a glycogen-like substance similar to that seen in Pompe disease.[40,41,46]

Myosin is the molecular motor that transduces energy from the hydrolysis of ATP into directed movement and that, by doing so, drives sarcomere shortening and muscle contraction. Cardiac myosin consists of two heavy chains (MyHC) and two pairs of light chains (MLC), referred to as essential (or alkali) light chains (MLC-1) and regulatory (or phosphorylatable) light chains (MLC-2).[68] The myosin molecule is highly asymmetric, consisting of two globular heads joined to a long rodlike tail. The light chains are arranged in tandem in the head-tail junction. Their function is not fully understood. Neither MLC-1 nor MLC-2 is required for the ATPase activity of the myosin head, but they probably modulate it in the presence of actin and contribute power stroke. Mutations have been found in the heavy chains and in the two types of ventricular light chains.

Concerning the heavy chains, β-MyHC is the major isoform of the human ventricle and of slow-twitch skeletal fibers. It is encoded by MYH7. This gene appears to be the most commonly mutated HCM gene, and hot spots for mutations have been identified.[30,66] Most mutations are missense mutations located either in the head or in the head-rod junction of the molecule. Based on their structural location in the myosin head, most mutations are likely to disrupt mechanical and catalytic components of actin-myosin interactin, resulting in reduced force generation. Sarcomere assembly also is likely to be disrupted. Mutations in the light meromyosin domain also have been identified, and Blair and colleagues[69] speculated that HCM develops in this case due to abnormalities of myosin filament assembly or interactions with thick filament binding proteins.

The myosin light chain isoforms are expressed in the ventricular myocardium and in the slow-twitch muscles and are MLC-2 s/v, encoded by MYL2, and MLC-1 s/v, encoded by MYL3. The myosin light chains are thought to influence the mechanical efficiency of cross-bridge cycling and speed of contraction. It is believed that these proteins regulate power output via a calcium-dependent mechanism, and disruption leads to the HCM phenotype.

MyBP-C is part of the thick filaments of the sarcomere, being located at the level of the transverse stripes, 43 nm apart, seen by electron microscopy in the sarcomere A band. Its function is uncertain, but evidence has existed since the 1990s to indicate structural and regulatory roles. Partial extraction of cMyBP-C from rat skinned cardiac myocytes and rabbit skeletal muscle fibers alters Ca²⁺-sensitive tension,[70] and it has been shown that phosphorylation of cMyBP-C alters myosin cross-bridges in native thick filaments, suggesting that cMyBP-C can modify force production in activated cardiac muscles. The cardiac isoform is encoded by the MYBPC3 gene.

The thin filament contains **actin**, the troponin complex, and tropomyosin. The troponin complex and tropomyosin constitute the Ca²⁺-sensitive switch that regulates the contraction of cardiac muscle fibers. Mutations have been found in α-TM and in two of the subunits of the troponin complex, cTnI, the inhibitory subunit, and cTnT, the tropomyosin-binding subunit.

α-TM is encoded by TPM1. The cardiac isoform is expressed in the ventricular myocardium and in fast-twitch skeletal muscles.[71] It shares the overall structure of other tropomyosins, which are rodlike proteins that possess a simple dimeric α-coiled-coil structure in parallel orientation along their entire length.[71] It is believed that some mutations in this gene could alter tropomyosin binding to actin.

cTnT is encoded by TNNT2. In human cardiac muscle, multiple isoforms of cTnT have been described, which are expressed in the fetal, adult, and diseased heart and which result from alternative splicing of the single gene TNNT2.[72,73] The precise physiologic relevance of these isoforms currently is poorly understood. Mutations in this gene are predicted to influence the inhibitory regulatory effect of the tropomyosin-troponin complex.

cTnI is encoded by TNNI3. The cTnI isoform is expressed only in cardiac muscles.[74] Cooperative binding of cTnI to actin-tropomyosin is a unique property of the cardiac variant. It is believed that mutations disrupt the calcium-sensitive switch mediated by this protein, resulting in increased calcium sensitivity and reduced maximum tension.

α-Cardiac actin mutations also cause familial HCM. Mogensen and coworkers[61] identified mutations in a family with heterogeneous phenotypes, ranging from asymptomatic with mild hypertrophy to pronounced septal hypertrophy and left ventricular outflow tract obstruction. Mutations in titin[62] and MLP[63] also have been identified, suggesting the Z-disc to be important in the development of HCM, although the mechanism is uncertain. In addition, mutations in caveolin-3 and unconventional myosin VI have been identified, but the functional abnormalities resulting in the clinical phenotype are currently unclear.[64,65]

The pattern and extent of left ventricular hypertrophy in patients with HCM vary greatly even in first-degree relatives. A high incidence of sudden death is reported in select families. An important issue is to determine whether the genotype heterogeneity observed in HCM accounts for the phenotypic diversity of the disease.

The results must be seen as preliminary, however, because the available data relate to only a few hundred individuals, and although a given phenotype may be apparent in a small family, examination of large or multiple families with the same mutation is required before drawing unambiguous conclusions.

Several concepts have been published for mutations in the *MYH7, TNNT2,* and *MYBPC3* genes. For *MYH7,* the prognosis for patients with different mutations has been shown to vary. The *R403Q* mutation was believed to be associated with markedly reduced survival,[75] whereas some others, such as *V606M,* seemed more benign. The disease caused by *TNNT2* mutations reportedly was associated with a 20% incidence of nonpenetrance, a relatively mild and sometimes subclinical hypertrophy, but a high incidence of sudden death, which occurred even in the absence of significant clinical left ventricular hypertrophy.[76,77] Mutations in *MYBPC3* have been characterized by specific clinical features with a mild phenotype in young subjects, a delayed age at the onset of symptoms, and a favorable prognosis before the age of 40.[78-81] Despite these assertions, however, the notion of mutation-specific clinical outcomes was challenged by Van Driest and colleagues,[51] who showed that "benign" mutations were uncommon (5 of 253), and that the mutations studied all had severe clinical disease.

Genetic studies also have revealed the presence of clinically healthy individuals carrying the mutant allele, which is associated in first-degree relatives with a typical phenotype of the disease. Several mechanisms could account for the large variability of the phenotypic expression of the mutations, including the roles of environmental differences and acquired traits (e.g., differences in lifestyle, risk factors, and exercise) and the existence of modifier genes or polymorphisms or both that could modulate the phenotypic expression of the disease. Significant results have been obtained so far regarding the influence of the angiotensin-converting enzyme (ACE) insertion/deletion polymorphism. Association studies showed that compared with a control population, the D allele is more common in patients with HCM and in patients with a high incidence of sudden cardiac death.[82,83] It also was shown that the association between the D allele and hypertrophy was seen in the case of *MYH7* R403 codon mutations, but not with *MYBPC3* mutation carriers,[84] raising the concept of multiple genetic modifiers in HCM.

Therapeutic Strategies

The mainstay of therapy in children with HCM has been pharmacologic approaches; the two major medication classes used include β-blockers and calcium channel blockers.[85-87] In small children, we have used propranolol as our drug of choice because of ease of access, liquid formulation, and low side-effect profile. Therapy in these children is monitored by heart rate response, with the goal being approximately 80 to 100 beats/min. Dosage typically is 2 to 5 mg/kg/day divided three times

daily. Verapamil has been popular in some institutions and reportedly results in good outcomes. In older children, we typically treat with atenolol; in children with excessive hypertrophy and severe outflow tract obstruction, we occasionally consider use of combination therapy (β-blocker plus calcium channel blocker), although this is not without risk. The risk-to-benefit ratio must be determined for each patient, however.

When standard pharmacologic therapy fails, there are limited options, although the size of the child plays a role. In small children, myomectomy is the only proved option,[88,89] but this is not without risk. In older patients, pacing protocols have been used, but are controversial.[90-92] In adults, alcohol septal ablation has been used, but this has not yet been championed in children because of the uncertainties regarding long-term outcomes associated with creating an infarct in a child.[93-96]

In patients with syncope, ventricular arrhythmias, or other presumed high risk, an implantable cardioverter defibrillator should be considered.[7] In some patients, pacing also is necessary. Heart failure in HCM occurs secondary to diastolic dysfunction or burned-out disease with resultant systolic dysfunction. In the case of diastolic dysfunction with heart failure and preserved systolic function, combination therapy with an ACE inhibitor and diuretic, with or without an angiotensin II receptor blocker, such as candesartan or losartan, is commonly used. In these patients, β-blockers, calcium channel blockers, and pacing also are considered, along with surgical relief.[9] In the case of systolic dysfunction, therapy is similar to that in patients with DCM and includes an ACE inhibitor plus β-blocker therapy, with or without a diuretic and digoxin.[9] Enalapril and carvedilol are the most common ACE inhibitor/β-blocker combination used. Finally, in children with metabolic or mitochondrial dysfunction underlying HCM, metabolic therapies occasionally have been successful. Similar to the therapy in DCM caused by these deficiencies, carnitine, coenzyme Q10, riboflavin, and thiamine may be considered.[11]

INFILTRATIVE FORMS OF HYPERTROPHIC CARDIOMYOPATHY

A variety of disorders that have apparent left ventricular hypertrophy and features of HCM occur as a result of infiltrative disorders. The classic form of infiltrative disease in this category is Pompe disease, a disorder typically presenting in the first weeks of life.[11] More recently, other forms of infiltrative disease have been identified with later onset disease, such as Fabry disease,[97] Danon disease,[98] and left ventricular hypertrophy resulting from mutations in AMP-activated protein kinase encoded by the *PRKAG2* gene.[40,41,46] These disorders, along with disorders caused by mitochondrial abnormalities and genetic dysmorphism syndromes, such as Noonan syndrome and LEOPARD syndrome (*l*entigines, *E*CG abnormalities, *o*cular hypertelorism, *p*ulmonary stenosis, *a*bnormalities of genitalia, *r*etardation of growth, and *d*eafness), are caused by abnormalities not primarily affecting the sarcomere.[11] Therapy is similar to the sarcomeric form of the disease, unless systolic dysfunction occurs, in which case heart failure therapy should be instituted.

Pompe Disease (Type II Glycogen Storage Disease)

Genetic deficiency of acid α-1,4-glucosidase, an enzyme involved in the breakdown of glycogen to glucose, results in a wide clinical spectrum ranging from the rapidly fatal infantile onset of type II glycogen storage disease to a slowly progressive adult-onset myopathy. The infantile-onset form (Pompe disease) typically manifests during the first 5 months of life, and patients usually die before their second birthday.[99] This rare inborn error of glycogen metabolism occurs in less than 1 per 100,000 births. Massive glycogen accumulation occurs, leading to the clinical findings of enlarged tongue, striking hepatomegaly, hypotonia with decreased deep tendon reflexes, and cardiomyopathy (usually HCM) with congestive heart failure. The glycogen accumulation can be noted histologically in the skeletal muscles, liver, and heart. Children usually die in the first 2 years of life. The diagnosis may be predicted from the pathognomonic ECG.[11,100] The disease has autosomal recessive inheritance; the gene coding for the lysosomal enzyme originally was mapped to chromosome 17 at sub-band 17q23-q25.[101]

Allelic variation at the acid α-glucosidase locus is presumed to be the most important factor in diversity of type II glycogen storage disease.[99,102] It has been shown that various combinations of homoallelic and heteroallelic mutant genotypes are the basis for this clinical heterogeneity. Zhong and associates[103] identified a missense mutation in one allele of a patient with Pompe disease. This base pair substitution resulted in a loss of restriction endonuclease sites, which allowed the investigators to show messenger RNA expression deficiency from the second allele using polymerase chain reaction–amplified RNA. This deficiency was the first evidence of single base pair missense mutations in patients with this disease. In addition to molecular analysis, the diagnosis can be made biochemically by analysis of α-glucosidase in blood lymphocytes or skin fibroblasts. Prenatal diagnosis is possible by amniocentesis or chorionic villus sampling by assay of α-glucosidase. Enzyme therapy is now possible and seems to reverse the cardiac phenotype.[104]

Fabry Disease

Fabry disease is an X-linked recessive disorder with mild expression occasionally seen in carrier females; it is caused by deficiency of the enzyme α-galactosidase and is found in 1 of 40,000 people. Young adults may be prone to renal failure and myocardial infarctions. Fabry disease usually has its onset in adolescence and usually manifests with sensations of burning pain in the hands and feet.[97,105] These sensations tend to be associated with fever, heart, cold, and exercise. With increasing age, multiple angiokeratomas become noticeable, especially around the umbilicus and genitalia. Corneal opacities are often noted. Progressive renal failure develops with age. CNS manifestations include seizures, headaches, and hemiplegia associated with an increased risk of stroke. Primary cardiac manifestations in affected males are HCM and mitral insufficiency, and the diagnosis depends on echocardiography.[106-108] The left ventricular myocardium and mitral valve tend to be areas of greatest storage of lipid material. On ECG, the PR interval is usually short. Deposition of sphingolipids in the coronary arteries leads to myocardial ischemia and infarction.[107,109]

The disease-causing gene originally was localized to the long arm of the X chromosome in the Xq22 region. The full-length complement DNA (cDNA) was isolated and sequenced,[110] showing a 1393-base pair cDNA with a 60-nucleotide 5′ untranslated region and encoding a precursor peptide of 429 amino acids. The gene was found to contain seven exons. Mutations and phenotypic correlation have been described.[111,112]

Nakao and colleagues[113] studied 1603 men by echocardiography and showed significant left ventricular hypertrophy in 230 subjects (14%), of whom 7 (3%) had proven α-galactoside deficiency. These patients had concentric left ventricular hypertrophy. Linhart and coworkers[114] studied 30 patients with Fabry disease and found 37% had concentric left ventricular hypertrophy, 10% had asymmetric septal hypertrophy, and 3% had an eccentric pattern of hypertrophy. Sachdev and associates[115] identified five patients with HCM diagnosed after age 40 and one with earlier onset (<40 years old) HCM, all with low α-galactoside activity. In five of the six patients, the hypertrophy was concentric, whereas one had asymmetric hypertrophy. In one case, left ventricular outflow tract obstruction was noted. Nonsustained ventricular tachycardia occurred in two patients, and another patient had second-degree atrioventricular block initially and then atrial fibrillation. It seems that these abnormalities in α-galactoside activity result in some cases of HCM or "unexplained" left ventricular hypertrophy.

Danon Disease

Danon disease is an X-linked dominant disorder characterized by intracytoplasmic vacuoles containing autophagic material and glycogen in cardiac and skeletal muscle cells, cardiomyopathy, and skeletal myopathy, with or without conduction defect, Wolff-Parkinson-White syndrome, or mental retardation.[116] The underlying abnormality affects lysosomal function and is due to mutations in the lysosomal associated membrane protein 2 (LAMP2).[117] The clinical phenotypic expression of Danon disease varies. Charron and associates[118] screened

50 cases of HCM for LAMP2 mutations and identified mutations in two patients with HCM and skeletal myopathy. Both of these individuals presented during their teenage years, and other, younger affected individuals in the family were identified, the youngest was 7 years of age.

Wolff-Parkinson-White syndrome and high-voltage QRS complexes on ECG were notable along with high creatine kinase plasma levels. In addition, late left ventricular dilation and dysfunction occurred with symptoms of heart failure. Atrial and ventricular arrhythmias and conduction disease were notable along with death of patients during their 20s. Visual acuity abnormality also was common, resulting from choriocapillary ocular atrophy. This disease seems to be underrecognized and may play a significant role in pediatric heart failure.

AMP-Activated Protein Kinase

AMP-activated protein kinase, encoded by the γ2 regulatory subunit of the *PRKAG2* gene on chromosome 7q31,[58] is an enzyme that modulates glucose uptake and glycolysis.[119,120] Dominant mutations in this gene first were identified by Gollob and associates[40] and Blair and colleagues[41] in 2001 in subjects with HCM, Wolff-Parkinson-White pre-excitation, and atrioventricular block. MacRae and coworkers[58] first described the genetic locus on chromosome 7q3 in 1995 in families with HCM and Wolff-Parkinson-White syndrome, and the affected individuals were believed to be clinically different from patients with other forms of adult HCM. Blair and colleagues[41] made the case that mutations in AMP-activated protein kinase resulted in HCM secondary to compromise of energy production and use, but Arad and colleagues[46] provided evidence that this disorder is a form of glycogen storage disease.

Cardiac pathology differed from other forms of HCM, with no myocyte and myofibrillar disarray seen, but instead pronounced vacuoles that were filled with glycogen-associated granules. The myocytes were enlarged, and interstitial fibrosis was minimal. Using a yeast system in which a similar enzyme is functional, Arad and associates[121] introduced the same mutations found in the patients and showed that the enzyme activity is persistent (i.e., does not turn off), leading to glycogen accumulation. The authors confirmed these findings by developing a murine model that mimics the human disorder.

ENERGY-DEPENDENT FORMS OF HYPERTROPHIC CARDIOMYOPATHY

Mitochondrial Cardiomyopathies

The human mitochondrial genome[122] is a small, circular DNA molecule that is maternally inherited. Mitochondrial DNA (mtDNA) encodes 13 of the 69 proteins required for oxidative metabolism and 22 transfer RNAs (tRNAs)

and 2 ribosomal RNAs (rRNAs) required for their translation. Because mtDNA has much less redundancy than the nuclear genome (in which essentially identical information is received from both parents), and tRNAs and rRNAs are present in multiple copies, the mitochondrial genome is an excellent target for mutations giving rise to human disease.[123-125] Mitochondria enjoy a symbiotic relationship with the cell. These subcellular organelles depend on nucleocytoplasmic mechanisms for most structural components, but contribute vital peptides that are central to cellular respiration. Mitochondria contain a permeable outer membrane and a highly restrictive inner membrane that guards the chemical microenvironment of the matrix compartment. Adaptive mechanisms exist for the passage of large and small molecules across the inner membrane. Translocases shuttle monocarboxylic acids, amino acids, acyl-carnitine conjugates, small ions, and other metabolites in and out of the mitochondrial matrix. Energy is required for importation of proteins into the mitochondria because the nuclear gene-synthesized mitochondrial proteins are precursor molecules that require presequence cleavage.

The 13 mtDNA genes are located in the respiratory chain[125-127] and include seven complex I subunits (ND1, 2, 3, 4L, 4, 5, and 6), one complex III subunit (cytochrome *b*), three complex IV subunits (COI, II, and III), and two complex V subunits (ATPase 6 and 8). Coordination must exist between nuclear and mitochondrial genomes to permit assembly of the complex holoenzymes. Each cell contains numerous mitochondria, and each mitochondrion contains multiple copies of mtDNA. This genetic material derives exclusively from the female gamete, and any mutation must be passed from the female parent to all progeny, male and female. The replicative segregation of mutant mtDNA copies within the cell determines whether this biologic disadvantage is expressed. In most mitochondrial disorders, patients carry a mix of mutant and normal mitochondria, a condition known as *heteroplasmy,* with the proportions varying from tissue to tissue and individual to individual within a pedigree in a manner correlating with severity of phenotype.[124,125]

Mitochondrial diseases often produce disturbances of brain and muscle function, presumably because these two organs are so metabolically active, and the metabolic demand is high during growth and development.[128] Cardiac disease is seen most commonly with respiratory chain defects.[129,130] Ragged red fibers are present in muscle biopsy specimens almost invariably when the molecular defect involves mtDNA (except in infants).[123] These defects represent the genetics of ATP production. The diverse clinical syndromes associated with various respiratory chain complexes are believed to result from involvement of tissue-nonspecific (generalized) subunits in other cases and the residual enzyme activity in affected tissues.[131]

The cardiac diseases associated with mitochondrial defects include HCM, DCM, and left ventricular non-compaction.[132] Although no theory has been advanced to explain the cause of these phenotypically different cardiac abnormalities, it is possible that the dilated form occurs after an initial hypertrophic response (i.e., it is a burned-out dilated form of HCM).

Respiratory Chain Abnormalities

Approximately 100 cases of **complex I deficiency** have been described,[133] with these cases including the myopathy syndrome and the encephalomyopathic syndrome. The latter includes a fatal infantile disorder with involvement of brain, muscle, and heart; a milder version with clinical manifestations later in childhood or early adulthood; and mitochondrial myopathy, encephalopathy, lactic acidosis, and stroke-like episodes (MELAS syndrome) believed to be secondary to reduced nicotinamide adenine dinucleotide coenzyme Q reductase abnormalities.[134]

Treatment of these disorders is limited. Riboflavin, succinate supplements (because the metabolite enters the respiratory chain at complex II), ubiquinone, and idebenone have been recommended for patients with MELAS. A mitochondrial mutation initially was described in a patient with MELAS and fatal infantile cardiomyopathy; this mutation was shown to be caused by an A-to-G transition in mtDNA of the isoleucine tRNA gene.[135] Analysis of enzyme activities and subunits in the heart revealed combined defects of complex I and complex IV of the respiratory chain. Similar mutations subsequently have been described.[136]

Complex II defects result in a myopathic or multisystemic disorder. Cardiomyopathy has been found alone and in conjunction with skeletal myopathy.[137] Encephalomyopathy also manifests with retinopathy, ataxia, spasticity, dementia, weakness, sensorineural hearing loss, and exercise intolerance.

Complex IV defects are similar clinically to complex I defects.[138] The mitochondrial genome encodes for three subunits of cytochrome-c oxidase, which represents the terminal portion of the respiratory chain and catalyzes conversion of molecular oxygen to water. A benign reversible infantile myopathy[139] that normalizes by early childhood may occur or a fatal infantile myopathy manifested by profound weakness, hypotonia, respiratory insufficiency, and death. This myopathy may occur alone or in association with severe renal tubular dysfunction or cardiomyopathy with red ragged fibers.

Kearns-Sayre syndrome is a mitochondrial myopathy that is characterized by ptosis, chronic progressive external ophthalmoplegia, abnormal retinal pigmentation, cardiac conduction defects, and DCM. Channer and coworkers[140] reported a case of rapidly developing progressive congestive heart failure and DCM requiring transplantation in a patient with Kearns-Sayre syndrome. Approximately 20% of Kearns-Sayre syndrome patients have cardiac involvement, and most usually

have conduction defects causing progressive heart block. These patients generally have large, heterogeneous deletions in the mitochondrial chromosome. Poulton and colleagues[141] showed germline deletions of mtDNA in a family with Kearns-Sayre syndrome using polymerase chain reaction to amplify across the deletion, with primers flanking these deletions. The patient was shown to have a deletion in muscle mtDNA and at low levels in blood that were identical to those found in the mother and sister. The probands had more deleted DNA, however, correlating with more severe symptoms. Other mutations also have been described.[142,143]

MERRF syndrome is a syndrome that is characterized by myoclonic epilepsy with ragged red muscle fibers (MERRF) and is caused by a single nucleotide substitution in tRNA LYS that apparently interferes with mitochondrial translation.[144,145] Shoffner and colleagues[146] showed an A-to-G transition mutation as the cause of the disease associated with defects in complexes I and IV. This abnormality causes decline in ATP-generating capacity, with onset of disease that includes cardiomyopathy. Other reports outline various disease-causing mutations.[147-149]

Hypoxemia Mitochondrial DNA Damage and Cardiac Disease

Because cardiac tissue relies on mitochondrial oxidative phosphorylation for energy production, it has been believed that deficiency of portions of this system or its end product can cause cardiac abnormalities.[150] Hypoxemia has been shown to increase oxygen radical production, which results in elevated mtDNA damage and altered oxidative phosphorylation gene expression. In addition, these enzymes have been shown to decline with age, whereas mtDNA deletions increase with age, especially deletion at the nucleotide 4977 base pair. Corral-Debrinski and coworkers[151] hypothesized that ischemic hearts would be likely to have increased chances of mtDNA deletion because of this effect of hypoxemia, and using polymerase chain reaction amplification across the deletion breakpoint of the common mtDNA[4977] deletion, these investigators showed that mtDNA damage was increased in chronically ischemic hearts and in some hearts with other forms of chronic cardiac disease (DCM and HCM). It is possible that oxidative phosphorylation gene induction may be part of a general response to chronic cardiac failure. Other reports support this view.[152,153] In addition, there is some support that endomyocardial biopsies should be performed in patients with HCM or DCM to increase the likelihood of detecting mitochondrial abnormalities.[154]

HYPERTROPHIC VERSUS RESTRICTIVE CARDIOMYOPATHY

RCM is a relatively rare form of cardiomyopathy, affecting only approximately 5% of individuals with heart muscle disease (see Chapter 19).[155] The disorder seems to have the worst outcome of all forms of cardiomyopathy (especially in children), however, with sudden death occurring within 2 to 5 years of diagnosis in more than one half of cases.[42] In some instances, ventricular tachycardia has been shown as the etiology of demise. In the remaining patients, congestive heart failure with or without pulmonary hypertension is notable.

Clinical Features

RCM most commonly manifests with syncope or sudden death in children.[42-44,156,157] Rarely does this disorder present in the first 2 years of life, with most children identified before puberty. Patients with later onset tend to present with signs and symptoms of congestive heart failure, particularly dyspnea, orthopnea, and abdominal pain. Chest pain and palpitations also may be prominent features. On physical examination, these children have a quiet precordium, regular rhythm, and nondisplaced apical impulse associated with a gallop rhythm, usually an S_4. If a murmur exists, it is usually due to atrioventricular valve regurgitation. The liver tends to be significantly enlarged and tender without splenomegaly. The lungs are usually clear to auscultation, and peripheral edema is rare.

Clinical Evaluation

The usual evaluation includes chest radiography, ECG, echocardiography, and Holter monitoring. Exercise testing

and cardiac catheterization also may be performed. Chest x-rays commonly show mild cardiomegaly and, in children with congestive heart failure, increased pulmonary vascular markings and Kerley B lines. As a result of the enlarged atria, pulmonary atelectasis is common. The ECG has classic features, including biatrial enlargement. Usually the QRS complexes, QT interval, and T wave morphology are normal, but atrial and ventricular arrhythmias may be noted along with ST-segment abnormalities.

RCM is characterized by atrial dilation bilaterally with normal sized ventricles (Fig. 20-6). Systolic function usually is preserved, but diastolic dysfunction is usually evident with abnormal mitral inflow patterns. Atrioventricular valve regurgitation is common, and evidence of elevated right heart pressures is typical. Cardiac hypertrophy, including asymmetric septal hypertrophy, occurs in some patients. Whether this condition is true RCM or HCM with restrictive physiology remains a conundrum. In some children, 24-hour Holter monitors show atrial or ventricular tachyarrhythmias. In addition, ST-segment abnormalities may occur, particularly at higher heart rates.

Elevated atrial and ventricular end-diastolic pressures are typical and worsen with volume challenge. A so-called square root sign confirms restrictive physiology. Pulmonary hypertension may be identified, and atrioventricular valve regurgitation is commonly seen on angiography. Coronary angiography and contractile function also are normal. In some patients, endomyocardial

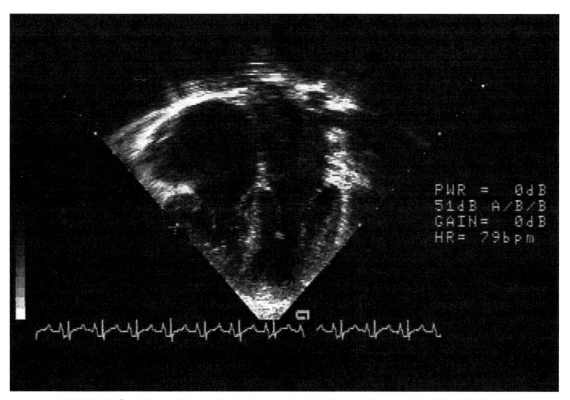

FIGURE 20-6 ■ Echocardiographic features of restrictive cardiomyopathy. There is biatrial enlargement with normal ventricular size and thickness.

biopsy may be performed. Myocyte hypertrophy and fibrosis may occur, but, in contrast to in adults, infiltrative processes (e.g., amyloid and sarcoid) are not seen.

Although a normal exercise test may be seen, this test may be dangerous in some individuals because of the propensity for ST-segment changes, particularly at higher heart rates, which may lead to serious ventricular arrhythmias. Reduced exercise capacity and abnormal oxygen consumption also are common.

Genetic Aspects

When RCM is inherited, autosomal dominant inheritance is most common, although autosomal recessive transmission has been reported.[45,67] Inherited disease seems to occur in less than 10% of cases, however. Two genes have been identified in autosomal dominant RCM so far, troponin I[158] and desmin.[159] In the cases with troponin I mutations, interventricular septal hypertrophy consistent with HCM with restrictive physiology was seen in several patients, whereas others had normal septal and wall thicknesses.[158] The patients with desmin mutations had pure RCM. Normal skeletal muscle function was found clinically in subjects with these gene defects. Other genes exist that cause this disorder, but these remain elusive. In some cases, RCM coexists with skeletal myopathy or conduction system disease or both.[159,160] In these cases, mutations in desmin have been described.[159,160] Mouse models of desmin knockouts are confirmatory.[47,161,162] In elderly patients with RCM, mutations in the prealbumin gene, transthyretin, have been described.[163,164]

Therapeutic Strategies

Children with RCM are possibly the highest risk population in pediatrics for sudden cardiac death. Therapy tends to be unsuccessful. Based on treatment results in patients with HCM, the other disorder associated with predominant diastolic dysfunction, β-blockers or calcium channel blockers initially were believed to be the treatment of choice. These agents have had little impact on outcome, however, and in some children have added to the symptoms. The use of β-blockers has caused hypoglycemia with associated seizures and syncope in several children.

No other pharmacologic agents have been useful in children without congestive heart failure; therapy of congestive heart failure in this subgroup is efficacious, however. The use of antiarrhythmic agents and implantable cardioverter defibrillators may protect some children at risk for arrhythmogenic sudden death. Most of these approaches have not reduced mortality, and in our institution children are listed for transplantation at the time of diagnosis with extremely good outcomes occurring. In patients waiting for transplantation in whom evidence of heart rate–related ischemia is noted, IV esmolol infusion has been useful.

LEFT VENTRICULAR NONCOMPACTION

Left ventricular noncompaction has been considered to be a rare disease and has been identified by a variety of names, including spongy myocardium, fetal myocardium, and noncompaction of the left ventricular myocardium.[39,165-168] The abnormality is believed to represent an arrest in the normal process of myocardial compaction, the final stage of myocardial morphogenesis, resulting in persistence of multiple prominent ventricular trabeculations and deep intertrabecular recesses. This cardiomyopathy is difficult to diagnose, unless the physician has a high level of suspicion during echocardiographic evaluation. On careful review of echocardiograms and other clinical data, it seems that left ventricular noncompaction is relatively common in children and is seen in adults.[39,67]

Two forms of left ventricular noncompaction occur: (1) isolated noncompaction and (2) noncompaction associated with congenital heart disease, such as septal defects (ventricular or atrial septal defect), pulmonic stenosis, and hypoplastic left heart syndrome.[67,165-169] In the isolated form and the form associated with congenital heart disease, metabolic derangements may be notable.[138,166]

Clinical Features

Left ventricular noncompaction most commonly manifests in infancy with signs and symptoms of heart failure, but some patients are identified during later childhood, adolescence, or adulthood. Pignatelli and associates[39] reported the findings on 36 children identified over a 5-year period, with the median age at presentation being 90 days (range 1 day to 17 years). In this study, 40% of the children presented with low cardiac output or congestive heart failure, and only one child (3%) presented with syncope. The most common presenting symptom other than heart failure was asymptomatic ECG or radiographic abnormalities, with 42% being asymptomatic. In addition, 14% of children had associated dysmorphic features, whereas 19% of affected children had first-degree relatives with cardiomyopathy. The children with dysmorphic features were diagnosed with DiGeorge syndrome ($n = 1$) and congenital adrenal hyperplasia ($n = 1$).

Clinical Evaluation

The usual evaluation includes an ECG, chest radiograph, echocardiogram, Holter monitoring, blood and urinary studies, and skeletal muscle biopsy. These studies, in addition to the clinical evaluation and a high degree of suspicion, should lead to a higher likelihood of correct diagnosis. Chest x-rays commonly show cardiomegaly (20%) or signs of heart failure, such as increased pulmonary vascular markings (40%). Blood and urine studies and muscle biopsy with biochemical analysis are important diagnostic tests in patients with left ventricular noncompaction.

Because of the association of left ventricular noncompaction with Barth syndrome,[169] mitochondrial syndromes, or other metabolic syndromes,[138,166] abnormalities may be notable with all such studies. These may include cyclic neutropenia (Barth syndrome), lactic acidosis (Barth syndrome, mitochondrial or metabolic disorders), 3-methylglutaconic acidemia (Barth syndrome, mitochondrial disease), and carnitine or fatty acid oxidation defects. Skeletal muscle biopsy specimens are commonly abnormal, showing evidence of mitochondrial proliferation and morphology abnormalities (with or without inclusions). Electron transport chain biochemistry also may be abnormal with deficiencies identified in complexes I through IV of the respiratory chain in association with elevated citrate synthase and succinate dehydrogenase. Cytochrome-c deficiencies also have been reported.

A high prevalence of ECG abnormalities (possibly ≥75%) is noted. The most prominent features seen are marked biventricular hypertrophy with extreme QTS voltage similar to that seen in Pompe disease (approximately 30%), T wave inversion (20%), pre-excitation (15% to 20%), and premature atrial and ventricular contractions (approximately 10%). Rarely, children present with supraventricular or ventricular tachycardia.

Two-dimensional echocardiography shows the classic features of noncompaction, including noncompaction morphology of deep trabeculations and intertrabecular recesses and ventricular hypertrophy (especially apical hypertrophy) with or without dilation (Fig. 20-7). In nearly 90% of patients, systolic dysfunction is noted at presentation.[4] Most commonly, the left ventricle alone is affected (80%), whereas biventricular noncompaction occurs in approximately 20% of children. Congenital heart disease occurs in 10% to 20% of children and should be specifically evaluated. Doppler interrogation identifies abnormal mitral inflow velocities consistent with restrictive physiology (decreased early-to-late diastolic filling ratio) in approximately one half of cases. Several children present with increased hypertrophy, and systolic function normalizes (or becomes hypercontractile) before reverting to the initial phenotype. Rarely, thrombi (particularly in the intertrabecular apical recesses) are noted.

Genetic Aspects

When left ventricular noncompaction is inherited, it can be transmitted as an X-linked, mitochondrial, autosomal recessive, or autosomal dominant trait.[67] In approximately 20% to 30% of cases, familial inheritance has been identified. The X-linked form usually is associated with isolated noncompaction and a mutation in the G4.5 (tafazzin) gene located on chromosome Xq28.[169] This gene also has been identified in patients with Barth syndrome.

In autosomal dominant inherited cases, mutations in the Z line protein encoding ZASP, located on chromosome 10q22, have been identified in isolated noncompaction,[170] whereas mutations in the gene encoding α-dystrobrevin, a cytoskeletal protein located on chromosome 18q12, have been identified in patients with noncompaction associated with congenital heart disease.[169] No genes have been identified so far for autosomal

LV Noncompaction

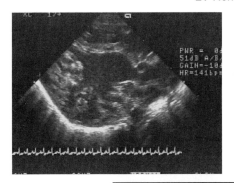
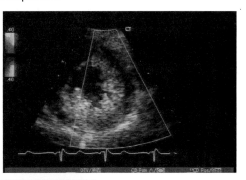
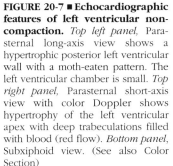
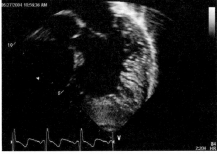

FIGURE 20-7 ■ Echocardiographic features of left ventricular noncompaction. *Top left panel,* Parasternal long-axis view shows a hypertrophic posterior left ventricular wall with a moth-eaten pattern. The left ventricular chamber is small. *Top right panel,* Parasternal short-axis view with color Doppler shows hypertrophy of the left ventricular apex with deep trabeculations filled with blood (red flow). *Bottom panel,* Subxiphoid view. (See also Color Section)

recessive–inherited noncompaction; mutations in mtDNA have been seen in patients with noncompaction.[138,166]

Therapeutic Strategies

The specific therapy depends on the clinical and echocardiographic findings. In patients with systolic dysfunction and heart failure, anticongestive therapy identical to therapy for patients with DCM is appropriate. In particular, ACE inhibitors, such as captopril and enalapril, and β-adrenergic blockers, such as metoprolol and carvedilol, are useful. Diuretics also may be needed. In patients exhibiting findings more consistent with HCM or diastolic dysfunction physiologic phenotype, β-blocker therapy alone with propranolol or atenolol is more appropriate. In patients with either of these forms of noncompaction with associated mitochondrial or metabolic dysfunction, some investigators add a "vitamin cocktail" to the cardiac therapy, with coenzyme Q10, carnitine, riboflavin, and thiamine commonly used alone or in combination.

In patients having associated congenital heart disease, appropriate therapeutic approaches may include simple pharmacologic therapy with diuretics for volume overload associated with left-to-right shunts, more complex pharmacologic therapy for patients with restrictive physiology and pulmonary hypertension, or invasive therapy with catheter intervention or surgical repairs, depending on the lesions. Intimate understanding of the cardiac function abnormalities, evidence of thrombi (which should be treated with anticoagulation), and the metabolic status of the patient is required by the interventional cardiologist, cardiac anesthesiologist, and surgeon approaching these patients invasively. In addition, cardiac rhythm disturbances need to be identified, and therapies such as pacemakers, implantable defibrillators, and intracardiac ablations need to be considered.

The clinical outcomes of patients with noncompaction have been reported to be poor with death occurring as a result of heart failure or sudden death presumably arrhythmia related or stroke related due to embolization of left ventricular thrombi.[168] Pignatelli and associates[39] showed a 5-year survival rate of 86%, however; when transplanted patients were added, the 5-year survival rate free of death or transplantation was 75%.

CURRENT STATUS AND FUTURE TRENDS

Familial HCM of adults is considered a disease of the sarcomere.[56,66,67] Similarly, patients with other cardiac disorders, such as familial DCM and familial ventricular arrhythmias (i.e., long QT syndromes and Brugada syndrome) have been shown to have mutations in genes encoding a consistent family of proteins.[67,171] In familial ventricular arrhythmias, ion channel (or ion channel modifier) gene mutations (i.e., ion channelopathy) have been found in all cases reported so far.[171,172] In familial DCM, cytoskeletal protein-encoding genes and sarcomeric proteins have been speculated to be causative (i.e., cytoskeletal/sarcomyopathy).[67,173,174] The final common pathways of these disorders include ion channels and cytoskeletal proteins, similar to the sarcomyopathy in HCM.[175] Intermediate disorders, such as arrythmogenic right ventricular dysplasia/cardiomyopathy, (ARVD/ARVC) seem to connect the primary electrical and primary muscle disorders mechanistically.[176-178] Although it is not yet certain what the underlying pathways and targets are for RCM, hints have been forthcoming. Desmin and other intermediate filament proteins seem to be at play in RCM, as has been shown in animal models, whereas the sarcomere is an additional target. In addition, it seems that cascade pathways are involved directly in some cases (i.e., mitochondrial abnormalities in HCM, DCM), whereas secondary influences are likely to result in the wide clinical spectrum seen in patients with similar mutations.

In HCM, mitochondrial and metabolic influences are probably important. Additionally, molecular interactions with such molecules as calcineurin, sex hormones, and growth factors probably are involved in the development of clinical signs, symptoms, and age of presentation. In the future, these factors are expected to be uncovered, allowing for development of new therapeutic strategies. HCM and overlap disorders that masquerade as HCM are important causes of heart failure and sudden death. The responsible genes and functional mechanisms are becoming clarified, and targeted therapies are on the near horizon. It is hoped that this new level of knowledge will lead to better outcomes in the near term, particularly in the childhood forms of the disease.[179,180]

Key Concepts

■ HCM is defined by its wall thickening—hence the term *hypertrophic heart disease*. The major impact of this disorder on human health is based on its predilection to be inherited; its reputation as the most common cause of sudden death in young, healthy, athletic individuals; and its potential to develop heart failure.

■ In the pediatric age range, the underlying etiologies responsible for HCM and the variable age range of onset differentiate the childhood form of the disease from the adult form.

■ Voltage-gated sodium channels colocalize with dystrophin, β-spectrin, ankyrin, and syntrophins, whereas potassium channels interact with the sarcomeric Z-disc and intercalated discs.[23-25] Because arrhythmias and conduction system diseases are common in children and adults with all forms of cardiomyopathy, this interaction could play an important role.

■ Disruption of the links from the sarcolemma to extracellular matrix at the dystrophin C-terminus and to the sarcomere and nucleus via N-terminal dystrophin interactions could lead to a "domino effect" disruption of systolic function, diastolic dysfunction, and development of arrhythmias.

■ HCM is considered to occur secondary to diastolic dysfunction, a disease of relaxation of the ventricular myocardium. Systolic function is preserved, or hypercontractile and left ventricular outflow tract obstruction may occur.

■ HCM is a primary myocardial disorder with an autosomal dominant pattern of inheritance that is characterized by hypertrophy of the left ventricle (with or without the right ventricle) with histologic features of myocyte hypertrophy, myofibrillar disarray, and interstitial fibrosis.

■ Studies of kindreds with HCM have shown that the distribution and severity of left ventricular hypertrophy may vary considerably, that asymmetric hypertrophy is no longer an essential requirement for the diagnosis of this disorder, and that even within the same family the features may differ.

■ Risk stratification has been reported with the use of exercise testing, with blunting or reduction of blood pressure or blunting of heart rate response to exercise being associated with increased risk. In particular, blood pressure reduction by more than 15 mm Hg or failure to increase blood pressure by more than 25 mm Hg is associated with increased risk. Other associated risk factors include syncope, nonsustained ventricular tachycardia, severe left ventricular hypertrophy on echocardiography (>3 cm in adults), and family history of premature death.

■ Various mechanisms for sudden death have been proposed, including ventricular bradyarrhythmias secondary to sinus node and atrioventricular conduction abnormalities and tachyarrhythmias triggered by reentrant depolarization pathways related to myofibrillar disarray and fibrosis, abnormal Ca^{2+} homeostasis, myocardial ischemia, left ventricular diastolic dysfunction, and left ventricular outflow tract obstruction.

■ Various risk stratification algorithms based on clinical parameters have been proposed to identify individuals with an increased propensity for sudden death. Given the complexity of mechanisms that may precipitate sudden death, it is not surprising that no single risk factor has been identified.

■ Genetic studies also have revealed the presence of clinically healthy individuals carrying the mutant allele, which is associated in first-degree relatives with a typical phenotype of the disease. Several mechanisms could account for the large variability of the phenotypic expression of the mutations, including the roles of environmental differences and acquired traits (e.g., differences in lifestyle, risk factors, and exercise) and the existence of modifier genes or polymorphisms or both that could modulate the phenotypic expression of the disease.

■ In small children, we have used propranolol as our drug of choice because of ease of access, liquid formulation, and low side-effect profile.

■ When standard pharmacologic therapy fails, there are limited options, although the size of the child plays a role. In small children, myomectomy is the only proven option, but this is not without risk. In older patients, pacing protocols have been used, but are controversial.

■ Heart failure in HCM occurs as a result of diastolic dysfunction or burned-out disease with resultant systolic dysfunction. In the case of diastolic dysfunction with heart failure and preserved systolic function, combination therapy with ACE inhibitors and diuretics, with or without angiotensin II receptor blockers, such as candesartan or losartan, commonly are used. In these patients, β-blockers, calcium channel blockers, and pacing also are considered, along with surgical relief. In the case of systolic dysfunction, therapy is similar to therapy for patients with DCM, including ACE inhibitors plus β-blocker therapy, with or without diuretics and digoxin. Enalapril and carvedilol is the most common ACE inhibitor/β-blocker combination used.

■ A variety of disorders that have apparent left ventricular hypertrophy and features of HCM occur secondary to infiltrative disorders. The classic form of infiltrative disease in this category is Pompe disease, a disorder typically presenting in the first weeks of life. More recently, other forms of infiltrative disease have been identified with later onset disease, such as Fabry disease, Danon disease, and left ventricular hypertrophy secondary to mutations in AMP-activated protein kinase encoded by the *PRKAG2* gene.

■ The cardiac diseases associated with mitochondrial defects include HCM, DCM, and left ventricular noncompaction. Although no theory has been advanced to explain the cause of these phenotypically different cardiac abnormalities, it is possible that the dilated form occurs after an initial hypertrophic response (i.e., it is a burned-out dilated form of HCM).

■ Left ventricular noncompaction has been considered to be a rare disease and has been identified by a variety of names, including spongy myocardium, fetal myocardium, and noncompaction of the left ventricular myocardium. The abnormality is believed to represent an arrest in the normal process of myocardial compaction, the final stage of myocardial morphogenesis, resulting in persistence of multiple prominent ventricular trabeculations and deep intertrabecular recesses.

■ Two forms of left ventricular noncompaction occur: (1) isolated noncompaction and (2) noncompaction associated with congenital heart disease, such as septal defects.

REFERENCES

1. Maron BJ: Hypertrophic cardiomyopathy: A systemic review. JAMA 2002;287:1308-1320.
2. Elliott P, McKenna WJ: Hypertrophic cardiomyopathy. Lancet 2004;363:188-189.
3. Ommen SR, Nishimura RA: Hypertrophic cardiomyopathy. Curr Probl Cardiol 2004;29:239-291.
4. McKenna WJ, Behr ER: Hypertrophic cardiomyopathy: Management, risk stratification, and prevention of sudden death. Heart 2002;87:169-176.
5. Frenneaux MP: Assessing the risk of sudden cardiac death in a patient with hypertrophic cardiomyopathy. Heart 2004;90:570-575.
6. Maron BJ, Carney KP, Lever HM, et al: Relationship of race to sudden cardiac death in competitive athletes with hypertrophic cardiomyopathy. J Am Coll Cardiol 2003;41:974-980.
7. Maron BJ: Hypertrophic cardiomyopathy and sudden death: New perspective on risk stratification and prevention with the implantable cardioverter-defibrillator. Eur Heart J 2000;21:1979-1983.
8. Spirito P, Maron BJ, Bonow RO, Epstein SE: Occurrence and significance of progressive left ventricular wall thinning and relative cavity dilation in hypertrophic cardiomyopathy. Am J Cardiol 1987;60:123-139.
9. Aurigemma GP, Gaasch WH: Diastolic heart failure. N Engl J Med 2004;351:1097-1105.
10. Gaasch WH, Zile MR: Left ventricular diastolic dysfunction and diastolic heart failure. Annu Rev Med 2004;55:373-394.
11. Towbin JA, Lipshultz SE: Genetics of neonatal cardiomyopathy. Curr Opin Cardiol 1999;14:250-262.
12. Schwartz SM, Duffy JY, Pearl JM, Nelson DP: Cellular and molecular aspects of myocardial dysfunction. Crit Care Med 2001;29:S214-S219.
13. Gregorio CC, Antin PB: To the heart of myofibril assembly. Trends Cell Biol 2000;10:355-362.
14. Squire JM: Architecture and function in the muscle sarcomere. Curr Opin Struct Biol 1997;7:247-257.
15. Clark KA, McElhinny AS, Beckerle MC, Gregorio CC: Striated muscle cytoarchitecture: An intricate web of form and function. Annu Rev Cell Dev Biol 2002;18:637-706.
16. Vigoreaux JO: The muscle Z band: Lessons in stress management. J Muscle Res Cell Motil 1994;15:237-255.
17. Barth AL, Nathke IS, Nelson WJ: Cadherins, catenins and APC protein: Interplay between cytoskeletal complexes and signaling pathways. Curr Opin Cell Biol 1997;9:683-690.
18. Burridge K, Chrzanowska-Wodnicka M: Focal adhesions, contractility, and signaling. Annu Rev Cell Dev Biol 1996;12:463-518.
19. Capetanaki Y: Desmin cytoskeleton: A potential regulator of muscle mitochondrial behaviour and function. Trends Cardiovasc Med 2002;12:339-348.
20. Stewart M: Intermediate filament structure and assembly. Curr Opin Cell Biol 1993;5:3-11.
21. Sharp WW, Simpson DG, Borg TK, et al: Mechanical forces regulate focal adhesion and costamere assembly in cardiac myocytes. Am J Physiol 1997;273:H546-H556.
22. Straub V, Campbell KP: Muscular dystrophies and the dystrophin-glycoprotein complex. Curr Opin Neurol 1997;10:168-175.
23. Furukawa T, Ono Y, Tsuchiya H, et al: Specific interaction of the potassium channel beta-subunit minK with the sarcomeric protein T-cap suggests a T-tubule-myofibril linking system. J Mol Biol 2001;313:775-784.
24. Kucera JP, Rohr S, Rudy Y: Localization of sodium channels in intercalated disks modulates cardiac conduction. Circ Res 2002;91:1176-1182.
25. Ribaux P, Bleicher F, Couble ML, et al: Voltage-gated sodium channel (SkM1) content in dystrophin-deficient muscle. Pflugers Arch 2001;441:746-755.
26. Maron BJ, Gardin JM, Flack JM, et al: Prevalence of hypertrophic cardiomyopathy in a general population of young adults: Echocardiographic analysis of 411 subjects in the CARDIA study. Circulation 1995;92:785-789.
27. Zile MR, Brutsaert DL: New concepts in diastolic dysfunction and diastolic heart failure: Part I. Diagnosis, prognosis, and measurements of diastolic function. Circulation 2002;105:1387-1393.
28. Redfield MM, Jacobsen SJ, Burnett JC Jr, et al: Burden of systolic and diastolic ventricular dysfunction in the community: Appreciating the scope of the heart failure epidemic. JAMA 2003;289:194-202.
29. Vulpian A: Contribution à l'étude des rétrécissements de l'orifice ventriculo-aortique. Arch Physiol 1868;3:220-222.
30. Watkins H: Genetic clues to disease pathways in hypertrophic and dilated cardiomyopathies. Circulation 2003;107:1344-1346.
31. Moolman JC, Corfield VA, Posen G, et al: Sudden death due to troponin T mutations. J Am Coll Cardiol 1997;29:549-555.
32. Watkins H, McKenna WJ, Thierfelder L, et al: Mutations in the genes for cardiac troponin T and α-tropomyosin in hypertrophic cardiomyopathy. N Engl J Med 1995;332:1058-1064.
33. Kimura A, Harada H, Park JE, et al: Mutations in the cardiac troponin I gene associated with hypertrophic cardiomyopathy. Nat Genet 1997;16:379-382.
34. Olson TM, Doan TP, Kishimoto NY, et al: Inherited and de novo mutations in the cardiac actin gene cause hypertrophic cardiomyopathy. J Mol Cell Cardiol 2000;32:1687-1694.
35. Poetter K, Jiang H, Hassanzadeh S, et al: Mutations in either the essential or regulatory light chains of myosin are associated with a rare myopathy in human heart and skeletal muscle. Nat Genet 1996;13:63-69.
36. Nagueh SF, Bachinski LL, Meyer D, et al: Tissue Doppler imaging consistently detects myocardial abnormalities in patients with hypertrophic cardiomyopathy and provides a novel means for an early diagnosis before and independently of hypertrophy. Circulation 2001;104:128-130.
37. Nagueh SF, Kopelen HA, Lim DS, et al: Tissue Doppler imaging consistently detects myocardial contraction and relaxation abnormalities, irrespective of cardiac hypertrophy, in a transgenic rabbit model of human hypertrophic cardiomyopathy. Circulation 2000;102:1346-1350.
38. McMahon CJ, Nagueh SF, Pignatelli RH, et al: Characterization of left ventricular diastolic function by tissue Doppler imaging and clinical status in children with hypertrophic cardiomyopathy. Circulation 2004;109:1756-1762.
39. Pignatelli RH, McMahon CJ, Dreyer WJ, et al: Clinical characterization of left ventricular noncompaction in children: A relatively common form of cardiomyopathy. Circulation 2003;108:2672-2678.
40. Gollob MH, Green MS, Tang AS, et al: Identification of a gene responsible for familial Wolff-Parkinson-White syndrome. N Engl J Med 2001;344:1823-1831.
41. Blair E, Redwood C, Ashrafian H, et al: Mutations in the gamma(2) subunit of AMP-activated protein kinase cause familial hypertrophic cardiomyopathy: Evidence for a central role of energy compromise in disease pathogenesis. Hum Mol Genet 2001;10:1215-1220.
42. Rivenes SM, Towbin JA, Gajarski RJ, et al: Sudden death and cardiovascular collapse in children with restrictive cardiomyopathies. Circulation 2000;102:876-882.
43. Denfield SW: Sudden death in children with restrictive cardiomyopathy. Card Electrophysiol Rev 2002;6:163-167.
44. Cetta F, O'Leary PW, Seward JB, Driscoll DJ: Idiopathic restrictive cardiomyopathy in childhood: Diagnostic features and clinical course. Mayo Clin Proc 1995;70:634-640.
45. Lewis AB: Clinical profile and outcome of restrictive cardiomyopathy in children. Am Heart J 1992;123:1589-1593.
46. Arad M, Benson DW, Perez-Atayde AR, et al: Constitutively active AMP kinase mutations cause glycogen storage disease mimicking hypertrophic cardiomyopathy. J Clin Invest 2002;107:357-362.

47. Wang X, Osinska H, Gerdes AM, Robbins J: Desmin filaments and cardiac disease: Establishing causality. J Card Fail 2002; 8(6 Suppl):S287-S292.

48. Niimura H, Bachinski LL, Sangwatanaroj S, et al: Mutations in the gene for cardiac myosin-binding protein C and late-onset familial hypertrophic cardiomyopathy. N Engl J Med 1998;338:1248-1257.

49. Vikstrom KL, Leinwand LA: Contractile protein mutations and heart disease. Curr Opin Cell Biol 1996;8:97-105.

50. Watkins H, Rosenweig A, Hwang DS, et al: Characteristics and prognostic implications of myosin missense mutations in familial hypertrophic cardiomyopathy. N Engl J Med 1992;326:1108-1114.

51. Van Driest SL, Ackerman MJ, Ommen SR, et al: Prevalence and severity of "benign" mutations in the β-myosin heavy chain, cardiac troponin T, and α-tropomyosin genes in hypertrophic cardiomyopathy. Circulation 2002;106:3085-3090.

52. Zile MR, Baicu CF, Gaasch WH: Diastolic heart failure-abnormalities in active relaxation and passive stiffness of the left ventricle. N Engl J Med 2004;350:1953-1959.

53. Jarcho JA, McKenna W, Pare JA, et al: Mapping a gene for familial hypertrophic cardiomyopathy to chromosome 14q1. N Engl J Med 1989;321:1372-1378.

54. Solomon SD, Jarcho JA, McKenna WJ, et al: Familial hypertrophic cardiomyopathy is a genetically heterogeneous disease. J Clin Invest 1990;86:993-999.

55. Watkins H, MacRae C, Thierfelder L, et al: A disease locus for familial hypertrophic cardiomyopathy maps to chromosome 1q3. Nat Genet 1993;3:333-337.

56. Thierfelder L, MacRae C, Watkins H, et al: A familial hypertrophic cardiomyopathy locus maps to chromosome 15q2. Proc Natl Acad Sci U S A 1993;90:6270-6274.

57. Carrier L, Hengstenberg C, Beckmann JS, et al: Mapping of a novel gene for familial hypertrophic cardiomyopathy to chromosome 11. Nat Genet 1993;4:311-313.

58. MacRae CA, Ghaisas N, Kass S, et al: Familial hypertrophic cardiomyopathy with Wolff-Parkinson-White syndrome maps to a locus on chromosome 7q3. J Clin Invest 1995;96:1216-1220.

59. Poetter K, Jiang H, Hassanzadeh S, et al: Mutation in either the essential regulatory light chains of myosin are associated with a rare myopathy in human heart and skeletal muscle. Nat Genet 1996;13:63-69.

60. Kimura A, Harada H, Park JE, et al: Mutations in the cardiac troponin I gene associated with hypertrophic cardiomyopathy. Nat Genet 1997;16:379-382.

61. Mogensen J, Klausen IC, Pederson AK, et al: α-Cardiac actin is a novel disease gene in familial hypertrophic cardiomyopathy. J Clin Invest 1999;103:R39-R43.

62. Satoh M, Takahashi M, Sakamoto T, et al: Structural analysis of the titin gene in hypertrophic cardiomyopathy: Identification of a novel disease gene. Biochem Biophys Res Commun 1999;2625:411-417.

63. Geier C, Perrot A, Ozcelik C, et al: Mutations in the human muscle LIM protein gene in families with hypertrophic cardiomyopathy. Circulation 2003;107:1390-1395.

64. Mohiddin SA, Ahmed ZM, Griffith AJ, et al: Novel association of hypertrophic cardiomyopathy, sensorineural deafness and a mutation in unconventional myosin VI (MYO6). J Med Genet 2004;41:309-314.

65. Hayashi T, Armimura T, Ueda K, et al: Identification and functional and of caveolin-3 mutation associated with familial hypertrophic cardiomyopathy. Biochem Biophys Res Commun 2004;313:178-184.

66. Seidman JG, Seidman C: The genetic basis for cardiomyopathy from mutation identification to mechanistic paradigms. Cell 2001;108:557-567.

67. Towbin JA, Bowles NE: The failing heart. Nature 2002;415:227-233.

68. Schiaffino S, Reggiani C: Molecular diversity of myofibrillar proteins: Gene regulation and functional significance. Physiol Rev 1996;76:371-423.

69. Blair E, Redwood C, de Jesus Oliveira M, et al: Mutations of the light meromyosin domain of the β-myosin heavy chain rod in hypertrophic cardiomyopathy. Circ Res 2002;90:263-269.

70. Hofmann PA, Hartzell HC, Moss RL: Alterations in Ca²⁺ sensitive tension due to partial extraction of C-protein from rat skinned cardiac myocytes and rabbit skeletal muscle fibers. J Gen Physiol 1991;97:1141-1163.

71. Lees-Miller JP, Helfman DM: The molecular basis for tropomyosin isoform diversity. Bioessays 1991;13:429-437.

72. Mesnard L, Logeart D, Taviaux S, et al: Human cardiac troponin T: Cloning and expression of new isoforms in the normal and failing heart. Circ Res 1995;76:687-692.

73. Townsend P, Barton P, Yacoub M, Farza H: Molecular cloning of human cardiac troponin T isoforms: Expression in developing and failing heart. J Mol Cell Cardiol 1995;27:2223-2236.

74. Hunkeler NM, Kullman J, Murphy AM: Troponin I isoform expression in human heart. Circ Res 1991;69:1409-1414.

75. Watkins H, Rosenzweig T, Hwang DS, et al: Characteristics and prognostic implications of myosin missense mutations in familial hypertrophic cardiomyopathy. N Engl J Med 1992;326:1108-1114.

76. Moolman JC, Corfield VA, Posen B, et al: Sudden death due to troponin T mutations. J Am Coll Cardiol 1997;29:549-555.

77. Nakajima-Taniguchi C, Matsui H, Fujio Y, et al: Novel missense mutation in cardiac troponin T gene found in Japanese patient with hypertrophic cardiomyopathy. J Mol Cell Cardiol 1997;29:839-843.

78. Bonne G, Carrier L, Bercovici J, et al: Cardiac myosin binding protein-C gene splice acceptor site mutation is associated with familial hypertrophic cardiomyopathy. Nat Genet 1995;11:438-440.

79. Watkins H, Conner D, Thierfelder L, et al: Mutations in the cardiac myosin binding protein-C gene on chromosome 11 cause familial hypertrophic cardiomyopathy. Nat Genet 1995;11:434-437.

80. Niimura H, Bachinski LL, Sangwatanaroj S, et al: Mutations in the gene for cardiac myosin-binding protein C and late-onset familial hypertrophic cardiomyopathy. N Engl J Med 1998;338:1248-1257.

81. Charron P, Dubourg O, Desnos M, et al: Clinical features and prognostic implications of familial hypertrophic cardiomyopathy related to cardiac myosin-binding protein C gene. Circulation 1998;97:2230-2236.

82. Yoneya K, Okamoto H, Machida M, et al: Angiotensin-converting enzyme gene polymorphism in Japanese patients with hypertrophic cardiomyopathy. Am Heart J 1995;130:1089-1093.

83. Tesson F, Dufour C, Moolman JC, et al: The influence of the angiotensin I converting enzyme genotype in familial hypertrophic cardiomyopathy varies with the disease gene mutation. J Mol Cell Cardiol 1997;29:831-838.

84. Ortlepp JR, Vosberg HP, Reith S, et al: Genetic polymorphisms in the renin-angiotensin-aldosterone system associated with expression of left ventricular hypertrophy in hypertrophic cardiomyopathy: A study of five polymorphic genes in a family with a disease causing mutation in the myosin binding protein C gene. Heart 2002;87:270-275.

85. Doiuchi J, Hamada M, Ito T, Kokubu T: Comparative effects of calcium-channel blockers and beta-adrenergic blocker on early diastolic time intervals and A-wave ratio in patients with hypertrophic cardiomyopathy. Clin Cardiol 1987;10:26-30.

86. Lorell BH: Use of calcium channel blockers in hypertrophic cardiomyopathy. Am J Med 1985;78:43-54.

87. Moran AM, Colan SD: Verapamil therapy in infants with hypertrophic cardiomyopathy. Cardiol Young 1998;8:310-319.

88. Nagueh SF, Ommen SR, Lakkis NM, et al: Comparison of ethanol septal reduction therapy with surgical myectomy for the treatment of hypertrophic obstructive cardiomyopathy. J Am Coll Cardiol 2001;38:1701-1706.

89. Maron BJ, Dearani JA, Ommen SR, et al: The case for surgery in obstructive hypertrophic cardiomyopathy. J Am Coll Cardiol 2004;44:2043-2053.

90. O'Rourke RA: Cardiac pacing: An alternative treatment for selected patients with hypertrophic cardiomyopathy and adjunctive therapy for certain patients with dilated cardiomyopathy. Circulation 1999;100:786-788.

91. Maron BJ: Appraisal of dual-chamber pacing therapy in hypertrophic cardiomyopathy: Too soon for a rush to judgment? J Am Coll Cardiol 1996;27:431-432.

92. Begley D, Mohiddin S, Fananapazir L: Dual chamber pacemaker therapy for mid-cavity obstructive hypertrophic cardiomyopathy. Pacing Clin Electrophysiol 2001;24:1639-1644.

93. Chang SM, Lakkis NM, Franklin J, et al: Predictors of outcome after alcohol septal ablation therapy in patients with hypertrophic obstructive cardiomyopathy. Circulation 2004;109:824-827.

94. Nielsen CD, Killip D, Spencer WH 3rd: Nonsurgical septal reduction therapy for hypertrophic obstructive cardiomyopathy: Short-term results in 50 consecutive procedures. Clin Cardiol 2003;26:275-279.

95. Park TH, Lakkis NM, Middleton KJ, et al: Acute effect of nonsurgical septal reduction therapy on regional left ventricular asynchrony in patients with hypertrophic obstructive cardiomyopathy. Circulation 2002;106:412-415.

96. Hess OM, Sigwart U: New treatment strategies for hypertrophic obstructive cardiomyopathy. J Am Coll Cardiol 2004;44:2054-2055.

97. Cable WJ, Kolodny EH, Adams RD: Fabry disease: Impaired autonomic function. Neurology 1982;32:498-502.

98. Sugie K, Yamamoto A, Murayama K, et al: Clinicopathological features of genetically confirmed Danon disease. Neurology 2002;58:1773-1778.

99. Hers HG, van Hoof F, de Barsy T: Glycogen storage diseases. In Scriver CR, Beaudet AL, Sly WS, Valle D (eds): The Metabolic Basis of Inherited Disease, 6th ed. New York, McGraw-Hill, 1989, pp 425-452.

100. Towbin JA:. Molecular genetic aspects of cardiomyopathy. Biochem Med Metab Biol 1993;49:283-320.

101. D'Ancona GG, Wurm J, Croce CM: Genetics of type II glycogenosis: Assignment of the human gene for acid α-glucosidase to chromosome 17. Proc Natl Acad Sci U S A 1979;76:4526-4529.

102. Beratis NG, LaBadie GU, Hirschhorn K: Genetic heterogeneity in acid α-glucosidase deficiency. Am J Hum Genet 1983;35:21-33.

103. Zhong N, Martiniuk F, Tzall S, Hirschhorn R: Identification of a missense mutation in one allele of a patient with Pompe disease and use of endonuclease digestion of PCR-amplified RNA to demonstrate lack of mRNA expression from the second allele. Am J Hum Genet 1991;49:635-645.

104. Raben N, Danon M, Gilbert AL, et al: Enzyme replacement therapy in the mouse model of Pompe disease. Mol Genet Metab 2003;80:159-169.

105. Masson C, Cisse I, Simon V, et al: Fabry disease: A review. Joint Bone Spine 2004;71:381-383.

106. Colucci WS, Lorell BH, Schoen FJ, et al: Hypertrophic obstructive cardiomyopathy due to Fabry's disease. N Engl J Med 1982;307:926-928.

107. Becker AE, Schoorl R, Balk AG, van der Heide RM: Cardiac manifestations of Fabry's disease: Report of a case with mitral insufficiency and electrocardiographic evidence of myocardial infarction. Am J Cardiol 1975;36:829-835.

108. Goldman ME, Cantor R, Schwartz MF, et al: Echocardiographic abnormalities and disease severity in Fabry's disease. J Am Coll Cardiol 1986;7:1157-1161.

109. Broadbent JC, Edwards WD, Gordon H, et al: Fabry cardiomyopathy in the female confirmed by endomyocardial biopsy. Mayo Clin Proc 1981;56:623-628.

110. Bishop DF, Calhoun DH, Bernstein HS, et al: Human alpha galactosidase A: Nucleotide sequence of a cDNA clone encoding the mature enzyme. Proc Natl Acad Sci U S A 1986;83:4859-4863.

111. Eng CM, Desnick RJ: Molecular basis of Fabry disease: Mutations and polymorphisms in the human α-galactosidase A gene. Hum Mutat 1994;3:103-111.

112. Okumiya T, Ishii S, Kase R, et al: α-Galactosidase gene mutations in Fabry disease: Heterogeneous expressions of mutant enzyme proteins. Hum Genet 1995;95:557-561.

113. Nakao S, Takenaka T, Maeda M, et al: An atypical variant of Fabry's disease in men with left ventricular hypertrophy. N Engl J Med 1995;333:288-293.

114. Linhart A, Palecek T, Bultas J, et al: New insights in cardiac structural changes in patients with Fabry's disease. Am Heart J 2000;139:1101-1108.

115. Sachdev B, Takenaka T, Teraguchih H, et al: Prevalence of Anderson-Fabry disease in male patients with late onset hypertrophic cardiomyopathy. Circulation 2002;105:1407-1411.

116. Danon MJ, Oh SJ, DiMauro S, et al: Lysosomal glycogen storage disease with normal acid maltase. Neurology 1981;31:51-57.

117. Nishino I, Fu J, Tanji K, et al: Primary LAMP-2 deficiency causes X-linked vascular cardiomyopathy and myopathy (Danon disease). Nature 2000;406:906-909.

118. Charron P, Villard E, Sebillon P, et al: Danon's disease as a cause of hypertrophic cardiomyopathy: A systematic survey. Heart 2004;90:842-846.

119. Cheung PC, Salt IP, Davies SP, et al: Characterization of AMP-activated protein kinase gamma-subunit isoforms and their role in AMP binding. Biochem J 2000;346:659-669.

120. Kemp BE, Mitchelhill KI, Stapleton D, et al: Dealing with energy demand: The AMP-activated protein kinase. Trends Biochem Sci 1999;24:22-25.

121. Arad M, Moskowitz IP, Patel VV, et al: Transgenic mice overexpressing mutant PRKAG2 define the cause of Wolff Parkinson-White syndrome in glycogen storage cardiomyopathy. Circulation 2003;107:2850-2856.

122. Attardi G: The elucidation of the human mitochondrial genome: A historical perspective. Bioessays 1996;5:34-39.

123. Wallace DC, Zheng X, Lott MT, et al: Familial mitochondrial encephalomyopathy (MERRF): Genetic, pathophysiological, and biochemical characterization of a mitochondrial DNA disease. Cell 1988;55:601-610.

124. Wallace DC: Mitochondrial DNA mutation and neuromuscular disease. Trends Genet 1989;5:9-13.

125. Clarke A: Mitochondrial genome: Defects, disease, and evolution. J Med Genet 1990;27:451-456.

126. Grivell LA: Small, beautiful and essential. Nature 1989;341:569-571.

127. Anderson S, Banker AT, Barrell BG: Sequence and organization of the human mitochondrial genome. Nature 1981;290:457-465.

128. Petty RKH, Harding AE, Morgan-Hughes JA: The clinical features of mitochondrial myopathy. Brain 1986;109:915-938.

129. Mariotti C, Tiranti V, Carrara F, et al: Defective respiratory capacity and mitochondrial protein synthesis in transformant cybrids harboring the tRNALeu(UUR) mutation associated with maternally inherited myopathy and cardiomyopathy. J Clin Invest 1994;93:1102-1107.

130. Vogel H: Mitochondrial myopathies and the role of the pathologist in the molecular era. J Neuropathol Exp Neurol 2001;60:217-227.

131. Capaldi RA, Halphen DG, Zhang YZ, Yanamura W: Complexity and tissue specificity of the mitochondrial respiratory chain. J Bioenerg Biomembr 1988;20:291-311.

132. Ozawa T, Tanaka M, Sugiyama S, et al: Multiple mitochondrial DNA deletions exist in cardiomyocytes of patients with hypertrophic or dilated cardiomyopathy. Biochem Biophys Res Commun 1990;170:830-836.

133. De Vivo DC, DiMauro S: Disorders of pyruvate metabolism, the citric acid cycle, and the respiratory chain. In Saudubray JM, Tada K, Fernandes J (eds): Inborn Metabolic Diseases. Berlin, Springer-Verlag, 1991, pp 125-167.

134. Kobayashi M, Morishita H, Sugiyama N, et al: Two cases of NADH-coenzyme Q reductase deficiency: Relationship to MELAS syndrome. J Pediatr 1987;110:223-227.

135. Tanaka M, Ino H, Ohno K, et al: Mitochondrial mutation in fatal infantile cardiomyopathy. Lancet 1990;336:1452.

136. Moraes CT, Ricci E, Bonilla E, DiMauro S: The mitochondrial tRNAleu(UUR) mutation in mitochondrial encephalopathy, lactic acidosis, and stroke-like episodes (MELAS): Genetic, biochemical, and morphological correlations in skeletal muscle. Am J Hum Genet 1992;50:934-949.

137. Papadimitriou A, Neustein HB, DiMauro S, et al: Histiocytoid cardiomyopathy of infancy: Deficiency of reducible cytochrome b in heart mitochondria. Pediatr Res 1984;18:1023-1028.

138. Scaglia F, Towbin JA, Craigen WJ, et al: Clinical spectrum, morbidity, and mortality in 113 pediatric patients with mitochondrial disease. Pediatrics 2004;114:925-931.

139. DiMauro S, Nicholson JF, Hays AP, et al: Benign infantile mitochondrial myopathy due to reversible cytochrome C oxidase deficiency. Ann Neurol 1983;14:226-234.

140. Channer KD, Channer JL, Campbell MJ, Rees JR: Cardiomyopathy in Kearns-Sayre syndrome. Br Heart J 1988;59:486-490.

141. Poulton J, Deadman ME, Ramacharan S, Gardiner RM: Germline deletions of mtDNA in mitochondrial myopathy. Am J Hum Genet 1991;48:649-653.

142. Moraes CT, DiMauro S, Zeviani M, et al: Mitochondrial DNA deletions in progressive external ophthalmoplegia and Kearns-Sayre syndrome. N Engl J Med 1989;320:1293-1299.

143. Moraes CT, Schon EA, DiMauro S, Miranda AF: Heteroplasmy of mitochondrial genomes in clonal cultures from patients with Kearns-Sayre syndrome. Biochem Biopsy Res Commun 1989;160:765-771.

144. Suomalainen A, Kollmann P, Octave J-N, et al: Quantification of mitochondrial DNA carrying tRNA8344Lys point mutation in myoclonus epilepsy and ragged-red fiber disease. Eur J Hum Genet 1993;1:88-95.

145. Tanno Y, Yoneda M, Nonaka I, et al: Quantitation of mitochondrial DNA carrying tRANLys mutation in MERRF patients. Biochem Biophys Res Commun 1991;179:880-885.

146. Shoffner JM, Lott MI, Lezza AM, et al: Myoclonic epilepsy and ragged-red fiber disease (MERRF) is associated with a mitochondrial DNA tRNA(Lys) mutation. Cell 1990;61:931-937.

147. Nakamura M, Nakano S, Goto Y, et al: A novel point mutation in the mitochondrial tRNASer(UCN) gene detected in a family with MERFF/MELAS overlap syndrome. Biochem Biophys Res Commun 1995;214:86-93.

148. Silvestri G, Moraes CT, Shanske S, et al: A new mtDNA mutation in the tRNA(Lys) gene associated with myoclonic epilepsy and ragged-red fibers (MERRF). Am J Hum Genet 1992;51:1213-1217.

149. Fukuhara N: Clinicopathologic features of MERRF. Muscle Nerve 1995;3:590-594.

150. Hatefi Y: The mitochondrial electron transport and oxidative phosphorylation system. Ann Rev Biochem 1985;54:1015-1069.

151. Corral-Debrinski M, Stepien G, Shoffner JM, et al: Hypoxemia is associated with mitochondrial DNA damage and gene induction: Implications for cardiac disease. JAMA 1991;266:1812-1816.

152. Dhalla NS, Afzal N, Beamish RE, et al: Pathophysiology of cardiac dysfunction in congestive heart failure. Can J Cardiol 1993;9:873-887.

153. Sabbah HN, Sharov V, Riddle JM, et al: Mitochondrial abnormalities in myocardium of dogs with chronic heart failure. J Mol Cell Cardiol 1992;24:1333-1347.

154. Rustin P, Lebidois J, Chretien D, et al: Endomyocardial biopsies for early detection of mitochondrial disorders in hypertrophic cardiomyopathies. J Pediatr 1994;124:224-228.

155. Tam JW, Shaikh N, Sutherland E: Echocardiographic assessment of patients with hypertrophic and restrictive cardiomyopathy: Imaging and echocardiography. Curr Opin Cardiol 2002;17:470-477.

156. Gewillig M, Mertens L, Moerman P, Dumoulin M: Idiopathic restrictive cardiomyopathy in childhood: A diastolic disorder characterized by delayed relaxation. Eur Heart J 1996;17:1413-1420.

157. Chen SC, Balfour IC, Jureidini S: Clinical spectrum of restrictive cardiomyopathy in children. J Heart Lung Transplant 2001;20:90-92.

158. Mogensen J, Kubo T, Duque M, et al: Idiopathic restrictive cardiomyopathy is part of the clinical expression of cardiac troponin I mutations. J Clin Invest 2003;111:209-216.

159. Perles Z, Bowles NE, Vatta M, et al: Familial restrictive cardiomyopathy caused by a missense mutation in the desmin gene: Possible role of apoptosis in disease pathogenesis. J Am Coll Cardiol 2002;39:45A.

160. Fitzpatrick AP, Shapiro LM, Rickards AF, Poole-Wilson PA: Familial restrictive cardiomyopathy with atrioventricular block and skeletal myopathy. Br Heart J 1990;63:114-118.

161. Wang X, Osinska H, Dorn GW 2nd, et al: Mouse model of desmin-related cardiomyopathy. Circulation 2001;103:2402-2407.

162. Mavroidis M, Capetanaki Y: Extensive induction of important mediators of fibrosis and dystrophic calcification in desmin-deficient cardiomyopathy. Am J Pathol 2002;160:943-952.

163. Jacobson DR, Pan T, Kyle RA, Buxbaum JN: Transthyretin ILE20: A new variant associated with late-onset cardiac amyloidosis. Hum Mutat 1997;9:83-85.

164. Hattori T, Takei Y, Koyama J, et al: Clinical and pathological studies of cardiac amyloidosis in transthyretin type familial amyloid polyneuropathy. Amyloid 2003;10:229-239.

165. Chin TK, Perloff JK, Williams RG, et al: Isolated noncompaction of left ventricular myocardium: A study of eight cases. Circulation 1990;82:507-513.

166. Stollberger C, Finsterer J, Blazek G: Left ventricular hypertrabeculation/ noncompaction and association with additional cardiac abnormalities and neuromuscular disorders. Am J Cardiol 2002;90:899-902.

167. Stollberger C, Finsterer J: Left ventricular hypertrabeculation/ noncompaction. J Am Soc Echocardiogr 2004;17:91-100.

168. Ichida F, Hamamichi Y, Miyawaki T, et al: Clinical features of isolated noncompaction of the ventricular myocardium: Long-term clinical course, hemodynamic properties and genetic background. J Am Coll Cardiol 1999;34:233-240.

169. Ichida F, Tsubata S, Bowles KR, et al: Novel gene mutations in patients with left ventricular noncompaction or Barth syndrome. Circulation 2001;103:1256-1263.

170. Vatta M, Mohapatra B, Jimenez S, et al: Mutations in Cypher/ZASP in patients with dilated cardiomyopathy and left ventricular noncompaction. J Am Coll Cardiol 2003;42:2014-2027.

171. Towbin JA: Cardiac arrhythmias: The genetic connection. J Cardiovasc Electrophysiol 2000;11:601-602.

172. Ackerman MJ: Cardiac channelopathies: It's in the genes. Nat Med 2004;10:463-464.

173. Towbin JA: Familial dilated cardiomyopathy. In Berul CI, Towbin JA (eds): The Molecular and Clinical Genetics of Cardiac Electrophysiological Disease. Kluwer Academic Publishers, Boston, 2000, pp 195-218.

174. Towbin JA: The role of cytoskeletal proteins in cardiomyopathies. Curr Opin Cell Biol 1998;10:131-139.

175. Bowles NE, Bowles KR, Towbin JA: The "final common pathway" hypothesis and inherited cardiovascular disease: The role of cytoskeletal proteins in dilated cardiomyopathy. Herz 2000;25:168-175.

176. Tiso N, Stephan DA, Nava A, et al: Identification of mutations in the cardiac ryanodine receptor gene in families affected with arrhythmogenic right ventricular cardiomyopathy type 2 (ARVD2). Hum Mol Genet 2001;10:189-194.

177. Rampazzo A, Nava A, Malacrida S, et al: Mutation in human desmoplakin domain binding to plakoglobin causes a dominant form of arrhythmogenic right ventricular cardiomyopathy. Am J Hum Genet 2002;71:1200-1206.

178. Gerull B, Heuser A, Wichter T, et al: Mutations in the desmosomal protein plakophilin-2 are common arrhythmogenic right ventricular cardiomyopathy. Nat Genet 2004;36:1162-1164.

179. Yetman AT, McCrindle BW: Management of pediatric hypertrophic cardiomyopathy. Curr Opin Cardiol 2005;20:80-83.

180. Arad M, Maron BJ, Gorham JM, et al: Glycogen storage diseases presenting as hypertrophic cardiomyopathy. N Engl J Med 2005;352:362-372.

CHAPTER 21

Valvular Insufficiency and Heart Failure

Beatriz Bouzas-Zubeldia
Michael A. Gatzoulis

Valvular heart disease is a mechanical problem in which stenotic or regurgitant lesions impose on the heart pressure overload, volume overload, or both. In many patients, valvular heart disease is associated with more complex cardiac anomalies, which has management and prognostic implications. Valvular insufficiency of any of the four cardiac valves in and of itself can be a cause of heart failure in children.

In valvular regurgitation, the heart has to cope with an increased volume of blood. The pathophysiologic sequence for valvular insufficiency is similar for the right and the left heart: increase in end-diastolic volume (EDV) first, followed by an increase in end-systolic volume, and finally a decrease in shortening and ejection fractions (Fig. 21-1). Different compensatory mechanisms and pathophysiologic adaptations develop to maintain the stroke volume for each type of valvular insufficiency, but heart failure eventually ensues. When symptoms of heart failure develop, irreversible ventricular dysfunction sometimes is established, and outcome after surgery ultimately may be compromised. Discerning the optimal time for intervention, before irreversible ventricular dysfunction develops, is a key point in the management of regurgitant valvular heart disease and is discussed in this chapter.

PULMONARY INSUFFICIENCY

Anatomic Considerations

Pulmonary regurgitation usually is not found as an isolated congenital lesion, although a small degree of pulmonary regurgitation can be a common echocardiographic finding in otherwise structurally normal hearts. Instead, most cases of pulmonary regurgitation are an undesirable result of surgical or catheter interventional procedures to relieve right ventricular outflow tract (RVOT) obstruction; the most common situations are after tetralogy of Fallot repair and surgical or balloon valvuloplasty of a stenotic pulmonary valve.

The **absent pulmonary valve syndrome** is a rare manifestation that comprises a wide range of congenital anomalies of the pulmonary valve that may lead to pulmonary regurgitation. There can be faulty development of one, two, or all three cusps of the valve; presence of dysplastic nodules, which are remnants of the valve cusps; or complete absence of the valve cusps.

The syndrome usually is associated with tetralogy of Fallot or ventricular septal defect, although it can also be found in isolation.[1]

Most patients with successful **tetralogy of Fallot** repair have an excellent prognosis.[2,3] Use of a transannular patch—more liberally practiced in an earlier era—to relieve the RVOT obstruction has been shown, however, to correlate with the development of residual pulmonary regurgitation in many patients. Transannular patch repair, RVOT reconstruction, and aggressive infundibulectomy also may lead to the formation of aneurysmal or akinetic regions in the RVOT. The presence of these aneurysmal and akinetic regions combined with chronic pulmonary regurgitation may contribute further to the development of right ventricular dysfunction.[4] As a result, routine and generous transannular patching has been abandoned, and limited transannular patching and preservation of the pulmonary valve function have become the current surgical goals, while adequately relieving RVOT obstruction.

Balloon valvuloplasty is the treatment of choice for patients with moderate or severe **pulmonary stenosis** except for patients with dysplastic valves or patients with primarily subvalvar or supravalvar pulmonary stenosis. For these patients, surgical relief of the obstruction is often required. Some degree of valvular incompetence of the pulmonary valve occurs in more than 70% of patients[5-9] after both procedures, although it seems to be less frequent after balloon valvuloplasty.[10] In the Second Natural History Study of Congenital Heart Defects, 87% of the operated patients had pulmonary regurgitation on echocardiography, which was more than moderate in 28% of the population.[7] Some discrepancies exist between the echocardiographic and the clinical findings; when clinical criteria are applied, 56% of the patients had clinical evidence of pulmonary regurgitation, but only 8% of the patients were classified as having severe regurgitation.[7]

Basic Pathophysiology

The adaptive response of the right ventricle to volume overload resulting from pulmonary regurgitation depends on the degree and duration of the regurgitant flow (Table 21-1).[11] More than moderate chronic pulmonary regurgitation produces right ventricular volume overload, with increased EDV followed in time by an increase of end-systolic ventricular volume and progressive

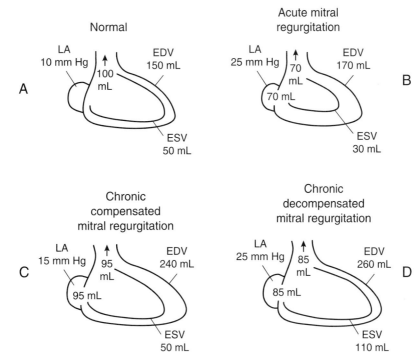

FIGURE 21-1 ■ **Pathophysiology of valvular insufficiency.** Stages of progressive valvular insufficiency and volume load on the ventricle are depicted. The pathophysiology illustrated is mitral regurgitation, but the sequential ventricular dimension changes leading to failure are similar with aortic insufficiency and with right-sided valvular insufficiency for the right ventricle. **A,** Normal. **B,** Acute mitral regurgitation leads to an increase in end-diastolic volume (EDV) with reductions in afterload and end-systolic volume (ESV). Although the ejection fraction is increased, the forward stroke volume is decreased because of regurgitant volume. The left atrial (LA) pressure is acutely elevated. **C,** Chronic compensated mitral regurgitation leads to eccentric hypertrophy and a further increase in EDV. This increased EDV results in increased afterload and increased ESV. The total and the forward stroke volumes are increased. The LA pressure decreases. The ejection fraction is above normal. Chronic decompensated mitral regurgitation (seen in **D**) leads to ventricular failure and an increase in ESV. Forward stroke volume is decreased, and the ejection fraction becomes normal or lower. The overall progression is an increase in EDV, followed by an increase in ESV, and finally a decrease in ejection fraction. (From Carabello BA, Crawford FA: Valvular heart disease. N Engl J Med 1997;337:36.)

TABLE 21-1

Pathophysiology of Chronic Pulmonary Regurgitation	
Substrates	Isolated congenital pulmonary regurgitation
	Absent pulmonary valve syndrome
	Postvalvotomy for pulmonary stenosis
	Postrepair of tetralogy of Fallot
Covariables	Peripheral pulmonary artery stenosis (−)
	Pulmonary hypertension (−)
	RVOT aneurysm/akinesia (−)
	RV restrictive diastolic physiology (+ in older patients)
Disease Progression	RV dilation (long compensatory phase)
	QRS prolongation (increased risk of VT/sudden cardiac death)
	Onset of tricuspid regurgitation
	RV systolic dysfunction
	Overt symptoms

(+) indicates positive influence on pulmonary regurgitation; (−) indicates negative influence on pulmonary regurgitation.

RV, right ventricular; RVOT, right ventricular outflow tract; VT, ventricular tachycardia.

deterioration of myocardial systolic function. Immediate postoperative pulmonary regurgitation is well tolerated after pulmonary repair of tetralogy of Fallot in infancy. In contrast, postoperative pulmonary regurgitation is poorly tolerated in an older child after late repair. This difference may relate to poor adaptation of a hypertrophied and poorly compliant right ventricle, further compromised with acute volume overload in the case of significant postoperative pulmonary regurgitation. Adult patients usually require pulmonary valve implantation at the time of repair.

Marked dilation of the right ventricle can lead to the development of secondary tricuspid regurgitation, which contributes to further dilation of the right ventricle and right atrium. The stretch and dilation of the right ventricle slows interventricular conduction and creates a mechanoelectrical substrate for reentry circuits, which may lead to sustained ventricular tachycardia. There is a correlation between QRS prolongation and right ventricular dilation. A QRS duration of 180 msec or more is shown to be a highly sensitive predictor of life-threatening ventricular arrhythmias in patients with previous repair of tetralogy.[12] Although a QRS lengthening seen soon after repair reflects a surgical injury to the myocardium or the right bundle branch, a late progressive QRS prolongation relates to right ventricular dilation, usually secondary to pulmonary regurgitation. Progressive QRS prolongation may have a greater prognostic effect than the absolute QRS values for sustained ventricular tachycardia and sudden cardiac death.

Different conditions leading to high pulmonary arterial pressure (e.g., distal pulmonary artery stenosis, pulmonary vascular disease, acquired bronchopulmonary disease, or left ventricular dysfunction) increase the degree of pulmonary regurgitation. In patients with repaired tetralogy of Fallot, the presence of residual distal pulmonary artery stenosis or residual shunts accelerates the development of right ventricular dilation.[13]

Many patients with repaired tetralogy of Fallot have restrictive right ventricular diastolic dysfunction, with decreased compliance of the right ventricle. Right ventricular diastolic physiology is defined with Doppler as antegrade laminar diastolic flow in the pulmonary artery during atrial systole, present throughout the respiratory cycle. In these patients, a stiff right ventricle is acting as a conduit between the right atrium and the pulmonary artery at the end of the diastole, and the antegrade late diastolic pulmonary flow contributes to cardiac output by shortening the duration of pulmonary regurgitation. Patients have a smaller right ventricle and better exercise tolerance.[14]

Clinical Presentation

Pulmonary regurgitation is usually well tolerated for many years. Patients remain symptom free until further right ventricular dilation and systolic dysfunction develop. Some patients with right ventricular dysfunction can be asymptomatic, although some degree of objective exercise intolerance can be found on exercise testing.[15] When patients become symptomatic, right ventricular dysfunction is usually well established and may be irreversible.

In patients with **isolated congenital pulmonary regurgitation** and otherwise normal hearts, symptoms are rare before the age of 30 years. After 40 years of age, patients develop right ventricular dysfunction and symptoms of right heart failure (Fig. 21-2).[16] Symptoms in patients with **repaired tetralogy of Fallot** appear at a younger age. This earlier occurrence of symptoms may relate to the associated lesions, early cyanosis, and the effect of surgery. Clinical manifestations include exercise intolerance, congestive heart failure,[15] atrial and ventricular arrhythmias,[17] and sudden cardiac death.

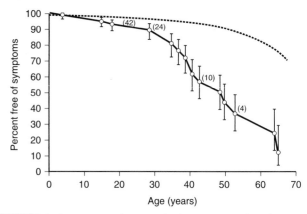

FIGURE 21-2 ■ Actuarial survival of patients with pulmonary insufficiency. Actuarial freedom from symptoms in patients with isolated congenital pulmonary valve regurgitation ($n = 72$, 17 events). The vertical bars enclose the 70% confidence limits (1 SD). The numbers in parentheses indicate the number of patients traced beyond the indicated age. The dashed line at the top is the actuarial survival of the U.S. general population starting at birth. (From Shimazaki Y, Blackstone EH, Kirklin JW: The natural history of isolated congenital pulmonary valve incompetence: Surgical implications. Thorac Cardiovasc Surg 1984;32:257.)

Clinical Assessment

Elevated jugular venous pressure, liver enlargement, and peripheral edema all can be present when there is right ventricular dysfunction with clinical heart failure. This presentation is uncommon, however. Most patients have a right ventricular heave, reflecting right ventricular dilation, best felt in the left sternal border. A dilated pulmonary trunk can be palpated as a systolic expansion in the second left intercostal space.

Auscultation reveals a normal S_1. S_2 can be single if there is no pulmonary component reflecting absent, defective, or stenotic pulmonary valve. If the pulmonary component is present, there is usually a wide splitting of S_2 because of delayed closure of the pulmonary valve. Splitting characteristically increases with inspiration. Congenital pulmonary valve regurgitation has a typical murmur, reflecting a low-pressure, low-velocity regurgitant flow.[18] It is a diamond-shaped, low- to medium-frequency diastolic murmur, best heard with the bell of the stethoscope at the second and third left intercostal spaces. The onset of the murmur is delayed after S_2, and its length is related to the degree of the pulmonary regurgitation. A relatively short diastolic murmur reflects the presence of severe regurgitation.[19] There is often an ejection systolic heart murmur reflecting augmented right ventricular stroke volume.

Clinical Evaluation

The ECG can be normal when the pulmonary regurgitation is mild to moderate. Most patients are in sinus rhythm, although atrial arrhythmias can be present. In patients with isolated pulmonary regurgitation, QRS prolongation, with rSR′ morphology in the right precordial leads, reflects volume overload of the right ventricle. Right bundle branch block is common, particularly in older patients with tetralogy of Fallot who underwent ventriculotomy, and it can make evaluation of right ventricular hypertrophy difficult. The duration of the QRS increases with time, reflecting right ventricular enlargement and potentially dysfunction. As discussed before, QRS duration and QRS change have prognostic implications for malignant arrhythmia and sudden cardiac death.

Patients with severe pulmonary regurgitation characteristically have on **chest radiographs** dilation of their pulmonary trunk, which can reach aneurysmal dimensions in patients with absent pulmonary valve syndrome. There is also right ventricular enlargement, usually proportional to the degree of pulmonary regurgitation.

Echocardiography permits the evaluation of pulmonary valve and RVOT morphology and the presence and degree of pulmonary regurgitation. When evaluated by Doppler, regurgitation of more than 53%[20] and the presence of a retrograde color flow from the distal pulmonary artery or its branches usually indicate severe regurgitation. A shorter duration of pulmonary regurgitant flow, expressed as a percentage of the total diastolic time on continuous-wave Doppler, and a pulmonary regurgitant jet diameter greater than 0.98 mm on color Doppler indicate independently severe pulmonary regurgitation (Fig. 21-3).[19] The size and function of the right ventricle also should be evaluated. Right ventricular systolic function in the presence of severe pulmonary regurgitation is often normal, but deteriorates with time after prolonged exposure to volume overload. Interventricular septal motion is usually abnormal during diastole, reflecting again volume overload. Adult patients with repaired tetralogy of Fallot may have restrictive right ventricular physiology, and this phenomenon can be detected easily with pulse-wave Doppler as a forward diastolic pulmonary flow coincident with atrial systole (see section on pathophysiology) and has prognostic implications.

Exercise testing is a useful adjunct for the evaluation of severity of pulmonary regurgitation and degree of right ventricular dysfunction. The test objectively documents the functional capacity of the patient and may reflect overall cardiac output. Changes in exercise capacity documented with serial testing may precede the onset of symptoms and could be used for defining the optimal timing for pulmonary valve surgery.

MRI has become the gold standard for the evaluation of biventricular mass, volume, and function; the evaluation of RVOT aneurysmal or akinetic regions; the quantification of pulmonary regurgitant fraction; and the identification of residual stenosis in the main pulmonary artery, the pulmonary branches, or right ventricle-to-pulmonary artery conduits.[4,21,22] **Cardiac catheterization** is reserved for patients whose hemodynamic assessment cannot be obtained accurately with

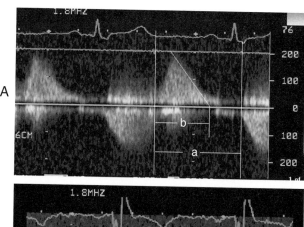

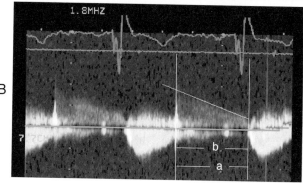

FIGURE 21-3 ■ Severity of pulmonary regurgitation assessed by continuous-wave Doppler. Continuous-wave Doppler echocardiographic recordings of pulmonary flow from patients with severe **(A)** and mild **(B)** pulmonary regurgitation. The duration of regurgitant flow *(b)* with respect to total diastole *(a)* is shorter in the patient with severe pulmonary regurgitation **(A)**. (From Li W, Davlouros PA, Kilner PJ, et al: Doppler-echocardiographic assessment of pulmonary regurgitation in adults with repaired tetralogy of Fallot: Comparison with cardiovascular magnetic resonance imaging. Am Heart J 2004;147: 165-172.)

noninvasive imaging (e.g., patients with a pacemaker) or for patients undergoing transcatheter interventions as a prelude to surgery if necessary.

Therapeutic Strategies

Diuretics are useful when patients develop symptoms of right-sided heart failure. There is evidence that patients with tetralogy of Fallot have neurohormonal activation and impaired cardiac autonomic nervous activity.[23,24] In this setting, administration of drugs that block neurohormonal activation, such as angiotensin-converting enzyme (ACE) inhibitors and β-blockers, and nonsurgical interventions, such as physical conditioning (known to affect the autonomic nervous system), may have prognostic and symptomatic benefits and delay the need for further surgery. Potential benefits of these therapies should be discerned with controlled trials, however.

Pulmonary valve replacement for pulmonary regurgitation is required in 14.7% of patients after tetralogy of Fallot repair.[25] Pulmonary valve replacement is a low-risk intervention with a perioperative mortality of 1.1% to 4%[26] and a good midterm survival (10-year survival of 86% to 95%).[26-28] Patients are likely to require further surgery because prostheses have a limited life span. Optimal timing of pulmonary valve implantation is important for preserving right ventricular function (not too late) and avoiding the need for early subsequent pulmonary valve implantation (not too early). Perioperative risk is higher in patients with established ventricular dysfunction by the time of pulmonary valve implantation.[28] Although such patients may still benefit from pulmonary valve implantation, they require optimal perioperative care. The rates of freedom from valve replacement are 81% at 5 years, 58% at 10 years, and 41% at 15 years.[29] Life span of pulmonary valve prostheses is longer in adult patients. Pulmonary valve replacement is best performed with bioprosthetic valves (homograft or porcine), with a lower rate of overall complications compared with mechanical prostheses, which are not employed for pulmonary valve replacement.[30,31]

Pulmonary valve implantation should be considered for patients with moderate-to-severe pulmonary regurgitation with symptoms and patients with clinical arrhythmia or progressive right ventricular dilation with early right ventricular dysfunction or new-onset tricuspid regurgitation or both. Symptomatic patients with moderate-to-severe pulmonary regurgitation with normal or mildly impaired right ventricular function improve clinically. In addition, these patients benefit in terms of ventricular function and propensity to arrhythmias.[28] Asymptomatic patients with right ventricular dilation also may benefit from pulmonary valve replacement by reducing ventricular volumes and preventing right ventricular dysfunction.[32] This approach needs further assessment, however.

Results are contradictory regarding the recovery of right ventricular function after pulmonary valve replacement. When replacement is performed in a timely manner, there is usually a reduction of the size of the right ventricle and an improvement in systolic function, when evaluated echocardiographically.[28,33,34] In contrast, pulmonary valve implantation, when performed late, may fail to lead to improved right ventricular dimensions and systolic function measured with radionuclide angiography.[35] In another study with a larger number of patients in whom ventricular dimensions were evaluated with echocardiography, an improvement in functional status and decreases in right ventricular dimensions after pulmonary valve implantation were reported.[28] Differences between imaging modalities may account in part for this discrepancy. In a more recent study, in which right ventricular function and degree of pulmonary regurgitation were evaluated with MRI, right ventricular volumes improved after pulmonary valve implantation.[32] It can be argued that to preserve right ventricular function, pulmonary valve replacement in adults should be considered before right ventricular dysfunction ensues.

After valve replacement, symptomatic patients experience subjective and objective improvements of exercise tolerance and overall clinical status relating to recovery of right ventricular function.[32-35] After pulmonary valve replacement, the progression of the QRS duration is stabilized, and this can be interpreted as a reduced risk of sustained ventricular tachycardia and sudden cardiac death. When pulmonary valve replacement was combined with intraoperative cryoablation, the incidence of atrial and ventricular arrhythmia also was reduced.[28]

Percutaneous implantation of a bovine valve mounted in a stent in the pulmonary position has been developed, albeit with relatively large-sized sheaths.[36] So far, it has been shown to be useful in relieving the obstruction in conduits without major complications and restoring competence of the RVOT. Follow-up is short, however, and patients with marked dilation of the RVOT may not be suitable for this approach. The issue of RVOT aneurysm or akinesia, which relates to sustained ventricular tachycardia, cannot be addressed solely with a transcatheter approach. Nevertheless, this is an important therapeutic advance, which may be applicable to other valve prostheses as well.

AORTIC INSUFFICIENCY

Anatomic Considerations

Aortic regurgitation can be a consequence of congenital malformations or acquired conditions involving the aortic valve, the aortic root, or the left ventricular outflow tract. It also is a common consequence of therapeutic procedures directed to relieve aortic valve stenosis and aortic valve replacement.

Bicuspid aortic valve is one of the most frequent congenital heart malformations. This anomaly may produce aortic stenosis, aortic regurgitation, or both.[37] Aortic regurgitation is mild in most cases, but can be severe in 12% of patients. Bicuspid aortic valve commonly is associated with aortic root dilation. Although severe aortic regurgitation can produce dilation of the aortic root secondary to an augmented stroke volume, aortic root dimensions in patients with bicuspid aortic valve are usually larger than expected for the degree of regurgitation. This situation suggests that an intrinsic abnormality of the aortic root wall may contribute at least in part to aortic dilation.[37] Aortic coarctation commonly is found in association with bicuspid aortic valve. In this situation, obstruction to distal aortic flow may aggravate the degree of the aortic regurgitation.

Aortic root dilation is a potential cause of aortic regurgitation. It can develop spontaneously or in association with congenital or acquired conditions. When the aortic root is dilated, the leaflets are displaced and fail to coapt. Progressive aortic dilation of the aortic root associated with aortic valve incompetence is a characteristic feature of Marfan syndrome. Dissection of the aortic wall is a potential complication that may aggravate the degree of regurgitation in these patients.

Ventricular septal defects, in particular the doubly committed juxta-arterial (also termed subpulmonary) ventricular septal defect type, can be complicated by aortic regurgitation. In this type of defect, there is a lack of fibrous continuity between the aortic media, the annulus, and the ventricular septum, which supports the aortic valve in normal conditions.[38] The lack of support of the aortic valve allows the coronary aortic cusp (usually right) to prolapse through the defect. The prolapsing cusp may experience progressive structural damage, resulting in aneurysmal dilation of the sinus of Valsalva. Aortic regurgitation is mild at first, but usually progresses with time, and the rate of progression varies. Patients with smaller ventricular septal defects usually have a faster progression to a more severe degree of aortic regurgitation as a result of the suction effect of a higher speed jet (Venturi effect). Aortic regurgitation is related less frequently to perimembranous ventricular septal defects.

Sinus of Valsalva aneurysm can be an acquired condition, secondary to bacterial endocarditis or trauma. Most cases are congenital, however, and are associated with a ventricular septal defect, as discussed earlier, or are due to a lack of fusion between the media of the aorta and the annulus of the aortic valve. The right coronary sinus is the most frequently affected. The rupture of the sinus of Valsalva aneurysm into the right atrium or ventricle is the most common complication, although rupture of the aneurysm into the left ventricle, producing acute aortic regurgitation, also can occur.[39,40]

Discrete subaortic stenosis is a progressive cardiac defect that consists of the presence of a fibrous shelf that encircles the outflow tract below the aortic valve. It is not present from birth and usually develops after the first 9 months of life. It commonly is found in association with other congenital or acquired heart defects.[41] During childhood, progression may be rapid, whereas in adults progression is usually slower.[42] Aortic regurgitation is common in this condition and has been related to the damage of the aortic valve cusps produced by the high-velocity jet originating from the subvalvar obstruction. Aortic regurgitation also can be secondary to infective endocarditis. The regurgitation is usually mild in children, but it can progress even after relief of the obstruction. During adult life, aortic regurgitation is often stable, and if it progresses, it does so at a slower rate.[42]

Aortic root dilation late after repair of **tetralogy of Fallot** has been reported in 16% of patients and can lead to aortic regurgitation severe enough to require valve replacement. Aortic root dilation in these patients relates in part to long-standing volume overload of the aorta. Patients with right ventricular outflow obstruction, pulmonary atresia being at the extreme, have augmented aortic flow resulting from an increased right-to-left shunting through the ventricular septal defect. A longer interval from palliation to repair also imposes volume overload on the left ventricle and aorta secondary to prolonged left-to-right shunting.[43] Histologic changes of the aortic root similar to Marfan syndrome, with cystic medial necrosis, have been reported in tetralogy of Fallot patients with dilated aorta. Whether these arterial wall anomalies are the cause or the consequence of aortic dilation needs further elucidation.[44]

Aortic regurgitation can be a complication of **surgical valvotomy** or **balloon valvuloplasty** for aortic valve stenosis. Aortic regurgitation also may develop after surgical procedures involving the creation of a **neoaortic valve** from the native pulmonary valve, such as the arterial switch operation, the Norwood procedure, and the Ross procedure. In this context, regurgitation is usually secondary to dilation of the neoaortic root.[45] In most patients, aortic regurgitation is mild, but occasionally progresses to become severe enough to require reintervention. Truncus arteriosus repair also can be complicated with **truncal valve incompetence** leading to aortic regurgitation.

Basic Pathophysiology

Acute aortic regurgitation may be a consequence of aortic root dissection, infective endocarditis, valve disruption after balloon dilation, or rupture of a sinus of Valsalva (Table 21-2). When acute aortic regurgitation develops, the normal left ventricle has no time to dilate to accommodate the sudden regurgitant flow. The acutely augmented EDV in a nondilated ventricle produces a rapid increase in the left ventricular end-diastolic pressure, which is transmitted to the left atrium and pulmonary veins. A high ventricular diastolic pressure

TABLE 21-2

Pathophysiology of Chronic Aortic Regurgitation	
Substrates	Bicuspid aortic valve
	Aortic root disease (Marfan syndrome, tetralogy of Fallot)
	Ventricular septal defect (aortic cusp prolapse)
	Sinus of Valsalva aneurysm
	Subaortic stenosis
	Common arterial trunk
	Acquired: postoperative, endocarditis
Covariables	Associated congenital heart conditions (coarctation of aorta) (−)
	Systemic hypertension (−)
	Aortic wall dissection (−)
	Coronary artery disease (−)
Disease Progression	LV dilation (eccentric hypertrophy)
	Concentric hypertrophy
	Myocardial ischemia
	LV dysfunction
	Onset of symptoms

(−) indicates negative influence on aortic regurgitation.
LV, Left ventricular.

exceeding left atrial diastolic pressure produces an early closure of the mitral valve in diastole, preventing backward transmission of the high diastolic left ventricular pressure, but also reducing the filling time of the ventricle. The failure of the left ventricle to dilate acutely precludes the use of the Frank-Starling mechanism, resulting in decreased systolic function. The adrenergic system is activated, and compensatory tachycardia develops, although this may be insufficient to increase the cardiac output. The elevation of the peripheral resistance secondary to catecholamine activation may be detrimental because the elevation of the afterload produces a further increase of the regurgitant volume.

In **chronic aortic regurgitation**, the left ventricle has to cope with an increased volume secondary to the diastolic regurgitant flow from the aorta. As a compensatory mechanism, the left ventricle dilates to accommodate the chronic volume overload, initially without a rise of its diastolic pressure. This dilation is achieved through eccentric hypertrophy of the left ventricle, with fiber enlargement and addition of new sarcomeres in series, which permit the sarcomeres to preserve a normal preload and contractility. The augmented diastolic volume in conjunction with a maintained myocardial contractility leads to an increase of the total stroke volume and a maintained forward stroke flow (total stroke volume minus regurgitant volume). As a result, left ventricular dilation leads to an increase of the systolic wall stress, explained by Laplace's law, which states that the parietal stress is proportional to the radius of the chamber and interventricular pressure and inversely related to wall thickness:

$$\text{Stress} = \frac{(\text{pressure} \times \text{radius})}{(2 \times \text{thickness})}$$

Consequently, there is an increase in left ventricular afterload because the dilated left ventricle has to achieve a higher level of systolic tension to develop any level of systolic pressure. The increased afterload stimulates the development of concentric hypertrophy, a compensatory mechanism that tries to diminish the wall stress of the ventricle. As aortic regurgitation progresses, the preload reserve and compensatory hypertrophy permit the ventricle to adapt to further increases of the diastolic volume. During this compensatory phase, which may last for many years, indices of left ventricular systolic function remain normal, and the patient remains asymptomatic. Compensatory mechanisms are not maintained indefinitely, however. An eventual exhaustion of preload reserve or an inadequate hypertrophic response leads to a continued increase in left ventricular afterload and reduction of ejection fraction. Initially, early left ventricular dysfunction may be reversible, and should aortic valve replacement be accomplished at this stage, suppression of afterload may be followed by improved systolic function and a reduction in left ventricular size. Later on, the enlarged ventricle develops irreversible myocardial injury, and systolic function may not recover after surgery.

In chronic severe aortic regurgitation, there may be some degree of myocardial ischemia secondary to increased myocardial oxygen consumption and augmented left ventricular mass and wall stress. At the same time, myocardial supply is impaired. Coronary blood flow and myocardial perfusion occur mainly during diastole, and in severe aortic regurgitation, the coronary perfusion pressure is reduced because diastolic pressure is low.

Clinical Presentation

In **acute aortic regurgitation**, there is a sudden elevation of the filling pressures of the left ventricle and impairment of the systolic function. Patients with acute aortic regurgitation usually present with pulmonary edema or cardiogenic shock or both, and the prognosis is ominous unless an urgent valve repair or replacement is performed.

During the initial compensated phase, patients with **chronic aortic regurgitation** may be symptom free for many years. When compensatory mechanisms are no longer effective, there is a progressive deterioration of left ventricular function. Even at this stage, patients may remain asymptomatic for some time. When symptoms develop, ventricular dysfunction, sometimes irreversible, is usually present. The symptoms include exertional dyspnea, orthopnea, and paroxysmal nocturnal dyspnea. Chest pain suggesting angina pectoris reflects the presence of myocardial ischemia. Some patients complain of palpitations and awareness of the heart beat secondary to a high stroke volume. In asymptomatic patients with chronic severe aortic regurgitation and normal left ventricular function, the rate of progression to symptoms or left ventricular dysfunction is approximately 4.3% per year. The rate of progression to asymptomatic left ventricular dysfunction is 1.3% per year, and the mortality is less than 0.2% per year.[46]

The best predictors for progression to symptoms, death, or left ventricular dysfunction are age, left ventricular end-diastolic dimension, and left ventricular end-systolic dimension.[47-49] Progression to symptoms in asymptomatic patients with depressed left ventricular dysfunction is around 25% per year.[50-52] When symptoms develop, there is a progressive reduction of survival. The mortality of patients with angina is higher than 10% per year and in patients with heart failure is more than 20% per year. All these data are derived from studies that mainly included adult patients with isolated aortic regurgitation. Patients with congenital heart conditions other than bicuspid aortic valve usually were excluded. A faster progression to left ventricular dysfunction and onset of symptoms is expected in patients with associated heart conditions.

Clinical Assessment

With **acute aortic regurgitation**, the clinical situation is usually critical. The patient is usually tachycardic and can present with signs of pulmonary edema or cardiogenic shock. The characteristic clinical signs of chronic aortic regurgitation are not as evident in this clinical setting. As a result of the early equalization of the diastolic pressure of the aorta and the left ventricle, the pulse pressure is not wide, and the diastolic murmur is short and hardly audible. The absence of evident clinical signs may lead to an underestimation of the degree of the regurgitation.

A wide pulse pressure is characteristic of severe **chronic aortic regurgitation**. The systolic pressure is high because of the elevated stroke volume, and the diastolic pressure is low because the regurgitation of blood from the aorta to the ventricle occurs during diastole. Several findings on examination that reflect wide pulse pressure include a collapsing arterial pulse (Corrigan sign), nodding of the head with the pulse (de Musset sign), a to-and-fro bruit over a partially collapsed femoral artery (Duroziez sign), visible capillary pulsations in the nail bed (Quincke sign), and a pulsatile uvula (Müller sign). Apex impulse is diffuse and displaced laterally and inferiorly. S_1 is usually normal. S_2 can be normal, accentuated when the cause of the regurgitation is aortic root disease, or diminished or absent when the problem is in the valve. S_3 may be present reflecting volume overload and is not an indicator of heart failure. There is a characteristic diastolic murmur that is best heard along the upper left sternal border when the cause of the regurgitation is valvular disease. When regurgitation is secondary to aortic root dilation, the murmur is best heard along the right sternal border. The murmur begins immediately after S_2 and is louder at the beginning with a decrescendo pattern. The duration of the murmur is related to the severity of the regurgitation, with a longer duration when the regurgitation is more severe. The diastolic murmur becomes louder after interventions directed to increase the arterial pressure, such as squatting or Valsalva manuver. When the regurgitation is severe, a mid-diastolic rumble can be heard (Austin Flint murmur). It is produced by a fast flow going across the mitral valve, which is relatively narrow because the aortic regurgitant jet impacting on the anterior leaflet of the mitral valve restricts its aperture. A systolic murmur is often present even if there is no aortic stenosis because of the augmented flow through the left ventricular outflow tract.

Clinical Evaluation

In chronic severe aortic regurgitation, the **ECG** usually shows sinus rhythm and left ventricular hypertrophy with strain. In acute aortic regurgitation, there is usually sinus tachycardia, and although hypertrophy is not always present, repolarization abnormalities are common.

In severe long-standing aortic regurgitation, the **chest radiograph** shows cardiac enlargement. There may be aneurysmal dilation of the ascending aorta when the cause of the regurgitation is aortic root disease. In acute aortic regurgitation, the size of the heart can be normal, but signs of pulmonary congestion or pulmonary edema are usually present.

Echocardiography is useful to confirm the presence and etiology of aortic regurgitation. The morphology of the aortic valve must be assessed and the size of the aortic root. The severity of the regurgitation can be evaluated with color Doppler by measuring the width or the area of the regurgitant jet. Indirect measurements of severe regurgitation are the presence of reversal of flow in the descending aorta, a fast decline of the slope of diastolic flow velocity (Fig. 21-4), and a high-velocity flow in the outflow tract.[53] The size and function of the left ventricle also must be evaluated. Serial measurements of left ventricular end-systolic and end-diastolic dimensions and volumes and systolic function indices are essential for deciding the optimal time for valve replacement. Diastolic vibration of the anterior leaflet of the mitral valve due to the diastolic regurgitant jet impacting on the valve can be appreciated. In acute aortic regurgitation, there may be an early closure of the mitral valve. Transesophageal echocardiography is useful for the diagnosis of aortic root disease and endocarditis when they are suspected as the cause of regurgitation.

Exercise testing can be useful to assess functional capacity and symptomatic response to exercise in patients with a history of equivocal symptoms. Although left ventricular response to exercise is usually abnormal, this has no independent diagnostic or prognostic value.[54,55] **Radionuclide angiography** usually is performed to assess left ventricular dimensions and systolic function when echocardiography is of suboptimal quality. It also can be useful for assessing left ventricular ejection fraction before recommending surgery in an asymptomatic patient with borderline left ventricular dysfunction on echocardiography. When available, **MRI** is an accurate test to quantify the severity of aortic

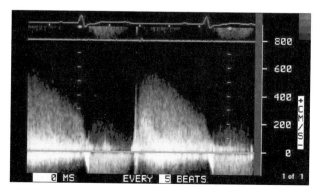

FIGURE 21-4 ■ **Aortic regurgitation.** Continuous-wave Doppler echocardiographic recording of aortic flow from a patient with severe aortic regurgitation. Note steep descent of regurgitant Doppler envelope.

regurgitation and ventricular volumes and function. It also can provide an accurate assessment of the aortic valve, aortic root, ascending and descending aorta, and aortic arch. **Angiography** may be necessary when noninvasive tests are not conclusive regarding the severity of aortic regurgitation and status of the left ventricle.[46] Angiography also should be done when surgery is planned in patients with risk of coronary disease or patients older than 40 years of age.

Therapeutic Strategies

Patients with more than trivial aortic regurgitation should have periodic follow-up. The objective of serial assessment in patients with chronic aortic regurgitation is to detect early onset of symptoms or preferably changes in left ventricular size and function, which may indicate the need for surgical intervention. After a patient with aortic regurgitation is seen for the first time, a subsequent assessment should be done early to rule out a subacute process with rapid progression. Frequency of follow-up depends on the degree of regurgitation, left ventricular size and function, and rates of progression of the size of the left ventricle and its systolic function compared with previous studies. Asymptomatic patients with mild regurgitation, no left ventricle dilation, and normal systolic function can be seen infrequently with an echocardiogram performed every 2 or 3 years. Asymptomatic patients with more severe dilation of the left ventricle have a high risk of developing symptoms or left ventricular dysfunction and should be assessed every 4 or 6 months.[46] Patients with dilation of the aortic root should be assessed at least annually. Indications for surgery are based not only on symptoms and left ventricular dimensions and function, but also on aortic root size.

Therapy with **vasodilating agents** in patients with aortic regurgitation may reduce cardiac afterload and consequently improve forward stroke volume and reduce aortic regurgitation. This activity is translated into reductions of EDV, wall stress, and afterload, which result in a reduction of ventricular mass and preservation of systolic function.[56] In patients with acute regurgitation, vasodilator therapy is useful in stabilizing patients while intervention is arranged. In the setting of chronic aortic regurgitation, the aim of the treatment is to improve the natural history of the disease. Long-term vasodilator therapy with nifedipine reduces or delays the need for surgery from 34% to 15% in asymptomatic patients with severe aortic regurgitation and normal left ventricular function.[57] Long-term treatment with ACE inhibitors has been shown to reduce regurgitant fraction and ventricular size and to increase ejection fraction,[58,59] but to date, no trials have evaluated the impact of vasodilation with ACE inhibitors on long-term natural history in children. Treatment with vasodilators could be useful in asymptomatic patients with severe aortic regurgitation with volume overload and normal systolic

function in delaying time to surgery. Patients with severe aortic regurgitation with symptoms or left ventricular dysfunction, who are not candidates for surgery, either for cardiac or noncardiac reasons, also may experience some symptomatic benefit from vasodilators. Vasodilator therapy is not an alternative to surgery in patients with left ventricular dysfunction, whether symptomatic or not. Patients with mild aortic regurgitation and normal left ventricular function without hypertension have an otherwise good long-term outcome, and vasodilator therapy is not recommended.[46]

β-Blocker therapy has been shown to slow the rate of aortic root dilation and reduce the development of aortic complications in patients with Marfan syndrome. This effect is mediated by a reduction in the systolic ejection impulse.[60] Whether this therapy is applicable to patients with aortic root dilation secondary to other etiologies, such as tetralogy of Fallot, is unknown.

The presence of symptoms, left ventricular end-diastolic and end-systolic dimensions, and systolic function are the major determinants of survival and postoperative left ventricular function.[47,49,61,62] If associated congenital abnormalities are present, all hemodynamically significant lesions should be repaired whenever possible. Smaller body size and younger age at presentation must be taken into account regarding indications, and indexed measurements of left ventricular dimensions and function should be used.

Surgery should be deferred in asymptomatic patients with mild ventricular enlargement and good systolic function because the outcome in this situation is excellent. These patients should undergo serial assessments, however, to detect any change in ventricular dimensions reflecting a relative deterioration of left ventricular function. Asymptomatic patients with severe ventricular enlargement (by Z-score criteria) should undergo operation, even if the ventricular function is normal. Most of these patients develop symptoms or left ventricular dysfunction or both, and surgical outcomes are better when surgery is performed before ventricular dysfunction develops. Asymptomatic patients also should be operated on when the resting ejection fraction is less than 50% or 55%.[47,63,64] When patients develop symptoms, they should undergo surgery.[65] Symptomatic patients with severe aortic regurgitation and either normal systolic function or moderate ventricular dilation should be operated on when no other cause for dyspnea is found. Outcome after surgery is better in patients with less advanced symptoms. Most patients with severe left ventricular dysfunction (ejection fraction <25%) and prolonged left ventricular dysfunction have developed irreversible myocardial dysfunction. The surgical risk in this setting and the mortality after surgery are high. Aortic valve replacement is usually a better alternative, however, than medical management alone.[66]

The choice of surgical approach is influenced by the cause of the regurgitation and individual patient factors.

Whenever possible, **valve repair** should be attempted. **Aortic homograft** degeneration is accelerated in pediatric patients. **Mechanical prostheses** have been widely used because of their longer durability. More recently, the **Ross procedure**, which consists of implantation of the native pulmonary valve in the aortic position and replacement of the pulmonary valve with a homograft, has been used for children and young adults because of its growth potential, optimal hemodynamic performance, and avoidance of long-term anticoagulation. When performed by skilled surgeons, the operative mortality is low, and the midterm results are good,[45,67,68] although complications related to autograft or homograft dysfunction can develop. The new porcine stentless valves have been shown to have good durability, and this may be a good alternative.[69]

When aortic regurgitation is secondary to a ventricular septal defect, early closure of the defect, before the aortic cusp is irreversibly damaged and the left ventricle dilates, is strongly recommended. When advanced changes are established, operative results are less good, and recurrence or persistence of regurgitation is frequent. When a patient presents with mild regurgitation, frequent echocardiographic follow-up is warranted. If there is any increase in the degree of regurgitation with time, surgery should be undertaken. Subaortic stenosis should be repaired early during childhood, before high-pressure gradients are established to avoid progressive left ventricle outflow obstruction and development of significant aortic regurgitation. In adults, because of the slow progression of the left ventricular outflow obstruction and regurgitation, surgery should be considered on the basis of clinical and hemodynamic findings.[42] In patients with aortic root dilation, including patients with Marfan syndrome, elective replacement of the aortic root has a low mortality. In contrast, emergency repair for acute aortic dissection is associated with high mortality. Prophylactic aortic root replacement associated with valve replacement or repair is recommended before aortic root diameters reach 55 to 60 mm in size. In patients with a family history of dissection, replacement should be performed when the aortic root measures 50 mm.[70] Although to date no aortic dissection has been reported in patients with tetralogy of Fallot with aortic root dilation, root replacement should be considered in patients when the aortic root diameter exceeds 55 mm, in patients with aortic regurgitation, and in patients referred for pulmonary valve implantation.[46,71]

TRICUSPID REGURGITATION

Anatomic Considerations

Most cases of tricuspid regurgitation in children and adolescents are congenital, with **Ebstein anomaly** being the most frequent malformation. Ebstein anomaly is an uncommon congenital heart abnormality characterized by apical displacement of the attachments of the septal and inferior (mural) leaflets from the atrioventricular junction into the right ventricular cavity.[72] The leaflets usually fail to coapt, producing tricuspid regurgitation. Some degree of tricuspid stenosis also can be present, although this is uncommon. The anterosuperior leaflet is usually elongated and may be abnormally tethered to the endocardium of the right ventricular free wall, which constrains the leaflet movement, contributing to valve incompetence. The inlet portion of the right ventricle is atrialized and has a thin muscular wall. The apical trabecular and outlet portions compose the functional right ventricle, which is usually smaller than normal. Accessory atrioventricular pathways, sometimes multiple, are commonly associated with Ebstein anomaly and are potential substrates for supraventricular tachycardia. Associated defects are common in Ebstein malformation, mainly when the malformation is diagnosed early in life. The most common are the pulmonary valve abnormalities (pulmonary stenosis and atresia), which probably are related to the low antegrade flow through the RVOT during intrauterine development. Ebstein anomaly can be present in hearts with double discordance (congenitally corrected transposition of the great arteries). In this situation, the tricuspid valve is the systemic atrioventricular valve, and the hemodynamic effect of tricuspid regurgitation is greater. Intra-atrial communication is present in many patients with tricuspid regurgitation, in the form of either a patent foramen ovale or an atrial septal defect.

Tricuspid valve dysplasia is the second most common cause of congenital tricuspid regurgitation. It comprises a wide range of underdevelopment of the leaflets, chordae, and papillary muscles. The proximal atrioventricular attachment of the tricuspid valve is normal in this condition. Other congenital causes of tricuspid regurgitation are tricuspid agenesis; cleft anterior leaflet, which may or may not be related to atrioventricular septal defects (see later); and Uhl anomaly (absence of parietal right ventricular myocardium, which is transformed into a thin, passive unexcitable conduit). Acquired valve disease is an uncommon cause of tricuspid regurgitation in children. It may be related to thoracic trauma[73] or infective endocarditis.

Functional regurgitation is a common cause of tricuspid regurgitation. Dilation of the right ventricle and tricuspid annulus secondary to elevated right ventricular pressure or volume can produce tricuspid regurgitation in anatomically normal tricuspid valves. Elevation of right ventricular systolic pressure can be produced by different cardiac or pulmonary conditions, such as mitral stenosis, primary pulmonary hypertension, Eisenmenger syndrome, or RVOT obstruction.[74]

Basic Pathophysiology

In tricuspid regurgitation, there is volume overload of the right heart chambers (Table 21-3). The right atrium

TABLE 21-3

Pathophysiology of Chronic Tricuspid Regurgitation	
Substrates	Ebstein anomaly
	Tricuspid valve dysplasia
	Other congenital: tricuspid agenesis, cleft of anterior leaflet, Uhl anomaly
	Acquired valve disease: endocarditis
	Functional regurgitation, secondary to elevated RV pressure or increased volume
Covariables	Small functional right ventricle (Ebstein anomaly) (−)
	Pulmonary hypertension (−)
	Associated congenital heart conditions (RVOT obstruction) (−)
	WPW syndrome (Ebstein anomaly) (−)
Disease Progression	RV and RA dilation
	SVT, atrial flutter, atrial fibrillation
	RV dysfunction
	LV dysfunction (Ebstein anomaly)
	Overt symptoms

(−) indicates negative influence on tricuspid regurgitation.
LV, left ventricular; RA, right atrial; RV, right ventricular;
RVOT, right ventricular outflow tract; SVT, supraventricular tachycardia;
WPW, Wolff-Parkinson-White.

and right ventricle dilate to accommodate the augmented volume of blood with a normal pressure. Right ventricular dysfunction finally may develop, usually with symptoms of low cardiac output and systemic venous congestion being present.

The hemodynamic consequences of Ebstein malformation are related not only to the degree of regurgitation, but also to the size of the functional right ventricle and the presence of associated anomalies. If the right ventricle is very small, forward pulmonary flow is reduced. This flow is compromised further if right ventricular obstruction is present. In the neonatal period, the elevated pulmonary vascular resistance augments the right ventricular systolic pressure, worsening tricuspid regurgitation. When the regurgitation is severe, right atrial pressure increases above the left atrial pressure, and patients with an intra-atrial communication may have right-to-left shunting. The intra-atrial communication acts like a safety valve to maintain systemic cardiac output at the expense of cyanosis under these circumstances. Left ventricular dysfunction can be present in patients with Ebstein anomaly. The cause of myocardial impairment is unknown, but may be due to chronic cyanosis, right heart dilation, septal abnormalities,[75] and increased left ventricular fibrosis.[76]

The right atrium is almost universally enlarged in patients with tricuspid regurgitation or Ebstein anomaly. An extremely enlarged right atrium during fetal life could prevent normal development of the lung, leading to pulmonary hypoplasia and the "wall-to-wall heart" appearance. Atrial fibrillation and flutter are common when marked right atrial dilation is present.

Atrioventricular reentry tachycardias related to accessory atrioventricular pathways are a common feature of Ebstein anomaly. Ventricular arrhythmias also can develop because of abnormalities of the ventricular myocardium.

Clinical Presentation

Symptoms are secondary to right-sided heart congestion and low cardiac output. Congestive symptoms include ascites, hepatomegaly, and peripheral edema. Low cardiac output produces fatigue, weakness, and dyspnea. Supraventricular arrhythmias are manifest with palpitations. If the arrhythmia is sustained, it may lead to hemodynamic deterioration and heart failure.

Ebstein malformation has a highly variable clinical course. Clinical presentation depends on the degree of apical displacement of the leaflets, functional status of the tricuspid valve, and associated anomalies.[77-79] When leaflets are severely displaced and tricuspid regurgitation is severe, profound congestive heart failure and death during the neonatal or even intrauterine period can occur.[80,81] Patients with mild displacement of the leaflets with a competent tricuspid valve may remain asymptomatic for many years and usually are diagnosed in adulthood because of a cardiac murmur or atrial arrhythmia. The initial clinical presentation varies according to the age of presentation. In fetal life, severe forms of Ebstein malformation usually are diagnosed during routine fetal scanning. The most common presentation in neonates is cyanosis. Infants usually present with congestive cardiac failure, whereas in older children the finding of an incidental murmur leads to the diagnosis. Arrhythmia is the most common presentation in adolescents and adults.[82]

Isolated tricuspid regurgitation, excluding Ebstein malformation, is uncommon, and the natural history is not well defined. Tricuspid regurgitation, in the absence of pulmonary hypertension, is usually well tolerated for many years, but some patients need surgical repair at some point. The associated morbidity and mortality are related mainly to hemodynamic problems and arrhythmias.

When Ebstein anomaly is detected early in life (fetal or neonatal period), the condition is usually severe or associated with other cardiac lesions or both. For patients requiring early surgery, the neonatal mortality is extremely high; neonates who survive the first month of life remain at high risk of late hemodynamic deterioration and sudden death. The 10-year actuarial survival in this group is 61%.[80,82] When Ebstein anomaly presents during late childhood or adulthood, the late outcome is far better. The annual risk of mortality decreases from 4% for the second year of life to 1.4% for ages 10 to 40. The main cause of death is heart failure followed by sudden death. Predictors of death in patients with Ebstein anomaly are a higher echocardiographic grade as per Celermajer and colleagues[82] (see later), cardiothoracic ratio greater than 60%, associated RVOT obstruction, and presentation in fetal life.

Clinical Assessment

Patients with severe tricuspid regurgitation and right ventricular dysfunction can have cachexia and jaundice. Cyanosis and clubbing can be present if a significant degree of right-to-left shunting is present. There can be asymmetry of the chest secondary to dilation of the right ventricle and atrium. Jugular veins are distended with abnormal systolic v waves. In patients with Ebstein malformation, jugular venous pressure can be normal owing to the elevated compliance of the dilated right atrium and atrialized right ventricle. The liver is usually enlarged and tender and may be pulsatile. At auscultation, there is a characteristic holosystolic murmur in the lower left sternal border, which is louder with inspiration (Carvallo sign). In Ebstein malformation, the first sound is widely split, with a loud tricuspid component resulting from the increased excursion of the anterosuperior leaflet (sail-like). The second sound may be widely split when a right bundle branch block is present. S_3 resulting from the opening of the enlarged anterosuperior leaflet and S_4 can be present.

Clinical Evaluation

The **ECG** sometimes shows atrial fibrillation and atrial flutter, right bundle branch block, and low voltage across the ECG leads. The right atrium may be enlarged with tall P waves. When Ebstein anomaly is present, one half of the patients have first-degree atrioventricular block. A short PR interval and a delta wave from early activation of the myocardium through an accessory pathway are present in 25% of the patients.[82,83]

On **chest radiograph**, there is cardiomegaly secondary to dilation of right cardiac chambers (mainly right atrium). In Ebstein anomaly, cardiac size varies from normal to extreme cardiomegaly. A globular cardiac silhouette with a narrow arterial pedicle is characteristic of this entity. If important right-to-left shunting is present, pulmonary vascular markings may be decreased.

Echocardiographic assessment permits the detection of tricuspid regurgitation, determination of its etiology, and estimation of severity. Right ventricular dimensions and function must be assessed. A paradoxical movement of the interventricular septum reflects volume overload. The morphologic features of Ebstein anomaly can be fully appreciated with echocardiography. An echocardiographic grading system permits prognostic stratification. The grade is obtained by calculating the ratio of the combined area of the right atrium and atrialized right ventricle to the area of the functional right ventricle and left chambers, obtained from a four-chamber view in diastole. Four grades of increased severity are defined: less than 0.5, 0.5 to 0.99, 1 to 1.49, and 1.5 or greater.[80,82] Pulmonary artery pressure determination is useful to discern the cause of tricuspid regurgitation. When systolic pulmonary arterial pressure is greater than 55 mm Hg, tricuspid regurgitation is usually functional. When systolic pulmonary arterial pressure is less than 40 mm Hg, the cause usually is related to valvar abnormality. Bubble contrast study can detect the presence of an interatrial communication and right-to-left shunting.

Exercise testing can be useful to evaluate functional capacity and the degree of oxygen desaturation with exercise. **MRI** permits the diagnosis of Uhl anomaly and right ventricular dysplasia. MRI also shows Ebstein anomaly of the tricuspid valve in older patients, in whom transthoracic echocardiography may be inconclusive. Echocardiography is diagnostic in most cases, and **cardiac catheterization** is rarely required, other than for electrophysiologic studies, investigation of associated cardiac defects, and evaluation when patients are considered for surgery.

Therapeutic Strategies

Management of tricuspid regurgitation depends on the etiology of the lesion, clinical features, and presence of associated defects. Most patients have a good functional class and do not need any therapy. Some patients with severe tricuspid regurgitation may require surgical intervention, however. Therapeutic strategies must be individualized for each patient.

When tricuspid regurgitation is functional, any intervention directed to decrease right ventricular pressure may result in an improvement of tricuspid regurgitation. Many neonates with Ebstein anomaly and cyanosis may show a spontaneous improvement when pulmonary vascular resistance decreases. In the meantime, treatment with oxygen, nitric oxide, and prostaglandin E_1 to maintain the patency of the arterial duct may be needed. When obstruction of the RVOT is present, surgical palliation is often required to improve cyanosis.

Symptoms of congestive heart failure can be treated with diuretics. Acute intravenous administration of antiarrhythmic agents in the face of severe tricuspid regurgitation may be affected by the poor antegrade flow to the circulation. In addition, although arrhythmias can be managed with medical treatment, some patients with poor response to antiarrhythmic therapy may require percutaneous radiofrequency ablation. Catheter ablation in patients with Ebstein anomaly and Wolff-Parkinson-White syndrome has not had as good results as in patients with normal hearts due to higher recurrence rates.[84] The higher recurrence rates are due to the frequent presence of multiple accessory pathways. When surgery is required for associated cardiac defects, ablation of accessory pathways can be performed perioperatively. When atrial fibrillation or atrial flutter or both are present, the maze procedure can be performed during surgery for hemodynamic reasons.[85]

Indications for surgical intervention in patients with tricuspid regurgitation are controversial. Patients with severe tricuspid regurgitation should undergo valve repair or replacement when one or more of the following conditions are present: (1) symptoms of heart failure, with New York Heart Association (NYHA) functional class III or IV despite medical therapy; (2) right-sided heart failure; (3) a right-to-left shunt producing progressive cyanosis with resting oxygen saturations of less than 90%; (4) asymptomatic cardiomegaly on chest x-ray (cardiothoracic ratio > 0.65%) or progressive right ventricular enlargement on echocardiography; and (5) recurrent supraventricular arrhythmias refractory to therapy.[86,87]

When surgery is necessary, **tricuspid valve repair** is preferred to valve replacement because of lower mortality and fewer long-term complications. Repair of the tricuspid valve has a perioperative mortality of 5% to 10%, depending on the series. The incidence of residual regurgitation is low, and most patients experience an improvement of functional capacity after surgery. Various surgical techniques have been used. In patients with Ebstein anomaly, it may be possible to create a monocusp valve from the anterosuperior tricuspid leaflet, provided that it is mobile and not tethered to the endocardium.[87-91] A transverse or longitudinal plication of the atrialized portion of the right ventricle also may be required.[87,89] Closure of the interatrial communication should be considered at the time of the surgery. A cleft of the anterior leaflet can be repaired with simple suture and annuloplasty. When the main problem is dilation of the tricuspid ring, an **annuloplasty** with a prosthetic ring (Carpentier) or without one (DeVega) has been shown to be effective.[92] When functional tricuspid regurgitation is mild, and relief of the cause of pulmonary hypertension is feasible (mitral stenosis), the regurgitation improves after surgery of the primary lesion without the need for tricuspid valve annuloplasty. Intraoperative transesophageal echocardiogram is indicated to assess the effect of annuloplasty or valve repair on valvular function. It may refine the surgical plan,[93] and when an annuloplasty is performed, it assists with determining the degree of adjustment of the leaflets to achieve a substantial reduction in residual regurgitation without creating valve stenosis.[94] Reconstruction of tricuspid leaflets, chordae, and papillary muscles after trauma may be possible. When the cause of the regurgitation is endocarditis, treatment with antibiotics may not be enough. Sometimes the valve needs to be excised completely, and a new valve can be reinserted some months later, when the infection is totally eradicated.

Tricuspid valve replacement is associated with high perioperative mortality (17% to 27%).[95-98] Patients with higher NYHA class and patients with congenital anomalies have a worse prognosis.[96] When valve replacement is necessary, bioprostheses are preferred because of the high rate of thrombotic complications of mechanical prostheses in the tricuspid position.[99,100] Newer mechanical prostheses have a better hemodynamic profile and low thrombogenicity, however, which can provide a good alternative to bioprosthetic valves and overcome the problem of high degeneration rate.[95-98]

Some patients with severe Ebstein anomaly may have a small functional right ventricle that is unable to perform as a right-sided pump. In this situation, the combination of **bidirectional cavopulmonary shunt (Glenn)** with valve repair to reduce the right ventricular preload may decrease operative mortality and improve symptoms.[101] Another alternative for these patients is the creation of a functional tricuspid atresia, with patching of the valve and excision of the atrial septum (Starnes approach),[102] followed by a total cavopulmonary connection (modified Fontan). Uhl anomaly also may require the exclusion of the right ventricle with either a cavopulmonary shunt or a Fontan operation. Some patients with severe tricuspid regurgitation and advanced right and left ventricular dysfunction require heart transplantation.

MITRAL REGURGITATION

Anatomic Considerations

Isolated **congenital mitral regurgitation** is an uncommon condition during childhood. Mitral regurgitation usually is associated with other congenital cardiac defects or connective tissue and metabolic or storage diseases. It also can be secondary to trauma; acquired inflammatory conditions, such as myocarditis or rheumatic fever; dilated cardiomyopathy; endocarditis; Kawasaki disease; and collagen vascular disorders.

Atrioventricular septal defect, a congenital abnormality caused by an abnormal development of the atrioventricular junction, is the most common congenital cardiac defect that is associated with mitral regurgitation. Atrioventricular septal defect comprises a combination of different anomalies, including ostium primum atrial septal defect, inlet ventricular septal defect (restrictive or nonrestrictive), and abnormalities of the atrioventricular valves. The uniform feature is a common atrioventricular junction with a trileaflet left atrioventricular valve (so-called cleft) (Fig. 21-5). There may be a common atrioventricular valve (complete atrioventricular septal defect) or separate left and right valves with three and four leaflets, respectively (partial atrioventricular septal defect). The morphology of the atrioventricular valves often leads to left or right atrioventricular valve regurgitation or both. Left atrioventricular valve regurgitation is also a common complication after surgical repair of atrioventricular septal defects.

Mitral valve prolapse is one of the most common forms of valvular disease. When current two-dimensional echocardiographic criteria are applied, the prevalence of mitral valve prolapse is 1.3%.[103] The mitral valve is myxomatous, with redundant leaflets and elongated chordae. During systole, there is an abnormal displacement of one or both mitral leaflets into the atrium.

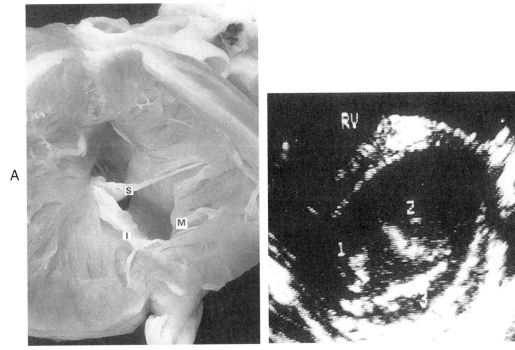

FIGURE 21-5 ■ **Left atrioventricular valve regurgitation.** Atrioventricular septal defect. Heart specimen **(A)** and two-dimensional echocardiography of a left atrioventricular valve **(B)**. The valve consists of three leaflets. The inferior *(1, I)* and superior *(2, S)* bridging leaflets cross the ventricular septum. The mural leaflet *(3, M)* is located laterally-posteriorly. (From SY Ho [ed]: Color Atlas of Congenital Heart Disease: Morphologic and Clinical Correlations. London, Mosby-Wolfe, 1995, p 68.)

Mitral valve prolapse is predominantly a benign condition, although some patients may have complications, such as cerebral embolic events, infective endocarditis, progression to severe mitral regurgitation requiring surgery, and even sudden cardiac death.

An **anomalous origin of the left coronary artery from the pulmonary trunk** may lead to ischemia and infarction of the anterolateral wall during the first few months of life. Mitral regurgitation is common, resulting from dilation of the left ventricle and the mitral valve ring or dysfunction of an infarcted anterior papillary muscle. The prognosis of this condition without surgery is generally poor; most children die during the first year of life from congestive heart failure. Reestablishment of a dual coronary artery supply system early in life, either by reimplanting the coronary artery or by creating a coronary to aortic tunnel with a pulmonary artery baffle, carries a good prognosis.[104,105] Mitral regurgitation usually improves without the need for mitral valve repair,[105,106] and left ventricular remodeling with marked improvement in ventricular function is common.

Basic Pathophysiology

In **chronic mitral regurgitation**, part of the stroke volume of the left ventricle, the regurgitant volume, is preferentially ejected back to the low-pressure left atrium (compared with this volume being ejected into the aorta in aortic regurgitation) (Table 21-4).

TABLE 21-4

Pathophysiology of Chronic Mitral Regurgitation	
Substrates	Atrioventricular septal defect (complete or partial)
	Mitral valve prolapse
	Isolated congenital mitral regurgitation
	Connective tissue, metabolic or storage diseases
	Acquired: trauma, inflammatory disorders (rheumatic fever, endocarditis, myocarditis, Kawasaki disease, collagen vascular disorders)
	Myocardial ischemia (CAD, ALCAPA)
	Dilated cardiomyopathy
Covariables	Systemic hypertension (−)
	Associated congenital heart conditions (LVOTO) (−)
Disease Progression	LA dilation
	LV dilation with enhanced contractility
	LV dysfunction with normal EF
	LV dysfunction with depressed EF
	Atrial arrhythmia
	Onset of symptoms

(−) indicates negative influence on mitral regurgitation.
ALCAPA, anomalous left coronary artery from pulmonary artery; CAD, coronary artery disease; EF, ejection fraction; LA, left atrial; LV, left ventricular; LVOTO, left ventricular outflow tract obstruction.

Chronic mitral regurgitation is characterized by volume overload with reduced afterload. The compensatory eccentric hypertrophy developed by the left ventricle permits the accommodation of the increased blood flow with a low filling pressure. The reduced ventricular afterload in conjunction with the increased EDV of the left ventricle leads to an enhanced contractility of myocardium. This condition results in an augmented total stroke volume to maintain forward systemic blood flow (total stroke volume minus regurgitant volume). During this initial compensated phase, the systolic function indices (ejection fraction or shortening fraction) are increased, and patients usually are asymptomatic.

This situation cannot be maintained in the long term. Further increases in the regurgitant volume or the ventricular dimension eventually lead to the development of left ventricular contractile dysfunction. End-systolic volumes and left ventricular filling pressures increase, and symptoms of pulmonary congestion and low cardiac output develop. Progressive dilation of the left atrium secondary to the increased volume results with time in atrial arrhythmias. Even at this stage, myocardial impairment of the left ventricle may be masked by low impedance to ejection provided by the left atrium, and systolic function indices may be within the normal range. Surgery should be performed before deterioration of ventricular function and not be delayed.

Acute mitral regurgitation usually is caused by rupture of a chorda or papillary muscle or is secondary to infective endocarditis. In this situation, the left ventricle has not had time to develop compensatory eccentric hypertrophy, and the sudden volume overload imposed on the left atrium and ventricle results in a rapid elevation of the filling pressure of both chambers and pulmonary congestion. The failure of the left ventricle to accommodate acutely to the diastolic volume also results in an acutely decreased forward systolic volume and to further pulmonary congestion.

Clinical Presentation

Patients with **chronic mitral regurgitation** usually remain asymptomatic for many years. Pediatric patients with mitral regurgitation become symptomatic earlier than adults.[107] Symptoms are those of pulmonary congestion, low cardiac output, and atrial arrhythmias. Patients may have dyspnea, fatigue, and weakness during exercise. In more advanced states, the patients may have orthopnea and nocturnal paroxysmal dyspnea.

Acute mitral regurgitation is a medical emergency. Patients usually present with pulmonary edema and cardiogenic shock. Urgent surgical treatment usually is required in this situation.

Available data on the natural history of mitral regurgitation are derived from studies that included a heterogeneous population with varied causes of mitral regurgitation and different definitions of severe mitral regurgitation, which makes the interpretation of these results difficult. Patients with severe mitral regurgitation may remain symptom free for many years. The development of symptoms of heart failure (NYHA class III or IV, even if transient) is an indicator of poor prognosis if surgical treatment is not performed immediately. Survival in symptomatic patients who do not undergo surgery may be around 33% at 8 years, with an average mortality of 5% per year.[108,109] The presence of myocardial impairment, even if the ejection fraction is normal, is also an indicator of a worse prognosis.

Clinical Assessment

In chronic severe mitral regurgitation, the apical impulse is enlarged and displaced. S_1 can be mild, and S_2 is loud if the patient develops pulmonary hypertension. S_3 may be present due to the rapid filling of the left ventricle, and this does not always reflect the presence of ventricular dysfunction.

There is a typical holosystolic murmur best heard at the apex with radiation to the axilla. In acute mitral regurgitation, the murmur is usually mild. In severe regurgitation, a diastolic murmur reflecting an augmented flow through the mitral valve can be present. The characteristic auscultatory finding in prolapse of the mitral valve is the midsystolic click resulting from the sudden tension of the mitral valve apparatus when the mitral leaflet prolapses into the atrium. It is frequently followed by an end-systolic murmur of mitral regurgitation.

Clinical Evaluation

The **ECG** usually shows left atrial enlargement and signs of left ventricular hypertrophy. The diagnosis of anomalous left coronary artery from the pulmonary artery should be excluded (Q waves in I and avL). In chronic severe mitral regurgitation, the size of the heart is enlarged on chest radiographs. When the regurgitation is acute, cardiomegaly is uncommon, and there are signs of pulmonary congestion.

The **echocardiogram** permits the evaluation of etiology and severity of mitral regurgitation and the structure of the mitral valve and its support apparatus. An anomalous coronary artery arising from the pulmonary trunk can be detected. The left ventricular end-diastolic and particularly end-systolic dimensions and the ejection fraction are the best estimates of the systolic performance of the left ventricle. During the compensatory phase of mitral regurgitation, the systolic function indices are higher than normal as a result of the favorable preload conditions and the normal afterload of the left ventricle. Serial assessment of these measurements and the atrial size and estimated pulmonary arterial pressure provide useful information in determining the optimal timing for surgery.

Cardiac catheterization should be performed when there is a discrepancy between clinical findings and noninvasive tests regarding the severity of the regurgitation or when the noninvasive tests are inconclusive.

It permits the evaluation of the severity of regurgitation, left ventricular volumes, systolic and diastolic function, and pulmonary artery pressure. It also is useful for identifying ischemic causes of mitral regurgitation, such as an anomalous origin of the left coronary artery from the pulmonary artery, although **MRI** can be useful for this disease.

Therapeutic Strategies

The rationale for the use of **vasodilating agents** drugs in chronic mitral regurgitation is that the reduction in the afterload may increase forward aortic flow and decrease the amount of regurgitant flow to the atria, preventing ventricular dilation and delaying surgery. In long term studies, vasodilator therapy has not been proved to be beneficial in asymptomatic patients, however. In severe mitral regurgitation secondary to primary valvular disease, afterload is not increased, and vasodilator therapy could mask the recognition of early myocardial dysfunction. Vasodilator therapy has no indication in asymptomatic patients with preserved left ventricular function and no systemic hypertension.[46] In contrast, vasodilator therapy has been shown to be beneficial in conditions in which mitral regurgitation is accompanied by increased afterload, such as dilated cardiomyopathy or coronary heart disease.[56] Although ACE inhibitors may reduce the size and mass of the left ventricle and improve the functional status in symptomatic patients,[110] medical treatment should not delay the time of surgery in symptomatic patients.

Vasodilator therapy is indicated in acute mitral regurgitation to stabilize patients before surgery is performed. Nitroprusside increases forward flow by diminishing regurgitant flow and the mitral valve annular dimensions.[111] Phosphodiesterase inhibitors, such as milrinone, also can be used to improve hemodynamic profile and cardiac output.

The most important preoperative predictors of outcome after surgery are ejection fraction together with end-systolic left ventricular dimensions[112,113] and the presence of symptoms.[114] Patients with myocardial impairment, even when ejection fraction is normal, may develop postoperative left ventricular dysfunction. Many of these patients have incomplete recovery of left ventricular function during follow-up.[115] Severely symptomatic patients (NYHA classes III and IV) may experience improvement of symptoms after surgery. Operative risk and late survival in these patients is worse, however, than in patients in NYHA functional classes I and II.[114] These findings support an early approach of performing surgical repair before the establishment of symptoms or left ventricular dysfunction or both.[116]

Determining the optimal time for surgical intervention is crucial for patients with severe mitral regurgitation. Symptomatic patients with severe mitral regurgitation have a poor prognosis and should undergo surgery without delay. If mild-to-moderate systolic impairment

is present, surgery could improve the symptoms and prevent further deterioration of left ventricular function. In contrast, when left ventricular ejection fraction is less than 30%, conventional surgery does not always lead to symptomatic improvement, and surgical outcomes are sometimes poor. In this situation, **heart transplantation** may be a preferred option. Surgery is indicated in asymptomatic patients when there is evidence of left ventricular dysfunction on echocardiogram (left ventricular ejection fraction ≤60%).[46,117] Asymptomatic patients with normal systolic function can be considered for surgery if valve repair can be performed with a low operative risk and good results to avoid left ventricular dilation and dysfunction.[118]

Surgery in children usually is delayed until the appearance of symptoms to avoid technical limitations (such as annular size) probable early reintervention to replace the valve because of somatic growth, and need for and the hazards of anticoagulation. This approach does not seem to increase significantly the risk of long-term ventricular dysfunction. In children, in contrast to adults, left ventricular dysfunction usually improves or even normalizes after surgery.[107]

Whenever possible, **mitral valve repair** is preferred to valve replacement. Mitral valve repair, when performed by a skilled surgeon, has a low perioperative risk and good long-term survival, with better preservation of systolic function and avoidance of complications derived from valve prostheses (deterioration of the biologic prostheses or long-term anticoagulation in mechanical prostheses).[119,120] Patients with a true cleft mitral valve, patients with a trileaflet left atrioventricular valve (in the setting of atrioventricular septal defects), and patients with mitral valve prolapse affecting the posterior leaflet are the best candidates for successful valve repair. When **mitral valve replacement** is performed, taking care to preserve the subvalvar apparatus results in better long-term function of the left ventricle and improved postoperative survival compared with mitral valve replacement with disruption of the subvalvar apparatus.[121,122]

CURRENT STATUS AND FUTURE TRENDS

Appropriate timing of surgery for valvular insufficiency is an essential part of the strategy in the care of these patients. Such a strategy entails proper understanding of the progression of ventricular adaptation and possible myocardial failure. Because the pathophysiologic process to heart failure in valvular disease can be insidious, vigilance for subtle unfavorable alterations in ventricular performance is of paramount importance. Research with newer methods of assessing myocardial performance will aid in the clinical follow-up of these patients. Surgical techniques, including bioengineered valves that prolong the longevity of these valve repairs or replacements, also are needed in the near future.[123]

Key Concepts

■ The pathophysiologic sequence for valvular insufficiency is similar for the right and the left heart: increase in EDV first, followed by an increase in end-systolic volume, and finally a decrease in shortening and ejection fractions.

■ Discerning the optimal time for intervention, before irreversible ventricular dysfunction develops, is a key point in the management of regurgitant valvular heart disease.

■ Immediate postoperative pulmonary regurgitation is well tolerated after pulmonary repair of tetralogy of Fallot in infancy. In contrast, postoperative pulmonary regurgitation is poorly tolerated in an older child after late repair. This difference may relate to poor adaptation of a hypertrophied and poorly compliant right ventricle, further compromised with acute volume overload in the case of significant postoperative pulmonary regurgitation.

■ Marked dilation of the right ventricle can lead to the development of secondary tricuspid regurgitation, which contributes to further dilation of the right ventricle and right atrium. The stretch and dilation of the right ventricle slows interventricular conduction and creates a mechanoelectrical substrate for reentry circuits, which may lead to sustained ventricular tachycardia.

■ When acute aortic regurgitation develops, the normal left ventricle has no time to dilate to accommodate the sudden regurgitant flow. The acutely augmented EDV in a nondilated ventricular produces a rapid increase in the left ventricular end-diastolic pressure, which is transmitted to the left atrium and pulmonary veins. The failure of the left ventricle to dilate acutely precludes the use of the Frank-Starling mechanism, resulting in decreased systolic function.

■ In chronic aortic regurgitation, the left ventricle has to cope with an increased volume because of the diastolic regurgitant flow from the aorta. As a compensatory mechanism, the left ventricle dilates to accommodate the chronic volume overload, initially without an increase of its diastolic pressure. This dilation is achieved through eccentric hypertrophy of the left ventricle, with fiber enlargement and addition of new sarcomeres in series, which permit the sarcomeres to preserve a normal preload and contractility.

■ Patients with severe tricuspid regurgitation should undergo valve repair or replacement when one or more of the following conditions are present: (1) symptoms of heart failure, with New York Heart Association (NYHA) functional class III or IV despite medical therapy; (2) right-sided heart failure; (3) a right-to-left shunt producing progressive cyanosis with resting oxygen saturations of less than 90%; (4) asymptomatic cardiomegaly on chest x-ray (cardiothoracic ratio >0.65%) or progressive right ventricular enlargement on echocardiography; and (5) recurrent supraventricular arrhythmias refractory to therapy.

■ In mitral regurgitation, part of the stroke volume of the left ventricle, the regurgitant volume, is preferentially ejected back to the low-pressure left atrium (compared with this volume being ejected into the aorta in aortic regurgitation). Chronic mitral regurgitation is characterized by volume overload with reduced afterload.

Acknowledgments

We thank Dr. Babu-Narayan for reviewing this chapter.

REFERENCES

1. Westaby S, Katsumata T: Congenital absence of a single pulmonary valve cusp. Ann Thorac Surg 1997;64:849.
2. Murphy JG, Gersh BJ, Mair DD, et al: Long-term outcome in patients undergoing surgical repair of tetralogy of Fallot. N Engl J Med 1993;329:593.
3. Nollert G, Fischlein T, Bouterwek S, et al: Long-term survival in patients with repair of tetralogy of Fallot: 36-year follow-up of 490 survivors of the first year after surgical repair. J Am Coll Cardiol 1997;30:1374.
4. Davlouros PA, Kilner PJ, Hornung TS, et al: Right ventricular function in adults with repaired tetralogy of Fallot assessed with cardiovascular magnetic resonance imaging: Detrimental role of right ventricular outflow aneurysms or akinesia and adverse right-to-left ventricular interaction. J Am Coll Cardiol 2002;40:2044.
5. Chen CR, Cheng TO, Huang T, et al: Percutaneous balloon valvuloplasty for pulmonic stenosis in adolescents and adults. N Engl J Med 1996;335:21.
6. Griffith BP, Hardesty RL, Siewers RD, et al: Pulmonary valvulotomy alone for pulmonary stenosis: Results in children with and without muscular infundibular hypertrophy. J Thorac Cardiovasc Surg 1982;83:577.
7. Hayes CJ, Gersony WM, Driscoll DJ, et al: Second natural history study of congenital heart defects: Results of treatment of patients with pulmonary valvar stenosis. Circulation 1993;87:I-28.
8. McCrindle BW: Independent predictors of long-term results after balloon pulmonary valvuloplasty. Valvuloplasty and Angioplasty of Congenital Anomalies (VACA) Registry Investigators. Circulation 1994;89:1751.
9. McCrindle BW, Kan JS: Long-term results after balloon pulmonary valvuloplasty. Circulation 1991;83:1915.
10. O'Connor BK, Beekman RH, Lindauer A, et al: Intermediate-term outcome after pulmonary balloon valvuloplasty: Comparison with a matched surgical control group. J Am Coll Cardiol 1992;20:169.
11. Laneve SA, Uesu CT, Taguchi JT: Isolated pulmonary valvular regurgitation. Am J Med Sci 1962;244:446.
12. Gatzoulis MA, Till JA, Somerville J, et al: Mechanoelectrical interaction in tetralogy of Fallot: QRS prolongation relates to right ventricular size and predicts malignant ventricular arrhythmias and sudden death. Circulation 1995;92:231.
13. Ilbawi MN, Idriss FS, DeLeon SY, et al: Factors that exaggerate the deleterious effects of pulmonary insufficiency on the right ventricle after tetralogy repair: Surgical implications. J Thorac Cardiovasc Surg 1987;93:36.
14. Gatzoulis MA, Clark AL, Cullen S, et al: Right ventricular diastolic function 15 to 35 years after repair of tetralogy of Fallot:

Restrictive physiology predicts superior exercise performance. Circulation 1995;91:1775.

15. Carvalho JS, Shinebourne EA, Busst C, et al: Exercise capacity after complete repair of tetralogy of Fallot: Deleterious effects of residual pulmonary regurgitation. Br Heart J 1992;67:470.

16. Shimazaki Y, Blackstone EH, Kirklin JW: The natural history of isolated congenital pulmonary valve incompetence: Surgical implications. Thorac Cardiovasc Surg 1984;32:257.

17. Marie PY, Marcon F, Brunotte F, et al: Right ventricular overload and induced sustained ventricular tachycardia in operatively "repaired" tetralogy of Fallot. Am J Cardiol 1992;69:785.

18. Bousvaros CA, Deuchar DC: The murmur of pulmonary regurgitation which is not associated with pulmonary hypertension. Lancet 1961;2:962.

19. Li W, Davlouros PA, Kilner PJ, et al: Doppler-echocardiographic assessment of pulmonary regurgitation in adults with repaired tetralogy of Fallot: Comparison with cardiovascular magnetic resonance imaging. Am Heart J 2004;147:165-172.

20. Goldberg SJ, Allen HD: Quantitative assessment by Doppler echocardiography of pulmonary or aortic regurgitation. Am J Cardiol 1985;56:131.

21. Helbing WA, Niezen RA, Le Cessie S, et al: Right ventricular diastolic function in children with pulmonary regurgitation after repair of tetralogy of Fallot: Volumetric evaluation by magnetic resonance velocity mapping. J Am Coll Cardiol 1996;28:1827.

22. Helbing WA, de Roos A: Optimal imaging in assessment of right ventricular function in tetralogy of Fallot with pulmonary regurgitation. Am J Cardiol 1998;82:1561.

23. Davos CH, Davlouros PA, Wensel R, et al: Global impairment of cardiac autonomic nervous activity late after repair of tetralogy of Fallot. Circulation 2002;106:I69.

24. Bolger AP, Sharma R, Li W, et al: Neurohormonal activation and the chronic heart failure syndrome in adults with congenital heart disease. Circulation 2002;106:92.

25. Gatzoulis MA, Elliott JT, Guru V, et al: Right and left ventricular systolic function late after repair of tetralogy of Fallot. Am J Cardiol 2000;86:1352.

26. Yemets IM, Williams WG, Webb GD, et al: Pulmonary valve replacement late after repair of tetralogy of Fallot. Ann Thorac Surg 1997;64:526.

27. Oechslin EN, Harrison DA, Harris L, et al: Reoperation in adults with repair of tetralogy of Fallot: Indications and outcomes. J Thorac Cardiovasc Surg 1999;118:245.

28. Therrien J, Siu SC, Harris L, et al: Impact of pulmonary valve replacement on arrhythmia propensity late after repair of tetralogy of Fallot. Circulation 2001;103:2489.

29. Caldarone CA, McCrindle BW, Van Arsdell GS, et al: Independent factors associated with longevity of prosthetic pulmonary valves and valved conduits. J Thorac Cardiovasc Surg 2000;120:1022.

30. Balaguer JM, Byrne JG, Cohn LH: Orthotopic pulmonic valve replacement with a pulmonary homograft as an interposition graft. J Card Surg 1996;11:417.

31. Kawachi Y, Masuda M, Tominaga R, et al: Comparative study between St. Jude Medical and bioprosthetic valves in the right side of the heart. Jpn Circ J 1991;55:553.

32. Vliegen HW, van Straten A, de Roos A, et al: Magnetic resonance imaging to assess the hemodynamic effects of pulmonary valve replacement in adults late after repair of tetralogy of Fallot. Circulation 2002;106:1703.

33. Warner KG, Anderson JE, Fulton DR, et al: Restoration of the pulmonary valve reduces right ventricular volume overload after previous repair of tetralogy of Fallot. Circulation 1993;88:II-189.

34. Bove EL, Kavey RE, Byrum CJ, et al: Improved right ventricular function following late pulmonary valve replacement for residual pulmonary insufficiency or stenosis. J Thorac Cardiovasc Surg 1985;90:50.

35. Therrien J, Siu SC, McLaughlin PR, et al: Pulmonary valve replacement in adults late after repair of tetralogy of Fallot: Are we operating too late? J Am Coll Cardiol 2000;36:1670.

36. Bonhoeffer P, Boudjemline Y, Qureshi SA, et al: Percutaneous insertion of the pulmonary valve. J Am Coll Cardiol 2002;39:1664.

37. Keane MG, Wiegers SE, Plappert T, et al: Bicuspid aortic valves are associated with aortic dilatation out of proportion to coexistent valvular lesions. Circulation 2000;102:III-350.

38. Yacoub MH, Khan H, Stavri G, et al: Anatomic correction of the syndrome of prolapsing right coronary aortic cusp, dilatation of the sinus of Valsalva, and ventricular septal defect. J Thorac Cardiovasc Surg 1997;113:253.

39. Kucukoglu S, Ural E, Mutlu H, et al: Ruptured aneurysm of the sinus of Valsalva into the left ventricle: A case report and review of the literature. J Am Soc Echocardiogr 1997;10:862.

40. Yoshida S, Togashi M, Chida A, et al: Ruptured sinus of Valsalva aneurysm into the left ventricle. Jpn Heart J 1978;19:954.

41. Khoshnevis R, Barasch E, Pathan A, et al: Echocardiographic diagnosis of left ventricular outflow tract obstruction caused by an acquired subaortic membrane after mitral valve replacement. J Am Soc Echocardiogr 1999;12:319.

42. Oliver JM, Gonzalez A, Gallego P, et al: Discrete subaortic stenosis in adults: Increased prevalence and slow rate of progression of the obstruction and aortic regurgitation. J Am Coll Cardiol 2001;38:835.

43. Niwa K, Siu SC, Webb GD, et al: Progressive aortic root dilatation in adults late after repair of tetralogy of Fallot. Circulation 2002;106:1374.

44. Niwa K, Perloff JK, Bhuta SM, et al: Structural abnormalities of great arterial walls in congenital heart disease: Light and electron microscopic analyses. Circulation 2001;103:393.

45. Paparella D, David TE, Armstrong S, et al: Mid-term results of the Ross procedure. J Card Surg 2001;16:338.

46. Bonow RO, Carabello B, de Leon AC, et al: Guidelines for the management of patients with valvular heart disease: A report of the American College of Cardiology/American Heart Association Task Force on Practice Guidelines (Committee on Management of Patients with Valvular Heart Disease). J Am Coll Cardiol 1998;32:1486.

47. Dujardin KS, Enriquez-Sarano M, Schaff HV, et al: Mortality and morbidity of aortic regurgitation in clinical practice: A long-term follow-up study. Circulation 1999;99:1851.

48. Siemienczuk D, Greenberg B, Morris C, et al: Chronic aortic insufficiency: Factors associated with progression to aortic valve replacement. Ann Intern Med 1989;110:587.

49. Bonow RO, Lakatos E, Maron BJ, et al: Serial long-term assessment of the natural history of asymptomatic patients with chronic aortic regurgitation and normal left ventricular systolic function. Circulation 1991;84:1625.

50. Henry WL, Bonow RO, Rosing DR, et al: Observations on the optimum time for operative intervention for aortic regurgitation: II. Serial echocardiographic evaluation of asymptomatic patients. Circulation 1980;61:484.

51. McDonald IG, Jelinek VM: Serial M-mode echocardiography in severe chronic aortic regurgitation. Circulation 1980;62:1291.

52. Bonow RO: Radionuclide angiography in the management of asymptomatic aortic regurgitation. Circulation 1991;84:I-296.

53. Cheitlin MD, Alpert JS, Armstrong WF, et al: ACC/AHA guidelines for the clinical application of echocardiography: A report of the American College of Cardiology/American Heart Association Task Force on Practice Guidelines (Committee on Clinical Application of Echocardiography). Developed in collaboration with the American Society of Echocardiography. Circulation 1997;95:1686.

54. Borer JS, Bacharach SL, Green MV, et al: Exercise-induced left ventricular dysfunction in symptomatic and asymptomatic patients with aortic regurgitation: Assessment with radionuclide cineangiography. Am J Cardiol 1978;42:35178.

55. Wilson RA, Greenberg BH, Massie BM, et al: Left ventricular response to submaximal and maximal exercise in asymptomatic aortic regurgitation. Am J Cardiol 1988;62:606.

56. Levine HJ, Gaasch WH: Vasoactive drugs in chronic regurgitant lesions of the mitral and aortic valves. J Am Coll Cardiol 1996;28:1083.

57. Scognamiglio R, Rahimtoola SH, Fasoli G, et al: Nifedipine in asymptomatic patients with severe aortic regurgitation and normal left ventricular function. N Engl J Med 1994;331:689.

58. Schon HR, Dorn R, Barthel P, et al: Effects of 12 months quinapril therapy in asymptomatic patients with chronic aortic regurgitation. J Heart Valve Dis 1994;3:500.

59. Alehan D, Ozkutlu S: Beneficial effects of 1-year captopril therapy in children with chronic aortic regurgitation who have no symptoms. Am Heart J 1998;135:598.

60. Shores J, Berger KR, Murphy EA, et al: Progression of aortic dilatation and the benefit of long-term beta-adrenergic blockade in Marfan's syndrome. N Engl J Med 1994;330:1335.

61. Carabello BA, Williams H, Gash AK, et al: Hemodynamic predictors of outcome in patients undergoing valve replacement. Circulation 1986;74:1309.

62. Carabello BA, Usher BW, Hendrix GH, et al: Predictors of outcome for aortic valve replacement in patients with aortic regurgitation and left ventricular dysfunction: A change in the measuring stick. J Am Coll Cardiol 1987;10:991.

63. Tornos MP, Olona M, Permanyer-Miralda G, et al: Clinical outcome of severe asymptomatic chronic aortic regurgitation: A long-term prospective follow-up study. Am Heart J 1995;130:333.

64. Bonow RO, Rosing DR, Kent KM, et al: Timing of operation for chronic aortic regurgitation. Am J Cardiol 1982;50:325.

65. Tornos MP, Olona M, Permanyer-Miralda G, et al: Heart failure after aortic valve replacement for aortic regurgitation: Prospective 20-year study. Am Heart J 1998;136:681.

66. Bonow RO, Nikas D, Elefteriades JA: Valve replacement for regurgitant lesions of the aortic or mitral valve in advanced left ventricular dysfunction. Cardiol Clin 1995;13:73.

67. Takkenberg JJ, Dossche KM, Hazekamp MG, et al: Report of the Dutch experience with the Ross procedure in 343 patients. Eur J Cardiothorac Surg 2002;22:70.

68. Elkins RC: The Ross operation: A 12-year experience. Ann Thorac Surg 1999;68:S14.

69. David TE, Bos J: Aortic valve replacement with stentless porcine aortic valve: A pioneer series. Semin Thorac Cardiovasc Surg 1999;11:9.

70. Gott VL, Greene PS, Alejo DE, et al: Replacement of the aortic root in patients with Marfan's syndrome. N Engl J Med 1999;340:1307.

71. Warnes CA, Child JS: Aortic root dilatation after repair of tetralogy of Fallot: Pathology from the past? Circulation 2002;106:1310.

72. Anderson RH, Ho SH: The anatomy of Ebstein's malformation. In Redington AN, Brawn WJ, Deanfield SE, Anderson RH (eds): The Right Heart in Congenital Heart Disease. London, Greenwich Medical Media LTD, 1998, pp 169-176.

73. van Son JA, Danielson GK, Schaff HV, et al: Traumatic tricuspid valve insufficiency: Experience in thirteen patients. J Thorac Cardiovasc Surg 1994;108:893.

74. Waller BF, Moriarty AT, Eble JN, et al: Etiology of pure tricuspid regurgitation based on anular circumference and leaflet area: Analysis of 45 necropsy patients with clinical and morphologic evidence of pure tricuspid regurgitation. J Am Coll Cardiol 1986;7:1063.

75. Benson LN, Child JS, Schwaiger M, et al: Left ventricular geometry and function in adults with Ebstein's anomaly of the tricuspid valve. Circulation 1987;75:353.

76. Celermajer DS, Dodd SM, Greenwald SE, et al: Morbid anatomy in neonates with Ebstein's anomaly of the tricuspid valve: Pathophysiologic and clinical implications. J Am Coll Cardiol 1992;19:1049.

77. Lev M, Liberthson RR, Joseph RH, et al: The pathologic anatomy of Ebstein's disease. Arch Pathol 1970;90:334.

78. Zuberbuhler JR, Allwork SP, Anderson RH: The spectrum of Ebstein's anomaly of the tricuspid valve. J Thorac Cardiovasc Surg 1979;77:202.

79. Anderson KR, Zuberbuhler JR, Anderson RH, et al: Morphologic spectrum of Ebstein's anomaly of the heart: A review. Mayo Clin Proc 1979;54:174.

80. Celermajer DS, Cullen S, Sullivan ID, et al: Outcome in neonates with Ebstein's anomaly. J Am Coll Cardiol 1992;19:1041.

81. Roberson DA, Silverman NH: Ebstein's anomaly: Echocardiographic and clinical features in the fetus and neonate. J Am Coll Cardiol 1989;14:1300.

82. Celermajer DS, Bull C, Till JA, et al: Ebstein's anomaly: Presentation and outcome from fetus to adult. J Am Coll Cardiol 1994;23:170.

83. Watson H: Natural history of Ebstein's anomaly of tricuspid valve in childhood and adolescence: An international co-operative study of 505 cases. Br Heart J 1974;36:417.

84. Cappato R, Schluter M, Weiss C, et al: Radiofrequency current catheter ablation of accessory atrioventricular pathways in Ebstein's anomaly. Circulation 1996;94:376.

85. Theodoro DA, Danielson GK, Porter CJ, et al: Right-sided maze procedure for right atrial arrhythmias in congenital heart disease. Ann Thorac Surg 1998;65:149.

86. Gentles TL, Calder AL, Clarkson PM, et al: Predictors of long-term survival with Ebstein's anomaly of the tricuspid valve. Am J Cardiol 1992;69:377.

87. Mair DD, Seward JB, Driscoll DJ, et al: Surgical repair of Ebstein's anomaly: Selection of patients and early and late operative results. Circulation 1985;72:II-70.

88. Hardy KL, May IA, Webster CA, et al: Ebstein's anomaly: A functional concept and successful definite repair. J Thorac Cardiovasc Surg 1964;48:927.

89. Carpentier A, Chauvaud S, Mace L, et al: A new reconstructive operation for Ebstein's anomaly of the tricuspid valve. J Thorac Cardiovasc Surg 1988;96:92.

90. Danielson GK, Fuster V: Surgical repair of Ebstein's anomaly. Ann Surg 1982;196:499.

91. Augustin N, Schmidt-Habelmann P, Wottke M, et al: Results after surgical repair of Ebstein's anomaly. Ann Thorac Surg 1997;63:1650.

92. Lambertz H, Minale C, Flachskampf FA, et al: Long-term follow-up after Carpentier tricuspid valvuloplasty. Am Heart J 1989;117:615.

93. Bajzer CT, Stewart WJ, Cosgrove DM, et al: Tricuspid valve surgery and intraoperative echocardiography: Factors affecting survival, clinical outcome, and echocardiographic success. J Am Coll Cardiol 1998;32:1023.

94. De Simone R, Lange R, Tanzeem A, et al: Adjustable tricuspid valve annuloplasty assisted by intraoperative transesophageal color Doppler echocardiography. Am J Cardiol 1993;71:926.

95. Van Nooten GJ, Caes F, Taeymans Y, et al: Tricuspid valve replacement: Postoperative and long-term results. J Thorac Cardiovasc Surg 1995;110:672.

96. Rizzoli G, De Perini L, Bottio T, et al: Prosthetic replacement of the tricuspid valve: Biological or mechanical? Ann Thorac Surg 1998;66:S62.

97. Scully HE, Armstrong CS: Tricuspid valve replacement: Fifteen years of experience with mechanical prostheses and bioprostheses. J Thorac Cardiovasc Surg 1995;109:1035.

98. Ratnatunga CP, Edwards MB, Dore CJ, et al: Tricuspid valve replacement: UK Heart Valve Registry mid-term results comparing mechanical and biological prostheses. Ann Thorac Surg 1998;66:1940.

99. Kiziltan HT, Theodoro DA, Warnes CA, et al: Late results of bioprosthetic tricuspid valve replacement in Ebstein's anomaly. Ann Thorac Surg 1998;66:1539.

100. Kawano H, Oda T, Fukunaga S, et al: Tricuspid valve replacement with the St. Jude Medical valve: 19 years of experience. Eur J Cardiothorac Surg 2000;18:565.

101. Chauvaud S, Fuzellier JF, Berrebi A, et al: Bi-directional cavopulmonary shunt associated with ventriculo and valvuloplasty in Ebstein's anomaly: Benefits in high risk patients. Eur J Cardiothorac Surg 1998;13:514.

102. Starnes VA, Pitlick PT, Bernstein D, et al: Ebstein's anomaly appearing in the neonate: A new surgical approach. J Thorac Cardiovasc Surg 1991;101:1082.

103. Freed LA, Levy D, Levine RA, et al: Prevalence and clinical outcome of mitral-valve prolapse. N Engl J Med 1999;341:1.

104. Takeuchi S, Imamura H, Katsumoto K, et al: New surgical method for repair of anomalous left coronary artery from pulmonary artery. J Thorac Cardiovasc Surg 1979;78:7.

105. Huddleston CB, Balzer DT, Mendeloff EN: Repair of anomalous left main coronary artery arising from the pulmonary artery in infants: Long-term impact on the mitral valve. Ann Thorac Surg 2001;71:1985.

106. Schwartz ML, Jonas RA, Colan SD: Anomalous origin of left coronary artery from pulmonary artery: Recovery of left ventricular function after dual coronary repair. J Am Coll Cardiol 1997;30:547.

107. Krishnan US, Gersony WM, Berman-Rosenzweig E, et al: Late left ventricular function after surgery for children with chronic symptomatic mitral regurgitation. Circulation 1997;96:4280.

108. Delahaye JP, Gare JP, Viguier E, et al: Natural history of severe mitral regurgitation. Eur Heart J 1991;12:5.

109. Otto CM: Clinical practice: Evaluation and management of chronic mitral regurgitation. N Engl J Med 2001;345:740.

110. Schon HR, Schroter G, Barthel P, et al: Quinapril therapy in patients with chronic mitral regurgitation. J Heart Valve Dis 1994;3:303.

111. Yoran C, Yellin EL, Becker RM, et al: Mechanism of reduction of mitral regurgitation with vasodilator therapy. Am J Cardiol 1979;43:773.

112. Crawford MH, Souchek J, Oprian CA, et al: Determinants of survival and left ventricular performance after mitral valve replacement. Department of Veterans Affairs Cooperative Study on Valvular Heart Disease. Circulation 1990;81:1173.

113. Enriquez-Sarano M, Tajik AJ, Schaff HV, et al: Echocardiographic prediction of left ventricular function after correction of mitral regurgitation: Results and clinical implications. J Am Coll Cardiol 1994;24:1536.

114. Tribouilloy CM, Enriquez-Sarano M, Schaff HV, et al: Impact of preoperative symptoms on survival after surgical correction of organic mitral regurgitation: Rationale for optimizing surgical indications. Circulation 1999;99:400.

115. Starling MR, Kirsh MM, Montgomery DG, et al: Impaired left ventricular contractile function in patients with long-term mitral regurgitation and normal ejection fraction. J Am Coll Cardiol 1993;22:239.

116. Ling LH, Enriquez-Sarano M, Seward JB, et al: Clinical outcome of mitral regurgitation due to flail leaflet. N Engl J Med 1996;335:1417.

117. Ross J Jr: Afterload mismatch in aortic and mitral valve disease: Implications for surgical therapy. J Am Coll Cardiol 1985;5:811.

118. Schlant RC: Timing of surgery for patients with nonischemic severe mitral regurgitation. Circulation 1999;99:338.

119. Enriquez-Sarano M, Schaff HV, Orszulak TA, et al: Valve repair improves the outcome of surgery for mitral regurgitation: A multivariate analysis. Circulation 1995;91:1022.

120. Corin WJ, Sutsch G, Murakami T, et al: Left ventricular function in chronic mitral regurgitation: Preoperative and postoperative comparison. J Am Coll Cardiol 1995;25:113.

121. David TE, Uden DE, Strauss HD: The importance of the mitral apparatus in left ventricular function after correction of mitral regurgitation. Circulation 1983;68:II-76.

122. Horskotte D, Schulte HD, Bircks W, et al: The effect of chordal preservation on late outcome after mitral valve replacement: A randomized study. J Heart Valve Dis 1993;2:150.

123. Rieder E, Seebacher G, Kasimir MT, et al: Tissue engineering of heart valves: Decellularized porcine and human valve scaffolds differ importantly in residual potential to attract monocytic cells. Circulation 2005;[Epub].

CHAPTER 22
Valvular Stenosis and Heart Failure

Wanda C. Miller-Hance

Valvular stenoses comprise a spectrum of abnormalities that impair ventricular filling or ejection, may alter hemodynamics significantly, and may have a profound impact on the physiology of affected children. These lesions may be congenital, acquired, or the result of prior surgical interventions. By compromising the ability of the individual to generate an adequate cardiac output to meet the systemic circulatory demands, valvular obstruction imparts a hemodynamic burden on the heart and may lead to right, left, or biventricular heart failure (Table 22-1). This chapter focuses on the cardiovascular malformations most commonly associated with valvular stenosis in the pediatric age group that lead to impaired heart function. Emphasis is on the pathophysiology of these lesions, the roles of diagnostic modalities, and medical and surgical management strategies in children and young adults. Although valvular obstruction is the subject of this chapter and other valvular pathologies are discussed elsewhere (see Chapter 21), it is important to consider that concomitant stenotic and regurgitant disease may be present in some children.

PULMONARY STENOSIS

Anatomic Considerations

Pulmonary valve stenosis is the predominant pathology in patients with right ventricular outflow tract (RVOT) obstruction (accounting for >80% of all lesions). Most cases are congenital in nature. Other, less common malformations that result in obstruction to pulmonary blood flow include infundibular pathology, muscle bundles within the body of the right ventricle, and alterations in the architecture of the pulmonary arterial bed. These lesions may be found in isolation or occur as part of more complex malformations; in tetralogy of Fallot, various anatomic levels of RVOT obstruction are encountered.

Pulmonary valve stenosis is reported in approximately 10% of patients with congenital heart disease.[1] In isolated or classic pulmonary valve stenosis, findings include systolic valvar doming, varying degrees of leaflet tethering and thickening, and commissural fusion resulting in the formation of peripheral raphes and narrowing of the valve. In the uncomplicated or pure form of pulmonary stenosis, the ventricular septum is intact. An interatrial communication in the form of a patent foramen ovale or secundum atrial septal defect is frequently identified. In a few patients (approximately 20% of all cases of pulmonary valve stenosis), a variant characterized by valvar dysplasia is recognized.[2] In this variant there is marked thickening of the valvar cusps, myxomatous or mucoid degeneration, and

TABLE 22-1

Pathophysiologic Alterations Associated with Valvar Stenosis	
Pulmonary stenosis	Systolic pressure gradient between right ventricle and pulmonary artery
	Impaired right ventricular emptying
	Right ventricular hypertension
	Right ventricular hypertrophy
	Tricuspid regurgitation
	Right atrial dilation
	Cyanosis in the presence of an interatrial communication
	Decreased stroke volume and cardiac output
Aortic stenosis	Systolic pressure gradient between left ventricle and aorta
	Increased left ventricular afterload
	Impaired left ventricular emptying
	Increased wall stress
	Left ventricular hypertrophy
	Increased end-systolic volume
	Increased end-diastolic volume
	Increased left ventricular end-systolic pressure
	Impaired coronary blood flow
	Decreased stroke volume and cardiac output
Tricuspid stenosis	Diastolic pressure gradient between right atrium and right ventricle
	Right atrial hypertension
	Cyanosis in the presence of an interatrial communication
	Systemic venous congestion
	Reduced right ventricular preload
	Decreased stroke volume and cardiac output
Mitral stenosis	Diastolic pressure gradient between left atrium and left ventricle
	Increased left atrial pressure
	Impaired left ventricular filling
	Decreased left ventricular end-diastolic volume
	Increased pulmonary venous and arterial pressures
	Decreased stroke volume and cardiac output

minimal if any commissural fusion.[2,3] In these patients, narrowing of the sinotubular junction, annular hypoplasia, short main pulmonary artery segment, and stenoses of the branched pulmonary arteries are commonly observed. The dysplastic valve is associated with Noonan syndrome.[3-7]

Neonates with **critical pulmonary stenosis**, the most severe form of pulmonary valve stenosis in infancy, display fused raphes associated with a restrictive eccentric pin-sized opening, significant degrees of right ventricular hypertrophy and either functional or anatomic hypoplasia. Tricuspid valve abnormalities are a common association. Endocardial fibrosis with or without right ventricular infarction also may be present.[8] **Infundibular stenosis** as an isolated entity occurs rarely. This lesion is characterized by pure fibromuscular narrowing of the subpulmonary infundibulum, creating a RVOT gradient. Occasionally, infundibular obstruction of the dynamic type may be seen after the relief of valvar stenosis, so-called suicide right ventricle; this is a consequence of the acute decrease in right ventricular afterload and the associated right ventricular hypertrophy.[9] The pathology in **double-chambered right ventricle**, a relatively rare anomaly that accounts for approximately 1% of all cases of congenital heart disease, is characterized by the presence of anomalous muscle bundles within the trabecular component of the right ventricle.[10] The result is the division of the right ventricle into two components, one high-pressure chamber proximal to the obstruction and a distal low-pressure compartment.[11] A ventricular septal defect is a commonly associated defect.[12,13] The RVOT obstruction in double-chambered right ventricle is considered by most investigators to be an acquired condition. **Branched or peripheral pulmonary artery stenosis** may occur in isolation or more commonly in association with other complex forms of structural heart disease. This condition is identified in 2% to 3% of patients with congenital heart disease. Peripheral pulmonary artery stenosis also may be a feature of syndromes such as congenital rubella, Noonan, Alagille, Williams, and cutis laxa. The obstruction may affect a single site, but multiple vessels are involved in most cases. The pathologic spectrum varies from discrete obstruction to more extensive vascular hypoplasia. The level of obstruction may be located anywhere from the proximal pulmonary bifurcation to regions within the subsegmental or more distal pulmonary arteries.

Basic Pathophysiology

The magnitude of RVOT obstruction in patients with pulmonary valve stenosis is related directly to the degree of valvar narrowing. The main pathophysiologic consequence is an elevation of right ventricular pressures, and the systolic pressure generated by the right ventricle may exceed that of the left ventricle. This situation results in pathologic alterations of the right-sided cardiac structures. Right ventricular hypertrophy, as a result of the chronically increased afterload, serves as a compensatory mechanism to maintain right ventricular output. If the infundibular region participates in the hypertrophic response, there is further aggravation of the outflow obstruction. This further aggravation also may contribute to a reduction in the right ventricular cavity size in severe cases.

In right-sided obstructive lesions, right ventricular dilation rather than hypertrophy occasionally may result from an increased afterload, eventually culminating in right ventricular dysfunction and heart failure. In addition, ventricular interdependence may affect left ventricular performance and lead to biventricular failure. Structural changes in the tricuspid valve lead to functional abnormalities, such as tricuspid regurgitation and associated right atrial dilation. Diminished right ventricular **compliance** in neonates with critical pulmonary stenosis and severe chamber hypertrophy is likely to be associated with diastolic dysfunction. Subendocardial ischemia resulting in myocardial infarction and fibrosis and the associated hypoxia may account for systolic impairment and eventual chamber dilation and congestive heart failure.[8] The presence of cyanosis in patients with RVOT obstruction usually reflects interatrial right-to-left shunting and reduced pulmonary blood flow; this is seen in association with severe right ventricular hypertrophy, fibrosis, or ventricular dysfunction.

Clinical Presentation

In general, mild-to-moderate degrees of valvar obstruction result in minimal or no symptoms, although this also may be the case in patients with severe obstruction. Most children present for evaluation of a cardiac murmur. Cyanosis suggests severe obstruction in association with an interatrial communication; this is a common presenting feature in infants with critical disease. In older children, symptoms associated with compromised cardiac output include dyspnea on exertion and fatigue. Chest pain and syncope are unusual findings. Overt right heart failure in the absence of significant tricuspid insufficiency is relatively uncommon in children because adequate stroke volume and cardiac output are maintained at the expense of right ventricular hypertrophy. In the current era, survival of children into adolescence and adulthood is the expectation.[14] Decompensation may occur in an adult with chronic severe obstruction with the development of right ventricular dilation or a reduction in cardiac output. Right ventricular failure in patients with more than moderate obstruction and no intervention generally occurs beyond the fourth decade and may be precipitated by rhythm disorders.[15]

Clinical Evaluation

In pulmonary valve stenosis, S_1 is usually normal. Auscultation is characterized by a harsh crescendo-decrescendo systolic murmur heard best at the upper left sternal border. The murmur may radiate to the back.

Occasionally an ejection click may be audible, but this finding is absent in supravalvar or subvalvar pathology. Findings consistent with severe valvar obstruction include a loud late peaking murmur and wide splitting of S_2 related to delayed pulmonary valve closure. In contrast to the fixed splitting of S_2 encountered in patients with an atrial septal defect, in pulmonary stenosis, respiratory variation is present. A tricuspid regurgitant murmur also may be appreciated. A thrill along the pulmonary outflow tract and a right ventricular heave over the precordium may be palpable.

The **ECG** may assist in the assessment of the severity of the outflow obstruction. A normal tracing is seen in nearly one half of patients with mild stenosis. Subtle findings include a right ventricular conduction delay and slight rightward deviation of the frontal plane QRS axis. With moderate or severe obstruction, an abnormal ECG is frequently the case. Features of moderate disease include right-axis deviation of the frontal plane QRS axis, prominent right-sided forces as suggested by an R-to-S ratio in the right precordium of 4:1, and R waves typically less than 20 mm. Severe pulmonary stenosis is associated with a right-axis or extreme right-axis deviation of the mean frontal QRS axis; a pure R, Rs, or qR pattern in the right chest leads; an R wave exceeding 20 mm in amplitude; and T wave inversion in the right precordial leads consistent with a strain pattern. Occasional ST changes suggesting ischemia have been identified. Tall, peaked P waves in lead II and the right precordial leads indicate associated right atrial enlargement.

The **chest radiograph** shows a normal cardiac contour in mild cases of valvar pulmonary stenosis. Poststenotic dilation results in a prominent main pulmonary trunk in most patients with valvar obstruction. Dilation of the left pulmonary artery also may be seen. A prominent right heart border related to right atrial dilation is observed in some patients. Normal pulmonary vascularity accompanied by a normal heart size is the rule except for rare cases of severe obstruction and associated cardiac decompensation. Cardiomegaly is present with pulmonary stenosis significant enough to cause tricuspid regurgitation or congestive heart failure.

Two-dimensional **echocardiography** and spectral and color flow Doppler mapping are routinely used to characterize the pathology and define the level and severity of obstruction. In valvar pathology, thickening of the leaflets, doming, and restricted systolic excursion may be appreciated. Valvar dysplasia is characterized by marked leaflet deformity and thickening.[16] Assessment of the main and branched pulmonary arteries for poststenotic dilation is feasible. In addition, associated pathology, such as narrowing of the sinotubular junction, may be readily identified. A complete examination includes assessment of the subpulmonary region; tricuspid and pulmonary valve competency; integrity and position of the interatrial septum; shape of the ventricular septum; and right ventricular size, function, and wall thickness. The size of the pulmonary annulus and degree of annular or pulmonary artery hypoplasia are determined. Interrogation of the proximal branch pulmonary arteries is generally possible, but distal assessment requires other imaging modalities, such as angiography or MRI.

Doppler echocardiography allows for quantitation of the transvalvar pressure gradient. The instantaneous pressure gradient across the pulmonary valve can be obtained by application of the modified Bernoulli equation (pressure gradient in mm Hg = 4 × squared peak Doppler velocity across the pulmonary valve). In cases of associated intracardiac shunting, this gradient may be exaggerated by the increased pulmonary blood flow. It is important to consider that gradients derived from Doppler echocardiography represent instantaneous gradients rather than peak-to-peak gradients measured at cardiac catheterization. These differences are not of great significance in this pathology, however, as they may be for aortic stenosis. In general, Doppler-derived estimates of pulmonary stenosis correlate well with pressure gradients measured at cardiac catheterization.[17] The right ventricular systolic pressure also can be predicted from the tricuspid regurgitation jet velocity.[18] Late diastolic forward pulmonary flow detected by Doppler echocardiography that occurs during atrial systole suggests restrictive right ventricular physiology and is associated with a hypertrophied, noncompliant right ventricle.

Exercise intolerance may be present in severe pulmonary stenosis and in patients who have undergone late intervention.[19,20] Formal **exercise testing** has not played a significant role in the clinical evaluation or follow-up of these patients and currently is not routinely used.

MRI provides detailed anatomic information and may aid in the evaluation of the location of the right ventricular obstruction, size of the right ventricle and main and branched pulmonary arteries, and determination of associated lesions. Functional assessment of the right ventricular myocardium also is feasible with quantitation of right ventricular volumes and ejection fraction. Most importantly, this modality may be particularly useful in the evaluation of distal pulmonary arterial pathology.

Most patients with pulmonary valvar stenosis currently undergo **cardiac catheterization** for therapeutic purposes because echocardiography allows for detailed definition of the anatomy and hemodynamics in most cases. Typical findings include elevation of the right ventricular systolic pressure in the presence of normal pulmonary artery pressures. The right ventricular end-diastolic pressure is usually normal, but may be elevated in cases of severe right ventricular obstruction or dysfunction. The determination of the transvalvar gradient, extent of right ventricular systolic hypertension, and ratio between the right and left ventricular systolic pressures

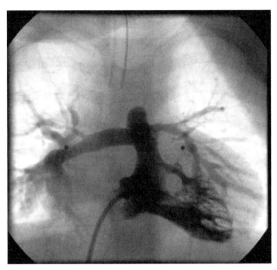

FIGURE 22-1 ■ Peripheral pulmonary artery stenosis. Pulmonary artery angiogram in the anteroposterior projection shows diffuse left pulmonary artery hypoplasia and multiple areas of narrowing throughout the pulmonary vasculature consistent with peripheral pulmonary artery stenoses.

establishes the degree and severity of the obstruction. Right ventricular angiocardiography in multiple projections defines the location of the obstruction, right ventricular size, and associated abnormalities. Angiographic delineation of obstructive pathology in the distal pulmonary arterial bed has been the standard diagnostic modality (Fig. 22-1). In the presence of an interatrial communication and moderate-to-severe right ventricular obstruction, bidirectional atrial level shunting may be observed. This shunting also is evident by oxymetric analysis showing left atrial desaturation in the presence of fully saturated pulmonary venous blood.

Therapeutic Strategies

Pulmonary stenosis of mild-to-moderate degree (peak systolic gradient <50 mm Hg) in children is generally well tolerated. Progression in the severity of the obstruction may develop, and careful follow-up is indicated, particularly in young infants. Need for intervention is based on clinical evidence and diagnostic assessment consistent with moderate-to-severe disease even in the absence of symptoms.

Percutaneous balloon valvuloplasty is considered the treatment of choice in patients with isolated valvar pulmonary stenosis.[21-23] Mid-term and long-term outcomes generally have been excellent using this approach.[24-26] Assessment of valve morphology may affect the management plan because dysplastic valves do not consistently respond favorably in the long-term to catheter-based interventions. This relates to the fact that commissural fusion is not a significant component of this pathology. For stenoses in distal locations, balloon angioplasty in combination with **intravascular stenting** plays a particularly important role. Numerous studies have reported on the safety of pulmonary valvuloplasty in children. Serious complications are rare, but pulmonary regurgitation may develop in some cases.[27,28]

Infants with critical pulmonary stenosis who present with cyanosis and ductal dependent pulmonary circulation usually require stabilization and prostaglandin E_1 therapy. Although catheter therapies may lead to effective relief of the obstruction in many cases, factors such as abnormal ventricular morphology, relatively small pulmonary/tricuspid annulus, hypoplasia of the branched pulmonary arteries, interatrial right-to-left shunting, and right ventricular noncompliance may not allow for immediate improvement in pulmonary blood flow in some infants, and discontinuation of prostaglandin infusion may not be possible. In cases of persistent cyanosis, an additional reliable source of pulmonary blood flow is established, usually in the form of a **systemic-to-pulmonary artery shunt.**

Surgical valvotomy or partial/total valvectomy, frequently accompanied by commissurotomy, is indicated for patients with dysplastic valves or patients who had an unfavorable result after balloon valvuloplasty. Although most surgeons prefer a controlled procedure under direct vision, in a few cases a closed technique has been used. Concomitant resection of infundibular obstruction or placement of a transannular patch may be necessary in patients with infundibular hypoplasia. **Valve replacement** with or without a homograft or heterograft conduit also may be required in patients with severe valvar stenosis, near atresia, or coexisting significant valvar regurgitation.

The infundibular hypertrophy that frequently accompanies pulmonary valvar stenosis may regress over time as the obstruction is relieved, and the ventricular myocardium remodels.[9,29,30] Occasionally, there is no regression of this pathology, or the obstruction may increase. In some cases, short-term β **blockade** has been recommended if a dynamic component of subvalvar obstruction becomes manifest after the relief of the valve stenosis.

AORTIC STENOSIS

Anatomic Considerations

Obstruction to left ventricular outflow can occur at the level of the aortic valve, above the valve (supravalvar), or below the valve (subvalvar). This obstruction may occur in isolation or as part of complex heart disease (e.g., Shone association, interrupted aortic arch). The pathology in most patients with left ventricular outflow tract obstruction involves stenosis of the aortic valve (one third to three quarters of patients), and numerous morphologic subtypes have been identified in aortic valve disease. Male gender predominance is recognized in this condition.

Abnormalities that account for **aortic valve stenosis** include annular hypoplasia, alteration in the number of leaflets and commissures, and abnormal valve mobility;

this represents approximately 3% to 5% of all patients with congenital heart disease.[31-33] The bicuspid or bicommissural aortic valve is the most common valvar anomaly and variant of congenital aortic valve stenosis.[34] This anomaly also is reported to be the most frequent of all congenital cardiac malformations and is known to occur in approximately 2% of the general population.[35] Familial clustering of aortic valve disease has been reported.[36,37] The pathology is frequently the result of commissural fusion leading to the finding of a raphe or "false" commissure. In most cases, the affected (deficient or absent commissure) involves the intercoronary commissure. This abnormality does not imply valvar stenosis. A bicuspid aortic valve may be found in asymptomatic individuals, within the context of associated left ventricular obstructive lesions, or as part of the spectrum of left ventricular hypoplasia. The prevalence of associated defects is relatively high ($\leq 20\%$) and frequently includes patent ductus arteriosus, aortic coarctation, and ventricular septal defect. Acquired aortic stenosis can be secondary to rheumatic heart disease with adhesion and fusion of the commissures and cusps. In adults, calcific degenerative aortic stenosis is a common cause of aortic stenosis.

Critical aortic stenosis is considered to be part of the spectrum of hypoplastic left heart syndrome. Ill neonates with this condition exhibit a primitive, malformed, thick, frequently unicuspid aortic valve with a restrictive central orifice. The aortic annulus, root, and ascending aorta are typically hypoplastic. In some cases, left ventricular dilation combined with severe systolic dysfunction and mitral regurgitation are seen. Atrophy and infarction of papillary muscles also may occur.[38] Varying degrees of left ventricular chamber underdevelopment, mitral and aortic arch hypoplasia, and endocardial fibroelastosis are observed in other infants. The endocardial pathology represents intrauterine fibrotic alterations to the left ventricular wall resulting from compromised subendocardial oxygen delivery secondary to myocardial ischemia. Aortic stenosis is a common cause of heart failure in infancy and without intervention carries a high mortality rate.[39]

Supravalvar aortic stenosis involves narrowing of the ascending aorta above the level of the aortic valve in the region of the sinotubular junction.[40] This malformation accounts for a few cases (1% to 2%) of aortic obstruction in children. It is considered to be the result of a mutation or alteration of the elastin gene.[41] Supravalvar aortic stenosis may follow an autosomal dominant pattern or may occur as part of Williams syndrome.[42,43] The arteriopathy found in these children also may involve the origin of the coronary arteries or other systemic and pulmonary vessels.[44] Diffuse narrowing of the abdominal aorta may occur in association with renal artery stenosis.

Subvalvar aortic stenosis may take a variety of forms, including a discrete fibromuscular ridge or membrane; a complex, tunnel-like obstruction; and hypertrophy of the interventricular septum as seen in hypertrophic cardiomyopathy. Discrete disease accounts for nearly 10% of cases of aortic outflow obstruction. The lesion typically extends to the base of the aortic leaflets and may involve the mitral valve. The shelf that encircles the outflow tract is considered to be an acquired pathology because it is rare in infancy. Less common forms of subaortic obstruction, such as complex tunnel-like narrowing, are observed in association with other malformations, including annular hypoplasia, aortic stenosis, and posterior malalignment of the ventricular septum (as may be the case in patients with aortic arch interruption).

Basic Pathophysiology

Impedance to left ventricular ejection in aortic stenosis results in elevation of left ventricular systolic pressure and a transvalvar pressure gradient; this leads to increased myocardial force and left ventricular wall stress. The hypertrophic response leads to an unfavorable mass-to-volume ratio, but serves an adaptive mechanism, allowing the left ventricle to generate increased systolic pressure, while normalizing wall stress and maintaining a normal ejection fraction (in accordance with the LaPlace equation). The diastolic compliance of the heart is often abnormal in aortic stenosis due to the increased mass and resultant diastolic stiffness of the ventricle. If the ventricular muscle mass acquisition is not adequate to normalize wall stress (resulting in an afterload mismatch), the muscle fails, and ejection fraction is depressed. Other chronic systemic compensatory responses include systemic vasoconstriction, increased blood volume, and increased heart rate, the last-mentioned leading to decreased diastolic pressure time index of myocardial oxygen supply (the area between the aortic and left ventricular pressure in diastole) (Fig. 22-2).

With chronic obstruction, the hypertrophied myocardium may be at risk for the development of subendocardial ischemia as a consequence of decreased coronary perfusion gradient and an imbalance in the ratio of myocardial oxygen supply and demand. The left atrial *A* wave is large because of increased contraction of a hypertrophied left atrium and decreased compliance of the hypertrophied left ventricle, and the right atrial *A* wave is enlarged because of suboptimal interventricular interaction. In addition, tachycardia results in shortened diastolic filling time, further compromising coronary blood flow in these patients, and may lead to significant myocardial ischemia. Throughout the adaptation process, the left ventricular end-diastolic volume remains normal. In aortic stenosis, factors such as increasing left ventricular afterload, inadequate hypertrophic remodeling (with loss of myofibrils and proliferation of fibroblasts and collagen fibers), and decreased myocardial systolic or diastolic performance may compromise stroke volume and contribute to cardiac

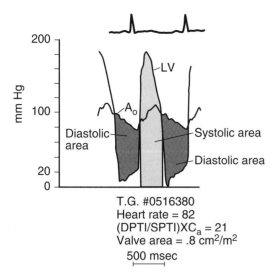

T.G. #0516380
Heart rate = 82
(DPTI/SPTI)XC$_a$ = 21
Valve area = .8 cm^2/m^2

500 msec

FIGURE 22-2 ■ Systolic and diastolic pressure time indices. The pressure curves show calculation for subendocardial flow index. The systolic pressure time index (SPTI) is the area under the left ventricular curve during aortic ejection. The diastolic pressure time index (DPTI) is the area under the aortic curve during the period when the aortic pressure is greater than the left ventricle (LV) minus the left ventricular end-diastolic pressure. The ratio of DPTI × arterial oxygen content to SPTI is proportional to myocardial oxygen consumption. Ao, aorta (From Freed MD: Aortic stenosis. In Allen HD, Clark EB, Gutgesell HP (eds), et al: Moss and Adams Heart Disease in Infants, Children, and Adolescents, 6th ed. Philadelphia, Lippincott Williams & Wilkins, 2001, p. 972.)

stenosis may increase with age, leading to clinical significance in adulthood or with advanced age. The most common symptoms during childhood are easy fatigue and dyspnea. Angina, chest pain, or syncope suggests significant pathology as the result of compromised coronary and systemic blood flow. Only 10% of patients with aortic stenosis develop clinical evidence of congestive heart failure early in life[45]; this is manifested by tachypnea, poor feeding, diaphoresis with feeds, failure to thrive, and hepatomegaly.

Aortic stenosis in the fetus frequently is associated with cardiac dysfunction and may lead to hydrops in some cases (see Chapter 25).[46-48] The hydrops is a consequence of ongoing subendocardial ischemia and severe myocardial dysfunction. A neonate with critical disease may exhibit signs and symptoms of severe heart failure or shock. Ductal dependency for systemic blood flow is a common feature in these neonates. Heart failure symptoms, such as dyspnea, hepatomegaly, and a gallop rhythm, may be prominent. A low cardiac output state characterized by poor peripheral perfusion, paleness, cool extremities, and lactic acidemia also may be present. Severe ventricular dilation and dysfunction often accompany the clinical presentation. In some neonates, papillary muscle infarction is part of the presentation.[49] Without intervention, the mortality rate for critical aortic valve stenosis is invariably high.

dysfunction and heart failure. The overall effects of aortic stenosis lead to increased myocardial oxygen consumption with decreased myocardial oxygen supply and ultimately myocardial ischemia, left ventricular systolic and diastolic dysfunction, and heart failure.

Aortic stenosis is a relatively common cause of heart failure in infancy. In the case of multiple sequential obstructions, although the magnitude of the obstruction may not be severe at any particular level, the combined effect of the pathologies may be clinically relevant and result in heart failure symptoms. Aortic stenosis in the neonatal period occurring in conjunction with endocardial fibroelastosis and left ventricular dilation and dysfunction carries a poor prognosis. The fibrotic myocardial changes lead to severe impairment of systolic and diastolic ventricular function and marked elevations of left ventricular end-diastolic and left atrial pressures. The physiologic alterations in these patients are complex and affect not only the cardiovascular system, but also other major organs.

Clinical Presentation

The morphologic diversity of aortic valve stenosis accounts for its variable presentation. Children with a bicuspid aortic valve or mild aortic valvar stenosis are generally asymptomatic, and growth and development are usually normal. This anomaly may go unrecognized or present as an incidental heart murmur. The severity of

Clinical Evaluation

In young infants with aortic stenosis, a hyperactive precordium, gallop rhythm, and right ventricular tap may be noted. On auscultation, a systolic ejection murmur is detected at the upper right sternal border that may be accompanied by an ejection click. The murmur is often harsh and of loud intensity radiating to the neck or suprasternal notch. The intensity and duration of the murmur may not correlate with the severity of the obstruction; if the obstruction is severe, the murmur may be minimal or even inaudible because there may be associated ventricular dysfunction and compromised cardiac output. Findings associated with moderate disease include a reduction in the pulse pressure (with slow rise in arterial pulse) and respiratory influence in the splitting of S$_2$.[50] In small infants, the **ECG** frequently displays criteria consistent with right ventricular hypertrophy (e.g., upright T waves, voltage criteria). T wave inversion, characteristic of a strain pattern, and ST-segment changes across the precordial leads are common. Older infants and children with severe stenosis show abnormally high R wave amplitudes in the left precordial leads and deep S waves over the right precordium consistent with left ventricular hypertrophy; this generally occurs in severe outflow obstruction. The presence of Q waves may suggest myocardial ischemia resulting from increased myocardial stress and subendocardial ischemia from the increased wall thickness. Atrial enlargement (right or left) may be seen. ECG findings may not always correlate with the severity of the disease, but progressive ECG changes usually reflect an increasing outflow gradient.

The **chest radiograph** findings in valvar aortic stenosis are age dependent. Although cardiomegaly is a frequent occurrence in patients with aortic stenosis who present in infancy, it is an uncommon finding in older children, in whom the heart size is normal to minimally enlarged. A cardiac silhouette showing rounding of the left heart border is consistent with left ventricular hypertrophy, and poststenotic dilation of the ascending aorta is frequently noted. An enlarged cardiac silhouette in older children suggests hemodynamic decompensation and the development of myocardial failure. Left atrial enlargement is consistent with severe pathology. Pulmonary vascular markings may be normal or increased. Frank pulmonary edema is found most commonly in infants with critical disease.

The **echocardiogram** in aortic stenosis provides detailed two-dimensional information of the aortic valve morphology. The parasternal long-axis and short-axis views in valvar aortic stenosis show abnormalities in the number and size of the valve cusps, abnormalities in the degrees of commissural fusion, and altered systolic excursion or doming. Inspection of the ascending aorta may show poststenotic dilation. Multiple levels of obstruction as seen in the Shone complex may not allow for the accurate determination of the severity of coexistent aortic valve disease. In patients with supravalvar aortic stenosis, an hourglass deformity of the ascending aorta is identified just above the level of the sinuses of Valsalva. In some cases, the area of narrowing may be diffuse and extend to the levels of the distal ascending aorta and arch vessels. Relevant data in all patients with ventricular outflow tract obstruction include assessment of left ventricular size and function, degree of wall thickness, and associated pathology (e.g., aortic regurgitation, mitral valve dysfunction, hypoplasia of left-sided structures, aortic arch obstruction). Measurements typically are performed in two planes, and the data are related to normal values for body surface area (Z-scores). In most patients with congenital valvar stenosis outside of the neonatal period, hyperdynamic systolic function is identified. Inspection of the endocardial surface and papillary muscles is important in infants with critical stenosis.

Spectral Doppler and color flow mapping allows for determination of the level and severity of the obstruction and is an important diagnostic tool in the initial assessment and follow-up of these patients. Disturbed aliased flow that originates at the level of the valve is characteristic of aortic valve disease. The gradient obtained by Doppler echocardiography reflects the peak instantaneous pressure difference, whereas the gradient measured at catheterization represents the peak-to-peak pressure gradient. It is well established that Doppler-derived mean gradients have a better correlation to transvalvar gradients obtained in the cardiac catheterization laboratory.[51] Alterations in cardiac output, catecholamine level, and sedation state may affect the measurement of valve gradients. In the presence of severe left ventricular dysfunction and reduced cardiac output, Doppler velocities may be normal or minimally increased and may not reflect the severity of the obstruction. This also may be the case in neonates with ductal patency or a substantial intracardiac shunt and relatively reduced forward flow across the aortic valve. Estimates of aortic valve area may be obtained from planimetry or by application of the continuity equation. New echocardiographic approaches using Doppler tissue imaging and myocardial strain rate may provide further insight in the quantitative assessment of ventricular function in these patients.[52-54] Although the identification of critical obstruction is feasible by fetal echocardiography, the impact of prenatal diagnosis on postnatal outcome has not been entirely defined.

Exercise testing in patients with aortic stenosis provides useful information during follow-up and objective evidence of the degree of obstruction. Parameters considered as potential correlates of the severity of the disease include symptoms, duration of exercise, systolic blood pressure changes, ventricular ectopy, and degree of ST-segment depression. Progressive increments in stroke volume associated with exertion lead to significant increases in the left ventricular outflow gradients.

The usefulness of **MRI** has been reported in the evaluation of patients with Shone complex and aortic stenosis and in the functional evaluation of valvular heart disease.[55-57] This imaging approach also may be beneficial in children with supravalvar obstruction in further delineating the anatomy (Fig. 22-3). More recent studies document the reliability and reproducibility of this modality in the determination of valve area in adults with aortic valve stenosis.[58,59]

Cardiac catheterization is used primarily as a therapeutic modality in patients with evidence of severe obstruction as suggested by symptoms, physical examination, and other diagnostic studies. The v wave of the left atrial pressure wave is usually the tallest in normal subjects, but the a wave is the predominant wave in patients with aortic stenosis secondary to decreased left ventricular compliance. Access into the left ventricle for determination of the ventricular to aortic pressure gradient is accomplished either in a prograde fashion by crossing an existing interatrial communication or using the transseptal approach or via the retrograde route. As in the case of echocardiography, pressure measurements may underestimate the severity of the pathology in conditions of low cardiac output, intracardiac shunts, and ductal patency with right-to-left shunting. Biplane left ventricular angiography shows the aortic jet and the valvar abnormalities. Any associated aortic regurgitation most commonly is determined angiographically after contrast injection into the aortic root. Cardiac output

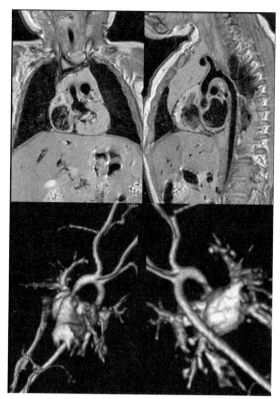

FIGURE 22-3 ■ Supravalvar aortic stenosis. *Top panel,* Coronal *(left)* and sagittal *(right)* spin MRI scans show the characteristic area of narrowing above the sinuses of Valsalva in supravalvar aortic stenosis. The discrete area of obstruction, just distal to the origin of the coronary arteries, is shown. *Bottom panel,* Three-dimensional rendered MRI scans from gadolinium-enhanced contrast injection in two different long-axis projections further define the aortic pathology and the anatomy of surrounding structures. (See also Color Section)

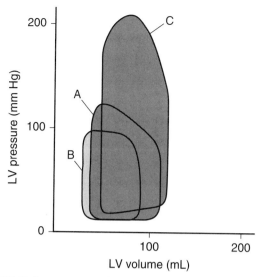

FIGURE 22-4 ■ Pressure volume loops in valvular stenosis. The relationships between left ventricular (LV) pressure and volume in the normal heart *(A)*, mitral stenosis *(B)*, and aortic stenosis *(C)*. (From Jackson JM, Thomas SJ, Lowenstein E: Anesthetic management of patients with valvular heart disease. Semin Anesth 1982;1:239.)

measurements can be obtained, and aortic valve area can be determined.

The use of sophisticated, high-fidelity catheters facilitates the generation of left ventricular pressure and simultaneously recorded volume curves at cardiac catheterization.[60] The pressure volume relationship is influenced greatly by compensatory mechanisms and adaptive responses triggered by the clinical condition. The pressure-volume loop analysis in valvular heart disease provides significant insight into ventricular function, pathophysiology of the disease, and potential therapies (see Chapters 7 and 8) (Fig. 22-4). Despite these benefits, the technical demands of the measurements have hindered the routine clinical application of this technique.

Therapeutic Strategies

All patients with aortic valve disease, including asymptomatic children with a bicuspid aortic valve, require antibiotic prophylaxis in view of the risk of bacterial endocarditis.[61,62] Patients with evidence of mild obstruction merit close follow-up because in a significant number progression of the disease may occur.[63,64]

The symptoms in infants with critical aortic stenosis who present with heart failure and a low output state are likely related to ductal constriction or closure.

Initiation of prostaglandin E_1 therapy in an effort to maintain systemic perfusion via right-to-left ductal shunting may be lifesaving. Concomitant therapy of ill patients frequently includes mechanical ventilatory support to reduce work of breathing, and diuretic therapy and infusion of inotropic agents to augment systemic output.

The medical management of congestive heart failure in children with aortic stenosis is limited and typically has included **diuretic** therapy aimed at reducing cardiac preload and improving symptoms; this should be instituted with caution because a sudden decrease in preload in the face of elevated ventricular end-diastolic pressure may be detrimental. **Digoxin** and **angiotensin-converting enzyme inhibitors** have been used in the ambulatory setting, and inotropic agents and inodilators have been used in hospitalized patients. The potential role of **vasodilator** therapy, traditionally considered contraindicated in patients with severe aortic obstruction, has been examined more recently in critically ill adults with aortic stenosis with favorable results.[65] Concerns regarding the detrimental effects of vasodilator therapy in this setting relate to the potential for acute reductions in systemic vascular resistance without compensatory increases in cardiac output that may result in significant hemodynamic instability. The report noted rapid, marked, and consistent improvement in patients with decompensated heart failure and left ventricular dysfunction as a result of nitroprusside therapy. Whether this favorable response also may be the case in children with aortic stenosis and heart failure remains to be determined.

Numerous publications have documented the usefulness of **percutaneous balloon valvuloplasty** in the management of critically ill infants with aortic stenosis.[66-69]

The benefits of this approach also have been shown in older children and adolescents with moderate-to-severe aortic valve obstruction.[70] The procedure most commonly involves the use of either single or double balloons placed in a retrograde fashion, although the antegrade or prograde approach also has been used.[71] Most interventions have resulted in a significant reduction of gradients with success rates similar to those obtained by means of open surgical valvotomies.[72] Potential complications of catheter-based interventions include bleeding, ventricular dysrhythmias, transient myocardial ischemia during balloon inflation, development of or increase in the severity of aortic regurgitation, and arterial compromise related to vascular access. Complication rates are known to be higher in infants. Although balloon dilation of supravalvar and subvalvar aortic stenoses has been reported, the preferred management strategy is considered by most to be surgical intervention.[73-79]

The surgical approach of aortic valve stenosis is mandated by the anatomic substrate; the size of the aortic annulus, root, and subaortic area; and the associated defects.[80,81] The adequacy of the mitral valve and left ventricle are crucial elements in the decision as to whether a biventricular circulation is achievable in neonates with severe pathology or multiple left-sided obstructions. Although an individualized approach is essential in the care of these patients, numerous factors have been correlated with poor outcomes, including a small left ventricle, hypoplastic mitral/aortic annulus, papillary muscle infarction, and the presence of endocardial fibroelastosis.[38,72,82-84] These variables have been incorporated into scoring systems that may assist in clinical decision making. Many surgical interventions, some of which are now of historic interest, have been used in the management of the heterogeneous group of patients that compose the spectrum of aortic stenosis. These include **aortic valvotomy** (open/closed), left ventricular apex to aortic conduit, **Ross procedure**, **Ross-Konno operation** or other root enlargement procedures, **aortic homograft placement**, Damus-Kaye operation, Norwood palliation, and **valve replacement**.[85-87] Intermediate and long-term outcomes after these procedures are influenced strongly by the initial pathology and severity of the lesion. In a few patients, cardiac transplantation may be the only feasible option. Mechanical circulatory support may be considered at several points during the care of these infants as a bridge to an intervention or for postcardiotomy failure.

Fetal congestive heart failure and hydrops related to critical aortic stenosis present a formidable challenge (see Chapter 25). Transplacental digitalization has been used in this setting with improvement or resolution of the manifestation of heart failure.[88] Some centers have opted for fetal interventions hoping to alter the natural history of this condition in utero and potentially avoid the progression of the disease.[89]

TRICUSPID STENOSIS

Anatomic Considerations

Congenital malformations of the tricuspid valve leading to isolated stenosis are exceedingly rare.[90] Only a few case reports of this anomaly have been published, including one that describes a familial occurrence.[91] Tricuspid stenosis is an extremely rare cause of right-sided heart failure. Variants of this pathology consist of valvar stenosis or hypoplasia of the valvular apparatus.[92] In the case of valvar stenosis, the annulus is of normal or near-normal size, and the leaflets exhibit thickening, commissural fusion, and shortened chordae. Conversely, hypoplasia of the valve apparatus is characterized by a reduced annular size, small but otherwise normal valve leaflets, and support apparatus.

In pediatric patients, tricuspid valve stenosis or hypoplasia occurs most commonly as part of **hypoplastic right heart syndrome** and associated with other structural abnormalities, such as right-sided obstructive lesions. Associated congenital malformations frequently include underdevelopment of the right heart and critical pulmonary stenosis or pulmonary atresia with intact ventricular septum. Some patients with Ebstein anomaly or patients with other forms of valve dysplasia also may exhibit a component of tricuspid stenosis.

In the presence of multivalvar disease, tricuspid stenosis is more likely to occur in association with tricuspid regurgitation than alone. Although the tricuspid valve is the least likely structure to be affected in **rheumatic heart disease**, this accounts for most cases of tricuspid stenosis in older patients. In rare cases, endocarditis may result in an acquired form of tricuspid stenosis. Right heart pathology, such as vegetations or tumors, in extremely rare cases may interfere with right atrial emptying and lead to functional tricuspid stenosis. This is also the case of cor triatriatum dexter, an unusual anomaly characterized by persistent venous valves that divide the right atrium into proximal and distal components. Acquired tricuspid stenosis also may be the result of surgical intervention for congenital heart disease. Such is the case of stenosis of the right-sided atrioventricular valve component after repair of an atrioventricular septal defect.

Basic Pathophysiology

Obstruction to right ventricular inflow results in increments of the right atrial pressure in the absence of an adequate source for egress of the right atrial blood. This situation leads to elevation of systemic venous pressures, passive venous congestion, and signs and symptoms of ascites and congestive heart failure. The atrial a wave may be very tall and approaches the systolic pressure in the right ventricle. The overall hemodynamic result is reduced cardiac output. In the presence of an interatrial communication, right-to-left atrial shunting results in cyanosis.

Clinical Presentation

The clinical features of tricuspid stenosis may closely mimic the features of tricuspid atresia, making the distinction between these two pathologies extremely challenging in some patients.[93] The severity of the associated lesions may dominate the clinical presentation in patients with tricuspid valve disease.

The clinical presentation in infants and children with severe tricuspid pathology and a restrictive interatrial communication may be that of a low cardiac output state. Conversely, mild-to-moderate disease may be difficult to identify because of the high compliance of the systemic capacitance vessels and right atrium accounting for a delayed diagnosis. Symptoms include hepatomegaly and anasarca and in most patients are related primarily to the effects of associated lesions. Cyanosis as a presenting symptom is typical of patients with atrial level shunting.

Clinical Evaluation

Right atrial hypertension is manifested by prominence of the a wave in the jugular venous pulse in the absence of an adequate interatrial communication. A slow y descent is related to delayed right ventricular filling. A presystolic impulse may be palpable in the right parasternal area and over the right upper quadrant corresponding to the region over the liver. The diastolic rumble of tricuspid stenosis is audible along the parasternal border, although an opening snap is uncommon in children. The combination of distended neck veins and hepatic congestion in the absence of pulmonary hypertension or increased pulmonary blood flow should raise the suspicion of right ventricular inflow obstruction. Overt right heart failure in tricuspid stenosis as manifested by evidence of peripheral edema or ascites is rare.

The **ECG** in isolated tricuspid stenosis shows high-amplitude P waves typical of right atrial enlargement. Left-axis deviation, paucity of right ventricular forces, and prominent posterior forces, findings commonly found in tricuspid atresia, also may be present. Additional alterations in the ECG correspond to the changes of associated pathology. The occurrence of left anterior fascicular block has been reported in patients with congenital tricuspid stenosis and a secundum atrial septal defect.[94]

The **chest radiograph** findings in these patients include cardiomegaly and prominence of the right heart border related to dilation of the superior vena cava and right atrium. No evidence of pulmonary artery enlargement is present, and oligemic lung fields can be seen. Coexisting malformations account for additional radiographic abnormalities.

Echocardiography provides information regarding annular size, leaflet morphology, and supporting structures. In the presence of valvar stenosis, two-dimensional imaging shows thickening of the leaflets and diastolic doming, commissural fusion, and reduced diastolic valve motion. The tricuspid annular size is determined, and the right ventricle is evaluated to assess the adequacy of the apical and outlet portions. Potential associated lesions are examined. Interrogation of the atrial septum is important to determine if it provides an acceptable outlet to the systemic venous return in case of severe inflow obstruction. The nature and severity of the right ventricular outflow obstruction, if present, are defined by spectral and color Doppler. Echocardiographic assessment of the tricuspid valve area, although reported in adults with tricuspid stenosis, has not been a consistent component of the evaluation in children. Increasing severity of tricuspid valve disease is characterized by increased flow acceleration and peak diastolic velocity across the right ventricular inflow. In contrast to the literature addressing the echocardiographic evaluation of mitral stenosis in children, data regarding the quantitative assessment of tricuspid stenosis in this age group are scant. In general, mean gradients obtained by Doppler echocardiography compare well with cardiac catheterization in the assessment of the severity of tricuspid stenosis.[95] The presence of tricuspid stenosis in association with right ventricular hypoplasia in infants with pulmonary atresia and intact ventricular septum present management dilemmas regarding the feasibility of a biventricular repair. Criteria used to identify patients suitable for a two-ventricle repair include tricuspid valve Z-scores (>-3) and tricuspid-to-mitral annulus ratio (>0.5).

Exercise testing in combination with echocardiography may provide supportive evidence for the diagnosis of tricuspid stenosis as the diastolic gradient increases secondary to increases in transvalvar blood flow. In older children, it also could be a modality to evaluate functional capacity.

Although there is a paucity of information regarding the usefulness of **MRI** in the evaluation of isolated congenital tricuspid valve disease, the high definition structural and functional information provided by this modality should be expected to be beneficial in the diagnostic assessment of these patients.

A diastolic pressure gradient between the right atrium and the right ventricle is characteristic of tricuspid stenosis at **cardiac catheterization**. The transvalvar gradient may be amplified by a fluid challenge, deep inspiration, or exercise but can be as little as 2 mm Hg. Elevations of the right atrial pressure and particularly the *A* wave are seen; a slow *y* descent is consistent with altered right ventricular filling. Angiography shows the degree of right atrial enlargement and the narrow diastolic jet.[96] Diastolic doming of the tricuspid valve is seen along with reduced mobility of the leaflets, resulting in delayed emptying of contrast material from the right atrium into the right ventricle.

Therapeutic Strategies

The role of medical therapy is limited in patients with tricuspid stenosis. In patients with mild disease or anticipating intervention, diuretic therapy and fluid and sodium restriction may be indicated to ameliorate symptoms related to systemic venous congestion. Patients in whom the primary pathology is commissural fusion, with a relatively normal annulus, subvalvular apparatus, and right ventricular cavity, may be amenable to **percutaneous tricuspid balloon valvuloplasty**.[97-99] The intervention results in splitting of the commissures and enhancement in the mobility of the leaflets.

Patients with tricuspid stenosis may allow for surgical strategies that generally are not feasible in patients with tricuspid atresia, thus the importance of the differentiation between these two pathologies. Surgical options in tricuspid stenosis include **leaflet commissurotomy**, **valvotomy**, and **valve replacement**.[100-102] The selection of a mechanical versus a bioprosthetic valve depends on many factors, including surgeon preference.[102] Coexisting disease also may need to be addressed. In severe cases of malformed valves and valves associated with marked right ventricular hypoplasia, single ventricle palliation may be the only option. A potential approach in patients with mild-to-moderate tricuspid stenosis and hypoplasia and a mildly hypoplastic right ventricle is the so-called **one-and-a-half ventricle repair**. In this procedure, a bidirectional cavopulmonary connection is created to allow for a portion of the systemic venous return to bypass the right ventricle, and associated lesions are addressed.[103,104] The need for intervention in younger patients is mandated by intractable heart failure and severe disease.

MITRAL STENOSIS

Anatomic Considerations

Congenital mitral stenosis includes a broad spectrum of structural abnormalities that result in obstruction to left ventricular inflow. The congenital form of this malformation occurs rarely in isolation, with a reported incidence of less than 0.4% among patients with congenital heart disease. Mitral inflow obstruction is more prevalent in the presence of coexisting left-sided abnormalities or in association with other defects. Acquired forms of mitral stenosis resulting from rheumatic disease, endocarditis, mucopolysaccharidoses, repair of atrioventricular septal defects, and other pathologies are seen more commonly than the congenital form of mitral valve disease.

A wide variety of structural derangements account for the morphologic spectrum of congenital mitral stenosis,[105] and the valvar structures may exhibit dysplastic features or hypoplasia or both. Abnormalities of the valve itself or supporting structures are classic findings. Deformities may include annular hypoplasia, leaflet thickening, and shortened and thickened chordae. The support apparatus may display obliteration of interchordal spaces and hypoplasia or absence of papillary muscles resulting in the anatomic or functional form of a **parachute mitral valve**. Less common anatomic types of mitral inflow obstruction include mitral arcade (so-called hammock valve), stenosing supravalvar mitral ring, parachute mitral valve, and double-orifice mitral valve.

In some patients, more than one anatomic abnormality leading to mitral stenosis may coexist. Such is the case of patients with **Shone complex**, characterized by aortic coarctation, subaortic obstruction, parachute mitral valve, and supravalvar mitral ring.[106] The abnormalities identified in patients with an anomalous mitral arcade include thickened and immobile leaflets, fused commissures, and shortened and thickened chords.[107] Direct insertion on the valve leaflets into the papillary muscle without intervening chordal structures may be seen in some patients. Thickened papillary muscles may contribute to the subvalvar obstruction.[108,109] The pathology typically results in a mixed disorder characterized by mitral stenosis and regurgitation.[107,110] In addition, pathologies such as cor triatriatum, left atrial thrombus, or tumor may mimic the features of mitral stenosis.

Supravalvar mitral ring is a rare anomaly characterized by the presence of a partial or complete shelflike fibrous ring in the left atrial aspect of the mitral valve[111]; this membrane is frequently in close proximity to the valve. In contrast to cor triatriatum, the obstructive ring does not divide the left atrium into proximal and distal structures, and the membrane immediately adjacent to the mitral valve is located below the left atrial appendage (as opposed to above the atrial appendage in cor triatriatum). The reported incidence of this malformation in cases of congenital mitral stenosis is 9% to 20%. The size of the ring orifice and impact on the mobility of the mitral valve leaflets determine the severity of the obstruction. This lesion is usually part of the Shone complex.

In **rheumatic mitral stenosis**, the characteristic features are commissural fusion and chordal thickening, shortening, and calcification. The anatomic type of mitral valve obstruction plays a major role in the selection of therapeutic options.

Basic Pathophysiology

Mitral valve obstruction results in an increased diastolic pressure gradient and delayed egress of pulmonary venous blood from the left atrium into the left ventricle; this is associated with left atrial pressure elevation and increased pulmonary venous and arterial pressures. Engorgement of pulmonary capillaries leads to increases in hydrostatic pressures that result in pulmonary edema if plasma oncotic pressure is exceeded (see Chapter 9).

The pulmonary edema accounts for ventilation-perfusion mismatching and pulmonary venous desaturation. The respiratory symptoms in patients with mitral inflow obstruction are related primarily to pulmonary congestion secondary to increased lung water and interstitial edema. In addition, increased airway resistance in long-standing mitral stenosis is due to encroachment of congested bronchial veins on the smaller airways and left bronchial distortion secondary to left atrial dilation. The elevations in pulmonary artery pressure are caused by a backward transmission of elevated left atrial pressure, a reactive element of pulmonary vasoconstriction, and morphologic changes in the pulmonary vascular tree.

In the presence of an interatrial communication decompressing the left atrium, the clinical manifestations of mitral stenosis may be subtle. Associated with significant inflow obstruction is heart failure, however, as the end result of altered loading conditions in the left atrium and left ventricle, pulmonary venous hypertension, and decreased systemic forward flow. In mitral stenosis, compensatory mechanisms triggered by the reduced ventricular filling and low cardiac output state, such as peripheral vasoconstriction, may contribute further to the failing heart as the left ventricular myocardial performance may be negatively affected by the increased systemic afterload. In addition, any increase in flow (e.g., hypervolemia or exercise) in mitral stenosis quadruples the pressure gradient because the transvalvar gradient is a function of the square of the transvalvar flow rate. The right ventricle initially responds to the increased pressure load of pulmonary hypertension by muscle hypertrophy; however, with ongoing mitral valve obstruction, there can be progressive right ventricular chamber dilation and dysfunction with insufficiency of the tricuspid and pulmonary valves.

Clinical Presentation
The marked variability within each anatomic type of mitral inflow obstruction accounts for the age at presentation and symptoms. The clinical presentation also is influenced by the presence of associated pathology. The features of mitral stenosis vary with the severity of inflow obstruction. In infants, symptoms of congestive heart failure frequently include increased work of breathing, diaphoresis, feeding difficulties, and failure to thrive. These symptoms are manifested by hypoxemia, hypercapnea, and pulmonary congestion. In older children, fatigue associated with exercise intolerance is observed as the transpulmonary gradient increases in response to the increased transmitral flow. Recurrent respiratory infections also may be seen. Conditions such as anemia, fever, and mitral regurgitation may increase the transmitral pressure gradient further, leading to clinical decompensation.

Severe left atrial dilation in some cases may be associated with left bronchial compression and symptoms related to either atelectasis or air trapping.

Significant pulmonary vascular changes have been reported in patients with pulmonary venous obstruction,[112] including progressive medial thickening and intimal fibrosis of the pulmonary arteries and veins in addition to lymphangiectasia. Some of these changes may be reversible as the pulmonary vasculature remodels in response to the relief of pulmonary venous obstruction.

Clinical Evaluation
In general, auscultation of a patient with congenital mitral stenosis shows the intensity of S_1 to be normal or decreased. In contrast, in the case of rheumatic mitral stenosis, an accentuated S_1 is frequently identified. The classic finding in adult patients of a diastolic opening snap in mitral stenosis is rarely appreciated in children; this is likely due to faster heart rates in children and the limited mobility of the leaflets. A low-frequency, mid-diastolic to late-diastolic murmur at the apex, which increases with expiration, is often auscultated. Elevations of pulmonary artery pressures account for a loud pulmonary component of S_2 and a right ventricular impulse.

The **ECG** displays a rightward frontal plane QRS axis, biphasic P wave consistent with left atrial enlargement, and increased right-sided forces consistent with right ventricular hypertrophy. A strain pattern may be seen in pulmonary arterial hypertension. Rhythm disturbances in chronic mitral stenosis in older children and young adults are unusual, but may include atrial flutter or fibrillation or both.

The **chest radiograph** in moderate-to-severe mitral stenosis is characterized by cardiomegaly and prominent pulmonary vascular markings. The increased pulmonary vascularity is the result of pulmonary venous congestion. This is evident by the presence of Kerley B lines and redistribution of blood to the upper pulmonary segments. Findings consistent with left atrial enlargement include straight upper left heart border, double atrial shadow, elevated left main stem bronchus, and posterior displacement of the cardiac silhouette. Enlargement of the main pulmonary artery is consistent with pulmonary hypertension. Cardiac decompensation related to right heart failure is evident by dilation of the right atrium and ventricle.

Cross-sectional **echocardiography** plays a key role in the evaluation of mitral valve disease in children.[113-117] Two-dimensional imaging defines the anatomy of the mitral valve and support apparatus. A comprehensive study includes cross-sectional examination of the mitral valve in a series of planes from the base of the heart to the apex. This study allows for interrogation of the supravalvar and subvalvar structures. Important data include determination of annular size and of mitral valve area, evaluation of diastolic excursion of the valvar leaflets, examination of the chordae tendinae, and assessments of the number and distribution of papillary muscles. Spectral and color flow Doppler interrogation are essential in the evaluation of the location and severity of the obstruction (Fig. 22-5). Pulsed-wave and continuous-wave Doppler allows for assessment of the peak and mean transvalvar diastolic pressure gradient[118]; this in combination with the pressure half-time and left atrial size are the major

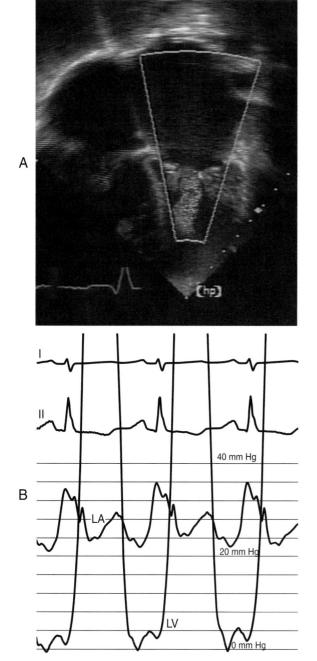

FIGURE 22-5 ■ Mitral stenosis. A, Four-chamber transthoracic echocardiogram in a child with rheumatic mitral stenosis displaying aliased, disturbed flow across the restrictive valvar orifice by color Doppler interrogation. **B,** Pressure tracings obtained at cardiac catheterization during transcatheter intervention. A large diastolic pressure gradient is identified between the left atrium (LA) and left ventricle (LV). (See also Color Section)

echocardiographic parameters considered in the determination of the severity of the obstruction. Additional information includes evaluation of the pulmonary veins and pulmonary arteries. Associated pathology, such as mitral regurgitation or other structural anomalies, also should be investigated. The assessment of left atrial thrombi is relevant in patients with a history of chronic atrial dysrhythmias. The tricuspid or pulmonary regurgitation velocity jet, if present, is used to estimate pulmonary artery pressures.

Features consistent with a supravalvar mitral ring include diastolic evidence of ridges in the mitral annulus immediately above the valve. Because the membrane may become firmly adherent to the valvar leaflets, the distinction between obstructive ring and valve may become more difficult to the point where the diagnosis of this condition may be nearly impossible. The parachute mitral valve is characterized by unifocal attachment of the mitral valve support apparatus to a single or dominant papillary muscle, causing subvalvar obstruction. The outlet of blood from the left atrium is primarily through the restrictive interchordal spaces.[119]

Exercise testing and pharmacologic stress assessment have been found to be useful in adults with mitral stenosis for evaluation when symptoms have not correlated with echocardiographic data, for prognostic evaluation, for guidance of heart failure therapy, and for risk stratification.[120-123] The application of this modality to mitral valve disease in children has not been well defined.

MRI has been used in the assessment of mitral valve obstruction because it provides anatomic and functional information regarding valve motion, papillary muscles, and coexistent abnormalities of the left ventricular outflow tract and aortic arch.[55] The angiographic features of the various types of left ventricular inflow obstruction have been well characterized.[124] **Cardiac catheterization** in mitral stenosis shows a measurable gradient between the left atrial *A* wave and the left ventricular end-diastolic pressure (transmitral pressure gradient) (see Fig. 22-5). This pressure gradient also can be derived from the assessment of the pulmonary capillary wedge pressure. A tall *A* wave characterizes the left atrial pressure tracing; a gradual pressure decline after the mitral valve opening also is seen (*y* descent). In patients with mild mitral stenosis, the pulmonary artery pressure and pulmonary vascular resistance can be normal at rest.

Therapeutic Strategies

Close observation and follow-up are warranted for patients with mild mitral stenosis and minimal or no symptoms. Pharmacologic agents are indicated in the treatment of congestive heart failure. **Diuretic** therapy is used in most cases of moderate or severe disease to decrease left atrial pressure and alleviate symptoms related to pulmonary vascular congestion. Infants with symptomatic congenital mitral stenosis present a significant therapeutic challenge. Additional interventions in the forms of catheter or surgical therapies are indicated for moderate-to-severe disease and for patients failing maximal medical therapy; efforts usually are made to intervene before onset of pulmonary hypertension.

Although there is considerable literature regarding the role of **balloon valvuloplasty** of the rheumatic mitral valve, data are limited regarding the application of catheter-based interventions in congenital mitral valve disease.[125-128] Balloon dilation of the stenotic mitral valve has been reported in infants with varying success rates. One retrospective review of the management of severe mitral stenosis in infants reported no procedure-related mortality in 18 infants (age 8.7 ± 5.7 months; weight 5.9 ± 1.9 kg) who had undergone balloon dilation.[129] In most patients, sequential dilations were performed to an average final balloon diameter 0.9 times the mitral annulus diameter. Successful dilation was accomplished in 15 patients, as judged by a greater than 30% decrease in left ventricular *A* wave to left ventricular end-diastolic pressure gradient. In 44% of infants who had minimal reductions in the transmitral gradient, sustained clinical improvement was associated with a lesser need for medical therapy of heart failure. An intermediate and mid-term outcome review of balloon mitral valvotomy in children and adolescents documented a success rate of nearly 97% and no mortality related to the procedure or during follow-up.[130] Mitral regurgitation may complicate interventional therapy.

Strategies for the surgical management of mitral stenosis are influenced by the morphologic type of obstruction.[131-135] The procedures typically include **valvotomy**, **commissurotomy**, **resection of supravalvar obstruction**, and **mitral valve repair/reconstruction or replacement** as indicated and determined by the pathology. In cases of subvalvar obstruction related to a parachute mitral valve, splitting of the chords and papillary muscles may be considered. The reported operative mortality in a report of 13 infants undergoing mitral valve surgery was shown to be quite significant (in the range of 30%).[129] Although others have reported no to minimal operative mortality in the infant group, reoperation rates are high and predicated by the complexity of the mitral abnormalities and associated anomalies.[132,133] In cases in which mitral valve repair is not feasible, alternative approaches include mitral valve replacement with mechanical or xenograft valves and placement of conduits from the left atrium to the left ventricle.[136,137] Replacement of the mitral valve with a pulmonary autograft, also known as the **Ross II procedure** with Kananni modification, has been proposed as a safe alternative in select patients.[138] This intervention obviates the need for anticoagulation. Many studies have addressed the issue of outcomes in children undergoing surgical interventions for congenital mitral stenosis.[105,133,135,139-141] The varying pathologies, age at intervention, operative approaches, and follow-up

periods make an overall assessment of surgical results difficult, however.

Despite significant medical and surgical advances, the management of patients with Shone complex continues to present a challenge. A study by Bolling and colleagues of 30 patients with this anomaly reported the presence of a supravalvar mitral ring in 22 patients and mitral valve abnormalities (e.g., a parachute mitral valve, fused chordae, or single papillary muscle) in 26 patients.[142] One third of the patients required mitral valve interventions (repair or replacement). Although no perioperative mortality was noted during the initial surgical procedure, mortality increased to 25% after the second intervention primarily related to mitral valve disease. Another study focusing on the late outcome of this patient population noted a significant impact of the mitral valve pathology and the presence of pulmonary hypertension.[143]

CURRENT STATUS AND FUTURE TRENDS

The remarkable disease spectrum of valvular stenosis in children is related to a great extent to the frequent occurrence of inflow and outflow obstruction in association with other structural abnormalities and complex pathologies. It is well established that valvular stenosis results in pathophysiologic alterations that may be well compensated in mild-to-moderate disease or may lead to significant morbidity and even mortality in severe cases.

Diagnostic improvements in the identification and follow-up of valvular heart disease in children have been largely due to the major role of echocardiography in defining anatomy and function and new developments in noninvasive imaging modalities.[144] The medical and surgical management of these patients has undergone advances, but pediatric studies still lack the scientific sophistication of adult studies.[145] Many of the therapeutic innovations relate to catheter-based techniques and other procedures in interventional cardiology. The care of these children has been facilitated by improvements of perfusion, anesthetic, and surgical strategies and a multidisciplinary approach in perioperative care. Despite these achievements, the outcomes of pediatric patients are difficult to determine because of the heterogeneity of the anatomic substrates and fewer follow-up studies compared with adults.[146] Important questions remain unanswered regarding the appropriate timing of interventions (medical and surgical), optimal strategies for patients with complex disease, and the long-term impact of approaches widely employed today.[147] As our understanding of the key mechanisms and molecular basis of heart failure continues to improve, and advances in the clinical assessment and therapy of heart failure continue to evolve, our ability to care for these patients will undoubtedly be enhanced.

Key Concepts

- In right-sided obstructive lesions, right ventricular dilation rather than hypertrophy occasionally may result from an increased afterload, eventually culminating in right ventricular dysfunction and heart failure. In addition, ventricular interdependence may affect left ventricular performance and lead to biventricular failure.

- Diminished right ventricular compliance in neonates with critical pulmonary stenosis and severe chamber hypertrophy is likely to be associated with diastolic dysfunction. Subendocardial ischemia resulting in myocardial infarction and fibrosis and the associated hypoxia may account for systolic impairment and eventual chamber dilation and congestive heart failure.

- Overt right heart failure in the absence of significant tricuspid insufficiency is relatively uncommon in children because adequate stroke volume and cardiac output are maintained at the expense of right ventricular hypertrophy.

- Impedance to left ventricular ejection in aortic stenosis results in elevation of left ventricular systolic pressure and a transvalvar pressure gradient; this leads to increased myocardial force and left ventricular wall stress. The hypertrophic response leads to an unfavorable mass-to-volume ratio, but serves as an adaptive mechanism allowing the left ventricle to generate increased systolic pressure, while normalizing wall stress and maintaining a normal ejection fraction (in accordance to the Laplace equation).

- The diastolic compliance of the heart is often abnormal in aortic stenosis due to the increased mass and resultant diastolic stiffness of the ventricle. If the ventricular muscle mass acquisition is not adequate to normalize wall stress (resulting in an afterload mismatch), the muscle fails, and ejection fraction is depressed.

- Other chronic systemic compensatory responses include systemic vasoconstriction, increased blood volume, and increased heart rate, the last-mentioned leading to decreased diastolic pressure time index of myocardial oxygen supply (the area between the aortic and the left ventricular pressure in diastole).

- In aortic stenosis, factors such as increasing left ventricular afterload, inadequate hypertrophic remodeling (with loss of myofibrils and proliferation of fibroblasts and collagen fibers), and decreased myocardial systolic or diastolic performance may compromise stroke volume and contribute to cardiac dysfunction and heart failure. The overall effects of aortic stenosis lead to increased myocardial oxygen consumption with decreased myocardial oxygen supply and ultimately myocardial ischemia, left ventricular systolic and diastolic dysfunction, and heart failure.

- The potential role of vasodilator therapy, traditionally considered contraindicated in patients with severe aortic obstruction, has been examined more recently in critically ill adults with aortic stenosis with favorable results.

- A potential approach in patients with mild-to-moderate tricuspid stenosis and hypoplasia and a mildly hypoplastic right ventricle is the so-called one-and-a-half ventricle repair. In this surgery, a bidirectional cavopulmonary connection is created to allow for a portion of the systemic venous return to bypass the right ventricle, and associated lesions are addressed.

- In mitral stenosis, compensatory mechanisms triggered by the reduced ventricular filling and low cardiac output state, such as peripheral vasoconstriction, may contribute further to the failing heart because the left ventricular myocardial performance may be negatively affected by the increased systemic afterload. In addition, any increase in flow (e.g., hypervolemia or exercise) in mitral stenosis quadruples the pressure gradient because the transvalvar gradient is a function of the square of the transvalvar flow rate.

REFERENCES

1. Keith JD: Prevalence, incidence, and etiology. In Keith JD, Rowe RD, Vlad P (eds): Heart Disease in Infancy and Childhood. New York, Macmillan, 1978, pp 3-13.
2. Koretzky ED, Moller JH, Korns ME, et al: Congenital pulmonary stenosis resulting from dysplasia of valve. Circulation 1969; 40:43.
3. Linde LM, Turner SW, Sparkes RS: Pulmonary valvular dysplasia: A cardiofacial syndrome. Br Heart J 1973;35:301.
4. Noonan JA: Hypertelorism with Turner phenotype: A new syndrome with associated congenital heart disease. Am J Dis Child 1968;116:373.
5. Burch M, Sharland M, Shinebourne E, et al: Cardiologic abnormalities in Noonan syndrome: Phenotypic diagnosis and echocardiographic assessment of 118 patients. J Am Coll Cardiol 1993;22:1189.
6. Noonan J: Noonan syndrome: Then and now. Cardiol Young 1999;9:545.
7. Noonan JA: Noonan syndrome revisited. J Pediatr 1999;135:667.
8. Franciosi RA, Blanc WA: Myocardial infarcts in infants and children: I. A necropsy study in congenital heart disease. J Pediatr 1968;73:309.
9. Ben-Shachar G, Cohen MH, Sivakoff MC, et al: Development of infundibular obstruction after percutaneous pulmonary balloon valvuloplasty. J Am Coll Cardiol 1985;5:754.
10. Lucas RVJ, Varco RL, Lillehei CW, et al: Anomalous muscle bundle of the right ventricle: Hemodynamic consequences and surgical considerations. Circulation 1962;25:443.
11. Alva C, Ho SY, Lincoln CR, et al: The nature of the obstructive muscular bundles in double-chambered right ventricle. J Thorac Cardiovasc Surg 1999;117:1180.
12. Cabrera A, Martinez P, Rumoroso JR, et al: Double-chambered right ventricle. Eur Heart J 1995;16:682.
13. Cil E, Saraclar M, Ozkutlu S, et al: Double-chambered right ventricle: Experience with 52 cases. Int J Cardiol 1995;50:19.
14. Hayes CJ, Gersony WM, Driscoll DJ, et al: Second natural history study of congenital heart defects: Results of treatment of patients with pulmonary valvar stenosis. Circulation 1993;87:I-28.

15. Dore A: Pulmonary stenosis. In Gazoulis MA, Webb GD, Daubeney PEF (eds): Diagnosis and Management of Adult Congenital Heart Disease. London, Churchill Livingstone, 2003, pp 299-303.

16. Musewe NN, Robertson MA, Benson LN, et al: The dysplastic pulmonary valve: Echocardiographic features and results of balloon dilatation. Br Heart J 1987;57:364.

17. Currie PJ, Hagler DJ, Seward JB, et al: Instantaneous pressure gradient: A simultaneous Doppler and dual catheter correlative study. J Am Coll Cardiol 1986;7:800.

18. Currie PJ, Seward JB, Chan KL, et al: Continuous wave Doppler determination of right ventricular pressure: A simultaneous Doppler-catheterization study in 127 patients. J Am Coll Cardiol 1985;6:750.

19. Krabill KA, Wang Y, Einzig S, et al: Rest and exercise hemodynamics in pulmonary stenosis: Comparison of children and adults. Am J Cardiol 1985;56:360.

20. Driscoll DJ, Wolfe RR, Gersony WM, et al: Cardiorespiratory responses to exercise of patients with aortic stenosis, pulmonary stenosis, and ventricular septal defect. Circulation 1993;87 (2 Suppl);I:114-120.

21. Kan JS, White RI Jr, Mitchell SE, et al: Percutaneous balloon valvuloplasty: A new method for treating congenital pulmonary-valve stenosis. N Engl J Med 1982;307:540.

22. Kan JS, White RI, Mitchell SE, et al: Percutaneous transluminal balloon valvuloplasty for pulmonary valve stenosis. Circulation 1984;69:554.

23. Rao PS, Wilson AD, Thapar MK, et al: Balloon pulmonary valvuloplasty in the management of cyanotic congenital heart defects. Cathet Cardiovasc Diagn 1992;25:16.

24. Sullivan ID, Robinson PJ, Macartney FJ, et al: Percutaneous balloon valvuloplasty for pulmonary valve stenosis in infants and children. Br Heart J 1985;54:435.

25. Rao PS: Balloon pulmonary valvuloplasty: A review. Clin Cardiol 1989;12:55.

26. McCrindle BW, Kan JS: Long-term results after balloon pulmonary valvuloplasty. Circulation 1991;83:1915.

27. Lababidi Z, Wu JR: Percutaneous balloon pulmonary valvuloplasty. Am J Cardiol 1983;52:560.

28. Poon LK, Menahem S: Pulmonary regurgitation after percutaneous balloon valvoplasty for isolated pulmonary valvar stenosis in childhood. Cardiol Young 2003;13:444.

29. Fawzy ME, Galal O, Dunn B, et al: Regression of infundibular pulmonary stenosis after successful balloon pulmonary valvuloplasty in adults. Cathet Cardiovasc Diagn 1990;21:77.

30. Nakanishi T, Tsuji T, Nakasawa M, et al: Configurations of right ventricular pressure curves and infundibular stenosis after balloon pulmonary valvuloplasty. Cardiol Young 1995;5:44.

31. Campbell M, Kauntze R: Congenital aortic valvular stenosis. Br Heart J 1953;15:179.

32. Ferencz C, Rubin JD, McCarter RJ, et al: Congenital heart disease: Prevalence at livebirth. The Baltimore-Washington Infant Study. Am J Epidemiol 1985;121:31.

33. Kitchiner DJ, Jackson M, Walsh K, et al: Incidence and prognosis of congenital aortic valve stenosis in Liverpool (1960-1990). Br Heart J 1993;69:71.

34. Edwards JE: The congenital bicuspid aortic valve. Circulation 1961;23:485.

35. Roberts WC: The congenitally bicuspid aortic valve: A study of 85 autopsy cases. Am J Cardiol 1970;26:72.

36. McDonald K, Maurer BJ: Familial aortic valve disease: Evidence for a genetic influence. Eur Heart J 1989;10:676.

37. Clementi M, Notari L, Borghi A, et al: Familial congenital bicuspid aortic valve: A disorder of uncertain inheritance. Am J Med Genet 1996;62:336.

38. Moller JH, Nakib A, Edwards JE: Infarction of papillary muscles and mitral insufficiency associated with congenital aortic stenosis. Circulation 1966;34:87.

39. Lofland GK, McCrindle BW, Williams WG, et al: Critical aortic stenosis in the neonate: A multi-institutional study of management, outcomes, and risk factors. Congenital Heart Surgeons Society. J Thorac Cardiovasc Surg 2001;121:10.

40. Williams JC, Barratt-Boyes BG, Lowe JB: Supravalvular aortic stenosis. Circulation 1961;24:1311.

41. Nickerson E, Greenberg F, Keating MT, et al: Deletions of the elastin gene at 7q11.23 occur in approximately 90% of patients with Williams syndrome. Am J Hum Genet 1995;56:1156.

42. Morris CA: Genetic aspects of supravalvular aortic stenosis. Curr Opin Cardiol 1998;13:214.

43. Bruno E, Rossi N, Thuer O, et al: Cardiovascular findings, and clinical course, in patients with Williams syndrome. Cardiol Young 2003;13:532.

44. Rein AJ, Preminger TJ, Perry SB, et al: Generalized arteriopathy in Williams syndrome: An intravascular ultrasound study. J Am Coll Cardiol 1993;21:1727-1730.

45. Moller JH, Nakib A, Eliot RS, et al: Symptomatic congenital aortic stenosis in the first year of life. J Pediatr 1966;69:728.

46. Huhta JC, Carpenter RJJ, Moise KJJ, et al: Prenatal diagnosis and postnatal management of critical aortic stenosis. Circulation 1987;75:573.

47. McCaffrey FM, Sherman FS: Prenatal diagnosis of severe aortic stenosis. Pediatr Cardiol 1997;18:276.

48. Simpson JM, Sharland GK: Natural history and outcome of aortic stenosis diagnosed prenatally. Heart 1997;77:205.

49. Lewis AB, Heymann MA, Stanger P, et al: Evaluation of subendocardial ischemia in valvar aortic stenosis in children. Circulation 1974;49:978.

50. Hossack KF, Neutze JM, Lowe JB, et al: Congenital valvar aortic stenosis: Natural history and assessment for operation. Br Heart J 1980;43:561.

51. Bengur AR, Snider AR, Serwer GA, et al: Usefulness of the Doppler mean gradient in evaluation of children with aortic valve stenosis and comparison to gradient at catheterization. Am J Cardiol 1989;64:756.

52. Moreno R, Zamorano J, Almeria C, et al: Isovolumic contraction time by pulsed-wave Doppler tissue imaging in aortic stenosis. Eur J Echocardiogr 2003;4:279.

53. Kiraly P, Kapusta L, Thijssen JM, et al: Left ventricular myocardial function in congenital valvar aortic stenosis assessed by ultrasound tissue-velocity and strain-rate techniques. Ultrasound Med Biol 2003;29:615.

54. Nikitin NP, Witte KK: Application of tissue Doppler imaging in cardiology. Cardiology 2004;101:170.

55. Roche KJ, Genieser NB, Ambrosino MM, et al: MR findings in Shone's complex of left heart obstructive lesions. Pediatr Radiol 1998;28:841.

56. Caruthers SD, Lin SJ, Brown P, et al: Practical value of cardiac magnetic resonance imaging for clinical quantification of aortic valve stenosis: Comparison with echocardiography. Circulation 2003;108:2236.

57. Delhaas T, Kotte J, van der Toorn A, et al: Increase in left ventricular torsion-to-shortening ratio in children with valvular aortic stenosis. Magn Reson Med 2004;51:135.

58. Friedrich MG, Schulz-Menger J, Poetsch T, et al: Quantification of valvular aortic stenosis by magnetic resonance imaging. Am Heart J 2002;144:329.

59. Kupfahl C, Honold M, Meinhardt G, et al: Evaluation of aortic stenosis by cardiovascular magnetic resonance imaging: Comparison with established routine clinical techniques. Heart 2004;90:893.

60. McKay RG, Spears JR, Aroesty JM, et al: Instantaneous measurement of left and right ventricular stroke volume and pressure-volume relationships with an impedance catheter. Circulation 1984;69:703.

61. Dajani AS, Taubert KA, Wilson W, et al: Prevention of bacterial endocarditis: Recommendations by the American Heart Association. Circulation 1997;96:358.

62. Horstkotte D, Follath F, Gutschik E, et al: Guidelines on prevention, diagnosis and treatment of infective endocarditis executive

summary; the task force on infective endocarditis of the European Society of Cardiology. Eur Heart J 2004;25:267.

63. Campbell M: The natural history of congenital aortic stenosis. Br Heart J 1968;30:514.

64. Keane JF, Driscoll DJ, Gersony WM, et al: Second natural history study of congenital heart defects: Results of treatment of patients with aortic valvar stenosis. Circulation 1993;87:(2 Suppl):I:16-27.

65. Khot UN, Novaro GM, Popovic ZB, et al: Nitroprusside in critically ill patients with left ventricular dysfunction and aortic stenosis. N Engl J Med 2003;348:1756.

66. Lababidi Z, Weinhaus L: Successful balloon valvuloplasty for neonatal critical aortic stenosis. Am Heart J 1986;112:913.

67. Kasten-Sportes CH, Piechaud JF, Sidi D, et al: Percutaneous balloon valvuloplasty in neonates with critical aortic stenosis. J Am Coll Cardiol 1989;13:1101.

68. Egito ES, Moore P, O'Sullivan J, et al: Transvascular balloon dilation for neonatal critical aortic stenosis: Early and midterm results. J Am Coll Cardiol 1997;29:442.

69. Pass RH, Hellenbrand WE: Catheter intervention for critical aortic stenosis in the neonate. Catheter Cardiovasc Interv 2002;55:88.

70. Lababidi Z, Wu JR, Walls JT: Percutaneous balloon aortic valvuloplasty: Results in 23 patients. Am J Cardiol 1984;53:194.

71. Hausdorf G, Schneider M, Schirmer KR, et al: Anterograde balloon valvuloplasty of aortic stenosis in children. Am J Cardiol 1993;71:460.

72. Kugler JD, Campbell E, Vargo TA, et al: Results of aortic valvotomy in infants with isolated aortic valvular stenosis. J Thorac Cardiovasc Surg 1979;78:553.

73. Hazekamp MG, Quaegebeur JM, Singh S, et al: One stage repair of aortic arch anomalies and intracardiac defects. Eur J Cardiothorac Surg 1991;5:283.

74. Sharma BK, Fujiwara H, Hallman GL, et al: Supravalvar aortic stenosis: A 29-year review of surgical experience. Ann Thorac Surg 1991;51:1031.

75. Myers JL, Waldhausen JA, Cyran SE, et al: Results of surgical repair of congenital supravalvular aortic stenosis. J Thorac Cardiovasc Surg 1993;105:281.

76. Pinto RJ, Loya Y, Bhagwat A, et al: Balloon dilatation of supravalvular aortic stenosis: A report of two cases. Int J Cardiol 1994;46:179.

77. Lababidi Z: Balloon dilatation of discrete membranous subaortic stenosis. J Invasive Cardiol 1996;8:297.

78. Stamm C, Kreutzer C, Zurakowski D, et al: Forty-one years of surgical experience with congenital supravalvular aortic stenosis. J Thorac Cardiovasc Surg 1999;118:874.

79. Brown JW, Ruzmetov M, Vijay P, et al: Surgical repair of congenital supravalvular aortic stenosis in children. Eur J Cardiothorac Surg 2002;21:50.

80. Leung MP, McKay R, Smith A, et al: Critical aortic stenosis in early infancy: Anatomic and echocardiographic substrates of successful open valvotomy. J Thorac Cardiovasc Surg 1991;101:526.

81. Rychik J, Murdison KA, Chin AJ, et al: Surgical management of severe aortic outflow obstruction in lesions other than the hypoplastic left heart syndrome: Use of a pulmonary artery to aorta anastomosis. J Am Coll Cardiol 1991;18:809.

82. Mocellin R, Sauer U, Simon B, et al: Reduced left ventricular size and endocardial fibroelastosis as correlates of mortality in newborns and young infants with severe aortic valve stenosis. Pediatr Cardiol 1983;4:265.

83. Parsons MK, Moreau GA, Graham TP Jr, et al: Echocardiographic estimation of critical left ventricular size in infants with isolated aortic valve stenosis. J Am Coll Cardiol 1991;18:1049.

84. Rhodes LA, Colan SD, Perry SB, et al: Predictors of survival in neonates with critical aortic stenosis. Circulation 1991;84:2325.

85. Keane JF, Bernhard WF, Nadas AS: Aortic stenosis surgery in infancy. Circulation 1975;52:1138.

86. Gula G, Wain WH, Ross DN: Ten years' experience with pulmonary autograft replacements for aortic valve disease. Ann Thorac Surg 1979;28:392.

87. Hraska V, Krajci M, Haun C, et al: Ross and Ross-Konno procedure in children and adolescents: Mid-term results. Eur J Cardiothorac Surg 2004;25:742.

88. Schmider A, Henrich W, Dahnert I, et al: Prenatal therapy of non-immunologic hydrops fetalis caused by severe aortic stenosis. Ultrasound Obstet Gynecol 2000;16:275.

89. Tworetzky W, Marshall AC: Balloon valvuloplasty for congenital heart disease in the fetus. Clin Perinatol 2003;30:541.

90. Morgan JR, Forker AD, Coates JR, et al: Isolated tricuspid stenosis. Circulation 1971;44:729.

91. Davachi F, McLean RH, Moller JH, et al: Hypoplasia of the right ventricle and tricuspid valve in siblings. J Pediatr 1967; 71:869.

92. Svane S: Congenital tricuspid atresia: A report on 8 autopsied cases. Scand J Thorac Cardiovasc Surg 1971;5:227.

93. Shore DF, Rigby ML, Lincoln C: Severe tricuspid stenosis presenting as tricuspid atresia: Echocardiographic diagnosis and surgical management. Br Heart J 1982;48:404.

94. Cohen ML, Spray T, Gutierrez F, et al: Congenital tricuspid valve stenosis with atrial septal defect and left anterior fascicular block. Clin Cardiol 1990;13:497.

95. Fawzy ME, Mercer EN, Dunn B, et al: Doppler echocardiography in the evaluation of tricuspid stenosis. Eur Heart J 1989;10:985.

96. Calleja HB, Hosier DM, Kissane RW: Congenital tricuspid stenosis: The diagnostic value of cineangiocardiography and hepatic pulse tracing. Am J Cardiol 1960;6:821.

97. Khalilullah M, Tyagi S, Yadav BS, et al: Double-balloon valvuloplasty of tricuspid stenosis. Am Heart J 1987;114:1232.

98. Lokhandwala YY, Rajani RM, Dalvi BV, et al: Successful balloon valvotomy in isolated congenital tricuspid stenosis. Cardiovasc Intervent Radiol 1990;13:354.

99. Krishnamoorthy KM: Balloon dilatation of isolated congenital tricuspid stenosis. Int J Cardiol 2003;89:119.

100. Smith MD, Sagar KB, Mauck HP, et al: Surgical correction of congenital tricuspid stenosis. Ann Thorac Surg 1982;34:329.

101. Scully HE, Armstrong CS: Tricuspid valve replacement: Fifteen years of experience with mechanical prostheses and bioprostheses. J Thorac Cardiovasc Surg 1995;109:1035.

102. Hayashi J, Saito A, Yamamoto K, et al: Is a bioprosthesis preferable in tricuspid valve replacement. Thorac Cardiovasc Surg 1996;44:230.

103. Muster AJ, Zales VR, Ilbawi MN, et al: Biventricular repair of hypoplastic right ventricle assisted by pulsatile bidirectional cavopulmonary anastomosis. J Thorac Cardiovasc Surg 1993; 105:112.

104. Clapp SK, Tantengco MV, Walters HL, et al: Bidirectional cavopulmonary anastomosis with intracardiac repair. Ann Thorac Surg 1997;63:746.

105. Carpentier A, Branchini B, Cour JC, et al: Congenital malformations of the mitral valve in children: Pathology and surgical treatment. J Thorac Cardiovasc Surg 1976;72:854.

106. Shone JD, Sellers RD, Anderson RC, et al: The developmental complex of "parachute mitral valve," supravalvular ring of left atrium, subaortic stenosis, and coarctation of aorta. Am J Cardiol 1963;11:714.

107. Layman TE, Edwards JE: Anomalous mitral arcade: A type of congenital mitral insufficiency. Circulation 1967;35:389.

108. Castaneda AR, Anderson RC, Edwards JE: Congenital mitral stenosis resulting from anomalous arcade and obstructing papillary muscles: Report of correction by use of ball valve prosthesis. Am J Cardiol 1969;24:237.

109. Frech RS, White RIJ, Bessinger FB, et al: Anomalous mitral arcade with enlarged papillary muscles: Angiographic study of two cases. Radiology 1972;103:633.

110. Parr GV, Fripp RR, Whitman V, et al: Anomalous mitral arcade: Echocardiographic and angiographic recognition. Pediatr Cardiol 1983;4:163.

111. Macartney FJ, Scott O, Ionescu MI, et al: Diagnosis and management of parachute mitral valve and supravalvar mitral ring. Br Heart J 1974;36:641.

112. Endo M, Yamaki S, Ohmi M, et al: Pulmonary vascular changes induced by congenital obstruction of pulmonary venous return. Ann Thorac Surg 2000;69:193.

113. LaCorte M, Harada K, Williams RG: Echocardiographic features of congenital left ventricular inflow obstruction. Circulation 1976;54:562.

114. Celano V, Pieroni DR, Morera JA, et al: Two-dimensional echocardiographic examination of mitral valve abnormalities associated with coarctation of the aorta. Circulation 1984;69:924.

115. Grenadier E, Sahn DJ, Valdes-Cruz LM, et al: Two-dimensional echo Doppler study of congenital disorders of the mitral valve. Am Heart J 1984;107:319.

116. Vitarelli A, Landolina G, Gentile R, et al: Echocardiographic assessment of congenital mitral stenosis. Am Heart J 1984;108: 523.

117. Banerjee A, Kohl T, Silverman NH: Echocardiographic evaluation of congenital mitral valve anomalies in children. Am J Cardiol 1995;76:1284.

118. Hatle L, Brubakk A, Tromsdal A, et al: Noninvasive assessment of pressure drop in mitral stenosis by Doppler ultrasound. Br Heart J 1978;40:131.

119. Schaverien MV, Freedom RM, McCrindle BW: Independent factors associated with outcomes of parachute mitral valve in 84 patients. Circulation 2004;109:2309.

120. Bach DS: Stress echocardiography for evaluation of hemodynamics: Valvular heart disease, prosthetic valve function, and pulmonary hypertension. Prog Cardiovasc Dis 1997;39:543.

121. Decena BF, Tischler MD: Stress echocardiography in valvular heart disease. Cardiol Clin 1999;17:555.

122. Omede P, Bucca C, Rolla G, et al: Cardiopulmonary exercise testing and exhaled nitric oxide in the assessment of patients with mitral stenosis. Min Cardioangiol 2004;52:29.

123. Reis G, Motta MS, Barbosa MM, et al: Dobutamine stress echocardiography for noninvasive assessment and risk stratification of patients with rheumatic mitral stenosis. J Am Coll Cardiol 2004;43:393.

124. Macartney FJ, Bain HH, Ionescu MI, et al: Angiocardiographic/pathologic correlations in congenital mitral valve anomalies. Eur J Cardiol 1976;4:191.

125. Alday LE, Juaneda E: Percutaneous balloon dilatation in congenital mitral stenosis. Br Heart J 1987;57:479.

126. Chen GY, Tseng CD, Chiang FT, et al: Congenital mitral stenosis: Challenge of percutaneous transvenous mitral commissurotomy. Int J Cardiol 1997;60:99.

127. Abdul Aziz B, Alwi M: Balloon dilatation of congenital mitral stenosis in a critically ill infant. Cathet Cardiovasc Interv 1999;48:191.

128. Spevak PJ, Bass JL, Ben-Shachar G, et al: Balloon angioplasty for congenital mitral stenosis. Am J Cardiol 1990;66:472.

129. Moore P, Adatia I, Spevak PJ, et al: Severe congenital mitral stenosis in infants. Circulation 1994;89:2099.

130. Kinsara AJ, Fawzi ME, Sivanadam V: Immediate and midterm outcome of balloon mitral valvotomy in children and adolescents. Can J Cardiol 2002;18:967.

131. Coles JG, Williams WG, Watanabe T, et al: Surgical experience with reparative techniques in patients with congenital mitral valvular anomalies. Circulation 1987;76:(3 Pt 2);III:117-122.

132. Barbero-Marcial M, Riso A, De Albuquerque AT, et al: Left ventricular apical approach for the surgical treatment of congenital mitral stenosis. J Thorac Cardiovasc Surg 1993;106:105.

133. Uva MS, Galletti L, Gayet FL, et al: Surgery for congenital mitral valve disease in the first year of life. J Thorac Cardiovasc Surg 1995;109:164.

134. McCarthy JF, Neligan MC, Wood AE: Ten years' experience of an aggressive reparative approach to congenital mitral valve anomalies. Eur J Cardiothorac Surg 1996;10:534.

135. Zias EA, Mavroudis C, Backer CL, et al: Surgical repair of the congenitally malformed mitral valve in infants and children. Ann Thorac Surg 1998;66:1551.

136. Laks H, Hellenbrand WE, Kleinman C, et al: Left atrial-left ventricular conduit for relief of congenital mitral stenosis in infancy. J Thorac Cardiovasc Surg 1980;80:782.

137. Corno A, Giannico S, Leibovich S, et al: The hypoplastic mitral valve: When should a left atrial-left ventricular extracardiac valved conduit be used? J Thorac Cardiovasc Surg 1986;91:848.

138. Brown JW, Ruzmetov M, Turrentine MW, et al: Mitral valve replacement with the pulmonary autograft: Ross II procedure with Kabanni modification. Pediatr Card Surg Annu Semin Thorac Cardiovasc Surg 2004;7:107.

139. Kadoba K, Jonas RA, Mayer JE, et al: Mitral valve replacement in the first year of life. J Thorac Cardiovasc Surg 1990;100:762.

140. Adatia I, Moore PM, Jonas RA, et al: Clinical course and hemodynamic observations after supraannular mitral valve replacement in infants and children. J Am Coll Cardiol 1997;29:1089.

141. Serraf A, Zoghbi J, Belli E, et al: Congenital mitral stenosis with or without associated defects: An evolving surgical strategy. Circulation 2000;102:III-166.

142. Bolling SF, Iannettoni MD, Dick MN, et al: Shone's anomaly: Operative results and late outcome. Ann Thorac Surg 1990;49:887.

143. Brauner RA, Laks H, Drinkwater DCJ, et al: Multiple left heart obstructions (Shone's anomaly) with mitral valve involvement: long-term surgical outcome. Ann Thorac Surg 1997;64:721.

144. DiBello V, Giorgi D, Viacava P, et al: Severe aortic stenosis and myocardial function: Diagnostic and prognostic usefulness of ultrasonic integrated backscatter analysis. Circulation 2004;110: 849-855.

145. Popovic ZB, Khot UN, Novaro GM, et al: Effects of sodium nitroprusside in aortic stenosis associated with severe heart failure: Pressure volume loop analysis using a numerical model. Am J Physiol Heart Circ Physiol 2005;288:H416-423.

146. Ruel M, Rubens FD, Masters RG, et al: Late incidence and predictors of persistent or recurrent heart failure in patients with mitral prosthetic valves. J Thorac Cardiovasc Surg 2004;128: 278-283.

147. Fawzy ME, Stefadouros MA, Hegazy H, et al: Long-term clinical and echocardiographic results of mitral balloon valvotomy in children and adolescents. Heart 2005;91:743-748.

Single Ventricle and Ventricular Performance

Mark A. Fogel

Although heart failure is a clinical diagnosis, with the definition covered in other chapters, assessment of cardiac function is a key element in the management and care of these patients. In patients with a single ventricle, assessment of heart failure presents an enormous challenge for the following reasons: (1) Single ventricles are a heterogeneous group anatomically and functionally, and nearly all patients require either reconstructive surgery or heart replacement; (2) physiology varies from a volume loaded ventricle to a volume unloaded one leading to the Fontan procedure,[1] although even that is arguable at certain stages[2]; (3) the systemic circulation varies from a runoff lesion physiology (into the pulmonary circulation as in the Norwood stage I reconstrucion[3]) to one without a runoff lesion as in the final Fontan reconstruction[1]; (4) the aorta may or may not undergo aortic reconstruction (e.g., aortic-to-pulmonary anastomosis as in Norwood stage I for hypoplastic left heart syndrome[3]); and (5) passive flow into the lungs in the final stage of Fontan reconstruction is still poorly understood, and optimizing this flow is continually discussed in the literature.[4,5] For all these reasons, assessment of the performance of the single-ventricle heart is complicated, and unifying themes across the entire patient population are difficult. This chapter discusses some of the issues behind single ventricular function, and a short background on the physiology of the single ventricle and the reconstructive surgery is presented. Many of these issues are unique to the single ventricle and sometimes, as shown in this chapter, may offer insights into the functioning of the normal "dual-chambered" circulation.

SINGLE VENTRICLE AND SURGICAL STRATEGIES

The anatomy of single ventricles varies: (1) systemic right ventricle versus left ventricle; (2) D-loop variety versus L-loop variety[6]; (3) true single ventricle (i.e., an atrioventricular valve-to-ventricle connection in which both atrioventricular valves or a common atrioventricular valve enters one ventricle in the presence of only one sinus portion of the heart) versus a "functional" single ventricle (any type of ventricular arrangement, such as a malaligned atrioventricular canal, in which from a "functional" standpoint, the ventricle acts like a single pumping chamber). Arising from these numerous complex combinations is the unifying theme that only one usable ventricle is present, or both ventricles are connected in such a way that separating them into two pumping chambers is impossible.

There may be outflow obstruction or hypoplasia of one of the great vessels, and blood flow to the obstructed circulation can be maintained by flow in the ductus arteriosus, flow through a stenotic pulmonary valve (allowing just enough blood to enter the pulmonary circulation[7]), or flow through a ventricular septal defect if one or both great vessels arises from the hypoplastic ventricle.[8] Surgical reconstruction separates the systemic and pulmonary circulations by allowing passive blood flow into the pulmonary circulation, while the functional single ventricle pumps to the systemic circulation. This type of surgical reconstruction is performed in stages today, and the physiology changes with each stage.

Before bidirectional cavopulmonary anastomosis, surgery may or may not be necessary. There may be adequate but restricted pulmonary blood flow in a patient with tricuspid atresia, normally related great arteries, and a ventricular septal defect.[8] Patients with hypoplastic left heart syndrome need immediate surgery, however— the Norwood stage I procedure:[3] (1) transection of the main pulmonary artery and anastomosis with the hypoplastic aorta with homograft augmentation of the arch, (2) atrial septectomy, and (3) placement of a systemic-to-pulmonary artery shunt. A right ventricular-to-pulmonary artery conduit (Sano procedure)[9,10] has been substituted for the systemic-to-pulmonary artery shunt in some institutions; this has the theoretical advantage of better coronary perfusion because of little diastolic runoff. Whether surgical reconstruction is needed or not, the single ventricle pumps blood to the systemic and pulmonary circulation in parallel, causing a volume overload.

When pulmonary vascular resistance has decreased adequately (approximately 3-6 months of age), the **hemi-Fontan procedure** or the **bidirectional cavopulmonary anastomosis** is performed.[2,11,12] This is a superior vena cava-to-pulmonary artery anastomosis with exclusion of this blood flow to the atrium and ligation of the systemic-to-pulmonary artery shunt. The ventricle does not have direct access to the pulmonary circulation in this setup and is volume unloaded. It is not clear, however, that it remains volume unloaded throughout the time the patient is in this physiology.[2] Cardiac output is maintained at the expense of cyanosis because only part of the systemic venous return enters

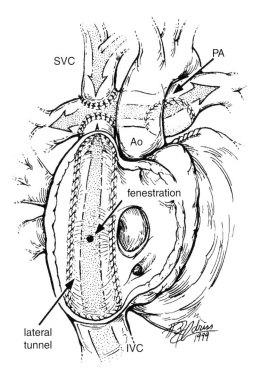

FIGURE 23-1 ■ **The lateral atrial tunnel type of Fontan.** The lateral atrial tunnel is made of a gusset of polytetrafluoroethylene and of the native right atrial wall. A fenestration can be seen in the baffle. Ao, aorta; IVC, inferior vena cava; PA, pulmonary artery; SVC, superior vena cava. (From Jacobs ML: *The functional single ventricle and Fontan's operation.* In Mavroudis C, Backer CL (eds): *Pediatric Cardiac Surgery.* Philadelphia, Mosby, 2003, p. 506.)

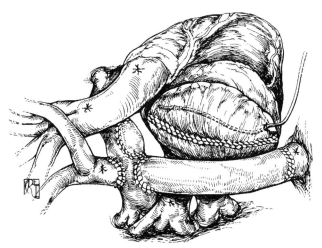

FIGURE 23-2 ■ **The extracardiac conduit type of Fontan.** A right-sided superior cavopulmonary anastomosis is seen with an interposition of a polytetrafluoroethylene graft conduit between the inferior vena cava and the underside of the pulmonary artery. (From Mavroudis C, Deal B, Backer CL, et al: *The favorable impact of arrhythmia surgery on total cavopulmonary artery Fontan conversion. Semin Thorac Cardiovasc Surg Pediatr Card Surg Annu* 1999;2:143-156.)

HEMODYNAMIC FACTORS AND SINGLE VENTRICULAR PERFORMANCE

Before the bidirectional cavopulmonary anastomosis, the major factor in this stage is the chronic ventricular volume overload on the single ventricle.[2,11,13] The anatomic single ventricle, especially that of the morphologically right ventricle with its abnormal fibrous architecture, may be poorly suited to handle such a volume abnormality on a long-term basis. There are other factors at play as well—systemic arterial desaturation, ventricular hypertrophy,[2] and altered afterload as the systemic and pulmonary circulations are in parallel.

The physiology of **volume overload** in a single ventricle increases wall stress via Laplace's law with increases in myocardial hypertrophy to compensate partially for this overload (Fig. 23-3). In the face of decreased systemic arterial oxygen saturation, this in turn increases myocardial oxygen demand. In addition, alterations in the Starling curve[14] may lead to further cardiac enlargement, which would increase myocardial oxygen demand further. Overall, the volume load may come from more than just pumping to two circulations—atrioventricular valve and, much more rarely, semilunar valve insufficiency also can add to the hemodynamic burden. Of patients with hypoplastic left heart syndrome, 50% to 60% have tricuspid regurgitation preoperatively, which is one of the risk factors for outcome.[15]

The increased myocardial oxygen consumption translates into **increased coronary blood flow**. In a 1997 study,[12] 22 patients with hypoplastic left heart syndrome and aortic atresia were studied by transesophageal

the lungs. This intermediate procedure was instituted when some studies noted that the ventricular wall thickness-to-chamber dimension ratio acutely increased when the Fontan procedure was performed without this step.[2,11] Diastolic ventricular compliance issues were believed to be at play because low output, tachycardia, and hemodynamic deterioration were present after the Fontan procedure. A form of bidirectional cavopulmonary anastomosis that is definitely not volume unloaded is one in which an additional source of pulmonary blood flow is left in place, such as a systemic-to-pulmonary artery shunt or forward flow through a stenotic pulmonary valve.

At approximately 2 years of age, the circulations are separated via the **Fontan operation** by directing inferior vena cava blood into the lungs by placement of a patch along the lateral wall of the atria ("lateral wall tunnel") (Fig. 23-1) or by the use of an extracardiac conduit (Fig. 23-2). All blood must traverse the lungs by passive flow to maintain cardiac output. A communication (a "fenestration") is purposely created between the systemic and the pulmonary venous pathways to allow for shunting between the circulations when there is increased pulmonary vascular resistance. The cardiac output can be maintained in this fashion at the expense of cyanosis. The fenestrations generally close spontaneously. Because the circulations are now separated, the ventricle is volume unloaded.

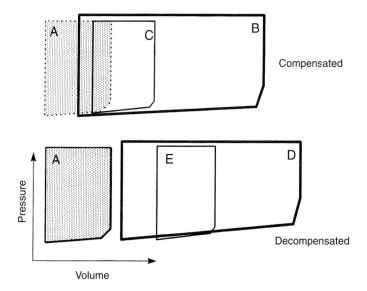

FIGURE 23-3 ■ **Pressure-volume loop in single ventricle with volume overload. Top**, Diagram illustrates the normal pressure-volume relationship (loop **A**) and the pressure-volume relationship of the chronic volume overloaded but compensated ventricle (loop **B**). Loop **C** represents the pressure-volume loop after removal of the chronic volume overload but with different characteristics. **Bottom**, Diagram shows a decompensated ventricle and its pressure-volume loop (loop **D**). Loop **E** illustrates the dilated single ventricle with high end-diastolic pressures even after removal of the volume overload. (From Lawrenson J, Gewillig M: *The ventricle in the functionally univentricular heart*. In Redington A, Brawn WJ, Deanfield JE, Anderson RH [eds]: *The Right Heart in Congenital Heart Disease*. London, Greenwich Medical Media, 1998, p. 128.)

echocardiography immediately before and after bidirectional cavopulmonary anastomosis and immediately before and after Fontan procedure to measure coronary blood flow. Preoperative bidirectional cavopulmonary anastomosis patients had higher coronary blood flow, velocity time integral, and peak velocity than postoperative bidirectional cavopulmonary anastomosis patients and patients after Fontan procedure. Coronary flow in patients with hypoplastic left heart syndrome after stage I Norwood reconstruction was similar to the physiology of aortic insufficiency.[16,17] In both, the ventricle is volume loaded, and systemic diastolic blood pressure is low. Flow changed from predominately systolic in preoperative bidirectional cavopulmonary anastomosis to systolic and diastolic at the other time points. Compare this flow with the normal left ventricle, where most coronary blood flow occurs during diastole, whereas in the normal right ventricle, flow is continuous throughout the cardiac cycle (systolic flow greater than diastolic flow). Right ventricular coronary flow can change, however, to a more left ventricle like profile when right ventricular pressure becomes systemic.[17] In patients with hypoplastic left heart syndrome, the right ventricle is systemic, but it does not become left ventricle like. The flow pattern is more consistent with the patterns in aortic regurgitation.[16,17]

Neurohumoral changes also occur at this volume loaded stage, which may lead to congestive heart failure. The atria and the ventricle synthesize brain and atrial natriuretic peptides, which are released by myocardial stretch and have emerged as markers of heart failure.[18] Brain and atrial natriuretic peptides were measured in a study comparing single ventricle patients before bidirectional cavopulmonary anastomosis and after bidirectional cavopulmonary anastomosis and normal individuals.[19] Patients before bidirectional cavopulmonary anastomosis showed an increase in natriuretic peptides over patients after bidirectional cavopulmonary anastomosis and over

normal controls. These elevated levels were in the absence of qualitatively decreased ventricular shortening by echocardiography and may represent a precursor to heart failure.

To determine the optimal hemodynamic parameters to maximize oxygen delivery, mathematical models have been created[20,21] with crucial variables, such as cardiac output and pulmonary venous oxygen saturation. Among the findings were (1) optimal pulmonary-to-systemic flow ratio for systemic oxygen delivery is ≤1; (2) with increasing pulmonary-to-systemic flow ratio, systemic oxygen delivery initially increases, reaches a peak, then decreases; and (3) as the cardiac output and pulmonary venous saturation increase, the optimal pulmonary-to-systemic flow ratio decreases.

Because the single ventricle is faced with chronic volume overload, which has been documented by numerous techniques,[2,22,23] **global ventricular performance** parameters differ from normal hearts. A study using cardiac MRI documented significantly increased ventricular output, end-diastolic volume, ventricular mass, and ejection fraction (66%) in the pre-bidirectional cavopulmonary anastomosis ventricle compared with the volume unloaded Fontan stage.[2] Angiography and radionuclide techniques[22] found a significantly increased end-diastolic volume compared with controls, but found a smaller ejection fraction (51% to 52%), ventricular output, and ventricular mass compared with the MRI study. These studies did not produce similar results because (1) hypoplastic left heart syndrome was the diagnosis in most patients in the cardiac MRI study, whereas the angiography and radionuclide studies were performed on patients with many types of univentricular hearts that were of the left ventricle type, and (2) the angiography and radionuclide studies were performed on older patients (mean age 6.4 years versus 5.7 months). Age is an important consideration; in a study by echocardiography, ejection fraction was 59% for patients 2 to 10 years old and 52% for patients older than 10, and end-diastolic volume and dimensions ranged from 245% to 283% and 145% to 149% of normal.[23]

Before bidirectional cavopulmonary anastomosis, the degree of **ventricular hypertrophy**[2,22,23] plays an important clinical role in the univentricular heart. In the era when bidirectional cavopulmonary anastomosis was not routinely performed, increased preoperative left ventricular muscle mass was found to be a significant risk factor for poor outcome in patients undergoing Fontan procedure.[24] Even after Fontan, Kirklin and coworkers[25] found ventricular hypertrophy to be a significant risk factor for death.

A measure of the integrated function of the heart is **total heart volume** (i.e., volume of atria and ventricles), which changes little during the cardiac cycle (<5%)[26]; this occurs by reciprocating volume changes in the atria and ventricles and minimizes the wasted energy expenditure to move extracardiac structures. Intracycle constancy of the center of mass of the entire heart volume also is true for the reasons just stated.[27,28] It has been shown that 4 of 10 patients before bidirectional cavopulmonary anastomosis had total heart volumes vary by greater than 5% (threshold for normal individuals),[28] and the center of mass of the total heart volume moved significantly in the superoinferior and anteroposterior planes, all indicating that pre-bidirectional cavopulmonary anastomosis single ventricles not only perform more volume work, but also waste energy by unnecessarily displacing extracardiac structures.

Pre-bidirectional cavopulmonary anastomosis single ventricles show **regional ventricular dysfunction** and global functional abnormalities. Using angiocardiography, 2 of 18 patients showed regional wall motion abnormalities.[29] Using cardiac MRI tagging,[30] the inferior wall of 11 of 13 patients with hypoplastic left heart syndrome before bidirectional cavopulmonary anastomosis showed the largest compressive strain of all wall regions. Counterclockwise and clockwise wall motions were noted in the ventricular short axis (the normal systemic ventricle shows uniform rotation in the short axis), meeting in an area of no twist, which showed the greatest strain.

Bidirectional Cavopulmonary Anastomosis

Because there is no direct access to the pulmonary circulation from the univentricular heart in a typical bidirectional cavopulmonary anastomosis, the ventricle pumps one cardiac output to the body, and whatever flow goes to the brain and upper body becomes the pulmonary blood flow via the superior vena cava. Blood flow from the rest of the body enters the heart via the inferior vena cava; volume loading of the ventricle is not present. The decrease in **ventricular volume** immediately after bidirectional cavopulmonary anastomosis has

been documented in many studies. Immediately after bidirectional cavopulmonary anastomosis, ventricular end-diastolic volume was found to have decreased by 33% in a study by echocardiography.[11] Another echocardiography investigation in the early postoperative period showed decreases in the end-diastolic volume from 20% to 25% with preserved ejection fraction.[31,32] This volume unloading can have significant adverse clinical impact and affect ventricular function; subaortic obstruction may occur in patients with a bulboventricular foramen caused by narrowing of the outlet.[33]

There is some evidence to suggest that volume unloading may change during the time when the patient is in bidirectional cavopulmonary anastomosis physiology, or that it does not occur in all patients. Bidirectional cavopulmonary anastomosis patients were evaluated 6 to 9 months after surgery by cardiac MRI[2] and were found to have ventricular end-diastolic volumes that were not statistically different from patients before bidirectional cavopulmonary anastomosis with the cardiac index remaining high. This finding may have resulted in part from a redistribution of blood flow to the brain (increased perfusion) to meet the needs of the pulmonary blood flow. Development of aortopulmonary collaterals may be another cause, which have been shown to develop in 65% of patients, imposing a volume load.[34]

Not all univentricular heart patients may benefit from volume unloading in bidirectional cavopulmonary anastomosis.[32] During the early postoperative bidirectional cavopulmonary anastomosis period, a study by echocardiography found a significant decrease in ventricular volumes in the overall study population. Subgroup analysis showed no significant decrease in the subgroup with a pulmonary artery band, but a significant decrease in ventricular volumes in patients with a systemic-to-pulmonary artery shunt. To complicate matters further, the study also suggested that ventricular morphology may play a role—morphologic left ventricles did have a significant decrease in ventricular volumes postoperatively, but morphologic right ventricles did not. In another study,[35] patients who were older (>10 years old) also did not seem to benefit from volume unloading by bidirectional cavopulmonary anastomosis and had a decreased ejection fraction, whereas patients younger than 3 years old had a decreased ventricular volume and a greater ejection fraction. Prior palliative surgery, ventricular morphology, and age of the patient all can influence the degree of volume unloading to the single ventricle.

Whether there is a decrease in **ventricular mass** after bidirectional cavopulmonary anastomosis surgery is uncertain. In the immediate postoperative period after the bidirectional cavopulmonary anastomosis procedure, an echocardiographic study[11] showed only an 11% to 13% increase in ventricular wall thickness by echocardiography, which was not statistically significant. Cardiac MRI showed no significant change in mass 6 to

9 months after surgery. Forbes and colleagues[35] did show a significant decrease in ventricular mass after bidirectional cavopulmonary anastomosis, although this effect was seen only in patients younger than 3 years old.

Before routine use of the bidirectional cavopulmonary anastomosis, the acute change in **mass/volume relationship** during volume unloading by the Fontan procedure was believed to play a major adverse role in outcome.[2,11,24] Preoperative mass/volume was greater in patients with poor outcomes than patients with good outcomes after the Fontan procedure.[24] The rationale with the creation of the bidirectional cavopulmonary anastomosis surgery was to allow a significant amount of the systemic venous return to fill the ventricle without first passing through the lungs, then the single ventricle could tolerate the mass/volume change better. Although insertion of the bidirectional cavopulmonary anastomosis may improve clinical outcome, it did not change the mass/volume postoperatively because an increase of 103% to 111% in wall thickness-to-ventricular volume was found by echocardiography.[11] The increase in the mass/volume may self-correct because a cardiac MRI study showed no difference in mass/volume between patients before and 6 to 9 months after bidirectional cavopulmonary anastomosis surgery.[2]

Similar to the work done on patients before bidirectional cavopulmonary anastomosis, a mathematical model to optimize the **pulmonary-to-systemic flow** ratio after bidirectional cavopulmonary anastomosis was created. The key findings in this physiology included the following: (1) As the superior-to-inferior vena cava flow ratio increases, total body oxygen delivery and arterial and superior vena caval saturations increase; (2) with increasing superior-to-inferior vena cava flow ratio, lower body oxygen delivery and inferior vena cava oxygen saturation initially increase, reach a peak, then decrease; (3) for a given oxygen delivery, bidirectional cavopulmonary anastomosis decreases the amount of cardiac output required; and (4) as the percentage of lower body oxygen consumption increases, oxygen delivery and saturation decrease.

Single-ventricle **regional wall function** changes after bidirectional cavopulmonary anastomosis surgery, although the pattern of wall twisting remains unchanged. Cardiac MRI[2] showed that patients after bidirectional cavopulmonary anastomosis had the smallest compressive strains and the largest heterogeneity of compressive strains in all four wall regions studied at two short-axis slice levels throughout staged reconstruction. Similar to patients before bidirectional cavopulmonary anastomosis, however, wall twisting around the short axis exhibited similar motion.

A "hybrid bidirectional cavopulmonary anastomosis" circulation also has been created—the superior vena cava is connected to the pulmonary artery, excluding the right atrium from superior vena caval flow, but additional sources of pulmonary blood flow are left, such as a systemic-to-pulmonary artery shunt or antegrade flow from the ventricle, as in pulmonic stenosis.[37] This circulation clearly adds another dimension to the physiology and places a volume load on the ventricle.

Fontan Operation

The Fontan operation is the final phase of reconstruction that separates the circulation in single-ventricle patients; the operation has evolved over the years, and this evolution has had an impact on ventricular function. There was the era before and after bidirectional cavopulmonary anastomosis, the era before and after the use of fenestration in the Fontan, and the era at present of various types of Fontan operations. This section provides a brief overview of ventricular function in the single ventricle after Fontan.

Fontan reconstruction was the principal **volume reduction** surgery before the bidirectional cavopulmonary anastomosis era by placing the circulations in series rather than in parallel. This step should decrease wall stress, ventricular size, and hypertrophy. In addition, cardiac efficiency and peripheral perfusion should improve with the elimination of shunting to the low-resistance pulmonary vascular bed and normalization of sympathetic tone. By placing the circulations in series, however, total systemic resistance increases relative to the previous stage. To complicate things further, it has been suggested that the noncompliant baffle attached to the ventricle may increase afterload as well.[2,28,30] All of these physiologic parameters have an impact on the ultimate ventricular performance of the single ventricle. The possible alterations in Fontan mechanics include systolic and diastolic myocardial dysfunction, altered venous and arterial hemodynamics, conduction system trauma with ensuing arrhythmias, and valvar dysfunction.

It has been known that the single ventricle after Fontan has relatively low cardiac output[2,22,34] and diminished exercise capacity. The low cardiac output is the result of numerous altered states, including elevated systemic vascular resistance[22] and abnormal venous mechanics. Senzaki and associates[37] compared the impedance, hemodynamics, and power in a normal dual-chambered circulation in patients with single ventricle after Fontan and in patients with single ventricle after a systemic-to-pulmonary artery shunt. Pulsatile and nonpulsatile components of ventricular afterload were separated out, and the authors related these changes as **ventricular-vascular coupling**. This comparison was performed at rest and with dobutamine stress. The Fontan patients were found, at rest and with β-adrenergic stimulation, to have an elevation of the pulsatile component of ventricular afterload ("low-frequency impedance") and vascular resistance ("nonpulsatile" load on the ventricle); these findings were associated closely with decreased cardiac index. Wave reflection in the Fontan circuit was found to be the major contributor to

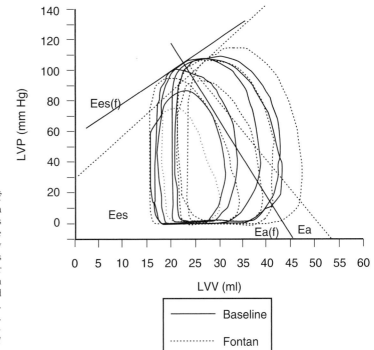

FIGURE 23-4 ■ End-systolic pressure volume (Eesf versus Ees) and arterial elastances (Eaf versus Ea) with control and after Fontan operation (f). Diagram shows ventriculoarterial mechanics after the Fontan operation. As the curves illustrate, the end-systolic pressure-volume trajectory (index of ventricular contractility) becomes flatter (Ees_f versus Ees), whereas the arterial elastance curve (index of vascular loading) becomes steeper (Ea_f versus Ea) after the Fontan operation. This unfavorable combination results in increased ventriculoarterial coupling and reduced mechanical efficiency. LVP, left ventricular pressure; LVV, left ventricular volume. (From Szabo G, Buhmann V, Graf A, et al: *Ventricular energetics after the Fontan operation: Contractility afterload mismatch.* J Thorac Cardiovasc Surg 2003;125:1061-1069.)

the increased ventricular afterload; this was unique to the Fontan circuit, as it was not found in single-ventricle patients after systemic to pulmonary artery shunt. In addition, hydraulic power cost per unit of forward flow was 40% lower in the dual-chambered circulation than in the single-ventricle circulation, which was attributed to the lack of a pulmonary pumping ventricle. The conclusion was that Fontan physiology is associated with disadvantageous ventricular power and afterload profiles.

An animal study of the Fontan circulation using pressure-volume and impedance spectrum analysis showed that after the Fontan operation, there exists a contractility-afterload mismatch secondary to increased impedance caused by the additional connection of the pulmonary vascular bed to the systemic vasculature with deterioration of the myocardial contractility (Fig. 23-4). This study showed that an increased ventriculoarterial coupling ratio and concomitant reduced mechanical efficiency with limited cardiac reserve occur after the Fontan circulation is established. In short, the single ventricle is not able to use heterometric (Frank-Starling mechanism) autoregulation, homeometric (Anrep effect) autoregulation, or even increased mean filling pressure (Guytonian relationship) to counter the increased afterload after the Fontan operation. Finally, an interim bidirectional cavopulmonary anastomosis preceding the Fontan operation can improve the ventricular energetics after the procedure (Fig. 23-5).

The noncompliant baffle in the atria may be another potential source of increased afterload in the Fontan patient. The restriction of systolic atrioventricular valve

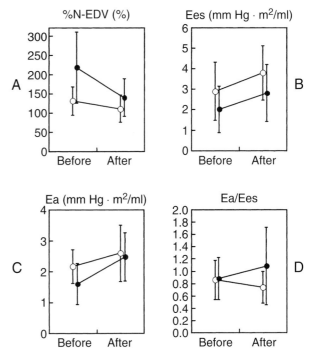

FIGURE 23-5 ■ Cardiac performance comparing staged (interim bidirectional cavopulmonary anastomosis) (*open circles*) **and primary** (*filled circles*) **Fontan groups. A,** The %N-EDV (percent of normal systemic ventricular end-diastolic volume) decrease was greater in the primary group. **B,** The end-systolic pressure volume (Ees) (contractility or end-systolic elastance) increased in the staged and primary groups. **C,** The arterial elastance (Ea) (afterload or effective arterial elastance) increased in both groups as well, but the increment of Ea was greater in the primary group. **D,** The Ea/Ees (mechanical efficiency-ventriculoarterial coupling) ratio (ventriculoarterial coupling) decreased in the staged group, whereas it increased in the primary group. (From Tanoue Y, Sese A, Ueno Y, et al: *Bidirectional Glenn procedure improves the mechanical efficiency of total cavopulmonary connection in high-risk Fontan candidates. Circulation* 2001;103:2176-2180.)

plane motion toward the apex as seen with atrial fibrillation has been believed to occur because of the loss of atrial compliance and disrupts the constancy of total heart volume and center of mass motion.[38,39] A noncompliant baffling material is attached to the atria in many types of Fontan reconstructions and could act similarly, disrupting normal cardiac mechanics. A study that measured the **constancy of total heart volume and center of mass** in Fontan patients[28] showed that a significant number of Fontan patients (71%) did not have constant total heart volume throughout the cardiac cycle, disrupted in part by baffle placement. Correlations existed between the lateral plane and the anteroposterior and superoinferior planes ($r^2 = 0.51$ to 0.91) of the heart's center of mass motion, presumably because these planes are linked by the lateral wall tunnel baffle sewn into the lateral and posterior walls of the atria. Differences in lateral wall motion between Fontan patients and patients before and after bidirectional cavopulmonary anastomosis were shown, regardless of whether the heart maintained constant total heart volume, using two-factor analysis of variance.

Although the Fontan ventricle is ideally volume unloaded, certain factors, such as atrioventricular and semilunar valve insufficiency, may play a role to place a **volume load** on the single ventricle. Of patients who have hypoplastic left heart syndrome, 61% have neoaortic insufficiency, which was found in a 21-year follow-up, and 49% had progressed over time.[40] Aortopulmonary collaterals may be another source of volume load on the ventricle because 30% of Fontan patients had these collaterals by angiography.[34]

Another contributor to the overall detriment of cardiac efficiency after Fontan is altered **venous mechanics**. There is reduced venous capacitance in these patients, with decreased pooling of blood in the legs as well. In addition, there is increased venous tone, which limits the ability to mobilize blood from the capacitance vessels, impairing cardiac output. Lastly, there is a loss of the normal augmentation in portal venous flow that takes place with expiration, and there are elevated hepatic venous wedge pressures reflecting elevated splanchnic venous pressures (which are moderated by fenestration of the baffle).

These hemodynamic alterations all may be tied into elevated levels of **circulating vasoactive substances** after Fontan, which also may affect the single-ventricle myocardium directly. There is an elevation of atrial natriuretic peptide, which increases sodium excretion and promotes diuresis; decreases blood pressure and total peripheral resistance; and markedly inhibits renin, aldosterone, and vasopressin secretion. Angiotensin II, a potent vasoconstrictor that modulates vascular tone, glomerular and tubular function, and aldosterone secretion, and endothelin-1, which is a potent endothelium-derived vasoconstrictor (especially of the pulmonary vascular bed), are elevated after Fontan.

These major external factors combine with **intrinsic myocardial factors** to decrease rest and exercise ventricular performance. At rest, cardiac index in Fontan patients ranges from 2.4 to 3 L/min/m²,[2,22,34] and ejection fraction ranges from 50% to 56%[2,22,41] even 10 years after surgery. In the immediate postoperative period, wall thickness increases, but this does not persist; nearly 2 years after Fontan completion, the ventricular mass[2] by MRI decreases much below the other stages of surgical reconstruction. This decrease in wall thickness is clinically important because ventricular hypertrophy is associated with increased risk of death after Fontan.[25] Even 10 years after Fontan reconstruction, myocardial mass was found to be 75 g/m² by MRI, not significantly different from a normal control group.[41]

Age of operation in Fontan patients is strongly associated with ventricular shape, wall stress, and other systolic indices of ventricular performance.[23] With increasing age (>10 years old), patients with single left ventricles after Fontan repair had a greater end-systolic wall stress than patients who were repaired at 2 to 10 years old. Other indices, such as velocity of circumferential fiber shortening, fractional shortening, and ejection fraction, were not better than the palliated group who did not have a Fontan operation or bidirectional cavopulmonary anastomosis. Velocity of circumferential fiber shortening, fractional shortening, and ejection fraction all were negatively correlated with age of operation ($r = -0.41$ to -0.54; $P < .01$). Age of operation older than 10 years was associated with a more normal ventricular ellipsoidal shape, however, than age of operation between 2 and 10 years.

Regional ventricular wall function also is abnormal in patients after Fontan reconstruction. The inferior and superior walls near the base in short axis showed increased compressive strains (hyperfunctioning) compared with other wall regions in patients (mostly hypoplastic left heart syndrome) who had undergone Fontan completion around 2 years of age.[30] In general, strain is greater near the base than the apex. Endocardial compressive strain is less than epicardial strain, which is opposite the normal human left ventricle.[30] Eleven of 25 patients with tricuspid atresia after Fontan completion, at an average age of 6.5 years, were found to have hypokinesia of various wall regions.[29] In short axis, using cardiac MRI,[30] there was paradoxical inferior wall systolic motion, and the greatest radial systolic motion was found in the superior wall. From a rotational standpoint, in short axis, there were wall regions of clockwise and counterclockwise twist that met in a zone of no twist, which showed the greatest compressive strains, similar to other stages of reconstruction.

Diastolic function also is impaired in the single ventricle after Fontan. Peak filling rate, diastolic filling time, and time to peak filling rate were measured using radionuclide techniques in patients with mostly single left ventricle morphology after Fontan procedure.[22]

Diastolic filling time was longer and the time to peak filling rate was shorter in patients after Fontan than before Fontan. Peak filling rate was smaller in Fontan patients than in a control group of patients with a normal two-ventricle circulation. Echocardiographic serial diastolic assessment after Fontan surgery shows that isovolumic relaxation time is significantly longer, and E wave deceleration time, E and A wave velocities, and E:A velocity ratio were reduced compared with normal early and late after the procedure.

CURRENT STATUS AND FUTURE TRENDS

The study of ventricular function in single-ventricle patients is an extremely complex evaluation because of numerous factors, including the variability in reconstructive techniques and the types of single ventricles. Much progress has been made in understanding the complicated pumping action of the heart, but much more needs to be accomplished. In addition to the stages of surgery and impact on single ventricular function, there are other important factors that determine ventricular performance. Ventricular morphology plays a role in ventricular function of the univentricular heart. Single ventricular morphology is related to exercise capacity, atrioventricular valve regurgitation, hypoxia, and impaired heart rate response with exercise. Coronary blood flow also can be compromised in patients with single ventricles. One example is hypoplastic left heart syndrome, which has an abnormal coronary artery morphology. Another example is pulmonary atresia with intact ventricular septum, which sometimes must undergo single ventricle reconstructive surgery, where coronary cameral fistulas and the so-called right ventricle–dependent coronary circulation may exist.

Another important consideration in single-ventricle function is ventricular-ventricular interaction. It has been known for many years that the normal right ventricle and left ventricle do not act independently of each other, and that ventricular-ventricular interaction occurs. Mechanical coupling of the ventricles is the presumed mechanism of ventricular interdependence and is shown by a contribution of the left ventricle-to-right ventricle pressure generation and the right ventricle-to-left ventricle pressure generation. In single ventricles, there is by definition no second ventricle to augment ventricular function, and this absence may adversely affect ventricular mechanics and ultimately the long-term viability of the single ventricle. A comparison of ventricular mechanics in single ventricles with the mechanics in a dual-chambered circulation has been studied by cardiac MRI, and the regional function has been delineated.[42,43] Finally, it is known that by any measure, exercise capacity in single-ventricle patients who have undergone Fontan reconstruction is significantly

decreased compared with normal individuals matched for age and gender. Maximal work rates and oxygen consumption are 50% to 60% of what would be expected from normal individuals. Reasons for this impairment vary and include abnormal chronotropic response, the inability to augment stroke volume when the demand of the body increases, the heterogeneity of the patient population including age at operation, anatomic and surgical subtypes, and elevated neurohormones. The need to help Fontan patients exercise well, especially considering that many are children, is clear.

The study of single ventricular function in aggregate was presented in this chapter under the framework of stages of reconstruction. Numerous complicating factors play a role in determining ventricular function, however, and teasing out differences among these will be a difficult task for future research. The Sano procedure (ventricular-to-pulmonary artery conduit creation) is a newer technique to provide pulmonary blood flow in these patients,[9,10] and the results in terms of ventricular function and clinical outcome of this change in surgical approach remain to be determined. Because there is no systemic-to-pulmonary artery shunt, diastolic pressure is higher and should provide better coronary perfusion. A ventriculotomy is performed, which could affect ventricular performance. In the future, the fate of the single ventricle in young adults and older patients will rely on innovative investigations and clinical vigilance.[45-47]

Key Concepts

■ Before bidirectional cavopulmonary anastomosis, the major factor in this stage is the chronic ventricular volume overload on the single ventricle. The anatomic single ventricle, especially that of the morphologically right ventricle with its abnormal fibrous architecture, may be poorly suited to handle such a volume abnormality on a long-term basis. There are other factors at play as well—systemic arterial desaturation, ventricular hypertrophy, and altered afterload as the systemic and pulmonary circulations are in parallel.

■ Prior palliative surgery, ventricular morphology, and age of the patient all can influence the degree of volume unloading to the single ventricle.

■ An animal study of the Fontan circulation using pressure-volume and impedance spectrum analysis showed that after the Fontan operation, a contractility-afterload mismatch exists secondary to increased impedance caused by the additional connection of the pulmonary vascular bed to the systemic vasculature with deterioration of the myocardial contractility.

■ An increased ventriculoarterial coupling ratio and concomitant reduced mechanical efficiency with limited cardiac reserve after the Fontan circulation is established. In short, the single ventricle is not able to use heterometric (Frank-Starling mechanism) autoregulation, homeometric (Anrep effect) autoregulation, or even increased mean filling pressure (Guytonian relationship) to counter the increased afterload after the Fontan operation.

■ An interim bidirectional cavopulmonary anastomosis preceding the Fontan operation can improve the ventricular energetics after the procedure.

■ Although the Fontan ventricle is ideally volume unloaded, certain factors, such as atrioventricular and semilunar valve insufficiency, may play a role to place a volume load on the single ventricle.

■ Coronary blood flow also can be compromised in patients with single ventricles. One example is hypoplastic left heart syndrome, which has an abnormal coronary artery morphology. Another example is pulmonary atresia with intact ventricular septum, which sometimes must undergo single-ventricle reconstructive surgery, where coronary cameral fistulas and the so-called right ventricle dependent coronary circulation may exist.

■ Another important consideration in single-ventricle function is ventricular-ventricular interaction. It has been known for many years that the normal right ventricle and left ventricle do not act independently of each other, and that ventricular-ventricular interaction occurs. Mechanical coupling of the ventricles is the presumed mechanism of ventricular interdependence and is shown by a contribution of the left ventricle-to-right ventricle pressure generation and the right ventricle-to-left ventricle pressure generation. In single ventricles, there is by definition no second ventricle to augment ventricular function, and this absence may adversely affect ventricular mechanics and ultimately the long-term viability of the single ventricle.

REFERENCES

1. Fontan F, Baudet E: Surgical repair of tricuspid atresia. Thorax 1971;26:240-248.
2. Fogel MA, Weinberg PM, Chin AJ, et al: Late ventricular geometry and performance changes of functional single ventricle throughout staged Fontan reconstruction assessed by magnetic resonance imaging. J Am Coll Cardiol 1996;28:212-221.
3. Norwood WI, Lang P, Hansen D: Physiologic repair of aortic atresia: Hypoplastic left heart syndrome. N Engl J Med 1983;308:23-26.
4. Fogel MA, Weinberg PM, Rychik J, et al: Caval contribution to flow in the branch pulmonary arteries of Fontan patients using a novel application of magnetic resonance presaturation pulse. Circulation 1999;99:1215-1221.
5. Sharma S, Goudy S, Walker P, et al: In vitro flow experiments for determination of optimal geometry of total cavopulmonary connection for surgical repair of children with functional single ventricle. J Am Coll Cardiol 1996;27:1264-1269.
6. Van Praagh R: Terminology of congenital heart disease: Glossary and commentary. Circulation 1977;56:139-143.
7. Sondheimer HM, Freedom RM, Olley PM: Double outlet right ventricle: Clinical spectrum and prognosis. Am J Cardiol 1977;39:709.
8. Edwards JE, Burchell HB: Congenital tricuspid atresia: A classification. Med Clin North Am 1949;33:1117-1196.
9. Sano S, Ishino K, Kawada M, et al: Right ventricle-pulmonary artery shunt in first-stage palliation of hypoplastic left heart syndrome. J Thorac Cardiovasc Surg 2003;126:504-510.
10. Pizarro C, Malec E, Maher KO: Right ventricle to pulmonary artery conduit improves outcome after Stage I Norwood for hypoplastic left heart syndrome. Circulation 2003;108(Suppl II):II-155-II-160.
11. Seliem MA, Baffa JM, Vetter JM, et al: Changes in right ventricular geometry and heart rate early after hemi-Fontan procedure. Ann Thorac Surg 1993;55:1508-1512.
12. Fogel MA, Rychik J, Vetter J, et al: Effect of volume unloading surgery on coronary flow dynamics in patients with aortic atresia. J Thorac Cardiovasc Surg 1997;113:718-727.
13. Pasque MK: Fontan hemodynamics. J Card Surg 1988;3:45-52.
14. Alyono D, Ring WS, Anderson MR, et al: Left ventricular adaptation to volume overload from large aortocaval fistula. Surgery 1984;96:360.
15. Weinberg PM, Peyser K, Hackney JR: Fetal hydrops in a newborn with hypoplastic left heart syndrome: Tricuspid valve stopper. J Am Coll Cardiol 1985;6:1365-1369.
16. Kisanuki A, Murayama T, Matsushita R, et al: Transesophageal Doppler echocardiographic assessement of left coronary blood flow velocity in chronic aortic regurgitation. Am Heart J 1997;131:101-106.
17. Hongo M, Goto T, Watanabe N, et al: Relation of phasic coronary flow velocity profile to clinical and hemodynamic characteristics of patients with aortic valve disease. Circulation 1993;88:953-960.
18. Muders R, Kromer EF, Griese DP, et al: Evaluation of plasma natriuretic peptides as markers for left ventricular dysfunction. Am Heart J 1997;134:442-449.
19. Wahlander H, Westerlind A, Lindstedt G, et al: Increased levels of brain and atrial natriuretic peptides after the first palliative operation, but not after a bidirectional Glenn anastomosis, in children with functionally univentricular hearts. Cardiol Young 2003;13:268-274.
20. Austin EH, Santamore WP, Barnea O: Balancing the circulation in hypoplastic left heart syndrome. J Cardiovasc Surg 1994;35:137-139.
21. Barnea O, Austin EH, Richman B: Balancing the circulations: Theoretic optimization of pulmonary/systemic flow ratio in hypoplastic left heart syndrome. J Am Coll Cardiol 1994;24:1376-1381.
22. Akagi T, Benson LN, Green M, et al: Ventricular performance before and after Fontan repair for univentricular atrioventricular connection: Angiographic and radionuclide assessment. J Am Coll Cardiol 1992;20:920-926.
23. Sluysmans T, Sanders SP, van der Velde M, et al: Natural history and patterns of recovery of contractile function in single left ventricle after Fontan operation. Circulation 1992;86:1753-1761.
24. Seliem M, Muster AJ, Paul MH, et al: Relation between preoperative left ventricular muscle mass and outcome of the Fontan procedure in patients with tricuspid atresia. J Am Coll Cardiol 1989;14:750-755.
25. Kirklin JK, Blackstone EH, Kirklin JW, et al: The Fontan operation: Ventricular hypertrophy, age and date of operation as risk factors. J Thorac Cardiovasc Surg 1986;92:1049-1064.
26. Hoffman EA, Ritman EL: Invariant total heart volume in the intact thorax. Am J Physiol 1985;249:H883-H890.
27. Hoffman EA, Rumberger J, Dougherty L: A geometric view of cardiac "efficiency." J Am Coll Cardiol 1989;13:86A.
28. Fogel MA, Weinberg PW, Fellows KE, et al: Magnetic resonance imaging of constant total heart volume and center of mass in patients with functional single ventricle before and after staged Fontan procedure. Am J Cardiol 1993;72:1435-1443.
29. Akagi T, Benson LN, Williams WG, et al: Regional ventricular wall motion abnormalities in tricuspid atresia after the Fontan procedure. J Am Coll Cardiol 1993;22:1182-1188.

30. Fogel MA, Gupta KB, Weinberg PW, et al: Regional wall motion and strain analysis across stages of Fontan reconstruction by magnetic resonance tagging. Am J Physiol 1995;269(Heart Circ Physiol 38):H1132-H1152.

31. Lemes V, Ritter SB, Messina J, et al: Enhancement of ventricular mechanics following bidirectional superior cavopulmonary anastomosis in patients with single ventricle. J Card Surg 1995;10:119-124.

32. Berman NB, Kimball TR: Systemic ventricular size and performance before and after bidirectional cavopulmonary anastomosis. J Pediatr 1993;122:S63-S67.

33. van Son JA, Falk V, Walther T, et al: Instantaneous subaortic outflow obstruction after volume reduction in hearts with univentricular atrioventricular connection and discordant ventriculoarterial connection. Mayo Clin Proc 1997;72:309-314.

34. Triedman JK, Bridges ND, Mayer JE, et al: Prevalence and risk factors for aortopulmonary collateral vessels after Fontan and bidirectional Glenn procedures. J Am Coll Cardiol 1993;22:207-215.

35. Forbes TJ, Gajarski R, Johnson GL, et al: Influence of age on the effect of bidirectional cavopulmonary anastomosis on left ventricular volume, mass and ejection fraction. J Am Coll Cardiol 1996;28:1301-1307.

36. Santamore WP, Barnea O, Riordan CJ, et al: Theoretical optimization of pulmonary-to-systemic flow ratio after a bidirectional cavopulmonary anastomosis. Am J Physiol 1998;274:H694-H700.

37. Senzaki H, Masutani S, Kobayashi J, et al: Ventricular afterload and ventricular work in Fontan circulation: Comparison with normal two-ventricle circulation and single ventricle circulation with Blalock-Taussig shunt. Circulation 2002;105:2885-2892.

38. Hoffman EA, Ritman EL: Law of constant volume disrupted by atrial fibrillation. Fed Proc 1986;45:776.

39. Hoffman EA: Constancy of total heart volume: An imaging approach to cardiac mechanics. In Sideman S, Beyer R (eds): Imaging Measurements and Analysis of the Heart. New York, Hemisphere Publishing, 1991, pp 3-19.

40. Cohen MS, Marino BS, McElhinney DB, et al: Neo-aortic root dilation and valve regurgitation up to 21 years after staged reconstruction for hypoplastic left heart syndrome. J Am Coll Cardiol 2003;42:533-540.

41. Eiken A, Fratz S, Gutfried C, et al: Hearts late after Fontan operation have normal mass, normal volume and reduced systolic function. J Am Coll Cardiol 2003;42:1061-1065.

42. Fogel MA, Weinberg PM, Fellows KE, et al: A study in ventricular-ventricular interaction: Single right ventricles compared with systemic right ventricles in a dual chambered circulation. Circulation 1995;92:219-230.

43. Fogel MA, Weinberg PM, Gupta KB, et al: Mechanics of the single left ventricle: A study in ventricular-ventricular interaction II. Circulation 1998;98:330-338.

44. Fogel MA, Weinberg PM, Hoydu A, et al: The nature of flow in the systemic venous pathway in Fontan patients utilizing magnetic resonance blood tagging. J Thorac Cardiovasc Surg 1997;114:1032-1041.

45. Szabo G, Buhmann V, Graf A, et al: Ventricular energetics after the Fontan operation: Contractility afterload mismatch. J Thorac Cardiovasc Surg 2003;125:1061-1069.

46. Mott AR, Feltes TF, McKenzie ED, et al: Improved early results with the Fontan operation in adults with functional single ventricle. Ann Thorac Surg 2004;77:1334-1340.

47. Vitarelli A, Conde Y, Cimino E, et al: Quantitative assessment of systolic and diastolic ventricular function with tissue Doppler imaging after Fontan type of operation. Int J Cardiol 2005;102:61-69.

CHAPTER 24

Dysrhythmias and Ventricular Dysfunction

Bryan C. Cannon
Naomi J. Kertesz

When the heart is at an inappropriate rate or in atrioventricular (AV) dyssynchrony (or both), hemodynamic compromise can occur, which eventually leads to ventricular dysfunction. Chronic sustained supraventricular tachycardia can lead to myocardial ischemia secondary to prolonged periods of decreased diastolic filling time. The ventricular dysfunction and ensuing heart failure with dysrhythmias depend on the dysrhythmia rate, duration of dysrhythmia, presence of AV synchrony, age of the patient, and underlying anatomy and function. Various cardiomyopathic states can be associated with tachydysrhythmias as well. This close interaction between arrhythmias and heart failure creates a chicken-egg dilemma in certain patients.[1]

This chapter discusses the various tachyarrhythmias and bradyarrhythmias that can be the primary etiology that leads to ventricular dysfunction and heart failure in children. This chapter also delineates the dysrhythmias more commonly associated with heart failure after cardiac surgery. The other half of the chicken-egg dilemma, the cardiomyopathies and associated dysrhythmias, is addressed in Chapter 43.

TACHYCARDIA-INDUCED VENTRICULAR DYSFUNCTION OR CARDIOMYOPATHY

Although patients with poor cardiac function are more prone to developing rhythm disturbances, occasionally the primary cause of ventricular dysfunction is a tachyarrhythmia (hence the term *tachycardiomyopathy*).[2,3] The ventricular dysfunction associated with tachyarrhythmias may be so severe that patients mistakenly may be diagnosed as having cardiomyopathy and listed for heart transplantation; it is imperative that such tachyarrhythmias are diagnosed correctly and in a timely fashion to avoid an unnecessary transplantation.[4] In a study by Zimmerman and colleagues,[5] incessant atrial tachycardia was present in 17% of patients listed for cardiac transplantation and accounted for 37% of patients initially diagnosed with idiopathic cardiomyopathy.

Tachyarrhythmias leading to cardiomyopathy are typically incessant. In adults, tachycardia-induced cardiomyopathy can be secondary to AV nodal reentry tachycardia or atrial flutter or fibrillation, whereas in children, tachydysrhythmias more commonly associated with cardiomyopathy are atrial ectopic tachycardia (AET)

and permanent junctional reciprocating tachycardia (PJRT). Although the minimal heart rate necessary to develop tachycardia is unknown, most studies suggest that patients who develop tachycardia-induced cardiomyopathy have heart rates greater than 140 beats/min.[6] An animal study also revealed that rapid ventricular pacing for only 3 weeks can lead to heart failure.[7] Recovery of heart function after a dysrhythmia is terminated may take weeks to months, depending on the clinical situation and duration of the dysrhythmia.[8]

Although tachycardia may be atrial or ventricular in origin and may have an automatic focus or reentrant mechanism, supraventricular tachycardias (Fig. 24-1) are the most common cause of tachycardia-induced cardiomyopathy.[9] A hemodynamic study of prolonged supraventricular tachycardia and its effects showed that after 12 weeks of chronic supraventricular tachycardia and 12 weeks of recovery, ejection fraction recovered, and end-diastolic volume remained significantly elevated (Fig. 24-2). The stroke volume increased because the ejection fraction returned to normal, while the end-diastolic volume remained elevated.

Fetal Tachydysrhythmias

Incessant tachycardias may be present in utero and may be detected by fetal echocardiography.[10] It is frequently possible for a trained fetal ultrasonographer to distinguish atrial tachycardias (e.g., atrial flutter), reentrant tachycardias, and ventricular tachycardias. Research tools such as magnetocardiography may aid in the diagnosis of arrhythmias and may be specific enough to diagnose Wolff-Parkinson-White syndrome.[11] Patients with fetal tachyarrhythmias may have severe myocardial dysfunction with fetal hydrops (see Chapter 25). The disturbances may be so severe as to cause fetal demise.

In a study by Krapp and associates,[12] despite medical treatment of the arrhythmias, the overall mortality rate of fetuses with atrial flutter or incessant supraventricular tachycardia was around 9%. Treatment of the mother, with subsequent transplacental passage of the medication to the fetus, has been successful in many cases. Although digoxin, sotalol, flecainide, and amiodarone all have been used in the treatment of fetal tachycardias,[13] transplacental passage of these medications may be impaired by fetal hydrops. Injection of adenosine directly into the fetal umbilical vein also has been reported as a method of terminating reentrant fetal tachyarrhythmias.[14]

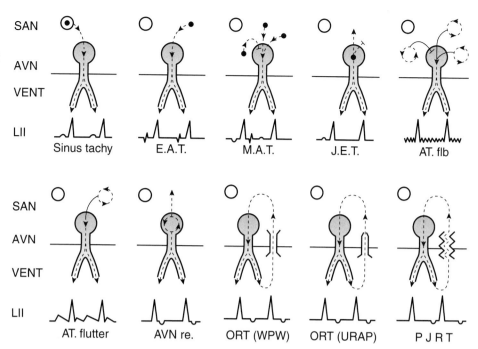

FIGURE 24-1 ■ **Mechanisms of supraventricular tachycardias.** The diagrams depict the various mechanisms of narrow QRS tachycardia, and the ECGs at the bottom of each diagram depict the axis and the timing of the P wave. AT, atrial; AVN, atrioventricular node; EAT, ectopic atrial tachycardia; JET, junctional ectopic tachycardia; MAT, multifocal atrial tachycardia; ORT, orthodromic reciprocating tachycardia; PJRT, permanent form of reciprocating tachycardia; SAN, sinoatrial node; URAP, unidirectional retrograde accessory pathway; VENT, ventricle; WPW, Wolff-Parkinson-White. (From Walsh EP: *Clinical approach to diagnosis and acute management of tachycardias in children. In Walsh EP, Saul JP, Triedman JK [eds]: Cardiac Arrhythmias in Children and Young Adults with Congenital Heart Disease.* Lippincott, Williams & Wilkins, Philadelphia, 2001, p. 99.)

Careful monitoring of the mother while receiving these drugs is important because occasionally drug toxicity or proarrhythmic effects occur.

Atrial Ectopic Tachycardia

AET, also known as ectopic atrial tachycardia or automatic atrial tachycardia, may cause tachycardia-induced heart failure or cardiomyopathy.[15] AET results when an abnormal focus of cells in the atrium distinct from the sinus node spontaneously depolarizes faster than the sinus node. AET may be incessant and may increase or decrease its rate based on sympathetic tone and catecholamine state. Distinct P waves are typically visible, although the P waves may have an abnormal morphology or be notched (Fig. 24-3). The P wave axis is frequently abnormal on the surface ECG, unless the focus of the tachycardia is near the sinus node. First-degree AV block or Mobitz type I second-degree AV block (Wenckebach) may be present and give a clue to the presence of an abnormal tachycardia. The focus of AET is more likely to be in the right atrium than the left atrium,[16] and frequently the focus of AET coming from the high right

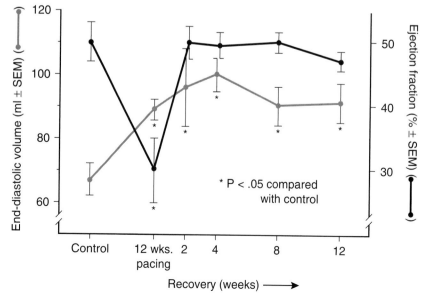

FIGURE 24-2 ■ **Hemodynamic changes in prolonged supraventricular tachycardia.** Changes in end-diastolic volume *(gray line)* and ejection fraction *(black line)* are plotted after 12 weeks of supraventricular tachycardia and during 12 weeks of recovery. The ejection fraction returned to baseline, while the end-diastolic volume remained elevated. (From Fyfe DA, Lowe JE, Damiano RZJ, et al: *Hemodynamic function in arrhythmias. In Gillette P, Garson A [eds]: Pediatric Arrhythmias: Electrophysiology and Pacing.* Philadelphia, WB Saunders, 1990, p. 508.)

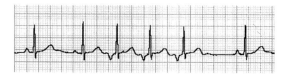

FIGURE 24-3 ■ Atrial ectopic tachycardia. ECG shows bursts of slow atrial tachycardia with a different P wave axis and a compensatory pause after termination of the tachycardia.

atrium is the right atrial appendage. Although this origin results in an upright P wave in leads I and aVF (normal P wave axis), the P wave is frequently completely negative in lead V1, giving a clue to the presence of an ectopic atrial focus. In one third of cases, there may be multiple atrial foci as the source of the tachycardia.[17] Prolonged AET also can occur in a postoperative patient.[18]

Treatment of AET is challenging because pharmacologic control may be difficult to achieve. β-Blockers in combination with digoxin are effective in some patients and are typically the first line of therapy. β-Blockers help control the arrhythmias, whereas digoxin helps to increase vagal tone, preventing rapid conduction through the AV node to the ventricles. Atenolol may be used in older patients.

If intravenous medications are indicated, procainamide also may be used. Procainamide is a class IA agent that prolongs the effective refractory period and duration of action potential via inhibition of the fast sodium channel. It slows conduction in the atrium; QRS and QT intervals are prolonged. Procainamide levels should be checked frequently. In addition, because of the side effects of procainamide (e.g., a lupus-like syndrome), transitioning to a different oral agent when converting to oral therapy is preferred.

Caution also must be used when transitioning to an antiarrhythmic that prolongs the QT interval (e.g., sotalol or amiodarone) because procainamide is a QT interval–prolonging agent. Sotalol, a class III agent with β-blocking properties, prolongs the effective refractory period in atrial and ventricular tissues and action potential duration of Purkinje fibers. It can be used safely and effectively, but hypotension and reduction in ventricular function can rarely occur.[19]

Flecainide also has had success in the treatment of AET.[20] Flecainide is a class IC agent, which inhibits the fast sodium channels but have no significant effects on the refractory period. Class IC agents also shorten the duration of Purkinje action potential and inhibit conduction in the His-Purkinje system. Caution should be exercised when using flecainide or propafenone in patients with congenital heart disease because of the proarrhythmia potential. Although there are no data in pediatric patients, results of the Cardiac Arrhythmia Suppression Trial (CAST) indicated a higher mortality

rate in patients who received flecainide after a myocardial infarction.[21] These data have been extrapolated to the pediatric population, and children with structural congenital heart disease may be at increased risks for arrhythmias and sudden death with flecainide.

Amiodarone, a unique antiarrhythmic agent with class III properties (prolongation of action potential by blocking potassium channels, lengthening the action potential duration and effective refractory period) can be used for AET.[22] This agent is a structural analogue of thyroid hormone and may have effects on the thyroid hormone receptor and lead to hyper- or hypothyroidism. It has a long half-life because of its lipid solubility. In a study by Naheed and colleagues,[23] amiodarone, alone or in combination with a β-blocker, was effective at controlling AET in most patients.

Because these drugs have proarrhythmic action, especially in the face of cardiomyopathy, it may be appropriate to admit children to the hospital for drug initiation of all drugs except β-blockers. In children older than age 3 years, spontaneous resolution of AET is unlikely[24]; cardiac catheterization with ablation techniques may be one of the first lines of therapy in these patients although medical therapy is preferred until the child is older. In children younger than 6 months, there is a high incidence of spontaneous resolution of tachycardia with a low long-term incidence of recurrence. Medical control should be attempted in these patients until the tachycardia resolves.

Junctional Ectopic Tachycardia

Junctional ectopic tachycardia (JET) is more commonly a tachyarrhythmia seen acutely and transiently after cardiac surgery (likely a result of trauma near the bundle of His), but it can be seen as an isolated congenital tachyarrhythmia in a child, which could lead to ventricular dysfunction.[25] JET is a narrow complex tachyarrhythmia usually with AV dissociation, although retrograde conduction can occur; it is believed to have an automatic or ectopic focus that originates at the AV junction (Fig. 24-4). There is an association between JET and residual lesions.[26]

In the postoperative setting, immediate treatment is warranted because this tachyarrhythmia almost always is associated with hemodynamic compromise and low cardiac output syndrome. This tachyarrhythmia, being automatic in nature, is unresponsive to adenosine or cardioversion. First-line treatment includes corporal hypothermia to 34°C (sometimes with concomitant paralysis with nonvagolytic paralytic agents to avoid shivering), correction of electrolytes, and cessation of catecholamines and vasodilators (both of which may maintain catecholamines and the ectopic rhythm).

If JET is refractory to the above-mentioned measures, intravenous agents may be useful in slowing the rate to

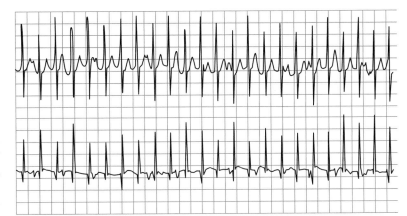

FIGURE 24-4 ■ Junctional ectopic tachycardia. A narrow QRS tachycardia with atrioventricular dissociation is seen. If the P waves are not readily discernible, atrial wire recordings can be made if available after cardiac surgery. (From Zipes DP, Jalife J [eds]: *Cardiac Electrophysiology: From Cell to Bedside.* Philadelphia, WB Saunders, p. 842, 1995.)

achieve AV synchrony with sequential AV pacing. Perry and coworkers[27] reported a 93% efficacy rate in children with JET when treated with amiodarone. Other agents that have shown efficacy include procainamide and propafenone. Use of a modified, commercially available temporary pacemaker for R wave synchronized atrial pacing in postoperative JET has been reported.[28]

Congenital JET is rare, but also can be associated with ventricular dysfunction; long-term pharmacologic therapy is needed. One therapeutic strategy involves β-blockers. As in postoperative JET, children with congenital JET also responded to amiodarone. In addition, propafenone has shown efficacy in the treatment of congenital JET.[29] Lastly, as a last resort in patients with JET and depressed ventricular function, a more invasive treatment strategy involves ablation of the AV node–His bundle region (with pacemaker therapy if AV block occurs)[30]; such a selective ablation strategy yielded a successful ablation of JET in a 10-month-old infant without AV block.[31]

Permanent Junctional Reciprocating Tachycardia and Accessory Pathways

Accessory pathway–mediated tachycardia also may result in cardiomyopathy. One accessory connection associated with ventricular dysfunction is the permanent form of junctional reciprocating tachycardia (PJRT),[32] which results from a slowly conducting accessory pathway that is located most commonly in the posteroseptal region. Because the pathway conducts slowly, tachycardia rates are most commonly 140 to 220 beats/min with some correlation with catecholamine state. The characteristic finding on surface ECG is a tachycardia with a long RP interval with deeply negative P waves in leads II, III, and aVF (Fig. 24-5). Because of its slower rate and presence of P waves on surface ECG (although the P waves have

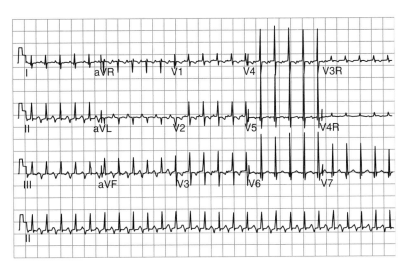

FIGURE 24-5 ■ Permanent form of junctional reciprocating tachycardia. ECG shows relatively normal-appearing P waves in lead I, but deeply negative P waves in leads II, III, and avF, which are associated with this tachyarrhythmia. The RP interval is longer than the PR interval.

an abnormal axis), PJRT may not be recognized until signs of ventricular dysfunction manifest. PJRT tends to be incessant, but temporarily terminates with maneuvers that cause AV block (e.g., adenosine, vagal stimulation); the tachycardia usually reinitiates shortly after termination. Spontaneous resolution of PJRT is rare.

Because of its incessant nature, medical management for PJRT typically is required. In children older than 3 to 4 years of age, cardiac catheterization with ablation techniques is the preferred method of treatment because it may provide a definitive cure.[33] In small children and infants in whom catheter ablation has a higher risk of complications, medical treatment is typically a first-line option, although catheter ablation has been successful in infants as young as 3 weeks old.[34]

Rarely, PJRT may respond to digoxin and β-blockers. In our experience, flecainide with or without the addition of a β-blocker is an effective drug to control PJRT. In refractory patients, sotalol or amiodarone may be necessary.

Ventricular Tachycardia

Although much less common than atrial tachyarrhythmias as a cause of cardiomyopathy, incessant ventricular arrhythmias also may result in cardiomyopathy if the rate is rapid, and the tachycardia is prolonged. Deal and associates[35] reported elevated left ventricular end-diastolic volumes and regional wall abnormalities in children with ventricular tachycardia without congenital heart disease. These ventricular rhythms usually have an automatic focus and frequently originate from the right or left ventricular outflow tract.[36] Some children with incessant ventricular tachycardia develop heart failure,[37] and 36% of children with ventricular tachycardia have evidence of left ventricular dysfunction.[38] Slowing the rate of the ventricular tachycardia potentially can improve the degree of congestive heart failure in these patients; total obliteration of the ventricular tachycardia may not be achievable.

Pharmacologic control of the arrhythmia occasionally may be achieved with a β-blocker alone, although sotalol and amiodarone are more effective at suppressing the tachycardia focus. Cardiac catheterization with ablation techniques also can be used to eliminate the tachycardia focus in patients with ventricular tachycardia. Techniques such as three-dimensional mapping, noncontact mapping, and mapping tachycardia based on a single ectopic beat have aided in the ability to localize and eliminate abnormal tachycardia foci in the cardiac catheterization laboratory.[39] Some arrhythmias that are difficult to control with medical therapy also can be treated by intraoperative cryothermic technique.[40]

Some of the lesions are due to hamartomas within the myocardium; if good control of the arrhythmia can be obtained, these hamartomas frequently spontaneously regress.[41] In rare cases, the only way to control these arrhythmias is with surgical excision of the tumor.[42]

These tumors are frequently visible to the naked eye as pale-colored areas of the myocardium and can be precisely excised.

When an arrhythmia causing tachycardia-induced cardiomyopathy is under good control by either medication or by means of catheter ablation techniques, the ventricular function typically normalizes. Many patients show a marked improvement 3 weeks after normalization of heart rate, although it may take 21 months to see a full recovery.[43]

CONGENITAL COMPLETE HEART BLOCK AND HEART FAILURE

Similar to tachyarrhythmias, complete AV block may result in ventricular dysfunction. Complete AV block results when an atrial impulse is not propagated to the ventricle. The incidence of congenital complete AV block is around 1 in 20,000 live births.[44] Around one third of these infants have associated congenital heart disease, with the most common lesion being corrected transposition of the great arteries. In comparison, around 50% of fetuses diagnosed in utero with congenital complete AV block have associated congenital heart disease, with the most common lesion being heterotaxy with left atrial isomerism.[45] Many of these patients have a poor outcome and die in utero.[46] In patients without structural heart disease, there is a strong correlation with the presence of SS-A/Ro and SS-B/La autoantibodies in the mother and congenital heart block in the infant.[47] Despite the presence of these antibodies, the mothers are frequently asymptomatic, and the first indication of the presence of an autoimmune disorder in a mother may be the birth of an infant with congenital AV block.

The presentation of patients with congenital complete AV block varies, as does the degree of ventricular dysfunction at presentation.[48] The degree of AV block may be progressive within the first 6 months after birth. Although uncommon, patients with first-degree AV block after birth may progress to higher degrees of AV block, and patients with second-degree AV block may progress to complete AV block.[49] Ventricular dysfunction may manifest at any time in patients with congenital AV block. In utero, ventricular dysfunction can be so severe that it results in fetal hydrops and even fetal demise. Other patients develop ventricular dysfunction at an older age, and some patients never have evidence of poor ventricular function. Even if patients are asymptomatic in childhood, 50% of these children develop symptoms in adulthood,[50] although the symptoms are usually minor. Infants with coexistent congenital heart disease tend to be more symptomatic at presentation. Almost all patients with congenital complete AV block have some degree of ventricular dilation, presumably from the increased stroke volume from their slow heart rates. Dilated cardiomyopathy develops in around 6% of patients diagnosed in utero or at birth, and the early initiation of pacemaker therapy does not change the incidence of development of late-onset cardiomyopathy.[51]

In addition to ventricular dysfunction, patients with congenital complete AV block are at risk for sudden death; patients who have slow ventricular rates or ventricular escape rhythms (or both) or ventricular ectopy have the highest risk for sudden death. In the landmark study by Michaelsson and Engle,[52] there were no sudden deaths in patients who had a ventricular rate greater than 60 beats/min and an atrial rate less than 140 beats/min. A study in older infants showed that no infant or child with a ventricular rate greater than 50 beats/min had syncope or sudden death.[53] A fetus exhibiting evidence of heart failure (fetal hydrops, poor ventricular function on fetal echocardiography) should be delivered as soon as it is feasible from an obstetric standpoint. Chronotropic drugs have limited long-term success in increasing the heart rate and cardiac output of patients with congenital complete AV block.

For this reason, permanent pacemaker implantation is the therapy of choice in patients who require treatment.[54] Class I indications for pacemaker placement (conditions for which there is evidence or general agreement that pacemaker implantation is beneficial, useful, and effective) include advanced symptomatic second-degree or third-degree AV block associated with symptomatic bradycardia, ventricular dysfunction, or low cardiac output; congenital third-degree AV block with a wide QRS escape rhythm, complex ventricular ectopy, or ventricular dysfunction; and congenital third-degree AV block in an infant with a ventricular rate less than 50 beats/min or with congenital heart disease and a ventricular rate less than 70 beats/min.[55] Class IIa indications for pacemaker placement (conditions for which there is conflicting evidence or divergence of opinion about the usefulness or efficacy of a procedure or treatment, but the weight of evidence or opinion is in favor of usefulness or efficacy) include congenital third-degree AV block in the first year of life with an average heart rate greater than 50 beats/min and abrupt pauses in ventricular rate that are two or three times the basic cycle length or associated with symptoms secondary to chronotropic incompetence.[56] A follow-up study showed that pacemaker therapy reduced morbidity and mortality in children with congenital complete AV block with and without congenital heart disease.[57]

ARRHYTHMIAS AND POSTOPERATIVE VENTRICULAR DYSFUNCTION AND HEART FAILURE

Patients with poor ventricular function may present with arrhythmias after cardiac surgery, and these arrhythmias may present immediately after surgery or many years after the operation. Some patients are at risk

because they already possess the basic substrate for having an arrhythmia. Patients with congenitally corrected transposition of the great arteries, Ebstein anomaly of the tricuspid valve, and hypertrophic cardiomyopathy have an increased incidence of accessory pathways (Wolff-Parkinson-White syndrome) and are at increased risks for having supraventricular arrhythmias and ventricular dysfunction.[58] In addition, electrolyte abnormalities, acidosis, ionotropes, and the cardiac surgery itself may cause arrhythmias in postoperative patients. Other morphologic substrates for arrhythmias after cardiac surgery include scarring, hypertrophy, and dilation of cardiac chambers, especially with concomitant heart failure.

Similar to patients who develop myocardial dysfunction and heart failure from persistent tachyarrhythmias, postoperative patients have hemodynamic derangements associated with dysrhythmias. The interplay between dysrhythmias and heart failure is probably even more essential in patients with congenital heart disease after cardiac surgery. A few common clinical situations of dysrhythmias in postoperative patients are discussed subsequently. Although data on the onset of arrhythmias and the predictive value of these arrhythmias of ventricular function are sparse, the data that do exist seem to indicate a possible mechanoelectric relationship because atrial fibrillation or flutter and ventricular tachycardia may portend ventricular dysfunction.[59]

Fontan Procedure and Intra-atrial Reentrant Tachycardia

After the Fontan procedure, patients have an increased incidence of arrhythmias associated with compromised ventricular function. Kurer and associates[60] reported that more than one half of patients after the Fontan procedure had some type of postoperative arrhythmias, with 27% of patients having hemodynamic compromise. In this study, the most common arrhythmia, and the one associated with the most compromise to cardiac output, was junctional ectopic tachycardia. Accelerated junctional rhythm also may be present (Fig. 24-6). About 20% of Fontan patients develop atrial arrhythmias (including AET, atrial flutter, and atrial fibrillation) in the postoperative period.[61]

Atrial arrhythmias also may manifest in long-term follow-up of Fontan patients. Atrial flutter or intra-atrial reentrant tachycardia (Fig. 24-7) is characterized by the

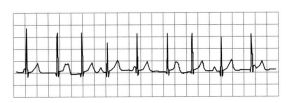

FIGURE 24-6 ■ Accelerated junctional rhythm. ECG shows accelerated junctional rhythm with an occasional sinus capture beat.

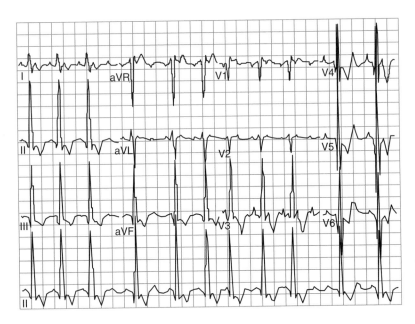

FIGURE 24-7 ■ Intra-atrial reentry tachycardia. Intra-atrial reentry tachycardia shows a 2:1 atrioventricular conduction. There is a complete return to baseline between successive P waves.

following: aberrant but uniform P wave or flutter wave morphology, constant rate with variable cycle lengths, variable AV block or 1:1 conduction, minimal rate variability, and sudden onset and offset.[62] This atrial tachyarrhythmia after the Fontan procedure may be difficult to control, and even with aggressive drug and antitachycardia pacemaker therapy, tachycardia is controlled in only about one half of the patients.[63] Systemic AV valve regurgitation and biatrial enlargement are commonly observed in patients who develop atrial tachycardia after the Fontan procedure, and these patients are more likely to develop right atrial thrombus and progressive heart failure.[64]

Medical management of Fontan patients with atrial tachycardia can be challenging because many of the patients have sinus node dysfunction and bradycardia, limiting the choices of antiarrhythmic therapy. Class III agents, such as sotalol and amiodarone, seem to have the best efficacy with a reasonable risk profile in treating this tachydysrhythmia. Another strategy involves the use of antitachycardic pacing as a means to terminate intra-atrial reentrant tachycardia, but this often is limited by the Fontan atrial anatomy and poor atrial thresholds.[65] Cardiac catheterization with radiofrequency ablation has a low long-term success rate in eliminating atrial arrhythmias after the Fontan operation.[66] This low success rate is likely due to multiple reasons, including limited venous access to the heart and thickened and enlarged atria with an inability to place complete transmural and linear lesions.

Fontan conversion with ablation lines placed at the time of an operation can treat medically refractory intra-atrial reentrant tachycardia successfully (Fig. 24-8).[67] This approach uses the concept that corridors of atrial tissue to create and sustain reentrant circuits need to be divided. Some centers advocate arrhythmia therapy with

any planned surgical revision in any patient with complex congenital heart disease, regardless if the patient has a history of atrial tachycardia.[68] Atrial pacing also can decrease the occurrence of atrial tachyarrhythmias.

Atrial arrhythmias and poor hemodynamics play significant roles in ventricular dysfunction after the Fontan operation, especially in patients with atriopulmonary Fontan operations. Some patients may present with severe compromise of ventricular function; in these patients, conversion to a lateral tunnel Fontan with radiofrequency or cryoablation lines placed in the atria to decrease the incidence of atrial arrhythmias may improve ventricular function significantly. In a study by Weinstein and coworkers,[69] there was a reduced

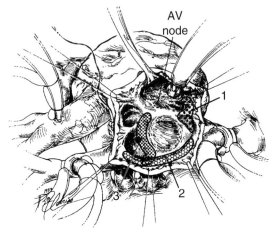

FIGURE 24-8 ■ Intraoperative right atrial maze ablation during Fontan conversion. The cryogenic lesions are placed where the numbers indicate (*1, 2,* and *3*). This procedure serves as therapy for intra-atrial reentrant tachycardia during the Fontan conversion surgery. AV, atrioventricular. (From Mavroudis C, Deal BJ, Backer CL, et al: *The favorable impact of arrhythmia surgery on total cavopulmonary artery Fontan conversion. Semin Thorac Cardiovasc Surg* 1999;2:143-156.)

incidence of atrial arrhythmias and improvement in New York Heart Association classification in all surviving patients after Fontan conversion, cryoablation, and pacemaker placement. There also is objective evidence of improved ventricular function with an increase in ejection fraction on follow-up echocardiograms in these patients.[70]

Other Operations

In a study of 122 postmortem cases from Boston Children's Hospital, the cause of death in 5% of patients after the **modified Norwood procedure** was likely a result of an arrhythmia.[71] In cases of a functional single ventricle, atrial tachyarrhythmias are especially poorly tolerated when there are coexisting hemodynamic alterations and are an important source of morbidity and mortality.[72] Many of the arrhythmias seen after the Norwood procedure are associated with poor ventricular function in a failing single ventricle and may be a marker for the need for intensified follow-up and therapy, additional surgery, or heart transplantation. As with any child with ventricular tachycardia after cardiac surgery, coronary ischemia or ventricular dysfunction or both should be considered a cause of the ventricular dysrhythmia.

Patients with **Ebstein anomaly of the tricuspid valve** also are at risk for arrhythmias. Because of the dilated right atrium and increased incidence of accessory pathways, these patients are at risk for atrial flutter, atrial fibrillation, AET, and reentrant supraventricular tachycardia,[73] all of which can lead to heart failure. In addition, because of the already compromised pulmonary blood flow in these patients, tachycardia is frequently poorly tolerated, and patients may have symptoms of compromised ventricular output even with brief episodes of tachycardia. Catheter ablation may be successful in eliminating reentrant tachycardias secondary to Wolff-Parkinson-White syndrome, although ablation is more difficult because of the displacement of the tricuspid valve and the presence of multiple accessory pathways in many of these patients. Atrial debulking during surgery with or without pacemaker placement may help to control other atrial dysrhythmias in these patients.

The development of ventricular arrhythmias has a large impact on the morbidity and mortality of patients after **tetralogy of Fallot repair**. The source of the ventricular tachycardia is frequently around the ventricular septal defect patch or right ventricular outflow tract. Ventricular tachycardia is more common in patients with poor hemodynamics after surgery, especially patients with pulmonary regurgitation and a markedly dilated or poorly functioning right ventricle.[74] In these patients, it is less likely that the arrhythmia per se is the cause of heart failure.

Atrial arrhythmias also may be associated with ventricular dysfunction after repair of tetralogy of Fallot. In a study by Harrison and colleagues,[75] the incidence of atrial tachycardias after tetralogy of Fallot repair was 12%, and the presence of an atrial tachycardia was associated with substantial morbidity, including congestive heart failure, reoperation, subsequent ventricular tachycardia, stroke, and death. In the same study, the development of atrial tachycardia in an adult late after tetralogy of Fallot repair was associated with older age at repair and a higher frequency of hemodynamic abnormalities (particularly right ventricular dilation and poor right ventricular function).

The most concerning long-term complication after tetralogy of Fallot repair is the risk of sudden death. The exact etiology of sudden death in these patients is not well understood. Atrial flutter and agonal bradycardia with advanced AV block have been proposed as arrhythmic mechanisms for sudden death.[76] A more accepted hypothesis is that ventricular tachyarrhythmias are the cause.[77] Ventricular dysfunction places patients at higher risk for sudden death presumably because of the increased risk of ventricular arrhythmias.[78] Another factor that has been associated with sudden death is QRS duration on a resting ECG. In a study by Gatzoulis and coworkers,[79] a QRS duration of greater than 180 msec was a sensitive marker for life-threatening arrhythmias. An increased QT dispersion combined with a QRS duration of greater than 180 msec further improved the risk stratification of postoperative tetralogy of Fallot patients.[80] These two markers also have been shown to correlate with a positive electrophysiology test for ventricular tachycardia.[81]

Arrhythmias also may be seen in association with ventricular dysfunction after an **atrial baffle repair** of D-transposition of the great arteries (Mustard or Senning operations) with two thirds of patients having arrhythmias during their lifetime.[82] Sinus node dysfunction is a common finding after the Mustard or Senning operation.[83] In a study from Toronto, 77% of patients were in normal sinus rhythm 5 years after their operation, but only 40% of patients were in normal sinus rhythm 20 years after their surgery.[84] Tachyarrhythmias also are an important cause of morbidity and mortality, including heart failure, in postoperative Mustard and Senning patients. In one study, with an average of 8 years of follow-up, arrhythmias occurred in 70% of Mustard and Senning patients, with 21% of the arrhythmias being ventricular dysrhythmias.[85] Ventricular arrhythmias are becoming a more prominent issue in patients as they grow older and are a significant problem greater than 10 years after the initial operation.[86] These arrhythmias are likely due to the inability of the right ventricle to function as a systemic ventricle with subsequent right ventricular failure. The right ventricular dysfunction and tricuspid regurgitation likely increase the risk of ventricular arrhythmias, which are the likely causes of the increased incidence of sudden death in these patients (see Chapter 27).

Implantable cardioverter defibrillators may be placed transvenously in these patients if they have no residual shunting. Care must be exercised not to obstruct the superior limb of the baffle with the leads causing superior

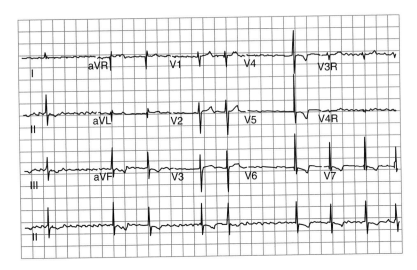

FIGURE 24-9 ■ Atrial fibrillation. ECG shows the chaotic baseline with an irregularly irregular rhythm that is typical for atrial fibrillation.

vena cava syndrome. The ventricular lead may be placed through the baffle into the left ventricle (pulmonary ventricle). Occasionally a second coil is required in the superior or inferior vena cava to obtain adequate defibrillation thresholds. In a study by Janousek and coworkers,[87] 4.2% of 359 Mustard or Senning patients experienced sudden death. In this study, severe tricuspid regurgitation or right ventricular dysfunction and uncontrolled supraventricular tachyarrhythmias were identified as the two significant risk factors for sudden death. These sudden deaths most commonly occur at least 8 to 15 years after the initial operation.[88] Chronic postoperative tachycardia after the Mustard or Senning operation is most commonly due to intra-atrial reentry tachycardia, although AV node reentry tachycardia and sinus node reentry tachycardia have also been documented.[89] Supraventricular tachycardia after age 18 years is associated with heart failure, whereas in patients younger than 18 years, pulmonary hypertension, systemic ventricular dysfunction, and junctional rhythm are independent risk factors for supraventricular tachycardia.[90]

In younger patients, consideration may be given to an arterial switch procedure with an atrial baffle takedown. These patients typically require banding of the pulmonary artery to retrain the left ventricle to pump against systemic pressures. No long-term results currently are available for these patients. It is not clear if this operation would decrease the incidence of atrial or ventricular arrhythmias or decrease the risk of sudden death.

Patients who have received an **orthotopic heart transplant** also are at risk of arrhythmias during episodes of ventricular dysfunction, which may or may not be related to graft rejection. In the immediate postoperative period, transplant recipients may have atrial or ventricular tachycardias, presumably as a result of the long ischemic times of the donor organs. These arrhythmias may result in severe circulatory embarrassment requiring immediate therapy. There is no correlation of arrhythmias in the immediate postoperative period and the long-term incidence of arrhythmias or ventricular dysfunction.[91] In adults, acute rejection with or without ventricular dysfunction may cause atrial fibrillation (Fig. 24-9) or flutter.[92] Atrial arrhythmias may occur in 50% of patients after transplantation, but atrial fibrillation is the only atrial arrhythmia that has been associated with an increased mortality in adult patients.[93] Ventricular dysfunction caused by acute rejection and transplant coronary artery disease may result in ventricular arrhythmias.[94]

After orthotopic heart transplantation, stable or progressive conduction system damage on the ECG may be associated with left ventricular dysfunction, increased mortality, and sudden death.[95] Patients with sinus node dysfunction or Wenckebach at least 6 months after cardiac transplantation may have an increased incidence of transplant coronary artery disease and may be at risk for ventricular dysfunction and sudden death.[96]

CURRENT STATUS AND FUTURE TRENDS

The specific mechanisms of ventricular dysfunction secondary to tachyarrhythmias are not well understood. As more information is obtained on a molecular level about the interactions of ion channels in the heart, however, more insight may be gained as to the specific mechanisms for the combination of myocardial dysfunction and arrhythmias. Mutations in the cardiac ryanodine receptor (cardiac sarcoplasmic reticulum calcium release channel) have been associated with chronic heart failure and triggered ventricular arrhythmias that respond to β-blockers (see also Chapter 2).[97]

Arrhythmias, especially tachyarrhythmias, can be one of the most frequently unrecognized causes of heart failure and even cardiomyopathy.[98] The emerging role of arrhythmogenesis and heart failure is being studied in great detail. In addition to a better understanding of the interaction between arrhythmia pathogenesis and heart failure,[99] new mapping (e.g., multielectrode catheter arrays and virtual activation sequencing) and therapeutic strategies are essential in eliminating arrhythmias as an etiology for heart failure in children.[100,101]

Key Concepts

■ The ventricular dysfunction and ensuing heart failure with dysrhythmias depend on the dysrhythmia rate, duration of dysrhythmia, presence of AV synchrony, age of the patient, and underlying anatomy and function.

■ The ventricular dysfunction associated with tachyarrhythmias may be so severe that patients mistakenly may be diagnosed as having cardiomyopathy and listed for heart transplantation; it is imperative that such tachydysrhythmias are diagnosed correctly and in a timely fashion to avoid an unnecessary transplantation.

■ Tachyarrhythmias leading to a cardiomyopathy are typically incessant. In adults, tachycardia-induced cardiomyopathy can be secondary to AV intranodal reentry tachycardia or atrial flutter or fibrillation, whereas in children, the tachydysrhythmias more commonly associated with cardiomyopathy are AET and PJRT.

■ Although the origin of tachycardia may be atrial or ventricular and may have an automatic focus or reentrant mechanism, supraventricular tachycardias are the most common cause of tachycardia-induced cardiomyopathy.

■ Treatment of AET can be challenging because pharmacologic control may be difficult to achieve. β-Blockers in combination with digoxin are effective in some patients and are typically the first line of therapy.

■ In children older than age 3 years, spontaneous resolution of AET is unlikely; cardiac catheterization with ablation techniques may be one of the first lines of therapy in these patients, although medical therapy is preferred until the child is older. In children younger than 6 months, there is a high incidence of spontaneous resolution of tachycardia with a low long-term incidence of recurrence. Medical control should be attempted in these patients until the tachycardia resolves.

■ Junctional ectopic tachycardia is more commonly a tachyarrhythmia seen acutely and transiently after cardiac surgery (likely a result of trauma near the bundle of His), but it can be seen as an isolated congenital tachyarrhythmia in a child, which could lead to ventricular dysfunction.

■ Because of its slower rate and presence of P waves on surface ECG (although the P waves have an abnormal axis), PJRT may not be recognized until signs of ventricular dysfunction manifest.

■ Although much less common than atrial tachyarrhythmias as a cause of cardiomyopathy, incessant ventricular arrhythmias also may result in cardiomyopathy if the rate is rapid, and the tachycardia is prolonged.

■ In addition to ventricular dysfunction, patients with congenital complete AV block are at risk for sudden death; patients who have slow ventricular rates or ventricular escape rhythms or ventricular ectopy have the highest risk for sudden death.

■ Class I indications for pacemaker placement (conditions for which there is evidence or general agreement that pacemaker implantation is beneficial, useful, and effective) include advanced symptomatic second-degree or third-degree AV block associated with symptomatic bradycardia, ventricular dysfunction, or low cardiac output; congenital third-degree AV block with a wide QRS escape rhythm, complex ventricular ectopy, or ventricular dysfunction; and congenital third-degree AV block in an infant with a ventricular rate less than 50 beats/min or with congenital heart disease and a ventricular rate less than 70 beats/min.

■ Although data on the onset of arrhythmias and the predictive value of these arrhythmias of ventricular function are sparse, the data that do exist seem to indicate a possible mechanoelectric relationship because atrial fibrillation or flutter and ventricular tachycardia may portend ventricular dysfunction.

■ Atrial arrhythmias and poor hemodynamics play significant roles in ventricular dysfunction after the Fontan operation, especially in patients with atriopulmonary Fontan operations. Some patients may present with severe compromise of ventricular function; in these patients, conversion to a lateral tunnel Fontan with radiofrequency or cryoablation lines placed in the atria to decrease the incidence of atrial arrhythmias may improve ventricular function significantly.

REFERENCES

1. Gallagher JJ: Tachycardia and cardiomyopathy: The chicken-egg dilemma revisited. J Am Coll Cardiol 1985;6:1172-1173.
2. Arunjo F, Ducla-Aoares JL: Tachycardiomyopathies. Rev Port Cardiol 2002;21:585-592.
3. Fenelon G, Wijns W, Andries E, et al: Tachycardiomyopathy: Mechanisms and clinical implications. Pacing Clin Electrophysiol 1996;19:95-106.
4. Walker NL, Cobbe SM, Birnie DH: Tachycardiomyopathy: A diagnosis not to be missed. Heart 2004;90:e7.
5. Zimmerman FJ, Pahl E, Rocchini AP, et al: High incidence of incessant supraventricular tachycardia in pediatric patients referred for cardiac transplantation. Pacing Clin Electrophysiol 1996;19:663.
6. Gelb BD, Garson A Jr: Noninvasive discrimination of right atrial ectopic tachycardia from sinus tachycardia in "dilated cardiomyopathy." Am Heart J 1990;120:886-891.
7. Coleman HN, Taylor RR, Pool PE, et al: Congestive heart failure following chronic tachycardia. Am Heart J 1971;81:790-798.
8. Rabbani LE, Wang PJ, Couper GL, et al: Time course of improvement in ventricular function after ablation of incessant automatic atrial tachycardia. Am Heart J 1991;121:816-819.
9. Gillette PC, Smith RT, Garson A Jr, et al: Chronic supraventricular tachycardia: A curable cause of congestive cardiomyopathy. JAMA 1985;253:391-392.

10. Oudijk MA, Stoutenbeek P, Sreeram N, et al: Persistent junctional reciprocating tachycardia in the fetus. J Matern Fetal Neonatal Med 2003;13:191-196.

11. Weismuller P, Abraham-Fuchs K, Schneider S, et al: Biomagnetic noninvasive localization of accessory pathways in Wolff-Parkinson-White syndrome. Pacing Clin Electrophysiol 1991;14(11 Pt 2):1961-1965.

12. Krapp M, Kohl T, Simpson JM, et al: Review of diagnosis, treatment, and outcome of fetal atrial flutter compared with supraventricular tachycardia. Heart 2003;89:913-917.

13. Khositseth A, Ramin KD, O'Leary PW, et al: Role of amiodarone in the treatment of fetal supraventricular tachyarrhythmias and hydrops fetalis. Pediatr Cardiol 2003;24:454-456.

14. Dangel JH, Roszkowski T, Bieganowska K, et al: Adenosine triphosphate for cardioversion of supraventricular tachycardia in two hydropic fetuses. Fetal Diagn Ther 2000;15:326-330.

15. Khongphatthanayothin A, Chotivitayatarakorn P, Lertsupcharoen P, et al: Atrial tachycardia from enhanced automaticity in children: Diagnosis and initial management. J Med Assoc Thai 2001;84:3121-3128.

16. Tracy CM, Swartz JF, Fletcher RD, et al: Radiofrequency catheter ablation of ectopic atrial tachycardia using paced activation sequence mapping. J Am Coll Cardiol 1993;21:910-917.

17. Koike K, Hesslein PS, Finlay CD, et al: Atrial automatic tachycardia in children. Am J Cardiol 1988;61:1127-1130.

18. Rosales AM, Walsh EP, Wessel DL, et al: Postoperative ectopic atrial tachycardia in children with congenital heart disease. Am J Cardiol 2001;88:1169-1172.

19. Tanel RE, Walsh EP, Lulu JA, et al: Sotalol for refractory arrhythmias in pediatric and young adult patients: Initial efficacy and long term outcome. Am Heart J 1995;130:791-797.

20. Mehta AV, Sanchez GR, Sacks EJ, et al: Ectopic automatic atrial tachycardia in children: Clinical characteristics, management and follow-up. J Am Coll Cardiol 1988;11:379-385.

21. Cardiac Arrhythmia Suppression Trial (CAST) Investigators: Preliminary report: Effect of encainide and flecainide on mortality in a randomized trial of arrhythmia suppression after myocardial infarction. The Cardiac Arrhythmia Suppression Trial (CAST) Investigators. N Engl J Med 1989;321:406-412.

22. Luedtke SA, Kuhn RJ, McCaffrey FM: Pharmacologic management of supraventricular tachycardias in children. Ann Pharmacother 1997;31:1227-1243.

23. Naheed ZJ, Strasburger JF, Benson DW Jr, et al: Natural history and management strategies of automatic atrial tachycardia in children. Am J Cardiol 1995;75:405-407.

24. Salerno JC, Kertesz NJ, Friedman RA, et al: Clinical course of atrial ectopic tachycardia is age-dependent: Results and treatment in children < 3 or > or = 3 years of age. J Am Coll Cardiol 2004;43:438-444.

25. Villain E, Vetter VL, Garcia JM, et al: Evolving concepts in the management of congenital junctional ectopic tachycardia: A multicenter study. Circulation 1990;81:1544-1549.

26. Gillette PC: Diagnosis and management of postoperative junctional ectopic tachycardia. Am Heart J 1989;118:192-194.

27. Perry JC, Fenrich AL, Hulse JE, et al: Pediatric use of intravenous amiodarone: Efficacy and safety in critically ill patients from a multicenter protocol. J Am Coll Cardiol 1996;27:1246-1250.

28. Janousek J, Vojtovid P, Gebauer RA: Use of a modified commercially available temporary pacemaker for R wave synchronized atrial pacing in postoperative junctional ectopic tachycardia. Pacing Clin Electrophysiol 2003;26:579-586.

29. Paul T, Reimer A, Janousek J, et al: Efficacy and safety of propafenone in congenital junctional ectopic tachycardia. J Am Coll Cardiol 1992;20:911-914.

30. Gillette PC, Garson A, Porter CJ, et al: Junctional automatic ectopic tachycardia: A new proposed treatment by transcatheter His bundle ablation. Am Heart J 1983;106:619-623.

31. VanHare G, Velvis H, Langberg J: Successful transcatheter ablation of congenital junctional ectopic tachycardia in a ten month old infant using radiofrequency energy. Pacing Clin Electrophysiol 1990;13:730-735.

32. McGuire MA, Lau KC, Davis LM, et al: Permanent junctional reciprocating tachycardia misdiagnosed as a cardiomyopathy. Aust N Z J Med 1991;21:239-241.

33. Semizel E, Ayabakan C, Ceviz N, et al: Permanent form of junctional reciprocating tachycardia and tachycardia-induced cardiomyopathy treated by catheter ablation: A case report. Turk J Pediatr 2003;45:338-341.

34. Noe P, Van Driel V, Wittkampf F, et al: Rapid recovery of cardiac function after catheter ablation of persistent junctional reciprocating tachycardia in children. Pacing Clin Electrophysiol 2002;25:191-194.

35. Deal BJ, Miller SC, Scagliotti D, et al: Ventricular tachycardia in young population without overt heart disease. Circulation 1986;73:1111-1118.

36. Umana E, Solares CA, Alpert MA: Tachycardia-induced cardiomyopathy. Am J Med 2003;114:51-55.

37. Tsuji A, Nagashima M, Hasegawa S, et al: Long term followup of idiopathic ventricular arrhythmias in otherwise normal children. Jpn Circ J 1995;59:654-662.

38. Pfammatter JP, Paul T: Idiopathic ventricular tachycardia in infancy and childhood: A multicenter study on clinical profile and outcome. J Am Coll Cardiol 1999;33:2067-2072.

39. Fung JW, Chan HC, Chan JY, et al: Ablation of nonsustained or hemodynamically unstable ventricular arrhythmia originating from the right ventricular outflow tract guided by noncontact mapping. Pacing Clin Electrophysiol 2003;26:1699-1705.

40. Zeigler VL, Gillette PC, Crawford FA, et al: New approaches to treatment of incessant ventricular tachycardia in the very young. J Am Coll Cardiol 1990;16:681-685.

41. Abushaban L, Denham B, Duff D: 10 year review of cardiac tumours in childhood. Br Heart J 1993;70:166-169.

42. Gharagozloo F, Porter CJ, Tazelaar HD, et al: Multiple myocardial hamartomas causing ventricular tachycardia in young children: Combined surgical modification and medical treatment. Mayo Clin Proc 1994;69:262-267.

43. Packer DL, Bardy GH, Worley SJ, et al: Tachycardia-induced cardiomyopathy: A reversible form of left ventricular dysfunction. Am J Cardiol 1986;57:563-570.

44. Landtmann B, Linder E, Hjelt L, et al: Congenital complete heart block: 1. A clinical study of 27 cases. Ann Paediatr Fenn 1964;10:99-104.

45. Schmidt KG, Ulmer HE, Silverman NH, et al: Perinatal outcome of fetal complete atrioventricular block: A multicenter experience. J Am Coll Cardiol 1991;17:1360-1366.

46. Eronen M, Heikkila P, Teramo K: Congenital complete heart block in the fetus: Hemodynamic features, antenatal treatment, and outcome in six cases. Pediatr Cardiol 2001;22:385-392.

47. Reed BR, Lee LA, Harmon C, et al: Autoantibodies to SS-A/Ro in infants with congenital heart block. J Pediatr 1983;103:889-891.

48. Buyon JP, Hiebert R, Copel J, et al: Autoimmune-associated congenital heart block: Demographics, mortality, morbidity and recurrence rates obtained from a national neonatal lupus registry. J Am Coll Cardiol 1998;31:1658-1666.

49. Askanase AD, Friedman DM, Copel J, et al: Spectrum and progression of conduction abnormalities in infants born to mothers with anti-SSA/Ro-SSB/La antibodies. Lupus 2002;11:145-151.

50. Michaelsson M, Jonzon A, Riesenfeld T: Isolated congenital complete atrioventricular block in adult life: A prospective study. Circulation 1995;92:442-449.

51. Moak JP, Barron KS, Hougen TJ, et al: Congenital heart block: Development of late-onset cardiomyopathy, a previously underappreciated sequela. J Am Coll Cardiol 2001;37:238-242.

52. Michaelsson M, Engle MA: Congenital complete heart block: An international study of the natural history. Cardiovasc Clin 1972;4:85-101.

53. Karpawich PP, Gillette PC, Garson A Jr, et al: Congenital complete atrioventricular block: Clinical and electrophysiologic predictors of need for pacemaker insertion. Am J Cardiol 1981;48:1098-1102.

54. Breur JM, Udink Ten Cate TE, Kapusta L, et al: Pacemaker therapy in isolated congenital heart block. Pacing Clin Electrophysiol 2002;1685-1691.

55. Gregoratos G, Abrams J, Epstein AE, et al: ACC/AHA/NASPE 2002 Guideline Update for Implantation of Cardiac Pacemakers and Antiarrhythmia Devices—summary article: A report of the American College of Cardiology/American Heart Association Task Force on Practice Guidelines (ACC/AHA/NASPE Committee to Update the 1998 Pacemaker Guidelines). J Am Coll Cardiol 2002; 40:1703-1719.

56. Dewey RC, Capeless MA, Levy AM: Use of ambulatory electrocardiographic monitoring to identify high-risk patients with congenital complete heart block. N Engl J Med 1987;316:835-839.

57. Balmer C, Fasnacht M, Rahn M, et al: Long term follow up of children with congenital complete atrioventricular block and impact of pacemaker therapy. Europace 2002;4:345-349.

58. Levine JC, Walsh EP, Saul JP: Radiofrequency ablation of accessory pathways associated with congenital heart disease including heterotaxy syndrome. Am J Cardiol 1993;72:689-693.

59. Gatzoulis MA, Walters J, McLaughlin PR, et al: Late arrhythmia in adults with Mustard procedure for transposition of the great arteries: A surrogate marker for right ventricular dysfunction? Heart 2000;84:409-415.

60. Kurer CC, Tanner CS, Norwood WI, et al: Perioperative arrhythmias after Fontan repair. Circulation 1990;82(5 Suppl):IV-190-IV-194.

61. Gelatt M, Hamilton RM, McCrindle BW, et al: Risk factors for atrial tachyarrhythmias after the Fontan operation. J Am Coll Cardiol 1994;24:1735-1741.

62. Triedman JK: Atrial reentrant tachycardias. In Walsh EP, Saul JP, Triedman JK (eds): Cardiac Arrhythmias in Children and Young Adults with Congenital Heart Disease. Philadelphia, Lippincott, Williams & Wilkins, p. 137-160, 2001.

63. Balaji S, Johnson TB, Sade RM, et al: Management of atrial flutter after the Fontan procedure. J Am Coll Cardiol 1994;23:1209-1215.

64. Ghai A, Harris L, Harrison DA, et al: Outcomes of late atrial tachyarrhythmias in adults after the Fontan operation. J Am Coll Cardiol 2001;37:585-592.

65. Baeriswyl G, Zimmerman M, Adamec R: Efficacy of rapid atrial pacing for conversion of atrial flutter in medically treated patients. Clin Cardiol 1994;17:246-250.

66. Deal BJ, Mavroudis C, Backer CL, et al: New directions in surgical therapy of arrhythmias. Pediatr Cardiol 2000;21:576-583.

67. Deal BJ, Mavroudis C, Backer CL: Beyond Fontan conversion: Surgical therapy of arrhythmias including patients with associated complex congenital heart disease. Ann Thorac Surg 2003;76: 542-554.

68. Mavroudis C, Deal BJ, Backer CL: Arrhythmia surgery in association with complex congenital heart repairs excluding patients with Fontan conversion. Semin Thorac Cardiovasc Surg Pediatr Card Surg Annu 2003;6:33-50.

69. Weinstein S, Cua C, Chan D, et al: Outcome of symptomatic patients undergoing extracardiac Fontan conversion and cryoablation. J Thorac Cardiovasc Surg 2003;126:529-536.

70. Agnoletti G, Borghi A, Vignati G, et al: Fontan conversion to total cavopulmonary connection and arrhythmia ablation: Clinical and functional results. Heart 2003;89:193-198.

71. Bartram U, Grunenfelder J, Van Praagh R: Causes of death after the modified Norwood procedure: A study of 122 postmortem cases. Ann Thorac Surg 1997;64:1795-1802.

72. Kanter RJ, Garson A Jr: Atrial arrhythmias during chronic follow-up of surgery for complex congenital heart disease. Pacing Clin Electrophysiol 1997;20(2 Pt 2):502-511.

73. Oh JK, Holmes DR Jr, Hayes DL, et al: Cardiac arrhythmias in patients with surgical repair of Ebstein's anomaly. J Am Coll Cardiol 1985;6:1351-1357.

74. Harrison DA, Harris L, Siu SC, et al: Sustained ventricular tachycardia in adult patients late after repair of tetralogy of Fallot. J Am Coll Cardiol 1997;30:1368-1373.

75. Harrison DA, Siu SC, Hussain F, et al: Sustained atrial arrhythmias in adults late after repair of tetralogy of Fallot. Am J Cardiol 2001;87:584-588.

76. Silka MJ, Hardy BG, Menashe VD, et al: A population-based prospective evaluation of risk of sudden cardiac death after operation for common congenital heart defects. J Am Coll Cardiol 1998;32:245-251.

77. Gillette PC, Yeoman MA, Mullins CE, et al: Sudden death after repair of tetralogy of Fallot: Electrocardiographic and electrophysiologic abnormalities. Circulation 1977;56(4 Pt 1):566-571.

78. Chandar JS, Wolff GS, Garson A Jr, et al: Ventricular arrhythmias in postoperative tetralogy of Fallot. Am J Cardiol 1990;65: 655-661.

79. Gatzoulis MA, Till JA, Somerville J, et al: Mechanoelectrical interaction in tetralogy of Fallot: QRS prolongation relates to right ventricular size and predicts malignant ventricular arrhythmias and sudden death. Circulation 1995;92:231-237.

80. Gatzoulis MA, Till JA, Redington AN: Depolarization-repolarization inhomogeneity after repair of tetralogy of Fallot: The substrate for malignant ventricular tachycardia? Circulation 1997;95:401-404.

81. Balaji S, Lau YR, Case CL, et al: QRS prolongation is associated with inducible ventricular tachycardia after repair of tetralogy of Fallot. Am J Cardiol 1997;80:160-163.

82. Oechslin E, Jenni R: 40 years after the first atrial switch procedure in patients with transposition of the great arteries: Long-term results in Toronto and Zurich. Thorac Cardiovasc Surg 2000;48:233-237.

83. El-Said G, Rosenberg HS, Mullins CE, et al: Dysrhythmias after Mustard's operation for transposition of the treat arteries. Am J Cardiol 1972;30:526-532.

84. Gelatt M, Hamilton RM, McCrindle BW, et al: Arrhythmia and mortality after the Mustard procedure: A 30-year single-center experience. J Am Coll Cardiol 1997;29:194-201.

85. Janousek J, Paul T, Luhmer I, et al: Atrial baffle procedures for complete transposition of the great arteries: Natural course of sinus node dysfunction and risk factors for dysrhythmias and sudden death. Z Kardiol 1994;83:933-938.

86. Altman CA, Vick GW III, Perry JC, et al: Ventricular tachycardia after repair of congenital heart disease. Prog Pediatr Cardiol 1995;4:229-236.

87. Janousek J, Paul T, Luhmer I, et al: Atrial baffle procedures for complete transposition of the great arteries: Natural course of sinus node dysfunction and risk factors for dysrhythmias and sudden death. Z Kardiol 1994;83:933-938.

88. Gewillig M, Cullen S, Mertens B, et al: Risk factors for arrhythmia and death after Mustard operation for simple transposition of the great arteries. Circulation 1991;84(5 Suppl):III-187-III-192.

89. Gillette PC, Kugler JD, Garson A Jr, et al: Mechanisms of cardiac arrhythmias after the Mustard operation for transposition of the great arteries. Am J Cardiol 1980;45:1225-1230.

90. Puley G, Siu S, Connelly M, et al: Arrhythmia and survival in patients >18 years of age after the Mustard procedure for complete transposition of the great arteries. Am J Cardiol 1999;83:1080-1084.

91. Scott CD, Dark JH, McComb JM: Arrhythmias after cardiac transplantation. Am J Cardiol 1992;70:1061-1063.

92. Cui G, Tung T, Kobashigawa J, et al: Increased incidence of atrial flutter associated with the rejection of heart transplantation. Am J Cardiol 2001;88:280-284.

93. Pavri BB, O'Nunain SS, Newell JB, et al: Prevalence and prognostic significance of atrial arrhythmias after orthotopic cardiac transplantation. J Am Coll Cardiol 1995;25:1673-1680.

94. Park JK, Hsu DT, Hordof AJ, et al: Arrhythmias in pediatric heart transplant recipients: Prevalence and association with death, coronary artery disease, and rejection. J Heart Lung Transplant 1993;12(6 Pt 1):956-964.

95. Leonelli FM, Dunn JK, Young JB, et al: Natural history, determinants, and clinical relevance of conduction abnormalities following orthotopic heart transplantation. Am J Cardiol 1996;77:47-51.

96. Cannon BC, Denfield SW, Friedman RA, et al: Late pacemaker requirement after pediatric orthotopic heart transplantation may predict the presence of transplant coronary artery disease. J Heart Lung Transplant 2004;23:67-71.

97. Scoote M, Williams AJ: The cardiac ryanodine receptor (calcium release channel): Emerging role in heart failure and arrhythmia pathogenesis. Cardiovasc Res 2002;56:359-372.

98. Brugada P, Andries E: Tachycardiomyopathy: The most frequently unrecognized cause of heart failure? Acta Cardiol 1993;48: 165-169.

99. Scoote M, Williams AJ: The cardiac ryanodine receptor: Emerging role in heart failure and arrhythmia pathogenesis. Cardiovasc Res 2002;56:359-372.

100. Gaita F, Antonio M, Riccardi R, et al: Cryoenergy catheter ablation: A new technique for treatment of permanent junctional reciprocating tachycardia in children. J Cardiovasc Electrophysiol 2004;15:263-268.

101. Drago F, De Santis A, Grutter G, et al: Transvenous cryothermal catheter ablation of re-entry circuit located near the atrioventricular junction in pediatric patients: Efficacy, safety, and midterm follow-up. J Am Coll Cardiol 2005;45:1096-1103.

CHAPTER 25

Heart Failure in the Fetus

James C. Huhta
Gerald Tulzer

Fetal echocardiography can diagnose many forms of congenital heart disease and assess the prognosis of cardiac lesions based on their anatomy and presentation in utero. The presence of signs of fetal heart failure, such as hydrops or valvular regurgitation, makes the assessment of prognosis more difficult, however. A tool for this assessment is the cardiovascular profile score, which combines ultrasound markers of fetal cardiovascular illness based on univariate parameters that have been correlated with perinatal mortality. This profile could become the fetal heart failure score and potentially could be used in much the same way as and in combination with the biophysical profile score.[1] This chapter reviews the pathophysiology of heart failure prenatally and presents a straightforward method for rapid evaluation of a fetus that may have fetal congestive heart failure.

FETAL CIRCULATION

The fetal circulation is unique and significantly different from the circulation in a newborn, infant, or child. Knowledge of these morphologic and physiologic differences is crucial for the understanding and assessment of fetal cardiovascular function. Most of this knowledge is derived from experimental animal data and, more recently, ultrasonography, which allows direct observation of the circulation in normal and abnormal human fetuses.

In the fetus, the ventricles pump blood in parallel rather than in series, with the left ventricle pumping to the aorta and upper body and the right ventricle pumping to the ductus arteriosus and the lower body and placenta (Fig. 25-1). The lungs have a high resistance in utero, and the placenta fulfills the role of oxygenating the blood

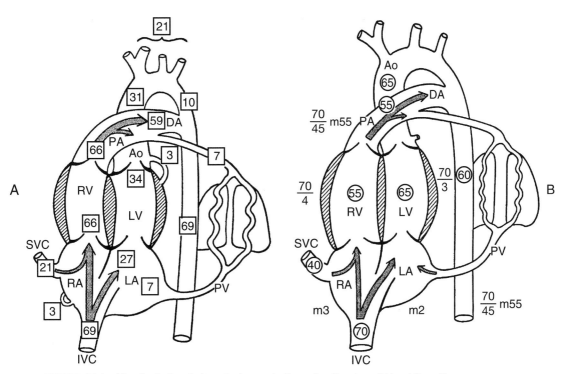

FIGURE 25-1 ■ **The fetal circulation. A,** Arrows indicate the direction of blood flow. Percentages of combined ventricular output in cardiac chambers and major vessels are presented in boxes. **B,** Oxygen saturations are presented in circles for cardiac chambers and major vessels (see text for description of the circulation). Ao, aorta; DA, ductus arteriosus; IVC, inferior vena cava; LA, left atrium; LV, left ventricle; PA, pulmonary artery; PV, pulmonary vein; RA, right atrium; RV, right ventricle; SVC, superior vena cava. (From Fineman JR, Soifer SJ: The fetal and neonatal circulations. In Chang AC, Hanley FL, Wernovsky G, et al [eds]: *Pediatric Cardiac Intensive Care.* Philadelphia, Williams & Wilkins, p. 18, 1998.)

and ridding the body of wastes. The highly oxygenated blood from the placenta passes to the ductus venosus, where a portion bypasses the liver and passes predominantly to the left atrium. The relatively deoxygenated blood from the upper body passes to the tricuspid valve, then to the ductus arteriosus and lungs. The deoxygenated blood from the inferior vena cava (IVC) and the right hepatic veins is directed to the right atrium and predominantly to the tricuspid valve. This distribution of lower body flow is accomplished by the posterior portion of the IVC connecting directly to the foramen ovale and the superior portion of the atrial septum, the crista dividens, which overlies the IVC, effectively dividing it into two streams.

The presence of three shunts (ductus venosus, foramen ovale, and ductus arteriosus) allows the fetal heart to work with two parallel circulations rather than one series circulation. Right and left atrial pressures are almost equal because of the presence of the foramen ovale, and right and left ventricular pressures are equal because of the ductus arteriosus. The left ventricle ejects into the upper body and cerebral circulation, and the right ventricle ejects into the pulmonary arteries and through the ductus arteriosus into the lower body and the placental circulation. The vascular beds of the upper and lower body are connected via the aortic isthmus. As a further consequence of the parallel arrangement of these circulations, ventricular outputs can be quite different. In the case of obstruction on one side of the heart, the other side is able to increase its work or even completely supply the whole circulation alone.

Fetal Cardiac Output

The cardiac ventricular output is the product of the heart rate and the stroke volume of the right and left ventricles. The stroke volume is determined by the preload, afterload, and myocardial contractility of each ventricle. An increase in the stretch of the ventricular chamber results in an increased contractility and stroke volume according to the Frank-Starling mechanism; this mechanism is now known to be present by 8 weeks of gestation in the human fetus. The Frank-Starling mechanism allows the cardiac output to be unchanged during periods of heart rate change ranging from 50 to 200 beats/min.

Distribution of cardiac output prenatally is quite different from that after birth and changes throughout gestation.[2] The fetal right ventricle always ejects more blood than the left ventricle (in the fetal lamb almost twice as much), and the lungs are perfused only by a small (7% to 25%) proportion of the combined ventricular output. Umbilical vein flow is divided at the entrance to the liver, where approximately 50% of its highly oxygenated blood is shunted through the ductus venosus directly to the IVC and right atrium and through the foramen ovale to the left atrium. The other 50% passes through the liver before reaching the IVC. Streaming within the IVC is such that the higher oxygenated blood, coming from the ductus venosus, is directed to the left atrium, whereas lower oxygenated blood from the hepatic circulation and superior vena cava preferentially enters the right ventricle. As a consequence, coronary arteries and brain are perfused with higher oxygenated blood. In the case of circulatory compromise, the fetus takes advantage of these shunts to shift more oxygenated blood to the left side of the heart, ensuring adequate perfusion of vital organs. Throughout gestation, distribution of combined ventricular output changes such that with increasing gestational age, lower body, lungs, gut, and brain receive a higher percentage, and placenta and kidneys receive a lower percentage.[3]

Because the pulmonary and systemic circulations are separate in the fetus, each ventricle has a stroke volume determined by the individual preload, afterload, and contractility of that chamber. Both ventricles are linked by the atrial pressures, which are similar owing to the presence of the foramen ovale. They also are linked by the ventricular septum, which is shared by each ventricle, and by the common arterial pressure, which is the result of the widely patent ductus arteriosus. The unique feature of the parallel nature of the ventricular ejection is that if there is increased afterload of one ventricle, the output of that ventricle decreases, and the output of the contralateral ventricle increases in a compensatory manner; this leads to the disproportionate growth of the normal side of the heart commonly associated with congenital heart disease. A functional separation of the ventricles at the level of the aortic isthmus has been observed such that any blood pressure change in the lower body causes increased right ventricular output without a change of ascending aortic pressure.

Fetal Heart Morphology and Function

The metabolic source of energy for the fetal myocardium is glucose almost exclusively. In adults, fatty acids are the major source of energy for the myocardium. Growth or increased workload in the fetus results in hyperplasia of the myocardium with an increased number of cells, whereas growth of the myocardium after birth is only by increased cell size or hypertrophy (increased protein content of each cell). Significant maturational changes occur during fetal life regarding size, shape and architecture of the ventricular myocyte.[4]

Myocardial **contractility** comparisons between fetal and adult animals have shown that the fetal myocardium develops less active tension than the adult at similar muscle lengths. Structural differences, such as fewer T tubules and less organized myofibrils, are observed, but there are also differences in calcium uptake into the sarcoplasmic reticulum. Decreased sympathetic innervations in the immature myocardium could influence the stress response of the myocardium. Fetal myocytes are smaller in size; have less mitochondria, sarcoplasmic reticulum, myofilaments, α/β-adrenoceptors, and T tubules; and have higher concentrations of DNA reflecting a larger number of nuclei. In contrast to postnatal life, myocardial growth is the result of an increase in the number of muscle cells rather than cell size. In the very immature heart, myofilaments are arranged in a more chaotic way, but they become better organized as gestation advances. These morphologic differences have been used to explain the reduced ability of the fetal myocyte to contract.

Besides the difference in contractility, the fetal heart reacts differently in response to **preload** and afterload changes. Several studies in isolated myocardium and intact hearts have shown a reduced compliance of the fetal myocardium.[5] Studies on the effect of preload changes on cardiac output in the fetus have shown that although reduction of preload resulted in a decrease of cardiac output, cardiac output increased only when filling pressures increased 2 to 4 mm Hg above resting pressures (but a further increase of atrial pressure did not result in a greater ventricular output).[6] This is in contrast to postnatal hearts, where a progressive increase in ventricular output is observed with an atrial pressure increase to 15 to 20 mm Hg. Increased **afterload** in the fetus is followed by a reduction in myocardial shortening and in stroke volume. If arterial pressures are kept constant, ventricular stroke volume increases even with atrial pressures of 10 to 15 mm Hg.[6] The Frank-Starling mechanism is present in the fetus, although it operates at the upper limit. In the fetus, one has to consider that right ventricular afterload is determined mainly by the vascular bed of the placenta, whereas left ventricular output is determined by the cerebral circulation. The effect of **heart rate** on combined ventricular output in the fetus is much more pronounced than postnatally.[7] As previously mentioned, the fetus has a range of heart rates from 50 to 200 beats/min at which the stroke volume of the ventricular chambers can adapt to maintain adequate combined ventricular output and tissue perfusion. Outside of this range, heart failure often results.

The major determinant of cardiac output is the afterload of the fetal ventricle. Any influence that increases the impedance to ejection inversely lowers the ventricular stroke volume by the effect on the systolic and diastolic functions of the heart. In growth restriction in the fetus secondary to placental dysfunction, the combined cardiac output decreases as a result of increased placental resistance.

HEART FAILURE IN THE FETUS AND HYDROPS FETALIS

The morphologic and functional differences described in this chapter affect the development and presentation of fetal heart failure. End-stage fetal heart failure results in hydrops fetalis. The reduced ability of the fetal heart to contract and to generate force, the lower myocardial compliance and the diminished Frank-Starling mechanism, the higher dependence of cardiac output on heart rate, and the lack of adrenoceptors all contribute to decreased cardiac reserve in response to stress and to a higher susceptibility of the fetus for the development of cardiac failure.

Factors Contributing to Hydrops

Several features are responsible for fluid accumulation in fetal tissue (Table 25-1). The final common pathway of many different conditions compromising the cardiovascular system is elevation of ventricular end-diastolic pressure, atrial pressure, and central venous pressure. In the fetus, even small increases in venous pressure have been shown to have significant physiologic effects.[8] In addition, the younger the fetus, the higher is its extracellular water content and the lower its tissue pressure. Fluid movement between the intravascular and extravascular space depends on intravascular and extravascular hydrostatic and oncotic pressures and the fluid filtration coefficient, which is determined by the capillary membrane (which is more permeable for fluid and protein in the fetus). Albumin concentration, largely responsible for oncotic pressure, is lower in the fetus and increases with gestational age. All of these factors favor fluid movement out of the capillary and into tissue. Lymphatic drainage of tissue seems to be much more important in the fetus; an elevated venous pressure may reduce lymphatic flow, however, further favoring the development of hydrops. Fall of arterial blood pressure and elevation of filling pressures additionally trigger hormonal responses, such as production of plasma arginine vasopressin (decreases urinary production), angiotensin II (increases fluid accumulation), and atrial natriuretic peptide (increases capillary permeability).[9]

Pulmonary edema as part of congestive heart failure usually does not occur in the fetus. Reasons include

TABLE 25-1

Factors Contributing to Edema Formation in the Fetus	
High compliance of interstitial space	Allows accommodation of large volume at low tissue pressure
High capillary filtration coefficient	Allows large water flux at low vascular pressure
Low colloidal osmotic pressure	Reduces fluid movement from interstitium to capillary
High capillary permeability to protein	
Sensitivity of lymphatic drainage to increased venous pressure	Decreases removal of fluid from interstitium via lymphatic channels

Adapted from Rudolph AM: Congenital Diseases of the Heart: Clinical-Physiological Considerations. New York, Futura, p. 18, 2001.

the following: (1) In the presence of a patent foramen ovale, left atrial hypertension does not develop; (2) the pulmonary arterioles are constricted; and (3) the lung is fluid-filled, and this is where the positive intra-amniotic pressure is transmitted. In the case of total anomalous pulmonary venous drainage with stenosis of the draining vessel or premature constriction or occlusion of the foramen ovale associated with left-sided obstructions, pulmonary venous hypertension can occur with secondary damage to the fetal lungs.[10]

When the clinician is faced with a fetus with hydrops fetalis, he or she first must determine if the hydrops is cardiac, inflammatory, or metabolic. Many cases of hydrops now are attributed to fetal systemic infection. New markers are identifying etiologic agents such as parvovirus and adenovirus. The associated hepatitis with these infections can compromise the protein-producing capability of the fetus, decreasing the fetal oncotic pressure in the vascular space and resulting in fluid loss out of the circulation. Immune hydrops always must be considered in the differential diagnosis, but other causes of anemia, such as hemoglobinopathies, can cause hydrops. Infections can cause hemolytic anemia, which can be treated by fetal transfusion. High central venous pressure may exceed the oncotic pressure of the interstitial space, causing fluid to pass into spaces such as the abdominal cavity (ascites), pleural or pericardial spaces (effusions), or any of the vital organs. In addition, multiple mechanisms of hydrops may coexist, and the primary cause may not be immediately obvious. More important is the determination of the prognosis of hydrops. This task would be aided by a semiquantitative measure of fetal heart failure.

The challenge of hydrops assessment and the diagnosis of heart failure can be summarized as the difficulty in knowing how well the fetal myocardium is performing under changing loading conditions. By combining information from the obstetric and cardiologic evaluations, the perinatal cardiologist can assess whether it is likely that the function abnormality is transient or permanent. The etiology cannot always be known, but the differential diagnosis often contains infectious, inherited, congenital, or toxic entities. After birth, the prognosis depends on the diagnosis and the evolution of the function abnormality over time. The long-term outcome depends on whether or not the insult is reversible and whether there were periods of ischemia, brain injury, or both. There are several possibilities for the cause of heart failure in the fetus after ruling out fetal infection (Table 25-2).

Markers of Fetal Mortality

The most useful predictor of perinatal death in fetal hydrops is the presence of umbilical venous pulsations.[11] The most common pathway of perinatal demise is compromised fetal cardiac output—fetal congestive heart failure. The following are requisite initial data that

TABLE 25-2

Causes of Fetal Congestive Heart Failure

Fetal arrhythmias
 Tachyarrhythmias (atrial flutter, supraventricular
  tachycardia)
 Bradyarrhythmias (complete heart block)
Anemia
Congenital heart disease with valvular regurgitation
 (see text)
Noncardiac malformations (e.g., diaphragmatic hernia or
 cystic hygroma)
Twin-to-twin transfusion recipient with volume and
 pressure overload
High cardiac output failure
 Sacrococcygeal teratoma, placental chorioangioma,
  aneurysm of the vein of Galen

should be collected during fetal echocardiography: (1) cardiac size-to-thoracic size ratio (cardiac divided by thoracic area ratio; normal 0.25 to 0.35) or cardiac-to-thoracic circumference ratio (normal <0.5); (2) venous Doppler (IVC or hepatic vein [increased atrial reversal] and umbilical cord vein [pulsations]); and (3) four-valve Doppler (any leak of the valves should be evaluated further). If there are abnormalities in any of these measurements, a cardiac cause or associated physiologic problem may be present, and detailed study is indicated to rule out serious cardiovascular involvement.

The cardiovascular system provides a large volume of information about the well-being of the fetus. It is currently readily accessible because of rapid developments in the technology of noninvasive techniques, particularly ultrasound. The fetus has become the new patient of the decade owing to the rapid changes in ultrasound technologies and other fetal assessment techniques. The fetal biophysical profile is useful to detect changes in fetal well-being, especially with heart failure resulting from abnormal heart rate.[1] The decision to deliver a fetus prematurely because of cardiac changes must be made in the context of the risks prenatally and postnatally and the risks to the mother and the fetus. Any assessment demands a coordinated team approach between perinatalogists, cardiologists, and neonatologists.[12]

The definition of fetal congestive heart failure is similar to congestive heart failure after birth—inadequate tissue perfusion. Inadequate cardiac output results in a series of complex reflexes and adaptations to improve forward flow to direct it to vital organs. This state can be described as a deficiency of flow of blood to the tissues such that certain reflexes are triggered for the survival of the fetus. One such response is that of the secretion of an excess of circulating catecholamines, which are produced in response to peripheral vascular detection of abnormal perfusion. Powerful hormonal reflexes that also are triggered include those that control salt and water retention (in an attempt to increase myocardial preload). It is now known that the fetus is capable of undergoing cytokine activation and the secretion of endothelin and troponin T.[13] The maturational changes of the systemic vascular bed with gestational age are unknown, but it is believed that vasoconstriction of the fetal systemic resistance vessels can occur in response to stress.

VENTRICULAR FUNCTION IN THE FETUS

Most attention has been paid to right ventricular function in the human fetus because this ventricle is most likely to show an abnormality during clinical situations associated with increased workload. Examples of right ventricular problems are summarized to illustrate an approach to ventricular function in the fetus. The right ventricle in the fetus is now understood to be a large contributor to the work output of the fetal myocardium because of the large volume and pressure work required of it. The earliest signs of altered function in the fetal heart are observed to be a reflection of right heart hemodynamics. Isolated right atrial enlargement is a sign of many abnormalities, especially early in gestation. This enlargement may occur because the right atrium is at the center of the fetal circulation. The normal flow from the right atrium to the left atrium reflects the normal right atrial-to-left atrial pressure gradient. Any increase in flow to the heart, such as with anemia or arteriovenous fistula, translates into enlargement of the right atrium. The right ventricle is pumping primarily to the lower body and placenta, and right atrial pressure elevation results from any increase in the resistance that is seen by this ventricle. Placental dysfunction later in gestation causes right ventricular dysfunction and secondary right atrial enlargement, whereas the left ventricle shows no signs of dysfunction.[14]

Right Ventricular Growth and Function
The geometry of the right ventricle in utero is different from the left ventricle. The right ventricle is tripartite with inflow, apical, and outflow portions. Calculating the volume of this chamber is difficult because of the complex shape of the chamber. In utero, it is more spherical and more like the left ventricle, but still must be measured with nongeometric techniques. After birth, the right ventricle atrophies, and the shape becomes more flattened and thinned. Right ventricular volume ejected is greater than left ventricular volume by echocardiographic measurements throughout gestation.[15] The right ventricle supplies the pulmonary arteries, the descending aorta, and the placenta via the ductus arteriosus. The high resistance of the pulmonary arteries is in parallel with the lower resistance of the lower body. The workload of the right ventricle is determined by the volume of blood pumped and the afterload. In general,

the work of the right ventricle can be described as the product of the afterload (blood pressure) × the stroke volume of ejection. The afterload of the right ventricle is unique because there are pressure reflections from the downstream resistance. These reflections from the proximal arterioles and, more importantly, from the proximal ductus arteriosus result in increased power expenditure for a given cardiac output. This increased power is illustrated by the shortened acceleration time in the pulmonary valve compared with the aortic valve. The right ventricle must perform the work of overcoming inertia, moving the mass of blood forward, and the oscillatory work resulting from the downstream pressure reflections that return to the pulmonary valve shortly after the onset of ejection. When the volume of blood pumped by a ventricle is reduced, the overall size of the ventricle becomes smaller than the contralateral side as a result of redistribution of flow at the atrial level. This finding of disproportion at the ventricular level is an excellent screening marker of ventricular dysfunction or congenital defect.

Another indication that the right ventricle is performing more work than the left ventricle is derived from data collected in fetal lambs measuring the coronary blood flow of both ventricles. The right ventricular coronary flow was consistently one third greater than the left ventricular flow.[16] Right ventricular size limits the volume of blood that is pumped with each systolic ejection. In situations with reduced right ventricular size with an intrinsically normal right ventricle, the right ventricular volume can be reduced by variables such as pericardial fluid or diastolic stiffness. A hypoplastic right ventricular chamber may limit its ejection volume if an increase in stroke volume is demanded of that chamber.

The heart rate also limits the volume of blood that can be ejected by the right or left ventricle by limiting the filling time of the ventricle. With fetal tachycardia, the cardiac output decreases with increasing heart rate. It is known from clinical experience that a fetus with a heart rate greater than 240 beats/min can become hydropic in 3 to 5 days during incessant tachycardia.

Right Ventricular Changes with Gestational Age
The inflow pattern of blood velocity can be useful to determine the diastolic characteristics of the right ventricle. The normal pattern is biphasic with an early filling wave (E wave) immediately after opening of the tricuspid valve, followed by a later atrial contraction wave (A wave). The atrial contraction augments right ventricular filling, and the filling waves sometimes can be used to assess the filling properties of the right ventricle. Tulzer and colleagues[17] and Harada and associates[18] analyzed longitudinally the filling patterns of the right ventricle and showed that the fetal circulation is right ventricular dominant. With increasing gestational age, the early filling wave increased in area, and the peak velocities showed increasing E waves and

decreasing A waves. Calculations of the distribution of cardiac output have shown that the right ventricle pumps more than the left ventricle. This distribution is maintained despite significant changes in the pulmonary vascular resistance and flow between 20 and 37 weeks of gestation.[19] Foramen ovale flow changes inversely with pulmonary blood flow, maintaining the net right ventricular output greater than that of the left ventricle.

Echocardiographic Assessment of Function

Because the right ventricle is complex in shape, techniques such as the calculation of the right ventricular function using nongeometric techniques using inflow and outflow time intervals are employed. The **myocardial performance index**, or so-called Tei index, of the right ventricle does not depend on geometric assumptions of the right ventricle and can be used as an afterload-independent parameter to follow changes in fetal right ventricular function over time. The Tei index is the isovolumic time divided by the ejection time. The isovolumic time is the sum of the two intervals— the isovolumic relaxation time and the isovolumic contraction time. This time can be measured by subtracting the ejection time from the time of inflow of the right ventricle (the time from tricuspid valve opening to closure). (See also Chapter 10)

Changes in the loading of the right ventricle result in hypertrophy of the chamber walls, and severe thickening can result in diastolic dysfunction (poor relaxation). The description of the right ventricular function requires that the loading conditions of the ventricle be known, and this is one of the most important goals in right ventricular assessment in the human fetus. The pulmonary vascular resistance has been estimated in the fetus and seems to decrease between 20 and 30 weeks of gestation, then increase again until term.[20]

The **tricuspid valve** is intimately associated with the right ventricular function. This valve is normally not regurgitant and maintains competence by a complex interaction with the right ventricular endocardium from which it arises early in fetal development. Any acute increase in right ventricular afterload, such as acute constriction of the ductus arteriosus, results in a small amount of tricuspid valve regurgitation within two heartbeats.[21] Sudden relief of this pressure work causes immediate cessation of the regurgitation; this implies that the shape and micromorphology of the right ventricular chamber are intimately associated with tricuspid valve function, and that there are constant instantaneous adjustments in the fetal right ventricle to maintain the workload. After examining more than 1000 normal fetuses, Respondek and coworkers[22] concluded that there is rarely any tricuspid regurgitation in the human fetus at anytime. Monitoring Tei function in the first trimester even before the development of the tricuspid valvular functional apparatus shows the same result—of not even a trace of leak. The marker of tricuspid regurgitation is a useful one clinically in detecting a right ventricle that may have early dysfunction. The time frame of the tricuspid regurgitation also is useful in deciding if the tricuspid regurgitation could be a sign of disordered myocardial function or is simply a result of normal adjustments to workload. The rapidity of the upstroke of the tricuspid regurgitation jet along with its peak velocity can provide valuable information about right ventricular function. A calculation of the change in pressure over time (dP/dt) can be performed with a good-quality tricuspid regurgitation jet.[23] A value of less than 400 mm Hg/sec was associated with death in hydropic fetuses. The peak velocity also can be used to assess the peak pressure in the right ventricle by using continuous-wave Doppler.

The most severe forms of right ventricular diastolic dysfunction are manifest by the finding of monophasic **inflow velocity**. The inability of the right ventricle to relax is shown dramatically in the rare patient with ductal occlusion. The right ventricle usually stays thick, small, and contracted before birth, but the ventricle relaxes and fills immediately after birth. Within days, the right ventricle may be able to change from a small thick ventricle to one that is supporting most of the circulation.

Systolic function also can be assessed by analyzing the ejection force of the fetal ventricles. This analysis is done at the outflow valves: The right and left ventricular force development is estimated by Newton's equation in which force is defined as the product of mass and acceleration, and the ejection force can be assessed using the shape of the ejection curve.[24,25] Such calculations show that the ejection forces of both ventricles are similar. Altered loading conditions can alter the force significantly.

The blood velocity pattern of the right ventricular ejection through the **pulmonary valve** can be used to learn whether or not the right ventricular afterload is increased. With decreasing right ventricular output, the time-velocity integral decreases, while the acceleration time shortens. The pulmonary valve function also is affected in relation to the underlying right ventricular function. Normally the pulmonary valve in the fetus is perfectly competent. With severe and end-stage right ventricular dysfunction, the valve may exhibit regurgitation, and this finding can have significant prognostic implications. This finding may be due to dysfunction of the infundibular muscle supporting the pulmonary valve.

The **ductus arteriosus** is a site where much can be learned about the left and right heart circulations. Flow is normally from the pulmonary artery to the descending aorta in systole and diastole. The peak velocity is between 0.8 and 2 m/sec and increases with increasing gestational age. The pulsatility index of the waveform (normal 1.9 to 3) does not change with gestational age.[26]

ABNORMAL RIGHT VENTRICULAR FUNCTION

Effects of Increased Afterload

Right ventricular dysfunction has been recognized more commonly in the most severe cases of **intrauterine growth restriction**.[27] Systemic and pulmonary vascular resistances are increased, and the placental resistance can be dramatically elevated. The marked decreases in oxygenation in this disease also may play a role in the compromise of right ventricular shortening. Dilation of the right ventricle and later decrease in right ventricular shortening demand prompt attention because these signs signal impending difficulty. Venous Doppler and presence of tricuspid valve regurgitation in this disease also portend compromised right ventricular function and the need for more detailed study.

The recipient larger twin in **twin-to-twin transfusion syndrome** can experience marked elevations in cardiac output and blood pressure. Typically the larger twin maintains a high cardiac output as a result of the volume transfusion plus a state of vasoconstriction as a result of vasoactive substances produced by the smaller twin.[28,29] With slow increases in the workload of the right ventricle, there is compensatory hypertrophy with minimal signs of hemodynamic decompensation. With more rapid onset of volume and pressure overload, however, the right ventricle stretches, and the tricuspid valve becomes insufficient. The coronary perfusion and subendocardial blood flow are progressively compromised by the hypertrophy and increased early systolic workload. These alterations probably are associated with an increase in the end-diastolic pressure of the right ventricle, and this is reflected in the end-diastolic pressure of the right atrium. The atrial contractions against an elevated pressure resistance produce retrograde flow during atrial systole in the hepatic veins and IVC. The ductus venosus is the earliest site to see altered flow patterns. With the onset of atrial reversal in this site or umbilical venous pulsations, the onset of metabolic acidosis can be imminent. Although many factors influence this outcome, one of the most important is the right ventricular myocardial reserve.

Ductal constriction is defined by the shape of the curve and the estimated mean velocity. Spontaneous or medication-induced constriction of the ductus arteriosus can be detected by the velocity, and the severity of ductal constriction can be estimated.[26] One of the most common clinical situations to observe right ventricular function changes is during fetal ductal changes. Either drug-induced or naturally occurring constriction or occlusion of the ductus arteriosus affects right ventricular shortening. In this situation, the overall right ventricular cross-sectional area changes with systole and diastole decreasing dramatically; although the right ventricle moves with contraction, there is little wall movement,

and the ejection volume is greatly decreased. The extent of this decrease was shown by Tulzer and colleagues,[21] and the total combined cardiac output may be normal. One of the most important observations from these data is that decreased shortening may not indicate abnormal contractility of the ventricle; this was shown by calculating dP/dt, the first derivative of the pressure change in the right ventricle using the tricuspid regurgitation jet. There is no reported case in the literature at this point of hydrops resulting from ductal occlusion or constriction without concomitant restriction of the foramen ovale. This is a reflection of the redistribution of cardiac output to the left ventricle. Monitoring of venous Doppler is most useful for assessing the impact of altered right ventricular function in this setting. In most cases, the pregnancy progresses without alteration in growth of the fetus, and the right ventricle becomes smaller and thicker. Rarely, congestive heart failure results.[30]

Effects of Increased Preload

An **arteriovenous fistula** with a shunt from the arterial to the venous circulation in the human fetus results in a large volume of blood returning to the right atrium. This large volume of blood results in dilated right heart structures and a high cardiac output. The fetal heart is well adapted to handle increasing volume loads if the overload is imposed gradually. If the shunt is increasing rapidly, as is seen sometimes with sacrococcygeal teratoma, cardiac decompensation and the development of hydrops fetalis can occur. An important sign of right ventricular decompensation in this scenario is valvular regurgitation. Early signs of even mild tricuspid regurgitation should signal an increase in fetal surveillance; subsequent development of mitral regurgitation is ominous and is a clear sign of a prehydropic state.

Congenital Heart Disease

Several abnormalities of the **pulmonary valve** exist. The most common right-sided heart abnormality is a bicuspid pulmonary valve. This anomaly usually results in trivial narrowing of the right ventricular outflow tract and no significant hemodynamic alteration. Less common is severe pulmonary stenosis with significant pressure increase in the right ventricle. In this lesion, the right ventricular pressure increases to suprasystemic levels only when it is most severe. At this point, a gradient is detected by an increased velocity across the pulmonary valve. One can estimate the degree to which the right ventricular pressure is greater than systemic pressure by converting the peak velocity to a gradient using the equation 4 × velocity squared. This gradient is associated with hypertrophy of the right ventricle and a decrease in the shortening fraction. More severe degrees of right ventricular outflow obstruction occur with pulmonary atresia. In this lesion, the pulmonary valve annulus is smaller than normal, and there are usually signs of endocardial change in the right ventricle, such as echogenic areas. In congenital heart defects with pulmonary stenosis or atresia and a ventricular septal defect, such as tetralogy of Fallot, the right ventricular size is maintained and is equal to the left ventricle because the pressures are equal. There is an uncommon form of pulmonary atresia with intact ventricular septum when infarction of the right ventricle occurs; there is sometimes severe tricuspid valve regurgitation. The right ventricle is larger than normal, and the right atrium may be massively enlarged. In the rare case of tetralogy of Fallot with absent valve syndrome, there is no ductus arteriosus, and the pulmonary arteries are enlarged. Pulmonary valve regurgitation is moderate or severe because there is no pulmonary valve (it is replaced by a fibrous ring). The right ventricle and the left ventricle experience the effects of the pulmonary regurgitant volume and are usually normal. Rarely, dysfunction of the right ventricle is indicated by disproportion of the ventricular sizes with right ventricular enlargement.

Tricuspid valve congenital abnormalities that result in significant amounts of tricuspid valve regurgitation are often fatal. One of the most common defects is tricuspid valve dysplasia.[31,32] In this lesion, the right ventricle and right atrium are massively dilated, and color Doppler shows that regurgitation is the cause. The key issue in this lesion is the nature of the right ventricular outflow tract. If there is no pulmonary stenosis, the lesion may have occurred later in gestation, and the prognosis is better. The degree of right ventricular cardiomyopathy can be assessed by measurement of the peak velocity of the tricuspid regurgitation jet. The lower the velocity, the worse the right ventricular dysfunction and prognosis. Ebstein malformation with varying severities of pulmonary stenosis or atresia in the fetus is the cancer of congenital heart disease.[31] The heart becomes enlarged to occupy more than 60% to 70% of the chest due to the right atrial and atrialized right ventricular enlargement. Pulmonary development can be altered irreversibly by compression of the heart, and associated pleural effusions often are present. Peak tricuspid regurgitation velocities of less than 2 m/sec are associated with a poor prognosis.

Primary cardiomyopathy of the right ventricle, such as Uhl anomaly or arrhythmogenic right ventricular dysplasia, has not been reported in the fetus. Any intractable ventricular arrhythmia in the fetus should prompt consideration of one of these diagnoses, however.

CARDIOVASCULAR PROFILE SCORE: AN INDEX OF FETAL HEART FAILURE

The diagnosis of fetal congestive heart failure must be addressed in a clinical approach similar to that after birth. The classic clinical tetrad of cardiomegaly, tachycardia, tachypnea, and hepatomegaly has been used in neonates and children. This clinical state in the fetus can be characterized by findings in at least five categories, which are obtained during the ultrasound examination. The five categories are each worth 2 points in a 10-point scoring system to assess the cardiovascular system. Abnormalities in the cardiovascular profile score may occur before the clinical state of hydrops fetalis. The five categories are as follows:

1. Hydrops
2. Umbilical venous Doppler
3. Heart size
4. Abnormal myocardial function
5. Arterial Doppler

Within specific disease entities, more emphasis is placed on certain areas by the physician to predict the prognosis. This information comprises only a portion of the total clinical picture and must be integrated by the physician into the diagnostic and treatment plans for the patient.

The cardiovascular profile score (Fig. 25-2) gives a semiquantitative score of the fetal cardiac well-being and uses known markers by ultrasound that have been correlated with poor fetal outcome. This profile is normal if the score is 10; signs of cardiac abnormalities result in a decrease of the score from 10. If there is hydrops with ascites and no other abnormalities, there would be a deduction of 1 point for hydrops (ascites but no skin edema) and no deductions for the other categories for a total score of 9.

Hydrops

Hydrops fetalis, in early stages, may manifest with ascites, pleural effusion, pericardial effusion, or a combination of these findings (Fig. 25-3). In advanced hydrops, there is generalized skin edema seen easily over the scalp and abdominal wall. In scoring hydrops for the cardiovascular profile score, 1 point is deducted for early hydrops and 2 points for skin edema.

Umbilical Venous Doppler

Fetal umbilical venous blood velocities have been examined, and investigations have been clinically promising.[33] Several studies have confirmed that normal flow in the IVC of the fetus has a pulsatile, triphasic pattern. The first forward wave begins to increase with atrial relaxation, reaches its peak during ventricular systole, then decreases to reach its nadir at the end of ventricular systole. The second forward wave occurs during early diastole, and a reverse flow is usually present in late diastole with atrial contraction. In normal pregnancy, the peak velocities obtained during the first wave of systole are greater than the early diastolic values. The systolic-to-diastolic ratios do not appear to change with advancing gestational age, but a significant decrease in flow reversal with atrial contraction is evident.

Studies in the fetal lamb have shown that this decrease in percentage of reversed flow seen in normal pregnancy is related to the pressure gradient between the right atrium and the right ventricle during end diastole.[33,34]

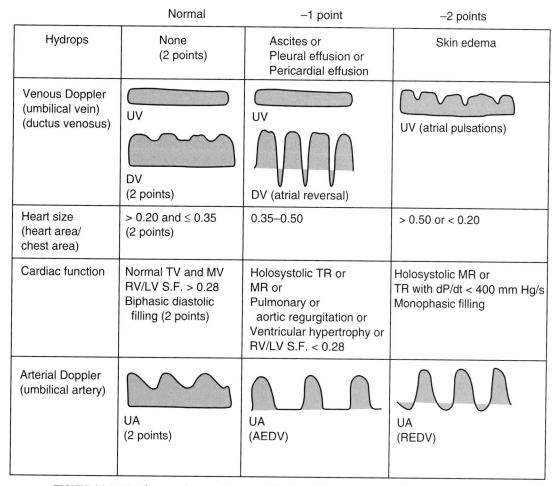

Hydrops	None (2 points)	Ascites or Pleural effusion or Pericardial effusion	Skin edema
	Normal	−1 point	−2 points
Venous Doppler (umbilical vein) (ductus venosus)	UV DV (2 points)	UV DV (atrial reversal)	UV (atrial pulsations)
Heart size (heart area/ chest area)	> 0.20 and ≤ 0.35 (2 points)	0.35–0.50	> 0.50 or < 0.20
Cardiac function	Normal TV and MV RV/LV S.F. > 0.28 Biphasic diastolic filling (2 points)	Holosystolic TR or MR or Pulmonary or aortic regurgitation or Ventricular hypertrophy or RV/LV S.F. < 0.28	Holosystolic MR or TR with dP/dt < 400 mm Hg/s Monophasic filling
Arterial Doppler (umbilical artery)	UA (2 points)	UA (AEDV)	UA (REDV)

FIGURE 25-2 ■ Cardiovascular profile score. The heart failure score is 10 if there are no abnormal signs and reflects 2 points for each of five categories: hydrops, venous Doppler, heart size, cardiac function, and arterial Doppler. AEDV, absent end-diastolic velocity; dP/dt, change in pressure over time of tricuspid regurgitation jet; DV, ductus venosus; LV, left ventricle; MR, mitral regurgitation; MV, mitral valve; REDV, reversed end-diastolic velocity; RV, right ventricle; s, second; S.F., ventricular shortening fraction; TR, tricuspid regurgitation; TV, tricuspid valve; UA, umbilical artery; UV, umbilical vein.

It seems to be related to ventricular compliance and ventricular end-diastolic pressure and reflects central venous pressure. Recording venous blood velocity might give important information on fetal cardiac pump function. Previous studies in humans have shown that alterations in central venous blood velocity patterns accurately reflect abnormalities in cardiac hemodynamics.[35] The abnormal pulsatility pattern of increased velocity of blood flow reversal away from the heart during atrial contraction has been reported in the fetus with congestive heart failure and may be a sign of increased end-diastolic pressure in the failing ventricles. Abnormal IVC flow velocity patterns have been described in several fetal pathologic conditions, including anemia, nonimmune hydrops, arrhythmias, and severe growth restriction, characterized by the absence of end-diastolic flow in the umbilical artery. A compromised fetus with acidosis is known to manifest abnormalities on venous Doppler, including increased atrial reversal in excess of normal in the IVC at the junction with the right atrium and increased pulsatility in the ductus venosus.

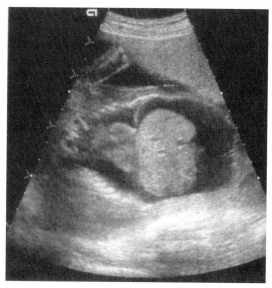

FIGURE 25-3 ■ Fetal hydrops. Longitudinal ultrasound section of the fetal chest and abdomen with the cephalic end of the fetus to the left. The image shows bilateral hydrothorax and ascites. (From Nicolini U: *Fetal hydrops and tumours.* In Rodeck CH, Whittle MJ [eds]: *Fetal Medicine.* London, Churchill Livingstone, p. 737, 1999.)

The prognostic importance of these abnormalities has been confirmed in fetuses with intrauterine growth restriction and with hydrops. An increased A/S ratio in the ductus venosus (peak atrial reversal divided by the peak filling wave during ventricular systole) seems to be the most useful sign in quantifying the increase of the atrial contraction in fetuses with growth retardation. Normally the ratio of the area of the atrial reversal to the entire forward flow area should be less than 7%. Transmission of the venous pulsations into the portal and umbilical circulation correlates with increasing degrees of cardiac compromise. Tulzer and coworkers[36] studied the cardiac factors related to prognosis in hydrops and noted that umbilical venous pulsations could stand in for many cardiac variables in predicting prognosis, including ventricular shortening fraction, ejection velocities and percentage, and IVC atrial reversal.

Abnormal venous Doppler findings progress retrograde from the heart in the following order:

1. Increased atrial reversal in the IVC
2. Ductus venosus atrial reversal
3. Portal venous atrial pulsations
4. Umbilical venous atrial pulsations

The end-stage finding of an abnormal venous Doppler is atrial pulsations in the umbilical cord vein. This finding of so-called diastolic block predicts perinatal mortality. Venous pulsations are abnormal in the portal vein, and such a finding may precede the progression to umbilical venous pulsations (Fig. 25-4). The most useful site for sampling in the abdomen is the ductus venosus, which can be identified by its location and color Doppler acceleration blood velocity pattern.

Venous Doppler was evaluated in a group of 41 fetuses diagnosed with congenital cardiac defects in utero and confirmed postnatally. The gestational age ranged from 18 to 38 weeks (mean gestational age 27.5 weeks). The fetuses were grouped into those with ventricular septal defects ($n=11$), those with tricuspid atresia or hypoplasia ($n=4$), those with hypoplastic left heart syndrome ($n=19$), and others ($n=7$), and all the venous Doppler patterns were analyzed. Abnormal IVC waveforms were present only in fetuses with tricuspid atresia or other right heart lesions where the returning flow to the heart all passed through the foramen ovale to reach the heart. Umbilical waveforms were nonpulsatile in all patients. The authors concluded that venous Doppler in fetuses with congenital heart disease without heart failure is normal (with the exception of tricuspid atresia and pulmonary atresia with intact septum). When abnormal central venous flow patterns occurred in association with cardiac defects in utero, they were usually secondary to other processes occurring simultaneously, which affect ventricular compliance (e.g., endocardial fibroelastosis) or rhythm-related hemodynamics (e.g., complete heart block).

To assess the venous system consistently, pulsed Doppler sampling is obtained in the IVC, the ductus venosus, the umbilical vein in the abdomen, and the umbilical cord vein as part of each serial examination. Transmission of the atrial reversal into the ductus venosus and later into the portal and cord vein sites over time suggests progression of heart failure. The cardiovascular profile score has deductions for abnormal venous Doppler as follows:

1. Ductus venosus atrial reversal—1 point
2. Umbilical venous atrial pulsations—2 points
3. Maximum deduction in any category—2 points

Heart Size

Enlargement of the cardiac chambers is a universal sign of heart failure. This is true in the fetus as well, but few of the mechanisms are understood. It is likely that neurohumoral reflexes are triggered, resulting in retention of extracellular volume leading to increased end-diastolic volume of the ventricles. At some point, this increased ventricular size indicates increased end-diastolic pressure. In contrast to the postnatal human, however, it is uncommon to encounter persistent tachycardia with signs of catecholamine excess. It is possible that the levels of humoral agents are modified by the fetal-maternal exchange mechanisms, which exist when the placenta is functioning normally.

The most common cardiac chamber to express enlargement as a sign of impending cardiac failure is the right atrium. The reasons for this relate to the many causes for heart failure, but the right atrium is a final pathway for blood flow returning to the heart and manifests enlargement in situations of relative foramen obstruction, volume overload, tricuspid valve regurgitation, and increased afterload. Increased right atrial size may be due to increased right ventricular end-diastolic pressure that resulted from an increased afterload or

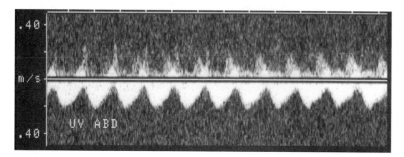

FIGURE 25-4 ■ Fetal tachycardia. Fetal tachycardia at a rapid rate produced pulsations in the umbilical vein in the abdomen (UV ABD).

coronary insufficiency. The right ventricle may be more susceptible to increased work because of the nature of the afterload and the resultant increased demands for oxygen in the face of increased chamber wall stress. It generally is believed that increased atrial wall stress without increased ventricular work does not lead to clinical difficulties in the fetus. Such a situation could be an early marker of cardiac decompensation and may predispose to supraventricular arrhythmias. Secretion of atrial natriuretic peptide could be a marker of this finding. In addition, slower than normal heart rate or persistent rapid heart rate leads to cardiomegaly. The time frame of the onset of the arrhythmia may be estimated by the effect on the cardiac size. An intermittent arrhythmia that has appeared recently would not be expected to cause cardiac enlargement.

Small heart size with external compression has been correlated with hydrops and poor outcome in fetuses with cystic adenomatoid malformation. When heart size is less than 20% of the chest area, fetal outcome is affected. In utero, the heart area can be compared easily with the area of the thorax, and the ratio should be less than one third and greater than one quarter in the presence of normal chest development.[37,38] In fetuses with cystic adenomatoid malformation, a small chest-to-thorax ratio (<0.2) is associated with a poor prognosis.[39] Cardiomegaly is a heart-to-chest area ratio greater than 0.35 at any time in gestation. Cardiac size calculations include the following:

1. Chest-to-thorax area ratio = cardiac area-to-chest area ratio (normal 0.2 to 0.35)
2. Chest-to-thorax circumference ratio = cardiac circumference-to-chest circumference ratio (normal <0.5)
3. Cardiac size: normal heart-to-chest area ratio is less than 0.35 and greater than 0.20
   Mild cardiomegaly: area ratio greater than 0.35–1 point
   Severe cardiomegaly: area ratio greater than 0.50–2 points
   Small heart ratio (<0.2)–2 points

Abnormal Myocardial Function

Cardiac function is assessed indirectly by the global shortening (and thickening) of the walls of the ventricles and by the function of the atrioventricular and semilunar valves. The right and left ventricles should shorten their diameters more than 28% in systole compared with diastole. Measurements of cardiac dimensions with time are performed using M-mode echocardiography. The **shortening fraction** of a ventricle is calculated by taking the difference between the diastolic (DD) and systolic dimensions (SD) and dividing by the diastolic dimension:

Fractional shortening = (DD − SD)/DD (normal >0.28)

An abnormal shortening fraction could reflect myocardial compromise or an increase in the fetal ventricular workload. Regardless, an increase in diastolic dimension often is related to a decrease in shortening fraction and should be regarded as an indication for more intensive monitoring.

The atrioventricular and semilunar valves are competent in the normal fetus, and if regurgitation is detected, it is usually a sign of altered cardiovascular physiology. Because **tricuspid valve regurgitation** is common after birth, it can be speculated that the fetal right ventricle is well adapted to systemic pressure work. Valvular competence is normal, and only in disturbances of cardiovascular physiology when there is increased ventricular wall stress is tricuspid valve regurgitation present. Trace tricuspid regurgitation, defined as nonholosystolic regurgitation lasting at least 70 msec, is not normal. Trace tricuspid regurgitation may be the first sign of a problem but has little prognostic importance. Holosystolic tricuspid regurgitation is abnormal and always indicates the need for further investigation.[22] When regurgitation is detected by color Doppler, it must be confirmed and graded by pulsed Doppler. With congenital diseases of the tricuspid valve, hydrops and fetal death can occur.[40] Regurgitation of other valves is usually a sign of more advanced congestive heart failure and may occur in a moribund fetus with acidosis and severe heart failure as a sign of myocardial compromise. Tricuspid valve regurgitation can be a reversible sign of heart failure, as observed in fetuses with successful in utero therapy for anemia or tachycardia. Progression to mitral valve regurgitation is always a sign of fetal congestive heart failure and usually means that a significant increase in left ventricular wall stress is present (Fig. 25-5). With severe myocardial failure, the support for the semilunar valves is compromised, and pulmonary or aortic valve regurgitation can occur.

Several disease states now are being identified in which thickening of the ventricular chambers (myocardial hypertrophy) occurs in the absence of congenital ventricular outflow obstruction. This thickening is assessed by measuring the **end-diastolic wall thickness** of the left ventricle and comparing it with the normal values for age. Any left ventricular posterior wall thickness greater than or equal to 4 mm is abnormal. The most severe cases of fetal hypertension that have been detected are in the larger of twins in the twin-to-twin transfusion syndrome,[29] in which a mortality of greater than 70% for the fetuses is common. Early identification of hypertrophy in the larger twin may be useful in patient management. Postnatally, neonatal hypertension can be severe and life-threatening. In utero interventions currently are being explored for this cause of congestive heart failure, including serial amniocentesis and laser ablation of the vascular communications.[28] Regardless of the etiology, thickening of the fetal ventricles could restrict the cardiac reserve before or after birth. Because cardiac hypertrophy can occur rapidly but takes weeks or months to resolve, its identification

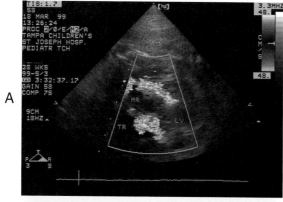

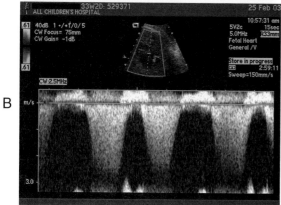

FIGURE 25-5 ▪ Mitral regurgitation (MR) and tricuspid regurgitation (TR) result in a massively enlarged heart. A, The atrioventricular valve regurgitation fills the entire chest. **B,** The slow upstroke of the MR jet is shown by continuous-wave Doppler in an apical view. LV, left ventricle. (See also Color Section)

is an important marker of a cardiovascular system at risk.

Abnormalities of diastolic function could be expected and should be excluded by comparing the **A and E wave filling patterns** of the ventricles using pulsed Doppler to standardized normal values. The filling pattern of the ventricles in diastole is an indicator of the diastolic function of the heart. Monophasic filling of the ventricles is a sign of compromised diastolic function and is a sign of fetal heart failure.[39] One rule of thumb is that the A wave of the ventricular filling is always greater than the E wave, and if it is higher or is indistinguishable, a detailed cardiac study should be performed. Monophasic filling of the ventricles occurs in severe diastolic dysfunction or with severe external cardiac compression. Studies using the myocardial performance index may be useful to reflect an abnormality of systolic and diastolic function and warrant more research.[40] Cardiac function maximal deduction is 2 points:

1. Right ventricular/left ventricular shortening fraction <0.28—1 point
2. Tricuspid regurgitation (holosystolic)–1 point
3. Mitral regurgitation–1 point
4. Monophasic ventricular filling–2 points
5. Pulmonary or aortic valve regurgitation–1 point

6. Valve regurgitation dP/dt <400 mm Hg/sec–2 points
7. Ventricular hypertrophy–1 point

Arterial Doppler

It is well established that the blood velocities measured by Doppler echocardiography in the umbilical artery and in other peripheral vascular beds can be used as an indirect indicator of the relative vascular impedances. An increased pulsatility index in the umbilical artery and descending aorta and a decreased index in the middle cerebral artery are noninvasive signs of redistribution of flow. A pulsed Doppler finding in one portion of the circulation is affected by changes in the rest of the circulation. If there is significant aortic valvular regurgitation in the fetus, the diastolic reversal in the descending aorta and the increased pulsatility index in the umbilical artery are secondary to this change in the heart and do not reflect peripheral resistance only.

The most common cause of elevated vascular resistance in the fetus is placental dysfunction secondary to vasculopathy leading to asymmetric growth restriction. This complex pathophysiologic state is poorly understood, but there is evidence that there is hypoxemia resulting from placental dysfunction and additional compromise of nutrition severe enough to impair growth. When the normal pattern of growth is disturbed (usually asymmetric, such that the brain continues growing but the body does not), the fetus is at risk of organ damage from hypoxemic-ischemic injury. The umbilical artery manifests this problem with a loss or reversal of diastolic blood flow. There is redistribution of flow to the brain (so-called brain sparing) resulting from reflex vasodilation of the cerebral vessels. This is manifested by a decrease in the pulsatility index in the middle cerebral artery such that diastolic flow is relatively increased (pulsatility index <2 standard deviations below the mean). In the fetus with hypoxemia, the peripheral fetal vessels are vasoconstricted, and the larger arteries are suspected to be noncompliant compared with normal fetuses with increased blood pressure.[41] This is a physiologic state characterized by increased vascular resistances and, at end stage, decreased cardiac output. Right ventricular enlargement occurs in some cases.

The vasoactive agents nitric oxide and prostacyclin are in decreased amounts with endothelial cell damage in the placenta. Preliminary studies in pregnant women with high pulsatility (impedance) indices during Doppler ultrasound measurement of umbilical blood flow velocity have revealed that maternal administration of the nitric oxide–donating drug glycerol trinitrate decreases the pulsatility index by reducing vasoconstriction in the fetal extracorporeal circulation. Further capability to treat placental vascular disease would benefit from advances in understanding endothelial cell function in pulmonary and other vascular beds. Altered vascular impedances can be a marker of impending heart failure in the fetus.

Fetal brain sparing is a marker of cardiac output redistribution that is sensitive for the detection of significant hypoxemia and placental dysfunction. Whether it would be useful for detecting the presence of acidosis in the fetus is being investigated.[42] There is evidence, however, that reversal of diastolic flow in the umbilical artery, if confirmed, may be a significant risk factor for abnormal outcomes. As a sign of fetal heart failure, the vasoconstriction resulting from decreased cardiac output and the compensatory sign of vasodilation in the brain can be included in the cardiovascular profile score, as follows:

1. Absent end-diastolic flow in the umbilical artery plus brain sparing*−1 point
2. Reversed end-diastolic flow in the umbilical artery −2 points

Summary of Cardiovascular Profile Score

The cardiovascular profile score is composed of 2 points in each of the five categories used in serial studies to provide a method of uniform physiologic assessment. By taking a multivariate approach, this type of multifactorial score can combine assessments of direct and indirect markers of cardiovascular function. Initial validation of the cardiovascular profile score in hydrops was shown by Falkensammer and Huhta.[43] Seven fetuses with hydrops, including three with congenital heart disease, had correlation of the cardiovascular profile score with the myocardial performance index (Tei index). Right ventricular and left ventricular Tei indices were assessed in normals and showed no change with gestational age. Hofstaetter and Huhta[44] measured the cardiovascular profile score in 59 fetuses with hydrops. Mortality was 21 of 59. The average score in the fetuses that died prenatally or postnatally was 4.9, whereas the average score in the survivors was 6.5.

TREATMENT OF FETAL HEART FAILURE

Treatment of fetal cardiovascular problems can be classified into five subgroups based on the etiology of congestive heart failure: (1) abnormal peripheral impedances causing redistribution of flow and growth failure, (2) high output resulting from anemia or arteriovenous fistula, (3) primary or secondary valvular regurgitation, (4) heart failure secondary to myocardial dysfunction, and (5) tachycardia and bradycardia. Interventions aimed at improving the effective cardiac output also are aimed at prolonging the pregnancy and preventing prematurity and prenatal asphyxia.

Echocardiography has long depended on the shortening of the ventricles to assess the systolic function. It is known, however, that the shortening is inversely proportional to the afterload of the heart, and intense vasoconstriction and redistribution of flow are often observed in fetal congestive heart failure. Better methods for the assessment of cardiac work, including pressure and flow data, are needed. Fetal dP/dt measurement is feasible when valvular regurgitation is present, and Doppler assessment of diastolic function may be useful in detecting compromise of myocardial function.

The rapidity with which a disease progresses determines the urgency of the treatment. The myocardial response to increased wall stress is either adequate or inadequate depending on the severity and timing and duration of the insult, the coronary perfusion, the nutritional state of the fetus, and other problems in the pregnancy.

The usual treatment of **placental dysfunction** is designed to improve the vascular impedance of the placenta and to increase the flow of oxygenated blood to the fetus. With bedrest, improved nutrition, or maternal oxygen, there may be improvement in placental function. Tocolytic medications may relax the placenta and improve its function. Myocardial support for growth restriction has not been proposed, partly because the validation of diagnostic methods is lacking. Studies of ventricular ejection force in growth restriction have shown that both ventricles have decreased ejection force. Advanced heart failure in this setting, with severely decreased arterial Pao_2 and poor nutrition, is manifested by nonspecific signs of increased right ventricular and right atrial size, atrial reversal in the venous Doppler pattern, and altered forward flow velocities.

Treatment with digoxin for evidence of **decreased ventricular shortening** is controversial. Digoxin is known to decrease the catecholamine response to congestive heart failure, and if there is diastolic dysfunction in the fetus, this may improve filling and lower filling pressures. If the afterload is high, an increase in oxygen consumption could result from increased inotropy without improved myocardial perfusion. Terbutaline seems to have promise as an inotropic and chronotropic agent,[45] but studies of the possible negative effects on the fetal myocardium are needed. At present, we use digoxin for fetal cardiac failure resulting from arrhythmias and high output states, such as fistula and anemia. In a case of acardiac twinning where the normal fetuses was supporting two circulations, digoxin seemed to improve cardiac function and resulted in a prolonged and successful gestation for the normal twin. Laser treatment of the twin-to-twin communications or cord ligation with acardiac twins can be applied to improve cardiac failure.

With **anemia**, it is possible to transfuse the fetus via the umbilical vein. The diagnosis of fetal anemia can be made using the middle cerebral artery peak velocity.[46] With anemia, the cardiac output is increased with a reduced oxygen carrying capacity. When there is cardiomegaly (see earlier for criteria), it is rational to use transplacental treatment of the fetus to support the

---

*Brain sparing is defined as an increase in the diastolic velocity in the middle cerebral artery for gestational age.

myocardium if the pregnancy will be continuing for enough time to get medication to therapeutic levels. Digoxin has been used in such circumstances because of its antiadrenergic benefits and the significant experience that has been gained about its safety in pregnancy. We use digoxin (Lanoxicaps), 0.2 mg orally two to four times per day based on maternal serum levels. We use a trough level of 1 to 2 ng/dL to avoid any maternal side effects. In fetuses with arteriovenous fistula and heart failure, we also use digoxin to support the heart.

When congenital **valvular regurgitation** is present in a fetus, it could be useful to decrease the afterload of the fetal ventricles as is done in infants with a similar problem. Medications that reduce the afterload, such as angiotensin-converting enzyme inhibitors, are known to be dangerous to the fetus, however. Reduction of catecholamine levels could have a similar effect, and digoxin could be useful in this situation. When **myocardial dysfunction** is seen without obvious reasons, and fetal infection has been excluded, an inherited form of cardiomyopathy of either the left ventricle or the right ventricle may be present in utero. We use digoxin for these patients as long as there is no sign of ventricular ectopy or tachycardia.

In pregnancies in which the mother has significant levels of anti-Rho and anti-La antibodies, we recommend dexamethasone if there are signs of valvular regurgitation, heart block, valvulitis, myocardial dysfunction, myocardial echogenicity, or effusion. Early use of this medication may prevent progression of heart block and myocardial injury.

Several postnatal forms of **congenital heart disease** may lead to fetal congestive heart failure or irreversible secondary damage to the fetal heart and lungs (e.g., right heart obstructive lesions such as tricuspid atresia, critical pulmonary stenosis or pulmonary atresia with intact ventricular septum with restrictive interatrial shunting, severe atrioventricular valve insufficiency, or premature constriction or occlusion of the foramen ovale associated with left heart obstructions). It was speculated that correcting or improving these anatomic problems in utero could prevent heart failure or fatal secondary damage or both.

The first intracardiac fetal interventions were reported in 1991.[47] Two fetuses with critical valvular aortic stenosis underwent an attempt in utero at percutaneous valvuloplasty with the goal to prevent irreversible myocardial damage of the left ventricle. In one of these fetuses, the aortic valve could be dilated successfully, but the fetus died postnatally as a result of persistent left ventricular dysfunction. Because of enormous technical difficulties and poor results (of 12 human fetuses, only 1 remained alive) and with increasingly better results for stage 1 Norwood palliation, this method was abandoned for several years.[48] More recently, this method has been used successfully again for fetuses with pulmonary atresia with an intact septum and signs of heart failure.[49] In these fetuses, relief of right ventricular outflow obstruction led to improvement of echocardiographic signs of heart failure. Because most fetuses with this anatomy do not develop heart failure in utero unless there is restrictive interatrial shunting or severe tricuspid regurgitation, this method should be limited to only a small subset. Whether prenatal decompression of small hypertensive right ventricles is able to establish growth, prevent coronary artery fistulas, and improve the chances of a biventricular repair postnatally has yet to be determined. It also remains unclear whether early dilation of critical stenotic aortic valves can prevent the development of hypoplastic left heart syndrome.

There is evidence that an intact atrial septum in hypoplastic left heart syndrome leads to morphologic changes of the pulmonary vasculature and pulmonary lymphangiectasia.[10] Creating an atrial communication and decompressing the left atrium should enable normal pulmonary venous drainage and prevent further damage to pulmonary vessels and parenchyma; this could become an additional goal for cardiac interventions.

To date, many technical problems regarding equipment, imaging, and access have not yet been solved in fetal intervention. Clinical indications for therapy have yet to be defined, and there is still a need for more natural history studies regarding in utero progression of congenital heart disease and congestive heart failure.

CURRENT STATUS AND FUTURE TRENDS

Fetal cardiac findings must be integrated into the clinical management of the fetus by the perinatologist. The cardiovascular profile score can be used to communicate between visits and between specialists to assess the urgency of abnormalities and the prognosis. Serial studies using the cardiovascular profile score are necessary to obtain the value from this test. With the cardiovascular profile score, uniform treatment strategies can be planned.[50]

Focused centers of excellence in fetal cardiac assessment are needed to investigate and achieve effective fetal treatment. Fetal diagnosis is impossible, however, unless ultrasound screening detects abnormalities during otherwise normal gestations. Each center of excellence in perinatal cardiology must accept the responsibility of education in the surrounding region. Good communication between heart screening sites and perinatal cardiology centers benefits all involved and allows progress to occur in this new field of cardiology, especially in the assessment and treatment of fetal heart failure.[51-53]

Key Concepts
■ The presence of three shunts (ductus venosus, foramen ovale, and ductus arteriosus) allows the fetal heart to work with two parallel circulations rather than one series circulation.
■ An increase in the stretch of the ventricular chamber results in an increased contractility and stroke volume

according to the Frank-Starling mechanism; this mechanism is now known to be present by 8 weeks gestation in the human fetus.

■ Because the pulmonary and systemic circulations are separate in the fetus, each ventricle has a stroke volume determined by the individual preload, afterload, and contractility of that chamber.

■ The unique feature of the parallel nature of the ventricular ejection is that if there is increased afterload of one ventricle, the output of that ventricle decreases, and the output of the contralateral ventricle increases in a compensatory manner.

■ Myocardial contractility comparisons between fetal and adult animals have shown that the fetal myocardium develops less active tension than the adult at similar muscle lengths. Structural differences, such as fewer T tubules and less organized myofibrils, are observed, but there are also differences in calcium uptake into the sarcoplasmic reticulum.

■ The major determinant of cardiac output is the afterload of the fetal ventricle. Any influence that increases the impedance to ejection inversely lowers the ventricular stroke volume by the effect on the systolic and diastolic functions of the heart

■ The reduced ability of the fetal heart to contract and to generate force, the lower myocardial compliance and the diminished Frank-Starling mechanism, the higher dependence of cardiac output on heart rate, and the lack of adrenoceptors all contribute to decreased cardiac reserve in response to stress and to a higher susceptibility of the fetus for the development of cardiac failure.

■ The most useful predictor of perinatal death in fetal hydrops is the presence of umbilical venous pulsations.

■ Most attention has been paid to the right ventricular function in the human fetus because this ventricle is most likely to show an abnormality during clinical situations associated with increased workload.

■ When the volume of blood pumped by a ventricle is reduced, the overall size of the ventricle becomes smaller than the contralateral side as a result of redistribution of flow at the atrial level. This finding of disproportion at the ventricular level is an excellent screening marker of ventricular dysfunction or congenital defect.

■ The myocardial performance index, or Tei index, of the right ventricle does not depend on geometric assumptions of the right ventricle and can be used as an afterload-independent parameter to follow changes in fetal right ventricular function over time.

■ Any acute increase in right ventricular afterload, such as acute constriction of the ductus arteriosus, results in a small amount of tricuspid valve regurgitation within two heartbeats.

■ The most severe forms of right ventricular diastolic dysfunction are manifested by the finding of monophasic inflow velocity.

■ Early signs of mild tricuspid regurgitation should signal an increase in fetal surveillance; subsequent development of mitral regurgitation is ominous and is a clear sign of a prehydropic state.

■ The cardiovascular profile score gives a semiquantitative score of the fetal cardiac well-being and uses known markers by ultrasound that have been correlated with poor fetal outcome. This profile is normal if the score is 10; signs of cardiac abnormalities result in a decrease of the score from 10.

■ Alterations in central venous blood velocity patterns accurately reflect abnormalities in cardiac hemodynamics. The abnormal pulsatility pattern of increased velocity of blood flow reversal away from the heart during atrial contraction has been reported in the fetus with congestive heart failure and may be a sign of increased end-diastolic pressure in the failing ventricles.

■ The most common cardiac chamber to express enlargement as a sign of impending cardiac failure is the right atrium. The reasons for this relate to the many causes for heart failure, but the right atrium is a final pathway for blood flow returning to the heart and manifests enlargement in situations of relative foramen obstruction, volume overload, tricuspid valve regurgitation, and increased afterload.

■ It is well established that the blood velocities measured by Doppler echocardiography in the umbilical artery and in other peripheral vascular beds can be used as an indirect indicator of the relative vascular impedances. An increased pulsatility index in the umbilical artery and descending aorta and a decreased index in the middle cerebral artery are noninvasive signs of redistribution of flow.

■ Treatment of fetal cardiovascular problems can be classified into five subgroups based on the etiology of congestive heart failure: (1) abnormal peripheral impedances causing redistribution of flow and growth failure, (2) high output resulting from anemia or arteriovenous fistula, (3) primary or secondary valvular regurgitation, (4) heart failure secondary to myocardial dysfunction, and (5) tachycardia and bradycardia.

REFERENCES

1. Manning FA Harman CR, Morrison I, et al: Fetal assessment based on fetal biophysical profile scoring. Am J Obstet Gynecol 1990; 162:703-709.
2. Fineman JR, Soifer SJ: The fetal and neonatal circulations. In Chang AC, Hanley FL, Wernovsky G, et al (eds): Pediatric Cardiac Intensive Care. Philadelphia, Lippincott Williams & Wilkins, pp. 17-24, 1998.
3. Rudolph AM: Distribution and regulation of blood flow in the fetal and neonatal lamb. Circ Res 1985;57:811-821.
4. Anderson PAW: Myocardial development. In Long W (ed): Fetal and Neonatal Cardiology. Philadelphia, WB Saunders, 1990, pp 17-38.
5. Friedman WF: The intrinsic properties of the developing heart. Prog Cardiovasc Dis 1972;15:87-111.

6. Thornburg KL, Morton MJ: Filling and arterial pressures as determinants of RV stroke volume in the sheep fetus. Am J Physiol 1983;244:H656-H663.

7. Rudolph AM, Heyman MA: Cardiac output in the fetal lamb: The effects of spontaneous and induced changes of heart rate on right and left ventricular output. Am J Obstet Gynecol 1976;124:183-192.

8. Johnson P, Sharland G, Allan LD, et al: Umbilical venous pressure in nonimmune hydrops fetalis: Correlation with cardiac size. Am J Obstet Gynecol 1992;167:1309-1313.

9. Rudolph AM: Congenital Diseases of the Heart: Clinical-Physiological Considerations. Armonk, NY, Futura, 2001.

10. Rychik J, Rome JJ, Collins MH, et al: The hypoplastic left heart syndrome with intact atrial septum: Atrial morphology, pulmonary vascular histopathology and outcome. J Am Coll Cardiol 1999;34:554-560.

11. Gudmundsson S, Huhta JC, Wood DC, et al: Venous Doppler ultrasonography in the fetus with non-immune hydrops. Am J Obstet Gynecol 1991;164:33-37.

12. Huhta JC: What is perinatal cardiology? (Editorial). Ultrasound Obstet Gynecol 1995;5:145-147.

13. Makikallio K, Vuolteenaho O, Jouppila P, Rasanen J: Association of severe placental insufficiency and systemic venous pressure rise in the fetus with increased neonatal cardiac troponin T levels. Am J Obstet Gynecol 2000;183:726-731.

14. Rasanen J, Huhta JC: Echocardiography in intrauterine growth restriction. In Divon MY (ed): Clinical Obstetrics and Gynecology. Philadelphia, Lippincott-Raven, 1997, pp 814-823.

15. Veille JC, Smith N, Zaccaro D: Ventricular filling patterns of the right and left ventricles in normally grown fetuses: A longitudinal follow-up study from early intrauterine life to age 1 year. Am J Obstet Gynecol 1999;180:849-858.

16. Thornburg KL, Reller MD: Coronary flow regulation in the fetal sheep. Am J Physiol 1999;277:R1249-R1260.

17. Tulzer G, Khowsathit P, Gudmundsson S, et al: Diastolic function of the fetal heart during second and third trimester: A prospective longitudinal Doppler-echocardiographic study. Eur J Pediatri 1994;153:151-154.

18. Harada K, Rice MJ, Shiota T, et al: Gestational age- and growth-related alterations in fetal right and left ventricular diastolic filling patterns. Am J Cardiol 1997;79:173-177.

19. Rasanen J, Wood DC, Weiner S, et al: Role of the pulmonary circulation in the distribution of human fetal cardiac output during the second half of pregnancy. Circulation 1996;94:1068-1073.

20. Rasanen J, Wood DC, Debbs RH, et al: Reactivity of the human fetal pulmonary circulation to maternal hyperoxygenation increases during the second half of pregnancy: A randomized study. Circulation 1998;97:257-262.

21. Tulzer G, Gudmundsson S, Rotondo KM, et al: Acute fetal ductal occlusion in lambs. Am J Obstet Gynecol 1991;165:775-778.

22. Respondek M, Kammermeier M, Ludomirsky A, et al: The prevalence and clinical significance of fetal tricuspid valve regurgitation with normal heart anatomy. Am J Obstet Gynecol 1994;171:1265-1270.

23. Tulzer G, Gudmundsson S, Rotondo KM, et al: Doppler in the evaluation and prognosis of fetuses with tricuspid regurgitation. J Matern Fetal Invest 1991;1:15-18.

24. Sutton MS, Gill T, Plappert T, et al: Assessment of right and left ventricular function in terms of force development with gestational age in the normal human fetus. Br Heart J 1991;66:285-289.

25. Rasanen J, Debbs RH, Wood DC, et al: Human fetal right ventricular ejection force under abnormal loading conditions during the second half of pregnancy. Ultrasound Obstet Gynecol 1997;10:325-332.

26. Tulzer G, Gudmundsson S, Sharkey AM, et al: Doppler echocardiography of fetal ductus arteriosus constriction versus increased right ventricular output. J Am Coll Cardiol 1991;18:532-538.

27. Rizzo G, Capponi A, Rinaldo D, et al: Ventricular ejection force in growth-retarded fetuses. Ultrasound Obstet Gynecol 1995;5:247-255.

28. Quintero RA, Morales WJ, Allen MH, et al: Staging of twin-twin transfusion syndrome. J Perinatol 1999;19:550-555.

29. Zosmer N, Bajoria R, Weiner E, et al: Clinical and echocardiographic features of in utero cardiac dysfunction in the recipient twin in twin-twin transfusion syndrome. Br Heart J 1994;72:74-79.

30. Hofstadler G, Tulzer G, Altmann R, et al: Spontaneous closure of the human fetal ductus arteriosus: A cause of fetal congestive heart failure. Am J Obstet Gynecol 1996;174:879-883.

31. Oberhoffer R, Cook AC, Lang D, et al: Correlation between echocardiographic and morphological investigations of lesions of the tricuspid valve diagnosed during fetal life. Br Heart J 1992;68:580-585.

32. Sharland GK, Chita SK, Allan LD: Tricuspid valve dysplasia or displacement in intrauterine life. J Am Coll Cardiol 1991;17:944-949.

33. Hecher K, Ville Y, Nicolaides KH: Fetal arterial Doppler studies in twin-twin transfusion syndrome. J Ultrasound Med 1995;14:101-108.

34. Reuss ML, Rudolph AM, Dae MW: Phasic blood flow patterns in the superior and inferior venae cavae and umbilical vein of fetal sheep. Am J Obstet Gynecol 1983;145:70-78.

35. Rizzo G, Arduini D, Romanini C: Inferior vena cava flow velocity waveforms in appropriate-and-small-for-gestational-age fetuses. Am J Obstet Gynecol 1992;166:1271-1280.

36. Tulzer G, Gudmundsson S, Wood DC, et al: Doppler in non-immune hydrops fetalis. Ultrasound Obstet Gynecol 1994;4:279-283.

37. Chaoui R, Bollmann R, Goldner B, et al: Fetal cardiomegaly: Echocardiographic findings and outcome in 19 cases. Fetal Diagn Ther 1994;9:92-104.

38. Respondek M, Respondek A, Huhta JC, Wilczynski J: 2D echocardiographic assessment of the fetal heart size in the 2nd and 3rd trimester of uncomplicated pregnancy. Eur J Obstet Gynecol Reprod Biol 1992;44:185-188.

39. Mahle WT Rychik J, Tian ZY, et al: Echocardiographic evaluation of the fetus with congenital cystic adenomatoid malformation. Ultrasound Obstet Gynecol 2000;16:620-624.

40. Eidem BW, Edwards JM, Cetta F: Quantitative assessment of fetal ventricular function: Establishing normal values of the myocardial performance index in the fetus. Echocardiography 2001;18:9-13.

40. Hornberger LK, Sahn DJ, Kleinman CS, et al: Tricuspid valve disease with significant tricuspid insufficiency in the fetus: Diagnosis and outcome. J Am Coll Cardiol 1991;17:167-173.

41. Stale H, Marsal K, Genner G, et al: Aortic diameter pulse waves and blood flow velocity in the small for gestational age fetus. Ultrasound Med Biol 1991;17:471-478.

42. Hecher K, Snijders R, Campbell S, Nicolaides K: Fetal venous, intracardiac, and arterial blood flow measurements in intrauterine growth retardation: Relationship with fetal blood gases. Am J Obstet Gynecol 1995;173:10-15.

43. Falkensammer CB, Huhta JC: Fetal congestive heart failure: Correlation of Tei-Index and Cardiovascular-Score. J Perinat Med 2001;29:390-398.

44. Hofstaetter C, Huhta JC: Outcome assessment in hydrops fetalis using a cardiovascular score. Abstract presented at the Society for Pediatric Research, May 2002, Baltimore.

45. Sharif DS, Huhta JC, Moise KJ, et al: Changes in fetal hemodynamics with terbutaline treatment and premature labor. J Clin Ultrasound 1990;18:85-89.

46. Detti L, Mari G: Noninvasive diagnosis of fetal anemia. Clin Obstet Gynecol 2003;46:923-930.

47. Maxwell D, Allan L, Tynan MJ: Balloon dilatation of the aortic valve in the fetus: A report of two cases. Br Heart J 1991;65:256-258.

48. Kohl T, Sharland G, Allan LD, et al: World experience of percutaneous ultrasound-guided balloon valvuloplasty in human fetuses with severe aortic valve obstruction. Am J Cardiol 2000;85:1230-1233.

49. Tulzer G, Arzt W, Franklin RC, et al: Fetal pulmonary valvuloplasty for critical pulmonary stenosis or atresia with intact septum. Lancet 2002;360:1567-1568.

50. Huhta JC: Right ventricular function in the human fetus. J Perinat Med 2001;29:381-389.

51. Huhta JC: Guidelines for the evaluation of heart failure in the fetus with or without hydrops. Pediatr Cardiol 2004;14(Suppl 1) 22-26.

52. Trines J, Hornberger LK: Evolution of congenital heart disease in utero. Pediatr Cardiol 2004;25:287-298.

53. Fayn E, Chou HA, Park D, et al: Ultrasonic biophysical measurements in the normal human fetus for optimal design of the monolithic fetal pacemaker. Am J Cardiol 2005;95:1267-1270.

C H A P T E R   2 6

Heart Failure in the Neonate

Tarun Mahajan
Anthony C. Chang

Heart failure in the neonate presents daunting challenges. First, cellular structure and signaling in the neonatal myocardium differ substantially from the more mature heart. In addition, the developmental cardiovascular anatomy and physiology of the newborn are fundamentally different from the anatomy and physiology of the older child and adult and change dramatically over the first few days and weeks of life. Lastly, pharmacokinetics of intravenous and enteral agents used to treat heart failure in the neonate differs from the mature child and adult. These variations between the neonate and the older child and the role these differences play in the recognition and treatment of heart failure in the neonate are addressed in this chapter. The developmental aspects of cardiac anatomy and physiology also are discussed in other chapters (see Section I).

FETAL AND POSTNATAL CIRCULATIONS

Understanding the circulatory changes that occur soon after birth is vital to understanding heart failure in the neonate. This section provides a brief overview of fetal circulation (a more detailed discussion can be found in Chapter 25) and explores the circulatory changes that occur after birth.

Fetal Circulation
Fetal nutritional and metabolic requirements are met via the placental circulation as it supplies the fetus with necessary nutrients and oxygen and carries wastes and metabolites away from the fetus. The fetal circulation functions, in essence, as a conduit between the umbilical vein (which brings oxygenated blood from the placenta) and the umbilical artery (which carries blood from the fetus to the placenta). Substantial flow of blood to the fetal lungs is not necessary; instead a premium is placed on delivery of blood to the placenta. This pattern of blood flow is achieved via several adaptations unique to the fetal circulation. The ductus venosus is encountered soon after blood enters the fetus via the umbilical vein, and it passes through the liver parenchyma and joins the inferior vena cava (IVC) just below the diaphragm. The ductus venosus provides an effective shunt from the umbilical vein to the IVC, bypassing the liver and allowing oxygenated blood from the placenta to travel directly to the fetal heart.

Blood entering the fetal right atrium from the vena cavae separates into two paths to send oxygen-rich blood from the ductus venosus to the brain and coronary circulations. The free edge of the atrial septum (the crista dividens) is situated just opposite the IVC. More than one half of the blood that enters the atrium from the IVC (having previously traversed the ductus venosus) crosses the foramen ovale, which provides a direct path to the left atrium. This blood leaves the left ventricle and enters the aorta, supplying oxygenated blood to the coronary arteries and cerebral vasculature. The remainder of blood entering the right atrium from the IVC and almost all of the blood entering via the superior vena cava pass through the tricuspid valve and into the right ventricle, then into the pulmonary artery. Most blood passes directly from the pulmonary artery to the aorta via the ductus arteriosus, again bypassing the lungs. Some blood ejected from the right ventricle and into the lungs does enter the pulmonary circulation, however. Rudolph[1] showed that approximately 8% of combined ventricular output enters the pulmonary circulation.

Postnatal Adaptation
At birth, the fetal circulation undergoes a series of complex changes. As the infant separates from the placenta, the umbilical-placental circulation ceases to exist. Circulation to the infant lungs must be established to provide for oxygenation and removal of carbon dioxide. A reduction in **pulmonary vascular resistance** is initiated on the first breath, with resulting increase in pulmonary arterial flow (Fig. 26-1). By 24 hours of life, mean pulmonary artery pressure has decreased to approximately one half systemic, with progressive decline to adult levels at 2 to 6 weeks. The reduction in pulmonary vascular resistance is to some extent mechanical, as the filling of the lungs with air on the first breath reduces compression of pulmonary vessels.[2,3] Additional factors that contribute to reduction in pulmonary vascular resistance are the increasing oxygen concentration of the blood[4,5] and changing concentrations of vasoactive substances, such as bradykinin,[6] endothelin, prostaglandins, and nitric oxide.

Although pulmonary vascular resistance decreases immediately after birth, systemic vascular resistance increases. As a result of these hemodynamic alterations, additional changes occur. First, left atrial pressure increases secondary to increased pulmonary blood flow

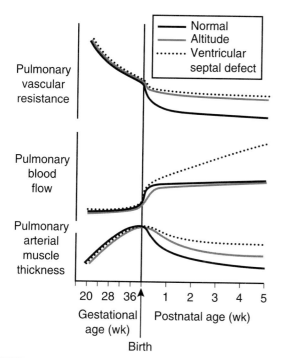

Pulmonary vascular resistance

Pulmonary blood flow

Pulmonary arterial muscle thickness

Legend:
— Normal
— Altitude
····· Ventricular septal defect

20 28 36↑ 1 2 3 4 5
Gestational age (wk) | Postnatal age (wk)

Birth

FIGURE 26-1 ■ Changes in pulmonary vascular resistance, pulmonary blood flow, and pulmonary arterial muscle thickness that occur after birth. Three curves are depicted in the graphs: normal fetus and neonate *(solid black line)*, fetus and neonate at altitude *(solid gray line)*, and fetus and neonate with a ventricular septal defect *(broken line)*. The last-mentioned curve has a different pattern of changes compared with normal. (From Heymann MA, Rudolph AM: *Effects of congenital heart disease on fetal and neonatal circulations. Prog Cardiovasc Dis* 1972;15:115-143.)

and subsequent increased pulmonary venous return to the left atrium. The septum primum apposes the crista dividens, resulting in closure of the **foramen ovale**. In the presence of elevated pulmonary vascular resistance, the foramen ovale can function as a communication that allows right-to-left shunting to decompress the right atrium. Second, the **ductus venosus** closes soon after birth. The precise mechanisms involved in the closure of the ductus venosus have not been elucidated, although it is suspected that cessation of umbilical venous return and resulting reduced flow through the ductus with contraction of a sphincter at the origin of the ductus venosus may play a role in closure.[7] Much current research involving closure of the ductus venosus centers on prostaglandins and their inhibitors. Studies on the fetal lamb have shown that administration of the prostaglandin synthesis inhibitor indomethacin induces constriction of the ductus venosus; administration of prostaglandin E_1 reversed the constriction.[8,9] Third, before birth, a right-to-left shunt occurs at the **ductus arteriosus**. After birth, as the pulmonary vascular resistance decreases, and the systemic vascular resistance increases, shunting through the ductus changes to left to right. Functional closure of the ductus arteriosus usually occurs at 12 to 15 hours,[10] although closure frequently is delayed in premature neonates.

Stimuli for postnatal duct closure include increased blood oxygen concentration[11,12] and changes in the concentrations of nitric oxide[13] and various prostaglandins.[14] Vasoactive agents, such as bradykinin[15] and norepinephrine,[16] also may play a role in the closure of the ductus arteriosus. Lastly, increased work is demanded of the left ventricle immediately after birth.

NEONATAL CARDIOVASCULAR ANATOMY AND PHYSIOLOGY

Neonatal Myocyte and Myocardium

After birth, the neonatal myocardium adjusts to circulatory changes with pressure and volume loading stimuli. The neonatal heart responds by parallel addition of myofibrils and by series addition of new sarcomeres. The neonatal heart shares with the heart of the older child and adult the ability to grow via hypertrophy. The growth demands faced by the neonatal heart are much greater, however, than the healthy adult heart. The hemodynamic alterations that occur immediately after birth require rapid increases in size and function of the left ventricle, which would be difficult to accomplish solely via physiologic hypertrophy.

The neonatal myocardium exhibits the ability to grow via hyperplasia, and this hyperplastic capability is believed to be stimulated by a stress-induced increase in the amount of fibroblast growth factors circulating within the neonate[17,18]; this capability for mitosis and rapid growth lasts 3 to 6 months[19] without returning later in life.[20] Myocyte replication[21] and hypertrophy[22] occurs at a much higher rate in the left ventricle than in the right ventricle, reflecting the greater postnatal growth needs of the left ventricle as it responds to the relatively high systemic vascular resistance.

The neonatal myocyte, in addition to possessing the ability to replicate, is structurally different from the myocyte of the adult; it is smaller, more rounded, and in general more primitive in appearance than the more mature myocyte. At an ultrastructural level, the neonatal myocyte possesses relatively few myofibrils,[23] which are disorganized and are situated at the periphery of the cell (Fig. 26-2).[24] During the postnatal period, the myofibrils grow in number and length, and widen and lengthen the myocyte. In addition, fewer mitochondria are present in the neonatal myocyte than in the mature myocyte[25]; the mitochondria that are present are disorganized, with varied shapes and sparse cristae, implying decreased aerobic capacity. T tubules, which are fundamental in the organization of muscle contraction, are not present initially in the newborn myocardium.[26] The density of contractile elements is lower in the neonatal myocyte than in the mature myocyte; animal studies have shown that 70% of neonatal myocyte is composed of noncontractile elements, whereas 30% of the adult myocyte is noncontractile.[27]

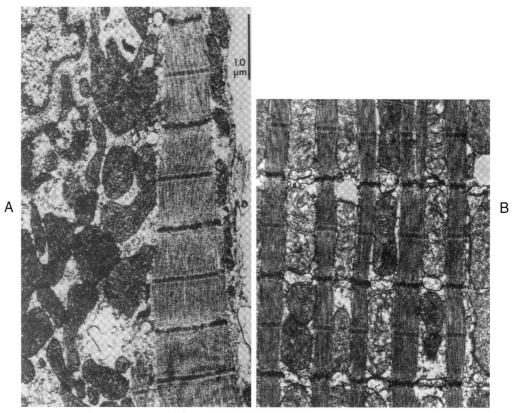

FIGURE 26-2 ■ **Electron micrograph of a longitudinal section from an isolated ventricular cell of a newborn and an adult animal. A,** A single myofibril is seen positioned adjacent to the cell surface on the right. Several mitochondria are seen in the central portion of the cell. **B,** The myofibrils and mitochondria are much better organized, forming rows of alternating myofibrils and mitochondria. (From Anderson PAW: *Myocardial development.* In Long WA [ed]: *Fetal and Neonatal Cardiology.* Philadelphia, WB Saunders, 1990, p. 18.)

Calcium handling also differs between immature and adult myocardium. Neonatal myocardium has reduced intracellular stores of calcium and a less organized sarcoplasmic reticulum compared with the adult myocardium.[28] Biochemical changes also exist between neonatal and mature myocardium; the concentrations of myosin ATPase and creatine kinase in lamb myocardium have been found to be lower in neonates than in adults.[29] The end result of the aforementioned differences between neonatal and mature myocardium is the reduced contractility of the neonatal myocardium.

During the first several months of life, the myocyte and the heart as a whole undergo a series of transformations to achieve the more mature form. Sarcomeres increase in number, density, and organization, achieving adult form by 5 months of age in the dog.[19] At the same time, mitochondria increase in number, size, and organization. During the early postnatal period, however, before these changes have taken place, the heart is different from the mature heart. As a result of the relatively decreased number, density, and organization of contractile proteins and the decreased intracardiac calcium stores, the contractility of the neonatal heart is limited. The immature myocardium is unable to generate as much tension per unit of cross-sectional area as the adult myocardium and is considerably less compliant,[30] whereas the adult myocardium consists of an intricately formed network of elongate myocytes that are connected end to end.

Neonatal Cardiac Physiology

The Frank-Starling curve of the neonatal myocardium shows a leftward shift and a decreased ascending limb compared with the adult heart, reflecting the decreased contractility and compliance of the neonatal heart.[31] On a microscopic level, maximal sarcomere length (and maximal contractility) is achieved at a lower filling volume in the neonate than in the adult.[32]

The neonatal heart functions at a relatively high **preload** (Fig. 26-3) with reduced preload volume reserve compared with the adult heart; as a result, the neonatal heart adjusts to increased volume load more poorly than does the heart of the older child[33] or adult.[34] Increasing preload above the optimal level does not improve cardiac output significantly; studies in the fetal lamb revealed that increasing filling pressures greater than 10 to 12 mm Hg resulted in little increase in stroke volume.[35] The ventricular interdependence in the neonate differs from the adult in that influence of left

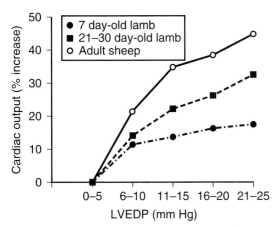

FIGURE 26-3 ■ **Response to volume loading in newborn versus adult sheep.** The response to volume loading with saline infusion is depicted in curves for a 7-day-old lamb *(solid circles)*, a 21- to 30-day old lamb *(solid squares)*, and an adult sheep *(open circles)*. The less mature animals are less able to generate additional cardiac output (y axis) at comparable left ventricular end-diastolic pressure (LVEDP) compared with the adult animal. (From Friedman WF, George BL: *Treatment of congestive heart failure by altering loading conditions of the heart. J Pediatr* 1985;106:697-704.)

ventricular pressure on right ventricular volume is evident at a pressure greater than 5 mm Hg (Fig. 26-4).

Afterload is related to numerous factors, including myocardial wall stress (σ) (defined as pressure × radius divided by twice the wall thickness, although the ellipsoidal left ventricle has two types of stresses, meridional and circumferential stresses), ejection pressure, impedance of the vasculature, and any potential mechanical outflow obstruction. In all hearts, an increase in afterload, with an unchanged preload and contractility, brings about a decrease in ventricular output. Because the neonatal myocardium has decreased contractility compared with the adult heart, the neonatal heart does not adjust as well as the adult heart to an increase in afterload. Studies examining the response of ventricular myocardium to changing afterloads revealed that neonatal myocardium shortens more slowly against the same load than adult myocardium.[36] In addition, studies examining the sarcomere shortening velocity in a single cardiac myocyte found that shortening velocities in the adult myocyte were greater than velocities in the neonatal myocyte.[37] Contractility and stroke volume in the immediate neonatal period also are constrained by extrinsic compression. Studies by Grant and colleagues[38] have shown that tissues surrounding the heart (chest wall, lungs, and pericardium) substantially increase pericardial pressure in the fetus and neonate, reducing stroke volume. On initiation of ventilation, pericardial pressure decreases, allowing for increasing left ventricular preload and stroke volume.[39]

The mature heart is able to respond to increasing afterload by increasing **contractility**, preserving cardiac output. The neonatal heart, for reasons described previously, is unable to augment contractility effectively.

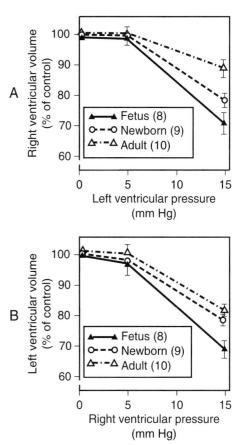

FIGURE 26-4 ■ **Ventricular interdependence in the fetus, newborn, and adult. A,** The influence of left ventricular filling on right ventricular volume in the fetus *(solid triangles)*, newborn *(open circles)*, and adult *(open triangles)*. At pressures greater than 5 mm Hg in the left ventricle, there is decrementally less right ventricular volume to 70% normal in the fetus. **B,** The influence of right ventricular filling on left ventricular volume in the fetus, newborn, and adult. Similar findings are seen in that the left ventricular volume is decreased with increasing right ventricular pressure more in the fetus than in the more mature myocardium. (From Romero T, Covell JW, Friedman WF: *A comparison of pressure volume relations of the fetal, newborn, and adult heart. Am J Physiol* 1972;222:1285-1293.)

The immature myocardium does not develop tension per unit cross-sectional area as well as the more mature myocardium (Fig. 26-5). Adjustment of cardiac output in the neonate, in response to increases in afterload, must be achieved almost exclusively via changes in heart rate. The neonatal myocardium is more sensitive to alterations in afterload than the mature myocardium and has a higher level of myocardial oxygen consumption. Judicious use of afterload reduction is an important part of neonatal heart failure management.

The neonatal myocardium is stiffer and less compliant than the more mature myocardium. The presence of specific neonatal isoforms of various structural proteins, including titin,[40,41] troponin I,[42] and myosin, may play a role in the stiffness of the neonatal myocardium. In addition, studies in fetal and neonatal hearts have revealed a mechanism for removal of calcium from troponin C specific to the neonatal heart.[43] Because the interaction

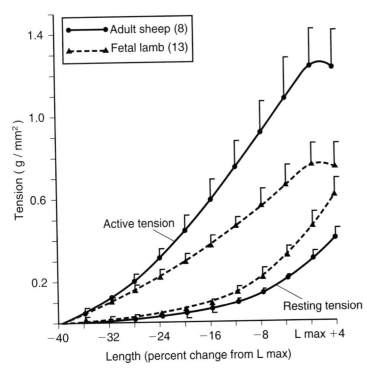

FIGURE 26-5 ■ **Isometric resting and active length-tension curves for fetal versus adult sheep.** The developed tension (y axis) and length (as % change from maximum length on the x axis) are plotted for fetal *(broken lines)* and adult *(solid lines)* sheep. The active tension generated by isometric contraction of the fetal cardiac muscle is significantly less than that of the adult myocardium. The fetal myocardium has diminished passive compliance. (From Friedman WF: *The intrinsic physiologic properties of the developing heart. Prog Cardiovasc Dis* 1973;15:87-111.)

between troponin C and calcium plays a key role in myocardial relaxation, the unique mechanism found in the neonate may play an important role in the differences in compliance between immature and mature myocardium.

Although the neonatal **coronary circulation** is adequate to accommodate the increase in work imposed on the left ventricle after birth, additional factors that often are associated with a neonate with congenital heart disease (e.g., hypoxemia, anemia, low diastolic pressure, tachycardia, and increased wall tension from volume and pressure overload) can compromise coronary oxygen

delivery and create an ischemic state. Overall, the neonatal myocardium can sustain periods of hypoxia better than the mature myocardium as a result of its capacity for anaerobic glycolysis.

Neonatal Autonomic Control of the Heart and Circulation

To understand neonatal heart failure, it is important to review briefly the autonomic control of the heart and circulation and examine the ways in which autonomic control differs between the neonatal and mature animal (Fig. 26-6). **Sympathetic innervation** begins with

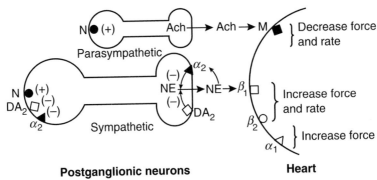

Postganglionic neurons   **Heart**

FIGURE 26-6 ■ **Sympathetic and parasympathetic innervations of the heart.** The cardiac neuroeffector junctions are depicted in this schematic representation. The sympathetic adrenergic efferent input is via norepinephrine (NE), whereas the parasympathetic cholinergic efferent input is via acetylcholine (Ach). The presynaptic autoregulatory α_2-receptors can exert a negative feedback control on NE release. Ach acts on the muscarinic receptor to decrease force and rate of contractions, but also can exert influence via inhibition of NE release from sympathetic nerves. DA, dopamine; M, muscarinic cholinergic receptor; N, nicotinic cholinergic receptor. (From Ruffolo RR, et al: *Drug, neurotransmitter and hormone receptors in the regulation of the cardiovascular system.* In Shoemaker WC, Thompson WL [eds]: Critical Care: State of the Art. Fullerton, Calif, Society of Critical Care Medicine, 1983.)

sympathetic fibers that originate from cell bodies located within the upper thoracic spinal cord. Preganglionic fibers travel from the cell bodies to bilateral paravertebral chains of ganglia, whereas longer postganglionic fibers extend from the paravertebral chains directly into the cardiac tissues. During neurotransmission, acetylcholine is released at the ganglion; interaction of acetylcholine with nicotinic cholinergic receptors on the postganglionic neuron stimulates release of norepinephrine at the neuroeffector junction. Norepinephrine then binds to β_1-receptors in the target cardiac tissue, triggering a series of conformational changes in regulatory G proteins. The conformational changes in these G proteins cause stimulation of the enzyme adenylate cyclase, which forms cAMP from ATP. The increased concentration of cAMP activates protein kinase A, an enzyme that activates numerous other regulatory proteins, affecting a variety of cardiac functions. Overall, cardiac effects of the binding of norepinephrine to the β_1-receptor include tachycardia and enhanced contractility and ventricular function (see Chapter 2).[44]

The α_1- and β_2-receptors play important roles in modifying heart rate and contractility and peripheral vascular tone; the α_2-receptor plays an important inhibitory role. Sympathetic activity induces increases in heart rate, contractility, and cardiac output, whereas **parasympathetic innervation** and action are inhibitory. Presympathetic parasympathetic nerves originate in the medulla oblongata, travel via the vagus nerves through the thorax, and synapse in the heart itself. Short postganglionic neurons synapse directly at the target tissues, where acetylcholine is released into the neuroeffector junction. Acetylcholine subsequently binds to cardiac muscarinic (M_2) receptors and causes a series of conformational changes in several regulatory proteins in a manner similar to that described for norepinephrine and the β_1-receptor. In contrast to the β_1-receptor, however, the M_2-receptor interacts with an inhibitory G protein. Stimulation of the M_2-receptor causes an inhibition of adenylate cyclase and resulting

decrease in cAMP production. In contrast to sympathetic stimulation, parasympathetic stimulation of the heart results in decreased heart rate and contractility.

Although the parasympathetic control of cardiac function in the neonate is relatively mature and is essentially similar to that in the adult, sympathetic control differs substantially between the neonate and the adult. In the more mature animal, little norepinephrine is found in preterminal nerve trunks, and most instead is found in the myocardium itself (Fig. 26-7).[45] In neonates, most norepinephrine is found in the nerve trunks because there is a relative paucity of sympathetic innervation in the neonatal myocardium. As a result, neonates depend more on circulating catecholamines for cardiocirculatory function than older children and adults.[46] Canine studies have revealed that circulating catecholamine levels in the neonate are 30 times greater than adult levels.[47] Analyses of catecholamine levels in neonates and older children have revealed that neonates have higher levels of catecholamines and neuropeptide Y, a marker of sympathetic activity, than their older counterparts.[48] Research also has revealed that neonates are not able to augment cardiac output in response to exogenous catecholamines as well as older children and adults.[49] It has been postulated that the relatively poor neonatal response to exogenous catecholamines results from the sparse sympathetic innervation in the neonatal myocardium.

As detailed elsewhere in this book, prolonged β-adrenoreceptor stimulation of the mature heart may cause receptor desensitization and down-regulation via protein kinase–mediated phosphorylation of agonist-occupied receptors. Studies have shown that children with reduced cardiac output and in heart failure have higher sympathetic tone than their normal counterparts, with resulting increases in concentrations of circulating catecholamines.[50,51] Children in heart failure have reduced numbers and densities of β-receptors compared with normal children; the reduction is seen chiefly with

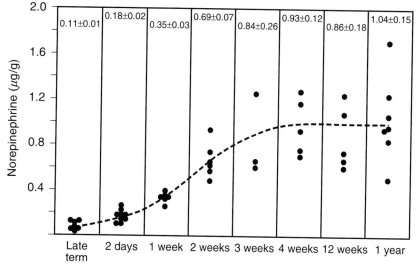

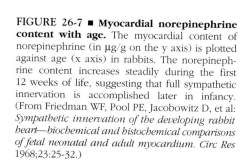

FIGURE 26-7 ■ **Myocardial norepinephrine content with age.** The myocardial content of norepinephrine (in $\mu g/g$ on the y axis) is plotted against age (x axis) in rabbits. The norepinephrine content increases steadily during the first 12 weeks of life, suggesting that full sympathetic innervation is accomplished later in infancy. (From Friedman WF, Pool PE, Jacobowitz D, et al: *Sympathetic innervation of the developing rabbit heart—biochemical and histochemical comparisons of fetal neonatal and adult myocardium. Circ Res* 1968;23:25-32.)

respect to the β_1-receptor.[52,53] In addition, studies of children in severe heart failure have revealed that adenylate cyclase may become uncoupled from adrenergic receptors in this population, reducing the effectiveness of sympathetic stimulation.[54] A study of patients with pulmonary stenosis examined the densities of adrenoreceptors before and after balloon valvuloplasty of the pulmonary valve. Before valvuloplasty, the children with pulmonary stenosis had 23% fewer β-receptors than the control group, a statistically significant difference. Within 10 minutes after valvuloplasty, the difference in β-receptor density had essentially resolved, however.[55] Lastly, chronic hypoxia has been shown to cause receptor desensitization.[56] The reduction in number and function of adrenergic receptors in children in heart failure contribute to the difficulty in treating these children with catecholamines.

This attenuation of adrenergic response is believed to be an important mechanism in the maintenance of cellular homeostasis.[57] In studies involving mammalian neonates of several species, however, this receptor desensitization has not been seen. Long-term β-agonist therapy in neonatal mammals has been shown to enhance, and not desensitize, adrenergic response.[58] This enhancement of function, unique to the neonate, is believed to occur via an increase in adenylate cyclase activity after β-receptor stimulation,[59] which is believed to occur through alterations in G protein activity.[60] It has been hypothesized that the absence of desensitization in the neonate may serve as a useful mechanism in the period during and immediately after birth, when surges in adrenergic activity are seen, and maintenance of β-receptor activity is required for proper adaptation to the postnatal environment.[61]

The sympathetic innervation of the vasculature is also less abundant in the neonate compared with the adult, providing an explanation for the vascular instability observed in neonates. Neurogenic control of the vasculature via the neuroeffector junction is not discussed in detail here.

ETIOLOGY AND PRESENTATION OF HEART FAILURE IN THE NEONATE

Heart failure presenting at birth is relatively rare and usually presents as hydrops fetalis; studies indicate that 26% of all cases of hydrops fetalis are associated with cardiac causes.[62] Heart failure presenting at birth (Table 26-1) can result from structural lesions that cause right atrial overload (pressure or volume), such as tricuspid atresia, pulmonary atresia, or Ebstein anomaly; tachyarrhythmias; tumors; myocarditis; and idiopathic calcification of coronary arteries. Cardiac lesions that cause heart failure on the first day of life include hypoplastic left heart syndrome, obstructed total anomalous pulmonary venous return (typically subdiaphragmatic), and severe tricuspid or pulmonary regurgitation (see also Chapter 14).

TABLE 26-1

Etiologies for Heart Failure in the Neonate
Cardiac Disease
Volume Overload
Tricuspid regurgitation
Arteriovenous fistula
Patent ductus arteriosus
Ventricular septal defect
Common atrioventricular canal
Truncus arteriosus
Pressure Overload
Aortic stenosis
Coarctation of the aorta
Interruption of the aortic arch
Systemic hypertension
Single-Ventricle Lesions with Excessive Pulmonary Blood Flow
Hypoplastic left heart syndrome
Tricuspid atresia
Miscellaneous
Myocarditis or cardiomyopathy
Supraventricular tachycardia
Complete heart block
Cardiac tumors
Idiopathic calcinosis of coronary arteries
Noncardiac Disease
Metabolic
Hypoxia
Hypoglycemia
Hypocalcemia and other electrolyte abnormalities
Miscellaneous
Anemia or polycythemia
Sepsis

Heart failure presenting at age 1 to 3 days typically results from left-sided obstructive lesions, including critical aortic stenosis, interrupted aortic arch, and severe aortic coarctation. Left-to-right shunts in which the blood is shunted into low-resistance areas, such as arteriovenous malformation and patent ductus arteriosus, frequently cause heart failure during the first week of life, especially in premature neonates. Left-to-right shunts (e.g., patent ductus arteriosus in a term infant, ventricular septal defect) produce heart failure in weeks 2 to 4 of life, unless the pulmonary vascular resistance is low earlier in life as observed with premature neonates. There are also instances in which neonates who had palliative surgeries in the first week of life develop heart failure in the ensuing weeks, such as a neonate with hypoplastic left heart syndrome after the Norwood palliative operation with significant right ventricular dysfunction with or without significant tricuspid regurgitation.

Noncardiac conditions may cause heart failure during the neonatal period. Conditions that reduce preload, such as hemorrhage and sepsis, reduce cardiac output by reducing stretch of ventricular fibers, via the Frank-Starling mechanism. Increased afterload, as is seen in systemic hypertension and severe polycythemia, also reduces cardiac output. Conditions that impair delivery of nutrients and oxygen to the myocardium, such as anemia, hypoxia, and hypoglycemia, impair contractility and cardiac output. Lastly, derangements in pH, sodium, calcium, and magnesium directly affect myocardial contractility and can cause heart failure. Clinical assessment of heart failure in the neonate and potential etiologies for heart failure are described in much more detail in Chapter 14.

TREATMENT OF NEONATAL HEART FAILURE

Therapies of heart failure in children and young adults are discussed extensively in Chapters 32 through 37. A few special considerations of the hemodynamic and pharmacokinetic differences between the neonate and older child and the implications that these differences may have on treatment are discussed here.

Digoxin and diuretics have long been mainstays of heart failure in children and adults. **Digoxin** is a cardiac glycoside that acts via inhibition of the Na^+, K^+-ATPase pump and is theoretically an inotropic agent. Studies examining the use of digoxin in neonates and infants in heart failure have produced conflicting results, however. A study of 21 infants with congestive heart failure secondary to ventricular septal defect found that only 6 of the 21 patients had an inotropic response to digoxin as measured by echocardiogram.[63] Another study examining 41 infants with congestive heart failure secondary to ventricular septal defect showed that infants with relatively low baseline systemic or pulmonary vascular resistance showed a favorable hemodynamic response to digoxin; however, patients with high baseline systemic or pulmonary vascular resistance experienced increases in left atrial pressure and pulmonary blood flow after digoxin administration.[64] The role of digoxin in the management of heart failure in neonates is unclear. **Diuretics** also have been a mainstay of the treatment of heart failure in neonates and children and remain particularly useful in patients with systemic or pulmonary vascular congestion. Diuretics may cause undesired neurohormonal activation, however, and worsen the condition in patients who have heart failure that is not due to vascular congestion.[65] Loop diuretics, the most commonly used group of diuretics, produce a relatively blunted response in neonates secondary to immaturity of renal secretory mechanisms.

Catecholamines, such as norepinephrine, dopamine, and dobutamine, traditionally have been used as pressors in the setting of acute decompensated congestive heart failure. These pharmacologic agents work via stimulation of β-receptors, with subsequent increases in cAMP and cardiac contractility. It is well recognized that catecholamines increase myocardial oxygen consumption, heart rate, afterload, and risk of arrhythmia.[66] Because neonates have a relatively high baseline level of sympathetic neurohormonal activity, the neonatal myocardium is overall less responsive to exogenous catecholamines than the myocardium in older children.[67] In addition, the rate of catecholamine clearance seems to differ between the neonate and the more mature child.[68,69] Another consideration is that the neonate has a larger volume of distribution for water-soluble drugs than the older child.[70-72] The differences in clearance and volume of distribution play a role in the decreased efficacy of catecholamines in the neonate. Additional studies have shown that neonates require a greater plasma concentration of exogenous catecholamine to affect the same increase in cardiac output and blood pressure as achieved in older children.[73-75] This phenomenon indicates that the receptor structure and response, not simply clearance and volume of distribution, differ between the neonate and the older child.

The difficulties experienced in treating neonatal heart failure with current medications have led to research into new medications. The efficacy of β-**blockers** in heart failure may seem counterintuitive in children because heart failure treatment traditionally has centered on reducing afterload and augmenting contractility. It is hypothesized that even in neonates and children, β blockade attenuates the activation of the neurohormonal system that occurs in heart failure. β-Blockers first were investigated for use in the treatment of heart failure in adults in the mid-1970s,[76] and studies since have shown improved hemodynamic status in adults who have received β-blockers for congestive heart failure.[77,78] More recent studies in children with congestive heart failure, including neonates, have produced similar results. A retrospective study of infants in severe congestive heart failure secondary to left-to-right shunt and refractory to digoxin and diuretics found that treatment with metoprolol improved symptoms of heart failure and reduced activation of the neurohormonal system.[79] Another study specifically examining infants in heart failure secondary to left-to-right shunt found that infants who received propranolol in addition to diuretics and digoxin had greater hemodynamic improvement than their counterparts who were treated with diuretics and digoxin alone.[80] Lastly, carvedilol is a nonselective β-receptor antagonist and an α_1-receptor antagonist and possesses vasodilatory activity in addition to the β-blocking activity of the other medications. A preliminary multicenter study has shown that when added to digoxin and diuretics, carvedilol improves symptoms and ventricular function in children with heart failure secondary to a variety of etiologies.[81] A long-term prospective multicenter study is under way to assess better carvedilol as a treatment for heart failure in children.[82] Trials examining the use of carvedilol in neonates are forthcoming in the future.

Angiotensin-converting enzyme (ACE) inhibitors act via inhibition of the conversion of angiotensin I to angiotensin II, a potent vasoconstrictor, and act to prevent the degradation of bradykinin, a vasodilator. ACE inhibitors improve cardiac output by reducing systemic vascular resistance. Several studies have shown improvements in hemodynamic status and heart failure symptoms after the addition of captopril to the treatment regimens of infants in heart failure[83-85]; studies with enalapril have shown similar results.[86,87] A study comparing low-dose captopril with propranolol in infants with severe congestive heart failure resulting from left-to-right shunts found, however, that infants who had received propranolol had improved heart failure scores, decreased plasma renin levels, and improved hemodynamics compared with children who had received captopril.[88] Because of decreased glomerular filtration in the neonate, ACE inhibitors should be used with caution and with lowered dosages on initiation of therapy.

The **phosphodiesterase inhibitors** amrinone and milrinone work in a manner similar to catecholamines in that they increase contractility via an activation of adenylate cyclase with subsequent increase in cAMP. In contrast to catecholamines, phosphodiesterase inhibitors do not interact with β-receptors and do not cause the tachycardia, increased myocardial oxygen consumption, and increased afterload seen with catecholamines. Instead, phosphodiesterase inhibitors inhibit the enzyme phosphodiesterase III, inhibiting the degradation of cAMP. In addition to increasing myocardial contractility, the phosphodiesterase inhibitors produce vasodilatory (in the systemic and pulmonary vascular beds) and lusitropic effects, which make them theoretically ideal for management of heart failure in the postoperative neonate with low cardiac output syndrome and heart failure. Multiple studies[89,90] have shown the positive hemodynamic effects of phosphodiesterase inhibitors on neonates in the intensive care setting; these effects include increased cardiac index, reduced atrial pressures, reduced pulmonary and systemic vascular resistances, and decreased left ventricular end-systolic wall stress. A multicenter prospective study (PRIMACORPS) found that prophylactic milrinone given to neonates immediately after congenital heart surgery reduced the risk of low cardiac output syndrome.[91]

CURRENT STATUS AND FUTURE TRENDS

Heart failure in neonates requires special understanding of the myriad of anatomic and physiologic differences between neonates and adults. There is currently a paucity of information on the pathophysiologic and therapeutic aspects of heart failure in newborns. Advances in medical therapy for heart failure, including increasing use of β-blockers, ACE inhibitors, phosphodiesterase inhibitors, and the calcium-sensitizing agent levosimendan,[92] will continue to improve the outcomes of neonates in congestive heart failure. Future directions in basic science and clinical research need to focus on the special characteristics of heart failure in the neonate and insight into special therapeutic needs of the failing neonatal myocardium.[93,94]

Key Concepts

▣ The reduction in pulmonary vascular resistance is to some extent mechanical, as the filling of the lungs with air on the first breath reduces compression of pulmonary vessels. Additional factors that contribute to reduction in pulmonary vascular resistance are the increasing oxygen concentration of the blood and changing concentrations of vasoactive substances, such as bradykinin, endothelin, prostaglandins, and nitric oxide.

▣ The neonatal myocardium exhibits the ability to grow via hyperplasia, and this hyperplastic capability is believed to be stimulated by a stress-induced increase in the amount of fibroblast growth factors circulating within the neonate.

▣ The density of contractile elements is lower in the neonatal myocyte than in the mature myocyte; animal studies have shown that 70% of neonatal myocyte is composed of noncontractile elements, whereas 30% of the adult myocyte is noncontractile.

▣ Calcium handling also differs between immature and adult myocardium. Neonatal myocardium has reduced intracellular stores of calcium and a less organized sarcoplasmic reticulum compared with the adult myocardium.

▣ The Frank-Starling curve of the neonatal myocardium shows a leftward shift and a decreased ascending limb compared with the adult heart, reflecting the decreased contractility and compliance of the neonatal heart.

▣ The neonatal heart functions at a relatively high preload, with reduced preload volume reserve compared with the adult; as a result, the neonatal heart adjusts to increased volume load more poorly than does the heart of the older child or adult.

▣ Because the neonatal myocardium has decreased contractility compared with the adult heart, the neonatal heart does not adjust as well as the adult heart to an increase in afterload.

▣ Adjustment of cardiac output in the neonate, in response to increases in afterload, must be achieved almost exclusively via changes in heart rate.

▣ Although the neonatal coronary circulation is adequate to accommodate the increase in work imposed on the left ventricle after birth, additional factors that often are associated with the neonate with congenital heart disease (e.g., hypoxemia, anemia, low diastolic pressure, tachycardia, and increased wall tension from volume and pressure overload) can compromise coronary oxygen delivery and create an ischemic state.

■ Although the parasympathetic control of cardiac function in the neonate is relatively mature and is essentially similar to that in the adult, sympathetic control differs substantially between the neonate and the adult.

■ In the more mature animal, little norepinephrine is found in preterminal nerve trunks, and most instead is found in the myocardium itself. In neonates, however, most norepinephrine is found in the nerve trunks because there is a relative paucity of sympathetic innervation in the neonatal myocardium. As a result, neonates depend more on circulating catecholamines for cardiocirculatory function than older children and adults.

■ It has been hypothesized that the absence of desensitization in the neonate may serve as a useful mechanism in the period during and immediately after birth, when surges in adrenergic activity are seen, and maintenance of β-receptor activity is required for proper adaptation to the postnatal environment.

REFERENCES

1. Rudolph AM: Distribution and regulation of blood flow in the fetal and neonatal lamb. Circ Res 1985;57:811-821.
2. Teitel DF, Iwamoto HS, Rudolph AM: Changes in the pulmonary circulation during birth-related events. Pediatr Res 1990;27:372-378.
3. Teitel DF, Iwamotot HS, Rudolph AM: Effects of birth-related events on central blood flow patterns. Pediatr Res 1987;22:557-566.
4. Cook CD, Drinker PA, Jacobson HN, et al: Control of pulmonary blood flow in the foetal and newly born lamb. J Physiol 1963;169:10-29.
5. Lauer RM, Evans JA, Aoki M, Kittle CF: Factors controlling pulmonary vascular resistance in fetal lambs. J Pediatr 1965;67:568-577.
6. Campbell AGM, Dawes GS, Fishman AP, et al: The release of bradykinin-like pulmonary vasodilator substance in foetal and newborn lambs. J Physiol 1968;195:83-96.
7. Meyer WW, Lind J: The ductus venosus and the mechanism of its closure. Arch Dis Child 1966;41:597-605.
8. Morin FC: Prostaglandin E1 opens the ductus venosus in the newborn lamb. Pediatr Res 1987;21:225-228.
9. Adeagbo AS, Coceani F, Olley PM: The response of the lamb ductus venosus to prostaglandins and inhibitors of prostaglandin and thromboxane synthesis. Circ Res 1982;51:580-586.
10. Moss AJ, Emmanouilides GC, Duffie ER Jr: Closure of the ductus arteriosus in the newborn infant. Pediatrics 1963;32:25-30.
11. Clyman RI, Mauray F, Wong L, et al: The developmental response of the ductus arteriosus to oxygen. Biol Neonate 1978;34:177-181.
12. Oberhansli-Weiss I, Heymann MA, Rudolph AM, Melmon KL: The pattern and mechanisms of response to oxygen by the ductus arteriosus and umbilical artery. Pediatr Res 1972;6:693-700.
13. Clyman RI, Waleh N, Black SM, et al: Regulation of ductus arteriosus patency by nitric oxide in fetal lambs: The role of gestation, oxygen tension, and vasa vasorum. Pediatr Res 1998;43:633-644.
14. Friedman WF, Printz MP, Kirkpatrick SE, Hoskins EJ: The vasoactivity of the fetal lamb ductus arteriosus studied in utero. Pediatr Res 1983;17:331-337.
15. Bateson EA, Schulz R, Olley PM: Response of fetal rabbit ductus arteriosus to bradykinin: Role of nitric oxide, prostaglandins, and bradykinin receptors. Pediatr Res 1999;45:568-574.
16. Smith GC, McGrath JC: Interactions between indomethacin, noradrenaline and vasodilators in the fetal rabbit ductus arteriosus. Br J Pharmacol 1994;111:1245-1251.
17. Engelmann GL, Dionne CA, Jaye MC: Acidic fibroblast growth factor and heart development: Role in myocyte proliferation and capillary angiogenesis. Circ Res 1993;72:7-19.
18. Schneider MD, Kirshenbaum LA, Brand T, MacLellan WR: Control of cardiac gene transcription by fibroblast growth factors. Mol Reprod Dev 1994;39:112-117.
19. Zak R: Development and proliferative capacity of cardiac muscle cells. Circ Res 1974;35(Suppl II):17-26.
20. Zak R, Kizu A, Bugaisky L: Cardiac hypertrophy: Its characteristic as a growth process. Am J Cardiol 1979;44:941-946.
21. Anversa P, Olivetti G, Loud AV: Morphometric study of early postnatal development in the left and right ventricular myocardium of the rat. Circ Res 1980;46:495-512.
22. Legato MJ: Cellular mechanisms of normal growth in the mammalian heart: II. A quantitative and qualitative comparison between the right and left ventricular myocytes in the dog from birth to five months of age. Circ Res 1979;44:263-279.
23. Claycomb WC: DNA synthesis and DNA enzymes in terminally differentiating cardiac muscle cells. Exp Cell Res 1979;118:111-114.
24. Legato MJ: Cellular mechanisms of normal growth in the mammalian heart: I. Qualitative and quantitative features of ventricular architecture in the dog from birth to five months of age. Circ Res 1979;44:250-262.
25. Sheldon CA, Friedman WF, Sybers HD: Scanning electron microscopy of fetal and neonatal lamb cardiac cells. J Mol Cell Cardiol 1976;8:853-862.
26. Sommer JR: Ultrastructural considerations considering cardiac muscle. J Mol Cell Cardiol 1982;14(Suppl 3):77-83.
27. Marijianowski MH, Van Der Loos CM, Mohrschladt MF, Becker AE: The neonatal heart has a relatively high content of total collagen and Type I collagen, a condition that may explain the less compliant state. J Am Coll Cardiol 1994;23:1204.
28. Mahony L, Jones LR: Developmental changes in cardiac sarcoplasmic reticulum in sheep. J Biol Chem 1986;261:15257-15265.
29. Ingwall JS, Kramer MF, Woodman D, Friedman WF: Maturation of energy metabolism in the lamb: Changes in myosin ATPase and creatine kinase activities. Pediatr Res 1981;15:1128-1133.
30. Downing SE, Talner N, Gardner TH: Ventricular function in the newborn lamb. Am J Physiol 1965;208:931-937.
31. Thornburg KL, Morton MJ: Filling and arterial pressure as determinants of stroke volume in the sheep fetus. Am J Physiol 1983;244:H656-H663.
32. Spotnitz WD, Spotnitz HM, Truccone NJ, et al: Relation of ultrastructure and function: Sarcomere dimensions, pressure-volume curves, and geometry of the intact left ventricle of the immature canine heart. Circ Res 1979;44:679-691.
33. Klopfenstein HS, Rudolph AM: Postnatal changes in the circulation and responses to volume loading in sheep. Circ Res 1978;42:839-845.
34. Romero TE, Friedman WF: Limited left ventricular response to volume overload in the neonatal period: A comparative study with the adult animal. Pediatr Res 1979;13:910-915.
35. Kirkpatrick SE, Pitlick PT, Naliboff J, Friedman WF: Frank-Starling relationship as an important determinant of fetal cardiac output. Am J Physiol 1976;231:495-500.
36. Friedman WF: The intrinsic physiologic properties of the developing heart. Prog Cardiovasc Dis 1972;15:87-111.
37. Nassar R, Reedy MC, Anderson PAW: Developmental changes in the ultrastructure and sarcomere shortening of the isolated rabbit ventricular myocyte. Circ Res 1987;61:475-483.

38. Grant DA, Maloney JE, Tyberg JV, Walker AM: Effects of external constraint on the fetal left ventricular function curve. Am Heart J 1992;123:1601-1609.

39. Grant DA, Kondo CS, Maloney JE, et al: Changes in pericardial pressure during the perinatal period. Circulation 1992;86:1615-1621.

40. Lahmers S, Wu Y, Call DR, et al: Developmental control of titin isoform expression and passive stiffness in fetal and neonatal myocardium. Circ Res 2004;94:505-513.

41. Opitz CA, Leake MC, Makarenko I, et al: Developmentally regulated switching of titin size alters myofibrillar stiffness in the perinatal heart. Circ Res 2004;94:967-975.

42. Hunkeler NM, Kullman J, Murphy AM: Troponin I isoform expression in human heart. Circ Res 1991;69:1409-1414.

43. Mahony L: Calcium homeostasis and control of contractility in the developing heart. Semin Perinatol 1996;20:510-519.

44. Sarnoff SJ, Gilmore JP, Brockman SK, et al: Regulation of ventricular contraction by the carotid sinus: Its effect on atrial and ventricular dynamics. Circ Res 1960;8:1123-1136.

45. Friedman WF, Pool PE, Jacobowitz D, et al: Sympathetic innervation of the developing rabbit heart: Biochemical and histochemical comparisons of fetal, neonatal, and adult myocardium. Circ Res 1968;23:25-32.

46. Erath HG Jr, Boerth RC, Graham TP Jr: Functional significance of reduced cardiac sympathetic innervation in the newborn dog. Am J Physiol 1982;243:H20-H26.

47. Geis WP, Tatooles CJ, Priola DV, Friedman WF: Factors influencing neurohormonal control of the heart in the newborn dog. Am J Physiol 1975;228:1685-1689.

48. Candito M, Albertini M, Politano S, et al: Plasma catecholamine levels in children. J Chromatogr 1993;617:304-307.

49. Teitel DF, Sidi D, Chin T, et al: Developmental changes in myocardial contractile reserve in the lamb. Pediatr Res 1985;19:948-955.

50. Sun LS, Du F, Schechter WS, et al: Plasma neuropeptide Y and catecholamines in pediatric patients undergoing cardiac operations. J Thorac Cardiovasc Surg 1997;113:278-284.

51. Dzimiri N, Galal O, Moorji A, et al: Regulation of sympathetic activity in children with various congenital heart diseases. Pediatr Res 1995;38:55-60.

52. Wu JR, Chang HR, Huang TY, et al: Reduction in lymphocyte beta-adrenergic receptor density in infants and children with heart failure secondary to congenital heart disease. Am J Cardiol 1996;77:170-174.

53. Kozlik-Feldmann R, Kramer HH, Wicht H, et al: Distribution of myocardial beta-adrenoceptor subtypes and coupling to the adenylate cyclase in children with congenital heart disease and implications for treatment. J Clin Pharmacol 1993;33:588-595.

54. Reithmann C, Reber D, Kozlik-Feldmann R, et al: A post-receptor defect of adenylyl cyclase in severely failing myocardium from children with congenital heart disease. Eur J Pharmacol 1997;330:79-86.

55. Galal O, Dzimiri N, Moorji A, et al: Sympathetic activity in children undergoing balloon valvuloplasty of pulmonary stenosis. Pediatr Res 1996;39:774-778.

56. Rocha-Singh KJ, Honbo NY, Karliner JS: Hypoxia and glucose independently regulate the beta-adrenergic receptor-adenylate cyclase system in cardiac myocytes. J Clin Invest 1991;88:204-213.

57. Hausdorff WP, Caron MG, Lefkowitz RJ: Turning off the signal: Desensitization of β-adrenergic receptor function. FASEB J 1990;4:2881-2889.

58. Giannuzzi CE, Seidler FJ, Slotkin TA: Beta-adrenoceptor control of cardiac adenylyl cyclase during development: Agonist pretreatment in the neonate uniquely causes heterologous sensitization, not desensitization. Brain Res 1995;694:271-278.

59. Zeiders JL, Seidler FJ, Slotkin TA: Agonist-induced sensitization of beta-adrenoceptor signaling in neonatal rat heart: Expression and catalytic activity of adenylyl cyclase. J Pharmacol Exp Ther 1999;291:503-510.

60. Auman JT, Seidler FJ, Slotkin TA: β-Adrenoceptor control of G protein function in the neonate: Determinant of desensitization or sensitization. Am J Physiol Regul Integr Comp Physiol 2002;283:1236-1244.

61. Booker PD: Pharmacological support for children with myocardial dysfunction. Paediatr Anaesth 2002;12:5-25.

62. Machin GA: Hydrops revisited: Literature review of 1,414 cases published in the 1980s. Am J Med Genet 1989;34:366-390.

63. Berman W Jr, Yabek SM, Dillon T, et al: Effects of digoxin in infants with a congested circulatory state due to a ventricular septal defect. N Engl J Med 1983;308:363-366.

64. Seguchi M, Nakazawa M, Momma K: Further evidence suggesting a limited role of digitalis in infants with circulatory congestion secondary to a large ventricular septal defect. Am J Cardiol 1999;83:1408-1411.

65. Cohn JN: The management of chronic heart failure. N Engl J Med 1996;335:490-498.

66. Hoffman TM, Wernovsky G, Atz AM, et al: Efficacy and safety of milrinone in preventing low cardiac output syndrome in infants and children after corrective surgery for congenital heart disease. Circulation 2003;107:996-1002.

67. Park IS, Michael LH, Driscoll DJ: Comparative response of the developing canine myocardium to inotropic agents. Am J Physiol 1982;242:H13-H18.

68. Notterman DA, Greenwald BM, Moran F, et al: Dopamine clearance in critically ill infants and children: Effect of age and organ system dysfunction. Clin Pharmacol Ther 1990;48:134-147.

69. Allen E, Pettigrew A, Frank D, et al: Alterations in dopamine clearance and catechol-O-methyltransferase activity by dopamine infusions in children. Crit Care Med 1997;25:181-189.

70. Ramamoorthy C, Anderson GD, Williams GD, Lynn AM: Pharmacokinetics and side effects of milrinone in infants and children after open heart surgery. Anesth Analg 1998;86:283-289.

71. Wettrell G: Distribution and elimination of digoxin in infants. Eur J Clin Pharmacol 1977;11:329-11:335.

72. Lawless S, Burckart G, Diven W, et al: Amrinone in neonates and infants after cardiac surgery. Crit Care Med 1989;17:751-754.

73. Martinez AM, Padbury JF, Thio S: Dobutamine pharmacokinetics and cardiovascular responses in critically ill neonates. Pediatrics 1992;89:47-51.

74. Berg RA, Donnerstein RL, Padbury JF: Dobutamine infusions in stable, critically ill children: Pharmacokinetics and hemodynamic actions. Crit Care Med 1993;21:678-686.

75. Habib DM, Padbury JF, Anas NG, et al: Dobutamine pharmacokinetics and pharmacodynamics in pediatric intensive care patients. Crit Care Med 1992;20:601-608.

76. Waagstein F, Hjalmarson A, Varnauskas E, Wallentin I: Effect of chronic beta-adrenergic receptor blockade in congestive cardiomyopathy. Br Heart J 1975;37:1022-1036.

77. CIBIS-II Investigators: The cardiac insufficiency bisoprolol study II (CIBIS-II): A randomized trial. Lancet 1999;353:9-13.

78. MERIT-HF Study Group: Effect of metoprolol CR/XL in chronic heart failure: Metoprolol CR/XL randomized intervention trial in congestive heart failure (MERIT-HF). Lancet 1999;353:2001-2007.

79. Buchhorn R, Bartmus D, Siekmeyer W, et al: Beta-blocker therapy of severe congestive heart failure in infants with left to right shunts. Am J Cardiol 1998;81:1366-1368.

80. Buchhorn R, Hulpke-Wette M, Hilgers R, et al: Propranolol treatment of congestive heart failure in infants with congenital heart disease: The CHF-PRO-INFANT trial. Int J Cardiol 2001;79:167-173.

81. Bruns LA, Chrisant MK, Lamour JM, et al: Carvedilol as therapy in pediatric heart failure: An initial multicenter experience. J Pediatr 2001;138:505-511.

82. Shaddy RE, Curtin EL, Sower B, et al: The Pediatric Randomized Carvedilol Trial in Children with Heart Failure: Rationale and design. Am Heart J 2002;144:383-389.

83. Shaddy RE, Teitel DF, Brett C: Short-term hemodynamic effects of captopril in infants with congestive heart failure. Am J Dis Child 1988;142:100-105.

84. Scammell AM, Arnold R, Wilkinson JL: Captopril in treatment of infant heart failure: A preliminary report. Int J Cardiol 1987;16:295-301.

85. Shaw NJ, Wilson N, Dickinson DF: Captopril in heart failure secondary to a left to right shunt. Arch Dis Child 1988;63:360-363.

86. Leversha AM, Wilson NJ, Clarkson PM, et al: Efficacy and dosage of enalapril in congenital and acquired heart disease. Arch Dis Child 1994;70:35-39.

87. Sluysmans T, Styns-Cailteux M, Tremouroux-Wattiez M, et al: Intravenous enalaprilat and oral enalapril in congestive heart failure secondary to ventricular septal defect in infancy. Am J Cardiol 1992;70:959-962.

88. Buchhorn R, Ross RD, Hulpke-Wette M, et al: Effectiveness of low dose captopril versus propranolol therapy in infants with severe congestive heart failure due to left-to-right shunts. Int J Cardiol 2000;76:227-233.

89. Chang AC, Atz AM, Wernovsky G, et al: Milrinone: Systemic and pulmonary hemodynamic effects in neonates after cardiac surgery. Crit Care Med 1995;23:1907-1914.

90. Teshima H, Tobita K, Yamamura H, et al: Cardiovascular effects of a phosphodiesterase III inhibitor, amrinone, in infants: Non-invasive echocardiographic evaluation. Pediatr Int 2002;44:259-263.

91. Hoffman TM, Wernovsky G, Atz AM, et al: Efficacy and safety of milrinone in preventing low cardiac output syndrome in infants and children after corrective surgery for congenital heart disease. Circulation 2003;107:996-1002.

92. Turanlahti M, Boldt T, Palkama T, et al: Pharmacokinetics of levosimendan in pediatric patients evaluated for cardiac surgery. Pediatr Crit Care Med 2004;5:457-462.

93. Nelson DP, Schwartz SM, Chang AC: Neonatal physiology of the functionally univentricular heart. Cardiol Young 2004;14 Suppl 7: 52-60.

94. Fesseha AK, Eidem BW, Dibardino DJ, et al: Neonates with aortic coarctation and cardiogenic shock: Presentation and outcomes. Ann Thorac Surg 2005;79(5):1650-1655.

CHAPTER 27

Heart Failure in Adults with Congenital Heart Disease

Wayne J. Franklin
Gary D. Webb

Currently, there are an estimated 4 to 5 million people with heart failure in the United States and another estimated 10 million people in Europe.[1] In the United States, 400,000 new cases of heart failure are diagnosed each year, and it is the leading diagnosis in patients older than 64 years old who are discharged from the hospital. In the United Kingdom, estimates have shown that a city with 1 million people should expect to have 10,000 patients with heart failure (2000 to 3000 new cases each year) needing 5000 hospital admissions and about 140 inpatient beds.[2,3] Deaths from heart failure also are increasing, largely as a result of more patients surviving acute coronary syndromes who are left with depressed ventricular function and die from chronic cardiomyopathy (Fig. 27-1).

These large numbers of patients contribute to escalating health care costs. Heart failure costs in the United States were close to $40 billion per year in the early 1990s; the costs to health care systems worldwide have continued to increase as well. Most heart failure data in the United States involve patients with acquired heart disease, but the subset of heart failure secondary to congenital heart disease is steadily growing. The true incidence of heart failure in adults with congenital heart disease is not defined, and epidemiologic studies are difficult to perform. Nonetheless, clinicians who routinely care for such patients know that heart failure often develops in these patients, and that the treatment is not always straightforward. Several centers worldwide have made efforts to address heart failure in adult patients with congenital heart defects.

This chapter addresses the following questions: Do adults with congenital heart disease develop heart failure? What types of patients are predisposed to the heart failure syndrome? Do these patients die of heart failure? What kinds of treatments are available?

ADULT PATIENTS WITH CONGENITAL HEART DISEASE AND HEART FAILURE

To begin a discussion of the development of heart failure, one first must examine the conditions and anatomy that may cause certain cardiac defects to be predisposed to ventricular dysfunction. Traditionally the hemodynamic model taught that heart failure was caused by pump dysfunction, and therapies using this model focused on inotropes, vasodilators, and diuretics. Current practice defines the *heart failure syndrome* as a state of high neurohormonal imbalance which includes many novel features, such as cardiac remodeling, neuroendocrine activation, and cytokine release. Current therapies

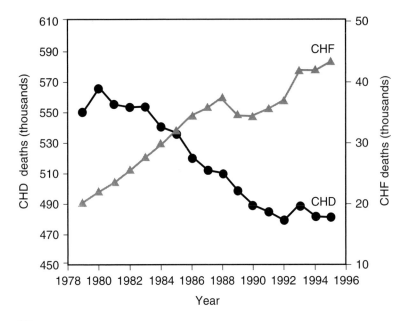

FIGURE 27-1 ■ Deaths in the United States from heart disease. Deaths secondary to coronary heart disease (CHD) are decreasing, whereas deaths secondary to chronic congestive heart failure (CHF) are increasing. (From Eichhorn EJ: *Prognosis determination in heart failure. Am J Med* 2001;110:7A.)

concentrate on some conventional drugs (diuretics, digoxin), but also add afterload reduction, β blockade, and newer neurohormonal agents.[4]

The broad etiologic categories for adults with congenital heart disease and heart failure include primary pump failure (systolic dysfunction) and hypertrophy (diastolic dysfunction) of the right, left, or single ventricle. In a study by Piran and colleagues[5] of 188 patients with systemic right ventricles or single ventricles, ventricular function was assessed by radionuclide angiography or echocardiography, and symptoms were graded according to the New York Heart Association (NYHA) classification. The authors found that 22% of Mustard patients, 32% of congenitally corrected transposition of the great arteries (cc-TGA) patients, and 40% of Fontan patients had heart failure using the original Framingham criteria.[6] Of these, 82.4% were in NYHA class I or II, 13.3% were in NYHA class III, and 4.3% were in NYHA class IV heart failure. Symptomatic patients also had significantly lower anaerobic thresholds and lower peak volume of oxygen usage measurements. At 15-year follow-up, mortality in the symptomatic group was higher (47.1%) than in the asymptomatic group (5%). The authors found that the best predictors of mortality were NHYA class, systemic ventricular ejection fraction, and age at operation.

A study by Oechslin and coworkers[7] retrospectively analyzed the cause of death in a large number (2609 consecutive) of adults with congenital heart disease. The authors concluded that over the 15-year study period, the mortality rate was 8%, and the mean age of death was 37 ± 15 years. The second most common mode of death was heart failure, which accounted for 21% of all deaths. This number is likely an underrepresentation because the leading cause of death—"sudden death"—undoubtedly included other patients with precedent heart failure. The highest mortalities by diagnoses were cc-TGA (26%), tricuspid atresia (25%), and single-ventricle physiology (23%). The study included 48 patients with Eisenmenger syndrome (4%), who had a 40% mortality rate. Studies such as these, in addition to clinical experience, confirm the belief that a significant percentage of congenital heart disease patients can and do develop heart failure over time. The next section delineates which congenital lesions are particularly predisposed to the development of heart failure. The development of heart failure is usually a chronic process. Aside from an acute myocardial infarction, patients usually experience an interval of asymptomatic ventricular dysfunction before the development of overt symptoms of cardiocirculatory decompensation. In acquired heart disease, heart failure often is triggered by an index event, such as a myocardial infarction or myocarditis. Some authors claim that congenital heart disease is "the original heart failure syndrome" that develops from abnormal cardiac pressure, volume, tension, and flow.[8] For congenital heart disease, the beginnings of the heart failure syndrome may lie in their cardiac anatomy, and this syndrome is most likely to occur in patients with systemic right ventricles and single ventricles.

Some patients with conditions with a pressure-loaded systemic right ventricle and patients with a functionally single ventricle may be particularly prone to develop heart failure. Right heart failure may occur in patients with Ebstein anomaly or with tetralogy of Fallot after corrective repair but with varying degrees of pulmonary insufficiency, and left heart failure can be a result of mitral or aortic insufficiency (see Chapters 16 and 21).

HEART FAILURE IN ADULT PATIENTS WITH SYSTEMIC RIGHT OR SINGLE VENTRICLES

Congenitally Corrected Transposition of the Great Arteries

Although the terminology for cc-TGA varies (L-transposition, atrioventricular [AV]/ventriculoarterial discordance, or congenitally corrected transposition), the development of systemic ventricular dysfunction is not usually anticipated. Heart failure is highly likely to develop during the lifetime of these patients, but the age of onset of right ventricular dysfunction varies and depends on the presence or absence of associated lesions. cc-TGA is rare (<1% of all congenital heart lesions), and isolated cc-TGA (i.e., without other associated cardiac anomalies) is even rarer. Other cardiac abnormalities (ventricular septal defect, 74%; valvar or subvalvar pulmonic stenosis, 74%; tricuspid [systemic AV] valve abnormalities with subsequent regurgitation, 38%; or complete heart block, 5%) are the rule.[9]

The onset of heart failure may be related to the interdependence of the associated defects with systemic ventricular function. Accurate prediction of the onset of heart failure in this population is complicated by the heterogeneity of the associated lesions, comorbidities (e.g., hypertension, diabetes, or coronary artery disease), and lifestyle (e.g., smoking or alcohol use). Large studies in these patients are lacking because of the relative infrequency of this lesion, but systemic ventricular dysfunction is known to occur.[10,11] Graham and associates[12] reported that 67% of cc-TGA patients with associated lesions and 25% with isolated cc-TGA had heart failure by age 45.

In a study by Presbitero and colleagues[13] on the natural history of isolated cc-TGA, heart failure was present in 24% of patients age 41 to 50 years and in 77% of patients age 51 to 60. A significant number of these patients had complete heart block in childhood (18% to 25%). Nearly 30% of these patients developed left AV valve regurgitation by age 31, a decade before heart failure was noted. As mentioned previously, cc-TGA patients frequently have an abnormal systemic tricuspid valve. In the Presbitero study of isolated cc-TGA, the onset of clinical left AV valve regurgitation was not seen until after age 20, however. In many instances, tricuspid regurgitation in cc-TGA patients reflects worsening systemic ventricular function. In other patients, primary systemic tricuspid regurgitation triggered ventricular dilation and dysfunction. In either case, clinicians should be aware that the development of left AV valve regurgitation in cc-TGA patients may be a sign of worsening systemic right ventricular function.

In the largest published study of cc-TGA, Rutledge and coworkers[14] found that 23 (19%) of 121 patients had documented heart failure. This study had few adults in its cohort (6 of 121), however. Congestive heart failure on presentation was documented in more than one half of the patients in all age groups (neonatal through adult). This study also showed that poor right ventricular function led to an earlier mortality compared with patients with normal right ventricular function (Fig. 27-2).

Connelly and associates[15] reviewed 52 patients over 15 years (all >18 years old) and assessed their functional status, surgical history, and mortality. In their cohort, 13 (25%) patients died, at a mean age of 38.5 years. Six of the 13 (46%) patients died of progressive heart failure; heart failure had been present in 60% of the deceased patients. Similar to other studies, this report found that significant systemic AV valve regurgitation was present in 26% of survivors (16% with "moderate," 10% with "severe") and was diagnosed in 24% of the patients who died (Fig. 27-3). In this study, heart failure had an even higher association with death than did AV valve regurgitation. In the Presbitero study, AV valve regurgitation was found earlier (beginning at age 21) than heart failure (first documented at age 41). In the

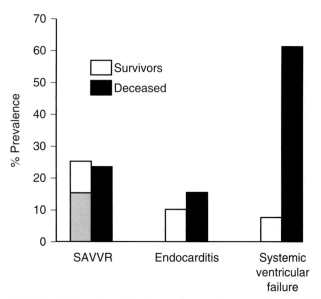

FIGURE 27-3 ■ Complications observed in patients with congenitally corrected transposition of the great arteries. Comparison of survivors and deceased patients in prevalence of systemic atrioventricular valve regurgitation (SAVVR), endocarditis, and systemic ventricular failure. Among survivors with SAVVR, shaded and open areas show patients who have moderate *(shaded)* and severe *(open)* regurgitation. (From Connelly MS, Liu PP, Williams WG, et al: *Congenitally corrected transposition of the great arteries in the adult: Functional status and complications. J Am Coll Cardiol* 1996; 27:1238-1243.)

study by Connelly, of the 39 remaining patients (age 18 to 54 years, mean age 32 years), all had at least one other cardiac anomaly, most commonly a systemic AV valve abnormality (15 patients) in addition to pulmonic stenosis or a ventricular septal defect or both. It is impossible to divide this heterogeneous group into patients with heart failure and select isolated lesions. Despite their heterogeneity, one still can conclude that patients with cc-TGA are at risk of heart failure, systemic AV valve regurgitation, heart block, and endocarditis. Heart failure is a predictor of poor outcome for cc-TGA patients. More than 60% of cc-TGA patients have developed heart failure by age 40.

Surgical options for these patients address the associated defects. Imamura and colleagues[16] reported that in 22 patients who underwent a double-switch procedure (see Chapter 42), age at operation ranged from 3 months to 55 years. Ten patients underwent arterial switch plus Senning procedures, and 12 underwent Rastelli plus Senning procedures. Before the double-switch procedure, 6 patients required pulmonary artery banding, and 10 had systemic-to-pulmonary artery or Glenn shunts. No early or late mortality was reported. In their series, this operation also improved systemic AV valve regurgitation in all patients except one. Moderate left ventricular systolic dysfunction developed 5 months postoperatively in one patient. The more traditional surgical approach is to patch the ventricular septal defect and bypass the pulmonary outflow obstruction with a valved conduit,

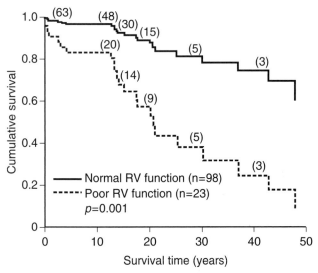

FIGURE 27-2 ■ Right ventricular (RV) function in congenitally corrected transposition of the great arteries. Kaplan-Meier curves for patients with congenitally corrected transposition of the great arteries show a better long-term survival pattern with normal RV function. (From Rutledge JM, Nihill MR, Fraser CD, et al: *Outcome of 121 patients with congenitally corrected transposition of the great arteries. Pediatr Cardiol* 2002;23:137-145.)

leaving the right ventricle supporting the systemic circulation. Sometimes, replacement of the systemic tricuspid valve is performed.

Mustard or Senning Operations

The Mustard and Senning atrial switch procedures for dextraposed TGA were a major breakthrough in congenital heart surgery. Before the development of these techniques, these cyanotic infants had a 90% mortality rate within the first year of life. With surgery, 90% could survive, although problems included arrhythmias, baffle leaks and obstruction, and systemic right ventricular dysfunction.

The incidence of systemic right ventricular dysfunction has been debated. Studies have shown that the incidence of right ventricular dysfunction varies, and that its age of onset is unpredictable.[17-19] The incidence of significant right ventricular systolic dysfunction ranges from 0% to 66%.[20] Although systolic dysfunction is the usual concern, Reich and associates[20] noted that the long-term ventricular performance may be dominated by diastolic and systolic dysfunction.[13] Right ventricular dysfunction was noted in 8% and left ventricular dysfunction in 10% of 153 atrial switch patients, without a significant increase at the 8-year follow-up. Reich and associates[20] found, however, that left ventricular diastolic filling was abnormal in 80% of patients as the rapid filling phase was markedly decreased, whereas the slow filling phase and filling resulting from atrial contraction were increased. In some patients, these differences were noted 1 week after operation. The left ventricular peak filling rate also was found to deteriorate over time. Reich and associates[20] hypothesized that the abnormal filling of the ventricles not only may be related to ventricular diastolic dysfunction, but also to the properties of the intra-atrial baffles. Interdependence of the right and left ventricles may play an important role. Interdependence involves not only the interventricular septum, but also other areas of the ventricles. About 20% to 40% of the normal right ventricular systolic pressure and stroke volume result from left ventricular contraction. Ventricular interdependence may help to determine the right ventricular response to changes in volume and pressure and even to myocardial ischemia.[21] There have been no studies on ventricular interdependence in atrial switch patients, but one can infer that the interaction between the left ventricle and systemic right ventricle in these patients is not normal.

Chang and colleagues[22] compared two surgical interventions for mainly pediatric atrial switch patients with right ventricular failure and found that 50% had some left ventricular dysfunction. Cochrane and colleagues[23] claimed that late failure of the systemic right ventricle occurs in 10% of patients who have undergone an atrial switch operation. In their experience, the mean interval from atrial switch to right ventricular failure was 7 years. In a large study of 358 atrial switch patients, Sarkar and coworkers[24] reported that clinical systemic right ventricular failure was uncommon, and 92% of the Senning patients and 89% of the Mustard patients were in NHYA functional class I. Although systemic right ventricular dysfunction is commonly seen in atrial switch patients, frank heart failure is relatively uncommon and certainly not inevitable.

Although several possible mechanisms of right ventricular dysfunction have been postulated, Lubiszewska and colleagues[25] offered additional insight. The authors' premise relates to an earlier hypothesis that right ventricular dysfunction may be related to a mismatch between right ventricular blood supply and demand.[26] Ventricular function and perfusion defects were measured using the modified Bruce protocol in 61 patients age 7 to 23 years using technetium-99m methoxyisobutyl isonitrile single-photon emission computed tomography (SPECT). Fifty-six patients were NYHA class I, and 5 were NYHA class II. Patients with right ventricular ejection fraction less than 33% were considered to have ventricular systolic dysfunction. Mean right ventricular ejection fraction was 36.1% ± 7.7%, mean left ventricular ejection fraction was 52.1% ± 9.4%, and 26% of patients had impaired right ventricular function by their definition. Moderate or severe perfusion abnormalities were noted on the rest images in 33% of patients and on the stress images in 21%. Reversible perfusion defects were associated with lower right ventricular and left ventricular ejection fractions and were more prevalent in the older patients in the study. Coronary anomalies and myocardial perfusion mismatch may play an important role in systemic right ventricular dysfunction.

Surgical management of the "failed" Mustard or Senning patient can involve orthotopic transplantation or a switch conversion procedure. The latter procedure is a two-stage operation in which a pulmonary artery band is placed to induce hypertrophy to "prepare" the left ventricle eventually to become the systemic ventricle. After the left ventricle has been adequately retrained, the intra-atrial baffles are taken down, and an arterial switch operation is performed. The time to retrain the left ventricle usually has been at least 6 to 12 months before moving to the second stage. Overall the switch conversion procedure has had mixed results. After the pulmonary artery band placement, some patients have an acutely decompensated subpulmonary left ventricle that can be difficult to manage postoperatively, and that may not recover systolic function. Death after placement of the pulmonary artery band occurred in the Chang study (the only death in this report) and in the Connelly study (one of three deaths). Cases of patients in their 30s who have had successful arterial switch conversion operations have been reported by Cetta and coworkers[27] and Padalino and associates.[28]

Cochrane and colleagues[23] reported the results of 24 patients on whom they had performed arterial switch conversions. Four patients underwent direct conversion to arterial switch with one operative death. The other 20 patients underwent pulmonary artery banding with one band-related operative death. Twelve patients went on to switch conversion 13 days to 5 years (mean 26 months) after band placement. The early mortality rate was 12.5% with one late death 1 year after operation. Including overall mortality, the 1-year actuarial survival rate after conversion was 80% in their series. Poirier and Mee[29] published the follow-up report to this series in 2000. Anatomic correction by changing the left ventricle over to the systemic circulation was performed in 84 patients, 43 of whom had received a pulmonary artery band. The overall mortality rate for this group was 15.4%. There were eight early and five late deaths; all of these patients had had a prior atrial switch operation. Older age and abnormal coronary anatomy were associated with higher operative mortality. Follow-up echocardiographic evaluation showed normal right ventricular function in 89% and normal left ventricular function in 91% of patients. The authors concluded that the switch conversion after left ventricular retraining produces good results in prepubescent patients, but in adult patients, the success of the operation is less predictable, and the early and late mortality rates are significantly higher. For adult patients with a failed atrial switch procedure, cardiac transplantation may be the preferred surgical option.

Single Ventricle and Fontan Operation

Survival into adulthood for patients with single ventricles (e.g., double-inlet left ventricle, tricuspid atresia, hypoplastic left heart syndrome) is now the trend since the development of the Fontan-type operation. Early experiences with right atrial-to-pulmonary connections now have been supplanted by the lateral tunnel or extracardiac conduit Fontan procedures. There are many patients with so-called "classic Fontan" operation who were operated on in the 1970s and 1980s who have reached adult age. These patients have diverse original and postoperative anatomies.

The term *failed Fontan* may be all-inclusive and be applied to various clinical scenarios in which these patients have cardiopulmonary compromise. When these palliated single-ventricle patients deteriorate, the etiology is often multifactorial. Complications such as atrial arrhythmias, Fontan-circuit pathway obstructions, ventricular dysfunction, worsening cyanosis, and protein-losing enteropathy are well described.[30-33]

Heart failure in Fontan patients is difficult to differentiate from the complex syndrome of cardiopulmonary deterioration to which these patients are predisposed. Pleural effusions may compromise respiratory function via atelectasis, which can worsen cyanosis. Hepatic dysfunction and hypoalbuminemia may lead to ascites, which can decrease lung volumes by limiting diaphragmatic excursion. Deep venous and atrial thrombi can cause conduit obstruction or pulmonary emboli, which

can increase pulmonary pressures and subsequently reduce pulmonary blood flow. These patients may present with what would be the equivalent of "right-sided" heart failure for biventricular hearts. These patients also can have pulmonary venous obstruction from the severely dilated atrium. Lastly, some patients have ventricular dysfunction that is severe with elevated end-diastolic pressures.

As mentioned earlier, the early Fontan procedures used direct atriopulmonary connections, which predisposed to atrial enlargement years later. This often massive atrial dilation could lead to even worse Fontan circuit hemodynamics and "lower flow" states as blood swirled inefficiently around in the enlarged right atrium, as seen on echocardiography and angiography. Surgical intervention for this failed Fontan condition involves revision of the Fontan circuit and concomitant intraoperative ablative surgery for atrial arrhythmias. Results have been promising. (See Chapter 42).

Data from Boston show that several factors were associated with an increased incidence of failure,[34] including a mean preoperative pulmonary artery pressure of 19 mm Hg or more, younger age at operation, heterotaxy syndrome, a right-sided tricuspid valve as the only systemic AV valve, pulmonary artery distortion, an atriopulmonary connection arising from the right atrial body or appendage, the absence of a baffle fenestration, and longer cardiopulmonary bypass time. The presence of a pacemaker was associated with late Fontan failure. A morphologic left ventricle with normally related great vessels or a single right ventricle was associated with a lower probability of late failure. It can be predicted from perioperative risk factors which patients are more likely to have early or late failure after the Fontan operation. This strategy may lead to more aggressive surveillance in higher risk patients.

At Texas Children's Hospital, we follow more than 200 postoperative adult Fontan patients, and nearly one third have at least mild ventricular systolic dysfunction as documented by echocardiography. As expected, a worse NYHA class is associated consistently with a lower survival and worse outcome.[35] Close observation for the development of heart failure combined with early initiation of medical or surgical therapy is appropriate. The current total cavopulmonary connections, improved techniques, and improved conduit material (i.e., Dacron or Gore-Tex) may mean that the current generation of Fontan patients will have improved hemodynamics and better functional outcomes. Although long-term data are unavailable, short-term and intermediate-term data are promising. Fontan revision procedures have become relatively common at our institution when a failed Fontan patient presents. When a high-functioning patient with a classic Fontan or variant presents, debate still exists as to when or if to revise the Fontan; individual patient evaluation on a case-by-case basis should be performed.

HEART FAILURE MANAGEMENT IN ADULTS WITH CONGENITAL HEART DISEASE

Adults with congenital heart disease and heart failure should be treated according to their specific anatomy and physiology and not as uniformly as adults with congestive heart failure sometimes are treated. Biventricular patients with failing systemic right ventricles can be treated as one would treat systemic left ventricle patients with severe left ventricular dysfunction, although data showing the efficacy of current cardiac medications on the failing right ventricle are limited. Until better data are available regarding the medical treatment of patients with systemic right ventricles, the adult trials involving patients with acquired heart disease may serve as best available evidence. Many more complex adult patients with congenital heart defects should be assessed at centers specializing in the care of these patients. The paradigm shift in thinking about heart failure pathophysiology has moved from the hemodynamic model of pump failure to a neurohormonal model. A report showed that neurohormonal changes in adults with congenital heart disease are similar to findings in adults with heart failure and acquired heart diseases (Fig. 27-4).[36] This section provides general guidelines for adult patients with congenital heart disease and heart failure (see also Chapters 32-40).

Outpatient Medical Management

Overall, few data are available on the management of heart failure in adults with congenital heart disease. Initial oral agents for these patients should include standard **diuretics** to control pulmonary edema and congestion. Particular care should be given to the use of diuretics in single-ventricle patients who have had Fontan-type palliation because these patients experience passive and nonpulsatile filling of their pulmonary vasculature; volume reduction and preload depletion also can have deleterious effects in an adult patient with Eisenmenger syndrome or outflow tract obstruction with secondary hypertrophy and diastolic dysfunction.

Adult studies such as the SOLVD, CONSENSUS II, and ATLAS trials have shown the benefit of **afterload reduction** with angiotensin-converting enzyme (ACE) inhibitors.[37-39] These drugs have been shown to improve left ventricular remodeling and ejection fraction and may reduce systemic AV valve regurgitation.

Data supporting **angiotensin II receptor antagonists** (ARBs) in left ventricular dysfunction also have been reported in the ELITE[40] and STRETCH[41] trials, and ARBs should be strongly considered as additive therapy or as monotherapy, especially if patients are intolerant of ACE inhibitors. ARBs make intuitive sense because ACE inhibitors block only about 15% to 20% of total body angiotensin production, and receptor blockade may provide more complete therapy. ACE inhibitor therapy should be included in first-line treatment, and ARB use should be considered early in treatment. Clinical trials of ARBs are lacking in children, but there are good safety and efficacy data in adults.

For patients in NYHA classes III and IV heart failure already receiving a loop diuretic and ACE inhibitor, the RALES trial showed mortality and morbidity benefits with the use of spironolactone, 25 mg daily.[42] There were fewer hospitalizations and an improvement in NYHA class with the use of this drug. Spironolactone works by being an **aldosterone receptor blocker**, the end product of the renin-angiotensin-aldosterone axis, which is highly active in heart failure. Caution should be used in patients with renal failure because the median creatinine increased by 0.05 to 0.10 mg/dL, and patients with a baseline creatinine of 2.5 mg/dL were excluded from this trial. The EPHESUS trial also showed the benefit of another aldosterone antagonist, eplerenone, in adult heart failure patients.[43]

Numerous trials on adult patients with normal intracardiac anatomy, such as CIBIS-II,[44] MERIT-HF,[45] and COPERNICUS,[46] have shown morbidity and mortality benefits with **β-blockers**. Although previously believed to be contraindicated in patients with depressed ventricular function because of negative inotropic effects, these drugs are now standard in adult heart failure therapy. These drugs act within the neurohormonal axis to combat the deleterious effects of the increased sympathetic tone that is prevalent in the heart failure syndrome. Low-dose β-blockers can be started in the outpatient setting and titrated to the therapeutic dose over several weeks. Monitoring is required during up-titration. A mild increase in shortness of breath or lower extremity edema may be related to the negative inotropic effect. In acute decompensated heart failure, β-blockers should be stopped to start therapy with the appropriate inotropes (see Appendix for clinical trial information).

Inpatient Medical Management

Standard intravenous adult heart failure therapy should be followed. Diuretics should be used judiciously when there is evidence of pulmonary congestion, but should be used sparingly in Fontan-palliated patients whose pulmonary blood flow depends on adequate preload. **Inotropic agents** should be used when treating acutely decompensated heart failure. First-line therapy should include dopamine or dobutamine for inotropic support. Other agents, such as epinephrine or norepinephrine, can be added if more α-tone and β-agonist effects are required. At Texas Children's Hospital, we have had good experience using the vasoconstrictor vasopressin for hypotension from decreased cardiac output. Vasopressin often allows an increase in α-tone without a direct increase in heart rate. Lastly, phosphodiesterase inhibitors should be included in the inotropic

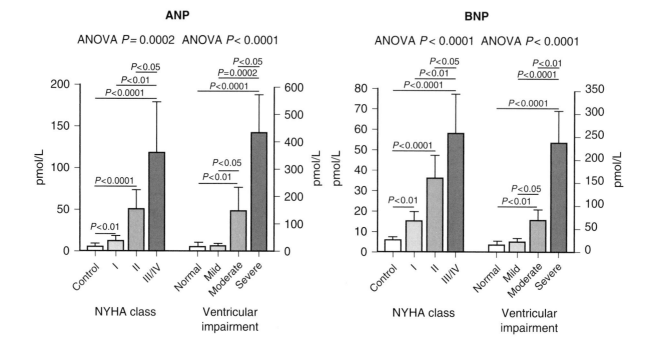

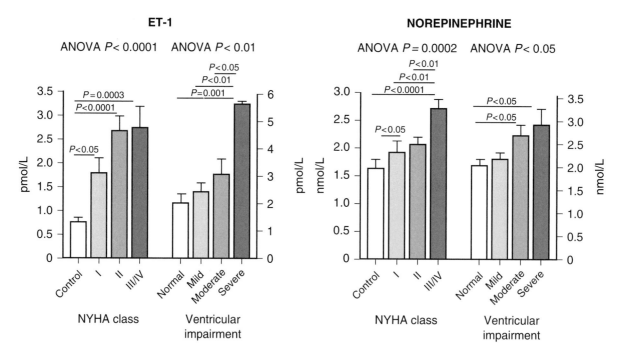

FIGURE 27-4 ■ Neurohormones in adults with congenital heart disease. Levels of atrial and brain natriuretic peptides (ANP and BNP), endothelin-1 (ET-1), and norepinephrine are found to correlate with degree of heart failure in these patients. NYHA, New York Heart Association. (From Bolger AP, Sharma R, Li W, et al: *Neurohormonal activation and the chronic heart failure syndrome in adults with congenital heart disease. Circulation* 2002;106:92-99.)

agents used for low cardiac output secondary to congestive heart failure.

Agents for pulmonary hypertension should be considered because biventricular patients can present with increased pulmonary artery pressure secondary to

systemic ventricular dysfunction. As heart failure progresses, these patients develop an increased left atrial pressure secondary to increased systemic ventricular end-diastolic pressure. Although treatment of the primary cause of the secondary pulmonary hypertension should be undertaken, other agents, such as oxygen and nitric oxide, may be implemented. Established agents, such as epoprostenol, have been used, although data on their utility in congenital heart disease and heart failure are limited, and one trial in adults with severe heart failure showed no benefit and increased mortality.[47] Other oral therapies, such as the endothelin receptor antagonist bosentan and the phosphodiesterase inhibitor sildenafil, are still undergoing trials for their use in heart failure. Newer agents, such as the calcium-sensitizing agent levosimendan and the intravenous endothelin-receptor antagonist tezosentan, are undergoing trials for their application in acute heart failure. (See Chapter 38).

Evaluation and Surveillance

Close monitoring of fluid balance, heart size, pulmonary congestion, and pleural or pericardial effusions should be performed. More invasive therapy, such as bedside pulmonary artery catheters, may not be possible or useful in congenital heart disease patients because of the presence of intracardiac shunts or limited venous access. Studies in adults have shown that continuous pulmonary artery catheters have increased morbidity, while not significantly improving clinical outcomes, and in many institutions they have fallen out of favor. Pulmonary artery pressure measurements can be taken from Doppler echocardiography or from cardiac catheterization. Ventricular function assessment is usually by transthoracic **echocardiography**, although these patients may have poor acoustic windows because of their repeated operations or increased girth. Pediatric cardiologists generally have reserved transesophageal echocardiography for the immediate preoperative setting in the operating room, but this modality may see greater use as more adult congenital patients present to echocardiography laboratories. Caution should be taken in sedating these patients for transesophageal echocardiograms; in addition, a consultation with a cardiac anesthesiologist should be considered, given the propensities for myocardial depression and arrhythmias with many anesthetic agents.

Another imaging option is **cardiovascular MRI**, which can provide excellent anatomic information and shunt quantification, stroke volume calculation, and right and left ventricular ejection fraction determination. MRI has become a preferred imaging modality because the images, in expert hands, can be remarkably detailed, and the hemodynamic information is becoming more and more extensive. Patients with pacemakers are not always able to undergo cardiac MRI. For these patients, a nuclear study (usually with technetium-99m) with gated SPECT imaging provides satisfactory quantitative assessment of ventricular function. Periodic assessment of ventricular function by one of the aforementioned imaging modalities is recommended. When more invasive hemodynamic and angiographic data are needed, cardiac catheterization can be arranged and is necessary as part of a cardiac transplantation evaluation. Many complex adult patients should be catheterized by clinicians who are trained in congenital heart disease and in laboratories familiar with adults.

Surgical Options

Although mechanical support is becoming more widespread, **ventricular assist devices** have been used sparingly in adults with heart failure and congenital heart disease. Some reasons for its limited use in congenital heart disease patients are smaller patient size, complex anatomy, and uncertain long-term experience with adult patients with noncongenital heart disease. The Thoratec ventricular assist device[48] has been used in patients with a body surface area of 1.3 m², however, and the placement of a BVS 5000 has been reported in a 22-kg child.[49] There are limited reports of assist devices used in adult congenital heart disease patients.[50,51] In 2003, at St. Luke's Episcopal Hospital, we also implanted ventricular assist devices in two adult congenital heart disease patients with end-stage heart failure as a bridge to successful heart transplantation. Given that many centers around the world are gaining experience with ventricular assist devices, it is likely that such mechanical support will be used in more congenital heart disease patients with heart failure. All modes of mechanical support are discussed at length in other chapters. (See Chapters 45-50).

Cardiac transplantation is another option for adults with congenital heart disease and heart failure. The United Network for Organ Sharing registry reported in 2001 that congenital heart disease constituted just 2% of all the diagnosis codes as the reason for cardiac transplantation. The challenge of cardiac transplantation in adult congenital heart disease patients differs from other adult heart disease patients in that the patients often have had previous thoracic operations, which increase the risks of bleeding and adhesions to cardiac structures and conduits. In addition, due to their multiple bypass runs, these patients have been exposed to multiple blood products, and finding a match in the face of elevated plasma reactive antigens may be difficult. (See Chapter 41 for more discussion).

Researchers from the Mayo Clinic reported that from 1991 to 1998, their institution performed 136 transplants, 16 (11.8%) of which were for congenital heart disease. Of these 16 transplants, 11 (69%) were in patients older than 18 years of age (mean age 26.1 years). The 1-year survival for the congenital heart disease patients was 86.2% ± 9.1% compared with 94.5% ± 2% for patients with acquired disease.[52] At the University of Pittsburgh from 1984 to 1999, 69 (5.4%) of the 1281 transplants were for congenital heart disease and had similar survival results to transplants in adults with noncongenital heart disease.[53]

CURRENT STATUS AND FUTURE TRENDS

The number of adults with congenital heart disease has surpassed the number of children and adolescents with congenital heart disease, and long-term complications in these patients can be expected. Heart failure, one of the most rapidly growing areas of adult cardiology, is a major long-term sequela for many adult congenital heart disease patients. Heart failure may be systolic or diastolic and may be a consequence of the original lesion or of the interventional treatments. Patients with systemic right ventricles or functional single-ventricle anatomy who have had a Fontan procedure are particularly prone to heart failure.

Currently, studies in adults with congenital heart disease and heart failure are sparse in number.[54] We should apply general adult heart failure medical and surgical data to these patients until more data on adult congenital heart disease patients are available. The future medical and surgical management of this new population of heart failure patients and their psychosocial well-being is crucial.[55,56]

Key Concepts

■ The broad etiologic categories for adults with congenital heart disease and heart failure include primary pump failure (systolic dysfunction) and hypertrophy (diastolic dysfunction) of the right, left, or single ventricle.

■ For congenital heart disease, the beginnings of the heart failure syndrome may lie in their cardiac anatomy, and this syndrome is most likely to occur in patients with systemic right ventricles and single ventricles.

■ Some patients with conditions with a pressure-loaded systemic right ventricle and patients with a functionally single ventricle may be particularly prone to develop heart failure. Right heart failure may occur in patients with Ebstein anomaly or with tetralogy of Fallot after corrective repair but with varying degrees of pulmonary insufficiency, and left heart failure can be a result of mitral or aortic insufficiency.

■ The term *failed Fontan* may be all-inclusive and be applied to various clinical scenarios in which these patients have cardiopulmonary compromise. When these palliated single-ventricle patients deteriorate, the etiology is often multifactorial. Complications such as atrial arrhythmias, Fontan-circuit pathway obstructions, ventricular dysfunction, worsening cyanosis, and protein-losing enteropathy are well described.

■ Neurohormonal changes in adults with congenital heart disease are similar to findings in adults with heart failure and acquired heart diseases.

■ Particular care should be given to the use of diuretics in single-ventricle patients who have had Fontan-type palliation because these patients experience passive and nonpulsatile fillings of their pulmonary vasculature; volume reduction and preload depletion also can have deleterious effects in adult patients with Eisenmenger syndrome or outflow tract obstruction with secondary hypertrophy and diastolic dysfunction.

■ Cardiovascular MRI can provide excellent anatomic information and shunt quantification, stroke volume calculation, and right and left ventricular ejection fraction determination.

REFERENCES

1. Heart Disease and Stroke Statistics. 2005 Update, American Heart Association. www.americanheart.org/downloadable/heart/1105390918119HDSStats2005Update.pdf.
2. Cleland JGF, Khand A, Clark AC: The heart failure epidemic: Exactly how big is it? Eur Heart J 2001;22:623-626.
3. Cleland JGG, Gemmel I, Khand A, Boddy A: Is the prognosis of heart failure improving? Eur Heart J 1999;1:229-241.
4. Francis GS: Pathophysiology of chronic heart failure. Am J Med 2001;110 Suppl 7A:37S-46S. Review.
5. Piran S, Veldtman G, Siu S, et al: Heart failure and ventricular dysfunction in patients with single or systemic right ventricles. Circulation 2002;105:1189-1194.
6. McKee PA, Castelli WP, McNamara PM, Kannel WB: The natural history of congestive heart failure: The Framingham study. N Engl J Med 1971;285:1441-1446.
7. Oechslin EN, Harrison DA, Connelly MS, et al: Mode of death in adults with congenital heart disease. Am J Cardiol 2000;86:1111-1116.
8. Bolger AP, Coats AJS, Gatzoulis MA: Congenital heart disease: The original heart failure syndrome. Eur Heart J 2003;24:970-976.
9. Garson AT, Bricker JT, Fisher DJ (eds): The Science and Practice of Pediatric Cardiology. Baltimore, Lippincott Williams & Wilkins, 66:1525-1534, 1998.
10. Hornung TS, Bernard EJ, Jaeggi ET, et al: Myocardial perfusion defects and associated systemic ventricular dysfunction in congenitally corrected transposition of the great arteries. Heart 1998;80:322-326.
11. Hornung TS, Bernard EJ, Celermajer DS, et al: Right ventricular dysfunction in congenitally corrected transposition of the great arteries. Am J Cardiol 1999;84:1116-1119.
12. Graham TP Jr, Bernard YD, Mellen BG, et al: Long-term outcome in congenitally corrected transposition of the great arteries: A multi-institutional study. J Am Coll Cardiol 2000;36:255-261.
13. Presbitero P, Somerville J, Rabajoli F, et al: Corrected transposition of the great arteries without associated defects in adult patients: Clinical profile and follow up. Br Heart J 1995;74:57-59.
14. Rutledge JM, Nihill MR, Fraser CD, et al: Outcome of 121 patients with congenitally corrected transposition of the great arteries. Pediatr Cardiol 2002;23:137-145.
15. Connelly MS, Liu PP, Williams WG, et al: Congenitally corrected transposition of the great arteries in the adult: Functional status and complications. J Am Coll Cardiol 1996;27:1238-1243.
16. Imamura M, Drummond-Webb JJ, Murphy DJ Jr, et al: Results of the double switch operation in the current era. Ann Thorac Surg 2000;70:100-105.
17. Graham TP Jr: Hemodynamic residua and sequelae following intraatrial repair of transposition of the great arteries: A review. Pediatr Cardiol 1982;2:203-213.
18. Graham TP Jr, Burger J, Bender HW, et al: Improved right ventricular function after intra-atrial repair of transposition of the great arteries. Circulation 1985;72(3 Pt 2):II-45-II-51.
19. Wong KY, Venables AW, Kelly MJ, Kalff V: Longitudinal study of ventricular function after the Mustard operation for transposition of the great arteries: A long term follow up. Br Heart J 1988;60: 316-323.

20. Reich O, Voriskova M, Ruth C, et al: Long-term ventricular performance after intra-atrial correction of transposition: Left ventricular filling is the major limitation. Heart 1997;78:376-381.

21. Santamore WP, Dell'Italia LJ: Ventricular interdependence: Significant left ventricular contributions to right ventricular systolic function. Prog Cardiovasc Dis 1998;40:289-308.

22. Chang AC, Wernovsky G, Wessel DL, et al: Surgical management of late right ventricular failure after Mustard or Senning repair. Circulation 1992;86(5 Suppl):II-140-II-149.

23. Cochrane AD, Karl TR, Mee RB: Staged conversion to arterial switch for late failure of the systemic right ventricle. Ann Thorac Surg 1993;56:854-862.

24. Sarkar D, Bull C, Yates R, et al: Comparison of long-term outcomes of atrial repair of simple transposition with implications for a late arterial switch strategy. Circulation 1999;100 (19 Suppl): II-176-II-181.

25. Lubiszewska B, Gosiewska E, Hoffman P, et al: Myocardial perfusion and function of the systemic right ventricle in patients after atrial switch procedure for complete transposition: Long-term follow-up. J Am Coll Cardiol 2000;36:1365-1370.

26. Turina MI, Siebenmann R, von Segesser L, et al: Late functional deterioration after atrial correction for transposition of the great arteries. Circulation 1989;80(3 Pt 1):I-162-I-167.

27. Cetta F, Bonilla JJ, Lichtenberg RC, et al: Anatomic correction of dextrotransposition of the great arteries in a 36-year-old patient. Mayo Clin Proc 1997;72:245-247.

28. Padalino MA, Stellin G, Brawn WJ, et al: Arterial switch operation after left ventricular retraining in the adult. Ann Thorac Surg 2000;70:1753-1757.

29. Poirier NC and Mee RB: Left ventricular reconditioning and anatomical correction for systemic right ventricular dysfunction: Semin Thorac Cardiovasc Surg Pediatr Card Surg Annu 2000;3:198-215.

30. Driscoll DJ, Offord KP, Feldt RH, et al: Five- to fifteen-year follow-up after Fontan operation. Circulation 1992;85:469-496.

31. Gewillig M, Wyse RK, de Leval MR, Deanfield JE: Early and late arrhythmias after the Fontan operation: Predisposing factors and clinical consequences. Br Heart J 1992;67:72-79.

32. Cromme-Dijkhuis AH, Hess J, Hahlen K, et al: Specific sequelae after Fontan operation at mid- and long-term follow-up: Arrhythmia, liver dysfunction, and coagulation disorders. J Thorac Cardiovasc Surg 1993;106:1126-1132.

33. Mertens L, Hagler DJ, Sauer U, et al: Protein-losing enteropathy after the Fontan operation: An international multicenter study. PLE study group. J Thorac Cardiovasc Surg 1998;115:1063-1073.

34. Gentles TL, Mayer JE, Gauvreau K, et al: Fontan operation in five hundred consecutive patients: Factors influencing early and late outcome. J Thorac Cardiovasc Surg 1997;114:376-391.

35. Driscoll DJ, Offord KP, Feldt RH, et al: Five-to fifteen-year follow-up after Fontan operation. Circulation 1992;85:469-496.

36. Bolger AP, Sharma R, Li W, et al: Neurohormonal activation and the chronic heart failure syndrome in adults with congenital heart disease. Circulation 2002;106:92-99.

37. The SOLVD Investigators: Studies of left ventricular dysfunction: Effect of enalapril on survival in patients with reduced ventricular ejection fractions and congestive heart failure. N Engl J Med 1991; 325:293-302.

38. Packer M, Poole-Watson PA, Armstrong PW, et al: Comparative effects of low and high doses of ACE inhibitor, lisinopril, on morbidity and mortality in chronic heart failure. Circulation 1999;100: 2312-2318.

39. Swedberg K, Held P, Kjekhus J, et al: Effects of the early administration of enalapril on mortality in patients with acute myocardial infarction: Results of the Cooperative New Scandinavian Enalapril Survival Study II. N Engl J Med 1992;327:678-684.

40. Pitt B, Martinez FA, Meurers GG, et al: Randomized trial of losartan vs. captopril in patients > 65 with heart failure (Evaluation of Losartan in the Elderly). Lancet 1997;349:747-752.

41. Riegger GAJ, Bouzo H, Petr P, et al: Improvement in exercise tolerance and symptoms of congestive heart failure during treatment with candesartan cilexetil. Circulation 1999;100: 2224-2230.

42. Pitt B, Zannad F, Remme WJ, et al, for the Randomized Aldactone Evaluation Study Investigators: The effect of spironolactone on morbidity and mortality in patients with severe heart failure. N Engl J Med 1999;341:709-717.

43. David KL, Nappi JM: The cardiovascular effects of eplerenone: A selective aldosterone receptor antagonist. Clin Ther 2003;25: 2647-2668.

44. CIBIS-II Investigators and Committees: The cardiac insufficiency study II (CIBIS): A randomized trial. Lancet 1999;353:9-13.

45. Hjalmarson A, Goldstein S, Fagerberg B, et al, the MERIT-HF Study Group: Effect of metoprolol CR/XL in chronic heart failure: Metoprolol CR/XL randomized intervention in congestive heart failure. JAMA 2000;283:1295-1302.

46. Fowler MB: Carvedilol prospective randomized cumulative survival (COPERNICUS) trial: Carvedilol in severe heart failure. Am J Cardiol 2004;93:35-39B.

47. Califf RM, Adams KF, McKenna WJ: A randomized controlled trial of epoprostenol therapy for severe congestive heart failure: The Flolan International Randomized Survival Trial (FIRST). Am Heart J 1997;134:44-54.

48. Reinhartz O, Copeland JG, Farrar DJ: Thoratec ventricular assist devices in children with less than 1.3 m² of body surface area. ASAIO J 2003;49:727-730.

49. Sadeghi AM, Marelli D, Talamo M, et al: Short-term bridge to transplant using the BVS 5000 in a 22-kg child. Ann Thorac Surg 2000;70:2151-2153.

50. Petrofski JA, Hoopes CW, Bashore TM, et al: Mechanical ventricular support lowers pulmonary vascular resistance in a patient with congenital heart disease. Ann Thorac Surg 2003;75:1005-1007.

51. Merkle F, Boettcher W, Stiller B, Hetzer R: Pulsatile mechanical cardiac assistance in pediatric patients with the Berlin heart ventricular assist device. J Extra Corpor Technol 2003;35:115-120.

52. Speziali G, Driscoll DJ, Danielson GK, et al: Cardiac transplantation for end-stage congenital heart defects: The Mayo Clinic experience. Mayo Cardiothoracic Transplant Team. Mayo Clin Proc 1998;73: 923-928.

53. Pigula FA, Gandhi SK, Ristich J, et al: Cardiopulmonary transplantation for congenital heart disease in the adult. J Heart Lung Transplant 2001;20:297-303.

54. Hopkins WE, Chen Z, Fukagawa NK, et al: Increased atrial and brain natriuretic peptides in adults with cyanotic congenital heart disease: Enhanced understanding of the relationship between hypoxia and natriuretic peptide secretion. Circulation 2004;109(23):2872-2877.

55. Moons P, Marquet K, Budts W, et al: Validity, reliability, and responsiveness of the "Schedule for the Evaluation of Individual Quality of Life–Direct Weighting" (SEIQoL-DW) in congenital heart disease. Health Qual Life Outcomes 2004;2:27.

56. Book WM: Heart failure in the adult patient with congenital heart disease. J Card Fail 2005;11:306-312.

CHAPTER 28

Heart Failure in Pediatric Pulmonary Diseases

Felix R. Shardonofsky

The cardiovascular and pulmonary systems act in a concerted fashion to transport respiratory gases and metabolic byproducts to and from peripheral tissues under varying metabolic demands and physiologic constraints; all of this is determined by organ systems and developmental states, and health or disease. Disorders affecting either the cardiovascular or the pulmonary system may alter the function and structure of the other as a result of mechanical,[1] autonomic,[2] and neurohumoral[3] interactions. Congestive heart failure can induce changes in the lungs and the right ventricle (see Chapter 16), whereas pulmonary diseases can lead to biventricular dysfunction and congestive heart failure.

Respiratory-induced cardiovascular abnormalities are summarized in Table 28-1. The severity of these abnormalities is influenced by the functional status of the cardiovascular system before the occurrence of the respiratory disturbance, the nature and severity of the respiratory disease process, the organ system's developmental state,[4] and genetic factors.[5] The manifestations of altered cardiovascular physiology in pulmonary diseases can dominate the clinical presentation, as occurs in persistent pulmonary hypertension of the newborn (PPHN) or massive pulmonary embolism,[7] or can be relatively silent, as occurs in systemic arterial hypertension associated with sleep-disordered breathing.[8]

In any case, cardiovascular compromise secondary to respiratory disorders is usually clinically significant because it is associated with increased morbidity and mortality rates.[6-9] This chapter reviews mechanical interactions between the respiratory and cardiovascular systems, pulmonary hypertension resulting from altered respiratory structure and function, right ventricular responses to acute increases in afterload, and pediatric respiratory disorders that most frequently cause heart failure.

CARDIOPULMONARY INTERACTION AND HEMODYNAMIC EFFECTS

Spontaneous Respiration

Breathing modulates the heart's loading conditions[1]; generates demands for oxygen, substrates, and blood flow as a result of respiratory muscle activity[10]; induces variations of autonomic regulation of cardiovascular physiology[11]; and influences the neuroendocrine control of sodium and water balance.[3] During spontaneous inspirations, pleural pressure (Ppl) decreases, causing an elevation in transpulmonary pressure (P_L), which increases the lung volume.[1] On expiration, the lung elastic recoil drives the lung volume back to its functional residual capacity (FRC). The inspiratory decrease in Ppl may range from a few centimeters of water during resting normal inspirations to a maximum of about -80 cm H_2O during loaded inspirations caused by extrathoracic or intrathoracic airway obstruction, airspace or interstitial lung disorders, or chest wall abnormalities.

The **cardiopulmonary interaction** is represented in a two-compartment model of the circulation in Figure 28-1. A decrease in Ppl causes a proportional increase in left ventricular transmural pressure and a decrease in right atrial pressure (P_{RA}).[12] Small decreases in P_{RA} during unloaded inspirations increase the pressure gradient for venous return, increasing the systemic venous return and the right ventricular preload and right ventricular stroke volume. In addition, the descent of the diaphragm increases intra-abdominal pressure, which further increases the venous pressure gradient between the thorax and the periphery. Larger decreases in P_{RA} associated with loaded inspirations produce no further increases in systemic venous return, however, because the venous system achieves a state of flow limitation in which venous flow is independent of P_{RA}.[13] This mechanical coupling between the ventilatory pump and the back pressure for venous return is physiologically significant in patients with congenital heart disease with cavopulmonary anastomoses because it allows the inspiratory muscles to promote pulmonary blood flow and cardiac output.[14]

TABLE 28-1

Cardiovascular Abnormalities Arising from Respiratory System Disorders
Alterations in right ventricular and left ventricular loading conditions
Ventricular systolic or diastolic dysfunction or both
Structural remodeling of the heart
Arrhythmias
Heart failure
Systemic arterial hypertension
Pulmonary vascular disease
Development of systemic-to-pulmonary collateral circulation
Hypertrophy of the systemic arterial supply to the lungs
Lung edema

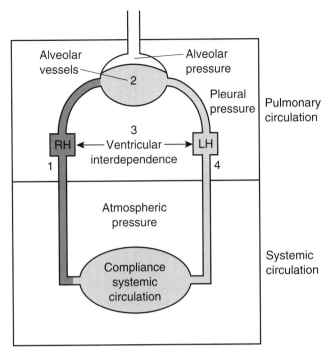

FIGURE 28-1 ■ **Cardiopulmonary interaction.** The two-compartment model of the circulation is shown. The right heart (RH) and the left heart (LH) are influenced by pleural (intrathoracic) pressure. The respiratory cycle alters cardiac output through the effect of intrathoracic pressure preload at (1) and afterload at (4) via change of alveolar pressure (2). Ventricular interaction also is seen at (3). (From Bohn D: *Cardiopulmonary Interaction*. In Chang AC, Hanley FL, Wernowsky G, et al [eds]: *Pediatric Cardiac Intensive Care*. Philadelphia, Williams & Wilkins, 1998.)

As the right ventricular end-diastolic volume (EDV) increases, the interventricular septum shifts to the left of its neutral position, and the left ventricular elastance increases as a result of **ventricular interdependence**, causing a reduction in left ventricular EDV.[15] Under conditions of severe airway obstruction, lung hyperinflation, and hypoxia, further increase in right ventricular EDV secondary to an enhanced right ventricular afterload, impaired left ventricular relaxation secondary to hypoxia,[16] or compression of the heart by stiff and hyperinflated lungs[17] can produce marked reductions in left ventricular preload and stroke volume. Although the transmission of Ppl to the left ventricular wall is attenuated by the pericardium,[18] the left ventricular transmural pressure and maximal systolic wall stress increase in proportion to the inspiratory descent in Ppl, causing a decrease in left ventricular stroke volume and an increase in myocardial oxygen consumption.[19] If severe, increases in systolic wall stress may decrease coronary perfusion, promoting an imbalance between myocardial oxygen consumption and oxygen supply that can cause myocardial hypoxia if the coronary flow reserve is limited. During normal inspirations, changes in left ventricular loading conditions decrease the systemic arterial pressure by about 10 mm Hg. On loaded inspirations, these mechanisms along with the transmission

of Ppl to the arterial system promote a greater decrease in arterial pressure, which is referred to as **pulsus paradoxus**.[20]

Although the mechanical load imposed by physiologic inspirations on normal ventricles causes only minor variations of heart function, it can produce a decrease in left ventricular output and myocardial ischemia under conditions of impaired inotropic function, decreased coronary blood flow, or increased peripheral oxygen consumption. These settings can be encountered in sepsis, myocardial infarction complicated with lung edema, myocardial disease, and weaning from mechanical ventilation.[21-23] In addition, an overwhelming increase in left ventricular afterload and hypoxia brought about by extrathoracic or intrathoracic airway obstruction can produce left ventricular dysfunction in a previously normal heart.[12,16,19] Lastly, an expiratory increase in Ppl resulting from dynamic lung hyperinflation secondary to intrathoracic flow limitation can decrease the systemic venous return and promote severe hypotension if hypovolemia or peripheral vasodilation concomitantly occurs.

Because the pulmonary vascular bed and the right ventricle exist within the thorax, changes in Ppl at constant lung volume (Mueller or Valsalva maneuver) do not alter the pressure gradient between the pulmonary vascular bed and the right ventricle.[1] Variations in lung volume cause passive elevations in **pulmonary vascular resistance (PVR)** and right ventricular afterload, however, which reflect variations in the pressure acting on the outer surface of lung vessels (Px).[1] For vessels within connective bronchovascular sheaths (i.e., extra-alveolar vessels), Px is a distending interstitial pressure proportional to the magnitude of Ppl.[25] Because extra-alveolar vascular transmural pressures and diameters are small at low lung volumes and increase with increasing volumes, the resultant flow resistance peaks at lung volumes less than FRC and decreases as lung volume rises above FRC.[26] For vessels within alveolar septa (i.e., alveolar vessels), Px is a compressive pressure equal to alveolar pressure (Palv),[25] and blood flow depends on the relative magnitudes of pulmonary artery (Ppa), left atrial (P_{LA}), and alveolar pressures.[26]

In regions where Ppa > Palv > P_{LA} (zone II state), alveolar vessels behave as Starling resistors, in which the back pressure to right ventricular ejection is Palv rather than P_{LA}.[1,25] An increase in lung volume increases the back pressure to right ventricular ejection because it requires an increase in Palv relative to Ppl, as P_L = Palv − Ppl. Accordingly, the magnitudes for Ppa and right ventricular systolic stress are increased. In regions where Palv > Ppa (zone state I), flow does not occur except in alveolar corner vessels, where Px < Palv, whereas in regions where P_{LA} > Palv, blood flow is determined by Ppa − P_{LA}, being independent of lung volume. As a result of serial resistance contributions, PVR reaches its nadir at FRC and increases as lung

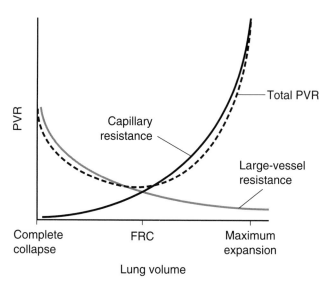

FIGURE 28-2 ■ Pulmonary vascular resistance (PVR) and lung volume relationship. PVR depends on the lung volume. As seen in the graph, the sum of the resistance (total PVR) is contributed by the large vessel resistance and the capillary resistance. At lung volumes less than functional residual capacity (FRC), the lungs are atelectatic, and the PVR increases as a result of compression of the larger vessels. As lung volume increases, and the alveoli become more expanded, PVR increases secondary to compression of the pulmonary capillaries. (From Meliones JN, Cheifetz IM: *Pulmonary physiology and heart lung interactions.* In Garson A, Bricker JT, Fisher DJ, et al [eds]: *The Science and Practice of Pediatric Cardiology.* Philadelphia, Williams & Wilkins, 1998, p. 298.)

volume departs from FRC in either direction (hypoinflation or hyperinflation) (Fig. 28-2).[26] These mechanisms explain in part the occurrence of passive elevations of PVR and right ventricular afterload in conditions associated with a decreased FRC, as seen in acute respiratory distress syndrome, and explain increases in PVR and right ventricular afterload in disorders that feature dynamic lung hyperinflation resulting from a severe asthma attack[27] or exercise in subjects with chronic airflow limitation.[28] During severe airway obstruction, marked decreases in Ppl, hypoxic pulmonary vasoconstriction, and left ventricular dysfunction[16,19] may alter the forces governing the fluid exchange in the lung microvasculature[29-31] and may induce stress failure of pulmonary capillaries,[32] causing lung edema (see Chapter 9).

Mechanical Ventilation

Mechanical ventilation can elicit beneficial or detrimental cardiovascular effects depending on a patient's cardiovascular and pulmonary states (i.e., the circulating blood volume, vascular resistances, myocardial reserve, autonomic control, lung volumes, intrathoracic pressures, and metabolic rate).[33] In the setting of a critical imbalance between oxygen consumption and oxygen supply, such as in circulatory shock or hypoxemic respiratory failure, mechanical ventilation can improve the oxygen delivery to peripheral tissues by abolishing spontaneous ventilation and reducing the oxygen cost from work of breathing. Provided that the cardiac output remains constant, a decrease in total oxygen consumption increases the values for mixed

venous and arterial partial pressure of oxygen even if the magnitude of the right-to-left shunting of blood is unchanged. Resumption of spontaneous inspirations during weaning from mechanical ventilation represents an exercise stress that increases left ventricular afterload and oxygen consumption, causing left ventricular failure or myocardial ischemia or both in patients with limited cardiovascular reserve.[23,24] Just as general muscle wasting can be observed with chronic heart failure, weakness of the respiratory muscles (including the diaphragm) alters respiratory mechanics. In this regard, it is likely that the current difficulty to predict weaning success using measurements of ventilatory and gas exchange function is due to the limited ability to assess a patient's cardiopulmonary reserve at the bedside.[33,34]

During inspirations produced by the delivery of positive pressure at the airway opening (i.e., **intermittent positive-pressure ventilation [IPPV]**), P_L increases as a result of an elevation in Palv relative to Ppl. Increases in Ppl depend on the compliances of the lung and chest wall.[35] The hemodynamic effects of IPPV are roughly proportional to the increase in airway pressure (Paw), but also depend on the magnitudes of Ppl, pericardial pressure, and lung volume, which vary in a complex manner, and the mechanical properties of the lung, chest wall, and pericardium. The analyses of the relationships between intrathoracic pressures and lung volume exceed the scope of this chapter but can be found in an excellent review.[33] An increase in Ppl causes an increase in P_{RA}, which promotes a decrease in systemic venous return,[12,13] and a decrease in left ventricular transmural pressure, which unloads the left ventricle. The latter can be reflected by an inspiratory increase in stroke volume and blood pressure, which is referred to as *reversed pulsus paradoxus.*[36,37]

When PVR is enhanced as a consequence of decreased lung volume and hypoxic pulmonary vasoconstriction, the institution of IPPV and **positive end-expiratory pressure (PEEP)** corrects alveolar hypoxia, promotes alveolar recruitment, and decreases sympathetic tone, resulting in a decrease in PVR and right ventricular afterload. Marked lung volume elevations as a result of the prescription of high PEEP levels or dynamic lung hyperinflation can increase the magnitudes for PVR and right ventricular afterload, however, and promote a decrease in right ventricular output and right ventricular ischemia.[38] A decreased systemic venous return secondary to Ppl and P_{RA} elevations, ventricular interdependence, and an increased diastolic ventricular elastance reflecting a restriction in diastolic ventricular expansion imposed by hyperinflated and stiff lungs all can contribute to decreasing the cardiac output further. Ultimately, these mechanisms reduce the effectiveness of IPPV as a life-sustaining intervention.[33] In this setting, a decrease in cardiac output is exacerbated by a decrease in stressed venous blood volume and mitigated by fluid administration.[39] The deleterious effects of IPPV and PEEP on right ventricular function and systemic venous returns can be attenuated by prescribing pressure-controlled ventilation, low tidal volumes, and prolonged expiratory times; avoiding prolonged high-PEEP levels; and restoring the intravascular volume.[40] Diverse modes of mechanical ventilation that produce similar changes in relevant intrathoracic pressures and work of breathing result in similar hemodynamic effects.

IPPV and PEEP promote the secretion of atrial natriuretic peptide and antidiuretic hormone by the right atrium and sympathetic activation, causing retention of water and electrolytes by the kidney.[3] During the course of these neurohormonal responses, the administration of hypotonic electrolyte solutions can produce severe hyponatremia, which can induce brain edema, lung edema, and death.[41,42] The institution of IPPV improves cardiac output in subjects and experimental animals with congestive heart failure.[24,36,43] In addition, therapy with **continuous positive airway pressure (CPAP)** in patients with acute congestive heart failure improves oxygenation, decreases the work of breathing, and, in some cases, increases the cardiac output.[44] CPAP therapy in patients with congestive heart failure and sleep-disordered breathing is associated with improved survival and functional capacity and decreased levels of neurohumoral activation, as reflected by decreased circulating norepinephrine and endothelin-1 (ET-1) concentrations.[45]

Because IPPV and high PEEP levels alter the mechanical coupling between inspiratory muscle activation and backpressure for venous return and dissociate the P_{RA} from right ventricular EDV,[33] positive-pressure ventilation has potential detrimental effects in patients with restrictive right ventricular physiology. This is a low cardiac output state that may occur after surgical repair of tetralogy of Fallot and is characterized by antegrade diastolic pulmonary arterial flow that is coincident with right atrial systole. The cardiac output in these patients is highly sensitive to the effects of increased Ppl, filling pressures and sinus rhythm. In this setting, negative extrathoracic pressure ventilation significantly increases the cardiac output by increasing systemic venous return.[46] Similar to spontaneous inspirations, inspirations achieved by mechanical delivery of subatmospheric (negative) pressure on the outer surface of the chest wall produce an increase in P_L as a result of a decrease in Ppl relative to Palv, which remains close to atmospheric pressure.

PULMONARY DISEASES AND THE CARDIOVASCULAR SYSTEM

Right Ventricular Function and Failure

Under physiologic postnatal conditions, the right ventricle pumps systemic venous blood returning to the heart into a low-resistance, high-capacitance pulmonary circulation, while keeping a low atrial pressure to optimize the rate of venous return. Left ventricular contraction provides significant assistance to the right ventricle, with about two thirds of the magnitudes of right ventricular pressure and volume output being accounted for by the left ventricular contraction.[47,48] The right ventricular function is pivotal to cardiovascular homeostasis when the right ventricular afterload is enhanced. This notion is exemplified by clinical data showing that the functional capacity and survival of patients with idiopathic pulmonary arterial hypertension are related to the values for cardiac output rather than to the magnitudes of Ppa and PVR. In this setting, the failure of the right ventricle reflects a mechanical uncoupling of the right ventricle from the pulmonary vascular bed.[49,50]

In the cardiac catheterization laboratory, the ventricular contractile properties and arterial input impedance can be assessed in terms of ventricular end-systolic elastance (Ees) and effective arterial elastance (Ea). Ees and Ea are estimated from the slopes of the end-systolic ventricular pressure-volume relationship and of systolic arterial pressure-stroke volume relationship, with the Ees-to-Ea ratio reflecting the degree of ventricular-arterial coupling efficiency.[50] A maximal mechanical efficiency (or the highest stroke work per myocardial oxygen consumption per beat) is achieved under physiologic loading conditions, in which the value for Ees doubles that for Ea. Decreasing Ees-to-Ea ratios reflect a progressive decline in ventricular-arterial coupling efficiency, with values for Ees/Ea less than 1 indicating a ventricle's inability to produce forward blood flow (see Chapters 7 and 8 for more detailed discussions).[50-52]

The forces opposing myocardial shortening or afterload include flow-resistive, elastic, inertial, and pulse-wave reflective components.[49] The right ventricular work can be partitioned into a steady component required to maintain a forward flow across the pulmonary vascular bed and a pulsatile component spent in the production of pulsatile waves in large pulmonary arteries. It has been shown in experimental animals that a proximal lesion of the pulmonary vascular bed, such as a reduction in main pulmonary artery diameter, can increase the pulmonary Ea and pulsatile component of right ventricular work, causing an increase in right ventricular afterload that is greater than that observed in animals with lung microvascular injury, despite the fact that both lesions produce similar elevations in Ppa.[53]

The right ventricular adaptation to an enhanced afterload depends on the rate of increase, the magnitude and duration of the afterload elevation, and the age of the patient. Increases in right ventricular afterload imposed perinatally are tolerated better than increases occurring after the physiologic remodeling of the right ventricle that turns the right ventricle into a thin-walled chamber, highly susceptible to acute afterload elevations.[54-56] When the right ventricular afterload is chronically enhanced, the right ventricle hypertrophies and is able to generate systolic pressures equal to or greater than systemic pressures for many years. In this condition, the right ventricular pressure volume relationship displays features that are similar to those pertaining to the left ventricle.[57]

An acute increase in right ventricular afterload that leads to right ventricular dysfunction can occur in disease states, such as acute pulmonary embolism,[7,58] PPHN,[6] pulmonary hypertensive crisis,[59] septic shock,[60-62] or acute respiratory distress syndrome.[63] The hemodynamic consequences of these conditions depend on the magnitude of the afterload and the underlying cardiopulmonary status.[64] Right ventricular dysfunction, heart failure, and eventually death may occur as a result of an augmented right ventricular wall stress, myocardial ischemia, ventricular interdependence, and impaired left ventricular output.[7,38,47,64]

As the right ventricular stroke volume declines in response to an elevated afterload, homeostatic mechanisms, including homeometric or heterometric myocardial regulation and endogenous catecholamine-mediated tachycardia and vasoconstriction, maintain the cardiac output and systemic arterial blood pressure within physiologic limits temporarily.[7] The right ventricular systolic pressure increases, attaining a maximum value of about approximately 40 mm Hg.[64] This increase and a prolongation of the right ventricular mechanical ejection cause an inversion of the transseptal pressure gradient,[65] resulting in flattening and a leftward shift of the interventricular septum at end systole.[66] Because the right ventricle has a low diastolic elastance,[67] a sudden increase in right ventricular afterload produces a marked dilation of the right ventricle and tricuspid regurgitation. The right ventricular end-systolic volume increases more than the right ventricular EDV, reflecting a decrease in right ventricular ejection fraction.[64] The left ventricular preload is reduced as a consequence of a decrease in right ventricular stroke volume, a diminished left ventricular compliance secondary to diastolic ventricular interdependence, and a decrease in the left ventricular systolic pressure and stroke volume.[47] The ventricular interdependence produces a positive feedback that progressively worsens cardiac function, as right ventricle–dependent reductions in left ventricular filling diminish the magnitude of the left ventricular systolic pressure, which decreases the left ventricular assistance to right ventricular function, further increasing the right ventricular volume and impairing left ventricular filling.[7,47] When homeostatic mechanisms become exhausted, aortic hypotension ensues,[7] promoting subendocardial ischemia in a setting of increased myocardial oxygen demand and increased ventricular wall stress.[38] During an acute increase in afterload, the maximal right ventricular function is determined by the right ventricular coronary perfusion and the left ventricular systolic function through mechanical interdependence.[47]

The clinical manifestations of these acute hemodynamic disturbances vary from subclinical right ventricular dysfunction to sudden death.[66,68,69] Classic signs of right ventricular failure include right ventricular heave; accentuated P₂; systolic murmur of tricuspid regurgitation; and, in some pediatric patients, jugular venous distention, edema, ascites, and hepatomegaly. Chest radiography is sometimes not useful in assessing pulmonary hypertension and right heart failure because right ventricular hypertrophy is not easily discernible. ECG can show right axis deviation and right ventricular hypertrophy. Echocardiography has been more useful in delineating cardiopulmonary interaction in pulmonary hypertension, with characteristic findings such as tricuspid valve regurgitation with a high velocity and flattening or paradoxical motion of the interventricular septum. Lastly, MRI also is essential in measuring ventricular dimensions.

In patients with right ventricular failure resulting from major **pulmonary embolism**, cardiac arrest, systemic arterial hypotension, and tissue hypoperfusion are associated with high mortality rates.[7] Acute and severe right ventricular dysfunction may be clinically silent until catastrophic complications ensue.[7,68] Cardiac biomarkers of right ventricular dysfunction, including serum concentrations of troponin and brain natriuretic peptide, which likely reflect the presence of myocardial microinfarctions and an enhanced ventricular wall stress, are being used along with echocardiography to identify patients with pulmonary embolism who may benefit from specific therapeutic interventions.[69] In **septic shock**, the right ventricular afterload typically is increased as a result of acute lung injury and cardiopulmonary interactions secondary to aggressive mechanical ventilation,[60] whereas the right ventricular mechanical efficiency is altered secondary to mechanisms that impair homeometric myocardial regulation, such as systemic hypotension, maldistribution of coronary blood flow, and decreased contractility secondary to inflammatory mediators and oxidative stress.[62]

Pulmonary Hypertension in the Neonatal Period

At birth, mechanical stresses caused by lung expansion and the increased alveolar pressure of oxygen associated with the onset of alveolar ventilation activate endothelium signaling pathways, which release vasodilator substances[70,71] to cause calcium-sensitive potassium channel activation[72] and pulmonary vasodilation. This sequence produces a decrease in PVR and an increase in pulmonary blood flow,[73] allowing pulmonary gas exchange. Concomitantly the cytoskeleton of endothelial and vascular smooth muscle cell remodels so that cells become thinner and spread around larger vascular lumens.[74] These physiologic processes can be perturbed by adverse stimuli or disease processes that cause lung vascular injury, lung developmental abnormalities, or congenital cardiovascular defects,[6,75] resulting in the syndrome referred to as **Persistent Pulmonary Hypertension of the Neonate (PPHN)** (Table 28-2).

Occasionally, PPHN occurs in the absence of abnormal obstetric history and concomitant cardiopulmonary disease. The syndrome of PPHN features pulmonary

TABLE 28-2

Factors Associated with Pulmonary Vascular Disease in Neonates

Pulmonary
    Aspiration of meconium, amniotic fluid, or blood
    ARDS due to surfactant deficiency
    Transient tachypnea
    Pulmonary hemorrhage
    Developmental abnormalities
        Pulmonary hypoplasia
        Congenital diaphragmatic hernia
        Cystic adenomatoid malformation
        Phrenic nerve agenesis
        Alveolar capillary dysplasia
        Pulmonary lymphangiectasia
    Pneumonia
    Thromboemboli
    Surfactant protein B deficiency
Infectious
    Group B streptococcus
    Listeria monocytogenes
    Escherichia coli
    Haemophilus influenzae
    Bordetella pertussis
Metabolic
    Hypoglycemia
    Hypocalcemia
    Acidosis
    Severe intrauterine or intrapartum hypoxia
Hematologic
    Polycythemia
    Thrombocytopenia
    Acute hemorrhage
    Anemia
Gastrointestinal
    Omphalocele
    Gut perforation
    Gastroschisis
Gestational
    Chronic asphyxia
    Postmaturity
    Premature ductal closure
    Maternal hypoxia, hemorrhage, hypotension
Drug induced
    Aspirin, indomethacin, naproxen
Cardiovascular disease
    Obstructive pulmonary venous drainage[75]
    LV inflow or outflow tract obstruction
    LV dysfunction

ARDS, acute respiratory distress syndrome; LV, left ventricular.
Modified from Kinsella JP, Abman SH: *Persistent pulmonary hypertension of the newborn: Strategies in clinical management*. In Peacock AJ (ed): *Pulmonary Circulation: A Handbook for Clinicians*. Chapman & Hall Medical, London, 1996, pp 437-448.)

hypertension, enhanced vascular reactivity, severe hypoxemia secondary to an increased PVR and varying degrees of intrapulmonary and extrapulmonary right-to-left shunting of blood, and structural vascular remodeling characterized by neomuscularization and hypertrophy of the media and adventitia of preacinar arteries.[6,74] Frequently, hypovolemia, systemic hypotension, and

impaired inotropic function secondary to hypoxia or sepsis may worsen the infant's hemodynamic status.[6,76]

The **mechanisms** of PPHN are not entirely understood. Experimentally, intrauterine hypoxia,[4] inflammation,[6] and pulmonary hypertension[77] have been shown to alter the expression of genes and signaling pathways that are crucial for normal pulmonary vascular adaptation to extrauterine life. Prenatal pulmonary hypertension caused by closure of the ductus arteriosus in fetal lambs decreases the expression of calcium-sensitive potassium channel mRNA[78] and vascular endothelial growth factor (VEGF).[79] The activation of calcium-sensitive potassium channels is required for a sustained postnatal pulmonary vasodilation,[72] whereas VEGF signaling pathway is pivotal for lung vascular growth during late gestation and normal endothelial cell function.[79] The arginine–nitric oxide (NO)–cGMP and prostacyclin pathways that mediate the oxygen-dependent and lung distention–induced pulmonary vasodilation are altered in PPHN.[4,6]

A diminished NO production may result from a decreased expression of endothelial NO synthase secondary to reduced VEGF expression[79] or neonatal hypoxia,[80] decreased serum arginine concentration,[81] or increased rate of cGMP inactivation by phosphodiesterase type 5. In a lamb model of congenital diaphragmatic hernia–induced lung hypoplasia, the NO-cGMP pathway was found to be intact, whereas the activation of ET-1 receptors was increased.[82] These data along with reported elevations in ET-1 serum concentrations in infants with PPHN[83] suggest that ET-1, which possesses potent lung vascular constrictor and promitogenic properties, could have a pathogenic role in PPHN. The release of other vaso-constrictor/promitogen substances, such as leukotrienes and thromboxane A_2, along with an enhanced endothelial cell adhesion to circulating white blood cells and the activation of endogenous vascular elastase likely contribute to produce this neonatal lung vascular disease.[6,84]

A **diagnosis** of PPHN is established in infants with hypoxic respiratory failure by the presence of a right-to-left or bidirectional ductal shunt, increased systolic Ppa, signs of enhanced right ventricular afterload, and absence of congenital heart defect on echocardiography.[6,85] Etiologic factors must be investigated thoroughly and addressed efficiently. Initial life-sustaining strategies include conventional mechanical ventilation with high fractions of oxygen, sedation, correction of hypovolemia and acidosis, and infusion of vasoactive and inotropic drugs.[85] A better knowledge of the molecular mechanisms regulating the transitional lung circulation has led to the development of inhaled NO therapy. This treatment improves oxygenation by reverting the extrapulmonary right-to-left shunting of blood and improving the matching of lung perfusion to alveolar ventilation, decreasing the degree of required ventilatory support and the need for extracorporeal support,[85-87] which is a last resort option.[88] In some cases, delivery of NO can be maximized by lung volume recruitment, accomplished by use of high-frequency oscillatory ventilation.[85] Some infants, particularly infants with congenital diaphragmatic hernia or sepsis, show a suboptimal or absent therapeutic response to NO despite an optimal delivery of the drug. In these cases, the addition of phosphodiesterase inhibitors,[89] adenosine (which activates A2 receptors and potassium-ATP channels),[90] or inhaled prostacyclin[91] may be beneficial.

Despite therapeutic advances, PPHN accounts for significant morbidity and mortality rates. Patients with **congenital diaphragmatic hernia** pose a major challenge because they have not experienced decrease in mortality rates or in extracorporeal membrane oxygenation use in response to inhaled NO therapy. A subset of infants with congenital diaphragmatic hernia who have a protracted course or late onset of pulmonary hypertension requiring prolonged mechanical ventilation or a second course of extracorporeal membrane oxygenation may benefit from noninvasive delivery of inhaled NO.[92] Lethal **lung dysplasias**, such as surfactant protein B deficiency, alveolar capillary dysplasia, or pulmonary lymphangiectasis, may mimic PPHN and should be suspected in infants who have dysmorphic features, organ system malformations, or failure to improve after 10 to 14 days on extracorporeal membrane oxygenation.[93]

"Pulmonary hypertension occurs in **surfactant deficiency-induced acute respiratory distress syndrome** as a result of alveolar hypoxia and a passive increase in PVR secondary to a decreased FRC.[94] Although pulmonary hypertension typically resolves with the resolution of the basic disease process, persistent pulmonary hypertension contributes to the morbidity and mortality of infants who develop severe **chronic lung disease of infancy (CLDI)**. The administration of low-dose inhaled NO to premature infants with acute respiratory distress syndrome caused significant decreases in mortality rate and occurrence of CLDI.[95]

Pulmonary Hypertension Beyond the Neonatal Period

Table 28-3 presents a diagnostic classification of disorders associated with pulmonary hypertension based on common physiologic features and pathobiologic mechanisms.[96] In adult patients with respiratory system disorders or hypoxemia, pulmonary hypertension generally is defined by the presence of resting values for mean or systolic Ppa greater than the corresponding 95% confidence intervals, or 20 mm Hg or 35 mm Hg.[97,98] Pulmonary vascular disease may occur in a wide variety of pediatric respiratory disorders (Table 28-4). Infants with CLDI typically show severe Ppa elevations, which may be exacerbated by hypoxia, acute lung inflammation triggered by infection, gastroesophageal reflux, or aspiration.

The pulmonary vascular disease resulting from **pediatric respiratory disorders** features varying degrees of vasoconstriction, enhanced vascular reactivity,[99-101]

TABLE 28-3

Classification of Pulmonary Hypertension
Pulmonary Arterial Hypertension
Idiopathic
Familial
Associated with
Collagen vascular disease
Congenital systemic-to-pulmonary shunts
Portal hypertension
HIV infection
Drugs and toxins
Others (thyroid disorders, glycogen storage disease, Gaucher disease, hereditary hemorrhagic telangiectasia, hemoglobinopathies, myeloproliferative disorders, splenectomy)
Associated with significant venous or capillary involvement
Pulmonary veno-occlusive disease
Pulmonary capillary hemangiomatosis
Persistent pulmonary hypertension of the newborn
Pulmonary Venous Hypertension
Left-sided atrial or ventricular heart disease
Left-sided valvular heart disease
Pulmonary Hypertension Associated with Lung Diseases or Hypoxemia or Both
Chronic obstructive pulmonary disease
Interstitial lung disease
Sleep-disordered breathing
Alveolar hypoventilation disorders
Chronic exposure to high altitude
Developmental abnormalities
Pulmonary Hypertension Due to Chronic Thrombotic or Embolic Disease or Both
Thromboembolic obstruction of proximal pulmonary arteries
Thromboembolic obstruction of distal pulmonary arteries
Nonthrombotic pulmonary embolism (tumor, parasites, foreign material)
Miscellaneous
Histiocytosis
Sarcoidosis
Takayasu arteritis
POEMS syndrome
Lymphangiomatosis
Compression of pulmonary vessels (adenopathy, tumor, fibrosing mediastinitis)

POEMS, Polyneuropathy, Organomegaly, Endocrinopathy, M protein, Skin changes
From Simonneau G, Galiè N, Rubin LJ, et al: *Clinical classification of pulmonary hypertension*. J Am Coll Cardiol 2004;43:5S-12S.

altered vascular structure, and impaired vascular growth[102,103] or loss of pulmonary vascular bed.[104] These abnormalities result from multiple mechanisms, among which alveolar hypoxia and endothelial cell injury are paramount (Table 28-5). Alveolar hypoxia results from hypobaric conditions, alveolar hypoventilation, or mismatching of ventilation to lung perfusion. Regardless of duration, alveolar hypoxia causes vasoconstriction of lung arterioles and venules by various mechanisms,

TABLE 28-4

Chronic Pulmonary Hypertension Associated with Disorders of the Respiratory System or Hypoxemia in Pediatric Patients

Obstructive ventilatory incapacity
   Chronic lung disease of infancy
      Bronchopulmonary dysplasia
      Congenital diaphragmatic hernia
      Meconium aspiration
      Persistent pulmonary hypertension of the newborn
      Neonatal pneumonia, sepsis
      Tracheoesophageal fistula
      Neuromuscular diseases
   Cystic fibrosis
   Bronchiectasis
   Bronchiolitis obliterans
   Langerhans histiocytosis
Restrictive ventilatory incapacity
   Lung hypoplasia
   Interstitial lung disorders, extrinsic allergic alveolitis
   Lung fibrosis
   Neuromuscular disease
   Kyphoscoliosis
Abnormalities of respiratory drive
   Central alveolar hypoventilation
   Sleep-disordered breathing
      Hypertrophy of tonsils and adenoids
      Craniofacial abnormalities
   Obesity-hypoventilation syndrome
Hypobaric hypoxemia

including a decrease in voltage-gated potassium channel conductance in vascular smooth muscle cells that induces cell membrane depolarization, opening of voltage-gated calcium channels, and increases of cytosolic calcium.[105] Hypoxia promotes the release of vasoconstrictor substances, such as ET-1 and serotonin from non–vascular smooth muscle cells.[106] Hypoxic pulmonary vasoconstriction improves the matching of ventilation to perfusion when alveolar hypoxia involves discrete fractions of lung, being a homeostatic mechanism to optimize

TABLE 28-5

Mechanisms Causing Pulmonary Hypertension or Modulating the Severity of Pulmonary Hypertensive Responses in Pediatric Respiratory Disorders or Both

Vasoconstriction (hypoxic and nonhypoxic)
Endothelial dysfunction
Alterations in vascular structure (remodeling)
Thrombosis in situ
Developmental abnormalities of pulmonary vasculature
Loss of pulmonary vascular bed
Lung volume–related changes in pulmonary vascular
   resistance
Genetic background
Development of systemic-pulmonary arterial collaterals
Left ventricular dysfunction

pulmonary gas exchange. Widespread alveolar hypoxia may cause maladaptive vascular responses, however, causing pulmonary hypertension or worsening of pulmonary hypertension unrelated to respiratory disorders. The magnitude of hypoxic pulmonary vasoconstriction is enhanced by decreases in blood pH.

Chronically, hypoxia modulates the transcription of an array of genes encoding for cytokines (interleukin [IL]-1, IL-8), growth factors (VEGF, platelet-derived growth factor, fibroblast growth factor), vasoactive substances (ET-1, NO, prostacyclin, angiotensin II), receptors (ET-1_A), and extracellular matrix proteins (fibronectin, tropoelastin) in lung vascular cells.[106-112] These cellular responses, which are influenced by the degree of lung development, cause structural arterial remodeling characterized by muscularization of nonmuscular precapillary arterioles, hypertrophy of the tunica media, intimal proliferation, adventitial thickening, and enhanced vasa vasorum density.[111-114] The hypertensive response to hypoxia is modulated by genetic polymorphisms[5] and is partially reversible when hypoxia is resolved.

Diverse noxious stimuli (including hypoxia, enhanced shear stress brought about by hypoxic pulmonary vasoconstriction, circulating proinflammatory mediators, and circulating reactive oxygen species) produced in lung disorders such as cystic fibrosis or CLDI may induce lung endothelial injury, which alters synthetic, cell adhesive, permeability, and hemostatic functions of endothelial cells. As a result, a functional imbalance occurs in pulmonary hypertension in which the endothelial production of vasoconstrictor, promitogenic, and prothrombotic molecules, such as ET-1, thromboxane A_2, leukotrienes, platelet-activating factor, and angiotensin II, is increased in detriment of the synthesis of vasodilator, antiproliferative, and antithrombotic products, such as NO and prostacyclin.[106-108] Alterations in endothelial permeability allow blood-borne substances to reach vascular tissues and activate the endogenous vascular elastase; this releases growth factors bound to extracellular matrix proteins, inducing cell proliferation and deposition of extracellular tissue matrix within vascular walls.[84] It has been shown that the expression of angiopoietin-1 mRNA, a protein involved in the recruitment of vascular smooth muscle cells around blood vessels, and the phosphorylation of TIE2, the endothelial receptor for angiopoietin-1, are up-regulated in lung tissues obtained from patients with pulmonary hypertension of diverse etiology.[115] Because angiopoietin-1 shuts off the expression of bone morphogenetic protein receptor 1A, a transmembrane protein required for bone morphogenetic protein receptor 2 signaling in pulmonary endothelial cells, this signaling pathway would provide a molecular link for all forms of pulmonary hypertension.

A reduced alveolar capillary density shown in autopsied lungs from patients with congenital diaphragmatic hernia, CLDI,[102,103] and cystic fibrosis[104] could increase the magnitude of the PVR and decrease the recruitment capacity of the lung vascular bed. A reduced vascular density in CLDI likely reflects an impaired angiogenesis secondary to premature birth and chronic inflammation resulting from life-support treatments,[102,103] whereas in cystic fibrosis it could be due to altered vascular development or apoptosis of alveolar septa secondary to chronic lung inflammation.[104] Apoptosis of alveolar septa could result from a disruption of VEGF signaling pathways between alveolar epithelial and endothelial cells[79] or may occur through VEGF-independent mechanisms, as shown in a murine model of acute malnutrition.[116]

Additional mechanisms, such as the development of systemic-to-pulmonary arterial collaterals,[100,117] left ventricular dysfunction,[118,119] and passive increases in PVR produced by changes in lung volume, may contribute to increase the magnitude of Ppa in select cases. Pulmonary hypertension can complicate the course of **interstitial lung disorders** resulting from systemic sclerosis, systemic lupus erythematosus, mixed connective tissue disorder,[120] hypersensitivity pneumonitis, sarcoidosis,[121] and Langerhans cell histiocytosis.[122] In some patients with systemic sclerosis, the severity of pulmonary hypertension seems to be proportional to the magnitude of the restrictive ventilatory defect as reflected by the occurrence of proportional decreases in forced vital capacity and carbon monoxide diffusion in the lung. In other cases, pulmonary hypertension severity exceeds that of the lung parenchymal involvement, as indicated by decreases in carbon monoxide diffusion in the lung greater than those of vital capacity. The clinical course of the latter group of patients is more severe than the course experienced by the former, being similar to that reported for patients with idiopathic pulmonary hypertension. Therapy with bosentan,[123] a dual ET-1 receptor antagonist, and treprostinil,[124] a prostacyclin analogue, has been shown to produce short-term improvement in patients with pulmonary hypertension associated with connective tissue disorders.

Bronchopulmonary dysplasia or CLDI represents the final pathway of a heterogeneous group of pulmonary disorders that start in the neonatal period.[117] In most cases, bronchopulmonary dysplasia results from premature birth with injury to the immature lung caused by life-sustaining therapies.[102,103] CLDI is defined by the presence of persistent respiratory symptoms and signs, hypoxemia, and abnormal findings on chest radiography at 36 weeks' corrected age.[117] The epidemiology of CLDI has changed over time. Classic bronchopulmonary dysplasia typically occurs in infants born in the late saccular or alveolar phase of airspace development and features varying degrees of lung fibrosis, atelectasis, and alveolar overexpansion; marked remodeling of the airways; and vascular involvement with hypertrophy and peripheral extension of vascular smooth muscle. Advances in perinatal care since the 1980s have led to the survival of preterm infants born in the early

saccular phase of airspace development, and as a consequence of the injury in severely immature lungs, the bronchopulmonary dysplasia that develops is characterized by less severe fibrosis and cellular proliferation and marked arrest of alveolar development.[102,114] Cardiovascular abnormalities in CLDI include pulmonary hypertension, marked lung vascular reactivity,[99,101] impaired vascular permeability, remodeling of the lung vascular bed, development of systemic-to-pulmonary collateral vessels, atrioventricular valve incompetence, biventricular hypertrophy, progressive ventricular dysfunction, subendocardial ischemia, and systemic hypertension.[100]

Severe pulmonary hypertension contributes to the morbidity and mortality of patients with CLDI.[17] In patients with CLDI who require prolonged mechanical ventilation, close follow-up with ECG and echocardiogram looking for evidence of unresolved or worsening of pulmonary hypertension is warranted. In patients with severe pulmonary hypertension, cardiac catheterization studies are indicated to rule out undiagnosed congenital heart defects, assess the severity of the pulmonary hypertension and the degree of lung vascular reactivity to oxygen and vasodilator drugs, and determine whether large systemic-to-pulmonary collaterals are present.[100] Select patients may benefit from closure of an atrial septal defect (which in a healthy patient would be hemodynamically insignificant) and long-term therapy with vasodilator agents.[125]

Cystic fibrosis is a multisystemic disorder produced by mutations of the gene that encodes the cystic fibrosis transmembrane regulator protein. It typically causes a persistent endobronchial infection and inflammation that bring about airflow limitation, altered gas exchange, and bronchiectasis; ultimately, respiratory insufficiency and death ensue. Similar to bronchopulmonary dysplasia, hypoxemia as a result of small airway obstruction is a common feature.

Cardiovascular complications resulting from cystic fibrosis-related lung disease include hypertrophy of the systemic arterial supply to the lung, pulmonary hypertension, and ventricular dysfunction. Hypertrophy of the systemic arterial supply to the lung can cause life-threatening hemoptysis. Current treatment involves a diagnostic angiographic examination of the systemic arteries of the lungs followed by selective embolization of dysplastic arteries exposed to systemic blood pressure.[126]

Chronic pulmonary hypertension in cystic fibrosis likely develops after temporary elevations of Ppa during exacerbations of lung inflammation, sleep-induced hypoxemia, and exercise.[127,128] The prevalence of pulmonary hypertension increases with lung disease progression, as reflected by measurements of ventilatory capacity[118,129] and indices of oxygenation.[9] The pathogenesis of pulmonary hypertension in cystic fibrosis–related lung disease has not been investigated systematically. The aforementioned mechanisms of pulmonary hypertension likely have a pathogenic role in cystic fibrosis–induced pulmonary hypertension.

Right ventricular hypertrophy and heart failure with its ominous prognosis were recognized in early studies.[129-131] Since the 1980s, the incidence of overt heart failure in cystic fibrosis has declined as a result of the treatment of chronic hypoxia with supplemental oxygen. Subclinical heart abnormalities, such as reductions in right ventricular ejection fraction,[132] right ventricular free wall excursion amplitude,[133] and systolic Doppler tissue velocities,[134] have been shown in stable patients with moderate-to-severe cystic fibrosis–related lung disease studied at rest. These changes likely reflect an increased right ventricular afterload, rather than right ventricular systolic dysfunction,[133] because the resting cardiac index[118,128,129] and right ventricular end-systolic pressure volume relationships[135] have been reported to be within normal ranges in cystic fibrosis patients studied at rest. During submaximal exercise, patients having values for forced expiratory volume in 1 second greater than 56% of predicted showed a limited stroke volume recruitment and an enhanced chronotropic response.[136] In some patients with advanced lung disease, prolonged right ventricular isovolumic relaxation times[133] and diastolic Doppler tissue velocities[119] and elevated pulmonary capillary wedge pressure values[118,129] reflect the occurrence of diastolic right or left ventricle dysfunction or both. These sequelae could be a consequence of chronic hypoxemia, circulating inflammatory mediators secondary to lung inflammation,[134,137] activation of the renin-angiotensin-aldosterone system,[138,139] ventricular interdependence, malnutrition, hypovitaminosis,[140] and microvascular complications of poorly controlled cystic fibrosis–related diabetes mellitus.

The diagnosis and treatment of sleep-related hypoxia resulting from ventilation-perfusion mismatch or **obstructive sleep-disordered breathing (OSDB)** are the most important interventions to minimize the development of pulmonary hypertension in cystic fibrosis. In select patients with advanced cystic fibrosis–induced lung disease and severe pulmonary hypertension, the administration of inhaled vasodilator drugs, such as iloprost, which allow a more selective pulmonary vasodilation than that achieved by vasodilator substances delivered intravenously, may be beneficial as a bridge for lung transplantation.[141]

The etiologic factors of obstruction to airflow in the upper airway of children include craniofacial disorders, subglottic stenosis, choanal atresia, neuromuscular weakness, and hypertrophy of the tonsillar adenoids. OSDB and **Cheyne-Stokes respiration-central sleep apnea (CSR-CSA)** syndrome embody a spectrum of abnormalities involving the control of breathing during sleep that may cause cardiovascular disease and increased morbidity and mortality of patients with underlying cardiovascular pathology.[8,142] **OSDB** is a common condition that features repetitive episodes of inspiratory flow limitation or cessation of inspiratory flow (i.e., obstructive sleep apnea [OSA]), resulting from altered upper airway geometry, impaired upper airway muscle function during sleep, and genetic factors.[143] CSR-CSA events, which occur in about 40% of adult subjects with congestive heart failure, represent a form of periodic breathing in which apnea and hypopnea alternate with ventilatory periods, having a crescendo and decrescendo pattern of tidal volume.[143] OSDB events cluster during rapid-eye-movement sleep, whereas CSR-CSA events typically occur during non–rapid-eye-movement sleep, a state in which metabolic-chemical mechanisms are the main influence on the control of ventilation.

In patients with congestive heart failure, concerted effects of stimulation of vagal receptors by increased left ventricular volumes, increased left ventricular end-diastolic pressure (EDP), passive lung congestion, enhanced chemoreceptor sensitivity, hypoxia, variations in sleep state and arousals, prolonged circulatory time, and upper airway instability promote respiratory control system instability. This instability causes fluctuations of $Paco_2$ below and above the apneic threshold that result in apnea alternating with hyperventilation (Fig. 28-3).[144] OSA and CSR-CSA may coexist in patients with congestive heart failure, in whom physiologic stresses imposed by OSA during the beginning of the night may worsen left ventricular function, setting the stage for the occurrence of CSR-CSA later in the same night.[143]

The mechanisms linking OSDB and cardiovascular disease include alterations in the heart's loading conditions, blood gas composition, cardiovascular autonomic regulation, hemostatic and endocrine functions, and inflammation.[143] These changes often operate in conjunction with other risk factors for cardiovascular disease, such as obesity, hypertension, and diabetes mellitus. Episodes of obstructive hypoventilation and OSA are associated with inspiratory efforts against a narrowed (obstructive hypoventilation) or occluded (OSA) upper airway (see loaded inspiration in this chapter), hypoxia with or without hypercapnia, and arousals from sleep (Fig. 28-4). These mechanisms along with chemoreceptor and baroreceptor activation increase the sympathetic neural outflow, producing peripheral vasoconstriction, hypertension, tachycardia, and increased myocardial oxygen consumption.[143] These cardiovascular stresses increase left ventricular afterload[145]; impair myocardial relaxation, which raises left ventricular EDP[16]; and alter the matching of myocardial oxygen supply to oxygen demand. As a result, the cardiac output decreases during OSA, tachycardia and hypertension occur by the end of apnea and early postapnea ventilatory period,[143] and myocardial ischemia may develop in subjects with coronary flow limitation.[146] Hypoxia, hypercapnia, acidosis, and, in some cases, the transmission of an elevated left ventricular EDP to the pulmonary arterial bed[147] all increase the Ppa and right ventricular afterload, which contribute to decrease the cardiac output.

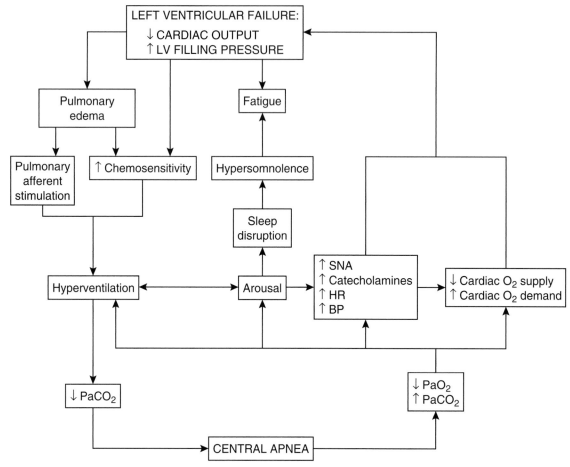

FIGURE 28-3 ■ Mechanisms causing central sleep apnea in congestive heart failure (see text for details). BP, blood pressure; HR, heart rate; LV, left ventricular; SNA, sympathetic nerve activity. (From Leung RST, Bradley TD: *Sleep apnea and cardiovascular disease. Am J Respir Crit Care Med* 2001;164: 2147-2165.)

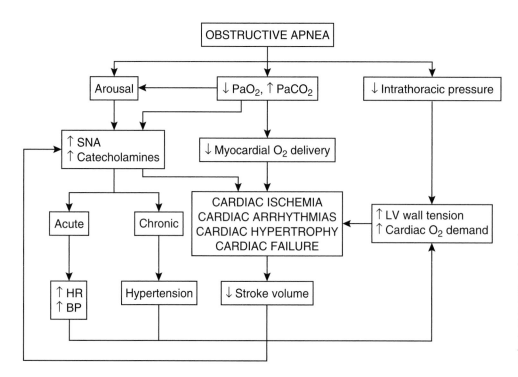

FIGURE 28-4 ■ Effects of obstructive disordered breathing on the cardiovascular system (see text for details). BP, blood pressure; HR, heart rate; LV, left ventricular; SNA, sympathetic nerve activity. (From Leung RST, Bradley TD: *Sleep apnea and cardiovascular disease. Am J Respir Crit Care Med* 2001;164: 2147-2165.)

OSDB events are ended by arousals from sleep, which activate dilator upper airway muscles, restore airway patency and alveolar ventilation, and bring resolution to acute functional changes elicited by OSA and obstructive hypoventilation events.[143] Changes of enhanced sympathetic nervous system activity[148,149] and altered chemoreceptor and baroreceptor sensitivities.[150] are sustained into wakefulness, promoting a decrease in heart rate variability and increase in blood pressure variability.[148,151] Recurrent hypoxia and reoxygenation bring about conditions resembling ischemia-reperfusion[152] and induce the production of radical oxygen species and proinflammatory substances, such as tumor necrosis factor-α, IL-6 and IL-1β, and platelet aggregation and up-regulation of vascular adhesion molecules.[153] This proinflammatory state may promote myocardial dysfunction and remodeling, atherosclerosis, and endothelial dysfunction. The last mentioned is reflected by enhanced production of ET-1,[154] decreased production of NO,[155] and impaired endothelium-dependent vasodilation.[156] OSDB also causes a prothrombotic state that features blood hyperviscosity; platelet activation; elevated levels of fibrinogen, thrombin-antithrombin complexes, and tissue plasminogen inhibitor-1[157]; insulin resistance; and altered release of growth hormone, corticosteroids, and adipokines.[158]

Sustained systemic arterial hypertension, which is the most important risk factor for the development of coronary artery disease, heart failure, and stroke, may develop in children[159-161] and adults with OSDB.[162,163] A causative association between OSDB and hypertension is supported by results obtained in animal models[164] and the reductions in blood pressure and neural sympathetic activity experienced in response to treatments for OSDB.[163,165,166] Enhanced arterial stresses induced by OSDB may be particularly deleterious in patients with connective tissue disorders, such as Marfan syndrome, in whom treatment of OSDB may arrest the progression of aortic root dilation.[167]

In infants and children, OSDB has been shown to cause sustained elevations in Ppa that may bring about hypertrophy, dysfunction, and failure of the right ventricle.[168-173] In most of these cases, tonsillectomy or adenoidectomy (or both) or continuous positive airway pressure therapy produces a rapid improvement of pulmonary hemodynamics, suggesting that hypoxia-induced vasoconstriction is pivotal in the pathogenesis of pulmonary hypertension associated with OSDB in pediatric patients. In adults, a link between OSDB and daytime pulmonary hypertension has been questioned because of confounding factors in many studies. Studies have confirmed that mild elevations of Ppa may occur during wakefulness in adult subjects with OSA in the absence of lung disease. The prevalence of resting pulmonary hypertension ranges from 17% to 53%[174-177] whereas exertional pulmonary hypertension may occur in 80% of cases.[174] Notably, more than one half of these cases had

elevated values for pulmonary capillary wedge pressure at rest and during exercise. Continuous positive airway pressure treatment for 6 months reduces the values for mean Ppa in normotensive and hypertensive subjects.[174]

Systemic hypertension is the most frequent cause of left ventricular hypertrophy in these patients. In patients with OSA, left ventricular hypertrophy also may occur in the absence of hypertension,[168,178] however, as a result of cumulative effects of loaded inspirations, episodic hypoxia,[179] sympathetic activation, and increased circulating concentrations of IL-6 and IL-1β.[180] Asymptomatic left ventricular systolic[181] and diastolic[182] dysfunction during wakefulness have been reported in 7% and 37% of adults with OSA in the absence of coronary artery disease. Among patients with congestive heart failure and systolic dysfunction, the prevalence of OSA seems to be higher than that in healthy adults,[183] ranging from 11% to 37%.[184,185] A high prevalence of OSA also is reported in adults having congestive heart failure and diastolic left ventricular failure in whom a nadir value for pulse oximetry less than 70% was an independent predictor of an abnormal myocardial relaxation pattern.[182] Nighttime pulmonary edema or recurrent pulmonary edema can be a sign of OSDB-induced left ventricular failure and hypoxia in adult[186] and pediatric patients.[187] Systemic hypertension, hypoxia, myocardial ischemia, elevated neural sympathetic output, and humoral factors associated with OSDB are believed to cause cardiomyocyte injury[143] and contribute to worsen coexisting heart disease.[188,189]

Treatment of OSDB in patients with dilated cadiomyopathy and congestive heart failure[189,190] produces significant improvement in left ventricular ejection fraction and functional capacity.[188] Collectively, these data indicate that OSDB contributes to the pathophysiology and progression of heart failure. Although CSR-CSA is not associated with loaded inspirations, its physiologic burden is similar to that imposed by OSA in several respects. Episodes of CSR-CSA elicit profound hypoxemia, arousals from sleep, sleep fragmentation, sympathetic nervous activation, and oscillations of heart rate and blood pressure.[143] The last mentioned are related to oscillations in ventilation, reflecting a phase linking central sympathetic neuronal output to central respiratory drive. The heart rate and blood pressure variations are dominated by low-frequency contents that reflect an impaired autonomic regulation and sympathetic activation and portends an increased risk of death in congestive heart failure. Atrial overdrive pacing in patients with sleep-disordered breathing who were not in heart failure significantly decreased the prevalence of OSA and CSR-CSA, suggesting that stimuli originating from the heart are important in the control of breathing during sleep.[191] Cardiovascular stresses elicited by CSR-CSA predispose to malignant arrhythmias and sudden death, which occur in approximately 25% of patients with congestive heart failure.[192] Because CSR-CSA is an

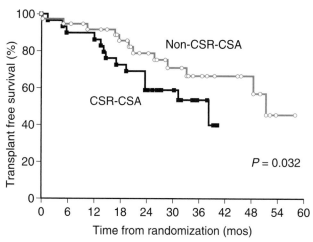

FIGURE 28-5 ■ Heart failure and Cheyne-Stokes respiration–central sleep apnea (CSR-CSA). Kaplan-Meier plots obtained in patients with congestive heart failure. The curves indicate that patients experiencing CSR-CSA had a significantly shorter survival than patients without CSR-CSA. (From Sin DD, Logan AG, Fitzgerald FS, et al: *Effects of continuous positive airway pressure on cardiovascular outcomes in heart failure patients with and without Cheyne-Stokes respiration.* Circulation 2000;102:61-66.)

independent risk factor for increased risk of death and heart transplantation (Fig. 28-5), it should be a therapeutic target after pharmacologic management has been maximized. Continuous positive airway pressure therapy has been shown to increase the functional capacity, left ventricular ejection fraction, and survival of patients with congestive heart failure (Fig. 28-6).[45]

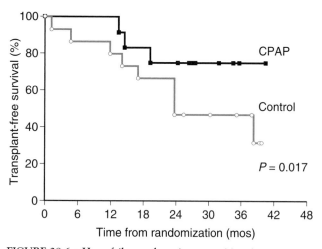

FIGURE 28-6 ■ Heart failure and continuous positive airway pressure (CPAP) treatment. Kaplan-Meier plots obtained in patients with congestive heart failure and Cheyne-Stokes respiration–central sleep apnea show that patients who were treated with CPAP and complied with therapy experienced a greater rate of heart transplant–free time than patients who did not receive treatment of sleep-disordered breathing. (From Sin DD, Logan AG, Fitzgerald FS, et al: *Effects of continuous positive airway pressure on cardiovascular outcomes in heart failure patients with and without Cheyne-Stokes respiration.* Circulation 2000;102:61-66.)

CURRENT STATUS AND FUTURE TRENDS

Heterogeneous disease processes involving the respiratory system can alter the heart's loading conditions, autonomic cardiovascular regulation, structure and function of the systemic and pulmonary vascular beds, hemostasis, and inflammation. These mechanisms can induce a wide range of unfavorable cardiovascular responses, depending on baseline cardiovascular status, developmental state of organ systems involved, nature of the morbid condition, and genetics.

In general terms, cardiovascular involvement significantly increases morbidity and mortality rates in patients with respiratory disorders. In some cases, the diagnosis of cardiovascular compromise requires a high index of suspicion and allows the implementation of therapeutic strategies based on physiologic principles. Therapy has been limited to oxygen, diuretics, and pharmacologic agents directed at lowering PVR, such as prostanoids, calcium channel blockers, angiotensin-converting enzyme inhibitors, and nitrates. Lung transplantation is the last therapeutic option. Much more insight needs to be developed via clinical investigations in the clinical realms of cardiopulmonary interaction and disease states in children.[193,194]

Key Concepts

■ The manifestations of altered cardiovascular physiology in pulmonary diseases can dominate the clinical presentation, as occurs in PPHN or massive pulmonary embolism, or can be relatively silent, as occurs in systemic arterial hypertension associated with sleep-disordered breathing.

■ As the right ventricular EDV increases, the interventricular septum shifts to the left of its neutral position, and the left ventricular elastance increases as a result of ventricular interdependence, causing a reduction in left ventricular EDV. Under conditions of severe airway obstruction, lung hyperinflation, and hypoxia, further increases in right ventricular EDV secondary to an enhanced right ventricular afterload, impaired left ventricular relaxation secondary to hypoxia, or compression of the heart by stiff and hyperinflated lungs can produce marked reductions in left ventricular preload and stroke volume.

■ Although the mechanical load imposed by physiologic inspirations on normal ventricles causes minor variations of heart function, it can produce a decrease in left ventricular output and myocardial ischemia under conditions of impaired inotropic function, decreased coronary blood flow, or increased peripheral oxygen consumption.

■ As a result of serial resistance contributions, PVR reaches its nadir at FRC and increases as lung volume departs from FRC in either direction (hypoinflation or hyperinflation).

■ The deleterious effects of IPPV and PEEP on right ventricular function and systemic venous returns can be attenuated by prescribing pressure-controlled ventilation, low tidal volumes, and prolonged expiratory times; avoiding prolonged high PEEP levels; and restoring the intravascular volume.

■ The institution of IPPV improves cardiac output in subjects and experimental animals with congestive heart failure. In addition, therapy with continuous positive airway pressure in patients with acute congestive heart failure improves oxygenation, decreases the work of breathing, and, in some cases, increases cardiac output.

■ As the right ventricular stroke volume declines in response to an elevated afterload, homeostatic mechanisms, including homeometric or heterometric myocardial regulation and endogenous catecholamine-mediated tachycardia and vasoconstriction, maintain cardiac output and systemic arterial blood pressure within physiologic limits temporarily.

■ Because the right ventricle has a low diastolic elastance, a sudden increase in right ventricular afterload produces a marked dilation of the right ventricle and tricuspid regurgitation.

■ The pulmonary vascular disease resulting from pediatric respiratory disorders features varying degrees of vasoconstriction, enhanced vascular reactivity, altered vascular structure, and impaired vascular growth or loss of pulmonary vascular bed. These abnormalities result from multiple mechanisms, among which alveolar hypoxia and endothelial cell injury are paramount.

■ A functional imbalance occurs in pulmonary hypertension in which the endothelial production of vasoconstrictor, promitogenic, and prothrombotic molecules, such as ET-1, thromboxane A_2, leukotrienes, platelet-activating factor, and angiotensin II, is increased in detriment of the synthesis of vasodilator, antiproliferative, and antithrombotic products, such as NO and prostacyclin.

■ CLDI is defined by the presence of persistent respiratory symptoms and signs, hypoxemia, and abnormal findings on chest radiography at 36 weeks' corrected age. Cardiovascular abnormalities in CLDI include pulmonary hypertension, marked lung vascular reactivity, impaired vascular permeability, remodeling of the lung vascular bed, development of systemic-to-pulmonary collateral vessels, atrioventricular valve incompetence, biventricular hypertrophy, progressive ventricular dysfunction, subendocardial ischemia, and systemic hypertension.

■ Cardiovascular complications resulting from cystic fibrosis–related lung disease include hypertrophy of the systemic arterial supply to the lung, pulmonary hypertension and ventricular dysfunction.

In patients with congestive heart failure, concerted effects of hypocapnia secondary to stimulation of vagal receptors by increased left ventricular volumes, increased left ventricular EDP, passive lung congestion, enhanced chemoreceptor sensitivity, hypoxia, variations in sleep state and arousals, prolonged circulatory time, and upper airway instability promote respiratory control system instability.

■ Sustained systemic arterial hypertension, which is the most important risk factor for the development of coronary artery disease, heart failure, and stroke, may develop in children and adults with OSDB.

REFERENCES

1. Permutt S, Wise RA, Brower RG: How changes in pleural pressure cause changes in afterload and preload. In Scharf SM, Cassidy SS (eds): Heart-Lung Interactions in Health and Disease. Lung Biology in Health and Disease, vol 42. New York, Marcel Dekker, 1989, pp 243-250.

2. De Burgh Daly M: Interactions between respiration and circulation. In Fishman A, Cherniack NS, Widdicombe JG (eds): Handbook of Physiology, Sect 3, vol II. American Physiological Society, Baltimore, 1986, pp 529-594.

3. Said SM: Neurohumoral aspects of respiratory-cardiovascular interactions. In Scharf SM, Pinsky MR, Magder S (eds): Respiratory- Circulatory Interactions in Health and Disease. Lung Biology in Health and Disease, vol 157. New York, Marcel Dekker, 2001, pp 427-445.

4. Haworth SG, Hislop AA: Lung development: The effects of chronic hypoxia. Semin Neonatol 2003;8:1-8.

5. Eddahibi S, Chaouat A, Morrell N, et al: Polymorphism of the serotonin transporter gene and pulmonary hypertension in chronic obstructive pulmonary disease. Circulation 2003;108:1839-1841.

6. Morin FC III, Stenmark KR: Persistent pulmonary hypertension of the newborn. Am J Respir Crit Care Med 1995;151:2010-2032.

7. Wood KE: Major pulmonary embolism: Review of a pathophysiolgic approach to the golden hour of hemodynamically significant pulmonary embolism. Chest 2002;121:877-905.

8. Shahar E, Whitney CW, Redline S, et al: Sleep-disordered breathing and cardiovascular disease: Cross-sectional results of the Sleep Heart Disease Health Study. Am J Respir Crit Care Med 2001;163:19-23.

9. Fraser KL, Tullis DE, Sasson Z, et al: Pulmonary hypertension and cardiac function in adult cystic fibrosis. Chest 1999;115:1321-1328.

10. Roussos C, Macklem PT: The respiratory muscles. N Engl J Med 1982;307:786-797.

11. Taha BH, Simon PM, Dempsey JA, et al: Respiratory sinus arrhythmia in humans: An obligatory role for vagal feedback from the lungs. J Appl Physiol 1995;78:638-645.

12. Bronberger-Barnea B: Mechanical effects of inspiration on heart function: A review. Fed Proc 1981;40:2172-2177.

13. Guyton AC, Lindsey AW, Abernathy B, Richardson T: Venous return at various right atrial pressures and the normal venous return curve. Am J Physiol 1957;189:609-615.

14. Redington AN, Penny D, Shinebourne EA: Pulmonary blood flow after total cavopulmonary shunt. Br Heart J 1991;65:213-217.

15. Santamore WP, Dell'Italia LJ: Ventricular interdependence: Significant left ventricular contributions to right ventricular systolic function. Prog Cardiovasc Dis 1998;40:289-308.

16. Cargill RI, Kiely DG, Lipworth BJ: Adverse effects of hypoxaemia on diastolic filling in humans. Clin Sci (Lond) 1995;89:165-169.

17. Cassidy SS, Wead WB, Seibert GB, Ramanathan M: Changes in left ventricular geometry during spontaneous breathing. J Appl Physiol 1987;63:803-811.

18. Takata M, Mitzner W, Robotham JL: Influence of the pericardium on ventricular loading during respiration. J Appl Physiol 1990;68:1640-1650.

19. Buda AJ, Pinsky MR, Ingels NB Jr, et al: Effect of intrathoracic pressure on left ventricular performance. N Engl J Med 1979;301:453-459.

20. Viola AR, Puy RJ, Goldman E: Mechanisms of pulsus paradoxus in airway obstruction. J Appl Physiol 1990;68:1927-1931.

21. Beach T, Millen E, Grenvik A: Hemodynamic response to discontinuance of mechanical ventilation. Crit Care Med 1973;1:85-90.

22. Hurford WE, Lynch KE, Strauss HW, et al: Myocardial perfusion as assessed by thallium-201 scintigraphy during the discontinuation of mechanical ventilation in ventilator-dependent patients. Anesthesiology 1991;74:1007-1016.

23. Lemaire F, Teboul JL, Cinotti L, et al: Acute left ventricular dysfunction during unsuccessful weaning from mechanical ventilation. Anesthesiology 1988;69:171-179.

24. Beach T, Millen E, Grenvick A: Hemodynamic response to discontinuance of mechanical ventilation. Crit Care Med 1973;1:85-90.

25. Permutt S, Brower RG: Mechanical support of blood vessels. In Crystal R, West JB, Barnes PJ, Weibel ER (eds): The Lung: Scientific Foundations, vol II. Philadelphia, Lippincott-Raven, 1997, pp 1447-1445.

26. Fishman A: Pulmonary circulation: Interactions between respiration and circulation. In Fishman A, Fisher AB (eds): Handbook of Physiology, Sect 3, vol I. American Physiological Society, Baltimore, 1985, pp 931-965.

27. Permutt S: Relation between pulmonary artery pressure and pleural pressure during acute asthmatic attack. Chest 1973;63:S25-S28.

28. Butler J, Schirijen F, Henriquez A, et al: Cause of the raised wedge pressure on exercise in chronic obstructive pulmonary disease. Am Rev Respir Dis 1988;138:350-354.

29. Stalcup SA, Mellins RB: Mechanical forces producing pulmonary edema in asthma. N Engl J Med 1977;297:592-956.

30. Lee KW, Downes JJ: Pulmonary edema secondary to laryngospasm in children. Anesthesiology 1983;59:347-349.

31. Oswalt CE, Gates GA, Holmstrom MG: Pulmonary edema as a complication of acute airway obstruction. JAMA 1977;238:1833-1835.

32. West JB: Pulmonary capillary stress failure. J Appl Physiol 2000; 89:2483-2489.

33. Pinsky MR: Hemodynamic effects of ventilation and ventilatory maneuvers. In Scharf SM, Pinsky MR, Magder S (eds): Respiratory-Circulatory Interactions in Health and Disease. Lung Biology in Health and Disease, vol 157. New York, Marcel Dekker, 2001, pp 183-218.

34. Michard F, Chemla D, Richard C, et al: Clinical use of respiratory changes in arterial pulse pressure to monitor the hemodynamic effects of PEEP. Am J Respir Crit Care Med 1999;159:935-939.

35. Jardin F, Genevray G, Bru-Ney D, Bourdarais JP: Influence of lung and chest wall compliances on transmission of airway pressure to the pleural space in critically ill patients. Chest 1985;88:653-658.

36. Pinsky MR, Summer WR, Wise RA, et al: Augmentation of cardiac function by elevation of intrathoracic pressure. J Appl Physiol 1983;54:950-955.

37. Abel JG, Salerno TA, Panos A, et al: Cardiovascular effects of positive pressure ventilation in humans. Ann Thorac Surg1987; 43:36-43.

38. Johnston WE, Vinten-Johansen J, Shugart HE, Santamore WP: Positive-end expiratory pressure potentiates the severity of canine right ventricular ischemia-reperfusion injury. Am J Physiol 1992; 262:H168-H176.

39. Berglund JR, Halden E, Jakobson S, Landelius J: Echocardiographic analysis of cardiac function during high PEEP ventilation. Intensive Care Med 1994;20:174-180.

40. Vieillard-Baron A, Loubieres Y, Schimitt JM, et al: Cyclic changes in right ventricular output impedance during mechanical ventilation. J Appl Physiol 1999;87:1644-1650.

41. Ayus JC, Arief AI: Pulmonary complications of hyponatremic encephalopathy: Noncardiogenic pulmonary edema and hypercapnic respiratory failure. Chest 1995;107:517-521.

42. Moritz ML, Ayus JC: Hospital-acquired hyponatremia: Why are there still deaths? Pediatrics 2004;113:1395-1396.

43. Pinsky MR, Marquez J, Martin D, Klein M: Ventricular assist by cardiac cycle-specific increase in intrathoracic pressure. Chest 1987;91:709-715.

44. Scharf SM: Ventilatory support in the failing heart. In Scharf SM, Pinsky MR, Magder S (eds): Respiratory-Circulatory Interactions in Health and Disease. Lung Biology in Health and Disease, vol 157. New York, Marcel Dekker, 2001, pp 519-550.

45. Sin DD, Logan AG, Fitzgerald FS, et al: Effects of continuous positive airway pressure on cardiovascular outcomes in heart failure patients with and without Cheyne-Stokes respiration. Circulation 2000;102:61-66.

46. Shekerdemian LS, Bush A, Shore DF, et al: Cardiorespiratory responses to negative pressure ventilation after tetralogy of Fallot repair: A hemodynamic tool for patients with a low-output state. J Am Coll Cardiol 1999;33:549-555.

47. Santamore WP, Dell'Italia LJ: Ventricular interdependence: Significance of left ventricular contributions to right ventricular systolic function. Prog Cardiovasc Dis 1998;40:289-308.

48. Damiano RJ Jr, La Follette P Jr, Cox JL, et al: Significant left ventricular contribution to right ventricular systolic function. Am J Physiol 1991;261:1514-1524.

49. Dell'Italia LJ, Santamore WP: Can indices of left ventricular function be applied to the right ventricle? Prog Cardiovasc Dis 1998; 40:309-324.

50. Asanoi H, Sasayama S, Kameyama T: Ventriculoarterial coupling in normal and failing heart in humans. Circ Res 1989;65:483-493.

51. Piene H, Sund T: Does normal pulmonary impedance constitute the optimal load for the right ventricle? Am J Physiol 1982;242: H154-H160.

52. Wauthy P, Pagnamenta A, Vassalli F, et al: Right ventricular adaptation to pulmonary hypertension: Interspecies comparison. Am J Physiol Heart Circ Physiol 2004;286:H1141-H1147.

53. Calvin JE, Baer RW, Glantz SA: Pulmonary artery constriction produces a greater right ventricular dynamic afterload than lung microvascular injury in the open chest dog. Circ Res 1985;56:40-56.

54. Redington AN, Gray HH, Hodson ME, et al: Characterisation of the normal right ventricular pressure-volume relation by bi-plane angiography and simultaneous micromanometer pressure measurements. Br Heart J 1988;59:23-30.

55. Granton JT, Rabinovitch M: Pulmonary arterial hypertension and congenital heart disease. Cardiol Clin 2002;20:441-457.

56. Hopkins WE, Waggoner AD: Severe pulmonary hypertension without right ventricular failure: The unique hearts of patients with Eisenmenger syndrome. Am J Cardiol 2002;89:34-38.

57. Redington AN, Rigby ML, Shinebourne EA, Oldershaw PJ: Changes in the pressure-volume relation of the right ventricle when its loading conditions are modified. Br Heart J 1990;63:45-49.

58. Wald M, Kirschner L, Lawrenz K, Amann G: Fatal air embolism in an extremely low birth weight infant: Can it be caused by intravenous injections during resuscitation? Intensive Care Med 2003;29:630-633.

59. Schulze-Neick I, Li J, Penny DJ, Redington AN: Pulmonary vascular resistance after cardiovascular bypass in infants: Effect on postoperative recovery. J Thorac Cardiovasc Surg 2001;121: 1033-1039.

60. Sibbald WJ, Paterson NA, Holliday RL, et al: Pulmonary hypertension in sepsis: Measurement by the pulmonary arterial diastolic pulmonary wedge pressure gradient and the influence of active and passive factors. Chest 1978;73:583-591.

61. Kimchi A, Ellrodt AG, Berman DS, et al: Right ventricular performance in septic shock: A combined radionuclide and hemodynamic study. Am J Coll Cardiol 1984;4:945-951.

62. Lambermont B, Ghuysen A, Kohl P, et al: Effects of endotoxic shock on right ventricular systolic function and mechanical efficiency. Cardiovasc Res 2003;59:412-418.

63. Vieillard-Baron A, Schmitt JM, Augarde R, et al: Acute core pulmonale in acute respiratory distress syndrome submitted to protective ventilation: Incidence, clinical implications and prognosis. Crit Care Med 2001;29:1551-1555.

64. Calvin JE Jr: Acute right heart failure: Pathophysiology, recognition, and pharmacological management. J Cardiothorac Vasc Anesth 1991;5:507-513.

65. Elzinga G, Pienne H, De Jong J: Left and right pump function and consequences of having two pumps in one heart: A study on isolated cat heart. Circ Res 1980;46:564-574.

66. Vieillard-Baron A, Prin S, Chergui K, et al: Echo-Doppler demonstration of acute cor pulmonale at the bedside in the medical intensive care unit. Am J Respir Crit Care Med 2002;166:1310-1319.

67. Laks M, Gardner D, Swan SHC: Volumes and compliances measured simultaneously in the right and left ventricle in the dog. Cir Res 1967;66:612.

68. Wojczak JA, Szalados JE: Right heart function: Neither silent nor passive. Crit Care Med 2002;30:2601-2603.

69. Konstantinides S, Geibel A, Olschewski M, et al: Importance of cardiac troponin I and T in risk stratification of patients with acute pulmonary embolism. Circulation 2002;106:1263-1268.

70. Abman SH, Chatfield BA, Hall SA, McMutry IF: Role of endothelium-dependent relaxing factor activity during transition of pulmonary circulation at birth. Am J Physiol Heart Circ Physiol 1990;259: H1921-H1927.

71. Leffler CW, Hessler JR, Green RS: The onset of breathing at birth stimulates pulmonary vascular prostacyclin synthesis. Pediatr Res 1984;18:928-942.

72. Tristani-Firouzi M, Martin EB, Tolarova S, et al: Ventilation-induced pulmonary vasodilatation at birth is modulated by potassium channel activity. Am J Physiol Lung Cell Mol Physiol 1999;276:L220-L228.

73. Emmanouilides GC, Moss AJ, Duffie ER, Adams FH: Pulmonary artery pressure changes in newborn infants from birth to 3 days of age. J Pediatr 1964;65:327-333.

74. Haworth SG: Pulmonary hypertension in childhood. In Askin FB, Langston C, Rosenberg HS, Bernstein J (eds): Pulmonary Disease. Perspectives on Pediatric Pathology, vol 18. Karger, Basel, Switzerland, 1995, pp 71-110.

75. Holcomb RG, Tyson RW, Ivy DD, et al: Congenital pulmonary venous stenosis presenting as persistent pulmonary hypertension of the newborn. Pediatr Pulmonol 1999;28:301-306.

76. Donnelly WH: Ischemic myocardial necrosis and papillary muscle dysfunction in infant and children. Am J Cardiovasc Pathol 1987;1:173-188.

77. Abman SH, Shanley PF, Accurso FJ: Failure of postnatal adaptation of the pulmonary circulation after chronic intrauterine pulmonary hypertension in fetal lambs. J Clin Invest 1989;83: 1849-1858.

78. Cornfield DN, Resnik ER, Herron JM, Abman SH: Chronic intrauterine pulmonary hypertension decreases calcium-sensitive potassium channel mRNA expression. Am J Physiol Circ Physiol 2000;279:L857-L862.

79. Grover TR, Parker TA, Zenge JP, et al: Intrauterine hypertension decreases lung VEGF expression and VEGF inhibition causes pulmonary hypertension in the ovine fetus. Am J Physiol Lung Cell Mol Physiol 2003;284: L508-L517.

80. Hislop AA, Springall DR, Oliveira R, et al: Endothelial nitric oxide synthase in hypoxic newborn porcine pulmonary vessels. Arch Dis Child 1997;77:F16-F22.

81. Vosakta RJ, Kashyap S, Trifiletti RR: Arginine deficiency accompanies persistent pulmonary hypertension of the newborn. Biol Neonate 1994;66:65-70.

82. Thébaud B, De Legausie P, Forgues D, et al: ET$_A$-receptor blockade and ET$_B$-receptor stimulation in experimental congenital diaphragmatic hernia. Am J Physiol Lung Cell Mol Physiol 2000; 278:L923-L932.

83. Endo A, Ayusawa M, Minato M, et al: Endogenous nitric oxide and endothelin-1 in persistent pulmonary hypertension of the newborn. Eur J Pediatr 2001;160:217-222.

84. Maruyama K, Ye C, Woo M, et al: Chronic hypoxic pulmonary hypertension in rats and increased elastolytic activity. Am J Physiol 1991;261:H1716-H1726.

85. Kinsella JP, Abman SH: Persistent pulmonary hypertension of the newborn: Strategies in clinical management. In Peacock AJ (ed): Pulmonary Circulation: A Handbook for Clinicians. Chapman & Hall Medical, London, 1996, pp 437-448.

86. Sadiq HF, Mantych G, Benawra, et al: Inhaled nitric oxide in the treatment of moderate persistent pulmonary hypertension of the newborn: A randomized, controlled, multicenter trial. J Perinatol 2003;23:98-103.

87. Canadian Inhaled Nitric Oxide Study Group and the NICHD Neonatal Research Network: The neonatal inhaled nitric oxide study in term and near-term infant with hypoxic respiratory failure: A multicenter randomized trial. N Engl J Med 1997; 336:597-604.

88. Clark HR, Yoder B, Sell MS: Prospective, randomized comparison of high-frequency oscillation and conventional ventilation in candidates for extracorporeal membrane oxygenation. J Pediatr 1994;123:447-454.

89. Kinsella JP, Torielli F, Ziegler JW, et al: Dipyridmole augmentation of response to nitric oxide. Lancet 1995;346:647-648.

90. Ng C, Franklin O, Vaidya M, et al: Adenosine infusion for the management of persistent pulmonary hypertension of the newborn. Pediatr Crit Care Med 2004;5:10-13.

91. Kelly LK, Porta NFM, Goodman DM, et al: Inhaled prostacyclin for term infants with persistent pulmonary hypertension refractory to inhaled nitric oxide. J Pediatr 2002;141:830-832.

92. Kinsella JP, Parker TA, Ivy DD, Abman SH: Noninvasive delivery of inhaled nitric oxide therapy for late pulmonary hypertension in newborn infants with congenital diaphragmatic hernia. J Pediatr 2003;142:397-401.

93. Inwald D, Brown K, Gensini F, et al: Open lung biopsy in neonatal and pediatric patients referred for extracorporeal membrane oxygenation. Thorax 2004;59:328-333.

94. Walther FJ, Benders MJ, Leighton JO: Persistent pulmonary hypertension in premature neonates with severe respiratory distress syndrome. Pediatrics 1992;90:899-904.

95. Schreiber MD, Gin-Mestan K, Marks JD, et al: Inhaled nitric oxide in premature infants with respiratory distress syndrome. N Engl J Med 2003;349:2099-2107.

96. Simonneau G, Galiè N, Rubin LJ, et al: Clinical classification of pulmonary hypertension. J Am Coll Cardiol 2004;43:5S-12S.

97. Weitzenblum E: Chronic cor pulmonale. Heart 2003;89:225-230.

98. Davidson CJ, Fishman RF, Bonow RO: Cardiac catheterization. In Braunwald E (eds): Heart Disease: A Textbook of Cardiovascular Medicine. Philadelphia, WB Saunders, 1997, pp 177-203.

99. Abman SH, Wolfe RR, Accurso FJ, et al: Pulmonary vascular response to oxygen in severe BPD. Pediatrics 1985;75:80-84.

100. Abman SH, Sondheimer HM: Pulmonary circulation and cardiovascular sequelae of bronchopulmonary dysplasia. In Weir EK, Archer SL, Reeves JT (eds): The Diagnosis and Treatment of Pulmonary Hypertension. Mount Kisco, NY, Futura Publishing, 1992, pp 155-180.

101. Mourani PM, Ivy DD, Gao D, Abman SH: Pulmonary vascular effects of inhaled nitric oxide and oxygen tension in bronchopulmonary dysplasia. Am J Respir Crit Care Med 2004; 170:1006-1113.

102. Tomashefski JF, Opperman HC, Vawter GF: BPD: A morphometric study with emphasis on the pulmonary vasculature. Pediatr Pathol 1984;17:469-487.

103. Coalson JJ: Pathology of new bronchopulmonary dysplasia. Semin Neonatol 2003;8:73-81.

104. Ryland D, Reid L: The pulmonary circulation in cystic fibrosis. Thorax 1975;30:285-292.

105. Post J, Hume J, Archer S, Weir EK: Direct role for potassium channel inhibition in hypoxia pulmonary vasoconstriction. Am J Physiol 1992;262:C882-C890.

106. Li H, Chen SJ, Chen YF, et al: Enhanced endothelin-1 expression and endothelin receptor gene expression in chronic hypoxia. J Appl Physiol 1994;77:1451-1459.

107. Stenmark KR, Mecham RP: Cellular and molecular mechanisms of pulmonary vascular remodeling. Annu Rev Physiol 1997; 59:89-144.

108. Voelkel NF, Tuder RM: Hypoxia-induced pulmonary vascular remodeling: A model of what human disease? J Clin Invest 2000;106:733-738.

109. Tuder RM, Flook B, Voelkel NF: Increased gene expression for VEGF and VEGF receptor KDR/Flt and Flt in lungs of chronically hypoxic rats. J Clin Invest 1995;95:1798-1807.

110. Durmowicz AG, Parks WC, Hyde DM, et al: Persistence, re-expression, and induction of pulmonary arterial fibronectin, tropoelastin, and type I procollagen mRNA expression in neonatal hypoxic pulmonary hypertension. Am J Pathol 1994;145: 1411-1420.

111. Stenmark KR, Bouchey D, Nemenoff R, et al: Hypoxia-induced pulmonary vascular remodeling: Contribution of adventitial fibroblasts. Physiol Res 2000;49:503-517.

112. Stenmark KR, Gerasimovskaya E, Nemenoff RA, Das M: Hypoxic activation of adventitial fibroblasts: Role in vascular remodeling. Chest 2002;122:326S-334S.

113. Davie NJ, Crossno JT, Frid MG, et al: Hypoxia-induced pulmonary adventitial remodeling and neovascularization: Contribution of progenitor cells. Am J Physiol Lung Cell Mol Physiol 2004;268: L668-L678.

114. Parker TA, Abman SH: The pulmonary circulation in bronchopulmonary dysplasia. Semin Neonatol 2003;8:51-62.

115. Du L, Sullivan CC, Chu D, et al: Signaling molecules in nonfamilial pulmonary hypertension. N Engl J Med 2003;348:500-509.

116. Massaro D, Massaro GD, Baras A, et al: Calorie-related rapid onset alveolar loss, regeneration, and changes in mouse lung gene expression. Am J Physiol Lung Cell Mol Physiol 2003;286:L896-L906.

117. American Thoracic Society: Statement on the care of the child with chronic lung disease of infancy and childhood. Am J Respir Crit Care Med 2003;168:356-396.

118. Stern RC, Borkat G, Hirschfeld SS, et al: Heart failure in cystic fibrosis. Am J Dis Child 1980;134:267-272.

119. Koelling TM, Dec GW, Ginns LC, Semigran MJ: Left ventricular diastolic function in patients with advanced cystic fibrosis. Chest 2003;123:1488-1494.

120. McGoon M, Gutterman D, Steen V, et al: Screening, early detection, and diagnosis of pulmonary arterial hypertension: ACCP evidence-based clinical practice guidelines. Chest 2004;126:13S-34S.

121. Solomon M, Anderson E: Sarcoidosis-associated pulmonary hypertension: A case successfully treated with corticosteroids. Chest 2001;120:361S-362S.

122. Fartouk H, Humbert M, Capron F, et al: Severe pulmonary hypertension in histiocytosis X. Am J Respir Crit Care Med 2000; 161:216-223.

123. Rubin LJ, Badesch DB, Barst RJ, et al: Bosentan therapy for pulmonary arterial hypertension. N Engl J Med 2002;346:896-903.

124. Oudiz RJ, Schilz RJ, Barst RJ, et al; Treprostinil study group: Treprostinil, a prostacyclin analogue, in pulmonary hypertension associated with connective tissue disease. Chest 2004;126: 420-427.

125. Abman SH: Monitoring cardiovascular function in infants with chronic lung disease of prematurity. Arch Dis Child Fetal Neonatal Educ 2002;87:F15-F18.

126. Brinson GM, Noone PG, Mauro MA, et al: Bronchial artery embolization for the treatment of patients with cystic fibrosis. Am J Crit Care Med 1998;157:1951-1958.

127. Kessler R, Faller M, Fourgaut G, et al: "Natural history" of pulmonary hypertension in a series of 131 patients with chronic obstructive pulmonary disease. Am J Respir Crit Care Med 2001;164:219-224.

128. Goldring RM, Fishman AP, Turino GM, et al: Pulmonary hypertension and cor pulmonale in cystic fibrosis of the pancreas. J Pediatr 1964;65:501-523.

129. Moss AJ, Harper WH, Dooley RR, et al: Cor pulmonale in cystic fibrosis of the pancreas. J Pediatr 1965;67:797-807.

130. May CD, Lowe CU: Fibrosis of the pancreas in infants and children. J Pediatr 1949;34:663-687.

131. Royce SW: Cor pulmonale in infancy and early childhood. Pediatrics 1951;8:255-274.

132. Matthay RA, Berger HJ, Loke J, et al: Right and left ventricular performance in ambulatory adults with cystic fibrosis. Br Heart J 1980;43:474-480.

133. Florea VG, Florea ND, Sharma R, et al: Right ventricular dysfunction in adult severe cystic fibrosis. Chest 2000;118: 1063-1068.

134. Ionescu AA, Ionescu AA, Payne N, et al: Subclinical right ventricular dysfunction in cystic fibrosis. Am J Respir Crit Care Med 1999;163:1212-1218.

135. Burghuber OC, Salzer-Muhar U, Bergmann H, Gotz M: Right ventricular performance and pulmonary hemodynamics in adolescent and adult patients with cystic fibrosis. Eur J Pediatr 1988;148:187-192.

136. Pianosi P, Pelech A: Stroke volume during exercise in cystic fibrosis. Am J Respir Crit Care Med 1996;153:1105-1109.

137. Kelly RA, Smith TW: Cytokines and cardiac contractile function. Circulation 1997;95:778-781.

138. Brilla CG, Rupp H, Funck R, Maisch B: The renin-angiotensin-aldosterone system and myocardial collagen matrix remodelling in congestive heart failure. Eur Heart J 1995;16(Suppl O):107-109.

139. Ramires FJA, Sun Y, Weber KT: Myocardial fibrosis associated with aldosterone or angiotensin II administration: Attenuation by calcium channel blockade. J Mol Cell Cardiol 1998;30:475-483.

140. Wiebicke W, Artlich A, Gerling I: Myocardial fibrosis: A rare complication of in patients with cystic fibrosis. Eur J Pediatr 1993;152:694-696.

141. Tissière P, Nicod L, Barazzone-Argiroffo C, et al: Aerosolized iloprost as a bridge to lung transplantation in a patient with cystic fibrosis and pulmonary hypertension. Ann Thorac Surg 2004;78:e48-e50.

142. Hung J, Whitford EG, Parsons RW, Hillman DR: Association of sleep apnea with myocardial infarction in men. Lancet 1990; 336:261-264.

143. Leung RST, Bradley TD: Sleep apnea and cardiovascular disease. Am J Respir Crit Care Med 2001;164:2147-2165.

144. Bradley TD, Floras JS: Pathophysiologic and therapeutic implications of sleep apnea in congestive heart failure. J Card Fail 1996;2:223-240.

145. Parker JD, Brooks D, Kozar LF, et al: Acute and chronic effects of airway obstruction on left ventricular performance. Am J Respir Crit Care Med 1999;160:1888-1896.

146. Mooe T, Franklin KA, Wiklund U, et al: Sleep-disordered breathing and myocardial ischemia in patients with coronary artery disease. Chest 2000;117:1597-1602.

147. Buda AJ, Schroeder JS, Guilleminault C: Abnormalities in pulmonary artery wedge pressure in sleep-induced apneas. Int J Cardiol 1981;1:67-74.

148. Somers KV, Dyken ME, Clary MP, Abboud FM: Sympathetic neural mechanisms in obstructive sleep apnea. J Clin Invest 1995;96:1897-1904.

149. Fletcher EC, Miller J, Schaaf JW, Fletcher JG: Urinary catecholamines before and after tracheostomy in patients with obstructive sleep apnea and hypertension. Sleep 1987;10:35-44.

150. Kara T, Narkiewicz K, Somers VK: Chemoreflexes: Physiology and clinical implications. Acta Physiol Scand 2003;177:377-384.

151. Narkiewicz K, Montano N, Cogliati C, et al: Altered cardiovascular variability in obstructive sleep apnea. Circulation 1998;98: 1071-1077.

152. Lavie L: Obstructive sleep apnoea syndrome: An oxidative stress disorder. Sleep Med Rev 2003;7:35-51.

153. Yokoe T, Minoguchi K, Matsuo H, et al: Elevated levels of C-reactive protein and interleukin-6 in patients with obstructive sleep apnea syndrome are decreased by nasal continuous positive airway pressure. Circulation 2003;107:900-908.

154. Phillips BG, Narkiewicz K, Pesek CA, et al: Effects of obstructive sleep apnea on endothelin-1 and blood pressure. J Hypertens 1999;17:61-66.

155. Ip MSM, Lam B, Chan L-Y, et al: Circulating nitric oxide is suppressed in obstructive sleep apnea and is reversed by nasal continuous positive airway pressure. Am J Respir Crit Care Med 2000;162:2166-2171.

156. Kato M, Roberts-Thompson P, Phillips BG, et al: Impairment of endothelium-dependent vasodilatation of resistance vessels in patients with obstructive sleep apnea. Circulation 2000;102:2607-2610.

157. Rangemark C, Hedner JA, Carlson JT, et al: Platelet function and fibrinolytic activity in hypertensive and normotensive sleep apnea patients. Sleep 1995;18:188-194.

158. Vgontzas AN, Chrouos GP: Sleep, the hypothalamic-pituitary-adrenal axis, and cytokines: Multiple interactions and disturbances in sleep disorders. Endrocrinol Metab Clin North Am 2002;31:15-36.

159. Marcus CL, Greene MG, Carroll JL: Blood pressure in children with obstructive sleep apnea. Am J Crit Care Respir Med 1998;157:1098-1103.

160. Enright PL, Goodwin JL, Sherrill DL, Quan SF: Blood pressure elevation associated with sleep-related breathing disorder in a community sample of white and Hispanic children: The Tucson Children's Assessment of Sleep Apnea Study. Arch Pediatr Adolesc Med 2003;157:901-904.

161. National High Blood Pressure Education Program Working Group on High Blood Pressure in Children and Adolescents: The fourth report on diagnosis, evaluation, and treatment of high blood pressure in children and adolescents. Pediatrics 2004;114(3 Suppl):555-576.

162. Peppard PE, Young T, Palta M, Skatrud J: Prospective study of the association between sleep-disordered breathing and hypertension. N Engl J Med 2000;342:1378-1384.

163. Nieto FJ, Young TB, Lind BK, et al: Association of sleep-disordered breathing, sleep apnea, and hypertension in a large community-based study. JAMA 2000;283:1829-1836.

164. Brooks D, Horner RL, Kozar LF, et al: Obstructive sleep apnea as a cause of systemic hypertension: Evidence from a canine model. J Clin Invest 1997;99:106-109.

165. Logan AG, Tkacova R, Perilowski SM, et al: Refractory hypertension and sleep apnea: Effects of CPAP on blood pressure and baroreflex. Eur Respir J 2003;21:241-247.

166. Fletcher EC, Miller J, Schaaf JW, Fletcher JG: Urinary catecholamines before and after tracheostomy in patients with obstructive sleep apnea and hypertension. Sleep 1987;10:35-44.

167. Cistulli PA, Wilcox I, Jeremy R, Sullivan CE: Aortic root dilatation in Marfan's syndrome: A contribution fro obstructive sleep apnea? Chest 1997;111:1763-1766.

168. Amin RS, Kimball TR, Bean JA, et al: Left ventricular hypertrophy and abnormal ventricular geometry in children and adolescent with obstructive sleep apnea. Am J Crit Care Respir Med 2002;165:1395-1399.

169. Tal A, Leiberman A, Margulis G, Sofer S: Ventricular dysfunction in children with obstructive sleep apnea: Radionuclide assessment. Pediatr Pulmonol 1988;4:139-143.

170. Chan D, Li AM, Yam MC, et al: Hurler's syndrome with cor pulmonale secondary to obstructive sleep apnoea treated with continuous positive airway pressure. J Paediatr Child Health 2003;39:558-559.

171. Brown OE, Manning SC, Ridenour B: Cor pulmonale secondary to tonsillar and adenoidal hypertrophy: Management considerations. Int J Pediatr Otorhinolaryngol 1988;16:131-139.

172. Sofer S, Weinhouse E, Tal A, et al: Cor pulmonale due to adenoidal or tonsillar hypertrophy or both in children. Chest 1988;93:119-122.

173. Sie KCY, Perkins JA, Clarke WR: Acute right heart failure due to adenotonsillar hypertrophy. Int J Pediatr Otorhinolaryngol 1997;41:53-58.

174. Hetzel W, Kochs M, Marx N, et al: Pulmonary hemodynamics in obstructive sleep apnea: Frequency and causes of pulmonary hypertension. Lung 2003;181:157-166.

175. Sanner BM, Doberauer C, Konermann M, et al: Pulmonary hypertension in patients with obstructive sleep apnea syndrome. Arch Intern Med 1997;157:2483-2487.

176. Alchanatis M, Tourkohoriti G, Kakouos S, et al: Daytime pulmonary hypertension in patients with obstructive sleep apnea. Respiration 2001;68:566-572.

177. Atwood CW, McCrory D, Garcia JGN, et al: Pulmonary arterial hypertension and sleep-disordered breathing: ACCP evidence-based clinical practice guidelines. Chest 2004;126:72S-77S.

178. Hedner J, Ejnell H, Caidahl K: Left ventricular hypertrophy independent of hypertension in patients with obstructive sleep apnea. J Hypertens 1990;8:941-946.

179. Fletcher EC, Lesske J, Behm R, et al: Carotid chemoreceptors, systemic blood pressure, and chronic episodic hypoxia mimicking sleep apnea. J Appl Physiol 1992;72:1978-1984.

180. Barth W, Deten A, Bauer M, et al: Differential remodeling of the left and right heart after norepinephrine treatment in rats: Studies on cytokines and collagen. J Mol Cell Cardiol 2000;32:273-284.

181. Laaban JP, Pascal-Sebaoun S, Bloch E, et al: Left ventricular systolic dysfunction in patients with obstructive sleep apnea syndrome. Chest 2002;122:1113-1138.

182. Fung JWH, Li TST, Choy DKL, et al: Severe obstructive sleep apnea is associated with left ventricular diastolic dysfunction. Chest 2002;121:422-429.

183. Young T, Palta M, Dempsey J, et al: The occurrence of sleep-disordered breathing among middle-aged adults. N Engl J Med 1993;328:1230-1235.

184. Sin DD, Fitzgerald F, Parker JD, et al: Risk factors for central and obstructive sleep apneas in 450 men and women with congestive heart failure. Am J Respir Crit Care Med 1999;160:1101-1106.

185. Javaheri S, Parker TJ, Liming JD, et al: Sleep apnea in 81 ambulatory male patients with stable heart failure: Types and their prevalences, consequences, and presentation. Circulation 1998;97:2154-2159.

186. Chan HS, Chiu HF, Tse LK, Woo KS: Obstructive sleep apnea presenting with nocturnal angina, heart failure, and near-miss sudden death. Chest 1991;99:1023-1025.

187. Chowdary YC, Patel JP: Recurrent pulmonary edema: An uncommon presenting feature of childhood obstructive sleep apnea hypoventilation syndrome in an otherwise healthy child. Clin Pediatr 2001;40:287-290.

188. Malone S, Liu PP, Holloway R, et al: Obstructive sleep apnea in patient with dilated myocardiopathy: Effects of positive airway pressure. Lancet 1991;338:1480-1484.

189. Naughton MT: Impact of treatment of sleep apnoea on left ventricular function in congestive heart failure. Thorax 1998;53(Suppl 3):S37-S40.

190. Kaneko Y, Floras JS, Usui K, et al: Cardiovascular effects of continuous positive airway pressure in patients with heart failure and obstructive sleep apnea. N Engl J Med 2003;348:1233-1241.

191. Garrigue S, Bordier P, Jaïs P, et al: Benefit of atrial pacing in sleep apnea syndrome. N Engl J Med 2002;346:404-412.

192. Jahaveri S: Effects of continuous positive airway pressure on sleep apnea and ventricular irritability in patients with heart failure. Circulation 2000;101:392-397.

193. Blum RH, McGowan FX: Chronic upper airway obstruction and cardiac dysfunction: Anatomic pathophysiology and anesthetic implications. Pediatr Anaesth 2004;14:75-83.

194. Branchlin AE, Soccal PM, Rochat T, et al: Severe left ventricular dysfunction secondary to primary pulmonary hypertension: Bridging therapy with bosentan before lung transplantation. J Heart Lung Transplant 2005;74:777-780.

CHAPTER 29

The Failing Cardiovascular System in Sepsis

Joseph A. Carcillo

In 1963, before the advent of neonatal and pediatric critical care medicine, a study of 900 infants at the University of Minnesota reported a 97% mortality in children with gram-negative sepsis and septic shock.[1] In 1985, the Children's National Medical Center reported a 57% mortality in children with septic shock.[2] The same center later reported a 12% mortality when aggressive volume resuscitation was used in 1991.[3] Stoll and colleagues[4] examined U.S. vital statistics and found improving neonatal and infant outcomes with sepsis. Angus and Watson[5-7] examined hospital discharge data to estimate U.S. mortality rates in children with severe sepsis and reported that mortality rates improved from 10% in 1995 to 9% in 1999.

Randomized controlled trials of antithrombin III[8] and bactericidal permeability-increasing protein[9] for children with purpura fulminans and presumed meningococcal septic shock showed 10% mortality rates in the placebo groups. Three centers have reported outcomes in children with septic shock when using therapeutic approaches similar to those recommended in the 2002 American College of Critical Care Medicine (ACCM) Clinical Practice Parameters for Hemodynamic Support of Pediatric and Neonatal Patients in Septic Shock.[10] St Mary's Hospital in the United Kingdom reported a 5% mortality in children with meningococcal septic shock,[12] whereas New York Hospital in the United States reported a 10% mortality.[11] The New York Hospital investigators observed 0% mortality in previously healthy children, but 15% mortality in children with chronic illness (mostly cancer patients).[12] Similar findings were observed at Children's Hospital of Pittsburgh when ACCM guidelines were implemented, with a 6% mortality, 2% in previously healthy children and 12% in children with chronic illness. Nhan and colleagues[13] observed 0% mortality in a randomized dengue shock fluid resuscitation trial for dengue shock.

Although outcomes are improving, the burden of newborn and pediatric sepsis is increasing in the United States. More children die with severe sepsis than die from cancer, with an estimated yearly health care cost of $4 billion in the United States for patients with this condition.[7] One half are newborns with most of these being of low birth weight.[7] One half of children with severe sepsis have underlying chronic illness.[7] Neurologic and cardiovascular illnesses are most common in infants with severe sepsis, and cancer and immunodeficiency are most common in children with severe sepsis. Medical advances have affected etiology and epidemiology. In 1991, Jacobs and colleagues[14] reported that the most

common causes of septic shock in children were, in descending order, *Haemophilus influenzae* type b, *Neisseria meningitidis,* and *Streptococcus pneumoniae.* The 1995 and 1999 national estimates suggest changes in common causes of septic shock. *H. influenzae* type b is all but nonexistent,[15] *N. meningitidis* is prevalent in only a few regions of the United States, and group B streptococcus is decreasing.[16] The use of *S. pneumoniae* vaccine is reducing the incidence of this infection.[17] The Canadian government has implemented nation-wide immunization in children younger than 2 years old for *N. meningitidis* serotype C.[18] The most prevalent causes of severe sepsis and septic shock in the United States now seem to be staphylococcal and fungal infections.

Sepsis sometimes is characterized as a circulatory state in which there is diffuse microvascular injury with concomitant biventricular systolic and diastolic dysfunction. Although cardiovascular collapse is observed frequently in patients with sepsis, myocardial dysfunction in these patients is often underappreciated as an associated condition. This chapter discusses the salient features of myocardial dysfunction and the circulatory derangement that are seen in sepsis.

DIAGNOSIS OF SEPSIS AND SEPTIC SHOCK

Sepsis and septic shock should be suspected in any newborn with respiratory distress and reduced perfusion, particularly in the presence of a maternal history of chorioamnionitis or prolonged rupture of membranes. It is important to distinguish newborn septic shock from cardiogenic shock caused by closure of the patent ductus arteriosus in newborns with ductal-dependent complex congenital heart disease. Any newborn with shock and hepatomegaly, cyanosis, a cardiac murmur, or differential upper and lower extremity blood pressures or pulses should be started on prostaglandin E_1 until complex congenital heart disease is ruled out by echocardiographic analyses. Newborn septic shock typically is accompanied by increased pulmonary artery pressures, and persistent pulmonary hypertension of the newborn (PPHN) can cause right ventricular failure.

The inflammatory triad of fever, tachycardia, and vasodilation is common in children with benign infections. Pediatric septic shock is suspected when children with this triad have a change in mental status manifested as inconsolable irritability, lack of interaction with parents, or becoming unarousable. The clinical diagnosis of septic shock is made in children who (1) have a suspected infection manifested by hypothermia or hyperthermia and (2) have clinical signs of decreased perfusion, including decreased mental status, prolonged capillary refill longer than 2 seconds (cold shock) or flash capillary refill (warm shock), diminished (cold shock) or bounding (warm shock) peripheral pulses, mottled cool extremities (cold shock), or decreased urine output of less than 1 mL/kg/hr. Septic shock has multiple etiologies, such as hypovolemia (from capillary leak and venodilation), myocardial dysfunction, pulmonary hypertension, hypoperfusion, and cytotoxic shock from decreased peripheral use of oxygen. Hypotension is not necessary for the clinical diagnosis of septic shock; however, its presence in a child with clinical suspicion of infection is confirmatory.

Developmental Differences in Hemodynamic Response to Sepsis

The predominant cause of mortality in adult septic shock is vasomotor paralysis.[19] Adults have myocardial dysfunction manifested as a decreased ejection fraction; however, cardiac output usually is maintained or increased by two mechanisms—tachycardia and ventricular dilation. Adults who do not develop this adaptive process to maintain cardiac output have a poor prognosis.[20] Pediatric septic shock is associated with severe hypovolemia, and children frequently respond well to aggressive volume resuscitation; however, the hemodynamic response of fluid-resuscitated children seems diverse compared with adults. Contrary to the adult experience, low cardiac output, not low systemic vascular resistance (SVR), is associated with mortality in pediatric septic shock.[21-30] Attainment of the therapeutic goal of cardiac index 3.3 to 6 L/min/m² may result in improved survival.[22,30] Also contrary to adults, oxygen delivery, not oxygen extraction, is the major determinant of oxygen consumption in children.[23] Attainment of the therapeutic goal of oxygen consumption greater than 200 mL/min/m² also may be associated with improved outcome.[22]

In 1998, investigators reported outcome when aggressive volume resuscitation (60 mL/kg fluid in the first hour) and goal-directed therapies[22] (goal cardiac index 3.3 to 6 L/min/m² and normal pulmonary capillary wedge pressure) were applied to children with septic shock.[30] Ceneviva and coworkers[30] reported 50 children with fluid-refractory (≥60 mL/kg in the first hour), dopamine-resistant shock. Most children (58%) showed a low cardiac output/high SVR state, and 22% had low cardiac output and low SVR. Hemodynamic states frequently progressed and changed over the first 48 hours, and persistent shock occurred in 33% of the patients. There was a significant decrease in cardiac function over time, requiring the addition of inotropes and vasodilators. Although decreasing cardiac function

accounted for most patients with persistent shock, some showed a complete change from a low output state to a high output/low SVR state.[31-34] Inotropes, vasopressors, and vasodilators were directed to maintain normal cardiac index and SVR in the patients. Mortality from fluid-refractory, dopamine-resistant septic shock in this study (18%) was markedly reduced compared with mortality in the 1985 study (58%),[30] in which aggressive fluid resuscitation was not used.

Neonatal septic shock can be complicated by the physiologic transition from fetal to neonatal circulation. In utero, 85% of fetal circulation bypasses the lungs through the patent ductus arteriosus and foramen ovale; this flow pattern is maintained by suprasystemic pulmonary artery pressures prenatally. At birth, inhalation of oxygen triggers a cascade of biochemical events that ultimately result in reduction in pulmonary artery pressure and transition from fetal to neonatal circulation with blood flow now being directed through the pulmonary circulation. Closure of the patent ductus arteriosus and foramen ovale complete this transition. Pulmonary artery pressures can remain elevated and the ductus arteriosus can remain open for the first 6 weeks of life, and the foramen ovale may remain probe patent for years. Sepsis-induced acidosis and hypoxia can increase pulmonary artery pressure and maintain patency of the ductus arteriosus, resulting in PPHN and persistent fetal circulation. Neonatal septic shock with PPHN is associated with increased right ventricle work. Despite in utero conditioning, the thickened right ventricle may fail in the presence of systemic pulmonary artery pressures, and decompensated right ventricular failure can be clinically manifested by tricuspid regurgitation and hepatomegaly. Newborn animal models of group B streptococcal and endotoxin shock also have documented reduced cardiac output and increased pulmonary, mesenteric, and SVR.[35-39] Therapies directed at reversal of right ventricular failure, through reduction of pulmonary artery pressures, commonly are needed in neonates with fluid-refractory shock and PPHN.

The hemodynamic response in premature, very-low-birth-weight infants with septic shock (<32 weeks' gestation, <1000 g) is least understood in part because pulmonary artery catheterization is impossible in this population. Most information has been assessed from echocardiographic evaluation alone. There is a paucity of studies devoted to septic shock in these patients. Literature is available, for the most part, on the hemodynamic response in premature infants with respiratory distress syndrome or shock of undescribed etiology. Echocardiographic analysis has documented reduced right ventricular and left ventricular function in premature newborns.[40] This and other literature indicate that premature infants with shock can respond to volume and inotropic therapies with improvements in stroke volume, contractility, and blood pressure.

Several other developmental considerations influence therapies for shock. Relative initial deficiencies in the thyroid and parathyroid hormone axes have been appreciated and can result in the need for thyroid hormone or calcium replacement or both.[41,42] Hydrocortisone therapy also has been examined in this population.[43] Immature mechanisms of thermogenesis require attention to external warming; in addition, reduced glycogen stores and muscle mass for gluconeogenesis require attention to maintenance of serum glucose. Standard practices in resuscitation of premature infants in septic shock employ a more graded approach compared with resuscitation of term neonates and children. This more cautious approach is a response to anecdotal reports that premature infants at risk for intraventricular hemorrhage (<30 weeks' gestation) can develop hemorrhage after rapid shifts in blood pressure; however, some investigators now question whether long-term neurologic outcomes are related to periventricular leukomalacia (a result of prolonged underperfusion) more than to intraventricular hemorrhage.

Another complicating factor in very-low-birth-weight infants is the persistence of the patent ductus arteriosus. This condition can occur because immature muscle is unable to constrict. Most infants with this condition are treated medically with indomethacin or surgically with ligation. Rapid administration of fluid may cause left-to-right shunting through the ductus with congestive heart failure induced by ventricular overload. Studies of therapies specifically directed at premature very-low-birth-weight infants with septic shock are needed. One single-center, randomized controlled trial reported improved outcome with use of daily 6-hour pentoxifylline infusions in extremely premature infants with sepsis.[44] This promising therapy warrants evaluation in the multicenter trial setting.[45]

Hemodynamic Profile in Septic Shock

Septic shock can be recognized, before hypotension occurs, by a clinical triad that includes hypothermia or hyperthermia, altered mental status, and peripheral vasodilation (warm shock) or cool extremities (cold shock). Therapies should be directed toward restoring normal mental status and peripheral perfusion. Restoration of urine output also can be a reassuring measure of successful resuscitation. Shock also should be evaluated and resuscitated using hemodynamic variables. Flow (Q) varies directly with perfusion pressure (dP) and inversely with resistance (R). This is mathematically represented by Q = dP/R. For the whole body, this is represented by cardiac output = mean arterial pressure (MAP) − central venous pressure (CVP)/SVR. This relationship also is evident for organ perfusion. In the kidney, renal blood flow = mean renal arterial pressure − mean renal venous pressure/renal vascular resistance. Some organs, including the kidney and

brain, have vasomotor autoregulation, which maintains blood flow in low blood pressure (MAP or mean renal arterial pressure) states.

At some critical point, perfusion pressure is reduced below the ability of the organ to maintain blood flow. The purpose of treatment of shock is to maintain perfusion pressure above the critical point below which blood flow cannot be maintained effectively in individual organs. Because the kidney receives the second highest blood flow of any organ in the body, measurement of urine output (with the exception of patients with hyperosmolar states leading to osmotic diuresis) and creatinine clearance can be used as an indicator of adequate perfusion pressure. In this regard, maintenance of MAP with norepinephrine has been shown to improve urine output and creatinine clearance in hyperdynamic sepsis.[46] Reduction in perfusion pressure below the critical point necessary for adequate organ perfusion also can occur in disease states with increased intra-abdominal pressure (IAP), such as bowel wall edema, ascites, or abdominal compartment syndrome. Increased IAP is associated with increased CVP; if this is not compensated for by an increase in MAP, perfusion pressure is decreased. Therapeutic reduction of IAP (measured by intrabladder pressure) results in restoration of perfusion pressure and has been shown to improve renal function in children.[47,48]

Shock also should be treated according to oxygen use measures. Measurements of cardiac output and oxygen consumption (cardiac index × [arterial oxygen content − mixed venous oxygen content]) have been proposed as being beneficial in patients with persistent shock because a cardiac index between 3.3 L/min/m² and 6 L/min/m² and oxygen consumption greater than 200 mL/min/m² are associated with improved survival.[22] Assuming a hemoglobin concentration of 10 g/dL and 100% arterial oxygen saturation, a cardiac index greater than 3.3 L/min/m² would correlate to a mixed venous oxygen saturation of greater than 70% in a patient with a normal oxygen consumption of 150 mL/min/m² (oxygen consumption = cardiac index × arterial oxygen content × oxygen extraction, therefore 150 mL/min/m²= 3.3 L/min/m² × [1.36 × 10 g/dL × 100 + PaO$_2$ × 003] × [100% − 70%]) (Fig. 29-1).

Low cardiac output is associated with mortality in pediatric septic shock.[21-30] In one study, children with fluid-refractory, dopamine-resistant shock were treated with goal-directed therapy (cardiac index >3.3 and <6 L/min/m²) and found to have predicted improved outcomes compared with historical reports.[30] Low cardiac output is associated with increased oxygen extraction. In an emergency department study in adults with septic shock, maintenance of superior vena cava oxygen saturation at greater than 70% by use of blood transfusion to a hemoglobin of 10 g/dL and inotropic support resulted in a 50% reduction in mortality compared with a group

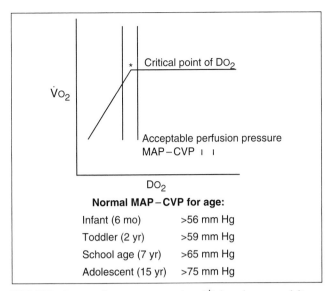

FIGURE 29-1 ■ Oxygen consumption ($\dot{V}o_2$) and oxygen delivery ($\dot{D}o_2$). Oxygen delivery is maintained at a level that ensures maximal oxygen consumption without increase in heart rate. The acceptable perfusion pressure ranges also are included. MAP–CVP, mean arterial pressure minus central venous pressure.

in whom mean arterial pressure minus central venous pressure (MAP–CVP) was maintained without attention to superior vena cava oxygen saturation.[49]

TREATMENT OF SEPTIC SHOCK

Monitoring and Fluid Resuscitation

Intravenous access for fluid resuscitation and inotrope/vasopressor infusion is more difficult to attain in newborns and children compared with adults. The American Heart Association and American Academy of Pediatrics have developed neonatal resuscitation program and pediatric advanced life support guidelines for emergency establishment of intravascular support.[50,51]

Two clinical case series have evaluated **fluid resuscitation** in pediatric septic shock.[13,52] The larger of the two case series used a combination of crystalloid and colloid therapies. There is only one randomized controlled trial comparing the use of colloid versus crystalloid resuscitation (dextran, gelatin, lactated Ringer solution, or saline) in children with dengue shock. All these children survived regardless of the fluid used, but the longest time to recovery from shock occurred in children who received lactated Ringer solution. Among patients with the narrowest pulse pressure, there was a suggestion that colloids were more effective than crystalloids in restoring normal pulse pressure. Based on these and other studies, the investigators agreed that fluid resuscitation with crystalloids and colloids is fundamentally important to survival from septic shock.[53-63] Debate on the efficacy of exclusive colloid resuscitation is ongoing.

In a clinical practice position paper, a group chosen for outstanding results in resuscitation of meningococcal septic shock (5% mortality) reported that they use 5% albumin exclusively (20 mL/kg boluses over 5 to 10 minutes) and intubate all patients who require greater than 40 mL/kg.[64] The Cochrane group meta-analysis, which implied harmful effects of colloid use in critical illness, evaluated no studies examining fluid resuscitation in children or newborns with septic shock.[65] Beneficial or harmful effects of colloid remain to be studied in this population.[66] The use of blood as a fluid expander was examined in two small pediatric studies, but no recommendations were given by the investigators.[67,68] There are no published studies or recommendations on targeted hemoglobin concentration in children. The last National Institutes of Health consensus conference recommended a target hemoglobin concentration of 10 g/dL in adults with cardiopulmonary compromise. An emergency department protocol directed toward maintenance of hemoglobin at 10 g/dL in adults with a superior vena cava oxygen saturation of less than 70% was associated with improved outcomes.[49]

Fluid infusion is best initiated with boluses of 20 mL/kg, titrated to clinical monitors of cardiac output, including heart rate, urine output, capillary refill, and level of consciousness. Large fluid deficits typically exist, and initial volume resuscitation usually requires 40 to 60 mL/kg, but can require 200 mL/kg. Cardiac patients with septic shock almost uniformly require lesser amounts of fluid, however. Fluid boluses of 10 mL/kg can be used in these children with titration to normal CVP and left atrial pressure (LAP).

Patients who do not respond rapidly to initial fluid boluses and patients with insufficient physiologic reserve should be considered for invasive hemodynamic monitoring. Filling pressures should be increased to optimize preload to attain maximal cardiac output; in most patients, this occurs with a pulmonary capillary wedge pressure of 12 to 15 mm Hg. Increases beyond this range usually do not enhance end-diastolic volume or stroke volume significantly and may be associated with decreased survival. Large volumes of fluid for acute stabilization in children have not been shown to increase the incidence of acute respiratory distress syndrome or cerebral edema. Increased fluid requirements may be evident for several days. Fluid choices include crystalloids (normal saline) and colloids (dextran, gelatin, or 5% albumin). Fresh frozen plasma may be infused to correct abnormal prothrombin time and partial thromboplastin time, but should not be pushed because it has hypotensive effects, likely caused by vasoactive kinins. It is reasonable to maintain hemoglobin concentration within the normal range for age in children with shock. Oxygen delivery depends significantly on hemoglobin concentration (oxygen delivery = cardiac index × [1.36 × % hemoglobin × % oxygen saturation + Pao$_2$ × 0.003), so hemoglobin should be maintained at a minimum of 10 g/dL.

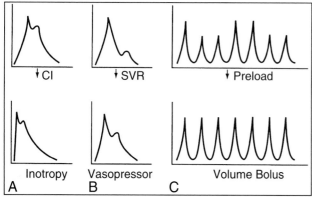

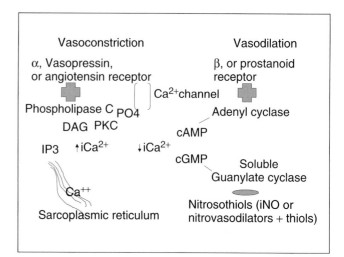

FIGURE 29-2 ■ Pulse-wave hemodynamics in sepsis. Diagrams predict responses to volume, inotropes, vasopressors, and vasodilators. **A,** The pressure over time is initially depressed (decreased cardiac index [↓CI]) as reflected by the slope of the upstroke and is improved with institution of inotropic support. **B,** With decreased systemic vascular resistance (↓SVR), the reflection wave is separated from the arterial wave. The vascular tone is increased with the use of a vasopressor as evidenced by summation of the arterial and reflection waves. **C,** The decreased preload (↓Preload) is shown by respiratory variation in the arterial waveform. This variation is lost with the augmentation of preload.

FIGURE 29-3 ■ Vasoconstrictors and vasodilators stimulate opposing second messenger systems. α-Adrenergic agonists, angiotensin, and vasopressin stimulate different receptors, which stimulate the production of inositol triphosphate (IP3) and diacylglycerol (DAG), leading to increased inducible calcium (iCa²⁺) and contraction. β₂-Agonists and vasodilator prostanoids stimulate cAMP production, and nitrosovasodilators and inducible nitric oxide (iNO) stimulate GMP production. These second messengers decrease iCa²⁺ and induce vasodilation. Type III and type V phosphodiesterase inhibitors can potentiate the effect of vasodilators. (See also Color Section)

Minimally invasive monitoring is necessary in children with fluid-responsive shock; however, central venous access and arterial pressure monitoring should be considered and used in children with fluid-refractory shock (Fig. 29-2). Maintenance of perfusion pressure (MAP−CVP or mean arterial pressure minus intra-abdominal pressure [MAP−IAP] if the abdomen is tense secondary to bowel edema or ascitic fluid) is necessary for organ (particularly renal) perfusion. Echocardiography is an appropriate noninvasive tool to assess myocardial function and rule out the presence of pericardial effusion. Superior vena cava oxygen saturation greater than 70% is associated with improved outcome during the first 6 hours of septic shock presentation. The decision to use pulmonary artery catheter monitoring should be reserved for patients who remain in shock despite therapies directed to clinical signs of perfusion, MAP−CVP, and superior vena cava oxygen saturation.[69]

Vasopressor Therapy

Dopamine remains the first-line vasopressor for high output and low SVR shock in adults. Although dopamine is the first-line drug for fluid-refractory hypotensive shock in the setting of low SVR, there is an age-specific insensitivity to dopamine.[70-78] Dopamine causes vasoconstriction by releasing norepinephrine from sympathetic vesicles. Immature animals and infants (<6 months old) may not have developed their full component of sympathetic vesicles. Dopamine-resistant shock responds to **norepinephrine** or **epinephrine**.[79,80] **Phenylephrine** is limited to use as a pure vasopressor because it has no β-adrenergic activity.[81] **Angiotensin** or **arginine vasopressin** can be effective in patients who are refractory to norepinephrine because it does not use the α-receptor, and its efficacy

is not affected by ongoing α-receptor down-regulation (Fig. 29-3).[82,83] Use of vasopressors can be titrated to end points of perfusion pressure (MAP−CVP) or SVR, which ensure optimal urine output and creatinine clearance. Nitric oxide inhibitors and methylene blue are considered to be investigational therapies.

Inotropic Therapy

As in adults, **dobutamine** or medium-dose dopamine can be used as the first line of inotropic support; however, children younger than age 12 months can be less responsive.[84-92] Dobutamine-refractory or dopamine-refractory shock secondary to low cardiac output can be reversed with **epinephrine** infusion.[93,94] Epinephrine is used more commonly in children than in adults. When pediatric patients remain in a normotensive low cardiac output/high SVR state, despite epinephrine and nitrosovasodilator therapy, the use of **milrinone** (if liver dysfunction is present) or **amrinone** (if renal dysfunction is present) should be strongly considered.[95-100] Phosphodiesterase inhibitors rarely are used in adults because catecholamine-refractory low cardiac output/high SVR is so uncommon; however, this hemodynamic state can represent a major proportion of children with fluid-refractory, dopamine-resistant shock.[20] Down-regulation of the β-receptors can be overcome by these drugs. Fluid boluses are likely to be required if amrinone or milrinone is administered with loading doses. Although recommended in the literature, it is not necessary to administer amrinone or milrinone as a bolus; the drugs are effective as a continuous infusion only, recognizing that it takes more than four half-lives to reach steady-state effect. Because of the long half-life elimination, these drugs should be discontinued at the first sign of tachyarrhythmias, hypotension, or diminished SVR. Hypotension-related toxicity with these drugs potentially can be overcome by stopping milrinone or amrinone and beginning norepinephrine. Norepinephrine counteracts the effects of increased cAMP in vascular tissue by stimulating the α-receptor. Norepinephrine accomplishes this without further β$_2$ stimulation.

Vasodilator Therapy

The use of vasodilators can reverse shock in pediatric patients who remain hypodynamic with a high SVR state despite fluid resuscitation and implementation of inotropic support.[100-102] Nitrosovasodilators (**nitroprusside** or **nitroglycerin** have a short half-life elimination) are a first-line therapy for children with epinephrine-resistant low cardiac output/elevated SVR shock because hypotension-associated toxicity can be reversed immediately by stopping the infusion. **Milrinone** or **amrinone** can be used for their vasodilating properties in patients with nitrosovasodilator-resistant low output syndrome or nitrosovasodilator-associated toxicity (cyanide or isothiocyanate toxicity from nitroprusside or methemoglobin toxicity from nitroglycerin). Other vasodilators used and reported in neonatal and pediatric septic shock include prostacyclin, phentolamine, pentoxifylline, and dopexamine.[103-106]

Miscellaneous Therapy

It is important to maintain metabolic and hormonal homeostasis in newborns and children. Hypoglycemia can cause neurologic devastation when missed. Hypoglycemia must be diagnosed rapidly and treated promptly. Hypocalcemia is a frequent, reversible contributor to cardiac dysfunction.[107,108] Calcium replacement should be directed toward normalizing ionized calcium levels. Replacement with thyroid or hydrocortisone or both can be lifesaving in children with thyroid or adrenal insufficiency and catecholamine-resistant shock.[109-122] Infusion therapy with triiodothyronine has been shown to be beneficial in postoperative congenital heart disease patients but has yet to be studied in children with septic shock.[123]

A randomized controlled trial has shown that a 7-day course of hydrocortisone plus fludrocortisone, maintaining a mean cortisol level around 100 μg/dL reduces mortality by 10% in adults with hypotension that persisted despite vasopressor therapy.[124] Until similar pediatric studies are performed, hydrocortisone (not methylprednisolone) therapy should be reserved for use in children with catecholamine resistance and suspected or proved drenal insufficiency. Adrenal insufficiency and particularly a low aldosterone state may be more common in septic shock than previously believed. Patients at risk include children with purpura fulminans and associated Waterhouse-Friderichsen syndrome, children who have previously received steroid therapies for chronic illness, and children with pituitary or adrenal abnormalities.

Adrenal insufficiency is defined in a patient with shock as a baseline cortisol level of less than 18 mg/dL in a patient with catecholamine requirements despite adequate volume status. Review of the pediatric literature reveals several case series[109-124] and two randomized trials that used "shock dose" hydrocortisone (50 mg/kg followed by the same dose over a 24-hour infusion) in children. The first randomized controlled trial showed improved outcome with hydrocortisone therapy in children with dengue shock. The second study was underpowered and showed no effect of hydrocortisone therapy on outcome in children with dengue shock. The reported shock dose of hydrocortisone is 25 times higher than the stress dose.

Although inhaled nitric oxide therapy is the treatment of choice for uncomplicated PPHN, metabolic alkalinization is an important initial resuscitative strategy during shock. PPHN in the setting of septic shock can reverse when acidosis is corrected. For centers with access to inhaled nitric oxide, this is the only selective pulmonary vasodilator reported to be effective in reversal of PPHN.[125-133] Extracorporeal membrane oxygenation (ECMO) remains the therapy of choice for patients with refractory PPHN and sepsis.

Extracorporeal Membrane Oxygenation Therapy

ECMO is not used routinely in adults (with the notable exception of the University of Michigan).[134] ECMO is a viable therapy for refractory shock in neonates, however.[135] The Extracorporeal Life Support Organization (ELSO) registry suggests that neonates have a similar outcome (approximate 80% survival) whether the indication for ECMO is refractory respiratory failure or refractory shock. Although the outcome is similar, neonates with septic shock have more complications (e.g., bleeding, infection) associated with therapy. The ELSO registry and other reports in the literature suggest outcome is less successful when ECMO is used for refractory pediatric septic shock (37% to 50% survival).[135-140] The committee agreed that use in pediatric septic shock is less successful, yet seems to be reasonable according to clinical judgment. ECMO is effective for pediatric cardiogenic shock.[141] It also is effective in adult Hantavirus victims with low cardiac output/high SVR shock.[142,143] The ELSO committee speculates that ECMO therapy is likely most successful in patients with refractory low cardiac output septic shock.

CURRENT STATUS AND FUTURE TRENDS

Sepsis is a common disease process that leads to an inflammatory process, which results in cardiovascular collapse and myocardial dysfunction. A myriad of inflammatory and anti-inflammatory markers that determine myocardial dysfunction are under investigation, including the inflammatory markers tumor necrosis factor, interleukin-1β, and interleukin-6 and the anti-inflammatory marker interleukin-13. In addition, adrenergic stimulation seems to influence inflammatory cytokine response in sepsis, but this process can lead to cardiomyocyte death via the reactive oxygen species–tumor necrosis factor-α–caspase signaling pathway.[144] One key component is nuclear factor κB, which is implicated in the regulation of multiple biologic reactions, including septic shock and myocardial dysfunction.[145] Lastly, more recent research indicates a role for natriuretic peptides (atrial natriuretic peptide and B-type natriuretic peptide) in the pathophysiology of septic shock and ventricular dysfunction.[146]

Much more investigative work needs to be done to elucidate the mechanisms of cardiac and vascular dysfunction in sepsis, particularly in neonates and children. Although the vasculature response in sepsis has been a focus of clinical investigations and guidelines (Figs. 29-4 and 29-5), there needs to be much more emphasis on the heart itself for future work in sepsis. Although there is little evidence for myocardial ischemia by echocardiography or ECG in sepsis, it is

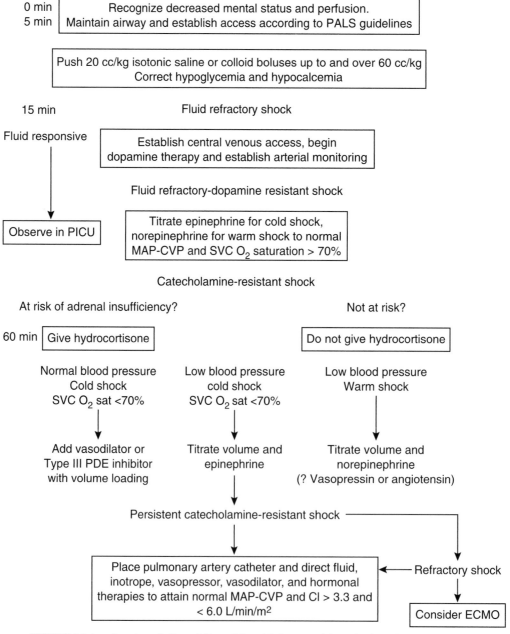

FIGURE 29-4 ■ American College of Critical Care Medicine guidelines for hemodynamic support of infants and children with septic shock. CI, cardiac index; ECMO, extracorporeal membrane oxygenation; MAP-CVP, mean arterial pressure minus central venous pressure; PALS, pediatric advanced life support; PDE, phosphodiesterase; PICU, pediatric intensive care unit; SVC, superior vena cava.

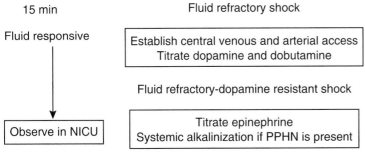

0 min
5 min

Recognize decreased perfusion, cyanosis, RDS
Maintain airway and establish access according to NRP guidelines

Push 10 cc/kg isotonic crystalloid or colloid boluses to 60 cc/kg
Correct hypoglycemia and hypocalcemia. Begin prostaglandin infusion until
echocardiogram shows no ductal-dependent lesion

15 min   Fluid refractory shock

Fluid responsive

Establish central venous and arterial access
Titrate dopamine and dobutamine

Fluid refractory-dopamine resistant shock

Observe in NICU

Titrate epinephrine
Systemic alkalinization if PPHN is present

Catecholamine-resistant shock

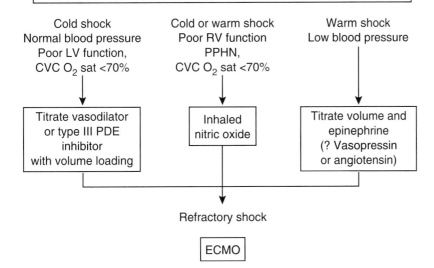

60 min   Direct therapies using echocardiogram and arterial and CVP monitoring

Cold shock
Normal blood pressure
Poor LV function,
CVC O$_2$ sat <70%

Cold or warm shock
Poor RV function
PPHN,
CVC O$_2$ sat <70%

Warm shock
Low blood pressure

Titrate vasodilator
or type III PDE
inhibitor
with volume loading

Inhaled
nitric oxide

Titrate volume and
epinephrine
(? Vasopressin
or angiotensin)

Refractory shock

ECMO

FIGURE 29-5 ■ American College of Critical Care Medicine guidelines for hemodynamic support of newborns with septic shock. CVC, central venous catheter; CVP, central venous pressure; ECMO, extracorporeal membrane oxygenation; LV, left ventricular; NICU, neonatal intensive care unit; NRP, neonatal resuscitation program; PDE, phosphodiesterase; PPHN, persistent pulmonary hypertension of the newborn; RDS, respiratory distress syndrome; RV, right ventricular.

now known that there is coronary vasoconstriction via leukotriene generation with resultant depressed myocardial function and myocardial necrosis.[147] In addition, nitric oxide– mediated stimulation of cGMP inhibits the adrenergic stimulated increase in slow inward calcium current and reduces the calcium affinity of the contractile machinery of the myocyte; nitric oxide can lead to direct cardiomyocyte injury via the formation of peroxynitrite in the presence of superoxide anion.[148] Current research has shown that ghrelin receptor, a potent vasoactive peptide, is up-regulated in the hyperdynamic phase of sepsis.[149] Lastly, the resuscitative philosophy in sepsis and septic shock needs to incorporate novel concepts, including use of novel agents, such as intravenous polyclonal immunoglobulin, granulocyte-macrophage colony- stimulating factor, or recombinant human activated protein C (an anticoagulant with anti-inflammatory properties), and

aggressive strategies, such as mechanical cardiopulmonary support.[150,151]

Key Concepts

■ Sepsis sometimes is characterized as a circulatory state in which there is diffuse microvascular injury with concomitant biventricular systolic and diastolic dysfunction. Although cardiovascular collapse is observed frequently in patients with sepsis, myocardial dysfunction in these patients is often underappreciated as an associated condition.

■ Septic shock has multiple etiologies, such as hypovolemia (from capillary leak and venodilation), myocardial dysfunction, pulmonary hypertension, hypoperfusion, and cytotoxic shock from decreased peripheral use of oxygen.

■ Pediatric septic shock is associated with severe hypovolemia, and children frequently respond well to aggressive volume resuscitation; however, the hemodynamic response of fluid-resuscitated children seems diverse compared with adults. Contrary to the adult experience, low cardiac output, not low SVR, is associated with mortality in pediatric septic shock.

■ When pediatric patients remain in a normotensive low cardiac output/high SVR state, despite epinephrine and nitrosovasodilator therapy, the use of milrinone (if liver dysfunction is present) or amrinone (if renal dysfunction is present) should be strongly considered.

■ Phosphodiesterase inhibitors rarely are used in adults because catecholamine-refractory low cardiac output/high SVR is so uncommon; however, this hemodynamic state can represent a major proportion of children with fluid-refractory, dopamine-resistant shock.

■ ECMO is not used routinely in adults. ECMO is a viable therapy for refractory shock in neonates. The ELSO registry suggests that neonates have a similar outcome (approximate 80% survival) whether the indication for ECMO is refractory respiratory failure or refractory shock.

■ Although there is little evidence for myocardial ischemia by echocardiography or ECG in sepsis, it is now known that there is coronary vasoconstriction via leukotriene generation with resultant depressed myocardial function and myocardial necrosis.

■ The resuscitative philosophy in sepsis and septic shock needs to incorporate novel concepts, including use of novel agents, such as intravenous polyclonal immunoglobulin, granulocyte-macrophage colony-stimulating factor, or recombinant human activated protein C (an anticoagulant with anti-inflammatory properties), and aggressive strategies, such as mechanical cardiopulmonary support.

REFERENCES

1. DuPont HL, Spink WW: Infections due to gram negative organisms: An analysis of 860 patients with bacteremia at University of Minnesota Medical Center. 1958-1966. Medicine 1968;48:307.
2. Pollack MM, Fields AI, Ruttimann UE: Distributions of cardiopulmonary variables in pediatric survivors and nonsurvivors of septic shock. Crit Care Med 1985;13:454-459.
3. Carcillo JA, Davis AL, Zaritsky A: Role of early fluid resuscitation in pediatric septic shock. JAMA 1991;266:1242-1245.
4. Stoll BJ, Holman RC, Shuchat A: Decline in sepsis-associated neonatal and infant deaths 1974-1994. Pediatrics 1998;102:E18.
5. Angus D, Linde-Zwirble WT, Lidicker J, et al: Epidemiology of severe sepsis in the United States: Analysis of incidence, outcome, and associated costs of care. Crit Care Med 2001;29:1303-1310.
6. Watson RS, Linde-Zwirble W, Lidicker J, et al: How does sepsis differ between children and adults? Am J Resp Crit Care Med 2001;163:A47.
7. Watson RS, Linde-Zwirble WT, Lidicker J, et al: The increasing burden of severe sepsis in U.S. children. Crit Care Med 2001;29:A8.
8. Brilli RJ, Jacobs BR, Lyons K, et al: Severe protein C deficiency in children who do not survive protein C deficiency. Crit Care Med 1999;27:A127.
9. Giroir BP, Scannon PJ, Levin M: Bactericidal permeability increasing protein: Lessons learned from the phase III randomized clinical trial of rBPI21 for adjuvant treatment of children with severe meningococcemia. Crit Care Med 2001;29(7 Suppl):S130-S135.
10. Carcillo JA, Fields AI; Task Force Members: Clinical practice parameters for hemodynamic support of pediatric and neonatal patients in septic shock. Crit Care Med 2002;30:1-13.
11. Pollard AJ, Britto J, Nadel S, et al: Emergency management of meningococcal disease. Arch Dis Child 1999;80:290-296.
12. Kutko MC, Calarco MP, Ushay M, et al: Mortality of pediatric septic shock may be less than previously reported. Crit Care Med 2000;28:T212.
13. Nhan NT, Phuong CXT, Kneen R, et al: Acute management of dengue shock syndrome: A randomized double-blind comparison of 4 intravenous fluid regimens in the first hour. Clin Infect Dis 2001;32:204-212.
14. Jacobs RF, Sowell MK, Moss MM, et al: Septic shock in children: Bacterial etiologies and temporal relationships. Pediatr Infect Dis J 1990;3:196-200.
15. Vadheim CM, Greenberg DP, Erikson E, et al: Eradication of Haemophilus influenzae B disease in Southern California Kaiser-UCLA vaccine study group. Arch Pediatr Adolesc Med 1994; 148: 51-56.
16. Adoption of hospital policies for prevention of perinatal group B streptococcal disease. MMWR Morb Mortal Wkly Rep 1998; 47: 665-670.
17. Lieu TA, Ray GT, Black SD, et al: Projected cost effectiveness of pneumococcal conjugate vaccination of healthy infants and children. JAMA 283:1460-1468, 2000.
18. MacLennan JM, Shackley F, Heath PT, et al: Safety, immunogenicity, and induction of immunologic memory by a serogroup C meningococcal vaccine in infants: A randomized controlled trial. JAMA 2000;283:2795-2801.
19. Parker MM, Shelhamer JH, Natanson C, et al: Serial cardiovascular variables in survivors and nonsurvivors of human septic shock: Heart rate as an early predictor of prognosis. Crit Care Med 1987; 15:923-929.
20. Parker MM, Shelhamer JH, Bacharach SL, et al: Profound but reversible myocardial depression in patients with septic shock. Ann Intern Med 1984;100:483-490.
21. Pollack MM, Fields AI, Ruttimann UE, et al: Sequential cardiopulmonary variables of infants and children in septic shock. Crit Care Med 1984;12:554-559.
22. Pollack MM, Fields AI, Ruttimann UE: Distributions of cardiopulmonary variables in pediatric survivors and nonsurvivors of septic shock. Crit Care Med 1985;13:454-459.
23. Carcillo JA, Pollack MM, Ruttimann UE, et al: Sequential physiologic interactions in cardiogenic and septic shock. Crit Care Med 1989;17:12-16.
24. Monsalve F, Rucabado L, Salvador A, et al: Myocardial depression in septic shock caused by meningococcal infection. Crit Care Med 1984;12:1021-1033.
25. Mercier JC, Beaufils F, Hartmann JF, et al: Hemodynamic patterns of meningococcal shock in children. Crit Care Med 1988; 16:27-33.
26. Simma B, Fritz MG, Trawoger R, et al: Changes in left ventricular function in shocked newborns. Intensive Care Med 1997;23: 982-986.
27. Walther FJ, Siassi B, Ramadan NA: Cardiac output in newborn infants with transient myocardial dysfunction. J Pediatr 1985;107: 781-785.
28. Ferdman B, Jureidini SB, Mink RB: Severe left ventricular dysfunction and arrhythmias as complication of gram positive sepsis: Rapid recovery in children. Pediatr Cardiol 1998;19:482-486.
29. Feltes TF, Pignatelli R, Kleinert S, et al: Quantitated left ventricular systolic mechanics in children with septic shock utilizing noninvasive wall stress analysis. Crit Care Med 1994;22:1647-1659.
30. Ceneviva G, Paschall JA, Maffei F, et al: Hemodynamic support in fluid refractory pediatric septic shock. Pediatrics 1998;102:e19.
31. Hoban LD, Paschal JA, Eckstein J, et al: Awake porcine model of intraperitoneal sepsis and altered oxygen utilization. Circ Shock 1991;34:252-262.

32. Green EM, Adams HR: New perspectives in circulatory shock: Pathophysiologic mediators of the mammalian response to endotoxemia and sepsis. J Am Vet Med Assoc 1992;200:1834-1841.

33. McDonough KH, Brumfield BA, Lang CH: In vitro myocardial performance after lethal and nonlethal doses of endotoxin. Am J Physiol 1986;250:H240-H246.

34. Natanson C, Fink MP, Ballantyne HK, et al: Gram-negative bacteremia produces both severe systolic and diastolic cardiac dysfunction in a canine model that simulates human septic shock. J Clin Invest 1986;78:259-270.

35. Dobkin ED, Lobe TE, Bhatia J, et al: The study of fecal E coli peritonitis-induced septic shock in a neonatal pig model. Circ Shock 1985;16:325-336.

36. Sosa G, Milstein JM, Bennett SH: E coli endotoxin depresses left ventricular contractility in neonatal lambs. Pediatr Res 1994;35:62-67.

37. Peevy KJ, Chartrand SA, Wiseman HJ, et al: Myocardial dysfunction in group B streptococcal shock. Pediatr Res 1994;19:511-513.

38. Meadow WL, Meus PJ: Unsuspected mesenteric hypoperfusion despite apparent hemodynamic recovery in the early phase of septic shock in piglets. Circ Shock 1985;15:123-129.

39. Meadow WL, Meus PJ: Early and late hemodynamic consequences of group B beta streptococcal sepsis in piglets: Effects on systemic, pulmonary, and mesenteric circulations. Circ Shock 1986;19:347-356.

40. Gill AB, Wendling AM: Echocardiographic assessment of cardiac function in shocked very low birthweight infants. Arch Dis Child 1993;68(1 Spec No):17-21.

41. Schonberger W, Grimm W, Gemp W, et al: Transient hypothyroidism associated with prematurity, sepsis, and respiratory distress. Eur J Pediatr 1979;132:85-92.

42. Roberton NR, Smith MA: Early neonatal hypocalcemia. Arch Dis Child 1975;50:604-609.

43. Osiovitch H, Phillipos E, Lemke RP: A short course of hydrocortisone in hypotensive neonates < 1250 grams in the first 24 hours of life: A randomized, double blind controlled trial. Pediatr Res 2000;47:2498.

44. Haque K, Mohan P: Pentoxifylline for neonatal sepsis. Cochrane Database Syst Rev 2003;(4):CD004205.

45. Zimmerman JJ: Appraising the potential of pentoxyfilline in septic premies. Crit Care Med 1999;27:695-697.

46. Redl-Wenzl EM, Armbruster C, Edelman G, et al: The effects of norepinephrine on hemodynamics and renal function in severe septic shock. Intensive Care Med 1993;19:151-154.

47. LeDoux D, Astiz ME, Carpati CM, et al: Effects of perfusion pressure on tissue perfusion in septic shock. Crit Care Med 2000;28:2729-2732.

48. Greenhalgh DG, Warden GD: The importance of intra-abdominal pressure measurements in burned children. J Trauma 1994;36:685-690.

49. Rivers E, Nguyen B, Havstad, et al: Early goal directed therapy in the treatment of severe sepsis and septic shock. New Engl J Med 2001;346:1368-1377.

50. Kanter RK, Zimmerman JJ, Strauss RH, et al: Pediatric emergency intravenous access: Evaluation of a protocol. Am J Dis Child 1986;140:132-134.

51. Idris AH, Melker RS: High flow sheaths for pediatric fluid resuscitation: A comparison of flow rates with standard pediatric catheters. Pediatr Emerg Care 1992;8:119-122.

52. Carcillo JA, Davis AI, Zaritsky A: Role of early fluid resuscitation in pediatric septic shock. JAMA 1991;266:1242-1245.

53. Carrol CG, Snyder JV: Hyperdynamic severe intravascular sepsis depends on fluid administration in cynomolgous monkey. Am J Physiol 1982;243:R131-R141.

54. Lee PK, Deringer JR, Kreiswirth BN, et al: Fluid replacement protection of rabbits challenged subcutaneous with toxic shock syndrome toxins. Infect Immun 1991;59:79-87.

55. Ottoson J, Dawidson I, Brandberg A, et al: Cardiac output and organ blood flow in experimental septic shock and treatment with antibiotics, corticosteroids, and fluid infusion. Circ Shock 1991;35:14-24.

56. Hoban LD, Paschall JA, Eckstein J, et al: Awake porcine model of intraperitoneal sepsis and altered oxygen utilization. Circ Shock 1991;34:252-262.

57. Wilson MA, Choe MC, Spain DA: Fluid resuscitation attenuates early cytokine mRNA expression after peritonitis. J Trauma 1996;41:622-627.

58. Boldt J, Muller M, Heesen M: Influence of different volume therapies and pentoxifylline infusion on circulating adhesion molecules in critically ill patients. Crit Care Med 1998;24:385-391.

59. Zadrobilek E, Hackl W, Sporn P, et al: Effect of large volume replacement with balanced electrolyte solutions on extravascular lung water in surgical patients with sepsis syndrome. Intensive Care Med 1989;15:505-510.

60. Powell KR, Sugarman LI, Eskenazi AE, et al: Normalization of plasma arginine vasopressin concentrations when children with meningitis are given maintenance plus replacement fluid therapy. J Pediatr 1990;117:515-522.

61. Pladys P, Wodey E, Betremieux P: Effects of volume expansion on cardiac output in the preterm infant. Acta Paediatr 1997;86:1241-1245.

62. Lambert HJ, Baylis PH, Coulthard MG: Central-peripheral temperature difference, blood pressure, and arginine vasopressin in preterm neonates undergoing volume expansion. Arch Dis Child Fetal Neonatal Educ 1998;78:F43-F45.

63. Bressack MA, Morton NS, Hortop J: Group B streptococcal sepsis in the piglet: Effects of fluid therapy on venous return, organ edema, and organ blood flow. Circ Res 1987;61:659-669.

64. Pollard AJ, Britto J, Nadel S, et al: Emergency management of meningococcal disease. Arch Dis Child 1999;80:290-296.

65. Cochrane Injuries Group: Human albumin administration in critically ill patients: Systematic review of randomized controlled trials. BMJ 1998;317:235-240.

66. Boldt J, Heesen M, Welters I: Does the type of volume therapy influence endothelial-related coagulation in the critically ill? Br J Anaesth 1995;75:740-746.

67. Lucking SE, Williams TM, Chaten FC: Dependence of oxygen consumption on oxygen delivery in children with hyperdynamic septic shock and low oxygen extraction. Crit Care Med 1990;18:1316-1319.

68. Mink RB, Pollack MM: Effect of blood transfusion on oxygen consumption in pediatric septic shock. Crit Care Med 1990;18:1087-1091.

69. McLuckie A, Murdoch IA, Marsh MJ, et al: Comparison of pulmonary artery and thermodilution cardiac indices in pediatric intensive care patients. Acta Paediatr 1996;85:336-338.

70. Padbury JF, Agata Y, Baylen BG, et al: Pharmacokinetics of dopamine in critically ill newborn infants. J Pediatr 1990;117:472-476.

71. Bhatt-Mehta V, Nahata MC, McClead RE, et al: Dopamine pharmacokinetics in critically ill newborn infants. Eur J Clin Pharmacol 1991;40:593-597.

72. Allen E, Pettigrew A, Frank D, et al: Alterations in dopamine clearance and catechol-O-methyltransferase activity by dopamine infusions in children. Crit Care Med 1997;25:181-189.

73. Outwater KM, Treves ST, Lang P: Renal and hemodynamic effects of dopamine in infants following cardiac surgery. J Clin Anesth 1990;2:253-257.

74. Lobe TE, Paone R, Dent SR: Benefits of high-dose dopamine in experimental neonatal septic shock. J Surg Res 1987;42:665-674.

75. Seri I, Tulassay T, Kiszel J, et al: Cardiovascular response to dopamine in hypotensive preterm neonates with severe hyaline membrane disease. Eur J Pediatr 1984;142:3-9.

76. Padbury JF, Agata Y, Baylen BG, et al: Dopamine pharmacokinetics in critically ill newborn infants. J Pediatr 1987;110:293-298.

77. Hentschel R, Hensel D, Brune T, et al: Impact on blood pressure and intestinal perfusion of dobutamine or dopamine in hypotensive preterm infants. Biol Neonate 1995;68:318-324.

78. Klarr JM, Faix RG, Pryce CJ: Randomized, blind trial of dopamine versus dobutamine for treatment of hypotension in preterm infants with respiratory distress syndrome. J Pediatr 1994;125:117-122.

79. Meadows D, Edwards JD, Wilkins RG, et al: Reversal of intractable septic shock with norepinephrine therapy. Crit Care Med 1988; 16:663-666.

80. Desjars P, Pinaud M, Potel G, et al: A reappraisal of norepinephrine therapy in human septic shock. Crit Care Med 1987;15: 134-137.

81. Gregory JS, Binfiglio NF, Dasta JF, et al: Experience with phenylephrine as a component of the pharmacologic support of septic shock. Crit Care Med 1991;19:1395-1400.

82. Yunge M, Petros A: Angiotensin for septic shock unresponsive to noradrenaline. Arch Dis Child 2000;82:388-389.

83. Rosenzweig EB, Starc TJ, Chen JM, et al: Intravenous arginine-vasopressin in children with vasodilatory shock after cardiac surgery. Circulation 1999;100(19 Suppl):11182-11186.

84. Harada K, Tamura M, Ito T, et al: Effects of low-dose dobutamine on left ventricular diastolic filling in children. Pediatr Cardiol 1996;17:220-225.

85. Stopfkuchen H, Schranz D, Huth R, Jungst BK: Effects of dobutamine on left ventricular performance in newborns as determined by systolic time intervals. Eur J Pediatr 1987; 146:135-139.

86. Stopfkuchen H, Queisser-Luft A, Vogel K: Cardiovascular responses to dobutamine determined by systolic time intervals in preterm infants. Crit Care Med 1990;18:722-724.

87. Habib DM, Padbury JF, Anas NG, et al: Dobutamine pharmacokinetics and pharmacodynamics in pediatric intensive care patients. Crit Care Med 1992;20:601-608.

88. Berg RA, Donnerstein RL, Padbury JF: Dobutamine infusions in stable, critically ill children: Pharmacokinetics and hemodynamic actions. Crit Care Med 1993;21:678-686.

89. Martinez AM, Padbury JF, Thio S: Dobutamine pharmacokinetics and pharmacodynamics and cardiovascular responses in critically ill neonates. Pediatrics 1992;89:47-51.

90. Perkin RM, Levin DL, Webb R, et al: Dobutamine: A hemodynamic evaluation in children with shock. J Pediatr 1982;100: 977-983.

91. Goto M, Griffin A: Adjuvant effects of beta-adrenergic drugs on indomethacin treatment of newborn canine endotoxic shock. J Pediatr Surg 1991;26:1156-1160.

92. Lopez SL, Leighton JO, Walther FJ: Supranormal cardiac output in the dopamine- and dobutamine-dependent preterm infant. Pediatr Cardiol 1997;18:292-296.

93. Bollaert PE, Bauer P, Audibert G, et al: Effects of epinephrine on hemodynamics and oxygen metabolism in dopamine-resistant septic shock. Chest 1990;98:949-953.

94. Meier-Hellman A, Reinhart K, Bredle DC, et al: Epinephrine impairs splanchnic perfusion in septic shock. Crit Care Med 1997;25:399-404.

95. Bailey JM, Miller BE, Kanter KR, et al: A comparison of the hemodynamic effects of amrinone and sodium nitroprusside in infants after cardiac surgery. Anesth Analg 1997;84:294-298.

96. Laitinen P, Happonen JM, Sairanae H, et al: Amrinone vs dopamine-nitroglycerin after reconstructive surgery for complete atrioventricular septal defect. J Cardiothorac Vasc Anesth 1997;11:870-874.

97. Sorenson GK, Ramamoorthy C, Lynn AM, et al: Hemodynamic effects of amrinone in children after Fontan surgery. Anesth Analg 1996;82:241-246.

98. Chang AC, Atz AM, Wernovsky G, et al: Milrinone: Systemic and pulmonary hemodynamics effects in neonates after cardiac surgery. Crit Care Med 1995;23:1907-1914.

99. Keeley SR, Bohn DJ: The use of inotropic and afterload-reducing agents in neonates. Clin Perinatol 1988;15:467-489.

100. Barton P, Garcia J, Kouatli A, et al: Hemodynamic effects of i.v. milrinone lactate in pediatric patients with septic shock: A prospective, double-blinded, randomized, placebo-controlled, interventional study. Chest 1996;109:1302-1312.

101. Lindsay CA, Barton P, Lawless S, et al: Pharmacokinetics and pharmacodynamics of milrinone lactate in pediatric patients with septic shock. J Pediatr 1998;132:329-334.

102. Irazusta JE, Pretzlaff RK, Rowin ME: Amrinone in pediatric refractory shock: An open label pharmacodynamic study. Pediatr Crit Care Med 2001;2:24-28.

103. Heyderman RS, Klein NJ, Shennan GI, et al: Deficiency of prostacyclin production in meningococcal shock. Arch Dis Child 1991;66:1296-1299.

104. Lauterbach R, Zembala M: Pentoxifylline reduces plasma tumor necrosis factor-alpha concentration in premature infants with sepsis. Eur J Pediatr 1996;155:404-409.

105. Kawczynski P, Piotrowski A: Circulatory and diuretic effects of dopexamine infusion in low-birth-weight infants with respiratory failure. Intensive Care Med 1996;22:65-70.

106. Habre W, Beghetti M, Roduit C, et al: Hemodynamic and renal effects of dopexamine after cardiac surgery in children. Anaesth Intensive Care 1996;24:435-439.

107. Drop LJ, Laver MB, Roberton NR, et al: Low plasma ionized calcium and response to calcium therapy in critically ill man. Anesthesiology 1975;43:300-306.

108. Cardenas-Rivero N, Chernow B, Stoiko MA, et al: Hypocalcemia in critically ill children. J Pediatr 1989;114:946-951.

109. Hatherill M, Tibby SM, Hilliard T, et al: Adrenal insufficiency in septic shock. Arch Dis Child 1999;80:51-55.

110. Ryan CA: Fatal childhood pneumococcal Waterhouse-Friderichsen syndrome. Pediatr Infect Dis J 1993;12:250-251.

111. Kohane DS: Endocrine, mineral, and metabolic disease in pediatric intensive care. In Rogers MC (ed): Textbook of Pediatric Intensive Care. Baltimore, Williams & Wilkins, 1996.

112. Matot I, Sprung CL: Corticosteroids in septic shock: Resurrection of the last rites? Crit Care Med 1998;26:627-629.

113. Briegel J, et al: Hemodynamic improvement in refractory septic shock with cortisol replacement therapy. Intensive Care Med 1992;18:318.

114. Moran JL, et al: Hypocortisolaemia and adrenocortical responsiveness at onset of septic shock. Intensive Care Med 1994; 20: 489-495.

115. Todd JK, Ressman M, Caston SA, et al: Corticosteroid therapy for patients with toxic shock syndrome. JAMA 1984;252:3399-3402.

116. Sonnenschein H, Joos HA: Hydrocortisone treatment of endotoxin shock: Another paradox in pediatrics. Clin Pediatr 1970;9: 251-252.

117. Hodes HL: Care of the critically ill child: Endotoxic shock. Pediatrics 1969;44:248-260.

118. Joosten KF, deKleign ED, Westerndorp J, et al: Endocrine and metabolic responses in children with meningococcal sepsis: Striking differences between survivors and nonsurvivors. J Clin Endocrinol Metab 2000;85:3746-3753.

119. Riordan FA: Admission cortisol and adrenocorticotropin hormone levels in children with meningococcal disease: Evidence of adrenal insufficiency? Crit Care Med 1999;27:2257-2261.

120. Soni A, Pepper GM, Wyrwinski PM, et al: Adrenal insufficiency occurring during septic shock, incidence, outcome, and relationship to peripheral cytokine levels. Am J Med 1995; 98: 266-271.

121. Migeon CJ, Kenny FM, Hung W, et al: Study of adrenal function in children with meningitis. Pediatrics 1967;40:163-181.

122. Sonnenschein H, Joos HA: Use and dosage of hydrocortisone in endotoxic shock. Pediatrics 1970;45:720.

123. Bettendorf M, Schmitt KG, Grulich Henn J, et al: Tri-iodothyronine treatment in children after cardiac surgery a double blind, randomized placebo controlled study. Lancet 2000;356:529-534.

124. Annane D, Sebille A, Charpentier C, et al: Effect of treatment with low doses of hydrocortisone and fludrocortisone on mortality in patients with septic shock. JAMA 2002;288:862-887.

125. Roberts JD Jr, Rinnai JR, Main FC 3rd, et al: Inhaled nitric oxide and persistent pulmonary hypertension of the newborn: The Inhaled Nitric Oxide Study Group. N Engl J Med 1997;336: 605-610.

126. Inhaled Nitric Oxide Study Group: Inhaled nitric oxide in full term and nearly full-term infants with hypoxic respiratory failure. N Engl J Med 1997;336:597-604.

127. Wung JT, James LS, Kilchevsky E: Management of infants with severe respiratory failure and persistence of the fetal circulation, without hyperventilation. Pediatrics 1985;76:488-494.

128. Drummond WH, Gregory GA, Heyman MA, et al: The independent effects of hyperventilation, tolazoline, and dopamine on infants with persistent pulmonary hypertension need to be taken into consideration when using these drugs. J Pediatr 1981; 98:603-611.

129. Drummond WH: Use of cardiotonic therapy in the management of infants with PPHN. Clin Perinatol 1984;11:715-728.

130. Gouyon JB, Francoise M: Vasodilators in persistent pulmonary hypertension of the newborn: A need for optimal appraisal of efficacy. Dev Pharmacol Ther 1992;19:62-68.

131. Meadow WL, Meus PJ: Hemodynamic consequences of tolazoline in neonatal group B streptococcal bacteremia: An animal model. Pediatr Res 1984;18:960-965.

132. Sandor GG, Macnab AJ, Akesode FA, et al: Clinical and echocardiographic evidence suggesting afterload reduction as a mechanism of action of tolazoline in neonatal hypoxemia. Pediatr Cardiol 1984;5:93-99.

133. Benitz WE, Malachowski N, Cohen RS, et al: Use of sodium nitroprusside in neonates: Efficacy and safety. J Pediatr 1985;106: 102-110.

134. Bartlett RH, Roloff DW, Custer JR, et al: Extracorporeal life support: The University of Michigan experience. JAMA 2000;283:904-908.

135. Meyer DM, Jessen ME: Results of extracorporeal membrane oxygenation in neonates with sepsis: The Extracorporeal Life Support Organization experience. J Thorac Cardiovasc Surg 1995; 109:419-425.

136. Bernbaum J, Schwartz IP, Gerdes M, et al: Survivors of extracorporeal oxygenation at 1 year of age: The relationship of primary diagnosis with health and neurodevelopmental sequalae. Pediatrics 1995;96(5 Pt 1):907-913.

137. The Collaborative UK ECMO (Extracorporeal Membrane Oxygenation) Trial: Follow-up to 1 year of age. Pediatrics 1998;101:E1.

138. Meyer DM, Jessen ME: Results of extracorporeal membrane oxygenation in children with sepsis: The Extracorporeal Life Support Organization. Ann Thorac Surg 1997;63:756-761.

139. Goldman AP, Kerr SJ, Butt W: Extracorporeal support for intractable cardiorespiratory failure due to meningococcal disease. Lancet 1997;349:466-469.

140. Beca J, Butt W: Extracorporeal membrane oxygenation for refractory septic shock in children. Pediatrics 1994;93:726-729.

141. Dalton HJ, Siewers RD, Fuhrman BP, et al: Extracorporeal membrane oxygenation for cardiac rescue in children with severe myocardial dysfunction. Crit Care Med 1997;21:1020-1028.

142. Hallin GW, Simpsom SQ, Crowell RE: Cardiopulmonary manifestations of Hantavirus pulmonary syndrome. Crit Care Med 1996;24:252-258.

143. Crowley MR, Katz RW, Kessler R, et al: Successful treatment of adults with Hantavirus pulmonary syndrome with ECMO. Crit Care Med 1998;26:409-414.

144. Fu YC, Chi CS, Yin SC, et al: Norepinephrine induces apoptosis in neonatal rat cardiomyocyte through a reactive oxygen species-TNF alpha-caspase signaling pathway. Cardiovasc Res 2004;62:558-567.

145. Brown MA, Jones WK: NF-kappaB action in sepsis: The innate immune system and the heart. Front Biosci 2004;9:1201-1217.

146. Witthaut R, Busch C, Fraunberger P, et al: Plasma atrial natriuretic peptide and brain natriuretic peptide in septic shock: Impact of interleukin-6 and sepsis-associated left ventricular dysfunction. Intensive Care Med 2003;29:1696-1702.

147. Dellinger RP: Cardiovascular management of septic shock. Crit Care Med 2003;31:946-955.

148. Marik PE: Cardiovascular dysfunction of sepsis: A nitric oxide and L-arginine deficient state? Crit Care Med 2003;31:971-974.

149. Wu R, Zhou M, Cui X, et al: Upregulation of cardiovascular ghrelin receptor occurs in the hyperdynamic phase of sepsis. Am J Physiol Heart Circ Physiol 2004;287:H1296–1302.

150. Dellinger RP, Carlet JM, Masur H, et al: Surviving sepsis campaign guidelines for management of severe sepsis and septic shock. Crit Care Med 2004;32:858-873.

151. Frommhold D, Birle A, Linderkamp O, et al: Drotrecogin alpha activated in neonatal septic shock. Scand J Infect Dis 2005;37:306–308.

CHAPTER 30

Outpatient Management of Pediatric Heart Failure

Jack F. Price

Congestive heart failure (CHF) in children is a clinical syndrome that challenges even the most adept pediatric cardiologist. Many of the standard physical examination findings that physicians are taught in medical school (e.g., rales, jugular venous distention, pedal edema) frequently are not applicable during the assessment of a child with heart failure. Well-known risk factors and comorbidities, such as smoking and diabetes, are rarely considered when taking a history of a child with ventricular dysfunction. Although attempts have been made to classify the symptoms and signs of heart failure in children, no standard functional classification exists for children with left ventricular dysfunction and CHF.[1] Despite the great advances in the understanding of heart failure management in adults, no large, randomized, placebo-controlled studies have been performed assessing the safety and efficacy of medical therapies for chronic heart failure in children. Much of the accepted practice comes by way of adult patients.

Just how does a pediatric cardiologist go about practicing "standard of care" medicine for a child with heart failure? Should children be treated like small adults? Is it appropriate to model a child's care after a paradigm that has evolved by assessing mortality rates among adult patients after myocardial infarction? The paucity of large clinical trials in children puts the pediatric cardiologist in the position of adopting proved methods of adult heart failure management and modifying them as they see fit, hoping they somehow will benefit the patient. Evidence-based medicine for the management of pediatric CHF does not exist at this time. Until large, multicenter trials of children with heart failure are performed, the best that pediatric cardiologists can do for their patients is to read the adult literature, cautiously introduce accepted therapies, and follow patients closely. This chapter reviews the outpatient management of children with ventricular dysfunction, with or without symptomatic heart failure. More detailed information on diagnosis, pathophysiology, and pharmacology can be found in other chapters and in the appendices.

TREATMENT FOR CHRONIC COMPENSATED HEART FAILURE

In 1995, the American Heart Association and the American College of Cardiology (AHA/ACC) formed a task force to recommend practice guidelines for the evaluation and management of heart failure in adults. These recommendations were made in collaboration with the International Society for Heart and Lung Transplantation (ISHLT) and were endorsed by the Heart Failure Society of America (HFSA). The guidelines were reassessed and updated in 2001.[2] The HFSA has established practice guidelines for the management of patients with heart failure caused by left ventricular dysfunction,[3] which can be accessed at the HFSA website (www.hfsa.org). The recommendations listed by each group are evidence based whenever possible; however, the strength of the evidence does not reflect the strength of the recommendation. That is, a strong recommendation may be based only on expert opinion and experience in certain instances, rather than on well-designed and adequately controlled clinical trials. Most of the following specific pharmacologic guidelines for heart failure management have been established by the HFSA or the AHA/ACC joint task force (See Appendix for select adult trials).

Angiotensin-Converting Enzyme Inhibitors

Inhibition of the angiotensin-converting enzyme (ACE) has been studied widely in adults with CHF and has come to be accepted as a mainstay of therapy for symptomatic and asymptomatic patients. Numerous studies have shown improved functional status, decreased hospitalization, and reduced mortality rates in heart failure patients, offering strong evidence for the use of ACE inhibitors as standard of care (Table 30-1).[4-9] The ACC/AHA executive summary recommends that ACE inhibitors be used in all adult patients with a reduced ejection fraction, with or without symptomatic heart failure.

The **Cooperative North Scandinavian Enalapril Survival Study (CONSENSUS)** randomized 253 patients with severe heart failure to receive either enalapril or placebo.[10] Mortality was reduced by 31% at 1 year (see Table 30-1). The entire reduction in total mortality was found to be in patients with progressive heart failure (a reduction of 50%), whereas no difference was seen in the incidence of sudden cardiac death. The study was prematurely discontinued because of the significant improvement in survival in the enalapril group. The **Studies of Left Ventricular Dysfunction (SOLVD)** trials examined the effect of enalapril on mortality in asymptomatic patients with reduced left ventricular ejection fraction and patients with symptomatic CHF.[11,12] Among the symptomatic patients (90%

TABLE 30-1

Select Clinical Trials of Angiotensin-Converting Enzyme Inhibitors in Heart Failure			
Trial	Drug	NYHA Class	Findings
CONSENSUS[10]	Enalapril	IV	31% reduction in mortality
SOLVD (Treatment)[11]	Enalapril	II-IV	16% reduction in mortality
SOLVD (Prevention)[12]	Enalapril	I	29% reduction in mortality or new-onset heart failure
V-HeFT II[13]	Enalapril versus hydralazine and isosorbide dinitrate	II-IV	28% reduction in mortality

NYHA, New York Heart Association.

of whom were New York Heart Association [NYHA] class II or III) randomized to enalapril or placebo in this multicenter trial, mortality was reduced by 16%. The largest reduction of deaths occurred in patients who died of progressive heart failure rather than patients who died suddenly. Among the patients with asymptomatic left ventricular dysfunction, 4228 were randomized to either enalapril or placebo and followed for an average of 37 months. No significant reduction in mortality alone occurred; however, when combined with patients who developed heart failure, a risk reduction of 29% was identified. In the **Vasodilator–Heart Failure Trial (V-HeFT II)**, the effects of hydralazine and isosorbide dinitrate were compared with the effects of enalapril in 804 men being treated with digoxin and diuretic for heart failure.[13] Two-year mortality was reduced by 28% in the enalapril arm with sudden death decreasing by 38%.

Little is known about the effect of ACE inhibition in children with ventricular dysfunction. Mortality may be reduced in infants and children with cardiomyopathy treated with ACE inhibitors. Enalapril may reduce left ventricular wall stress and improve function in children treated with chemotherapeutic agents.[14,15] There is evidence that captopril can increase cardiac output and stroke volume acutely in children with dilated cardiomyopathy, but long-term hemodynamic benefits have not been reported.[16] Lewis and Chabot[17] reported a significant improvement in survival 2 years after initiation of therapy in 27 patients treated with ACE inhibitors compared with children who received conventional medical therapy. Only one randomized, placebo-controlled study has been performed assessing the benefits of ACE inhibitors in children. Kouatli and colleagues[18] randomized 18 children who had undergone the Fontan procedure to receive either enalapril or placebo for 10 weeks. The authors concluded that exercise capacity, resting cardiac index, and diastolic function did not improve with enalapril therapy.

β-Adrenergic Receptor Blockers

Although previously viewed with skepticism, β-blocker therapy in patients with left ventricular dysfunction has become the standard of care and probably the most important addition to the current pharmacologic armamentarium of heart failure medical therapy. During the 1970s and 1980s, several small trials showed some hemodynamic and clinical benefits of β-blocker therapy.[19-22] Other large-scale studies have been performed since showing its safety and supporting its use for improving symptoms and reducing morbidity and mortality (Table 30-2).[23-33]

TABLE 30-2

Select Clinical Trials of β-Blockers in Heart Failure			
Trial	Drug	NYHA Class	Findings
Chronic heart failure (Packer et al)[35]	Carvedilol	II-IV	65% reduction in mortality; 27% reduction in hospitalization
PRECISE[36]	Carvedilol	III-IV	Small improvement in exercise tolerance; moderate symptomatic improvement
MOCHA[37]	Carvedilol	II-III	58% reduction in hospitalization; dose-related reduction in mortality
COPERNICUS[38]	Carvedilol	III-IV	24% combined risk reduction for morbidity and mortality
MERIT[41]	Metoprolol	II-IV	34% reduction in mortality

NYHA, New York Heart Association.

Consequently, β-blocker therapy is now recommended for most adult patients with CHF.

The HFSA recommends that "β-blocker therapy should be routinely administered to clinically stable patients with left ventricular systolic dysfunction (ejection fraction <40%) and mild to moderate heart failure symptoms who are on standard therapy, including ACE inhibitors, diuretics and digoxin." **Carvedilol** is the most studied and widely used β-blocker for the treatment of heart failure in adults. It is a third-generation β-adrenergic blocker and has vasodilatory and antioxidant properties. A landmark study evaluating the efficacy of carvedilol on morbidity and mortality in patients with CHF was performed by Packer and coworkers.[34] The investigators enrolled 1094 patients with chronic heart failure and randomized them to treatment protocols to receive either placebo or carvedilol. All participants had an estimated left ventricular ejection fraction of less than 35%, and they all received a 2-week trial of 6.25 mg of carvedilol twice daily before randomization to determine whether the drug would be tolerated. Baseline anti-CHF therapy was not discontinued. The dose was adjusted gradually upward over 2 to 10 weeks to the target level of 50 to 100 mg/day. Double-blinded therapy was maintained for 6 months, during which time patients' other drug therapies were kept constant. The study was stopped prematurely by the Data and Safety Monitoring Board based on the finding of a significant effect of carvedilol on survival. The risk of mortality with carvedilol was 65% less compared with placebo (3.2% carvedilol versus 7.8% placebo; $P < .001$), and there was a 27% reduction in the risk of hospitalization for cardiovascular causes (14.1% versus 19.6%; $P = .036$).

Data from the Prospective Randomized Evaluation of Carvedilol on Symptoms and Exercise **(PRECISE)** trial, which evaluated 278 patients with moderate-to-severe heart failure, revealed that patients treated with carvedilol had a greater frequency of symptomatic improvement (81% versus 53%), a greater increase in ejection fraction (8% versus 3%), and a decrease in incidence of mortality (4.5% versus 7.6%) compared with placebo-treated patients.[35] Similarly, the Multicenter Oral Carvedilol Heart Failure Assessment **(MOCHA)** trial showed clinical improvement in patients with chronic heart failure when treated with carvedilol.[36] A dose-dependent effect on left ventricular function and survival was noted with significant improvements in patients treated with 25 mg twice daily versus 6.25 mg twice daily. In addition, carvedilol lowered the hospitalization rate by 58%. The Carvedilol Prospective Randomized Cumulative Survival **(COPERNICUS)** trial examined the effect of carvedilol therapy in patients with advanced heart failure.[37] In this double-blinded, placebo-controlled study, 2289 patients who had symptoms at rest or with minimal exertion were evaluated for a mean duration of 10 months. Patients who required intensive care or intravenous vasodilators or inotropic agents were excluded. There were 190 deaths in the placebo group and 130 deaths

in the carvedilol group, indicating a 35% decrease in the risk of death with carvedilol. A total of 507 patients died or were hospitalized in the placebo group compared with 425 patients in the carvedilol group. This difference reflected a 24% decrease in the combined risk of death or hospitalization with carvedilol.

Krum and associates[38] assessed the clinical and hemodynamic effects of carvedilol in patients with severe heart failure. Forty-nine patients with advanced heart failure and a mean ejection fraction of 16% were treated with carvedilol or placebo for 14 weeks. The authors reported a marked improvement in symptoms and functional class in patients in the study group versus the placebo group. They also noted significant increases in ejection fraction and stroke volume and decreases in pulmonary capillary wedge pressure and systemic vascular resistance. β Blockade seemed to be well tolerated in this cohort of patients with advanced symptoms, although there was a higher incidence of first-degree and advanced heart block in patients treated with carvedilol.

Metoprolol is a second-generation β-adrenergic blocker lacking the additional vasodilatory and antioxidant properties of carvedilol. One of the earliest trials examining the efficacy of metoprolol in patients with heart failure was the **Metoprolol in Dilated Cardiomyopathy (MDC)** study.[39] In this multicenter study, morbidity and mortality were the primary end points. Among the 383 patients randomized to either metoprolol or placebo, there were 34% fewer primary end points in the metoprolol compared with the placebo group. The most significant finding was the reduced need for transplantation in metoprolol-treated patients (2 versus 19 patients). A larger, more definitive study was the Metoprolol CR/XL Randomized Intervention Trial in Congestive Heart Failure **(MERIT)** trial, which evaluated metoprolol CR/XL in 3991 patients with NYHA classes II through IV heart failure.[40] The primary end point was all-cause mortality. Patients were randomized to placebo or metoprolol at doses of 25 mg or 50 mg once daily. The target dose after an 8-week up-titration period was 200 mg once daily. Mortality was reduced in the metoprolol group by 34%, with an annual rate of 11% in the placebo group and 7.2% in the metoprolol group.

The largest study to compare carvedilol and metoprolol directly was the **Carvedilol Or Metoprolol European Trial (COMET)**.[41] This was a multicenter, double-blinded, randomized parallel group trial in which 3029 patients with chronic heart failure were randomized to either carvedilol (target dose 25 mg twice daily) or metoprolol (50 mg twice daily). Primary end points were all-cause mortality and hospital admissions. After a mean duration of therapy of 58 months, the all-cause mortality for carvedilol was 34% compared with 40% for the metoprolol group ($P = .0017$). Combined mortality and hospital admissions were different between the two groups. The authors concluded that carvedilol, used in heart failure patients optimally treated with diuretics and ACE inhibitors, had a significantly greater beneficial effect on survival than metoprolol.

The HFSA recommends that "β-blocker therapy should be initiated at low doses and up-titrated slowly, generally no sooner than at 2-week intervals." In general, adults are started on carvedilol at a dose of 3.125 mg twice daily with a target dose of 25 to 50 mg twice daily. The starting dose of metoprolol CR/XL is usually 25 mg once daily with an intended maintenance dose of 200 mg once daily. Heart failure patients need to be monitored closely for signs of intolerance of the β-blocker. The prescribing physician should evaluate for signs of worsening heart failure symptoms, including fatigue and diminished exercise tolerance, and vasodilatory side effects when used in combination with other cardiac medications. If the patient's clinical status seems to deteriorate during up-titration of the β-blocker, it may be necessary to adjust the other medications or down-titrate the β-blocker to the last tolerated dose.

Abrupt withdrawal is not recommended unless the patient develops cardiogenic shock. If a β-blocker is to be stopped, a period of slow down-titration of the drug dosage is recommended. A minimum period of 2 weeks should occur before further up-titration is attempted. When a β-blocker has been discontinued, reinstitution of the drug should be performed carefully in accordance with the following suggested guidelines:[42]

1. For patients who have been off the medication for less than 72 hours and who have not been in incipient cardiogenic shock, restart the β-blocker at the dose the patient was taking just before discontinuation.

2. For patients who have been off the medication for more than 72 hours but less than 7 days and who have not been in incipient cardiogenic shock, restart the β-blocker at one half the dose the patient was taking just before discontinuation.

3. For patients who have been off the medication for more than 7 days or have been in incipient cardiogenic shock recently, restart the medication at the starting (lowest) dose, orally twice daily, and retitrate.

In contrast to the adult literature, few data have been published showing the safety or efficacy of β-blocker therapy in children with heart failure. A few case reports and case series have indicated a possible benefit of β-blocker therapy in children with ventricular dysfunction, but no large, multicenter trials have been published. Shaddy and colleagues[43] described one of the earliest uses of metoprolol therapy in children with CHF. Fifteen patients with idiopathic cardiomyopathy were treated with metoprolol at a starting dose of 0.1 to 0.2 mg/kg/dose given twice daily. The dose was increased slowly over a period of weeks to a mean dose of 1.1 mg/kg/day. There was a significant increase in fractional shortening and ejection fraction after treatment with metoprolol for nearly 24 months. Bruns and colleagues[44] reported similar benefit using carvedilol. In a multi-institutional review, most of the 46 patients treated had been diagnosed with dilated cardiomyopathy and symptomatic heart failure. Carvedilol was given twice daily at an initial dose of 0.08 mg/kg, then up-titrated over several weeks to a mean dose of 0.46 mg/kg. After 3 months of therapy, functional classification improved, and shortening fraction increased modestly. Most patients developed side effects, most commonly dizziness, hypotension, and headache. Other reports also noted subjective and objective improvements in children with ventricular dysfunction treated with β-blockers.[45-53] The only large-scale randomized β-blocker study to be performed in children is the **Pediatric Randomized Carvedilol Trial in Children with Heart Failure**. This is a multicenter study in which the primary objective is to evaluate the efficacy of carvedilol in children with symptomatic ventricular dysfunction.[54] The investigators plan to enroll 150 patients younger than 17 years of age and determine efficacy of carvedilol therapy by assessing echocardiographic changes of ventricular performance and changes in neurohormone levels. In addition, the pharmacokinetics of carvedilol will be determined for this population.

At our institution, we use metoprolol predominantly in pediatric patients with heart failure because of its availability as a liquid compound. We select symptomatic and asymptomatic patients with isolated or globally depressed ventricular function. Occasionally, we use β-blocker therapy in patients with congenital heart disease and single-ventricle anatomy; however, data are lacking for safety and efficacy in this population. Most of our treated patients have been diagnosed with idiopathic or familial dilated cardiomyopathy, have a history of myocarditis, or have developed chemotherapy-induced ventricular dysfunction; a few have ischemic cardiomyopathy.

We typically initiate β-blocker therapy in clinically stable patients who already have been treated with an ACE inhibitor and usually digoxin or furosemide or both for at least 4 weeks. Sometimes patients are started on β-blocker therapy before hospital discharge after an episode of decompensation, we rarely begin therapy this soon. Our starting dose of metoprolol is 0.1 to 0.2 mg/kg per dose given twice daily. We monitor outpatients frequently while up-titrating the dose to a target level of approximately 1 mg/kg per dose given twice daily over several weeks or months. Before initiation of therapy, we advise the parents to watch for potential side effects. Side effects such as dizziness, fatigue, dyspnea, and hyperreactive airways disease are inquired about. Diarrhea is also a fairly common side effect in patients treated with carvedilol.

When using carvedilol, we usually start with a dose of 0.05 mg/kg per dose given twice daily with a target dose of 0.4 to 0.5 mg/kg per dose given twice daily for patients weighing less than 65 kg and 25 mg twice daily for patients weighing more than 65 kg. If a patient does not tolerate up-titration of the dose we usually reduce the dose to tolerable levels rather than discontinue the drug altogether because even small doses of β-blocker may have favorable effects. We rarely are required to reduce a dose or discontinue a medicine because of side effects. Maintenance therapy is continued while following patients at least once every 6 months.

Digoxin

Historically, digoxin has been used as a first-line therapy in children with ventricular dysfunction with or without symptoms of heart failure. This treatment approach seems rational given the purported benefits of digoxin, including enhanced inotropy, possible neurohormonal attenuation, and (in adults) ventricular rate control in patients with atrial fibrillation. There are no data showing decreased mortality in chronic heart failure patients treated with digoxin, however. In children, data are lacking for any type of benefit from digoxin when used in patients with ventricular dysfunction.

The HFSA recommends that "digoxin should be considered for patients who have symptoms of heart failure (NYHA classes II-III) caused by left ventricular systolic dysfunction while receiving standard therapy." The strength of this recommendation rests almost entirely on one trial, the **Digitalis Investigation Group (DIG) study**.[55] In the DIG study, 6800 patients with chronic heart failure who were treated with ACE inhibitors and diuretics were randomized to receive either digoxin (median starting dose 0.25 mg/day) or placebo. The primary end point of the study was all-cause mortality, assessed over an average follow-up of 3 years. Digoxin did not reduce all-cause mortality (34.8% in digoxin group and 35.1% in placebo group), but did reduce significantly the number of patient hospitalizations and cointerventions (e.g., increasing dose of diuretic or ACE inhibitor or adding new therapies) from 35% in the placebo group to 27% in the treatment group. A substudy of this group of patients evaluating the health-related quality of life revealed, however, that at 12 months there were no statistically significant differences in perceived health, physical functioning, depression, anxiety, anger, or the 6-minute walk between the digoxin and placebo groups.[56] Other studies have shown clinical improvement in patients treated with digoxin.[57,58]

More recent evidence has suggested that the dose of digoxin should be lower than what traditionally has been prescribed.[59] Adams and coworkers[60] examined the relationship between serum digoxin concentrations (SDC) and clinical efficacy in patients with symptomatic left ventricular dysfunction. The authors used the data from two randomized, double-blinded, placebo-controlled, digoxin-withdrawal trials: the **Prospective Randomized study Of Ventricular failure and Efficacy of Digoxin (PROVED)** and the **Randomized Assessment of Digoxin on Inhibitors of Angiotensin-Converting Enzyme (RADIANCE)**.[61,62] The trials randomized 266 patients with mostly NYHA class II functional classification and ejection fractions of 24% to 29%. Patients were classified into three groups by SDC (SDC <0.9 ng/mL, SDC 0.9 to 1.2 ng/mL, and

SDC >1.2 ng/mL). Multiple regression analysis failed to find a relationship between SDC and primary end points, such as worsening heart failure, change in left ventricular ejection fraction, and exercise tolerance.

In the heart failure and cardiomyopathy clinic at our institution, we routinely prescribe digoxin for patients with symptomatic ventricular dysfunction. We tend to treat at a lower dose (3 to 4 µg/kg per dose given twice daily) than what is usually recommended, and we do not follow serum digoxin levels. A loading dose is unnecessary. Frequently, we discontinue digoxin if a patient remains clinically stable for an extended period. These patients usually continue medical therapy with an ACE inhibitor and β-blocker.

Diuretic Agents

Although no large trials have been performed assessing the effect of diuresis on mortality, diuretic therapy remains a fundamental part of the outpatient management of heart failure.[63] Diuretics can reduce circulatory congestion effectively in patients with heart failure, but not all patients, especially children, develop symptomatic fluid retention as outpatients. The AHA/ACC guidelines for heart failure treatment recommend that "patients with evidence of fluid retention should be given a diuretic until a euvolumic state is achieved, and diuretic therapy should be continued to prevent the recurrence of fluid retention." Although the recommendation sounds reasonable, the benefits that might be gained from routine use of diuretics should be weighed against the potential risks and side effects. Electrolyte disturbances are common, including hyponatremia, hypokalemia, hypocalcemia, and hypomagnesemia. Metabolic abnormalities, such as metabolic alkalosis, dehydration, and nephrocalcinosis, also may occur.

Many physicians treating patients with CHF start with the least toxic drug, such as thiazides, in the lowest dose necessary to induce effective diuresis.[64] If fluid retention worsens, longer acting loop diuretics are prescribed. Other physicians start with a loop diuretic. A thiazide or potassium-sparing diuretic can be added if chronic resistance develops. A landmark study by Pitt and coworkers[65] showed the beneficial effects of the potassium-sparing diuretic spironolactone in patients with severe CHF. The **Randomized Aldactone Evaluation Study (RALES)** enrolled 1663 symptomatic patients with left ventricular systolic dysfunction and an ejection fraction of less than 35%. The patients were randomized to receive either 25 mg of spironolactone daily or placebo. After a mean follow-up of 24 months, there was a significant difference in mortality in patients treated with spironolactone (35%) compared with the placebo group (46%). This 30% reduction in the risk of death in patients in the spironolactone group was attributed to a lower risk of death from progressive heart failure and sudden death from cardiac causes. In addition, patients who received spironolactone had a significant improvement in the symptoms of heart failure (NYHA class). The exact reason that long-term antagonism of aldosterone provides such beneficial effects is not fully understood, but it is likely not due to the diuretic effect alone. Attenuation of myocardial interstitial fibrosis, treatment of hypertension, and inhibition of cytokine production also may play roles in reducing mortality.

At our institution, we generally treat newly diagnosed heart failure patients in the outpatient setting with a loop diuretic such as furosemide (1 mg/kg dose given twice daily). Patients with chronic heart failure who require hospitalization for exacerbation also are treated with diuretic therapy after discharge to home. Occasionally a patient who is refractory to loop diuretic therapy requires an alteration of his or her medication profile. We may add a thiazide diuretic or give metolazone once or twice a week with close follow-up. We rarely prescribe fluid restriction in children with chronic heart failure; however, some pediatric patients (usually adolescents) who remain edematous while treated with additional diuretics respond to fluid restriction or low sodium diet or both. We usually discontinue diuretic therapy in patients with chronic ventricular dysfunction once they have demonstrated clinical stability and no fluid retention. Almost always, these patients continue to be treated with an ACE inhibitor and a β-blocker. Discontinuing diuretic therapy in stable patients with heart failure can be done safely with appropriate follow-up.[66]

TREATMENT FOR CHRONIC DECOMPENSATED HEART FAILURE

Parenteral Inotropic Therapy

Despite maximal conventional medical therapy, some outpatients remain in a chronic decompensated state and require frequent hospital admissions or emergency department visits for treatment of heart failure exacerbations. A subpopulation of this ambulatory group may become inotrope dependent, experiencing a rapid recurrence of symptoms after they have been weaned from intravenous inotropic or vasodilator medications. Pediatric patients usually are referred for organ transplantation or mechanical assistance. In adult outpatients with end-stage heart failure, continuous or intermittent infusions of positive inotropic or vasodilatory agents often are used for symptomatic relief, as hospice care, or to bridge these patients to transplantation.[67]

In 1982, Leier and colleagues[68] described the first use of **dobutamine** infusion in ambulatory patients. In a controlled study, 15 adult outpatients received intermittent 4-hour infusions of dobutamine. Ventricular function, exercise tolerance, and overall clinical status improved at doses usually less than 10 μg/kg/min. One patient developed ventricular tachycardia. Subsequently, several case reports and case series were published describing the use of intravenous inotropic agents in patients with

intractable heart failure. Applefeld and associates[69] reported symptomatic improvement in three adults with chronic CHF treated with intermittent, continuous infusions of dobutamine. The inotrope was infused for 48 hours once weekly at dosages ranging from 1.5 to 8 μg/kg/min. Hodgson and colleagues[70] described their experience using intermittent dobutamine infusions in a 19-year-old man with presumed viral myocarditis and NYHA functional class IV symptoms. The patient was treated with 48-hour infusions of dobutamine at 6 μg/kg/min with 2 to 5 days between infusions. After 11 weeks of parenteral therapy, this patient underwent successful transplantation.

Roffman and associates[71] reported the use of intermittent dobutamine infusions in 11 patients with severe chronic CHF. All patients' symptoms had remained refractory to standard medical therapy when infusions were initiated at dosages of 1 to 2 μg/kg/min and titrated to a maximal dose of 15 μg/kg/min. The mean dose of dobutamine resulting in the maximum improvement in cardiac index was 9.4 μg/kg/min (range 1.5 to 15 μg/kg/min) with an increase in baseline cardiac index of 59%. All patients reported symptomatic improvement, and NYHA class was reduced by a mean of 1.2. Krell and coworkers[72] infused dobutamine weekly over 48 hours in 13 patients. A 25% increase in cardiac output occurred in all patients, although functional improvement was achieved in only seven patients. During the 26-week study period, only three patients survived. Six deaths occurred suddenly. The authors concluded that dobutamine infusions only partly improved symptoms, and that they probably did not prolong survival.

Applefeld and associates[73] later reported on another group of patients with severe chronic heart failure. Twenty-one patients were treated with either continuous (24 hours daily) or intermittent dobutamine. Four patients also received daily dopamine infusions. Cardiac index and NYHA functional class improved significantly during a mean of 7.8 months of parenteral therapy. Reported complications included bacteremia or cellulitis in 10 patients, drug extravasation in 3, and pump malfunction in 2. Mortality during this long-term period was high. Twenty patients died: 11 from heart failure, 4 suddenly, and 5 from noncardiac causes. Miller[74] described the use of intermittent infusions of dobutamine in 25 patients with refractory CHF as a bridge to transplantation. All patients were NYHA functional class IV and either could not be weaned from intravenous inotropic therapy in the hospital or could not be maintained on oral therapy alone. Most patients received a continuous infusion of 5 μg/kg/min, with duration of therapy ranging from 6 days to 11 months (mean duration 4.5 months). Thirteen patients underwent heart transplantation while receiving dobutamine as outpatients. All transplanted patients who had received dobutamine survived with an average follow-up of 27 months. Six of the patients died while waiting for a suitable organ.

Erlemeier and coworkers[75] reported a study comprising 20 patients in which participants with refractory heart failure were randomized to either dobutamine infusion at 9.25 μg/kg/min or placebo. In the treatment group, exercise duration and heart rate response to exercise increased, whereas body weight decreased. No significant changes were noted in the placebo group. Two patients died during the study; infusion therapy was tolerated in all patients without side effects. Other reports by Miller and colleagues[76] and Collins and associates[77] have shown similar hemodynamic or symptomatic benefits (or both) of outpatient parenteral inotropic therapy with dobutamine. The largest study was reported by Levine and coworkers,[78] in which 49 inotrope-dependent patients with end-stage heart failure were given dobutamine infusions as a bridge to the introduction or up-titration of ACE inhibitor/nitrate therapy. Continuous or intermittent outpatient infusions were tapered as much as possible while patients were treated with increasing doses of lisinopril and isosorbide nitrate. Over the course of 1 year, 14 patients required repeat dobutamine therapy with mean home therapy lasting 6.3 months. At 1 year, NYHA functional class and left ventricular ejection fraction improved, whereas yearly hospitalizations decreased significantly. Patients who were transplanted or died ($n = 22$) had no improvement in their ejection fraction and were hospitalized more frequently than the others.

To date, the largest case series of outpatients continuously supported on intravenous inotropes was reported by Hershberger and coworkers.[79] They reported on a cohort of 36 inotrope-dependent patients who were quite ill and in end-stage heart failure. Symptomatic hypotension, worsening dyspnea, renal insufficiency, and hypoperfusion most commonly prevented these patients from being weaned from inotropic support. There were 46 rehospitalizations (6 subjects accounted for 24 readmissions and 23 subjects had 0 or 1 readmission). Median survival was 3.4 months. Most patients died at home and chose not to be resuscitated.

Infusions of **milrinone** also have been used in the outpatient setting. Casario and colleagues[80] treated 10 end-stage heart failure patients with intermittent milrinone dosing in which infusions were given over 6 to 12 hours every 3 to 5 days. Patients tolerated the drug well, with no deaths and a fourfold decrease in hospitalizations during the study. Symptoms improved, and the mean number of reported hours of improvement after infusion therapy progressively increased during the study. Lopez-Candales and associates[81] described symptomatic improvement in 29 patients treated with milrinone for intractable heart failure. Study patients were randomized to treatment with milrinone, dobutamine, or placebo. Patients assigned to the milrinone arm required fewer treatment sessions. A significant reduction in quality-of-life scores and an increase in 6-minute walk assessments were noted in patients in the inotrope groups. No adverse events occurred.

The use of parenteral inotropic therapy in outpatients awaiting heart transplantation has been examined by Upadya and coworkers.[82] In their study, 21 patients listed as 1B status were treated with dobutamine, milrinone, or low-dose dopamine. Patients had improved functional capacity, improved renal function, and decreased number of hospitalizations during outpatient parenteral therapy compared with their pretreatment baseline. Actuarial survival to transplantation at 6 and 12 months was 84%. Inotropic outpatient therapy also has been used with favorable results in patients with end-stage heart failure in hospice and palliative care centers.[83]

In addition to improving symptoms, decreasing hospitalizations, and serving as a bridge to transplantation, outpatient inotropic therapy is cost-effective. Marius-Nunez and associates[84] reported their observations of cost containment in 36 patients treated with milrinone or dobutamine over a mean duration of 294 days. The number of emergency department visits, admissions, and days spent in the hospital decreased dramatically, and inpatient expenditures were reduced by 86%. Sindone and colleagues[85] also noted a cost savings, in 1997 dollars, of $370 for every day of home ambulatory inotropic drug therapy. The total amount saved for the 20 patients in their study, with more than 3000 days spent as outpatients, was $1,107,000, or an average of $55,350 per patient.

To date, data are lacking for the use of outpatient inotropic infusions in children with refractory heart failure. At our institution, we have used low-dose dopamine or milrinone or both in seven pediatric patients (mean age 14 years, none <8 years) as a bridge to transplantation. Six of these patients had been hospitalized or seen in the emergency department on multiple occasions before beginning parenteral therapy, and all had persistent symptoms of heart failure. The median duration of therapy was 10 weeks (range 4 to 84 weeks). Mean all-cause hospital admissions and emergency department visits significantly decreased during parenteral therapy, and mean ejection fraction significantly improved. One death and five catheter-related complications occurred in two patients. The only death occurred suddenly at home and was believed to be due to an arrhythmia. Despite the reported cases of success with such palliative care, no randomized controlled trials have been performed assessing the safety and efficacy of outpatient intermittent or continuous inotropic therapy. The conclusions of these investigators must be tempered by the risks of potential mortality and morbidity.[86,87]

Parenteral Vasodilator Therapy

Partly as a result of the reported safety, therapeutic success, and cost-effectiveness of ambulatory inotropic infusion therapy, investigators have evaluated the safety and feasibility of using serial infusions of **nesiritide** for the treatment of heart failure in the outpatient setting.[88] Nesiritide is a recombinant form of human B-type natriuretic peptide with several beneficial properties, including afterload reduction, diuresis, and reverse remodeling effects. It has been approved for the treatment of acutely decompensated heart failure in adults. In the **Follow-Up Serial Infusions of Nesiritide** pilot trial **(FUSION I)**, repeated infusions of nesiritide were administered in the ambulatory setting for the management of chronic decompensated heart failure. To date, FUSION I is the largest controlled study of outpatient intravenous therapy in patients with chronic heart failure. The objective was to determine the safety and tolerability of nesiritide in this setting. During the study, 210 patients were randomly assigned to usual care only or usual care plus weekly infusions of nesiritide at dosages of 0.005 µg/kg/min or 0.01 µg/kg/min for 12 weeks. Infusions were given over 4 to 6 hours after a bolus of 1 to 2 µg/kg. All patients were classified as NYHA class III or IV at enrollment, and all patients were receiving optimal oral therapy. A total of 1645 nesiritide infusions were administered; only 11 (<1%) were discontinued because of adverse events. The most commonly reported adverse events were symptomatic and asymptomatic hypotension. Two patients reported nausea, one patient became dehydrated, and one patient developed a myocardial infarction. The authors concluded that nesiritide, when given at these dosages, was safe and tolerated in outpatients with heart failure.

CURRENT STATUS AND FUTURE TRENDS

No large, randomized, controlled trials have been performed assessing the safety and efficacy of oral medications for the treatment of CHF in children. A multicenter trial using the β-blocker carvedilol in children has been undertaken with early results expected to be released in 2005. Until such studies are routinely performed in children, the pediatric cardiologist must rely on the conclusions made from large trials in adults and apply those findings cautiously to his or her patient population. Future strategies for outpatient therapy for children with heart failure need to address pertinent issues such as monitoring and access.[89]

Key Concepts

■ Despite the great advances in the understanding of heart failure management in adults, no large, randomized, placebo-controlled studies have been performed assessing the safety and efficacy of medical therapies for chronic heart failure in children.

■ The ACC/AHA executive summary recommends that ACE inhibitors be used in all adult patients with a reduced ejection fraction, with or without symptomatic heart failure.

■ Little is known about the effect of ACE inhibition in children with ventricular dysfunction. Mortality may be reduced in infants and children with cardiomyopathy treated with ACE inhibitors.

■ There is evidence that captopril can increase cardiac output and stroke volume acutely in children with

dilated cardiomyopathy, but long-term hemodynamic benefits have not been reported.

■ Although previously viewed with skepticism, β-blocker therapy in patients with left ventricular dysfunction has become the standard of care and probably the most important addition to the current pharmacologic armamentarium of heart failure medical therapy.

■ The only large-scale randomized β-blocker study to be performed in children is the Pediatric Randomized Carvedilol Trial in Children with Heart Failure.

■ In children, data are lacking for any type of benefit from digoxin when used in patients with ventricular dysfunction.

■ Although no large trials have been performed assessing the effect of diuresis on mortality, diuretic therapy remains a fundamental part of the outpatient management of heart failure.

■ In adult outpatients with end-stage heart failure, continuous or intermittent infusions of positive inotropic or vasodilatory agents are often used for symptomatic relief, as hospice care, or to bridge these patients to transplantation.

■ Despite the reported cases of success with such palliative care, no randomized controlled trials have been performed assessing the safety and efficacy of outpatient intermittent or continuous inotropic therapy.

REFERENCES

1. Ross RD, Bollinger RO, Pinsky WW: Grading the severity of congestive heart failure in infants. Pediatr Cardiol 1992;13:72-75.
2. Hunt SA, Baker DW, Chin MH, et al: ACC/AHA guidelines for the evaluation and management of chronic heart failure in the adult: Executive summary. A report of the American College of Cardiology/American Heart Association task force on practice guidelines. Circulation 2001;104:2996-3007.
3. Adams KF, Baughman KL, Dec WG, et al: HFSA guidelines for management of patients with heart failure caused by left ventricular dysfunction-pharmacologic approaches. J Card Fail 1999;5:357-382.
4. Captopril Multicenter Research Group: A placebo-controlled trial of captopril in refractory chronic congestive heart failure. J Am Coll Cardiol 1983;2:755-763.
5. Levine TB, Olivari MT, Garberg V, et al: Hemodynamic and clinical response to enalapril, a long-acting converting-enzyme inhibitor, in patients with congestive heart failure. Circulation 1984;69:548-553.
6. Uretsky BF, Shaver JA, Liang CS, et al: Modulation of hemodynamic effects with a converting enzyme inhibitor: Acute hemodynamic dose-response relationship of a new angiotensin converting enzyme inhibitor, lisinopril, with observations on long-term clinical, functional, and biochemical responses. Am Heart J 1988;116:480-488.
7. Riegger GA: Effects of quinapril on exercise tolerance in patients with mild to moderate heart failure. Eur Heart J 1991;12:705-711.
8. Packer M, Poole-Wilson PA, Armstrong PW, et al: Comparative effects of low and high doses of the angiotensin-converting enzyme inhibitor, lisinopril, on morbidity and mortality in chronic heart failure. ATLAS Study Group. Circulation 1999;100:2312-2328.
9. Van Veldhuisen DJ, Genth-Zotz S, Brouwer J, et al: High- versus low-dose ACE inhibition in chronic heart failure: A double-blind, placebo-controlled study of imidapril. J Am Coll Cardiol 1998;32:1811-1818.

10. Effects of enalapril on mortality in severe congestive heart failure: Results of the Cooperative North Scandinavian Enalapril Survival Study (CONSENSUS). The CONSENSUS Trial Study Group. N Engl J Med 1987;316:1429-1435.

11. The SOLVD Investigators: Effect of enalapril on survival in patients with reduced left ventricular ejection fractions and congestive heart failure: Results of the treatment trial of the Studies of Left Ventricular Dysfunction (SOLVD): A randomized double blind trial. N Engl J Med 1991;325:293-302.

12. The SOLVD Investigators: Effect of enalapril on mortality and the development of heart failure in asymptomatic patients with reduced left ventricular ejection fractions. N Engl J Med 1992;327:685-691.

13. Cohn JN, Johnson G, Ziesche S, Cobb F, et al: A comparison of enalapril with hydralazine-isosorbide dinitrate in the treatment of chronic congestive heart failure. N Engl J Med 1991;325:303-310.

14. Silber JH, Cnaan A, Clark BJ, et al: Enalapril to prevent cardiac function decline in long-term survivors of pediatric cancer exposed to anthracyclines. J Clin Oncol 2004;22:820-828.

15. Lipshultz SE, Lipsitz SR, Sallan SE, et al: Long-term enalapril therapy for left ventricular dysfunction in doxorubicin-treated survivors of childhood cancer. J Clin Oncol 2002;20:4517-4522.

16. Bengur AR, Beekman RH, Rocchini AP, et al: Acute hemodynamic effects of captopril in children with a congestive or restrictive cardiomyopathy. Circulation 1991;83:523-527.

17. Lewis AB, Chabot M: The effect of treatment with angiotensin-converting enzyme inhibitors on survival of pediatric patients with dilated cardiomyopathy. Pediatr Cardiol 1993;14:9-12.

18. Kouatli AA, Garcia JA, Zellers TM, et al: Enalapril does not enhance exercise capacity in patients after Fontan procedure. Circulation 1997;96:1507-1512.

19. Waagstein F, Hjalmarson A, Varnauskas E, et al: Effect of chronic beta-adrenergic receptor blockade in congestive cardiomyopathy. Br Heart J 1975;37:1022-1036.

20. Swedberg K, Hjalmarson A, Waagstein F, et al: Prolongation of survival in congestive cardiomyopathy by beta-receptor blockade. Lancet 1979;1:1374-1376.

21. Engelmeier RS, O'Connell JB, Walsh R, et al: Improvement in symptoms and exercise tolerance by metoprolol in patients with dilated cardiomyopathy: A double-blind, randomized, placebo-controlled trial. Circulation 1985;72:536-546.

22. Anderson JL, Lutz JR, Gilbert EM, et al: A randomized trial of low-dose beta-blockade therapy for idiopathic dilated cardiomyopathy. Am J Cardiol 1985;55:471-475.

23. Lechat P, Packer M, Chalon S, et al: Clinical effects of beta-adrenergic blockade in chronic heart failure: A meta-analysis of double-blind, placebo-controlled, randomized, trials. Circulation 1998;98:1184-1191.

24. Heidenreich PA, Lee TT, Massie BM: Effect of beta-blockade on mortality in patients with heart failure: A meta-analysis of randomized clinical trials. J Am Coll Cardiol 1997;30:27-34.

25. Pollock SG, Lystash J, Tedesco C, et al: Usefulness of bucindolol in congestive heart failure. Am J Cardiol 1990;66:603-607.

26. Woodley SL, Gilbert EM, Anderson JL, et al: β-Blockade with bucindolol in heart failure caused by ischemic versus idiopathic dilated cardiomyopathy. Circulation 1991;84:2426-2441.

27. Fisher ML, Gottlieb SS, Plotnick GD, et al: Beneficial effects of metoprolol in heart failure associated with coronary artery disease: A randomized trial. J Am Coll Cardiol 1994;23:943-950.

28. Bristow MR, O'Connell JB, Gilbert EM, et al: Dose-response of chronic β-blocker treatment in heart failure from either idiopathic dilated or ischemic cardiomyopathy. Circulation 1994;89:1632-1642.

29. CIBIS investigators: A randomized trial of β-blockade in heart failure: The Cardiac Insufficiency Bisoprolol Study. Circulation 1994;90:1765-1773.

30. Eichhorn EJ, Heesch CM, Barnett JH, et al: Effect of metoprolol on myocardial function and energetics in patients with nonischemic dilated cardiomyopathy: A randomized, double-blind, placebo-controlled study. J Am Coll Cardiol 1994;24:1310-1320.

31. Metra M, Nardi M, Giubbini R, et al: Effects of short- and long-term carvedilol administration on rest and exercise hemodynamic variables, exercise capacity and clinical conditions in patients with idiopathic dilated cardiomyopathy. J Am Coll Cardiol 1994; 24:1678-1687.

32. Olsen SL, Gilbert EM, Renlund DG, et al: Carvedilol improves left ventricular function and symptoms in chronic heart failure: A double-blind randomized study. J Am Coll Cardiol 1995;25: 1225-1231.

33. Krum H, Sackner-Bernstein JD, Goldsmith RL, et al: Double-blind, placebo-controlled study of the long-term efficacy of carvedilol in patients with severe chronic heart failure. Circulation 1995;92:1499-1506.

34. Packer M, Bristow MR, Cohn JN, et al: The effect of carvedilol on morbidity and mortality in patients with chronic heart failure. N Engl J Med 1996;334:1349-1355.

35. Packer M, Colucci WS, Sackner-Bernstein JD, et al: Double-blind, placebo-controlled study of the effects of carvedilol in patients with moderate to severe heart failure. The PRECISE Trial. Circulation 1996;94:2793-2799.

36. Bristow MR, Gilbert EM, Abraham WT, et al: Carvedilol produces dose-related improvements in left ventricular function and survival in subjects with chronic heart failure. Circulation 1996;94:2807-2816.

37. Packer M, Coats AS, Fowler MB, et al: Effect of carvedilol on survival in severe chronic heart failure. N Engl J Med 2001;344: 1651-1658.

38. Krum H, Sackner-Bernstein JD, Goldsmith R, et al: Double-blind, placebo-controlled study of the long-term efficacy of carvedilol in patients with severe heart failure. Circulation 1995;92:1499-1506.

39. Waagstein F, Bristow MR, Swedberg K, et al: Beneficial effects of metoprolol in idiopathic dilated cardiomyopathy. Lancet 1993; 342:1441-1446.

40. The MERIT-HF Study Group. Effect of metoprolol CR/XL in chronic heart failure: Metoprolol CR/XL randomized intervention trial in congestive heart failure. Lancet 1999;353:2001-2007.

41. Poole-Wilson PA, Swedberg K, Cleland JG, et al: Comparison of carvedilol and metoprolol on clinical outcomes in patients with chronic heart failure in the Carvedilol Or Metoprolol European Trial (COMET): Randomised controlled trial. Lancet 2003;362:7-13.

42. Eichhorn EJ, Bristow MR: Practical guidelines for initiation of β-adrenergic blockade in patients with chronic heart failure. Am J Cardiol 1997;79:794-798.

43. Shaddy RE, Tani LY, Gidding SS, et al: Beta-blocker treatment of dilated cardiomyopathy with congestive heart failure in children: A multi-institutional experience. J Heart Lung Transplant 1999;3: 269-274.

44. Bruns LA, Chrisant MK, Lamour JM, et al: Carvedilol as therapy in pediatric heart failure: An initial multicenter experience. J Pediatr 2001;138:505-511.

45. Shaddy RE: Beta-blocker therapy in young children with congestive heart failure under consideration for heart transplantation. Am Heart J 1998;136:19-21.

46. Gachara N, Prabhakaran S, Srinivas S, et al: Efficacy and safety of carvedilol in infants with dilated cardiomyopathy: A preliminary report. Indian Heart J 2001;53:74-78.

47. Williams RV, Tani LY, Shaddy RE: Intermediate effects of treatment with metoprolol or carvedilol in children with left ventricular systolic dysfunction. J Heart Lung Transplant 2002;21:906-909.

48. Horenstein MS, Ross RD, Singh TP, et al: Carvedilol reverses elevated pulmonary vascular resistance in a child with dilated cardiomyopathy. Pediatr Cardiol 2002;23:100-102.

49. Azeka E, Ramires JA, Valler C, et al: Delisting of infants and children from the heart transplantation waiting list after carvedilol treatment. J Am Coll Cardiol 2002;40:2034-2038.

50. Laer S, Mir TS, Behn F, et al: Carvedilol therapy in pediatric patients with congestive heart failure: A study investigating clinical and pharmacokinetic parameters. Am Heart J 2002;143:916-922.

51. Giardini A, Formigari R, Bronzetti G, et al: Modulation of neuro-hormonal activity after treatment of children in heart failure with carvedilol. Cardiol Young 2003;13:333-336.

52. Rusconi P, Gomez-Marin O, Rossique-Gonzalez M, et al: Carvedilol in children with cardiomyopathy: 3 year experience at a single institution. J Heart Lung Transplant 2004;23:832-838.

53. Australia/New Zealand Heart Failure Research Collaborative: Randomised, placebo-controlled trial of carvedilol in patients with congestive heart failure due to ischaemic heart disease. Lancet 1997;349:375-380.

54. Shaddy RE, Curtin EL, Sower B, et al: The pediatric randomized carvedilol trial in children with heart failure: Rationale and design. Am Heart J 2002;144:383-389.

55. The Digitalis Investigation Group: The effect of digoxin on mortality and morbidity in patients with heart failure. N Engl J Med 1997;336:525-533.

56. Lader E, Egan D, Hunsberger S, et al: The effect of digoxin on the quality of life in patients with heart failure. J Card Fail 2003;9:4-12.

57. DiBianco R, Shabetai R, Kostuk W, et al: A comparison of oral milrinone, digoxin, and their combination in the treatment of patients with chronic heart failure. N Engl J Med 1989;320:677-683.

58. The Captopril Multicenter Research Group: Comparative effects of therapy with captopril and digoxin in patients with mild to moderate heart failure. JAMA 1988;259:539-544.

59. Rathore SS, Curtis JP, Wang Y, et al: Association of serum digoxin concentration and outcomes in patients with heart failure. JAMA 2003;289:871-878.

60. Adams KF, Gheorghiade M, Uretsky BF, et al: Clinical benefits of low serum digoxin concentrations in heart failure. J Am Coll Cardiol 2002;39:946-953.

61. Uretsky BF, Young JB, Shahidi FE, et al: Randomized study addressing the effect of digoxin withdrawal in patients with mild to moderate chronic congestive heart failure: Results of the PROVED trial. J Am Coll Cardiol 1993;22:955-962.

62. Packer M, Gheorghiade M, Young JB, et al: Withdrawal of digoxin from patients with chronic heart failure treated with angiotensin-converting enzyme inhibitors. N Engl J Med 1993;329:1-7.

63. Rodkey SM, Young JB: The cardiovascular use of diuretics. Cardiol Clin Annu Drug Ther 1997;1:63-80.

64. Topol EJ, Young JB: Textbook of Cardiovascular Medicine. Philadelphia, Lippincott Williams & Wilkins, 2002.

65. Pitt B, Zannad F, Remme WJ, et al: The effect of spironolactone on morbidity and mortality in patients with severe heart failure. Randomized Aldactone Evaluation Study Investigators. N Engl J Med 1999;341:709-717.

66. Grinstead WC, Francis MJ, Marks GF, et al: Discontinuation of chronic diuretic therapy in stable heart failure patients. Am J Cardiol 1994;73:881-886.

67. Marius-Nenez AL, Heavey L, Fernandez RN, et al: Intermittent inotropic therapy in an outpatient setting: A cost-effective therapeutic modality in patients with refractory heart failure. Am Heart J 1996;132:805-808.

68. Leier CV, Huss P, Lewis RP, et al: Drug-induced conditioning in congestive heart failure. Circulation 1982;65:1382-1387.

69. Applefeld MM, Newman KA, Grove WE, et al: Intermittent, continuous outpatient dobutamine infusion in the management of congestive heart failure. Am J Cardiol 1983;51:455-458.

70. Hodgson JM, Aja M, Sorkin RP: Intermittent ambulatory dobutamine infusions for patients awaiting cardiac transplantation. Am J Cardiol 1984;53:375-376.

71. Roffman DSD, Appelfeld MM, Grove WR, et al: Intermittent dobutamine hydrochloride infusions in outpatients with chronic congestive heart failure. Clin Pharm 1985;4:195-199.

72. Krell MJ, Kline EM, Bates E, et al: Intermittent, ambulatory dobutamine infusions in patients with severe congestive heart failure. Am Heart J 1986;112:787-791.

73. Applefeld MM, Newman KA, Sutton FJ, et al: Outpatient dobutamine and dopamine infusions in the management of chronic heart failure: Clinical experience in 21 patients. Am Heart J 1987;114:589-595.

74. Miller LW: Outpatient dobutamine for refractory congestive heart failure: Advantages, techniques, and results. J Heart Lung Transplant 1991;10:482-487.

75. Erlemeier HH, Kupper W, Bleifeld W: Intermittent infusion of dobutamine in the therapy of severe congestive heart failure-long-term effects and lack of tolerance. Cardiovasc Drugs Ther 1992;6:391-398.

76. Miller LW, Merkle EJ, Herrman V: Outpatient dobutamine for end-stage congestive heart failure. Crit Care Med 1990;18:S30-S33.

77. Collins JA, Skidmore MA, Melvin DB, et al: Home intravenous dobutamine therapy in patients awaiting heart transplantation. J Heart Transplant 1990;9:205-208.

78. Levine TB, Levine AB, Elliott WG, et al: Dobutamine as bridge to angiotensin-converting enzyme inhibitor-nitrate therapy in end-stage heart failure. Clin Cardiol 2001;24:231-236.

79. Hershberger RE, Nauman D, Walker TL, et al: Care processes and clinical outcomes of continuous outpatient support with inotropes (COSI) in patients with refractory endstage heart failure. J Card Fail 2003;9:180-187.

80. Casario D, Clark J, Maisel A: Beneficial effects of intermittent home administration of the inotrope/vasodilator milrinone in patients with end-stage congestive heart failure: A preliminary study. Am Heart J 1998;135:121-129.

81. Lopez-Candales A, Vora T, Gibbons W, et al: Symptomatic improvement in patients treated with intermittent infusions of inotropes: A double-blind placebo controlled pilot study. J Med 2002;33:129-146.

82. Upadya S, Lee FA, Saldarriaga C, et al: Home continuous positive inotropic infusion as a bridge to cardiac transplantation in patients with end-stage heart failure. J Heart Lung Transplant 2004;23:466-472.

83. Candales AL, Carron C, Schwartz J: Need for hospice and palliative care services in patients with end-stage heart failure treated with intermittent infusions of inotropes. Clin Cardiol 2004;27:23-28.

84. Marius-Nunez AL, Heaney L, Fernandez RN, et al: Intermittent inotropic therapy in an outpatient setting: A cost-effective therapeutic modality in patients with refractory heart failure. Am Heart J 1996;132:805-808.

85. Sindone AP, Keogh AM, Macdonald PS, et al: Continuous home ambulatory intravenous inotropic drug therapy in severe heart failure: Safety and cost efficacy. Am Heart J 1997;134:889-900.

86. Thadani U, Roden DM: FDA panel report: January 1998. Circulation 1998;97:2295-2296.

87. Stevenson LW: Inotropic therapy for heart failure. N Engl J Med 1998;339:1848-1850.

88. Yancy CW, Saltzberg MT, Berkowitz RL, et al: Safety and feasability of using serial infusions of nesiritide for heart failure in an outpatient setting (from the FUSION I trial). Am J Cardiol 2004;94:595-601.

89. Cleland JG, Louis AA, Rigby AS, et al: Noninvasive home telemonitoring for patients with heart failure at high risk of recurrent admission and death: The Trans-European Network Home-Care Management System (TEN-HMS) Study. J Am Coll Cardiol 2005;45:1654-1664.

CHAPTER 31

Nursing and Psychosocial Aspects of Heart Failure

Sarah K. Clunie

Nurses provide an essential human resource in treating pediatric patients with heart failure. This chapter describes heart failure as it is seen from a nurse's perspective. Nurses specializing in heart failure contribute to optimal patient outcomes. Understanding the medical and psychosocial challenges for pediatric heart failure and heart transplantation allows caregivers to respond to the changing needs of patients over their life span. See other chapters for specific detailed discussions on the relevant topics.

NURSING ASSESSMENT OF HEART FAILURE AND CARDIOMYOPATHY

Heart failure is defined as an inability of the heart to pump an adequate amount of blood to the systemic circulation to meet the metabolic demands.[1] Although the etiologies of heart failure in children are diverse, the presentation of heart failure comprises a constellation of symptoms, signs, and physical findings. The pediatric patient exhibits signs of congestive heart failure (CHF) because of decreased myocardial contraction, increased preload, and increased afterload.

The signs and symptoms of heart failure fall into three categories: (1) impaired myocardial function, (2) pulmonary congestion, and (3) systemic venous congestion. In an infant, an inability to maintain growth secondary to either decreased nutritional intake or an increased catabolic state is a hallmark of heart failure.[2] The infant exhibits increased sympathetic tone with excessive diaphoresis and increased heart rate. Physical findings in the infant with heart failure include increased work of breathing, tachypnea, and hepatomegaly.[2] In older children, new-onset heart failure may be less overtly symptomatic. Malaise, decrease in level of daily activity, and weight loss may be present. Symptoms of abdominal pain, nausea, and anorexia can be present and sometimes divert attention from the real cardiac etiology.[2] Physical findings include rales and peripheral edema. Hepatomegaly, a gallop rhythm, and tachycardia also commonly are present.

Cardiomyopathy refers to abnormalities of the myocardium in which the ability of cardiac muscles to contract is impaired. Cardiomyopathies can be divided into three clinical categories according to the type of abnormal structure and dysfunction present: (1) dilated cardiomyopathy, (2) hypertrophic cardiomyopathy and (3) restrictive cardiomyopathy (Table 31-1). One of the most difficult adjustments with this diagnosis may be the realization of failing health and the need for restricted activity, especially for normal active youngsters. Children should be included in decisions regarding activity and allowed to discuss their feelings. Nurses play a key role in assisting patients to identify their lifestyle habits that require modifications, ultimately improving their quality of life and decreasing hospital admissions. Education focusing on self-care activities, diet, rest, and exercise enables patients to retain a sense of control in their lives.

SETTING UP A HEART FAILURE PROGRAM

Management of patients with heart failure in the 1990s increasingly moved from physician-directed, inpatient care to nurse-guided and nurse-coordinated care in the outpatient arena.[3] Benefits of outpatient management include enhanced quality of life for the patient, reduced costs, and avoidance of risks associated with hospitalization.[3,4] There is no universal definition or description of the ideal heart failure clinic. In some hospitals, the heart failure clinic consists of one nurse providing extra education during a consultation 1 hour per week. In other hospitals, the heart failure clinic can be a multidisciplinary heart failure team specialized in providing care for these chronically ill patients and their families, including regular follow-up, consulting hours, individualized education (e.g., computer-based education, group education sessions).[5] In optimizing clinical and economic management of heart failure, the use of a multidisciplinary outpatient clinic is on the leading edge of patient care. Patients and families benefit from participation in a heart failure clinic. The goal of the clinic is to manage early signs and symptoms of heart failure, decrease hospital admissions, and improve patient outcomes in heart failure.[6] Actions at the clinic must focus on chronic disease management rather than just episodic care.[7]

An integral part of any heart failure specialty program is evaluation, and every program should include a plan for evaluation of its effectiveness. Evaluation of the impact of a program allows for refinement to improve

TABLE 31-1

Classification of the Cardiomyopathies

Disorder	Description
Dilated cardiomyopathy	Dilation and impaired contraction of the left or both ventricles. Caused by familial/genetic, viral and/or immune, alcoholic/toxic, or unknown factors, or is associated with recognized cardiovascular disease
Hypertrophic cardiomyopathy	Left and/or right ventricular hypertrophy, often asymmetric, which usually involves the interventricular septum. Mutations in sarcoplasmic proteins cause the disease in many patients
Restrictive cardiomyopathy	Restricted filling and reduced diastolic size of either or both ventricles with normal or near normal systolic function. Is idiopathic or associated with other disease (e.g., amyloidosis, endomyocardial disease)
Arrhythmogenic right ventricular cardiomyopathy	Progressive fibrofatty replacement of the right, and to some degree left, ventricular myocardium. Familial disease is common
Unclassified cardiomyopathy	Diseases that do not fit readily into any category. Examples include systolic dysfunction with minimal dilation, mitochondrial disease, and fibroelastosis
Specfic Cardiomyopathies	
Ischemic cardiomyopathy	Manifests as dilated cardiomyopathy with depressed ventricular function not explained by the extent of coronary artery obstructions or ischemic damage
Valvular cardiomyopathy	Manifests as ventricular dyfunction that is out of proportion to the abnormal loading conditions produced by the valvular stenosis and/or regurgitation
Hypertensive cardiomyopathy	Manifests with left ventricular hypertrophy with features of cardiac failure due to systolic or diastolic dysfunction
Inflammatroy cardiomyopathy	Cardiac dysfunction as a consequence of myocarditis
Metabolic cardiomyopathy	Includes a wide variety of causes, including endocrine abnormalities, glycogen storage disease, deficiencies (e.g., hypokalemia), and nutritional disorders
General systemic disease	Includes connective tissue disorders and infiltrative diseases such as sarcoidosis and leukemia
Muscular dystrophies	Includes Duchenne, Becker-type, and myotonic dystrophies
Neuromuscular disorder	Includes Friedreich ataxia, Noonan syndrome, and lentiginosis
Sensitivity and toxic reactions	Includes reactions to alcohol, catecholamines, anthracyclines, irradiation, and others
Peripartal cardiomyopathy	First becomes manifest in the peripartum period, but it is likely a heterogeneous group

Derived from Richardson P, McKenna W, Bristow M, et al: Report of the 1995 World Health Organization/International Society and Federation of Cardiology Task Force on the Definition and Classification of Cardiomyopathies. Circulation 93:841, 1996. Copyright 1996, American Heart Association.

From Wayne J, Braunwald E: The cardiomyopathies and myocarditides. In Braunwald E (ed): Heart Disease, (6th ed.) Philadelphia, WB Saunders, 2001.

program effectiveness and provides data when seeking reimbursement for a program from managed care organizations and insurance companies. Schulman and colleagues[55] described the steps of evaluation of heart failure disease management programs: (1) define the patient population (i.e., the characteristics of patients eligible for the services), (2) define the goals of the program (i.e., improvements in functional status and quality of life and reductions in rehospitalizations and costs), (3) measure the effectiveness of the program, (4) analyze risk adjustment and outcomes, and (5) re-evaluate the program through continuous quality improvement.[15]

Heart Failure, Cardiomyopathy, and Transplant Clinic

The heart failure, cardiomyopathy, and transplant clinic at Texas Children's Hospital is composed of a multidisciplinary team. The **medical team** comprises four specially trained pediatric cardiologists who see patients on a weekly basis in the clinic. Every other month, a combined clinic with electrophysiology/pacemaker physicians is conducted to provide comprehensive total patient care. The patient population is composed of children with cardiomyopathies, heart transplants, end-stage heart disease, and children currently awaiting cardiac transplantation. A **nurse coordinator** heads the clinic and is a resource to the entire patient community and their families. The nurse coordinator screens all appointments that are made in the clinic to determine the appropriateness of the referral. The nurse coordinator also provides patient education, telephone follow-up, telephone counseling, and patient triaging. The nurse's role in providing support groups, communicating information, connecting patients and resources, and providing compassionate care for patients and their families are crucial to the adjustment of patients with heart failure.[8]

Advanced practice nurses also have a role in the heart failure clinic. They can play an integral role in the treatment of patients in varying stages of heart failure.[9] Through education, nurses learn to approach a patient holistically, integrating many aspects of care. This integration is key to the success of patient management and leads to positive outcomes.[9] The advanced practice nurse with prescription authority can direct heart failure care effectively for outpatients by using multidisciplinary resources of the hospital. Treatment strategies include titrating medications, symptom monitoring, tracking of medication and dietary compliance, telemonitoring, and providing aggressive multidisciplinary education.[10] The use of the advanced practice nurse is highly effective for reducing hospital admissions and improving quality of life and functional status for outpatients with heart failure.[10]

A **patient care assistant** prepares charts for the clinic, obtains medical records on referred patients, schedules needed tests, and provides continuity of care for the patients. A patient care assistant also may provide second language translation for patients. There is also a **dietitian** on the team. The dietitian participates in nutritional management and requirements for the patient and provides patient and family education regarding eating habits, a warfarin diet, and a diet high in protein and calories.[11] The dietitian also assesses the child's growth patterns. If a child is failing to thrive, the first step is to increase the caloric intake. If the child is still failing to thrive, enteral feeds via a gastrostomy tube or nasogastric tube are used frequently to create an optimal state while the child is waiting for a transplant or while the child's heart is getting better.

A clinical **social worker** is another active member of the clinic team. The social worker has the expertise and experience to help the child and family identify and discuss emotional, social, and financial issues and life changes that often accompany the disease process. At some point during the illness, the patient and family members may experience each of the following feelings: anxiety, uncertainty, and apprehension about the future; depression; stress; and frustration. Many concerns are raised regarding problems with siblings adjusting to having a critically ill sibling, bodily changes and their effects on self-esteem, resuming responsibility of self-care and roles that were established before the child's illness, family relationships and friendships, and going back to school or work. A **child life specialist** is another crucial member of the clinic team. Child life specialists help meet the developmental and emotional needs of children. The specialist's role is to help normalize the experience into concepts the child can understand, minimize anxiety, promote trust, and increase positive coping skills. The child life specialist can help the child and family by providing preparation and support before, during, and after the illness; providing preparation for various medical procedures; providing support and distraction during medical procedures; providing information and guidance on coping, relaxation, and distraction techniques for children to use during times of discomfort; providing information about the child's reaction to the hospital; and providing information on how to involve siblings in and teach them about their sibling's illness.

A chronic illness such as heart failure may result in an erosion of an individual's sense of self and lead to questions related to spirituality and life priorities.[8] Another important function of the clinic team is to provide pastoral care. The team is dedicated to the healing of the whole person and providing holistic care. The **chaplain** is available to the patient and family throughout the entire disease process. The chaplain identifies and serves the spiritual needs of patients with respect and compassion, honoring the diversity of their faith, traditions, and beliefs as resources for healing and growth.[12] The goal of spiritual support is to identify helpful ways for the child and family members to make sense out of what is happening. The spiritual assessment addresses their beliefs about being sick, the spiritual resources available to them, and their hope with treatment.[12] The chaplain is open to and supportive of the spiritual journey. As a result of the time involved and the intensity of the disease process, it is common for the patient and the family to develop a deep meaningful relationship with one or more of the chaplains. Because of the critical nature of the disease process and the twist of tragedy versus hope, many profound questions arise regarding the meanings of life and death. The chaplains are experienced in helping patients and their families work through these issues no matter what their religious or philosophical beliefs are.

Inpatient Heart Failure Service

Inpatient care consists of the heart failure team acting as a consult team for the patient. The team makes recommendations to the cardiology team following the patient. The team members deliver care while the patient is hospitalized, which makes the transition to outpatient management easier because a relationship is already established. See other chapters for more detailed discussions of treatment for heart failure in the acute inpatient setting.

PSYCHOSOCIAL ASPECTS OF HEART FAILURE CARE

Drug Compliance

Improvements in heart failure outcomes depend on patients' and parents' abilities to care for themselves and manage aspects of their condition. Patient self-management itself has become a measurable outcome.[13] Some behaviors, such as diet and fluid restriction, are prescribed, and self-management is often equated with adherence to the treatment regimen. The cost of outpatient medications is a significant factor in the lives of patients and families living with heart failure.[14] Costs and ability to pay for the medication regimen must be included in any teaching plan. Many patients and families do not volunteer information about their personal finances. Discharge planning should include a plan for paying for medications. Consultation with an appropriate health care professional, such as a social worker, may assist patients in securing services that deal with financial need.[14] If cost is a factor in noncompliance, suggestions for lower cost medication or financial assistance programs should be provided.[15] There are many reasons that patients may not comply with a therapeutic regimen. Lack of knowledge, poor motivation, decreased understanding, lower perceived self-efficacy, forgetfulness, and decreased support from family and other caregivers have been identified as factors that contribute to noncompliance. A patient may not comply with a prescribed medication regimen because he or she is unconvinced of the benefits of doing so or because he or she perceives that the side effects or inconvenience of following the regimen outweigh any benefits. Another factor that contributes to patient noncompliance and rehospitalizations for worsening heart failure is inadequate discharge planning and follow-up after discharge. To improve the compliance of heart failure patients, it is necessary to identify variables that affect the compliance of the patient, provider, and health care system levels and to develop strategies to improve, monitor, and sustain compliance at all levels. The promotion of patient compliance begins with discharge planning.

Patient and Parent Education

All patients with heart failure, regardless of etiology, and their families require education about the disease. A multidisciplinary approach should include teaching about dietary restrictions, reportable signs and symptoms, activity restrictions, medications and side effects, what to do in case of an emergency, and ability to cope with a chronic disease.[37] A clear and organized plan of patient education and counseling is crucial to the achievement of optimal outcomes.[15] To maintain a reasonable quality of life and reduce hospitalizations, patients and their families must receive a clear, understandable, and simple explanation of the pathophysiology of heart failure. The term *heart failure* must be explained with care, emphasizing that it is a decrease in the reserve power of the heart as a pump. A clarification between expected symptoms of heart failure and symptoms of worsening failure is important. Patients should be instructed to notify their health care provider immediately when they experience symptoms of worsening failure to prevent unnecessary hospitalizations or complications.

Patients should be taught the name of each drug and its purpose, dosage, frequency, and significant side effects to watch for. Patients should be instructed to bring all medications with them to clinic. During the clinic visit, information about each drug can be reviewed, and the patients' knowledge can be assessed. This assessment also helps to identify omissions, duplications, and confusion about drug dosages and drug interactions.

A written medication schedule is strongly recommended for all medications. When making the medication schedule, the schedule should be constructed to minimize the impact on the patient's daily activities and sleep schedule. Such knowledge enhances patients' ability to follow the recommendations of the health care team. The goals of education and counseling are to assist patients in compliance with their therapeutic regimen, to maintain clinical stability and function, and to improve quality of life.[16] These goals can be achieved best when the patient and family are knowledgeable about every aspect of the condition and treatment and are active participants in the plan of care (Table 31-2).

Psychosocial Issues

Sudden illness or diagnosis in a child who was previously healthy produces stress or crisis in family members. Difficulty in adjusting to the seriousness of the child's condition or feeling overwhelmed by the diagnosis is not unusual.[17] Assisting family members in finding ways to maintain their parental roles and learning about the medical therapies involved gives the nurse opportunities to develop a relationship with the family.[17] This relationship allows the nurse to provide psychosocial support of the ill child and the family.[17] Introduction of other multidisciplinary team members, such as social workers and chaplains, also may be useful.[17] The incidence of depression is greater in hospitalized patients with heart failure than in stabilized outpatients. Depression is associated with mortality in patients with heart failure. For patients with advanced heart failure, adjusting involves focusing on past decisions and regrets, dealing with present reality, and nurturing future hopes. The nurse's role in providing support groups, communicating information, connecting patients and resources, and providing compassionate care for patients and their families is crucial to the adjustment of patients with heart failure.[8] Creatively facilitating patient participation in leisure activities, hobbies, and work allows patients to reach out to others and enhance their own sense of meaning. Social support and enhancement of hope are important interventions for patients with heart failure. Specifically, hope is increased by the patient's spiritual values, medical treatment, health care providers, and family and friends. Dialogue regarding these sources of hope can be integral to the care of patients and provide potentially fruitful areas for research.

NURSING ROLE IN CARDIAC TRANSPLANTATION

Pediatric heart transplantation has become an effective therapeutic modality and a standard of care for infants and children with worsening heart failure and a limited life expectancy despite maximum medical and surgical management. In 1968, Dr. Denton Cooley in Houston,

TABLE 31-2

Desired Outcomes in Management of Patients with Heart Failure

Desired Outcome	Strategy
Patient will understand and follow medication regimen	Address financial concerns
	Discuss rationale behind each drug prescribed. Keep information basic and at patient's level of understanding
	Schedule frequent visits for increasing drug dosages and reinforcing education
Dietary modifications will be achieved	Use various forms of education—handouts, videos, charts, dietary logs
	Provide list of foods to avoid and teach how to read labels
	Teach what to do when patient has "cheated" (i.e., taken an extra dose of a diuretic)
	Consult dietitian
	Plan ahead by restricting sodium intake before special occasions
	Provide low-sodium recipes
Patient will begin to make appropriate lifestyle modifications	Incorporate exercise program, such as cardiac rehabilitation or home exercise prescription
	Refer patient to smoking cessation program if needed
	Explain adverse impact of alcohol on myocardial contractility
	Provide resources for cessation of alcohol consumption
Monitoring of signs and symptoms and weight will be understood	Provide tools for recording daily weights
	Have patient call health care provider if weight gain of ≥1.4 kg (≥3 lb) occurs
	Have patient call health care provider if changes occur in dyspnea on exertion, paroxysmal nocturnal dyspnea, or onset of shortness of breath
	Personalize patient's signs and symptoms by assessing specifically how they occur with fluid retention
Patient will seek care early when needed	Give patient permission to call when he or she has reportable signs or symptoms
	Provide handouts listing reportable signs and symptoms; be specific
	Call patients routinely to assess for signs and symptoms
	Provide contact person to call if needed
Social and emotional support will be provided	Address concomitant depression
	Provide information on education and support groups
	Include patient's family members in plan of care
	Arrange for spiritual care consultation
Care will be provided at lower cost with improved quality of life	Schedule frequent outpatient visits for better management of signs and symptoms leading to decreased readmissions
	Use established tools to evaluate patient's quality of life
	Involve a multidisciplinary team in patient's management
	Have resources available for patient when needed

From MacKlin M: Managing heart failure: A case study approach. Crit Care Nurse 2001;21:36–51

Texas, performed the first pediatric heart transplant. The operation was technically successful, and the patient did well initially; however, rejection occurred because there was no method to treat rejection.[18] In the early 1980s, cyclosporine became available, and there was a surge in pediatric heart transplantation. Indications for cardiac transplantation in children are cardiomyopathy and end-stage or inoperable congenital heart disease.[19] The challenge of organ transplantation is to maximize survival and improve quality of life. Transplantation is not a cure; it is trading one illness for another.

Transplantation Evaluation and Listing

Before transplantation, potential recipients are evaluated carefully to identify problems in other organ systems that might preclude or increase the risk of transplantation. Preoperative cardiac transplantation evaluations accomplish four objectives: (1) to establish the patient's diagnosis when necessary and to determine that cardiac transplantation is necessary, (2) to establish the course and prognosis of the patient's cardiac disease, (3) to identify the need for additional therapeutic interventions before transplantation, and (4) to educate the patient and family regarding the risks and benefits of cardiac transplantation.[20]

Review of the patient's medical history and complete physical examinations are used to determine the course and prognosis of the patient's cardiac disease. In addition to the cardiac evaluation, the immunologist and infectious disease specialist does a complete evaluation. Assessments done by social services personnel, nutritionists, and child life specialists are crucial to the patient's evaluation. Discussion with the referring physician allows the transplantation service to arrive at an assessment of the patient's current clinical status and the family's current level of understanding. Not all patients referred for transplantation are accepted because not all patients referred for transplantation actually need a heart transplant. The cardiothoracic surgeon, transplant cardiologist, transplant coordinator, and social worker perform the primary medical and psychosocial evaluations. Specialists from infectious diseases, psychiatry, nephrology, neurology, gastroenterology, dentistry, endocrinology, allergy/immunology, and pulmonology do ancillary medical evaluations if necessary. A psychosocial evaluation of the patient and family is done by the transplant social worker to identify potential problems in complying with the complex medical regimen after transplantation and in providing needed support systems.

A multitude of blood tests are done for evaluation, including blood typing; HLA typing; panel reactive antibodies; hematology (complete blood count dialysate-to-plasma ratio, and reticulocytes, prothrombin time/partial thromboplastin time/international normalized ratio); chemistries (liver function, renal function, immunoglobulins, complement, electrolytes, and nutritional function); and serologies (human immunodeficiency virus, cytomegalovirus, Epstein-Barr virus, parvovirus, Toxoplasma, human herpesvirus-6, herpes simplex virus, Mycoplasma, and hepatitis virus). Stool studies are sent for ova and parasites, culture and sensitivity, and α_1-antitrypsin, and urine studies are sent for urinalysis with microbiology, culture and sensitivity, and urine for cytomegalovirus. The child also requires a chest x-ray, ECG, echocardiogram, cardiac catheterization (right and left and coronary angiography), 24-hour Holter monitoring, and exercise stress test. Based on previous medical history, the child also may require CT scan, MRI, ultrasound, or a liver biopsy.

The multidisciplinary team includes physicians, nurses, and ancillary staff who specialize in the treatment of children with end-stage cardiac disease. The patient population ranges in age from newborns to 18 years. Patients accepted for cardiac transplant have end-stage disease, because of cardiomyopathy or congenital heart disease, which is not amenable to conventional surgery. The transplant team evaluates all referrals, manages outpatient care, and serves as consultants for inpatient care. When a patient completes the evaluation process, the medical, social, and financial information is presented to the medical review board. The responsibility of the board is to review each patient's case and to determine their candidacy for transplantation. The members of the board include the medical director, transplant immunologist, transplant surgeon, social worker, financial counselor, transplant coordinator, chaplain, psychiatrist, a representative from a nursing unit, hospital administrator, and chairman of the hospital ethics committee.

After a patient is evaluated and found to be a suitable cardiac transplant candidate, the appropriate forms are completed to allow the patient to be placed on the national **United Network of Organ Sharing (UNOS)** cardiac transplant waiting list. There are four different statuses at which a patient can be listed. Status 1A indicates a patient who is the sickest and requires a transplant immediately. These patients are intubated, are on an assist device, are on multiple inotropic support, are younger than 6 months old, or have life-threatening arrhythmias. Status 1B indicates a patient who is on a single inotrope, has growth failure (height or weight or both ≤5% on the growth chart), is on outpatient therapy with two inotropes, or is a fetus in utero with known cardiac disease that requires transplantation at time of birth. Status 2 indicates all other patients who currently need cardiac transplantation. Status 7 indicates patients who are temporarily rendered inactive on the transplant waiting list for reasons such as infection, financial problems, or too unstable. These patients do not accrue time at this status, but do not lose the time that they already have accrued. Changes in the UNOS status of a patient are made by the transplant service based on the clinical condition of the patient. If the patient's medical condition deteriorates, the UNOS status is reassessed and updated. Hearts are allocated to children based first on blood type and body size and then to the child in the highest priority status. During the waiting period, families must carry a pager to allow for immediate location at all times.

Transplant Nursing Care

The post-transplant course is complex (see Chapter 41). In the immediate postoperative phase, the patient is admitted to a private room in the cardiac intensive care unit. During the initial postoperative course, nurses who are skilled in the care of the heart transplant patient provide care. The patient-to-nurse ratio is 1:1 until the acuity allows for a 2:1 ratio. The initial goals of postoperative care are stabilization of hemodynamics, hemostasis, extubation, nutritional intake, ambulation, and freedom from infection (Table 31-3).[21]

Although heart function is greatly improved or normal after transplantation, the risk of rejection is serious. All patients are monitored closely for clinical symptoms of rejection. Signs and symptoms include fever, lethargy, decreased appetite, fluid retention, changes in vital signs, tachycardia, or an S_3 (gallop).[22] A change in the child's status should lead to immediate contact of the transplant physician. The diagnosis of rejection is based on clinical symptoms and confirmed by the endomyocardial biopsy specimen. Endomyocardial biopsy specimens are obtained on a routine basis, per institution-individualized schedule, to monitor closely for early rejection and to reduce the risk of severe rejection with subsequent graft damage. A scale for grading acute cellular rejection has been standardized by the International Society for Heart and Lung Transplant (Table 31-4).

Immunosuppressants must be taken for life and have many systemic side effects. The goal of immunosuppression is the prevention of acute rejection (Table 31-5).

TABLE 31-3

Desired System Goals After Cardiac Transplantation

Dysrhythmias
ECG will show (2) P waves due to recipient and donor sinus
nodes
  Can be mistaken for atrial dysrhythmias
Sinus node dysfunction (bradycardia) and tissue trauma
  Isoproterenol (Isuprel) can be used to drive the heart rate
  Less beat-to-beat variability
  Pacemakers should be kept at the bedside
Denervation
  Heart does not respond to stress in normal manner
  Inability to perceive chest pain
  Atropine is usually ineffective for bradycardia
  Drug of choice is epinephrine
  Adenosine should be used at low doses
  Heart rate must be accomplished via epicardial pacing or
    via intravenous stimulation of β-receptors
Atrial arrhythmias
  Can occur with mild electrolyte imbalances of K^+ and Mg^+

Systemic Hypertension*
Causes
Immunosuppression agents (cyclosporine and tacrolimus
[Prograf] therapy)
Steroid therapy
Presence of a new, efficient pump in the setting of a peripheral
  vascular bed that has been vasoconstricted in response to
  low cardiac output state
Donor-recipient size mismatch (big heart syndrome)
Renal artery vasoconstriction

Pulmonary Hypertension†
Causes
Increased pulmonary vascular resistance
Long-standing congenital heart disease and cardiomyopathy
Transient pulmonary vasoconstriction due to bypass such as
  atelectasis

Treatment
Isoproterenol
Sodium nitroprusside
Milrinone
Nitrous oxide
Prostaglandin E
Hyperventilation
Hyperoxygenation
Sedation

Low Cardiac Output Syndrome†
Impairment of myocardial function, which is caused by
  Decreased contractility caused by
    Cold ischemia/noncompliance
    Myocardial swelling
    Cardiac tamponade
    Dysrhythmias
  Increased afterload
    Increased pulmonary and systemic vascular resistance
    Pulmonary hypertension

Decreased preload
  Hypovolemia
  Decreased venous return
Medications
Anesthesia
Cardiopulmonary bypass

Fluid and Renal Management
Capillary leak syndrome
  Diuretics
  Nesiritide citrate (Natrecor)
Liberalize fluids as soon as patient allows
  Immunosuppressants are nephrotoxic
  Maintain strict intake and output
High risk for acute tubular necrosis
  Low cardiac output preoperatively
  Immunosuppression

Neurologic
At risk for seizures
  Prevent hypertension
  Minimize neurotoxic effects of cyclosporine
Pain management
Psychosocial
  Depression, anxiety, confusion, delirium
    ICU
    Steroids
    Overstimulation
    Sleep deprivation

Nutrition
Calories needed for
  Wound healing
  Prevent infection
Consult dietitian as soon as patient is extubated for dietary plan
Consult occupational therapist for feeding with infants
Daily weights when extubated

Infection
High risk due to immunosuppression
Susceptible to all forms of infection: bacterial, fungal,
  parasitic, and viral
Extubate patient as soon as patient is ready, and remove
  lines as soon as possible
Nothing per rectum
Close observation of all surgical incisions and intravenous
  lines for signs and symptoms of infection including
  fever, reddened tissue adjacent to the wound, drainage
  characteristics, wound odors, pain at wound site, and
  prolonged healing
Close attention to mucous membranes and presence of thrush
  Nystatin
  Good oral hygiene
Change electrodes daily
Aggressive pulmonary toilet
Early ambulation or parental holding
Good hand washing

*Close observation for the signs and symptoms of hypertension, including facial flushing, headache, abdominal pain, restlessness, tingling in the extremities, and blurred vision.
†Severe cases may require mechanical support.

TABLE 31-4

International Society for Heart and Lung Transplant (ISHLT) Standardized Grading Scale for Diagnosing Acute Rejection	
ISHLT Score	**Description**
0	No evidence of acute rejection
1A	Mild focal perivascular interstitial infiltrate
1B	Mild interstitial infiltrate
2	Moderate focal interstitial infiltrate
3A	Moderate multifocal lymphocytic infiltration with myocyte damage
3B	Diffuse inflammatory process with myocyte damage
4	Severe diffuse lymphocytic infiltration with hemorrhage, necrosis, and vasculitis

From Billingham ME, Cary NR, Hammond ME, et al: A working formulation for the standardization of nomenclature in the diagnosis of heart and lung rejection. Heart Rejection Study Group. J Heart Transplant 1990;9:587-593.

The heart transplant recipient is followed lifelong by a heart transplant institute. The child needs to take antirejection medications for the rest of his or her life. The longevity of the organ is unknown; the average life expectancy is 10 years for one heart. Children today can expect to need one or more heart transplants in their lifetime. The one limiting factor of the transplanted organ is the issue of transplant coronary artery disease. Currently the process by which the coronaries become infected is not completely understood. Many investigators postulate that low-grade chronic rejection over time causes coronary artery disease. The only treatment for transplant coronary artery disease currently in 2005 is retransplantation. Other potential long-term problems that may limit survival include cardiac rejection, renal dysfunction and nephrotoxicity, hypertension resulting from immunosuppression drugs, post-transplant lymphoproliferative disease, gingival hyperplasia, hirsutism, osteoporosis, obesity, hyperlipidemia, osteoporosis, diabetes mellitus, and infection.[23,24] These potential long-term problems have continued to limit long-term survival despite advances in immunosuppression. In the short-term after successful transplantation, children are able to return to full participation in age-appropriate activities and seem to adapt well to their new lifestyle. The long-term prognosis is unknown.

Nursing care after transplantation is demanding and complex, with careful attention to the physical needs of the child and the emotional needs of the child and family. Successful caring for a child after a heart transplant requires the expertise and dedication of many members of the health care team. Nurses play vital roles in assessment, coordination of care, psychosocial support, and patient and family education.[25] Transplantation is a treatment that has a much less negative impact on the

TABLE 31-5

Immunosuppression Drug Therapy			
Drug	**Action**	**Therapeutic Monitoring**	**Side Effects**
Calcineurin inhibitors: Cyclosporine (Sandimmune, Neoral, Gengraf)	Inhibits T cell proliferation by inhibiting calcineurin and blocking IL-2 production	Therapeutic drug levels; determined by time since transplant	Nephrotoxicity, hepatotoxicity, gingival hyperplasia, hirsutism, hypertension
Tacrolimus (Prograf)	Inhibits T cell proliferation by inhibiting calcineurin and blocking IL-2 production	Therapeutic drug monitoring; determined by time since transplant	Nephrotoxicity, hepatotoxicity, hyperglycemia, hair loss, hypertension
Antimetabolites: Mycophenolate mofetil (CellCept)	Inhibits T and B lymphocytes through blocking de novo purine biosynthesis	No approved therapeutic drug monitoring in pediatrics; monitor hemoglobin, hematocrit, white blood cells	Gastrointestinal symptoms, such as nausea, vomiting, and diarrhea; less frequently, bone marrow suppression occurs
Azathioprine (Imuran)	Inhibits all proliferating cells in the body; inhibits B and T cell proliferation	Monitor complete bood cell count	Pancytopenia, hepatotoxicity
Corticosteroids: Prednisone	Anti-inflammatory, inhibits margination and chemotactic function of lymphocytes	No therapeutic monitoring	Diabetes mellitus, hypertension, weight gain, osteoporosis, cataract formation, peptic ulcer disease, growth retardation

IL-2, interleukin-2.
From Berg A: Pediatric heart transplantation: A clinical overview. Crit Care Nurs Q 2002;25:79-87.

normal life activities of a child. Stresses remain for the child and the family, however, in relation to the uncertainty of the future, the child's health and well-being, social isolation, and financial burden.

Patient/parent education begins at the time of evaluation. The initial discussion with the transplant service averages 2 hours and gives a broad overview of cardiac transplantation. As the patient and family members proceed through the evaluation, subsequent listing, and follow-up, education is an ongoing process. After the cardiac transplant, education of the patient and parents continues. The transplant coordinator continuously provides patients and their families with education regarding transplantation. The nurse coordinator ensures the patient and their families are adequately prepared for discharge and ready to assume the responsibilities for day-to-day living after a cardiac transplant. The school nurse also plays an important role in the life of the heart transplant child. There are physical and psychological considerations for managing such students. Among the physical considerations are work capacity, appearance, organ rejection, and infection.[26] The psychological considerations are emotional, cognitive functioning, quality of life, and behavioral concerns. The school nurse is a key resource in informing staff about the unique concerns of pediatric heart recipients and in ensuring the child is integrated into the school setting.[26]

Family support is crucial to the success of the child with a heart transplant. Support does not end after discharge. The transplant coordinator and social worker are available 24 hours a day, 7 days a week, 365 days a year for support. The patient relations department is available to assist in patient and family needs. A child life specialist is dedicated to providing support for social and emotional needs and age-appropriate activities to the transplant patient, his or her siblings, and extended family. A chaplain also is available full-time and provides individualized care and counseling. The child recipient responds in a variety of ways to a heart transplant. The concept of having a foreign body inside the body is sometimes disturbing to children. They often speculate about the age, gender, personality, and physical characteristics of the donor. They may fear that the heart will wear out if it came from an older person. Some children are distressed that their heart came from a person of the opposite gender.

Corticosteroid therapy, necessary in cardiac transplants, creates undesirable side effects (growth failure, obesity, acne, and hirsutism) that are frequently sources of emotional and social problems for older children. The most frequent reason for noncompliance in childhood cardiac transplant recipients is dislike of undesirable side effects. The cosmetic implications of the side effects can be overwhelming, especially to adolescent girls. Deliberate discontinuation of the drugs most commonly is observed in teenage girls. Noncompliance also is seen frequently in children from families with poor

communication who are not supportive. Working with children and their families during the various stages of heart failure and transplantation is a difficult and challenging experience. Nurses must become familiar with the family; assess family strengths, weaknesses, and coping mechanisms; and be prepared to provide intensive support and guidance during the prolonged experience.[27] The child and family members need help in accepting what is happening to them; learning anticipatory guidance regarding predictable stresses; and dealing constructively with the physical, emotional, and financial burdens that are an ongoing part of this prolonged disability.

All patient's families meet with the transplant financial counselor during the pretransplant evaluation so that all parties are aware of the financial commitments on the part of the family and the hospital. The financial counselor assists the family in applications for any eligible support services not previously in place. The financial coordinator provides the transplant service with a written statement of available benefits from private insurance payers. Post-transplant, the hospital maintains a lifelong commitment to all patients who undergo cardiac transplantation.

Many different resources are available for transplant recipients. Housing can be provided for transplant patients and their immediate family at the Ronald McDonald House, which is a home-away-from home for families with children being treated at the medical center in the area. The Ronald McDonald House is a warm and friendly place, that encourages caring and sharing among the families in residence. At the Ronald McDonald House, parents find mutual comfort and support from each other, and children find playmates and friends with whom they can relate. The Ronald McDonald House is more like an individual residence than a hotel. There is a comfortable living room, a large family dining room, and several recreational areas. Families stay in one of the spacious bedrooms, each with a private bath. School-age children may study with a certified teacher. Cost per family per night varies according to different locations, but the average price is above $15 per night. Special arrangements and reduced rates are available for qualifying families.

NURSING ROLES IN DEATH AND DYING

The death of a child is viewed as outside the natural order of life.[54] Children represent hope, energy, and health. A dying child can challenge our understanding of life, faith, and certainty in the future. Little attention has been given to the palliative care needs of heart failure patients.[28] Sudden cardiac death with heart failure continues to be a prevalent problem and important health care challenge for clinicians. Sometimes the first sign of heart failure can be death. For children with progressive, life-threatening illness and their families, numerous compromises often are made when balancing between treatment and quality of life. The burden of chronic illness and the care it demands can exhaust a family financially, physically, and emotionally.

As the disease progresses, despite efforts at cure or control, the physician must weigh the cost of any proposed treatment with the impact that treatment would have on the child's comfort and quality of life. When it has been determined that the goals of care have shifted from attempts at cure or control of the disease to palliation and comfort, it is important to provide the family with all options available. The first goal is to determine the location of care that the family members feel is best for them and the child. Hospital care may provide the child and family members with the support and comfort of familiar staff and surroundings at a time when the child is very ill. Home care provides family members with the necessary medical equipment and medications and periodic nursing visits to maintain the child at home.

Hospice provides care to children with terminal illnesses. An interdisciplinary team of professionals skilled in caring for terminally ill patients provides support that enables family members to care for the child at home.[29] This team includes physicians, nurses, certified nursing assistants, social workers, chaplains, and volunteers. Hospice provides all the necessary equipment, supplies, and medications. Nursing visits are available 24 hours a day, 7 days a week. Emotional support is provided, such as listening, touching, expressing empathy, attending to the patients' and families wishes, comforting, encouraging, and being present.[30] Social workers and chaplains also make home visits to assist the family with the difficult emotional and spiritual issues that accompany the death of a child. Patients dying from heart failure experience a wide range of symptoms that are frequently distressing, including breathlessness, nausea, vomiting, and anxiety.[28] It is important that the patient receives supplemental oxygen if needed and antiemetic, antianxiety, and pain medications.

OTHER NURSING ISSUES IN HEART FAILURE

Mechanical Support

Mechanical support of cardiovascular function may be provided if conventional medical therapy fails to support effective systemic perfusion. Mechanical support can be provided through use of extracorporeal membrane oxygenation, an intra-aortic balloon pump (IABP), or a ventricular assist device. **Extracorporeal membrane oxygenation** therapy can support cardiac or pulmonary function through use of cardiopulmonary bypass with a membrane oxygenator. This device is used most commonly to treat severe respiratory failure in newborns, but it may be used to treat acute respiratory

failure or cardiac failure in older infants and children.[31] Extracorporeal membrane oxygenation should be considered for the treatment of acute, reversible cardiac or respiratory failure unresponsive to conventional medical management.[31] The **intra-aortic balloon pump** is another mechanical circulatory assist device that is used frequently in adult patients with myocardial failure.[32] There is limited experience in pediatric patients with the intra-aortic balloon pump.[56] It has limited effectiveness because of the need to match an appropriate-size balloon catheter to a small child or infant and the rapid heart rate, which minimizes the time for diastolic augmentation.[32]

The child in shock requires excellent medical and nursing management. The gravity of the child's condition and the complexity of care can be overwhelming and threatening for the child and family members. Several caveats apply: (1) Provide the patient and family members with essential information without overwhelming them with details; (2) assume that the child can hear everything said at the bedside, even if the child is receiving sedatives; (3) address the child by name, and always prepare the child before any touch and certainly before any painful procedures; (4) provide adequate sedation and analgesia for procedures and discomfort; and (5) encourage the parents to visit as much as possible and to touch the child.[33]

Ventricular assist devices are an option for patients whose hearts are in critical stages of failure. The purpose of a ventricular assist device is to provide mechanical circulation when the natural heart cannot maintain adequate cardiac output.[56] The benefits of mechanically unloading the injured ventricle are decrease in left ventricular mass, regression of left ventricular hypertrophy, reversal of ventricular dilation, improved efficiency of myocardial mitochondria, and reduction in neurohormonal derangements in heart failure.[34] The ventricular assist device can be either pulsatile or nonpulsatile flow.[58] The psychological support for children on mechanical support varies with the device used. Children with a body surface area of 0.1 to 0.7 m^2 usually are placed on a Biomedicus device.[57] Children with a body surface area of less than 0.7 m^2 are heavily sedated and most likely receiving a paralytic agent. Parental verbal and tactile stimulation is encouraged. Music therapy also has proved to be a positive intervention. Children with a body surface area greater than 0.7 m^2 can be placed on a Thoratec device. The psychological support provided for these patients is goal-oriented early ambulation, with the early period being with a physical therapist present and a member from the perfusion staff. Parents are encouraged to participate actively in their child's care. It is important to have a daily schedule/planner for all activities to prevent depression and boredom. Schooling with the child should begin as soon as is medically feasible. The nursing staff should provide frequent encouragement to the patient.

The dietitian should participate in nutritional management and requirements for the patient and provide patient education regarding bad eating habits, warfarin diet, and a diet high in protein to promote wound healing. It is important that the patient is provided with adequate analgesia, and nurses should cluster care to promote uninterrupted sleep. A child life specialist should work closely with the patient. The child life specialist can prepare siblings and friends before visiting the patient on the device and allow the patient to verbalize fears. The child life specialist also can discuss alterations in the family process, alteration in body image, and grieving related to the possibility of death.

Pharmacologic Agents

Nursing personnel who specialize in heart failure need to have a clear understanding of all pharmacologic agents used in heart failure (See Chapters 32 to 40). **Diuretics** are the mainstay of therapy in heart failure to mobilize edematous fluid, reduce pulmonary venous pressure, and reduce preload. If excess extracellular fluid is excreted, blood volume returning to the heart can be reduced, and cardiac function improves. The most commonly used agents are furosemide (Lasix), ethacrynic acid (Edecrin), spironolactone, and metolazone.

β-Blocker therapy has become standard therapy in adult patients with chronic heart failure resulting from systolic dysfunction.[35] Two of the most common β-blockers used today in heart failure are metoprolol and carvedilol. Both agents improve cardiac remodeling in patients with CHF. β-Blockers blunt activation of the sympathetic nervous system, which responds to low cardiac output by increasing circulating levels of catecholamines.[36] This blunting of neurohormonal activation improves left ventricular remodeling and cardiac functioning and decreases the occurrence of ventricular arrhythmias. β-Blockers initially may produce a worsening of signs and symptoms and should be started at low doses and increased slowly.[37] β-Blockers are indicated for the long-term management of chronic heart failure. β-Blockers should not be used in acutely ill patients ("rescue therapy"), including patients who are in an intensive care unit with refractory heart failure requiring intravenous inotropic therapy.[38]

Angiotensin-converting enzyme (ACE) inhibitors have become the vasodilator of choice in patients with mild-to-severe heart failure. ACE inhibitors block the conversion of angiotensin I to angiotensin II so that instead of vasoconstriction, vasodilation occurs. Vasodilation results in decreased pulmonary and systemic vascular resistance, decreased blood pressure, a reduction in afterload, and decreased right and left atrial pressures.[38] It also reduces the secretion of aldosterone, which reduces preload by preventing volume expansion from fluid retention and decreases the risk of hypokalemia. Renal blood flow is improved, which enhances diuresis. ACE inhibitors also exert a favorable effect on cardiac remodeling.[38] Captopril and enalapril are two examples

of ACE inhibitors used in children today. Children receiving therapy with ACE inhibitors should be advised that (1) side effects may occur early in therapy but do not generally prevent long-term use of the drug, (2) symptomatic improvement may not be seen until patients have received treatment for several weeks or months, and (3) ACE inhibitors may reduce the risk of the disease progression even if the symptoms of the patient have not responded favorably to treatment.[38]

Digoxin increases the force of contraction, decreases the heart rate, and slows the conduction of impulse through the atrioventricular node and indirectly enhances diuresis by increased renal perfusion.[38] The beneficial effects are increased cardiac output, decreased heart size, and decreased venous pressure and relief of edema.[38] It should be used in conjunction with diuretics, an ACE inhibitor, and a β-blocker.

Human **B-type natriuretic peptide** (nesiritide [Natrecor]) is indicated for intravenous treatment of patients with acutely decompensated heart failure who have dyspnea at rest or with minimal activity.[39] Endogenous human B-type natriuretic peptide (hBNP) is secreted by the ventricular myocardium in response to heart failure. Increased endogenous hBNP levels correlate with systolic dysfunction, diastolic dysfunction, increased left ventricular mass, and low ejection fraction.[40] hBNP has potent hemodynamic, diuretic, and natriuretic effects.[53] In in vitro and animal studies, hBNP produced cGMP-mediated vasodilation, systemic venous and arterial vasodilation, and coronary artery vasodilation. In human studies, hBNP decreased filling pressures, pulmonary capillary wedge pressure, right atrial pressure, and systemic vascular resistance; increased cardiac index; decreased aldosterone and norepinephrine; increased urine volume and sodium excretion; and increased coronary vasodilation.[41] Several essential components must be included in protocols for nesiritide, such as indications and restrictions for use and guidelines for monitoring hemodynamic parameters before and during infusion.[39] Specific dosing information also must be specified, including bolus dose, infusion, when to adjust the rate, and monitoring of hemodynamic parameters if needed.[39]

Biventricular pacing, or cardiac resynchronization therapy (CRT), is gaining increasing acceptance as a compelling treatment for individuals with advanced heart failure.[44] A prolonged PR interval, a wide QRS, and left bundle branch block are typical conduction disturbances associated with left ventricular dysfunction.[42,43] The interventricular conduction delays often lead to loss of synchronization of ventricular contraction, contributing to additional problems for heart failure patients.[43] CRT aims to re-establish normal electromechanical activity.[44] Reports from clinical trials have shown that CRT therapy improves functional status, exercise tolerance, and quality of life. CRT is accomplished using standard atrial and ventricular pacing leads. These leads are placed in the right atrium and right ventricle and used to pace the right side of the heart. A specially designed transvenous lead is inserted via the coronary sinus to a distal cardiac vein. The left ventricle is paced via this lead. With the three leads in place, the patient can receive traditional pacing therapy for bradycardic conditions along with CRT for optimal timing between atrial and ventricular contractions, improved coordination of the left ventricular septal and free wall, and coordinated contractile efforts of the left and right ventricular walls.[44]

Intermittent/long-term drug infusions on an outpatient basis have been used with increasing frequency in pediatric patients with advanced heart failure. The U.S. Food and Drug Administration has approved the use of parenteral positive inotropes for the short-term treatment of patients with acute, decompensated heart failure. Although inconsistent with the U.S. Food and Drug Administration recommendations for short-term use, continuous infusion of positive inotropes has been used successfully to support the circulation as a pharmacologic bridge to cardiac transplantation in patients with end-stage heart failure.[45] Available evidence indicates that positive inotropic infusion is associated with fewer heart failure symptoms, increased functional status, reduced health care cost, and decreased mortality.[45] Frequently used positive inotropes include dopamine, milrinone, and dobutamine. The risk-benefit analysis and the decision to use intermittent parenteral inotropic therapy in the management of end-stage heart failure can be made only by the individual patient and family members with the advice and support of the pediatric cardiologist. A patient who requires home infusions has advanced heart failure, and prognosis is poor without cardiac transplantation.[45]

Dietary Guidelines

Growth in children with heart failure is often compromised.[47] Patients with heart failure have symptoms that can affect their food intake, such as nausea, loss of appetite, and ascites.[46] Pharmacologic therapy can lead to loss of appetite, which makes the intake of food inadequate to fill the required energy and nutritional needs.[46] The caloric intake in infants and children may be adequate for age, but is inadequate to permit normal growth rates. Energy expenditure seems to be significantly elevated in this population relative to that of age-matched infants and children. Although caloric intake may be appropriate for age, increased energy expenditure leaves an infant or child with heart failure with little energy available for growth.

Decreased energy intake can involve deficiencies of specific nutrients or insufficient total caloric intake. Increased respiratory rate accompanying heart failure may be responsible for increased energy requirements. Most treatment strategies aim to facilitate catch-up growth, providing extra calories and protein that exceed the recommended dietary allowance for age. There is no generally accepted set of guidelines, however, that defines appropriate caloric intake for catch-up growth.[47] A 2-g sodium diet is frequently recommended, which can be achieved by avoiding salty foods and by not adding salt to foods after cooking. Frequent, small meals also may help alleviate unwanted symptoms of anorexia, caused by congestion of the gastrointestinal tract.[15]

Cardiac Rehabilitation

As the only major cardiovascular disease increasing in incidence and prevalence, CHF is a major health threat. Progression of the disease often leads to severe disability and requires intensive medical and psychological management.[48] Cardiac rehabilitation for CHF, the structured programming of exercise, and risk reduction teaching and counseling to promote healthy living with heart failure are grounded in a strong nurse-patient relationship that aims to improve a patient's functional ability; alleviate activity-related symptoms; improve quality of life; and restore and maintain physiologic, psychological, and social status.[49] The education and counseling components of cardiac rehabilitation for CHF address many issues, including maintenance of physical activity, recognition of activity limitations, conservation of energy, dietary modifications, adequate nutrition, psychological concerns, relaxation techniques, coping skills, medication schedule and side effects, lifestyle changes, and prognosis. In addition, emotional support and encouragement are provided. The expansion of home care services and advances in technology allow cardiac rehabilitation to take place in the patient's home, outpatient clinics, or school environment. Physical and occupational therapists work closely with the child to promote a structured regimen for a day-to-day schedule.

Quality of Life

Quality of life is defined as a multidimensional concept referring to a person's total well-being, including his or her functional capacity, psychological status, social functioning, physical health, and health perceptions.[50] In studies of quality of life in patients with heart failure, patients commonly report psychological distress, including depression, hostility, and anxiety; limitations in their activities of daily living; disruptions in work roles and social interactions with friends and family; and reduced sexual activity and satisfactions.[50] Quality of life is a relatively recent concept to be addressed in heart failure research. In addition to its importance as a research outcome, quality of life is emerging as a clinical outcome measure to guide treatment of patients with heart failure. This small but intriguing body of literature suggests that psychological factors are related to morbidity and mortality in patients with heart failure and that this relationship is independent of that of traditional medical risk factors. Quality of life is a dynamic continuum, relating to all aspects of one's life. Interventions aimed at reducing cardiovascular risk factors affect quality of life and patient satisfaction.[51] Understanding these interactions is important in achieving effective cardiovascular risk reduction. Quality of life must be viewed within the context of a person's emotional status; physical functioning; health status; family and social functioning; emotional, financial, and educational status; and cultural and religious beliefs.[51]

CURRENT STATUS AND FUTURE TRENDS

Pediatric heart failure is a challenging, lifelong set of circumstances for the child, family, health care team, and community. For cardiology nurses involved in the care of infants and children with heart failure, these are exciting times. An opportunity exists to provide leadership of the delivery of patient services and to strengthen the scope of the nurse's role as a direct care provider and collaborator. Coordinated efforts to provide high-quality care and age-appropriate education would enhance quality of life and decrease adverse outcomes.[52,60]

Key Concepts

- In an infant, an inability to maintain growth either secondary to decreased nutritional intake or an increased catabolic state is a hallmark of heart failure. The infant exhibits increased sympathetic tone with excessive diaphoresis and increased heart rate. Physical findings in the infant with heart failure include increased work of breathing, tachypnea, and hepatomegaly.

- In older children, new-onset heart failure may be less overtly symptomatic. Malaise, decrease in level of daily activity, and weight loss may be present. Symptoms of abdominal pain, nausea, and anorexia can be present and sometimes divert attention from the real cardiac etiology. Physical findings include rales and peripheral edema. Hepatomegaly, a gallop rhythm, and tachycardia also commonly are present.

- Management of patients with heart failure in the 1990s increasingly moved from physician-directed, inpatient care to nurse-guided and nurse-coordinated care in the outpatient arena. Benefits of outpatient management include enhanced quality of life for the patient, reduced costs, and avoidance of risks associated with hospitalization.

- The heart failure clinic can be a multidisciplinary heart failure team specialized in providing care for these chronically ill patients and their families, including regular follow-up, consulting hours, and individualized education (e.g., computer-based education, group education sessions).

- An integral part of any heart failure specialty program is evaluation, and every program should include a plan for evaluation of its effectiveness. Evaluation of the impact of a program allows for refinement to improve program effectiveness and provides data when seeking reimbursement for a program from managed care organizations and insurance companies.

- Improvements in heart failure outcomes depend on patients' and parents' abilities to care for themselves and manage aspects of their condition. Patient self-management itself has become a measurable outcome.

- All patients with heart failure, regardless of etiology, and their families require education about the disease. A multidisciplinary approach should include teaching about dietary restrictions, reportable signs and symptoms, activity restrictions, medications and side effects, what to do in case of an emergency, and ability to cope with a chronic disease.

- Preoperative cardiac transplantation evaluations accomplish four objectives: (1) to establish the patient's diagnosis when necessary and to determine that cardiac transplantation is necessary, (2) to establish the course and prognosis of the patient's cardiac disease, (3) to identify the need for additional therapeutic interventions before transplantation, and (4) to educate the patient and family regarding the risks and benefits of cardiac transplantation.

- Cardiac rehabilitation for CHF, the structured programming of exercise, and risk reduction teaching and counseling to promote healthy living with heart failure are grounded in a strong nurse-patient relationship which aims to improve a patient's functional ability; alleviate activity-related symptoms; improve quality of life; and restore and maintain physiologic, psychological, and social status.

REFERENCES

1. Albert N: Heart failure: The physiological basis for current therapeutic concepts. Crit Care Nurse 1999;19(3 Suppl):2-13.
2. Clark BJ 3rd: Treatment of heart failure in infants and children. Heart Dis 2000;2:354-361.
3. Von Rueden KT: Outpatient hemodynamic monitoring of patients with heart failure. J Cardiovasc Nurs 2002;16:62-71.
4. Paul S: Impact of a nurse-managed heart failure clinic: A pilot study. Am J Crit Care 2000; 9:140-146.
5. Jaarsma T, Stromberg A: Heart failure clinics in Europe. Prog Cardiovasc Nurs 2000;15:67-72.
6. Akosah KO, Schaper AM, Havlik P, et al: Improving care for patients with chronic heart failure in the community: The importance of a disease management program. Chest 2002;122:906-912.
7. Albert NM: Implementation strategies to manage heart failure outcomes. AACN Clin Issues 2000;11:396-411.
8. Westlake C, Dracup K: Role of spirituality in adjustment of patients with advanced heart failure. Prog Cardiovasc Nurs 2001;16:118-125.
9. Henrick A: Cost-effective outpatient management of persons with heart failure. Prog Cardiovasc Nurs 2001;16:30-56.
10. Crowther M: Optimal management of outpatients with heart failure using advanced practice nurses in a hospital-based heart failure center. J Am Acad Nurse Pract 2003;15:260-265.
11. Kuehneman T, Saulsburg D, Splett P, et al: Demonstrating the impact of nutrition intervention in a heart failure program. J Am Diet Assoc 2002;102:1790-1794.
12. Desai PP, Ng JB, Bryant SG: Care of children and families in the CICU: A focus on their developmental, psychological, and spiritual needs. Crit Care Nurs Q 2002;25:88-97.

13. Deaton C: Outcomes measurement. J Cardiovasc Nurs 2000;14:116-118.

14. Hussey LC, Hardin S, Blanchette C: Outpatient costs of medications for patients with chronic heart failure. Am J Crit Care 2002;11:474-478.

15. Grady KL, Dracup K, Kennedy G, et al: Team management of patients with heart failure: A statement for healthcare professionals from the Cardiovascular Nursing Council of the American Heart Association. Circulation 2000;102:2443-2457.

16. Svendsen A: Heart failure: An overview of consensus guidelines and nursing implications. Can J Cardiovasc Nurs 2003;13:30-34.

17. Suddaby EC: Viral myocarditis in children. Crit Care Nurse 1996;16:73-82.

18. Cooley D: Session I: Pediatric heart transplantation in historical perspective. J Heart Lung Transplant 1991;10:787-790.

19. Shaffer KM, Denfield SW, Schowengerdt KO, et al: Cardiac transplantation for pediatric patients with inoperable congenital heart disease. Texas Heart Inst J 1998;25:57-63.

20. Bricker JT, Frazier OH: Preoperative evaluation of the pediatric heart transplant candidate. Clin Transplant 1987;1:164-168.

21. Berg A: Pediatric heart transplantation: A clinical overview. Crit Care Nurs Q 2002;25:79-87.

22. Wade CR, Reith KK, Sikora JH, et al: Postoperative nursing care of the cardiac transplant recipient. Crit Care Nurs Q 2004;27:17-28.

23. Luikart H: Pediatric cardiac transplantation: Management issue. J Pediatr Nurs 2001;16:320-331.

24. Salyer J, Flattery MP, Joyner PL, et al: Lifestyle and quality of life in long-term cardiac transplant recipients. J Heart Lung Transplant 2003;22:309-321.

25. Hanton LB: Caring for children awaiting heart transplantation: Psychosocial implications. Pediatr Nurs 1998;24:214-221.

26. Duitsman DM, Suddaby EC, Masterson G: Unique considerations for the pediatric heart transplant recipient: The role of the school nurse. J School Nurs 1999;15:10-13.

27. Crone CC, Wise TN: Psychiatric aspects of transplantation: II. Preoperative issues. Crit Care Nurse 1999;19:51-63.

28. Davies N, Curtis M: Providing palliative care in end-stage heart failure. Prof Nurse 2000;15:389-392.

29. Coviello JS, Hricz-Borges L, Masulli PS: Accomplishing quality of life in end-stage heart failure: A hospice multidisciplinary approach. Home Healthcare Nurse 2002;20:195-198.

30. Kuuppelomaki M: Emotional support for dying patients: The nurses' perspective. Eur J Oncol Nurs 2003;7:120-129.

31. Suddaby EC, O'Brien AM: ECMO for cardiac support in children. Heart Lung 1993;22:401-407.

32. Veasy G, Webster H: Intra-aortic balloon pumping in infants and children. Cardiac Assists 1985;2:1-6.

33. Giganti AW: Families in pediatric critical care: The best option. Pediatr Nurs 1998;24:261-265.

34. McCafferty M, Sorbellini D, Cianci P: Telemetry to home: Successful discharge of patients with ventricular assist devices. Crit Care Nurse 2002;22:43-51.

35. Carter C: Beta blocker therapy for chronic heart failure. Am Fam Physician 2003;67:1793-1795.

36. Sadovsky R: Left ventricular dysfunction: Carvedilol vs. metoprolol. Am Fam Physician 2004;69:958-960.

37. MacKlin M: Managing heart failure: A case study approach. Crit Care Nurse 2001;21:36-51.

38. Tedesco C, Reigle J, Bergin J: Sudden cardiac death in heart failure. J Cardiovasc Nurs 2000;14:38-56.

39. Hachey DM, Smith T: Use of nesiritide to treat acute decompensated heart failure. Crit Care Nurse 2003;23:53-55.

40. Yamamoto K, Burnett JC, Jougasaki M, et al: The relative value of the natriuretic peptides as markers for detecting abnormal ventricular structure and function. J Am Coll Cardiol 1996;27:69A-70A.

41. Abraham WT, Lowes BD, Ferguson DA, et al: Systemic hemodynamic neurohormonal and renal effects of a steady state infusion of human brain natriuretic peptide in patients with hemodynamically decompensated heart failure. J Card Fail 1998;4:37-44.

42. Stone PH: Biventricular pacing offers a better life to some patients with chronic heart failure. Ann Intern Med 2003;138:485-487.

43. Lagrotteria JM: Biventricular pacing for congestive heart failure. Crit Care Nurs Q 2003;26:50-59.

44. Flanagan J, Horwood L, Bolin C, et al: Heart failure patients with ventricular dyssynchrony: Management with a cardiac resynchronization therapy device. Prog Cardiovasc Nurs 2003;18:184-191.

45. Levine BS: Intermittent positive inotrope infusion in the management of end-stage, low-output heart failure. J Cardiovasc Nurs 2000;14:76-93.

46. Jacobsson A, Pihl-Lindgren E, Fridlund B: Malnutrition in patients suffering from chronic heart failure: The nurse's care. Eur J Heart Fail 2001;3:449-456.

47. Forchielli ML, McColl R, Walker WA, et al: Children with congenital heart disease: A nutrition challenge. Nutr Rev 1994;52:348-353.

48. Goodwin BA: Home cardiac rehabilitation for congestive heart failure: A nursing care management approach. Rehabil Nurs 1999;24:143-147.

49. Liehr P, Leaverton R, Yepes A, et al: Addressing current challenges to cardiac rehabilitation care. AACN Clin Issues 2003;14:13-24.

50. Moser DK, Worster PL: Effect of psychosocial factors on physiologic outcomes in patients with heart failure. J Cardiovasc Nurs 2000;14:106-115.

51. Berra K: The effect of lifestyle interventions on quality of life and patient satisfaction with health and health care. J Cardiovasc Nurs 2003;18:319-325.

52. Lekan-Rutledge D: Heart failure. Am J Nurs 2004;104:15.

53. Mukoyama M, Nakao K, Hosoda K, et al: Brain natriuretic peptide as a novel cardiac hormone in humans: Evidence for an exquisite dual natriuretic peptide system, atrial natriuretic peptide and natriuretic peptide. J Clin Invest 1991 Apr;87(4):1402-1412.

54. Meert KL, Thurston CS, Briller SH: The spiritual needs of parents at the time of their child's death in the pediatric intensive care unit and during bereavement: A qualitative study. Pediatr Crit Care Med 2005 Jul;6(4):420-427.

55. Schulman KA, Mark DB, Califf RM: Outcomes and costs within a disease management program for advanced congestive heart failure. Am Heart J 1998 Jun;135(6 pt 2 Su):S285-S292.

56. Frazier OH, Bricker JT, Macris MP, Cooley DA: Use of a left ventricular assist device as a bridge to transplantation in a pediatric patient. Tex Heart Inst J 1989;16(1):46-50.

57. Scheinin SA, Radovancevic B, Parnis SM, et al: Mechanical circulatory support in children. Eur J Cardiothorac Surg 1994;8(10):537-540.

58. Louis PT, Bricker JT, Frazier OH, et al: Nonpulsative total left ventricular support in pediatric patients. Crit Care Med 1992 May;20(5):704-707.

59. Rosenthal D, Christant MR, Edens E, et al: International Society for Heart and Lung Transplantation: Practice guidelines for management of heart failure in children. J Heart Lung Transplant 2004 Dec;23(12):1313-1333.

60. Johansson P, Dahlstrom U, Brostrom A: Factors and interventions influencing health-related quality of life in patients with heart failure: A review of the literature. Eur J Cardiovasc Nurs 2005 Jun 18; [Epub ahead of print].

CHAPTER 32

Diuretics

Heather A. Dickerson
Anthony C. Chang

Since organic mercurial diuretics were first used in the 1920s, diuretic agents have become a mainstay of therapy for heart failure in adults and have shown a reduction in risk.[1] Despite the frequent use of these pharmacologic agents in children with heart disease, there remains a paucity of information on the clinical use and pharmacokinetic profiles of diuretic agents in pediatric patients.

To use diuretic agents effectively in the treatment of heart failure, it is essential for the clinician to understand developmental renal anatomy and physiology and to appreciate principles of renal adaptation to heart failure. An optimal strategy of diuretic use in the treatment of heart failure also requires clear understanding of classes of diuretics and their mechanisms of action and the concept of diuretic resistance. With the advent of myriad new diuretic agents now available for use in adults with heart failure, it is more important than ever to pursue investigative studies to validate the use of these pharmacologic agents in pediatric patients.

KIDNEY IN HEART FAILURE

Basic Renal Anatomy and Physiology

The **afferent and efferent arterioles** are regulated by various mediators to maintain glomerular hydrostatic pressure and filtration (Fig. 32-1). The fluid and electrolyte balance is controlled in the nephron at multiple sites with most of the glomerular ultrafiltrate being reabsorbed (Fig. 32-2).

The **proximal convoluted tubule** is involved with the reabsorption of sodium, chloride, bicarbonate, potassium, calcium, phosphate, glucose, and amino

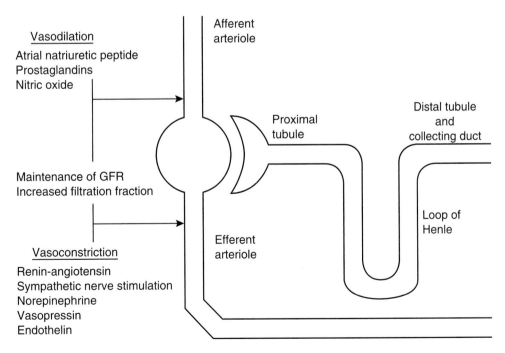

FIGURE 32-1 ■ Renovascular regulation. The afferent arterioles vasodilate and the efferent arterioles vasoconstrict in response to decreased renal plasma flow. These adaptive mechanisms enable the kidneys to maintain glomerular filtration rate (GFR). (From Lowrie L: *Diuretic therapy of heart failure in infants and children. Prog Pediatr Cardiol* 2000;12:45-55.)

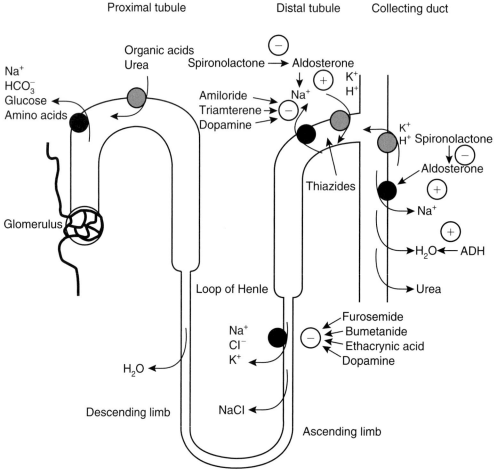

FIGURE 32-2 ■ The nephron and electrolyte management. Schematic diagram showing sections of the nephron, transporters important in electrolyte management by the kidney, and sites of action of the classes of diuretics. ADH, antidiuretic hormone. (From Shekerdemian LS, Redington, A: *Cardiovascular pharmacology.* In Chang AC, Hanley FL, Wernovsky G, et al [eds]: *Pediatric Cardiac Intensive Care.* Philadelphia, Williams & Wilkins, 1998, p 58.)

acids; it accounts for more than 50% of the resorption of filtered sodium. Fluid resorption is isosmotic, and carbonic anhydrase aids in the resorption of sodium bicarbonate. The **loop of Henle**, located in the inner medulla, also is involved in the reabsorption of water, sodium, chloride, and potassium. Greater than 90% of the filtered sodium that is reabsorbed in the nephron is absorbed mostly at the proximal convoluted tubule and the rest along the ascending loop of Henle. There is no solute transport in the descending limb of the loop of Henle, but this is where water leaves the nephron and enters the hyperosmotic interstitium surrounding the nephron. The **Na⁺/K⁺/2Cl⁻ cotransporter** is located in the thick ascending limb of the loop of Henle, and this is where ion transport occurs. The thick ascending limb of the loop of Henle also contacts the **macula densa**, a specialized epithelium that is involved in tubuloglomerular feedback that controls the amount of renin secretion and the amount of glomerular filtration. The **distal convoluted tubule**, where the **Na⁺/Cl⁻ transporter** is found, and the **collecting duct** control

the secretion of potassium and hydrogen ions and the reabsorption of sodium; these actions are influenced by aldosterone and antidiuretic hormone (vasopressin).

Renal Adaptations in Heart Failure

In heart failure, there are hemodynamic changes from ventricular dysfunction with resultant decreased cardiac output. The kidneys correct for this diminished perfusion by conservation of sodium and retention of water to expand the extracellular fluid volume. This reduced perfusion also causes decreased stimulation of vascular baroreceptors, which leads to activation of the adrenergic system causing peripheral vasoconstriction and release of vasopressin.[2,3]

With decrease in renal plasma flow, glomerular filtration rate (GFR) is preserved by (1) vasodilation of the afferent arterioles via atrial natriuretic peptide, prostaglandins, and nitric oxide and (2) vasoconstriction of the efferent arterioles via mediators such as norepinephrine, vasopressin, endothelin, and activation of the renin-angiotensin and sympathetic nervous systems.[4,5]

Because the vasoconstricting mediators are mainly responsible for maintaining GFR in heart failure, their effects can be neutralized in the presence of a vasodilator.

Renin secretion is increased as part of the renin-angiotensin-aldosterone system (RAAS) activation and results in **angiotensin II**–mediated increases in **aldosterone** (which increases sodium reabsorption in the collecting duct)[6] and **vasopressin** (which increases free water reabsorption in the collecting duct by various mechanisms, including up-regulation of the aquaporin-2 water channel).[7-9] In addition, angiotensin II directly increases proximal tubule sodium reabsorption. All of these mediators are involved in the derangement in fluid and solute balance in heart failure and are molecular targets for treatment of heart failure. Lastly, the resultant fluid expansion allows the heart to maintain cardiac output by operating at a higher level on the Frank-Starling curve at the expense of higher end-diastolic pressures and increased wall stress (Fig. 32-3).[10]

MECHANISMS OF ACTION AND CLASSES OF DIURETICS

Diuretics are agents that increase urine flow but specifically are pharmacologic agents that act directly on the kidneys to inhibit solute and water reabsorption. Most diuretics are inhibitors of the ion transporters in the renal tubules and are secreted mostly by proximal tubular cells via the organic acid transport systems; these drugs need to be in the tubular lumen to be effective. The relative potency of the diuretic is related partly to the proximal or distal location of the site of action; the more proximal the site of action, the more natriuresis is possible because of a larger capability for the diuretic agent to inhibit resorption of filtered sodium. The major classes of diuretics and their sites of action on the nephron are described subsequently in the format of the new molecular pharmacologic classification based on mechanisms of action (see drug formulary in the back of the book for dosages for diuretic agents).

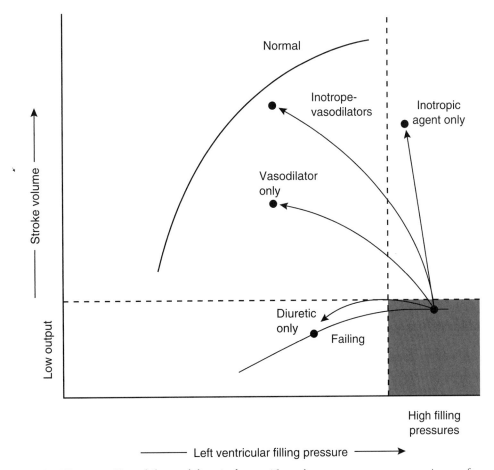

FIGURE 32-3 ■ Heart failure and diuretic therapy. The volume versus pressure curve is seen for normal hearts (*Normal*). The stroke volume is plotted along the y axis, and the left ventricular filling pressure is plotted along the x axis. In heart failure (*Failing*), the curve is shifted to the right and is lowered. Diuretic therapy alone lowers the filling pressure without any increase in cardiac output. The other therapies (inotropic agent only, inotrope-vasodilators, and vasodilator only) all increase stroke volume. (From Cohn JN, Franciosa JA: *Vasodilator therapy of cardiac failure. N Engl J Med* 1977;297:27-31.)

Sodium-Potassium-Chloride Cotransporter Inhibitors (Loop Diuretics)

Sodium-potassium-chloride ($Na^+/K^+/2Cl^-$) cotransporter inhibitors (loop diuretics) (Fig. 32-4A) act by reversibly inhibiting the $Na^+/K^+/2Cl^-$ cotransport system in the thick ascending limb of the loop of Henle and increase the excretion of sodium, potassium, chloride, hydrogen, and water. The increase in sodium excretion (25% of filtered sodium) overwhelms the distal nephron's capability to reabsorb sodium, resulting in natriuresis. In addition, there is increased excretion of magnesium and calcium. The Na^+/K^+-ATPase in the tubular cells exchanges sodium for potassium and creates the sodium gradient necessary for the $Na^+/K^+/2Cl^-$ cotransporter to function. Because there is less reabsorption of solute, there is less impetus for the reabsorption of water more distally in the collecting duct regardless of presence of vasopressin. The positive hemodynamic effects as a result of renal prostaglandin activation from furosemide administration include increased renal blood flow, decreased renal vascular resistance, and increased renin release with increased systemic vascular resistance (from activation of the renin-angiotensin system). These hemodynamic effects allow furosemide to retain some of its effectiveness in renal failure.

Examples of this class of potent diuretics include furosemide (Lasix), bumetanide (Bumex), ethacrynic acid (Edecrin), and torsemide (Demadex). There is wide experience with these agents for a myriad of clinical **indications** in pediatric patients. Loop diuretics are the mainstay of diuretic therapy for heart failure and are effective secondary to their relatively increased potency in sodium and water excretion over other classes of diuretics. In addition, these agents can increase venous capacitance and reduce left ventricular filling pressure. Furosemide has been associated with persistence of the patent ductus arteriosus, however, because of its prostaglandin stimulatory properties.[11] Loop diuretics (except ethacrynic acid) are effective even in patients with poor renal function because these agents are efficacious if there is decreased renal perfusion and diminished GFR. Loop diuretics also often are used for diuresis after cardiac surgery. These agents often are among the first-line pharmacologic agents for the treatment of systemic hypertension, particularly in patients with renal disease. Furosemide also has beneficial nondiuretic effects on pulmonary function with reduction in transvascular fluid filtration and improvement in lung function in children after cardiovascular surgery[12] and with movement of water from the interstitium and decrease in airway resistance in premature neonates with chronic lung disease and bronchopulmonary dysplasia.[13,14] There is limited reported pediatric experience with ethacrynic acid and torsemide.

Furosemide (and bumetanide) can be used effectively as a parenteral drug with peak effects at about 1 to 2 hours or as a continuous intravenous infusion.[15] Furosemide is also a weak carbonic-anhydrase inhibitor. The half-life of furosemide is prolonged in patients with renal failure as it undergoes significant renal metabolism, whereas the half-lives of bumetanide and torsemide are less affected secondary to their hepatic metabolism. Absorption of furosemide varies, and dosing should be based on the individual response to a dose[16]; bumetanide and torsemide are completely absorbed, and their dosing fluctuates to a lesser degree.[17] Furosemide also needs to be bound to albumin to achieve its effects.[18] Although ethacrynic acid and bumetanide are used much less frequently in children compared with furosemide, these agents can be considered as adjunctive therapy in cases of furosemide resistance.[19] Finally, there is preliminary evidence that torsemide-treated adult patients are less likely to be readmitted for heart failure compared with furosemide-treated patients.[20]

Loop diuretics (except ethacrynic acid) are contraindicated in patients with allergies to sulfonylureas/sulfonamides. Loop diuretics also displace warfarin from its protein-binding sites and increase its activity. These agents also increase the plasma levels of propranolol. The activity of loop diuretics is diminished when administered with probenecid (which competes for the receptors) or nonsteroidal anti-inflammatory drugs (which diminish glomerular filtrate formation).

The most frequent side effects seen with loop diuretics are electrolyte disturbances secondary to their loss in the urine and volume contraction with concomitant hypochloremic metabolic alkalosis. The latter is exacerbated by hydrogen ion secretion via H^+ ATPase in the collecting tubule secondary to aldosterone activation. Hypovolemia and hypotension also can be seen with overaggressive diuresis. Additional side effects include hypokalemia, hyponatremia, hypomagnesemia, hypocalcemia, and hyperglycemia. Hypokalemia is due to the kaliuretic effect in the ascending limb of the loop of Henle, but is worsened by aldosterone-mediated secretion of potassium in the collecting duct. Hypercalciuria can lead to nephrocalcinosis. Loop diuretics also can lead to secondary hyperparathyroidism. Furosemide and bumetanide also displace bilirubin from its protein-binding sites, further complicating its use in neonates.

Ototoxicity is a side effect that occurs more frequently with the use of higher doses or the concurrent use of other ototoxic drugs, such as aminoglycosides, and can range from tinnitus or vertigo to reversible or irreversible sensorineural hearing impairment. Ototoxicity may be due to the effects of the loop diuretics on the $Na^+/K^+/2Cl^-$ cotransporter in the endolymph causing electrolyte disturbances and potential endocochlear potential alterations in the inner ear.[21] Ethacrynic acid may have the highest ototoxic potential. Other side effects seen with the use of loop diuretics include arrhythmias/supraventricular tachycardia,[22] fever, headache, fatigue, myalgias, mental confusion, muscle

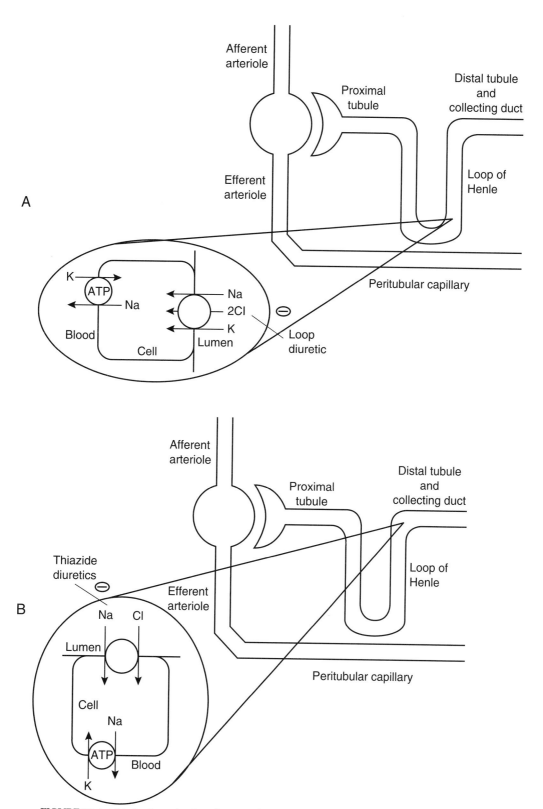

FIGURE 32-4 ■ Mechanisms of action of various classes of diuretic agents. A, Sodium-potassium-chloride ($Na^+/K^+/2Cl^-$) cotransporter inhibitors (loop diuretics). These agents act by reversibly inhibiting the $Na^+/K^+/2Cl^-$ cotransport system in the thick ascending limb of the loop of Henle and increase the excretion of sodium, potassium, chloride, hydrogen, and water. The Na^+/K^+-ATPase in the tubular cells exchanges sodium for potassium and creates the sodium gradient necessary for the $Na^+/K^+/2Cl^-$ cotransporter to function. **B,** Sodium-chloride (Na^+/Cl^-) cotransporter inhibitors (thiazide diuretics). This class of drugs inhibits the reabsorption of Na^+/Cl^- cotransporter in the distal convoluted tubule. In doing so, these agents prevent maximal dilution of the urine and increase the urinary excretion of sodium and chloride. Because of increased delivery of fluid, sodium, and chloride to the distal nephron, there is increased secretion of potassium and hydrogen ions into the urine as well. Similar to the loop diuretics, the Na^+/K^+-ATPase in the tubular cells exchanges sodium for potassium and creates the sodium gradient necessary for the Na^+/Cl^- cotransporter to achieve its function. The Na^+/Cl^- cotransporter inhibitors also possess carbonic anhydrase–inhibiting activity.

Continued

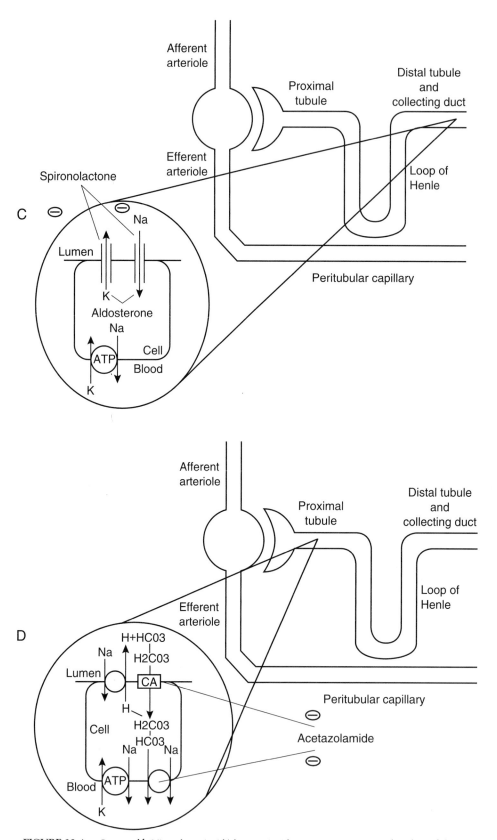

FIGURE 32-4 ■ C,—cont'd. Mineralocorticoid/glucocorticoid receptor antagonists. This class of diuretics, similar to the epithelial sodium channel inhibitors, is potassium sparing. This class of drugs inhibits the reabsorption of sodium in the distal convoluted tubule and collecting duct directly or via aldosterone. Spironolactone competitively inhibits aldosterone's effects on the distal convoluted tubule and collecting duct, decreasing the production of sodium channels, H^+/K^+-ATPase, and Na^+/K^+-ATPase. This action decreases the electrochemical gradient and decreases potassium and hydrogen ion secretion into the urine. **D,** Carbonic anhydrase inhibitor. Acetazolamide produces an alkaline diuresis by inhibiting hydrogen ion secretion by the proximal renal tubule, increasing the excretion of sodium, potassium, bicarbonate, and water. (From Lowrie L: *Diuretic therapy of heart failure in infants and children.* *Prog Pediatr Cardiol* 2000;12:45-55.)

cramps, nausea, gastrointestinal cramping and bleeding (especially with the concomitant use of steroids), pancreatitis, hyperuricemia, photosensitization, rash, agranulocytosis, thrombocytopenia, interstitial nephritis,[23] nephrocalcinosis,[24,25] and cholelithiasis in premature infants.[26]

Sodium-Chloride Cotransporter Inhibitors (Thiazide-like Diuretics)

Sodium-chloride (Na^+/Cl^-) cotransporter inhibitors, (thiazide-like diuretics) (Fig. 32-4B), inhibit the reabsorption of Na^+/Cl^- cotransporter in the distal convoluted tubule and increase the urinary excretion of sodium and chloride. Because the distal convoluted tubule is downstream from anatomic structures where most of the sodium reabsorption occurs and accounts for only about 5% to 10% of sodium to be reabsorbed, these diuretic agents have limited capability to prevent sodium reabsorption. With the increased delivery of fluid, sodium, and chloride to the distal nephron, there also is increased secretion of potassium and hydrogen ions into the urine. The electroneutral Na^+/Cl^- cotransporter inhibitors also possess carbonic anhydrase–inhibiting activity. Similar to the loop diuretics, the Na^+/K^+-ATPase in the tubular cells exchanges sodium for potassium and creates the sodium gradient necessary for the Na^+/Cl^- cotransporter to achieve its function.

This class of relatively weak diuretics includes chlorothiazide (Diuril), hydrochlorothiazide (Hydrodiuril) (a more potent analogue of chlorothiazide), and metolazone (Zaroxolyn). The **indications** of Na^+/Cl^- cotransporter inhibitors include use in combination with loop diuretics to increase diuresis in patients with heart failure. These agents also are efficacious as antihypertensive agents. Similar to loop diuretics, these diuretics are contraindicated in patients with allergies to sulfonamides. These diuretics have minimal effectiveness in the face of renal failure, and all but metolazone are ineffective in patients with a lowered creatinine clearance. Doses for these agents need to be increased to effect in renal failure because the drug must be excreted into the tubule in a sufficient amount to be effective.[27] Metolazone, a sulfonamide diuretic, has properties also consistent with $Na^+/K^+/2Cl^-$ cotransporter inhibitors and may be synergistic with these agents. Metolazone is particularly useful in diuretic-resistant fluid retention and in the presence of renal failure or diuretic resistance.[28,29] Metolazone has a long elimination half-life (2 days) and can have prolonged diuretic effects; pharmacokinetic data in children are sparse.

The most frequent side effects of Na^+/Cl^- cotransporter inhibitors are also electrolyte imbalances, including hyponatremia, hypokalemia, hypochloremia, hypercalcemia (from decreased renal calcium excretion), hypomagnesemia, and hyperglycemia. Hyperglycemia can be more pronounced with Na^+/Cl^- cotransporter inhibitors than with other classes of diuretics. Hypotension and prerenal azotemia can be issues

with aggressive diuresis, especially with the combination of a loop diuretic and metolazone. Other side effects include photosensitivity, impotence, bone marrow suppression, hemolytic anemia, headache, drowsiness, vertigo, nausea, vomiting, diarrhea, pancreatitis, and muscle weakness. Na^+/Cl^- cotransporter inhibitors also displace bilirubin from its protein-binding sites, and levels should be monitored.

Mineralocorticoid/Glucocorticoid Receptor Antagonists

Mineralocorticoid/glucocorticoid receptor antagonists (Fig. 32-4C), similar to the epithelial sodium channel inhibitors, are potassium sparing. Because aldosterone induces sodium reabsorption and facilitates potassium secretion, this class of drugs inhibits the reabsorption of sodium in the distal convoluted tubule and collecting duct. Spironolactone is a steroid-like compound that competitively inhibits the binding of aldosterone to the mineralocorticoid receptor, decreasing the production of Na^+ channels, H^+/K^+-ATPase and Na^+/K^+-ATPase.

Potassium-sparing diuretics are relatively weak diuretics and often are used as an adjunct in combination with the other diuretics to ameliorate the kaliuretic effects of the other diuretics. There is much experience with spironolactone as a long-term diuretic agent in adults with heart failure. A study in adults with stage C heart failure (the Randomized Aldactone Evaluation Study [RALES] trial) showed a decrease in mortality with the use of low-dose spironolactone. The RALES trial was a prospective, placebo-controlled trial of the use of low-dose spironolactone in adults with advanced heart failure. Most patients were on a 25-mg daily dose, and this dose seemed to have no diuretic or hemodynamic effect.[30] There was an overall 30% decrease in mortality combining sudden and pump failure deaths and a 35% decrease in hospitalizations. Patients had improvement in symptoms of heart failure based on New York Heart Association classification and improved exercise tolerance. The increased incidence of hyperkalemia could be predicted partly by baseline hyperkalemia, renal insufficiency, or angiotensin-converting enzyme (ACE) inhibitors. Further studies are necessary to validate this preliminary finding.[31]

There are many theoretical considerations and **indications** in the use of an aldosterone inhibitor such as spironolactone. First, spironolactone can block the excess aldosterone associated with heart failure that is not treated adequately with ACE inhibitors.[32] Second, aldosterone protects against potassium and magnesium depletion, which may be proarrhythmic and contribute to mortality in heart failure.[33] Third, there is the finding that spironolactone improves endothelial vasodilator dysfunction and suppresses vascular angiotensin conversion with favorable effects on left ventricular remodeling.[34,35] Lastly, treatment with spironolactone has been associated with decreased levels of B-type natriuretic peptide (BNP) and N-pro-atrial natriuretic factor by inducing favorable changes in left ventricular filling and compliance.[36]

There are some data on the use of spironolactone in pediatric patients. A small trial in children showed diuretic efficacy and safety of spironolactone but did not examine influence on mortality.[37] In addition, treatment with spironolactone in children after cardiac surgery did not seem to have an effect on the course of postoperative hyperaldosteronism.[38] Lastly, there was a report of a small case series with the use of high-dose spironolactone for patients who had a Fontan operation but developed protein-losing enteropathy.[39]

Spironolactone has **side effects** and should be used with caution in patients with hyponatremia, renal insufficiency, hyperkalemia, and hepatic disease. The electrolyte disturbances seen with potassium-sparing diuretics include hyperkalemia, hyponatremia, acidosis, hypercalcemia, and hypermagnesemia. Potassium levels should be monitored closely, especially with concurrent use of potassium supplementation or an ACE inhibitor, because injudicious use of spironolactone has led to renal failure and hyperkalemia. Potassium levels also should be monitored more closely in patients receiving β-blockers. Spironolactone also can diminish the excretion of digoxin. Spironolactone interferes with testosterone synthesis and may increase peripheral conversion of testosterone to estradiol, leading to gynecomastia, amenorrhea, and impotence. Other side effects include headache, vertigo, somnolence, depression, photosensitivity, rash, alopecia, nausea, vomiting, diarrhea, gastrointestinal bleeding, bone marrow suppression, weakness, muscle cramps, increased intraocular pressure, tinnitus, and dry mouth.

Carbonic Anhydrase Inhibitors

In the proximal tubule, hydrogen ion binds to bicarbonate to produce carbonic acid, which enters the tubular cell with the action of carbonic anhydrase. The class of carbonic anhydrase inhibitors (Fig. 32-4D) produces an alkaline diuresis by inhibiting membrane-bound and cytoplasmic carbonic anhydrase and blocking sodium bicarbonate reabsorption. This action results in increased excretion of sodium, potassium, bicarbonate, and water because there is less hydrogen ion available for Na^+/H^+ exchange.

The drug in clinical use in this category is acetazolamide (Diamox). Carbonic anhydrase inhibitors are weak diuretics and are used predominantly to treat the **metabolic alkalosis** caused by the other classes of diuretics.[40] As a result of its mechanism of action, another **indication** for acetazolamide may be congestive heart failure that is refractory to $Na^+/K^+/2Cl^-$ cotransporter inhibitors. Acetazolamide is ineffective in patients with renal failure. Its use also is avoided in patients with a hyperchloremic acidosis because this is worsened and in patients with severe lung disease because they are unable to correct for the acidosis. In addition to its use as a diuretic, acetazolamide has other clinical applications, such as treatment for altitude sickness, glaucoma, refractory seizures, and reduction of cerebrospinal fluid production in hydrocephalus. **Side effects** of acetazolamide include acidosis, hypokalemia, fatigue, muscle weakness, vertigo, depression, rash, photosensitivity, Stevens-Johnson syndrome, nausea, vomiting, gastrointestinal bleeding, bone marrow suppression, and renal calculi.

Epithelial Sodium Channel Inhibitors (Potassium-Sparing Diuretics)

Epithelial sodium channel inhibitors (potassium-sparing diuretics) directly block the sodium-selective channels and, similar to spironolactone, are potassium sparing. Amiloride (Midamor) and triamterene (Dyrenium) act directly on the sodium channels in the late distal convoluted tubule, cortical collecting tubule, and collecting duct, but are not direct aldosterone antagonists, such as spironolactone. Although amiloride is a distal sodium channel blocker, triamterene is a pteridine class agent that blocks sodium transport by inhibiting Na^+/K^+-ATPase distally.

Potassium-sparing diuretics block reabsorption of less than 3% of the filtered load of sodium and are weak natriuretic agents and so often are used in combination with more potent diuretics. These agents can lessen the degree of hypokalemia observed with loop or thiazide diuretic agents. Although amiloride is excreted by the kidneys, triamterene is metabolized by the liver and secreted into the tubular fluid of the kidney. There is no reported pediatric experience with these agents.

Osmotic Diuretics

Osmotic diuretics are freely filtered at the glomerulus and are poorly reabsorbed by the renal tubule. These drugs are pharmacologically inert and increase the osmotic pressure of the glomerular filtrate, which inhibits tubular reabsorption of water and electrolytes. The site of action is the proximal tubule and loop of Henle, and in contrast to the other diuretic agents described previously, osmotic agents are not secreted into the lumen by proximal tubular cells.

An example of an osmotic diuretic in clinical use is mannitol (Osmitrol). Part of the activity of mannitol may be due to the activation of vasodilatory prostaglandins. Mannitol increases the intravascular volume, and this may lead to unfavorable fluid shifts. Dosing with mannitol may cause worsening of congestive heart failure and pulmonary edema secondary to a sudden extracellular fluid volume expansion, especially in patients with renal insufficiency (because they are unable to filter it into the glomerular filtrate). For this reason, mannitol should be avoided in situations of intravascular fluid overload and decreased renal function and in premature neonates (because they have less tolerance for sudden fluid shifts and intraventricular hemorrhage). Mannitol also can cause hypovolemia, hypernatremia, hyperkalemia, convulsions, and headache. Mannitol is effective in decreasing intracranial and intraocular pressures. Other osmotic diuretics include glycerin, isosorbide, and urea.

Other Agents

Dopamine stimulates adrenergic and dopaminergic receptors at higher doses, but at low doses, its effects are mainly dopaminergic, and this results in renal and mesenteric vasodilation. In addition, D_1 receptors on luminal membranes of the proximal tubule can influence Na^+/K^+-ATPase and promote natriuresis. Even preterm infants seem to have dopamine receptor activity by 24 weeks of gestation.[41]

Dopamine can be used as a diuretic at a low dose (2.5 to 3 ug/kg/min continuous infusion).[42] Reports have shown inconsistent results with the use of low-dose dopamine for this indication because it has not always enhanced urinary sodium excretion.[43,44] Side effects include tachyarrhythmias, hypertension, headaches, nausea, and vomiting.

Fenoldopam (Corlopam) is a selective dopamine D_1 receptor agonist that causes vasodilation (systemic, renal, mesenteric, coronary, and pulmonary vasculatures), increased renal perfusion (dilates afferent and efferent renal arterioles), and increased natriuresis.[45] It has been shown to have renoprotective effects by maintaining renal blood flow, GFR, and natriuresis during ischemia.[46]

Information on the use of fenoldopam in children as an antihypertensive agent is preliminary.[47] Doses to increase the GFR (without a significant change in peripheral vascular resistance) range from 0.01 to 0.05 ug/kg/min without a preceding bolus. Tachyphylaxis may occur at about 48 hours. Fenoldopam is effective in patients with renal insufficiency and can reverse the vasoconstriction caused by angiotensin II and norepinephrine.[48] There is even evidence that fenoldopam aids in clearing pulmonary edema by direct effects on the pulmonary vasculature. At high doses (≥ 0.1 ug/kg/min), fenoldopam causes hypotension and a reflex tachycardia. Fenoldopam also can cause hypokalemia, headache, nausea, flushing, and an increase in intraocular pressure.

Other agents that can increase GFR include glucocorticoids, which can have mineralocorticoid activity, and theophylline, which inhibits sodium and chloride resorption in the proximal tubule.[49]

New Diuretic Agents

The new aldosterone antagonist **eplerenone** is a selective aldosterone antagonist. Effects of eplerenone in animal studies have included decreased left ventricular end-diastolic wall stress, decreased cardiomyocyte cross-sectional area, and reduced intracardiac fibrosis and remodeling.[50,51] Eplerenone is a more selective aldosterone blocker with less incidence of gynecomastia, secondary to its greater selectivity for the mineralocorticoid receptor compared with spironolactone.

In trials of patients with congestive heart failure, eplerenone has been shown to be associated with diminished deaths from cardiovascular causes and decreased hospitalizations for congestive heart failure.[52] Side effects include diminished blood pressure and hyperkalemia. There is no preliminary clinical experience with this agent in children with heart failure.

Natriuretic peptides include atrial natriuretic peptide, BNP, and urodilatin, a natriuretic peptide that comes from the renal distal tubular cells.[53,54] Natriuretic peptides cause afferent arteriolar dilation and efferent arteriolar constriction leading to an increase in the GFR; these agents also antagonize intrarenal vasoconstriction from catecholamines, angiotensin II, and renin.[55] In general, these natriuretic peptides do not activate the RAAS or the sympathetic nervous system and have specific effects, such as inhibition of vasopressin release by the pituitary gland and of aldosterone synthesis by the adrenal gland with decrease in collecting duct sodium reabsorption (see Chapter 6).[56]

With these combined effects, natriuretic peptides induce diuresis in patients with heart failure. With severe congestive heart failure, an infusion of BNP (recombinant human BNP [nesiritide]) increases urine output and urinary sodium excretion without significant changes in serum potassium; in addition, there is a vasodilating effect.[57] There is no clinical experience with natriuretic peptides in children.

Vasopressin release is stimulated by hypovolemia and increased serum osmolality.[58] Vasopressin elicits its effects through two separate receptors: V_1 receptors are on vascular smooth muscle and lead to the pressor effects of vasopressin, whereas V_2 receptors are located on cells in the collecting ducts and regulate the natriuretic and vasodilatory effects of vasopressin. Vasopressin activates V_2 receptors, causing translocation of aquaporin-2 water channels to the apical surface of the collecting duct, and increases their synthesis, promoting water retention. Vasopressin V_2 receptor **antagonists** increase free water clearance not only by inhibiting the action of vasopressin, but also via down-regulation of the aquaporin-2 water channel expression.[59]

These antagonists have good safety and hemodynamic profiles. Clinical use of vasopressin V_2 receptor antagonists has led to increased free water clearance, correction of hyponatremia, and increased urine output, while not affecting change in potassium handling.

Because neutral endopeptidase inactivates natriuretic peptides (endogenous and exogenously administered forms), the inactivation of this enzyme via inhibition can prolong the biologic half-life of natriuretic peptides.[60] These inhibitors, known as **vasopeptidase inhibitors**, can work in synergy with BNP.[61] There is even some evidence that this strategy can prevent adverse cardiac remodeling.[62]

PERITONEAL DIALYSIS AND HEMODIALYSIS (ULTRAFILTRATION)

When drug therapy for heart failure and diuresis fails, there is the possibility of using mechanical means, such as peritoneal dialysis or extracorporeal ultrafiltration, to ameliorate fluid overload.[63] These procedures can be done in an inpatient or ambulatory setting. Although some experts advocate the use of these methods as an adjunct when other modalities have failed to manage refractory fluid overload, others support using these mechanical means to remove fluid as a proactive line of treatment in patients with less severe heart failure. The overall benefits include mitigation of the neurohumoral stimulation, increase in urine output, and absorption of excessive extravascular fluid.[64,65] Peritoneal dialysis has been shown to reduce hospitalization rates and improve functional capacity in adults with heart failure.[66] Portability and safety of this mode of treatment have been increasing. Ultrafiltration also is a viable option in the treatment of patients with heart failure when diuretics are not effective or to augment their effectiveness and improve patient clinical status.[67]

PHARMACOLOGY OF DIURETIC USE IN HEART FAILURE

Diuretic Use in Heart Failure

The compensatory mechanism for the kidneys to respond to heart failure and diminished perfusion is via conservation of sodium and retention of water, which lead to congestion that can be relieved by diuretic use. Although the volume excess is relieved by diuretic agents, the resultant volume reduction can lead to reduced preload, reduced cardiac output and renal blood flow, and eventually a neurohumoral response to regain the fluid to expand intravascular volume. Excessive administration of diuretic agents can create a vicious cycle of diuretic use, followed by volume depletion, reduced preload and cardiac output, neurohumoral activation, and fluid retention.

Diuretics (except possibly spironolactone) do not directly affect the underlying mechanisms by which heart failure progresses, but treat the symptoms that occur as a result of the volume overload and congestion associated with heart failure. Diuretics diminish pulmonary congestion, decrease pulmonary vascular pressure, improve exercise intolerance, and decrease the respiratory distress and edema associated with heart failure. It is possible that decreasing the ventricular end-diastolic pressure may lessen ventricular hypertrophy and remodeling, but this has not been proved.

Other than studies involving spironolactone, no long-term studies have shown an improvement in mortality in heart failure with diuretics.[68] Short-term use has been associated with clinical benefits in terms of symptomatic relief. Diuretics should not be used as monotherapy for heart failure, but should be used as a component of multifaceted therapy targeted at symptoms and the underlying cause of heart failure.

Developmental Changes in Diuretic Response

The significant developmental milestones in increases in renal blood flow and GFR occur after 36 weeks' gestation and after the first week of the postnatal period; renal tubular function does not reach maximal levels until 1 to 2 years of age, which partly explains inability of neonates to excrete acid and their relatively higher fractional excretion of sodium.[69] Maturation of the tubular transporter systems is essential for appropriate secretion of the diuretic agents into the lumen. Neonates can be particularly vulnerable to certain diuretic agents that exacerbate certain renal deficiencies. Carbonic anhydrase inhibitors can lead to severe acidosis because neonates do not have enough reserve to excrete acid and have less intrinsic carbonic anhydrase activity. Age-appropriate strategy in the use of diuretics is essential for optimal clinical effects and minimal side effects.

These maturational changes and the developmental ontogeny of the kidney can affect the choice and dosing of the various diuretics in children, particularly in neonates and infants.[70] Infants have a lower GFR than older children and adults, and this deficit increases half-lives of filtered diuretics and decreases infants' ability to concentrate their urine. The half-life of furosemide is much longer (20 times longer) in premature neonates compared with older children or adults. This relatively decreased GFR also may contribute to the diminished ability of neonates to excrete sodium and water and eliminate drugs cleared by the kidney. In addition, children also have a larger volume of distribution than adults and lower serum albumin levels leading to prolonged drug half-lives and increased bioavailability. In addition, maturation of the gastrointestinal tract and the hepatic microsomal enzymes affects bioavailability of the diuretic agents. Lastly, neurohumoral changes in heart failure and pharmacokinetic and pharmacodynamic profiles of diuretics reflect the developmental changes during infancy and childhood.[71]

Clinical Strategy of Diuretic Use

The present strategy of diuretic use is to use as a first-line diuretic a $Na^+/K^+/2Cl^-$ cotransporter inhibitor, such as furosemide, followed by addition of another diuretic in the same class (e.g., ethacrynic acid) or a diuretic in a different class (e.g., a thiazide diuretic or spironolactone) if there is an insufficient response. Overall the major side effect and limitation of diuretics is electrolyte disturbance. Electrolytes must be monitored during the course of treatment with a diuretic because disturbances can lead to ineffectiveness of the diuretics or increase the risk of complications. Hypokalemia, seen most frequently with loop and thiazide diuretics, may lead to arrhythmias, which can increase mortality and may persist until coexisting electrolyte derangements are corrected. Electrolytes must be monitored more closely with concurrent use of an ACE inhibitor because an ACE inhibitor can increase serum potassium, and the effect can be cumulative with a potassium-sparing diuretic. In the adult SOLVD (Studies of Left Ventricular Dysfunction) trial, potassium-losing diuretics were associated with an increased risk of arrhythmic death, but potassium-sparing diuretics were not.[72] **Hyponatremia**, also observed most frequently with loop and thiazide diuretics, is secondary to increased renal excretion of sodium and excessive water retention and can be treated with a decrease in diuretic but not hypertonic saline solution (because aggressive supplementation counteracts the desired effect of the diuretic). The **metabolic alkalosis** with hypochloremia is partially a result of increased excretion of sodium and then potassium, which leads to increased secretion of hydrogen ion. This effect is exacerbated by contraction of extracellular fluid and loss of sodium chloride with increased reabsorption of sodium bicarbonate. This condition is treated with a decrease in the diuretic agent, supplementation of potassium and chloride if appropriate, judicious volume replacement, and use of acetazolamide.

The classes of diuretic agents with different mechanisms of action can potentiate one another. **Low-dose combinations** of different and synergistic diuretic classes may be preferable to monotherapy with loop diuretics because this prevents the compensatory mechanisms associated with long-term diuretic therapy (see later). In addition, low-dose combinations of diuretics with complementary mechanisms of action may cause less activation of the RAAS and fewer complications from electrolyte imbalances and toxicity from higher doses of a single drug.[73]

Combination diuretics that are used in adults are available and include Aldactazide (spironolactone, 25 mg, and hydrochlorothiazide, 25 mg), Dyazide and Maxzide (triamterene and hydrochlorothiazide), Moduretic (amiloride and hydrochlorothiazide), or any thiazide in addition to a loop diuretic. Most of these formulations are not available in doses suitable for smaller children and neonates, but can be considered in older children and adolescents as maintenance therapy after appropriate dosing has been determined.

Pharmacodynamic studies show that a maximally efficient diuretic dose for each patient and each diuretic exists, even in neonates (Fig. 32-5).[74] A **continuous infusion** strategy avoids troughs of diuretic concentration that render the drug less effective. Before starting an infusion, a bolus dose can be administered so that a therapeutic concentration of drug in the renal tubule can be reached early.

Infusions are more effective in improving diuresis than intermittent bolus doses and are effective in even some diuretic-resistant patients. The effect of diuresis is more easily titrated, and there are fewer hemodynamic fluctuations with continuous infusions.[75] There is

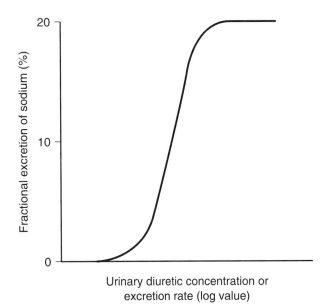

FIGURE 32-5 ■ **Pharmacodynamic curve of a diuretic agent.** Graph shows the fractional excretion of sodium on the y axis and the urinary diuretic concentration or excretion rate on the x axis. The sigmoid curve shows the relationship between the arrival of a diuretic agent at its site of action and its resultant natriuretic response. There is a threshold quantity of the diuretic agent that must be met for the drug to elicit a response. (From Brater DC: *Drug therapy: Diuretic therapy. N Engl J Med* 1998;339:387-395.)

theoretically less toxicity (ototoxicity and myopathies) with infusions secondary to lower peak levels.

Diuretic Resistance and Counterstrategy

There are myriad reasons as to why standard dosing of diuretics may be ineffective. Diuretic agents increase production of urine by blocking solute and water reabsorption and promoting excess salt and water excretion; these agents are less efficacious if there is decreased intravascular volume, decreased renal blood flow, decreased GFR, or decreased salt concentration. The clinical efficacy of diuretic agents depends on delivery of salt and water to the distal tubule.

Heart failure can reduce the bioefficacy of the diuretic agents for various reasons. **Renal insufficiency** causes standard doses of diuretics to be less efficacious because there is less secretion into the tubular lumen and less delivery of the drug to its site of action. Renal failure also increases the half-life of furosemide as its urinary excretion and renal conjugation are decreased. The decreased fractional excretion of sodium in patients with heart failure compared with normal individuals also may impair bioefficacy of diuretic agents. Measures to preserve renal blood flow and GFR (e.g., dopamine, fenoldopam, or natriuretic peptides) can minimize this negative influence. In patients with heart failure, there also may be **pharmacodynamic derangements** in diuretic agents that affect drug efficacy. There may be delayed absorption of the diuretic agents and inability to reach the optimal peak intraluminal levels of drug necessary to affect diuresis. Mesenteric congestion seems to affect drug absorption and dosing and can decrease the effectiveness of a standard dose. In addition, diuretics may be less effective in patients with hypoalbuminemia because there is less intravascular binding of the diuretics and less delivery to the proximal tubular cells for secretion. Lastly, there may be evidence for altered expression of the transporter gene that may influence the diuretic response to some agents.[76] Diuretics also may be ineffective secondary to **electrolyte abnormalities** from chronic diuresis. Hyponatremia can lead to secondary hyperaldosteronism; the decreased distal tubular sodium delivery can increase the stimulation of vasopressin production, leading to less free water excretion. In addition, with metabolic alkalosis, there is increased reabsorption of sodium in the proximal tubule and less distal delivery. Carbonic anhydrase inhibition can lead to increased delivery of sodium and chloride to the site of action of the loop diuretics, whereas concomitant dosing of spironolactone and an ACE inhibitor may potentiate the amount of sodium and volume excretion.

Concurrent dosing of **other medications** that can compromise the effectiveness of diuretics sometimes is overlooked. Nonsteroidal anti-inflammatory drugs (including aspirin) decrease the renal production of prostaglandins and block vasodilation with decreases in GFR and sodium excretion. In addition, probenecid and antibiotics such as trimethoprim and penicillin can decrease the proximal tubular secretion of diuretics, diminishing their effectiveness as the diuretic agents cannot reach the site of action. Accumulated organic acids in uremia also compete with diuretics for secretion into the renal tubule. Lastly, vasodilators may decrease renal blood flow, while they increase cardiac output and decrease GFR and efficacy of diuretic agents.

Two important phenomena, the braking effect and segmental nephron hypertrophy, can occur with long-term diuretic use, and both phenomena justify the use of combined diuretic regimens. The first phenomenon, called the **braking effect**, describes the decreased clinical responsiveness to diuretics with time. Although the exact mechanism of this phenomenon is not clear, the most likely etiology involves sodium retention secondary to volume changes and activation of the renin-angiotensin and adrenergic mechanisms. Combined diuretic therapy to increase sodium excretion and to diminish activation of the renin-angiotensin system may be warranted. There is a possible beneficial effect of the associated use of an ACE inhibitor with either loop diuretics or spironolactone to lessen the effects of RAAS stimulation. ACE inhibitors also block angiotensin II stimulation of thirst, vasopressin release, and tubular sodium reabsorption and enhance furosemide-induced natriuresis.

There is also a compensatory hypertrophy of the tubular epithelium distal to the site of action of loop diuretics that results in an increased ability for the tubule to reabsorb solutes. This phenomenon has been termed **sequential or segmental nephron hypertrophy**. This phenomenon occurs secondary to chronically increased exposure of the distal nephron to solute. For this reason, there is a synergism between loop and thiazide diuretics as thiazide diuretics block this distal site; this strategy is aptly termed *segmental nephron blockade*.[77]

Strategies to overcome diuretic resistance include use of more frequent administrations or a continuous infusion, use of combined diuretic therapy to block sodium resorption at multiple sites of action, and correction of electrolyte imbalance, metabolic derangements, and intravascular depletion.

CURRENT STATUS AND FUTURE TRENDS

Diuretic therapy is a mainstay in the treatment of congestive heart failure. Diuretics provide symptomatic relief, but the overall goal should be reduction of extracellular fluid volume with minimal stimulation of the neurohumoral systems. Loop diuretics are preferable to most other diuretics secondary to their effectiveness and potency. Combination therapy has been shown to be more effective than monotherapy with one class at escalating doses because sequential sites in the nephron can be blocked. Diuretic resistance also can be overcome by combination therapy or by continuous infusions.

New therapies are being investigated to increase the options for inducing diuresis, including selective aldosterone antagonists, natriuretic peptides, and vasopressin V_2 receptor antagonists. Ultrafiltration also is becoming a more viable option for therapy. Finally, novel diuretics in the future will eliminate side effects; these include adenosine A_1-receptor blockers, which would not perturb potassium homeostasis,[78] and aquaporin channel inhibitors (aquaretics), which would block the proximal tubule water channels to achieve natriuresis without reliance on sodium excretion altogether.[79,80]

Key Concepts
■ Despite the frequent use of these pharmacologic agents in children with heart disease, there remains a paucity of information on the clinical use and pharmacokinetic profiles of diuretic agents in pediatric patients.

■ With decrease in renal plasma flow, GFR is preserved by (1) vasodilation of the afferent arterioles via atrial natriuretic peptide, prostaglandins, and nitric oxide and (2) vasoconstriction of the efferent arterioles via mediators such as norepinephrine, vasopressin, endothelin, and activation of the renin-angiotensin and sympathetic nervous systems.

■ Most diuretics are inhibitors of the ion transporters in the renal tubules and are secreted mostly by proximal tubular cells via the organic acid transport systems; these drugs need to be in the tubular lumen to be effective.

■ The Na+/K+/2Cl− cotransporter inhibitors (loop diuretics) act by reversibly inhibiting the Na+/K+/2Cl− cotransport system in the thick ascending limb of the loop of Henle and increase the excretion of sodium, potassium, chloride, hydrogen, and water. The increase in sodium excretion (25% of filtered sodium) overwhelms the distal nephron's capability to reabsorb sodium, resulting in natriuresis.

■ The Na+/Cl− cotransporter inhibitors (thiazide diuretics) inhibit the reabsorption of Na+/Cl− cotransporter in the distal convoluted tubule and increase the urinary excretion of sodium and chloride. Because the distal convoluted tubule is downstream from anatomic structures where most of the sodium reabsorption occurs and accounts for only about 5% to 10% of sodium to be reabsorbed, these diuretic agents have limited capability to prevent sodium reabsorption.

■ Pharmacodynamic studies show that a maximally efficient diuretic dose for each patient and each diuretic exists, even in neonates. A continuous infusion strategy avoids troughs of diuretic concentration that render the drug less effective.

■ Two important phenomena, the braking effect and segmental nephron hypertrophy, can occur with long-term diuretic use, and both phenomena justify the use of combined diuretic regimens.

The first phenomenon, the braking effect, describes the decreased clinical responsiveness to diuretics with time. Although the exact mechanism of this phenomenon is not clear, the most likely etiology involves sodium retention secondary to volume changes and activation of the renin-angiotensin and adrenergic mechanisms.

There is also a compensatory hypertrophy of the tubular epithelium distal to the site of action of loop diuretics that results in an increased ability for the tubule to reabsorb solutes. This phenomenon has been termed sequential or segmental nephron hypertrophy.

■ Strategies to overcome diuretic resistance include use of more frequent administrations or a continuous infusion, use of combined diuretic therapy to block sodium resorption at multiple sites of action, and correction of electrolyte imbalance, metabolic derangements, and intravascular depletion.

REFERENCES

1. Faris R, Flather M, Purcell H, et al: Current evidence supporting the role of diuretics in heart failure: A meta-analysis of randomized controlled trials. Int J Cardiol 2002;82:149-158.
2. Cadnapaphornchai MA, Gurevich AK, Weinberger HD, et al: Pathophysiology of sodium and water retention in heart failure. Cardiology 2001;96:122-131.
3. Paul S: Balancing diuretic therapy in heart failure: Loop diuretics, thiazides, and aldosterone antagonists. CHF 2002;8:307-312.
4. Schrier RW, Abraham WT: Mechanisms of disease: Hormones and hemodynamics in heart failure. N Engl J Med 1999;341:577-585.
5. Williams JF, Bristow MR, Fowler MB, et al: Guidelines for the evaluation and management of heart failure. Circulation 1995;92:2764-2784.
6. Kramer BK, Schweda F, Riegger GAJ: Diuretic treatment and diuretic resistance in heart failure. Am J Med 1999;106:90-96.
7. Francis GS: Pathophysiology of chronic heart failure. Am J Med 2001;110:37S-46S.
8. Bristow MR, Port JD, Kelly RA: Treatment of heart failure: Pharmacological methods. In Braunwald E, Zipes DP, Libby P (eds): Heart Disease: A Textbook of Cardiovascular Medicine, 6th ed. Philadelphia, WB Saunders, 2001, pp 562-599.
9. Schrier RW, Martin PY: Recent advances in the understanding of water metabolism in heart failure. Adv Exp Med Biol 1998;449:415-426.
10. Kelly RA, Smith TW: Pharmacological treatment of heart failure. In Goodman LS, Hardman JG, Limbird LE, Gilman AG (eds): Goodman and Gilman's the Pharmacological Basis of Therapeutics. New York, McGraw-Hill, 2001, pp 809-838.
11. Green TP, Thompson TR, Johnson DE, et al: Furosemide promotes patent ductus arteriosus in premature infants with respiratory distress syndrome. N Engl J Med 1983;308:743-748.
12. Aufricht C, Votava F, Marx M, et al: Intratracheal furosemide in infants after cardiac surgery: Its effects on lung mechanics and urinary output, and its levels in plasma and tracheal aspirate. Intensive Care Med 1997;23:992-997.
13. Bancalari E, Gerhardt T: Bronchopulmonary dysplasia. Pediatr Clin North Am 1986;33:1-23.
14. Prandota J: Furosemide: Progress in understanding its diuretic, anti-inflammatory, and bronchodilating mechanisms of action, and use in the treatment of respiratory tract diseases. Am J Therap 2002;9:317-328.
15. Van der Vorst MM, Ruys-Dudok van Heel I, Kist-van Holthe JE, et al: Continuous intravenous furosemide in hemodynamically unstable children after cardiac surgery. Intenisve Care Med 2001;27:711-715.
16. Shankar SS, Brater DC: Loop diuretics: From the Na-K-2Cl transporter to clinical use. Am J Physiol Renal Physiol 2003;284:F11-F21.
17. Sullivan JE, Witte MK, Yamashita TS, et al: Dose-ranging evaluation of bumetanide pharmacodynamics in critically ill infants. Clin Pharmacol Ther 1996;60:424-434.
18. Inoue M, Okajima K, Itoh K, et al: Mechanism of furosemide resistance in analbuminemic rats and hypoalbuminemic patients. Kidney Int 1987;32:198-203.
19. Roberts RJ: Diuretics. In Roberts RJ (ed): Drug Therapy in Infants: Pharmacologic Principles and Clinical Experience. Philadelphia, WB Saunders, 1984, pp 226-249.
20. Murray MD, Deer MM, Ferguson JA, et al: Open-label randomized trial of torsemide compared with furosemide therapy for patients with heart failure. Am J Med 2001;111:513-520.
21. Rybak LP: Furosemide ototoxicity: Clinical and experimental aspects. Laryngoscope 1985;95(Suppl 38):1-14.
22. Wilson NJ, Adderley RJ, McEniery JA: Supraventricular tachycardia associated with continuous furosemide infusion. Can J Anaesth 1991;38:502-505.
23. Van der Vorst MM, Ruys-Dudok van Heel I, Kist-van Holthe JE, et al: Continuous intravenous furosemide in haemodynamically unstable children after cardiac surgery. Intensive Care Med 2001;27:711-715.
24. Alon US, Scagliotti D, Garola RE: Nephrocalcinosis and nephrolithiasis in infants with congestive heart failure treated with furosemide. J Pediatr 1994;125:149-151.
25. Witte MK, Stork JE, Blumer JL: Diuretic therapeutics in the pediatric patient. Am J Cardiol 1986;57:44A-53A.

26. Prandota J: Clinical pharmacology of furosemide in children: A supplement. Am J Therap 2001;8:275-289.

27. Brater DC: Diuretic therapy. N Engl J Med 1998;339:387-395.

28. Arnold WC: Efficacy of metolazone and furosemide in children with furosemide resistant edema. Pediatrics 1984;74:872-875.

29. Sica DA: Pharmacotherapy in congestive heart failure: Metolazone and its role in edema management. CHF 2003;9:100-105.

30. Pitt B, Zannad F, Remme WJ, et al: The effect of spironolactone on morbidity and mortality in patients with severe heart failure. N Engl J Med 1999;341:709-717.

31. Bozkurt B, Agoston I, Knowlton AA: Complications of inappropriate use of spironolactone in heart failure: When an old medicine spirals out of new guidelines. J Am Coll Cardiol 2003;41:215-216.

32. Bauersachs J, Fraccarollo D: Aldosterone antagonism in addition to angiotensin-converting enzyme inhibitors in heart failure. Min Cardioangiol 2003;51:155-164.

33. Richards AM, Nicholls MG: Aldosterone antagonism in heart failure. Lancet 1999;354:789-790.

34. Farquharson CA, Struthers AD: Spironolactone increases nitric oxide bioactivity, improves endothelial vasodilator dysfunction, and suppresses vascular angiotensinI/angiotensin II conversion in patients with chronic heart failure. Circulation 2000;101:594-597.

35. Rousseau MF, Gurne O, Duprez D, et al: Beneficial neurohormonal profile of spironolactone in severe congestive heart failure: Results from the RALES neurohormonal substudy. J Am Coll Cardiol 2002;40:1596-1601.

36. Biondi-Zoccai GG, Abbate A, Baldi A: Potential antiapoptotic activity of aldosterone antagonists in postinfarction remodeling. Circulation 2003;108:e26.

37. Kay JD, Colan SD, Graham TP: Congestive heart failure in pediatric patients. Am Heart J 2001;142:923-928.

38. Haschke F, Wimmer M, Parth K: Hyperaldosteronism after heart surgery in children: Part I. Treatment with aldosterone antagonist. Pediatr Padol 1981;16:317-326.

39. Ringel RE, Peddy SB: Effect of high-dose spironolactone on protein-losing enteropathy in patients with Fontan palliation of complex congenital heart disease. Am J Cardiol 2003;91:1031-1032.

40. Puschett JB: Pharmacological classification and renal actions of diuretics. Cardiology 1994;84(Suppl 2):4-13.

41. Van den Anker JN: Pharmacokinetics and renal function in preterm infants. Acta Paediatr 1996;85:1393-1399.

42. Bryan AG, Bolsin SN, Vianna PT, et al: Modification of the diuretic and natriuretic effects of a dopamine infusion by fluid loading in preoperative cardiac surgical patients. J Cardiothorac Vasc Anesth 1995;9:158-163.

43. Benmalek F, Behforouz N, Benoist JF, et al: Renal effects of low-dose dopamine during vasodepressor therapy for posttraumatic intracranial hypertension. Intensive Care Med 1999;25:399-405.

44. Vargo DL, Brater DC, Rudy DW, et al: Dopamine does not enhance furosemide-induced natriuresis in patients with congestive heart failure. J Am Soc Nephrol 1996;7:1032-1037.

45. Nussmeier NA: Improving perioperative outcomes in patients with end-stage heart failure. Rev Cardiovasc Med 2003;4(Suppl 1):S29-S34.

46. Halpenny M, Markos F, Snow HM, et al: Effects of prophylactic fenoldopam infusion on renal blood flow and renal tubular function during acute hypovolemia in anesthetized dogs. Crit Care Med 2001;29:855-860.

47. Strauser LM, Pruitt RD, Tobias JD: Initial experience with fenoldopam in children. Am J Therap 1999;6:283-288.

48. Garwood S, Swamidoss CP, Davis EA, et al: A case series of low-dose fenoldapam in seventy cardiac surgical patients at increased risk of renal dysfunction. J Cardiothorac Vasc Anesth 2003;17:17-21.

49. Bell M, Jackson E, Mi Z, et al: Low-dose theophylline increases urine output in diuretic-dependent critically ill children. Intensive Care Med 1998;24:1099-1105.

50. Pitt B: Do diuretics and aldosterone receptor antagonists improve ventricular remodeling? J Card Fail 2002;8(6 Suppl):S491-S493.

51. Suzuki G, Morita H, Mishima T, et al: Effects of long-term monotherapy with eplerenone, a novel aldosterone blocker, on progression of left ventricular dysfunction and remodeling in dogs with heart failure. Circulation 2002;106:2967-2972.

52. Pitt B, Remme W, Zannad F, et al: Eplerenone, a selective aldosterone blocker, in patients with left ventricular dysfunction after myocardial infarction. N Engl J Med 2003;348:1309-1321.

53. Meyer M, Wiebe K, Wahlers T, et al: Urodilatin as a new drug for the therapy of acute renal failure following cardiac surgery. Clin Exp Pharmacol Physiol 1997;24:374-376.

54. Seeman T, Meyer M, Schmitt CP, et al: Urinary excretion of urodilantin in healthy children and children with renal disease. Pediatr Nephrol 1998;12:55-59.

55. Stoupakis G, Klapholz M: Natriuretic peptides: Biochemistry, physiology, and therapeutic role in heart failure. Heart Dis 2003;5:215-223.

56. Costello-Boerrigter LC, Boerrigter F, Burnett JC: Revisiting salt and water retention: New diuretics, aquaretics, and natriuretics. Med Clin North Am 2003;87:475-491.

57. Moazami N, Damiano RJ, Bailey MS, et al: Nesiritide in the management of postoperative cardiac patients. Ann Thorac Surg 2003;75:1974-1976.

58. Jackson EK: Vasopressin and other agents affecting the renal conservation of water. In Hardman JG, Limbird LE, Gilman AG (eds): Goodman and Gilman's The Pharmacological Basis of Therapeutics, McGraw-Hill, New York, 2001, pp 789-809.

59. Xu DL, Martin PY, Ohara M, et al: Upregulation of aquaporin-2 water channel expression in chronic heart failure rat. J Clin Invest 1997;99:1500-1505.

60. Blaikley J, Sutton P, Walter M, et al: Tubular proteinuria and enzymuria following open heart surgery. Intensive Care Med 2003;29:1364-1367.

61. Chen HH, Lainchbury JG, Harty GJ, et al: Maximizing the natriuretic peptide system in experimental heart failure: Subcutaneous brain natriuretic peptide and acute vasopeptidase inhibition. Circulation 2002;105:999-1003.

62. Backlund T, Palojoki E, Saraste A, et al: Effect of vasopeptidase inhibitor omapatrilat on cardiomyocyte apoptosis and ventricular remodeling in rat myocardial infarction. Cardiovasc Res 2003;57:727-737.

63. Ronco C, Ricci Z, Bellomo R, et al: Extracorporeal ultrafiltration for the treatment of overhydration and congestive heart failure. Cardiology 2001;96:155-168.

64. Sharma A, Hermann DD, Mehta RL: Clinical benefit and approach of ultrafiltration in acute renal failure. Cardiology 2001;96:144-154.

65. Futterman LG, Lemberg L: Heart failure: Update on treatment and prognosis. Am J Crit Care 2001;10:285-293.

66. Mehrotra R, Khanna R: Peritoneal ultrafiltration for chronic congestive heart failure: Rationale, evidence, and future. Cardiology 2001;96:177-182.

67. Sheppard R, Panyon J, Pohwani AL, et al: Intermittent outpatient ultrafiltration for the treatment of severe refractory congestive heart failure. J Cardiol Fail 2004;10:380-383.

68. Klein L, O'Connor CM, Gattis WA, et al: Pharmacologic therapy for patients with chronic heart failure and reduced systolic function: Review of trials and practical considerations. Am J Cardiol 2003;91:18F-40F.

69. Sherbotie JR, Kaplan BS: Diuretics. In Yaffe SJ, Aranda J (eds): Pediatric Pharmacology: Therapeutic Principles in Practice. Philadelphia, WB Saunders, 1992, pp 524-534.

70. Kearns GL, Abdel-Rahman SM, Alander SW, et al: Developmental pharmacology: Drug disposition, action, and therapy in infants and children. N Engl J Med 2003;349:1157-1167.

71. Lowrie L: Diuretic therapy of heart failure in infants and children. Prog Pediatr Cardiol 2000;12:45-55.

72. Domanski M, Norman J, Pitt B, et al: Diuretic use, progressive heart failure, and death in patients in the Studies of Left Ventricular Dysfunction (SOLVD). J Am Coll Cardiol 2003;42:705-708.

73. Ellison DH: Diuretic therapy and resistance in congestive heart failure. Cardiology 2001;96:132-143.

74. Eades SK, Christensen ML: The clinical pharmacology of loop diuretics in the pediatric patient. Pediatr Nephrol 1998;12:603-616.

75. Luciani GB, Nichani S, Chang AC, et al: Continuous versus intermittent furosemide infusion in critically ill infants after open heart operations. Ann Thorac Surg 1997;64:1133-1139.

76. Shankar SS, Brater DC: Loop diuretic: From the Na-K-2Cl transporter to clinical use. Am J Physiol Renal Physiol 2003;284:F11-F21.

77. Knauf H, Mutschler E: Low-dose segmental blockade of the nephron rather than high-dose diuretic monotherapy. Eur J Clin Pharmacol 1993;44(Suppl 1):S63-S68.

78. Wilcox CS, Welch WJ, Schreiner GF, et al: Diuretic actions of a highly selective A1 receptor antagonist. J Am Soc Nephrol 1999;10:714-720.

79. Yamamoto T, Sasaki S: Aquaporins in the kidney: Emerging new aspects. Kidney Int 1998;54:1041-51.

80. Goldsmith SR: Current treatments and novel pharmacologic treatments for hyponatremia in congestive heart failure. Am J Cardiol 2005;95:14B-23B.

CHAPTER 33

Inotropic Agents in Heart Failure

Desmond Bohn

Myocardial dysfunction and reduced inotropy resulting in heart failure and low cardiac output are common findings in critically ill children. This condition may be due to pressure or volume overload in congenital heart disease, ischemic injury associated with cardiopulmonary bypass, or intrinsic disease of the heart muscle (cardiomyopathy or myocarditis). It is also an important, but less recognized, feature of septic shock (see Chapters 29).

The most common clinical manifestations of myocardial dysfunction are hypotension and poor peripheral perfusion, which usually lead the physician to start an inotropic agent to stimulate cardiac contractility and increase blood pressure. This simple and conventional clinical practice has many potential flaws, however. Blood pressure alone is a poor surrogate marker for cardiac function and should not be used as an index of myocardial contractility. Most inotropic agents used as intravenous infusions are catecholamines; in certain circumstances, these drugs may adversely affect myocardial function by increasing myocardial oxygen consumption, determined by myocardial tension, contractility, and heart rate. There is even a trend to use adrenergic blockade in the treatment of chronic heart failure in adults and children. In addition, reduced response to catecholamines in the failing myocardium can be observed as a result of **receptor down-regulation** and a process called **desensitization**, a decreased affinity of these receptors for circulating catecholamines. To make rational choices in the use of inotropic agents, one has to appreciate the potential benefits and the adverse effects; it is equally essential to correct potentially reversible factors that have negative influences over contractility, such as hypoxemia, acidosis, and other metabolic causes.

Much of the information in this chapter on inotropic agents comes from studies in either intact animals or in vitro studies on isolated myocardium. There are only a few studies on the effects of inotropes in children; of these existing studies, a significant number are in infants, in whom there are important age-related differences in myocardial performance compared with adults. This chapter focuses on catecholamines and digoxin; other inotropic agents (e.g., phosphodiesterase inhibitors and calcium-sensitizing agents) are discussed in Chapters 34 and 38.

MECHANISM OF ACTION OF INOTROPIC AGENTS

Adrenergic Receptors

The adrenergic receptors and alterations in heart failure are described in detail in Chapter 2 and they are reviewed briefly here. The adrenergic system has a predominant role in modulating the inotropic state of the myocardium. In the normal state, norepinephrine is released from sympathetic nerve endings in the heart. Epinephrine release from the adrenal medulla and overflow norepinephrine from noncardiac sympathetic nerve endings have little effect on the normal heart. Normal cardiac function at rest seems to be independent of adrenergic support. The situation changes in heart failure as circulating levels of epinephrine and norepinephrine are increased.[1]

The effects of the adrenergic system are mediated via **α-receptors (α-ARs)** and **β-receptors (β-ARs)**. β-ARs are found in myocardium and the smooth muscle of the vascular bed and the airways. To date, three types of β-ARs (β_1, β_2, and β_3) have been cloned and identified pharmacologically. These receptors can be stimulated by sympathetic neuronal activity, circulating catecholamines, or exogenously administered adrenergic agonists (Fig. 33-1).

The predominant β-AR in the mammalian heart is the **β_1-AR** (>75%). Activation of β_1-ARs results in increases in heart rate and contractility. Significant numbers of **β_2-ARs** also have been identified in the left ventricle in normal human hearts,[2] but the greatest concentration is found in vascular smooth muscle, where stimulation results in vasodilation. The effects are not confined to the periphery, however. In the transgenic mouse model, overexpression of β_2-ARs results in marked increases in contractility.[3] The hierarchy of relative densities of the β-ARs can change in heart failure, where β_1-ARs are down-regulated as a result of heightened sympathetic drive, whereas β_2-ARs have been shown to represent an increasing component of total β-AR activity.[4,5] In addition, the β_2-ARs are expressed in lymphocytes, which has been an area for investigators to measure adenylate cyclase as a manifestation β-AR desensitization.[6-12] The **β_3-ARs** also have been identified in the myocardium, but stimulation of these receptors is believed to promote a negative inotropic effect.[13] There is also a putative

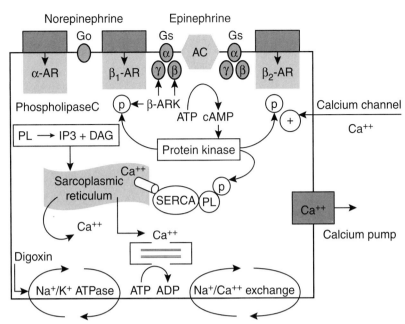

FIGURE 33-1 ■ The mechanism of action of catecholamines on the α and β receptors. Digoxin works by inhibiting the membrane-bound Na+,K+-ATPase and increasing intracellular calcium. Norepinephrine and epinephrine interact with adrenergic receptors and increase cyclic AMP, resulting in an increase in intracellular calcium and improved inotropy. An α-agonist can improve heart function because it can bind to α-adrenergic receptors on the cell membrane and stimulate phospholipase C via a coupling G protein. Phospholipase C promotes the release of intracellular messengers inositol triphosphate (IP3) and diacylglycerol (DAG). IP3 enhances the release of calcium from the sarcoplasmic reticulum, whereas DAG activates protein kinase C, leading to increased Ca^{2+} into the cell and an increased sensitivity of the contractile proteins to calcium (see text for more details). AC, adenylate cyclase; β-ARK, β-adrenergic receptor kinase; p, phosphorylation; PL, phospholamban; SERCA, sarcoplasmic reticulum Ca^{2+}-ATPase.

$β_4$-AR receptor, with stimulation resulting in a positive inotropic effect.[14]

There are two main types of α-**ARs** ($α_1$-AR and $α_2$-AR) with at least three subtypes ($α_{1A}$-AR, $α_{1B}$-AR, and $α_{1C}$-AR).[15] The $α_1$-**ARs** exist in the myocardium, where they produce increased contractility.[16-19] This contractility has been shown in ex vivo myocardial tissue from children with congenital heart defects.[20] In animal experimental models, the chronotropic and inotropic effects associated with $α_1$-AR stimulation seem to diminish in adult life.[21,22] $α_1$-ARs also are present in the coronary microcirculation, where they regulate coronary artery blood flow.[23] Stimulation of $α_2$-AR activity does not seem to produce any significant cardiovascular effect. α-ARs predominate in the periphery, where they modulate peripheral vascular tone via their action on vascular smooth muscle. The predominant peripheral $α_1$ effect is vasoconstriction via the presynaptic α-ARs, whereas activation of presynaptic $α_2$-ARs produces neurotransmitter release through a negative feedback mechanism.

Inotropic Agents and Interaction with Adrenergic Receptors

Most intravenous inotropic drugs in clinical use are sympathomimetic agents with action mediated via binding with adrenergic receptors in the myocardium and vascular smooth muscle. Although this action is the result of a series of complex biochemical reactions, it is important to review the mechanisms of action here (see Chapter 2).

The release of β-**agonists** stimulates membrane-bound G-protein receptor (Gs), which has three subunits, α, β, and γ, bound to GDP in its inactive state (see Fig. 33-1). The occupied receptor binds to the adjacent α subunit of the G protein, which is released and replaced by GTP. The GTP-α complex then binds to adenylate cyclase with the conversion of ATP to cyclic AMP (cAMP). The GTP is hydrolyzed to GDP and phosphate. The α-ADP complex then reattaches to its β-γ subunit on the G_s protein. The increase in cAMP concentration activates protein kinase, which causes the activation of many cellular proteins, including L-type Ca^{2+} channels, sarcoplasmic reticulum protein phospholamban, troponin I, and the ryanodine receptor. There is release of trigger Ca^{2+} into the cell with increased Ca^{2+} channel opening. cAMP enhances uptake and release of Ca^{2+} by the endoplasmic reticulum, enhancing cardiac contraction and relaxation. In addition, β-ARs can regulate other effects on voltage-sensitive calcium and sodium channels. Agonist-occupied β-ARs are phosphorylated by protein kinase, and β-AR kinases then become desensitized.[24-27] In heart failure, down-regulation and desensitization of these receptors occur because excessive catecholamines are present, from either persistent endogenous production or continued exogenous administration. In addition, many of the integral mechanisms of intracellular calcium and norepinephrine release and reuptake are rendered less effective in heart failure, limiting the efficacy of inotropic agents.

The mammalian heart also has $α_1$-ARs. An α-**agonist** can improve heart function because it can bind to α-ARs on the cell membrane and stimulate phospholipase C via a coupling G protein. Phospholipase C promotes the release of intracellular messengers inositol triphosphate and diacylglycerol. Inositol triphosphate enhances the release of calcium from the sarcoplasmic reticulum, whereas diacylglycerol activates protein kinase C, leading to increased Ca^{2+} into the cell and an increased sensitivity of the contractile proteins to calcium. Vascular tone is governed by flux of calcium and potassium in and out of the cell, local concentration of nitric oxide, activity of α-ARs and locally acting vasodilators. These α_1-AR effects result from increased cytosolic calcium independent of any changes in adenylate cyclase or cAMP activity.[28,29] α_2-AR activation is associated with inhibition of adenylate cyclase activity via G_i proteins with decreased intracellular cAMP levels. α_2-ARs do not have any recognized effect on vascular smooth muscle or the myocardium.[30]

There are two principal **dopaminergic receptors (DA$_1$ and DA$_2$)**, which produce different pharmacologic effects. The DA$_1$ receptors are located postsynaptically, and activation results in vasodilation in the mesentery and kidney. The increased renal blood flow results in a diuresis and natriuresis. The DA$_2$ receptors are located presynaptically on sympathetic nerve terminals, and activation inhibits angiotensin II–mediated aldosterone secretion of α-ARs.[30] Stimulation of these receptors also inhibits release of norepinephrine and prolactin and produces nausea and vomiting via the emetic center in the brain.

β-ADRENERGIC RECEPTOR AGONISTS

The most commonly used inotropes in critically ill patients are either naturally occurring (dopamine or epinephrine) or synthetic (dobutamine or isoproterenol) catecholamines, defined by a common 3,4-hydroxyl β-phenylethylamine structure. The catecholamines all bind to the β-ARs on cell surfaces and activate the G_s protein and increase cAMP, allowing Ca^{2+} influx into the cell (Fig. 33-2). Depending on the ratio of β_1 to β_2 properties, these agents have varying effects on myocardial contractility (inotropy), heart rate (chronotropy), and peripheral vascular resistance. There also are important, but less easily definable, effects on myocardial diastolic relaxation (lusitropy). All β-adrenergic agonists (except isoproterenol) have some α-agonist properties, which vary with dosage and produce a mixture of inotropic and vasoconstrictor effects (Table 33-1).

Epinephrine
Epinephrine is an endogenous catecholamine released from the adrenal medulla with the pharmacodynamic and hemodynamic actions mediated through β_1-ARs, β_2-ARs, and α-ARs. Epinephrine increases blood pressure, heart rate, and cardiac output in a dose-dependent fashion. At lower doses, the effect on the β_2-AR augments

TABLE 33-1

Catecholamines and Sites of Action				
Drug	**Site of Action**	**Dose Range (μg/kg/min)**	**Hemodynamic Effects**	**Adverse Effects**
Isoproterenol	β_1- and β_2-receptors No α_1 effects	0.05-0.5 (β only)	↑ inotropy, ↑ HR, ↓ MAP via β_1- and β_2-receptors Reduced PVR and SVR	Tachycardia and arrhythmias
Dopamine	β_1- and β_2-receptors α_1-receptors in periphery DA$_1$ and DA$_2$ receptors in the kidney	0.5-5 (dopaminergic); 5-10 (β and dopaminergic); >10 (α and β); >20 (α)	↑ inotropy, ↑ MAP, ↑ PVR. At <10 μg/kg, inotropic effects predominate Renal effects at <3 μg/kg	Tachycardia post-CPB Increasing α effects >10 μg/kg/min leads to increases in SVR and PVR. Tissue necrosis
Dobutamine	β_1- and β_2-receptors ($\beta_1 > \beta_2$) Minimal α_1 effects	5-10 (α and β)	↑ inotropy, ↑ HR via β_1- and β_2-receptors ↓ PVR and SVR Dilates coronary arteries	Tachycardia post-CPB. Vasodilator effects may result in reduced MAP
Epinephrine	β_1-, β_2-, and α_1-receptors	0.01-0.02 (β); 0.02-0.5 (α and β)	↑ inotropy, ↑ HR and MAP via β_1-receptors. Vasodilator at low doses via β_2-receptors	Tachycardia Vasoconstiction at higher doses via α-receptors Hyperglycemia Myocardial necrosis
Norepinephrine	α_1- and β_1-receptors Minimal β_2 effects	0.01-0.5 (α and β)	↑ MAP via α_1-receptors	Vasoconstriction and increased afterload

CPB, cardiopulmonary bypass; HR, heart rate; MAP, mean arterial pressure; PVR, pulmonary vascular resistance; SVR, systemic vascular resistance.

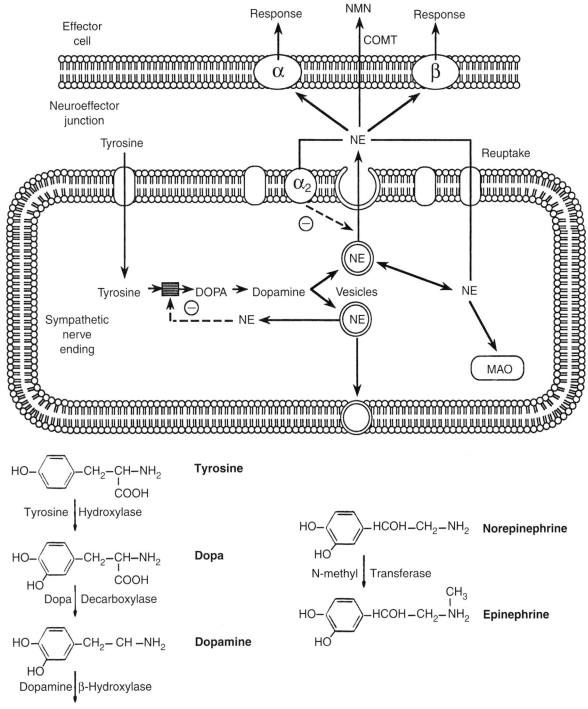

FIGURE 33-2 ■ Norepinephrine (NE) and catecholamines. NE is seen at the neuroeffector junction, where the effector cell can be either the myocyte or the vascular smooth muscle. Dopamine in the vesicles is converted to NE, which can be stored in vesicles or undergo exocytosis (and released into the neuroeffector junction). NE stimulates α- and β-receptors or is metabolized to normetanephrine (NMN) by catechol O-methyltransferase (COMT). NE can undergo reuptake and be either stored or broken down by monoamine oxidase (MAO) within the mitochondria. (From Helfaer MA, Wilson MD, Nichols DG: *Pharmacology of cardiovascular drugs.* In Nichols DG, Cameron DE, Greeley WJ, et al [eds]: *Critical Heart Disease in Infants and Children.* St Louis, Mosby, p. 187, 1995.)

skeletal muscle blood flow and lowers diastolic blood pressure.[31] It is a potent bronchodilator and causes renal and splanchnic vasoconstriction.[32,33] These potentially adverse effects may be less significant in the clinical setting, however, where the augmentation of cardiac output produces improved gut and renal perfusion.[34] Epinephrine increases plasma glucose levels, free fatty acid concentrations, and plasma renin activity[31] and decreases potassium and aldosterone levels.[35] Skin necrosis can occur with extravasation of the infusion, but can be treated with phentolamine, an α-adrenergic blocking agent.

The half-life of infused epinephrine is short (<3 minutes), and it is well absorbed when delivered into the lung via an endotracheal tube. Its principal use is during **cardiac resuscitation** because it increases left ventricular perfusion pressure and helps to augment myocardial perfusion. It is used increasingly in the management of **low cardiac output syndrome** after cardiopulmonary bypass (CPB) in adults. Epinephrine in doses of 0.01 μg/kg/min, 0.02 μg/kg/min, and 0.04 mg/kg/min increased cardiac index by 0.1 L/min/m², 0.7 L/min/m², and 1.2 L/min/m² and stroke volume by 2%, 12%, and 22% in one study of adult patients after CPB.[36] Compared with dobutamine, epinephrine produced less of an effect on heart rate for a given increase in stroke volume in adults after coronary artery bypass graft surgery;[37] there are no similar comparative studies in children.

Studies on the effect of epinephrine on contractility in newborn animals have shown that high doses (1.5 to 2 μg/kg/min) administered over 2 hours result in decreased contractility and ventricular compliance.[38,39] Epinephrine at a dose of 0.1 μg/kg/min has been shown to increase cardiac output in a newborn lamb model of single-ventricle physiology, whereas a large bolus dose (one half of that recommended for resuscitation) resulted in a marked increase in systemic vascular resistance (SVR) and a profound increase in pulmonary-to-systemic flow ratio.[40] Despite the lack of human data, there is an increasing trend to use low-dose epinephrine (<0.05 μg/kg/min) as a second-line inotropic agent (after dopamine) following CPB in children. At these dosages, the undesirable α-agonist effects are avoided while achieving the maximal β-adrenergic effects.

Isoproterenol

Isoproterenol is a synthetic catecholamine with exclusive β-adrenergic effects via $β_1$-ARs and $β_2$-ARs. Acting via the $β_2$ sites, isoproterenol dilates skeletal, renal, pulmonary, and mesenteric vascular beds and reduces diastolic blood pressure.[41] The net effect is a reduction in mean arterial pressure and renal blood flow.[42] The effect of the drug on the $β_1$-AR in the myocardium produces an increase in cardiac contractility together with a marked chronotropic effect, which is much more pronounced for an equivalent augmentation of cardiac output compared with dopamine and dobutamine[42]; this tachycardia also can lead to myocardial ischemia if prolonged or excessive. There may be important age-related differences to the response to isoproterenol.[43,44]

Studies in young animals have shown minor changes in cardiac output compared with mature animals in doses of up to 1.25 μg/kg/min but with a much more pronounced rate effect.[45] The increase in heart rate may be useful in the management of **atrioventricular block**, when a pacing option is not available. The combination

of tachycardia and reduced diastolic blood pressure produces an increased myocardial oxygen consumption and decreased coronary perfusion, both of which are highly undesirable in the postoperative period.[46,47] Another potential indication for the use of isoproterenol is for its chronotropic effect after **cardiac transplantation** because the newly transplanted heart often has a slow sinus mechanism. Isoproterenol, because of its low affinity for neuronal reuptake, is equally effective in innervated and denervated hearts. There is a tendency to develop tachyphylaxis with prolonged usage, and the chronotropic and inotropic effects are antagonized at low pH (<7.2).

The pulmonary vasodilator effects of isoproterenol have made it a useful option for the management of children with **pulmonary hypertension** or **right ventricular failure** or both and in situations of increased pulmonary vascular resistance after repair of congenital heart disease.[48] With the introduction of more selective pulmonary vasodilator therapy (e.g., inhaled nitric oxide), however, this indication has been rendered less useful.

Dopamine

Dopamine is an endogenous precursor of norepinephrine and is a central and peripheral nervous system transmitter. It acts on dopaminergic receptors (DA_1 and DA_2), β-ARs, and α-ARs and has a tyramine-like effect that causes release of norepinephrine, which is responsible for part of its inotropic effect. Its effects on adrenergic receptors are dose dependent: At doses of 3 to 5 μg/kg/min, the predominant effect is on β-ARs in the myocardium producing an inotropic and chronotropic response via the $β_1$-ARs; at doses of 5 to 10 μg/kg/min, α-agonist effects become increasingly significant. At doses greater than 10 μg/kg/min, the vasoconstrictor effects of α-AR stimulation predominate over the β-mediated vasodilator effects. Although dopamine also can increase flow to cerebral, coronary, renal, and splanchnic beds via postsynaptic DA_1 receptors, at higher doses this influence is minimal. Doses of less than 3 μg/kg/min have minimal effect on β-ARs; a study in adults using this dose showed no change in heart rate.[49]

There has been almost 20 years of experience in the use of dopamine in critical care medicine for the management of low cardiac output after CPB, after myocardial infarction, in association with cardiomyopathy, and in septic shock. There are many published studies on the use of dopamine for the failing myocardium, which span the age spectrum from preterm infants to adults. These studies generally have small patient numbers and varying hemodynamic end points, however.

In adults, the use of low-dose dopamine (<5 μg/kg/min) after CPB has been associated with increased myocardial contractility and a reduction in SVR, but with an increased measured myocardial oxygen consumption without an increase in coronary blood flow (may potentiate myocardial ischemia).[50] A similar potentially adverse effect has been noted with the use of dopamine after myocardial infarction with increased myocardial lactate production.[51] Dopamine at similar dosages increased cardiac output and stroke volume in patients with cardiomyopathy, but at higher doses, there were increases in heart rate, pulmonary capillary wedge pressure, and incidence of ectopy.[52] Because of these findings, the practice in adults after CPB is generally to limit dopamine dosages to less than 5 μg/kg/min.[36]

Numerous pediatric studies have been published since the 1970s. Many of the original studies that defined the pharmacodynamic properties of the drug in the pediatric age group were done by Driscoll and colleagues[42,45,53] using either the ex vivo model or intact animals. These investigators compared the effect of myocardium exposed to dopamine taken from young (<33 days old) versus adult animals and found that there were age-related differences in contractility with minimal effects shown in ventricular muscle taken from animals less than 7 days old. This effect could be significantly blocked by propranolol in all age ranges.[54] In a further series of studies in intact young animals comparing dopamine with dobutamine and isoproterenol, dopamine (2 to 50 μg/kg/min) increased cardiac output, blood pressure, and heart rate. The SVR was increased at high doses, and dopamine was the only drug that increased renal artery blood flow.[42]

Driscoll and colleagues[53,55] also published two studies on the use of dopamine in children. The first study was a retrospective review of 24 patients, including 20 with congenital heart disease and 4 with sepsis, with dopamine doses ranging from 0.3 to 25 μg/kg/min. In the 13 responders, there were increases in mean arterial pressure and urine output without a change in heart rate.[53] In the second series, children with congenital heart disease who were undergoing cardiac catheterization were infused with dopamine at doses of 2 and 7.5 μg/kg/min. There were increases in cardiac output and stroke volume and a reduction in SVR at both doses with no change in heart rate.[55]

Several studies have been published of the use of dopamine for prevention or amelioration of **low cardiac output syndrome** after repair of congenital heart disease using doses of 5 to 10 μg/kg/min. Stephenson and coworkers[56] used a dose of 8 μg/kg/min in 28 children after repair of a variety of different heart defects and found that cardiac output and stroke volume were increased with no change in SVR, and that these effects were augmented when nitroprusside was added. Williams and associates[57] found similar effects in patients after the Fontan operation using the same dose. The addition of nitroprusside in this instance resulted in the same increase in cardiac output at a lower right atrial pressure. In addition, Sakata and colleagues[58] compared dopamine and dobutamine, both at doses of 5 μg/kg/min and 10 μg/kg/min, after repair of congenital heart disease. Cardiac output, stroke volume, and blood pressure increased, and left atrial pressure and SVR decreased at both doses; there also was an increase in myocardial oxygen uptake. Finally, Girardin and coworkers[59] evaluated the effect of dopamine at 2.5 μg/kg/min and 5 μg/kg/min on hemodynamics and renal function in 14 children after repair of congenital heart disease and found that only the higher dose was associated with a significant change in hemodynamics (manifested by an increase in cardiac output and a reduction of left atrial pressure, but no change in heart rate or blood pressure). Changes in renal function also were seen only at the higher dose. Dopamine, acting via its effect on the splanchnic circulation, also has been shown to have significant effects on hepatic blood flow after CPB in children. Mitchell and colleagues[60] showed that a dose of 4 μg/kg/min of dopamine is associated with a 31% increase in the disappearance of indocyanine green.

There also are a few published studies on the use of dopamine in critically ill term and preterm infants with sepsis, transient myocardial ischemia, asphyxia, or lung disease of prematurity, but these studies contain less hemodynamic information. These studies, using Doppler technology for assessing cardiac output, showed that there is a significant incremental increase in cardiac output, blood pressure, and renal blood flow without a significant effect on heart rate at doses of 2 to 10 μg/kg/min.[61-66] In terms of pharmacokinetics, there may be important influences of age and disease on dopamine clearance. Notterman and associates[67] showed that dopamine clearance is increased in critically ill children younger than 2 years of age, and that it is reduced in hepatorenal failure.

Dopamine has a unique property among the inotropic agents in its selective action on the kidney via its effect on dopaminergic receptors. The DA_2 receptors are activated in the dose range of 0.2 to 0.4 μg/kg/min, whereas at slightly higher doses (0.5 to 3 μg/kg/min) recruit DA_1 receptors are recruited.[68] At these doses, dopamine increases renal perfusion and produces a diuresis and natriuresis with minimal effect on cardiac output or heart rate.[49] For these reasons, dopamine commonly is used to improve **renal function** after CPB or to increase renal perfusion in critically ill patients in situations where α-AR agonist therapy is being used to treat vasodilatory shock. The infusion of dopamine has been shown to increase renal plasma flow during the administration of norepinephrine in adults.[69,70] Comparing dopamine with dobutamine in critically ill adult patients, a study showed that dopamine induced a diuresis without changing creatinine clearance, whereas dobutamine improved creatinine clearance without producing a diuresis.[71]

The use of renal dose dopamine for renal perfusion also is common in pediatric practice. Girardin and colleagues[59] measured the effect of dopamine at 2.5 μg/kg/min and 5 μg/kg/min on renal function in children

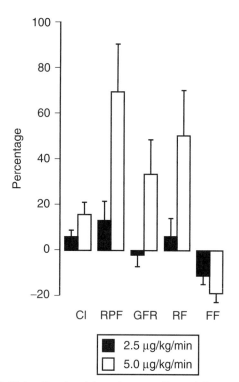

FIGURE 33-3 ■ **Renal and hemodynamic effects of dopamine.** Two doses of dopamine (2.5 μg/kg/min and 5 μg/kg/min) were studied, and increases in cardiac index (CI), renal plasma flow (RPF), glomerular filtration rate (GFR), renal fraction of cardiac output (RF), and filtration fraction (FF) were observed. (From Girardin E, Besner M, Rouge JC, et al: *Effect of low dose dopamine on hemodynamic and renal function in children. Pediatr Res* 1989;26:200-203.)

after CPB, renal plasma flow, glomerular filtration rate, and fractional sodium excretion, however, and found that these parameters were increased only at the higher dose (Fig. 33-3). These data suggest the dose for renal dose dopamine may be different in adults and children. Another study that compared dopamine at 2.5 μg/kg/min with dobutamine at the same dose after CPB in children found no difference in urine output, serum creatinine, fractional sodium excretion, or the need for diuretic therapy.[72] There also are several published studies on effects of dopamine on various indices of kidney function in premature newborns, which showed increased renal blood flow together with a diuresis and natriuresis.[61,73-75] Dopamine also has a similar beneficial effect in preventing some of the adverse renal effects associated with the use of indomethacin in the treatment of patent ductus arteriosus in premature neonates. These studies show similar findings without evidence that it has a beneficial effect on creatinine clearance.[75,76] A systematic review of all published renal dose dopamine studies in critically ill neonates and children when either creatinine clearance or glomerular filtration and urine output were used to measure improvement in renal function failed to find any supportive evidence for its use as a unique drug for increased renal perfusion.[77]

A large prospective, randomized, placebo-controlled trial in adults has confirmed this contention.[78]

Dobutamine

Dobutamine is a synthetic sympathomimetic agent that is an analogue of isoproterenol. The stimulation of α-ARs and β-ARs in the myocardium increases contractility, and the activation of β₂-ARs in the periphery produces vasodilation. The net effect is a reduction in SVR with only a modest increase in heart rate. At the time of its introduction into clinical practice in the 1970s, these hemodynamic effects made dobutamine a more attractive option than either dopamine or isoproterenol.

The initial experience in adults with cardiac failure showed that dobutamine in a dose of 2.5 to 15 μg/kg/min was associated with an increase in cardiac output and stroke volume and with a reduction in SVR and mean arterial pressure.[79] There is also a reduction in pulmonary artery pressure and pulmonary capillary wedge pressure. At doses greater than 10 to 15 μg/kg/min, excessive tachycardia and hypotension occurred.[30]

There have been numerous studies on the use of dobutamine in young animals. A study with intact newborn animals showed that cardiac output and heart rate increased with dobutamine, but that the heart rate effect was less than that of isoproterenol.[42] Compared with dopamine, there was no enhancement of renal blood flow. Another study showed that there were significant differences in hemodynamic responses to dobutamine between the newborn and older animals.[45] In an animal model of hypoplastic left heart syndrome, dobutamine at doses of 5 μg/kg/min and 15 μg/kg/min more than doubled the pulmonary-to-systemic flow ratio and resulted in a decrease in oxygen delivery, whereas epinephrine at 0.1 μg/kg/min decreased the pulmonary-to-systemic flow ratio and increased oxygen delivery.[80]

There is extensive experience with dobutamine in the management of **low cardiac output syndrome** after CPB in adults.[37,81,82] Doses of 5 to 6 μg/kg/min increase cardiac output and splanchnic blood flow. In the post-CPB situation, dobutamine at a dose of 5 μg/kg/min was reported to be associated with a greater degree of tachycardia, however, compared with epinephrine at a dose of 0.3 μg/kg/min with equivalent increases in cardiac output and stroke volume.[37] The net effect on contractility and heart rate increases myocardial oxygen consumption, whereas dobutamine itself has been shown to increase coronary blood flow.[50,83] These properties have favored the use of dobutamine as a challenge test in unmasking ischemic heart disease and in the assessment of the hemodynamic significance of gradients across the left ventricular outflow tract in aortic stenosis. In contrast to dopamine, dobutamine has no direct effect on renal blood flow, and changes in urine output occur indirectly via improved cardiac output.

The largest clinical experience with the use of dobutamine in cardiac disease has been in the treatment of low cardiac output syndrome in adults with severe **cardiomyopathy**. These studies tend to show short-term improvement in hemodynamics without increased long-term survival.[84,85] One large study comparing dobutamine with nitroprusside showed that the use of dobutamine was associated with increased mortality.[86] Dobutamine also has been shown to be associated with an increase in arrhythmogenicity and sudden death.[87] Dobutamine does seem to improve cardiac output and right ventricular ejection in adults with predominant right ventricular infarction.[88]

Comparative studies with dopamine suggest advantages for dobutamine in that dopamine produced limitation of coronary blood flow and an increase in pulmonary capillary wedge pressure (PCWP) and premature ventricular contractions.[50,52] Apart from patients with primary cardiac disease, dobutamine was widely used in critically ill adults in the 1990s based on studies that suggested maximizing tissue oxygen delivery could reduce the incidence of end-organ failure and improve survival.[89] Although high-dose dobutamine was effective in increasing oxygen delivery, it actually resulted in decreased survival.[90]

In pediatric studies, dobutamine has been shown to increase stroke volume and cardiac contractility in doses of 5 to 20 μg/kg/min in normal children.[91,92] Driscoll and colleagues[93] also studied the effect of the drug in children with congenital heart disease undergoing cardiac catheterization. Dobutamine at 2 μg/kg/min and 7.5 μg/kg/min resulted in increases in blood pressure, cardiac index, and stroke volume and a reduction in PCWP; there was no change in either pulmonary vascular resistance or SVR.

There are several published studies of the use of dobutamine for **low cardiac output syndrome** after cardiac surgery in children. We studied the effect of dobutamine at 1 μg/kg/min, 4 μg/kg/min, 7 μg/kg/min, and 10 μg/kg/min in 11 children (mean age 5 years, range 0.2 to 10.8 years).[94] Dose-dependent increases in cardiac output and blood pressure were observed with no change in stroke volume; there also was a significant increase in heart rate, which necessitated the discontinuation of the infusion in four patients. Important insights into lesion-specific effects of the drug have come from studies of Berner and colleagues,[95-97] who published a series of studies on the use of dobutamine for the management of low cardiac output syndrome after cardiac surgery. In the first study, they examined the effect of the addition of dobutamine to phentolamine in two groups of children after CPB: The first group had surgery for mitral valve disease, and the second group had repair of tetralogy of Fallot. Both groups received a continuous infusion of phentolamine (10 μg/kg/min). The addition of dobutamine at 5 μg/kg/min resulted in an increase in cardiac output in both groups, but the effect was more pronounced in the first group. There also was an increase in heart rate in both groups, but it was more significant in the second group. Stroke volume and blood pressure increased significantly only in the first group.[95] The inference they drew from this study was that left ventricular end-diastolic volume, which they measured preoperatively, was smaller than normal in patients with tetralogy, and changes in cardiac output with inotropes would be predominantly rate dependent.

In a second series, the same investigators compared dobutamine (2.5 μg/kg/min, 5 μg/kg/min, and 10 μg/kg/min) with isoproterenol (0.05 μg/kg/min, 0.1 μg/kg/min, and 0.2 μg/kg/min) administered in sequence in 12 children after repair of tetralogy of Fallot.[97] They found that there was no significant increase in either cardiac output or heart rate with dobutamine. There was no change in stroke volume with either drug. In a final, smaller series of eight children, Berner and colleagues[96] further investigated the effect of accelerating heart rate in patients with tetralogy of Fallot. They compared the effect of a 40% increase in heart rate produced by atrial pacing, dobutamine at 10 μg/kg/min (with and without atrial pacing), or isoproterenol at 0.1 μg/kg/min. They found that with dobutamine, there were small but significant increases in cardiac output, stroke volume, and shortening fraction. With isoproterenol, the changes in these parameters were more marked, in addition to reductions in SVR and left atrial pressure. There were no hemodynamic improvements with atrial pacing alone. Based on these studies, there seems to be little or no benefit to be derived from the use of dobutamine in patients with tetralogy of Fallot.

Several studies of the use of dobutamine in the management of pediatric patients with either **cardiomyopathy** or **septic shock** have been published.[98-102] In the largest of these studies, Perkin and associates[98] evaluated the effect of dobutamine at 2.5 μg/kg/min, 5 μg/kg/min, 7.5 μg/kg/min, and 10 μg/kg/min in 33 patients. They separately evaluated responses according to age (<12 months old versus >12 months old) and by underlying diagnosis (cardiogenic versus septic shock). Significant increases in cardiac output were seen with dobutamine at doses of 7.5 μg/kg/min and 10 μg/kg/min only in the older age group with significant increases in PCWP. There were no significant increases in heart rate or systemic or pulmonary artery pressures. The investigators also collected data on the incidence of adverse effects, defined as a greater than 25% increase in any vascular pressure or heart rate, and the incidence was 25%. The mortality rate also was high at 67% in septic and cardiogenic shock groups. Habib and coworkers[103] found increases in cardiac output and blood pressure with dobutamine at 7.5 μg/kg/min and 10 μg/kg/min in critically ill patients without congenital heart disease, whereas Martinez and associates[102] found modest increases in Doppler-derived cardiac output measurements, but no change in heart rate or blood pressure in a group of critically ill newborns at the same doses.

Norepinephrine

Norepinephrine is a catecholamine that serves as a local neurotransmitter in the adrenergic nervous system. It has predominant α-adrenergic actions, which cause vasoconstriction; this α-adrenergic effect overshadows its myocardial β1 effects. Norepinephrine also produces an inotropic effect through its action on the α1-AR in myocardium, but it has no effect on sinoatrial automaticity or on the rate of myocardial relaxation. There also are some significant β-adrenergic effects on the heart. Norepinephrine has been shown to dilate isolated human coronary arteries, an effect that is fully blocked by propanolol.[104] When administered to healthy patients, norepinephrine increases systolic and diastolic blood pressure, decreases renal blood flow, and increases afterload on the heart, although the adverse effect on renal blood flow can be reversed by the addition of low-dose dopamine.[69,70]

For these reasons, norepinephrine previously was believed to be a poor option in the treatment of either septic or cardiogenic shock. Its main use in clinical medicine is in the treatment of vasodilatory **septic shock**.[105-108] Studies have shown that doses of 0.4 to 2 μg/kg/min improve systemic pressure, oxygen delivery, and renal blood flow without any adverse effects on cardiac output.[109] A retrospective review of the outcome in septic shock has reported improved survival with the use of norepinephrine,[110] but there are no published studies in children. Norepinephrine and other vasopressors have been used to increase diastolic pressures associated with **vasodilatory shock** to preserve coronary and cerebral perfusion.

CARDIAC GLYCOSIDE: DIGOXIN

The use of cardiac glycosides in clinical medicine first was described by Withering in 1776, when he used the common foxglove plant (*Digitalis purpurea*) to treat patients with dropsy and irregular heartbeat. Since then, the popularity of using cardiac glycosides in the treatment of heart failure and atrial fibrillation has waxed and waned. This section discusses the pharmacokinetics, pharmacodynamics, and evidence for the efficacy of the most commonly used cardiac glycoside, digoxin, in the treatment of heart failure.

Digoxin is a semisynthetic compound made from the leaves of the plant *Digitalis lanata*. Each cardiac glycoside has three main components: a central steroid nucleus, an unsaturated lactone ring attached to carbon C_{17}, and one to four sugars attached at C_3. Digoxin increases the velocity and extent of the sarcomere shortening by decreasing the duration of contraction without changing muscle fiber tension. The pressure volume curve (Frank-Starling) of the ventricle is shifted upward and to the left. In addition to its inotropic properties, digoxin has important effects on heart rate through its action on the cardiac conduction and the autonomic nervous systems. Digoxin reduces sinoatrial node firing by increasing vagal tone and slows atrioventricular nodal conduction and increases its refractoriness,[111] but these effects can be abolished by atropine.[112]

Remote from the heart, digoxin also has important neurohormonal effects via its effects on sympathetic nervous system and baroreceptor function.[113] Abnormalities of carotid baroreceptor function and excess sympathetic nervous system activity are important components of heart failure. Digoxin has been shown to reduce circulating norepinephrine, renin, and aldosterone levels in this situation.[114-116] The net result of these various effects is increased inotropy without increased myocardial oxygen consumption.

The cellular mechanism of action of cardiac glycosides is via the sodium potassium pump in the cell membrane; this is a membrane protein responsible for pumping sodium into and potassium out of the cell. The exchange in ions is coupled to the hydrolysis of high-energy ATP with the formation of ADP (see Fig. 33-1). Cardiac glycosides inhibit this enzyme, which results in an accumulation of intracellular sodium, which limits the extrusion of intracellular Ca^{2+} via inhibition of the Na^+/Ca^{2+} exchanger. The increased Ca^{2+} is sequestered by the sarcoplasmic reticulum and is available during depolarization to increase myocardial contractility.[117-120]

Digoxin is extensively tissue bound and has an elimination half-life of 24 to 36 hours. The half-life is influenced by impairment of renal function as the drug is secreted and reabsorbed at glomerular level. There also is evidence that the steady-state volume of distribution of digoxin is reduced in renal failure.[121] For these reasons, the dosage should be reduced in patients with heart failure and reduced glomerular filtration rate and in patients with chronic renal failure.[120] Administration of amiodarone has been shown to increase steady-state digoxin levels, and the dosage should be reduced by 50% during concurrent administration.[122-124] Spirolactone, verapamil, propafenone, and flecainide used concomitantly all have been reported to increase digoxin levels and increase the potential risk of toxicity.[125-128] Toxicity also may be precipitated by the introduction of other drugs that adversely affect renal function (indomethacin, amphotericin, and aminoglycoside antibiotics).

Digoxin is well absorbed by the enteral route at similar rates in adults and children but is impaired in gastrointestinal disease and with increased gastrointestinal motility.[129-131] In neonates, peak serum levels are attained 30 to 90 minutes after oral administration. The window between maximal therapeutic effect and toxicity can be narrow with digoxin, and the incidence of toxicity has been reported to be high in premature infants.[132] Because the drug is predominantly tissue bound, serum levels are not a useful guide for therapeutic effect and should be measured only when toxicity is suspected. Endogenous digoxin-like substances can interfere with the therapeutic assay and give a spuriously high reading.[133,134] Myocardial concentrations of digoxin are significantly greater in infants compared with older children and adults and in the ventricles compared with the atria,[135,136] although the same differences were not found in animal models.[137]

Tissue binding is more extensive and the volume of distribution greater in infants; the elimination half-life and renal excretion also are enhanced, suggesting an alternative elimination pathway.[138] Maturity also has important effects on pharmacokinetics. Studies in infants have shown that in the preterm neonate, the half-life of digoxin is prolonged with a reduction in total body clearance and volume of distribution,[139,140] whereas the volume of distribution is increased in mature infants and older children. These data suggest that newborns are susceptible to overdose with digoxin and that the usual doses should be reduced in this age group.[141]

The clinical manifestations of toxicity include gastrointestinal (nausea and vomiting), neurologic (visual disturbances), and cardiac (arrhythmias) symptoms. Toxicity is potentiated by hypokalemia because it increases intracellular Na^+,K^+-ATPase sensitivity to digoxin. Hypomagnesemia also increases myocardial sensitivity to digoxin. Because both of these electrolyte abnormalities exist in patients with heart failure treated with diuretics, they are at increased risk of developing toxicity. The most hemodynamically significant toxic effects are due to rhythm disturbances, which include unifocal ventricular premature beats, first-degree atrioventricular block, or atrioventricular block accompanied by an accelerated junctional pacemaker. Minor degrees of atrioventricular block may respond to atropine administration, whereas ventricular rhythm disturbances and higher degrees of atrioventricular block may require the use of lidocaine or the insertion of a pacemaker. The effects of toxicity are mitigated by the correction of low serum potassium and magnesium levels. Apart from symptomatic treatment, the efficacy of digoxin-specific antibody fragments (Fab) has been established in adults and children.[142-146] Toxicity commonly is associated with serum levels greater than 2 ng/mL, but may occur at lower levels in the presence of hypokalemia or hypomagnesemia.

Most evidence of efficacy of digoxin in the treatment of heart failure comes from clinical trials in adults with ischemic or dilated cardiomyopathy. Uncontrolled trials have shown a reduction in PCWP and an improvement in cardiac output in patients with decompensated heart failure either as single therapy[147,148] or in combination with afterload reduction.[116,149-152] These were small studies with hemodynamic end points, and the

response was not uniform. The studies were underpowered to show clinically significant effects.

In two large randomized controlled trials of the use of digoxin in adults with stable mild-to-moderate heart failure (New York Heart Association class II or III) and systolic dysfunction (left ventricular ejection fraction <35%) either as single therapy or combined with captopril, patients showed symptomatic improvement.[153,154] In the largest published randomized trial to date of adult patients with mild-to-moderate heart failure (left ventricular ejection fraction <45%), there was no significant difference in mortality, but patients receiving digoxin had a significant decrease in the risk of hospitalization.[155] The commonly held belief that there is no relationship between serum levels and efficacy is now open to debate based on a post-hoc analysis from this study, which showed better outcomes in patients with serum levels of 0.5 to 0.8 ng/mL.[156]

There are only a few prospective studies of the use of digoxin in pediatric patients. Berman and associates[157] studied the effect of digoxin in 21 infants (mean age 2.7 months) with unrepaired ventricular septal defects. The effect was evaluated by M-mode and two-dimensional echocardiography and clinical response (e.g., change in heart size, weight gain). Six infants had an inotropic response as defined by improvement in function measured by echocardiographic findings, and an additional six infants had clinical improvement. The elimination half-life was 2 hours in this study with a volume of distribution of 9.8 L, values that are nearer to those found in adults rather than newborns. A study of the use of digoxin in low-birth-weight infants with patent ductus arteriosus showed no clear benefit and increased risk of toxicity.[132] There are no published randomized trials.

In the absence of any good published efficacy data for the use of digoxin in children, the only evidence comes from extrapolating from adult trials in dilated cardiomyopathy. Digoxin probably has a role in the treatment of children with **dilated cardiomyopathy** who have moderately reduced cardiac function after initial treatment with vasodilator therapy.[158] The use of digoxin in patients who present with acute cardiac decompensation secondary to dilated cardiomyopathy or myocarditis may accentuate any underlying degree of atrioventricular block with little beneficial effect on function. Its effect on the atrioventricular node makes it a useful drug in the treatment of patients with **atrial fibrillation** and a rapid ventricular response.[111]

LIMITATIONS OF EFFECTIVENESS AND ADVERSE EFFECTS OF INOTROPIC AGENTS

Although the commonly used inotropic agents are frequently effective in the treatment of low cardiac output state and decompensated heart failure, there are some important issues that may influence their effectiveness and in certain instances may worsen the situation. The desensitization mechanisms that reduce inotropic drug effectiveness include uncoupling of the receptor from the G protein, down-regulation of adrenergic receptors, and sequestration with internalization of the receptors.

Information obtained from studies in newborn animals suggests that there are **age-related differences** in the newborn myocardium compared with myocardium in older or adult animals in response to catecholamines; these differences involve density and function of adrenergic receptors, regulatory mechanisms of intracellular calcium, norepinephrine storage and reuptake, and ultrastructural and functional capacity. The myocardium in the normal neonate is less compliant and is preload limited and functions at near-maximum capacity because of high demands[159-164]; in addition, resting systolic indices are higher compared with adults.[165,166] Developmental age also has important effects on myocardial contractility: Studies in newborn animals have shown a decrease in resting contractility in the first few weeks of life, but with a progressive increase in maximal contractility in response to isoproterenol in vivo and in vitro over the same period.[54,167,168] These changes may be mediated partly by the fact that endogenous catecholamine levels are increased in normal newborns,[169,170] as are the levels of Y peptide (a marker of sympathetic nervous system activity).[171]

There also may be important **interspecies differences** that render the interpretation of the studies less than optimal. Studies in newborn compared with adult dogs have shown either no difference or enhanced response with increased adrenergic receptor density or in the response to inotropic drugs.[172,173] Caspi and associates[39] showed that the contractile state of the myocardium in pigs, as measured by left ventricular conductance catheters, was higher in newborn compared with adult animals. Baylen and colleagues[174] also showed that sympathetic activity and left ventricular contractility are increased in preterm lambs after acute increases in left ventricular afterload. Age-related changes in systolic and diastolic parameters also have been shown in humans and have been related to Ca^{2+}-dependent mechanisms.[175] There also are important maturation differences in ARs that may modify the response to exogenously administered catecholamines. In neonatal animal models, β_2-ARs seem to play a more important role in the inotropic response, whereas stimulation of the α_1-ARs changes from a positive chronotropic and inotropic effect from the neonate to the adult.[21,22,176-178] The adenylate cyclase activity of β-receptors in the myocardium also has been shown to decrease with increasing age in the human.[179]

The presence of **heart failure** and disease may have an important effect on the response to catecholamines in humans. In the normal heart, β_1 density is greater than β_2.[30] Bristow and coworkers,[180] in a study of explanted hearts of adults with end-stage cardiomyopathy,

showed that β_1-AR numbers were decreased and that isoproterenol-mediated adenylate cyclase contractile response was blunted compared with controls. Since then, other studies have shown that expression of β_1-ARs, but not β_2-ARs, are decreased in heart failure,[2,181,182] but that the β_2-ARs are uncoupled from activation of adenylate cyclase.[183-185] This phenomenon also is associated with increased levels of β-AR kinase.[186-189] In addition, neuronal reuptake of catecholamines is impaired in heart failure and can increase the efficacy of catecholamines with high reuptake affinity, such as epinephrine and dopamine. Finally, chronic elevation of norepinephrine, as is commonly seen in heart failure, results in a decrease in adenylate cyclase activation and uncoupling of the β-AR in association with decreased activity of the GTP coupling protein G_s.[190,191]

After **myocardial ischemia**, there also is an increase in circulating catecholamine levels together with increased β-AR density and elevated levels of cAMP.[24,186,192] Important changes occur with CPB when endogenous catecholamines also are elevated.[193-195] Despite this increased catecholamine stake, decreased β-AR coupling with adenylate cyclase in human lymphocytes has been noted in adults.[10,11,194] The significance of this finding is obscured by the fact that this measures only β_2-AR activity. Further studies using biopsy specimens have shown that despite increased catecholamine levels, isoproterenol-stimulated adenylate cyclase was decreased, implying an uncoupling between this and β-ARs.[195] In an animal study, this effect of CPB was blunted by the use of β-blockers.[196]

Numerous studies in children with **congenital heart disease** also suggest abnormal adrenergic receptor function.[5,7,8,178,197] Wu and coworkers[7,9] showed that there is a reduction in β-AR density and increased norepinephrine levels in children with heart failure. Dzimiri and associates[197] found increased norepinephrine levels, α-AR activity, and attenuated β-AR lymphocytic activity in children undergoing cardiac catheterization. A similar observation has been made in children with heart failure in whom higher norepinephrine levels and reduced β-AR density were found.[7] In children undergoing surgical repair, lymphocyte adenylate cyclase activity was increased during CPB and reduced in the postoperative period.[8] A more direct assessment using biopsy specimens of atrial tissue taken before and during aortic cross-clamping in children undergoing repair of congenital heart defects also showed uncoupling of β-ARs from the adenylate cyclase G_s protein complex.[198]

The most comprehensive study in patients with congenital heart disease was done by Kozlik-Feldmann and colleagues.[5] They found β-ARs were down-regulated, most commonly β_1-ARs, but there also was significant β_2-AR down-regulation in newborns with transposition of the great arteries and aortic valve stenosis. In patients with tetralogy of Fallot treated with propranolol, the reduction of β-AR activity was better preserved than in patients who were not treated. Studies that show down-regulation of β-ARs may provide a hypothesis for the decreased function after repair of congenital heart disease and the diminishing effect seen with increasing doses of catecholamines and phosphodiesterase inhibitors in this situation.

Attention has been focused more recently on the use of steroids to reverse the **down-regulation of ARs**. Studies have shown that ARs are transcriptionally regulated by glucocorticoids.[199] Davies and Lefkowitz[200] reported that corticosteroids increased β-ARs in circulating neutrophils in normal humans. Administration of methylprednisolone also up-regulates β-ARs in the myocardium in rats.[201] In a study of patients with severe sepsis, the administration of methylprednisolone to patients who had been treated with catecholamines for more than 72 hours was shown to result in an increase in cardiac index, whereas there was no effect on patients who had been on shorter term inotropic support.[202] This interval was the same period during which loss of effectiveness was observed in a study of adults with cardiomyopathy receiving continuous infusions of dobutamine.[203] In addition, samples of tissue taken from the left ventricle showed that receptor density was decreased in patients on long-term catecholamine treatment, whereas in patients treated with steroids, the AR density was increased.[202] Finally, in a retrospective review of critically ill children after repair of congenital heart disease who were being treated with high-dose (>0.1 μg/kg/min) epinephrine, the use of steroids was effective in enabling the dose of epinephrine to be reduced and the hemodynamic profile to be stabilized.[204]

The response to the potential limitations to the effectiveness of inotropic agents is usually to increase the dose to achieve the same hemodynamic effect; this concept is flawed because reduced or intermittent administration of catecholamines is the strategy necessary to reduce the down-regulation and desensitization process. Besides, increasing catecholamines is not risk-free because of the potential toxicity of catecholamines to the heart. The cardiotoxicities of isoproterenol and epinephrine include hypertrophy and necrosis of the myocardium.[205-208] The best illustration of these effects comes from a series of studies by Caspi and colleagues,[38,39,209,210] who evaluated the effect of exogenously administered epinephrine in animals. They used conductance catheters for the evaluation of changes in contractility and compliance of the left ventricle and examined the histology of the myocardium. In a first series of experiments, epinephrine at doses of 0.5 mg/kg/min and 2 μg/kg/min were infused for 2 hours into newborn and mature pigs.[39] The preinfusion cardiac output and contractile state were higher and left ventricular compliance was lower in newborns compared with adults. Low-dose epinephrine increased cardiac output in both groups, which was predominantly rate dependent in newborns with no change in contractility, returning to

baseline at the end of the infusion. High-dose epinephrine produced increases in heart rate, cardiac output, and contractility with a reduction in compliance in both groups. These effects returned to baseline in the mature animals but not in the newborns. With high-dose epinephrine, newborn animals had striking changes in the ultrastructure of the myocardium as assessed by electron microscopy: These changes included disruption of the sarcolemma with swelling of the mitochondria and deposition of calcium granules (Fig. 33-4). The investigators showed similar findings when a dose of 1.5 mg/kg/min was used.[38] In a further series of experiments, Caspi and colleagues[209,210] showed that these effects were not due to tachycardia alone because these findings could not be reproduced by rapid pacing, but the changes could be mitigated by magnesium. The significance of these findings, striking as they are, need to be interpreted in light of the fact that the doses of epinephrine used were significantly higher than would be used in clinical practice.

In addition to their potential to cause myocardial injury, all inotropic drugs can accelerate heart rate via their effect on adenylate cyclase and produce arrhythmias (particularly in the postoperative period). In a retrospective study, dopamine in a dose greater than 10 μg/kg/min was reported to be associated with dysrhythmias after repair of congenital heart disease.[211] The incidence of the most hemodynamically significant rhythm disturbance, junctional ectopic tachycardia, has been shown to be increased with the use of dopamine.[212]

CURRENT STATUS AND FUTURE TRENDS

The inotropic agents should not be the first-line treatment in the management of heart failure, especially in light of their well-documented adverse effects. First, reversible etiologies (e.g., hypoxia or acidosis) should be corrected to improve cardiac performance. In addition, preload should be optimized, especially in right-sided obstructive heart defects (pulmonary stenosis, tetralogy of Fallot) that exhibit restrictive right ventricular physiology. The physician also should be aware of the details of the cardiac anatomy, particularly the potential for left ventricular outflow tract obstruction, where inotropic therapy may increase the gradient. It would be unwise to use inotropic agents in children with aortic valvular or supravalvular stenosis or hypertrophic cardiomyopathy. Mixed venous oxygen saturations and arterial lactate measurements are useful guides to therapy.[213,214]

The future ideal inotropic agent is a drug that increases contractility without increasing heart rate and results in no increase in SVR or PVR. All current catecholamines have some of these unwanted effects. Low-dose epinephrine (<0.05 μg/kg/ min) has become a frequently used option in the post-CPB low cardiac

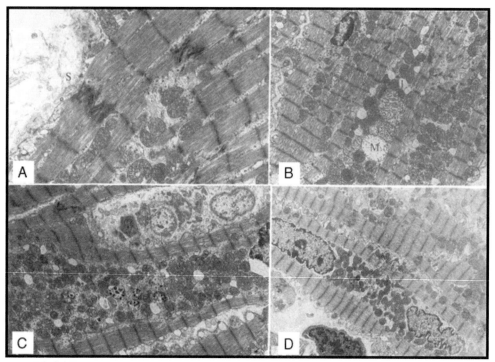

FIGURE 33-4 ■ **Epinephrine and myocardial ultrastructural changes.** Alterations in sarcolemma and mitochondria in myocardium of 3- to 5-day-old piglets after 2 hours of epinephrine intravenous infusion at 2 μg/kg/min. **A,** Electron micrograph of myocardium shows rupture of sarcolemma (S) (original magnification ×7000). **B,** Section through an area of myocardial damage shows mitochondrial (M) alterations, which consist of marked swelling, disruption of the cristae, and deposition of numerous lipid droplets (L) (original magnification ×3000). **C,** Swollen mitochondria that have lost many of their cristae are seen in the middle part of the field with the formation of vesicles that contain amorphous debris. **D,** Electron micrograph of the normal myocardium of a 3- to 5-day-old piglet (original magnification ×1500).

output state, but there are no comparative studies that show a significant beneficial effect compared with other inotropes. Dopamine at doses of less than 10 μg/kg/min is also an effective inotrope with a large cumulative experience in pediatric practice. Dobutamine has minimal vasoconstrictor effects, but the β effects may cause tachycardia, especially after repair of congenital heart disease in younger children.[94,95,215] The only comparative study of dopamine and dobutamine after repair of congenital heart disease, which used high doses, did not show any significant hemodynamic difference between drugs except for increases in pulmonary arterial pressure and pulmonary vascular resistance with dopamine.[216] This and other studies have used the logic of a combination of inotropes with vasodilators either in the form of α-blockers or nitroprusside.[56,95] This may be a useful technique when higher doses of inotropes are being used.

Most inotropic agents to date have a common final intracellular pathway of increased intracellular calcium, which may not be beneficial for the myocyte. A new generation of inotropic agents known as calcium-sensitizing agents achieve their positive inotropic effects without an increase in intracellular calcium or myocardial oxygen consumption.[217] In addition, future research in the treatment of heart failure with inotropic agents can be aimed at receptor resensitization strategies and at downstream signaling sites.[218] Lastly, a key direction should be focused on AR polymorphism and its role in responses of catecholamine response in heart failure in the neonatal and immature heart.[219-222]

Key Concepts

■ Reduced response to catecholamines in the failing myocardium can be observed as a result of receptor down-regulation and a process called desensitization, a decreased affinity of these receptors for circulating catecholamines.

■ The predominant β-AR in the mammalian heart is the β$_1$-AR (>75%). Activation of β$_1$-ARs results in increases in heart rate and contractility. Significant numbers of β$_2$-ARs also have been identified in the left ventricle in normal human hearts, but the greatest concentration is found in vascular smooth muscle, where stimulation results in vasodilation.

■ The hierarchy of relative densities of the β-ARs can change in heart failure, where β$_1$-ARs are down-regulated as a result of heightened sympathetic drive, whereas β_2-ARs have been shown to represent an increasing component of total β-AR activity.

■ The increase in cAMP concentration activates protein kinase, which causes the activation of many cellular proteins, including L-type Ca^{2+} channels, sarcoplasmic reticulum protein phospholamban, troponin I, and the ryanodine receptor.

■ Many of the integral mechanisms of intracellular calcium and norepinephrine release and reuptake are rendered less effective in heart failure, limiting the efficacy of inotropic agents.

■ There is an increasing trend to use low-dose epinephrine (<0.05 µg/kg/min) as a second-line inotropic agent (after dopamine) following CPB in children. At these dosages, the undesirable α-agonist effects are avoided while achieving the maximal β-adrenergic effects.

■ Digoxin increases the velocity and extent of the sarcomere shortening by decreasing the duration of contraction without changing muscle fiber tension. The pressure volume curve (Frank-Starling) of the ventricle is shifted upward and to the left. In addition to its inotropic properties, digoxin has important effects on heart rate through its action on the cardiac conduction and the autonomic nervous systems.

■ In the absence of any good published efficacy data for the use of digoxin in children, the only evidence comes from extrapolating from adult trials in dilated cardiomyopathy. Digoxin probably has a role in the treatment of children with dilated cardiomyopathy who have moderately reduced cardiac function after initial treatment with vasodilator therapy.

■ Down-regulation of β-ARs may provide a hypothesis for the decreased function after repair of congenital heart disease and the diminishing effect seen with increasing doses of catecholamines and phosphodiesterase inhibitors in this situation.

■ The cardiotoxicities of isoproterenol and epinephrine include hypertrophy and necrosis of the myocardium. With high-dose epinephrine, newborn animals had striking changes in the ultrastructure of the myocardium as assessed by electron microscopy: These changes included disruption of the sarcolemma with swelling of the mitochondria and deposition of calcium granules.

■ Most inotropic agents to date have a common final intracellular pathway of increased intracellular calcium, which may not be beneficial for the myocyte. A new generation of inotropic agents known as calcium-sensitizing agents achieves their positive inotropic effects without an increase in intracellular calcium or myocardial oxygen consumption.

REFERENCES

1. Colucci WS, Wright RF, Braunwald E: New positive inotropic agents in the treatment of congestive heart failure: Mechanisms of action and recent clinical developments: 1. N Engl J Med 1986;314:290-299.

2. Bristow MR, Ginsburg R: Beta 1 and beta 2-adrenergic-receptor subpopulations in nonfailing and failing human ventricular myocardium: Coupling of both receptor subtypes to muscle contraction and selective beta 1-receptor down-regulation in heart failure. Circ Res 1986;59:297-309.

3. Milano CA, Allen LF, Rockman HA, et al: Markedly enhanced myocardial function in transgenic mice with cardiac over-expression of the human beta 2-receptor adrenergic receptor. Science 1994; 264:582-586.

4. Bristow MR, Ginsburg R: Beta 2 receptors on myocardial cells in human ventricular myocardium. Am J Cardiol 1986;57:3F-6F.

5. Kozlik-Feldmann R, Kramer HH, Wicht H, et al: Distribution of myocardial beta-adrenoceptor subtypes and coupling to the adenylate cyclase in children with congenital heart disease and implications for treatment. J Clin Pharmacol 1993;33:588-595.

6. Brodde OE, Michel MC, Gordon EP, et al: Beta-adrenoceptor regulation in the human heart: Can it be monitored in circulating lymphocytes? Eur Heart J 1989;10(Suppl B):2-10.

7. Wu JR, Chang HR, Huang TM, et al: Reduction in lymphocyte beta-adrenergic receptor density in infants and children with heart failure secondary to congenital heart disease. Am J Cardiol 1996;77:170-174.

8. Sun LS, Pantuck CB, Morelli JJ, et al: Perioperative lymphocyte adenylyl cyclase function in the pediatric cardiac surgical patient. Crit Care Med 1996;24: 1654-1659.

9. Wu JR, Chang HR, Chen SS, et al: Circulating noradrenaline and beta-adrenergic receptors in children with congestive heart failure. Acta Paediatr 1996;85:923-927.

10. Smiley RM, Vulliemoz Y: Cardiac surgery causes desensitisation of the beta-adrenergic receptor system of human lymphocytes. Anesth Analg 1992;74:212-218.

11. Smiley RM, Pantuck CB, Chadburn A, et al: Down-regulation and densitisation of the beta-adrenergic receptor system of human lymphocytes after cardiac surgery. Anesth Analg 1993;77:653-661.

12. Brodde OE, Kretsch R, Ikezono K, et al: Human beta-adrenoceptors: Relation of myocardial and lymphocyte beta-adrenoceptor density. Science 1986;231: 1584-1585.

13. Gauthier C, Leblais V, Kobzik L, et al: The negative inotropic effect of beta 3-adrenoceptor stimulation is mediated by activation of a nitric oxide synthase pathway in human ventricle. J Clin Invest 1998;102: 1377-1384.

14. Post SR, Hammond HK, Insel PA: Beta-adrenergic receptors and receptor signaling in heart failure. Annu Rev Pharmacol 1999;39: 343-360.

15. Price DT, Lefkowitz RJ, Caron MG: Localisation of mRNA for three distinct alpha-1 adrenergic receptor subtypes in human species. Mol Pharmacol 1994;45:171-175.

16. Bruckner R, Meyer W, Mugge A, et al: Alpha-adrenoceptor-mediated positive inotropic effect of phenylephrine in isolated human ventricular myocardium. Eur J Pharmacol 1984;99:345-347.

17. Aass H, Skomedal T, Osnes JB: Demonstration of an alpha adrenoceptor-mediated inotropic effect of norepinephrine in rabbit papillary muscle. J Pharmacol Exp Ther 1983;226: 572-578.

18. Rosen MR, Hordof AJ, Ilvento JP, et al: Effects of adrenergic amines on electrophysiological properties and automaticity of neonatal and adult Purkinje fibers: Evidence for α- and β-adrenergic actions. Circ Res 1977;40:390-400.

19. Wagner J, Schumann H: Different mechanisms for the stimulation of myocardial alpha and beta-adrenergic receptors. Life Sci 1979; 40:390-400.

20. Borthne K, Haga P, Langslet A, et al: Endogenous norepinephrine stimulates both alpha 1- and beta-adrenoceptors in myocardium from children with congenital heart defects. J Mol Cell Cardiol 1995;27:693-699.

21. Sun LS, Rybin VO, Steinberg SF, et al: Characterization of the alpha 1-adrenergic chronotropic response in neuropeptide Y-treated cardiomyocytes. Eur J Pharmacol 1998;349:377-381.

22. Tanaka H, Manita S, Matsuda T, et al: Sustained negative inotropism mediated by alpha-adrenoceptors in adult mouse myocardia: Developmental conversion from positive response in the neonate. Br J Pharmacol 1995;114:673-677.

23. Chilian WM: Functional distribution of alpha 1- and alpha 2-adrenergic receptors in the coronary microcirculation. Circulation 1991;84:2108-2122.

24. Thandroyen FT, Muntz KH, Buja LM, et al: Alterations in beta-adrenergic receptors, adenylate cyclase, and cyclic AMP concentrations during acute myocardial ischemia and reperfusion. Circulation 1990;82(3 Suppl):II-30-II-37.

25. Zaugg M, Schaub MC, Parsch T, et al: Modulation of beta-adrenergic receptor subtype activities in perioperative medicine: Mechanisms and sites of action. Br J Anaesth 2002;88:101-123.

26. Scoote M, Poole-Wilson PA, Williams AJ: The therapeutic potential of new insights into myocardial excitation-contraction coupling. Heart 2003;89:371-376.

27. Bristow MR: Why does the myocardium fail? Insights from basic science. Lancet 1998;352(Suppl 1):SI-8-SI-14.

28. Autelitano DJ, Woodcock EA: Selective activation of alpha1A-adrenergic receptors in neonatal cardiac myocytes is sufficient to cause hypertrophy and differential regulation of alpha1-adrenergic receptor subtype mRNAs. J Mol Cell Cardiol 1998;30:1515-1523.

29. Hattori Y, Kanno M: Role of alpha1-adrenoceptor subtypes in production of the positive inotropic effects in mammalian myocardium: Implications for the alpha1-adrenoceptor subtype distribution. Life Sci 1998;62:1449-1453.

30. Chatterjee K, De Marco T: Role of nonglycosidic inotropic agents: Indications, ethics, and limitations. Med Clin North Am 2003;87:391-418.

31. Fitzgerald GA, Barnes P, Hamilton CA, et al: Circulating adrenaline and blood pressure: The metabolic effects and kinetics of infused adrenaline in man. Eur J Clin Invest 1980;10:401-406.

32. Zinner MJ, Kerr JC, Reynolds DG: Distribution and and arteriovenous shunting of gastric blood flow in the baboon: Effects of epinephrine and vasopressin infusions. Gastroenterology 1976;71:299.

33. Insel PA, Snavely MD: Catecholamines and the kidney: Receptors and renal function. Annu Rev Physiol 1981;43:625-636.

34. Coffin LH Jr, Ankeney JL, Beheler EM: Experimental study and clinical use of epinephrine for treatment of low cardiac output syndrome. Circulation 1966;33(4 Suppl):I-78-I-85.

35. Sternheim W, Dalakos TG, Streeten DP, et al: Action of L-epinephrine on the renin-aldosterone system and on urinary electrolyte excretion in man. Metabolism 1982;31:979.

36. Prielipp RC, Butterworth JF: Cardiovascular failure and pharmacological support after cardiac surgery. New Horiz 1999;7:472-488.

37. Butterworth JFT, Prielipp RC, Royster RL, et al: Dobutamine increases heart rate more than epinephrine in patients recovering from aortocoronary bypass surgery. J Cardiothorac Vasc Anesth 1992;6:535-541.

38. Caspi J, Coles JG, Benson LN, et al: Effects of high plasma epinephrine and Ca^{2+} concentrations on neonatal myocardial function after ischemia. J Thorac Cardiovasc Surg 1993;105:59-67.

39. Caspi J, Coles JG, Benson LN, et al: Age-related response to epinephrine-induced myocardial stress: A functional and ultrastructural study. Circulation 1991;84(5 Suppl):III-394-III-399.

40. Reddy VM, Liddicoat JR, McElhinney DB, et al: Hemodynamic effects of epinephrine, bicarbonate and calcium in the early postnatal period in a lamb model of single-ventricle physiology created in utero. J Am Coll Cardiol 1996;28:1877-1883.

41. Walters PA, Cooper PW, Denison AB, et al: Dilator responses to isoproterenol in cutaneous and skeletal muscle beds: Effects of adrenergic blocking drugs. J Pharmacol Exp Ther 1955;115:323-328.

42. Driscoll DJ, Gillette PC, Lewis RM, et al: Comparative hemodynamic effects of isoproterenol, dopamine, and dobutamine in the newborn dog. Pediatr Res 1979;13:1006-1009.

43. Buckley NM, Gootman PM, Yellin EL, et al: Age-related cardiovascular effects of catecholamines in anesthetized piglets. Circ Res 1979;45:282-292.

44. Driscoll DJ, Fukushige J, Hartley CJ, et al: The comparative hemodynamic effects of isoproterenol in chronically instrumented puppies and adult dogs. Dev Pharmacol Ther 1981;2:91-103.

45. Driscoll DJ, Gillette PC, Fukushige J, et al: Comparison of the cardiac actions of isoproterenol, dopamine and dobutamine in the neonatal and mature dog. Pediatr Cardiol 1980;1:307-314.

46. Holloway EL, Stinson EB, Derby GC, et al: Action of drugs in patients early after cardiac surgery: I. Comparison of isoproterenol and dopamine. Am J Cardiol 1975;35:656-659.

47. Kersting F, Follath F, Moulds R, et al: A comparison of cardiovascular effects of dobutamine and isoprenaline after open heart surgery. Br Heart J 1976;38:622-626.

48. Mentzer RM Jr, Alegre C, Nolan SP: Effect of dopamine and isoproterenol on pulmonary vascular resistance. Rev Surg 1976;33:433-436.

49. MacGregor DA, Prielipp RC, Black CS, et al: Renal dose dopamine does not alter the response to beta-adrenergic stimulation by isoproterenol in healthy human volunteers. Chest 1997;112:40-44.

50. Fowler MB, Alderman EL, Oesterle SN, et al: Dobutamine and dopamine after cardiac surgery: Greater augmentation of myocardial blood flow with dobutamine. Circulation 1984;70(3 Pt 2):I-103-I-111.

51. Mueller HS, Evans R, Ayres SM: Effect of dopamine on hemodynamics and myocardial metabolism in shock following myocardial infarction in man. Circulation 1978;57:361-365.

52. Leier CV, Heban PT, Huss P, et al: Comparative systemic and regional hemodynamic effects of dopamine and dobutamine in patients with cardiomyopathic heart failure. Circulation 1978;58:466-475.

53. Driscoll DJ, Gillette PC, McNamara DG: The use of dopamine in children. J Pediatr 1978;92:309-314.

54. Driscoll DJ, Gillette PC, Ezrailson EG, et al: Inotropic response of the neonatal canine myocardium to dopamine. Pediatr Res 1978;12:42-45.

55. Driscoll DJ, Gillette PC, Duff DF, et al: The hemodynamic effect of dopamine in children. J Thorac Cardiovasc Surg 1979;78:765-768.

56. Stephenson LW, Edmunds LH, Jr, Raphaely R, et al: Effects of nitroprusside and dopamine on pulmonary arterial vasculature in children after cardiac surgery. Circulation 1979;60(2 Pt 2):104-110.

57. Williams DB, Kieman PD, Schaff HV, et al: The hemodynamic response to dopamine and nitroprusside following right atrium-pulmonary artery bypass (Fontan procedure). Ann Thorac Surg 1982;34:51-57.

58. Sakata Y, Iijima T, Yoshida I, et al: (Effects of dopamine and dobutamine on systemic hemodynamics and myocardial metabolism in children after open heart surgery). Kyobu Geka 1991;44:461-466.

59. Girardin E, Berner M, Rouge JC, et al: Effect of low dose dopamine on hemodynamic and renal function in children. Pediatr Res 1989;26:200-203.

60. Mitchell IM, Pollock JC, Jamieson MP: Effects of dopamine on liver blood flow in children with congenital heart disease. Ann Thorac Surg 1995;60:1741-1744.

61. Seri I, Abbasi S, Wood DC, et al: Regional hemodynamic effects of dopamine in the sick preterm neonate. J Pediatr 1998;133:728-734.

62. Seri I: Circulatory support of the sick preterm infant. Semin Neonatol 2001;6:85-95.

63. Seri I, Tulassay T, Kiszel J, et al: Cardiovascular response to dopamine in hypotensive preterm neonates with severe hyaline membrane disease. Eur J Pediatr 1984;142:3-9.

64. Seri I, Rudas G, Bors Z, et al: Effects of low-dose dopamine infusion on cardiovascular and renal functions, cerebral blood flow, and plasma catecholamine levels in sick preterm neonates. Pediatr Res 1993; 34:742-749.

65. Padbury JF, Agata Y, Baylen BG, et al: Dopamine pharmacokinetics in critically ill newborn infants. J Pediatr 1987;110:293-298.

66. Walther FJ, Siassi B, Ramadan NA, et al: Cardiac output in new-born infants with transient myocardial dysfunction. J Pediatr 1985;107:781-785.

67. Notterman DA, Greenwald BM, Moran F, et al: Dopamine clearance in critically ill infants and children: Effect of age and organ system dysfunction. Clin Pharmacol Ther 1990;48:138-147.

68. Denton MD, Chertow GM, Brady HR: "Renal-dose" dopamine for the treatment of acute renal failure: Scientific rationale, experimental studies and clinical trials. Kidney Int 1996;50:4-14.

69. Richer M, Robert S, Lebel M: Renal hemodynamics during norepinephrine and low-dose dopamine infusions in man. Crit Care Med 1996;24:1150-1156.

70. Hoogenberg K, Smit AJ, Girbes AR: Effects of low-dose dopamine on renal and systemic hemodynamics during incremental norepinephrine infusion in healthy volunteers. Crit Care Med 1998;26:260-265.

71. Duke GJ, Briedis JH, Weaver RA: Renal support in critically ill patients: Low-dose dopamine or low-dose dobutamine? Crit Care Med 1994;22:1919-1925.

72. Wenstone R, Campbell JM, Booker PD, et al: Renal function after cardiopulmonary bypass in children: Comparison of dopamine with dobutamine. Br J Anaesth 1991;67:591-594.

73. Seri I: Effect of dopamine on indomethacin-induced impairment of renal function in preterm neonates. J Pediatr 1993;123:167-168.

74. Seri I: Cardiovascular, renal, and endocrine actions of dopamine in neonates and children. J Pediatr 1995;126:333-344.

75. Seri I, Tulassay T, Kiszel J, et al: The use of dopamine for the prevention of the renal side effects of indomethacin in premature infants with patent ductus arteriosus. Int J Pediatr Nephrol 1984;5:209-214.

76. Seri I, Abbasi S, Wood DC, et al: Regional hemodynamic effects of dopamine in the indomethacin-treated preterm infant. J Perinatol 2002;22:300-305.

77. Prins I, Plotz BB, Uiterwaal CS, et al: Low-dose dopamine in neonatal and pediatric intensive care: A systematic review. Intensive Care Med 2001;27:206-210.

78. Bellomo R, Chapman M, Finfer S, et al: Low-dose dopamine in patients with early renal dysfunction: A placebo-controlled randomised trial. Australian and New Zealand Intensive Care Society (ANZICS) Clinical Trials Group. Lancet 2000;356:2139-2143.

79. Leier CV, Webel J, Bush CA: The cardiovascular effects of the continuous infusion of dobutamine in patients with severe cardiac failure. Circulation 1977;56:468-472.

80. Riordan CJ, Randsbaek F, Storey JH, et al: Inotropes in the hypoplastic left heart syndrome: Effects in an animal model. Ann Thorac Surg 1996;62:83-90.

81. MacGregor DA, Butterworth JF, Zaloga CP, et al: Hemodynamic and renal effects of dopexamine and dobutamine in patients with reduced cardiac output following coronary artery bypass grafting. Chest 1994;106:835-841.

82. Ensinger H, Rantala A, Vogt J, et al: Effect of dobutamine on splanchnic carbohydrate metabolism and amino acid balance after cardiac surgery. Anesthesiology 1999;916:1587-1595.

83. Magorien RD, Unverferth DV, Brown GP, et al: Dobutamine and hydralazine: Comparative influences of positive inotropy and vasodilation on coronary blood flow and myocardial energetics in nonischemic congestive heart failure. J Am Coll Cardiol 1983;12(Pt 1):499-505.

84. Cody RJ: Do positive inotropic agents adversely affect the survival of patients with chronic congestive heart failure? I. Introduction. J Am Coll Cardiol 1988;12:559-561.

85. Packer M, Leier CV: Survival in congestive heart failure during treatment with drugs with positive inotropic actions. Circulation 1987;75(Suppl IV):55-63.

86. Capomolla S, Febo O, Opasich C, et al: Chronic infusion of dobutamine and nitroprusside in patients with end-stage heart failure awaiting heart transplantation: Safety and clinical outcome. Eur J Heart Fail 2001;3:601-610.

87. Pickworth KK: Long-term dobutamine therapy for refractory congestive heart failure. Clin Pharmacokinet 1992;11:618-624.

88. Dell'Italia LJ, Starling MR, Blumhardt R, et al: Comparative effects of volume loading, dobutamine, and nitroprusside in patients with predominant right ventricular infarction. Circulation 1985;72:1327-1335.

89. Boyd O, Grounds RM, Bennett ED: A randomized clinical trial of the effect of deliberate perioperative increase of oxygen delivery on mortality in high-risk surgical patients. JAMA 1993;270:2699-2707.

90. Hayes MA, Timmins AC, Yau EH, et al: Elevation of systemic oxygen delivery in the treatment of critically ill patients. N Engl J Med 1994;330:1717-1722.

91. Harada K, Tamura M, Ito T, et al: Effects of low-dose dobutamine on left ventricular diastolic filling in children. Pediatr Cardiol 1996;17:220-225.

92. Michelfelder EC, Witt SA, Khoury P, et al: Moderate-dose dobutamine maximizes left ventricular contractile response during dobutamine stress echocardiography in children. J Am Soc Echocardiogr 2003;16:140-146.

93. Driscoll DJ, Gillette PC, Duff DF, et al: Hemodynamic effects of dobutamine in children. Am J Cardiol 1979;43:581-585.

94. Bohn DJ, Boirier CS, Edmonds JF, et al: Hemodynamic effects of dobutamine after cardiopulmonary bypass in children. Crit Care Med 1980;8:367-371.

95. Berner M, Rouge JC, Friedli B: The hemodynamic effect of phentolamine and dobutamine after open-heart operations in children: Influence of the underlying heart defect. Ann Thorac Surg 1983;35:643-650.

96. Berner M, Oberhansli I, Rouge JC, et al: Chronotropic and inotropic supports are both required to increase cardiac output early after corrective operations for tetralogy of Fallot. J Thorac Cardiovasc Surg 1989;97:297-302.

97. Jaccard C, Berner M, Rouge JC, et al: Hemodynamic effect of isoprenaline and dobutamine immediately after correction of tetralogy of Fallot: Relative importance of inotropic and chronotropic action in supporting cardiac output. J Thorac Cardiovasc Surg 1984;87:862-869.

98. Perkin RM, Levin DL, Webb R, et al: Dobutamine: A hemodynamic evaluation in children with shock. J Pediatr 1982;100:977-983.

99. Schranz D, Stopfkuchen H, Jungst BK, et al: Hemodynamic effects of dobutamine in children with cardiovascular failure. Eur J Pediatr 1982;139:4-7.

100. Berg RA, Padbury JF, Donnerstein RL, et al: Dobutamine pharmacokinetics and pharmacodynamics in normal children and adolescents. J Pharmacol Exp Ther 1993;265:1232-1238.

101. Berg RA, Donnerstein RL, Padbury JF: Dobutamine infusions in stable, critically ill children: Pharmacokinetics and hemodynamic actions. Crit Care Med 1993;21:678-686.

102. Martinez AM, Padbury JF, Thio S: Dobutamine pharmacokinetics and cardiovascular responses in critically ill neonates. Pediatrics 1992;89:47-51.

103. Habib DM, Padbury JF, Anas NG, et al: Dobutamine pharmacokinetics and pharmacodynamics in pediatric intensive care patients. Crit Care Med 1992;20:601-608.

104. Sun D, Huang A, Mital S, et al: Norepinephrine elicits beta2-receptor-mediated dilation of isolated human coronary arterioles. Circulation 2002;106:550-555.

105. Marin C, Eon B, Saux P, et al: Renal effects of norepinephrine used to treat septic shock patients. Crit Care Med 1990;18:282-285.

106. Marik PE, Mohedin M: The contrasting effects of dopamine and norepinephrine on systemic and splanchnic oxygen utilization in hyperdynamic sepsis. JAMA 1994;272:1354-1357.

107. Martin C, Viviand X, Arnaud S, et al: Effects of norepinephrine plus dobutamine or norepinephrine alone on left ventricular performance of septic shock patients. Crit Care Med 1999;27:1708-1713.

108. Redl-Wenzl EM, Armbruster C, Edelmann G, et al: The effects of norepinephrine on hemodynamics and renal function in severe septic shock states. Intensive Care Med 1993;19:151-154.

109. Desjars P, Pinaud M, Bugnon D, et al: Norepinephrine therapy has no deleterious renal effects in human septic shock. Crit Care Med 1989;17:426-429.

110. Martin C, Viviand X, Leone M, et al: Effect of norepinephrine on the outcome of septic shock. Crit Care Med 2000;28:2758-2765.

111. Dec GW: Digoxin remains useful in the management of chronic heart failure. Med Clin North Am 2003;87:317-337.

112. Carlton RA, Miller PH, Grettinger JS: Effects of ouabain, atropine and ouabain and atropine on A-V nodal conduction in man. Circ Res 1967;20:283-288.

113. Gheorghiade M, Ferguson D: Digoxin: A neurohormonal modulator in heart failure? Circulation 1991;84:2181-2186.

114. Covit AB, Schaer GL, Sealey JE, et al: Suppression of the renin-angiotensin system by intravenous digoxin in chronic congestive heart failure. Am J Med 1983;75:445-447.

115. Kaye DM, Lambert GW, Lefkovits J, et al: Neurochemical evidence of cardiac sympathetic activation and increased central nervous system norepinephrine turnover in severe congestive heart failure. J Am Coll Cardiol 1994;23:570-578.

116. Ribner HS, Zuker MJ, Stisor C, et al: Vasodilators as first line therapy for congestive heart failure: A comparative hemodynamic study of hydralazine, digoxin and their combination. Am Heart J 1983;106:308-315.

117. McGarry SJ, Williams AJ: Digoxin activated sarcoplasmic reticulum Ca²⁺ release channels: A possible role in cardiac inotropy. Br J Pharmacol 1993;108:1043-1050.

118. Marban E, Tsien RW: Enhancement of cardiac calcium current during digitalis inotropy: Positive feedback regulation by intracellular calcium. J Physiol 1982;329:589-614.

119. Allen PD, Schmidt TA, Marsh JD, et al: Na,K-ATPase expression in normal and failing human left ventricle. Basic Res Cardiol 1992;87(Suppl 1):87-94.

120. Eichhorn EJ, Gheorghiade M: Digoxin. Prog Cardiovasc Dis 2002;44:251-266.

121. Cheng JW, Charland SL, Shaw LW, et al: Is the volume of distribution of digoxin reduced in patients with renal dysfunction? Determining digoxin pharmacokinetics by fluorescence polarization immunoassay. Pharmacotherapy 1997;17:584-590.

122. Moyser JO, Jaggaro NS, Grundy EN, et al: Amiodarone increases plasma digoxin concenrations. BMJ 1981;282:272.

123. Koren G, Soldin S, Macleod SM: Digoxin amiodarone interaction: In vivo and in vitro studies in rats. Can J Physiol Pharmacol 1983;61:1483-1486.

124. Koren G, Hesslein PS, MacLeod SM: Digoxin toxicity associated with amiodarone therapy in children. J Pediatr 1984;104:467-470.

125. Klein HO, et al: Verapamil-digoxin interaction. N Engl J Med 1980;303:160.

126. Klein HO, Lang R, Weiss E, et al: The influence of verapamil on serum digoxin concentration. Circulation 1982;65:998-1003.

127. Koren G, Soldin S, MacLeod SM: Digoxin-verapamil interaction: In vitro studies in rat tissue. J Cardiovasc Pharmacol 1983;5:443-445.

128. Zalzstein E, Koren G, Bryson SM, et al: Interaction between digoxin and propafenone in children. J Pediatr 1990;116:310-312.

129. Wettrell G, Andersson KE: Absorption of digoxin in infants. Eur J Clin Pharmacol 1975;9:49-55.

130. Hernandez A, Burton RM, Pagtakhan RD, et al: Pharmacodynamics of 3H-digoxin in infants. Pediatrics 1969;44:418-428.

131. Larese RJ, Mirkin B: Kinetics of digoxin: Absorption and relation of serum levels to cardiac arhythmias in children. Clin Pharmacol Ther 1974;15:387-396.

132. Berman W Jr, Dubynsky O, Whitman V, et al: Digoxin therapy in low-birth-weight infants with patent ductus arteriosus. J Pediatr 1978;93:652-655.

133. Koren G, Farine D, Maresky D, et al: Significance of the endogenous digoxin-like substance in infants and mothers. Clin Pharmacol Ther 1984;36:759-764.

134. Stone JG, Bentur Y, Zalstein G, et al: Effects of endogenous digoxin-like substances on the interpretation of high concentrations of digoxin in children. J Pediatr 1990;117:321-325.

135. Andersson KE, Bertler A, Wettrell G: Post-mortem distribution and tissue concentrations of digoxin in infants and adults. Acta Paediatr Scand 1975;64:497-504.

136. Park MK, Ludden T, Arom KU, et al: Myocardial vs serum digoxin concentrations in infants and adults. Am J Dis Child 1982;136:418-420.

137. Berman W Jr, Musselman J, Shortencarrier R: Localization of digoxin in sheep myocardium by immunofluorescent microscopy. Biol Neonate 1981;40:295-299.

138. Wettrell G, Andersson KE: Clinical pharmacokinetics of digixin in infants. Clin Pharmacol 1977;2:17-31.

139. Lang D, Von Bermuth G: Serum concentrations and serum half-life of digoxin in premature and mature infants. Pediatrics 1977;59:902-906.

140. Hastreiter AR, Simonton RL, van der Horst RL, et al: Digoxin pharmacokinetics in premature infants. Pediatr Pharmacol (New York) 1982;2:23-31.

141. Park MK: Use of digoxin in infants and children, with specific emphasis on dosage. J Pediatr 1986;108:871-877.

142. Antman EM, Wenger TL, Butler VP, et al: Treatment of 150 cases of life-threatening digitalis intoxication with digoxin-specific Fab antibody fragments: Final report of a multicenter study. Circulation 1990;81:1744-1752.

143. Smith TW, Butler VP, Haber E, et al: Treatment of life-threatening digitalis intoxication with digoxin-specific Fab antibody fragments. N Engl J Med 1982;307:1357-1362.

144. Kelly RA, Smith TW: Recognition and management of digitalis toxicity. Am J Cardiol 1992;69:108G-118G.

145. Hauptman PJ, Kelly RA: Digitalis. Circulation 1999;99:1265-1270.

146. Woolf AD, Wenger T, Smith TW, et al: The use of digoxin-specific Fab fragments for severe digitalis intoxication in children. N Engl J Med 1992;326:1739-1744.

147. Ribner B, Plucinski DA, Hseih AM, et al: Acute effects of digoxin on total systemic vascular resistance in congestive heart failure due to dilated cardiomyopathy: A hemodynamic-hormonal study. Am J Cardiol 1985;56:896-904.

148. Cohn K, Selzer A, Kersh ES, et al: Variability of hemodynamic responses to acute digitalization in chronic cardiac failure due to cardiomyopathy and coronary artery disease. Am J Cardiol 1975;35:461-468.

149. Gheorghiade M, Hall V, Lakier JB, et al: Comparative hemodynamic and neurohormonal effects of intravenous captopril and digoxin and their combinations in patients with severe heart failure. J Am Coll Cardiol 1989;13:134-142.

150. Tisdale JE, Gheorghiade M: Acute hemodynamic effects of digoxin alone or in combination with other vasoactive agents in heart failure. Am J Cardiol 1992;69:34G-47G.

151. Raabe DS: Combination therapy with digoxin and nitroglycerin in heart failure complicating acute myocardial infarction. Am J Cardiol 1979;43:990-994.

152. Cantelli I, Vitolo A, Lombardi G, et al: Combined hemodynamic effects of digoxin and captopril in patients with congestive heart failure. Curr Ther Res 1984;36:323-327.

153. Uretsky BF, Young JB, Shahida J, et al: Randomised study assessing the effect of digoxin withdrawl in patients with mild to moderate chronic congestive heart failure: Results of the PROVED trial. J Am Coll Cardiol 1993;22:955-962.

154. Packer M, Gherorghiade M, Young JB, et al: Withdrawl of digoxin from patients with chronic heart failure treated with angiotensin-converting-enzyme inhibitors. N Engl J Med 1993;329:1-7.

155. The effect of digoxin on mortality and morbidity in patients with heart failure: The Digitalis Investigation Group. N Engl J Med 1997;336:525-533.

156. Rathore SS, Curtis JP, Wong Y, et al: Association of serum digoxin concentration and outcomes in patients with heart failure. JAMA 2003;289:871-878.

157. Berman W Jr, Yabek SM, Dillon T, et al: Effects of digoxin in infants with congested circulatory state due to a ventricular septal defect. N Engl J Med 1983;308:363-366.

158. Venugopalan P, Agarwal AK, Worthing EA: Chronic cardiac failure in children due to dilated cardiomyopathy: Diagnostic approach, pathophysiology and management. Eur J Pediatr 2000;159:803-810.

159. Friedman WF: The intrinsic physiologic properties of the developing heart. Prog Cardiovasc Dis 1972;15:87-111.

160. Friedman WF, Pool PE, Jacobowitz D, et al: Sympathetic innervation of the developing rabbit heart: Biochemical and histochemical comparisons of fetal, neonatal, and adult myocardium. Circ Res 1968;23:25-32.

161. Romero TE, Friedman WF: Limited left ventricular response to volume overload in the neonatal period: A comparative study with the adult animal. Pediatr Res 1979;13:910-915.

162. Kirkpatrick SE, Pitlick PT, Naliboff J, et al: Frank-Starling relationship as an important determinant of fetal cardiac output. Am J Physiol 1976;231:495-500.

163. Klopfenstein HS, Rudolph AM: Postnatal changes in the circulation and responses to volume loading in sheep. Circ Res 1978;42:839-845.

164. Romero TE, Covell J, Friedman WF: A comparison of the pressure-volume relations of the fetal, newborn and adult heart. Am J Physiol 1972;222:1285-1290.

165. Riemenschneider TA, Brenner RA, Mason DT: Maturational changes in myocardial contractile state of newborn lambs. Pediatr Res 1981;15:349-356.

166. Berman W Jr, Musselman J: Myocardial performance in the newborn lamb. Am J Physiol 1979;237:H66-H70.

167. Teitel DF, Sidi D, Chin T, et al: Developmental changes in myocardial contractile reserve in the lamb. Pediatr Res 1985;19:948-955.

168. Park IS, Michael LH, Driscoll DJ: Comparative response of the developing canine myocardium to inotropic agents. Am J Physiol 1982;242:H13-H18.

169. Candito M, Albertini M, Politano S, et al: Plasma catecholamine levels in children. J Chromatogr 1993;617:304-307.

170. Eichler I, Eichler HG, Rotter M, et al: Plasma concentrations of free and sulfoconjugated dopamine, epinephrine, and norepinephrine in healthy infants and children. Klin Wochenschr 1989;67:672-675.

171. Kogner P, Bjork O, Theodorsson E: Plasma neuropeptide Y in healthy children: Influence of age, anaesthesia and the establishment of an age-adjusted reference interval. Acta Paediatr 1994;83:423-427.

172. Rockson SG, Homcy CJ, Quinn P, et al: Cellular mechanisms of impaired adrenergic responsiveness in neonatal dogs. J Clin Invest 1981;67:319-327.

173. Geis WP, Tatooles CJ, Priola DV, et al: Factors influencing neurohumoral control of the heart in the newborn dog. Am J Physiol 1975;228:1685-1689.

174. Baylen BG, Agata Y, Padbury JF, et al: Hemodynamic and neuroendocrine adaptations of the preterm lamb left ventricle to acutely increased afterload. Pediatr Res 1989;26:336-342.

175. Fisher DJ: The subcellular basis for the perinatal maturation of the cardiocyte. Curr Opin Cardiol 1994;9:91-96.

176. Kuznetsov V, Pak E, Robinson RB, et al: Beta 2-adrenergic receptor actions in neonatal and adult rat ventricular myocytes. Circ Res 1995;76:40-52.

177. Sun LS: Regulation of myocardial beta-adrenergic receptor function in adult and neonatal rabbits. Biol Neonate 1999;76:181-192.

178. Kozlik R, Kramer HH, Wicht H, et al: Myocardial beta-adrenoceptor density and the distribution of beta 1- and beta 2-adrenoceptor subpopulations in children with congenital heart disease. Eur J Pediatr 1991;150:388-394.

179. Brodde OE, Zerkowski H, Schranz D, et al: Age-dependent changes in the beta adrenergic-receptor-G-protein(s)-adenylyl cyclase system. J Cardiovasc Pharmacol 1995;26:20-26.

180. Bristow MR, Ginsburg R, Minobe WA, et al: Decreased catecholamine sensitivity and beta-adrenergic-receptor density in failing human hearts. N Engl J Med 1982;307:205-211.

181. Bristow MR, Minobe WA, Raynolds MV, et al: Reduced beta 1 receptor messenger RNA abundance in the failing human heart. J Clin Invest 1993;92:2737-2745.

182. Ungerer M, Bohm M, Elce JS, et al: Altered expression of beta-adrenergic receptor kinase and beta1-adrenergic receptors in the failing human heart. Circulation 1993;87:454-463.

183. Bohm M, Diet F, Feiler G, et al: Subsensitivity of the failing human heart to isoprenaline and milrinone is related to beta-adrenoceptor downregulation. J Cardiovasc Pharmacol 1988;12:726-732.

184. Bohm M, Flesch M, Schnabel P: Beta-adrenergic signal transduction in the failing and hypertrophied myocardium. J Mol Med 1997;75:842-848.

185. Bristow MR, Hershberger RE, Port JD, et al: Beta 1- and beta 2-adrenergic receptor-mediated adenylate cyclase stimulation in nonfailing and failing human ventricular myocardium. Mol Pharmacol 1989;35:295-303.

186. Strasser RH, Marquetant R, Kubler W: Adrenergic receptors and sensitization of adenylyl cyclase in acute myocardial ischemia. Circulation 1990;82(3 Suppl):II-23-II-29.

187. Ungerer M, Kessebohm K, Kronsbein K, et al: Activation of adrenergic-beta receptor kinase during myocardial ischemia. Circ Res 1996;79:455-460.

188. Dzimiri N: Regulation of beta-adrenoceptor signaling in cardiac function and disease. Pharmacol Rev 1999;51:465-501.

189. Lefkowitz RJ, Stadel JM, Caron MG: Adenylate cyclase-coupled beta adrenergic-receptors: Structure and mechanisms of activation and desensitisation. Annu Rev Biochem 1983;52:159-186.

190. Ross RD, Daniels SR, Schwartz DC, et al: Return of plasma norepinephrine to normal after resolution of congestive heart failure in congenital heart disease. Am J Cardiol 1987;60:1411-1413.

191. Vatner DE, Vatner SF, Nejima J, et al: Chronic norepinephrine elicits desensitization by uncoupling the beta-receptor. J Clin Invest 1989;84:1741-1748.

192. Maisel A, Motulsky H, Insel PA: Externalisation of beta-adrenergic receptors promoted by myocardial ischemia. Science 1985;230:183-186.

193. Reves J, Karp RB, Buttner E, et al: Neural and adrenomedullary catecholamine release in response to cardiopulmonary bypass in man. Circulation 1982;66:49-55.

194. Gerhardt MA, Booth JV, Chesnut LC, et al: Acute myocardial beta-adrenergic receptor dysfunction after cardiopulmonary bypass in patients with cardiac valve disease. Duke Heart Center Perioperative Desensitization Group. Circulation 1998;98(19 Suppl):II-275-II-281.

195. Booth JV, Landolfo KP, Chesnut LC, et al: Acute depression of myocardial beta-adrenergic receptor signaling during cardiopulmonary bypass: Impairment of the adenylyl cyclase moiety. Duke Heart Center Perioperative Desensitization Group. Anesthesiology 1998;89:602-611.

196. Booth JV, Spahn DR, McRae RL, et al: Esmolol improves left ventricular function via enhanced beta-adrenergic receptor signaling in a canine model of coronary revascularization. Anesthesiology 2002;97:162-169.

197. Dzimiri N, Galal O, Moorji A, et al: Regulation of sympathetic activity in children with various congenital heart diseases. Pediatr Res 1995;38:55-60.

198. Schranz D, Droege A, Broede A, et al: Uncoupling of human cardiac beta-adrenoceptors during cardiopulmonary bypass with cardioplegic cardiac arrest. Circulation 1993;87:422-426.

199. Collins S, Caron MG, Lefkowitz RJ: Beta-adrenergic receptors in hamster smooth muscle cells are transcriptionally regulated by glucocorticoids. J Biol Chem 1988;263:9067-9070.

200. Davies AO, Lefkowitz RJ: In vitro desensitization of beta adrenergic receptors in human neutrophils: Attenuation by corticosteroids. J Clin Invest 1983;71:565-571.

201. Sugiyama S, Hayashi K, Hanaki Y, et al: Effect of methylprednisolone on recovery of beta-adrenergic desensitisation in rat hearts. Drug Res 1991;41:439-443.

202. Saito T, Takanashi M, Gallagher E, et al: Corticosteroid effect on early beta-adrenergic down-regulation during circulatory shock: Hemodynamic study and beta-adrenergic receptor assay. Intensive Care Med 1995;21:204-210.

203. Unverferth DV, Blandford M, Kates RE: Tolerance to dobutamine after a 72-hour continuous infusion. Am J Med 1980;69:262-266.

204. Shore S, Nelson DP, Pearl JM, et al: Usefulness of corticosteroid therapy in decreasing epinephrine requirements in critically ill infants with congenital heart disease. Am J Cardiol 2001;88:591-594.

205. Tse J, Powell JR, Base CA, et al: Isoproterenol-induced cardiac hypertrophy: Modification in characteristics of beta-adrenergic receptor-adneylyl cyclase and ventricular contraction. Endocrinology 1979;105:246-255.

206. Varley KG, Dhalla NS: Excitation-contraction coupling in the heart: XII. Intracellular calcium in isoproterenol induced myocardial necrosis. Exp Mol Pathol 1973;19:94-105.

207. Ferrans VJ, Hibbs RG, Black WC, et al: Isoproterenol-induced myocardial necrosis: A histological and electron microscopic study. Am Heart J 1964; 69:71-90.

208. Ferrans VJ, Hibbs RG, Weily HS, et al: A histochemical and electron microscopic study of epinephrine-induced myocardial necrosis. J Mol Cell Cardiol 1970;1:11-22.

209. Caspi J, Coles JG, Benson LN, et al: Heart rate independence of catecholamine-induced myocardial damage in the newborn pig. Pediatr Res 1994;36(1 Pt 1):49-54.

210. Caspi J, Coles JG, Benson LN, et al: Dose-related effects of magnesium on myocardial function in the neonate. Hypertension 1994;23:174-178.

211. Guller B, Fields AI, Coleman MG, et al: Changes in cardiac rhythm in children treated with dopamine. Crit Care Med 1978; 6:151-154.

212. Hoffman TM, Bush DM, Wernovsky G, et al: Postoperative junctional ectopic tachycardia in children: Incidence, risk factors, and treatment. Ann Thorac Surg 2002;74:1607-1611.

213. Duke T, Butt W, South M, et al: Early markers of major adverse events in children after cardiac operations. J Thorac Cardiovasc Surg 1997;114:1042-1052.

214. Munoz R, Lausson PC, Palacio G, et al: Changes in whole blood lactate levels during cardiopulmonary bypass for surgery for congenital cardiac disease: An early indicator of morbidity and mortality. J Thorac Cardiovasc Surg 2000;119:155-162.

215. Innes PA, Frazer RS, Booker PD, et al: Comparison of the haemodynamic effects of dobutamine with enoximone after open heart surgery in small children. Br J Anaesth 1994;72:77-81.

216. Booker PD, Evans C, Franks R: Comparison of the haemodynamic effects of dopamine and dobutamine in young children undergoing cardiac surgery. Br J Anaesth 1995;74:419-423.

217. Kaheinen P, Pollesello P, Levijoki J, et al: Effects of levosimendan and milrinone on oxygen consumption in isolated Guinea-pig heart. J Cardiovasc Pharmacol 2004;43:555-561.

218. Lohse MJ, Engelhardt S, Eschenhagen T: What is the role of beta adrenergic signaling in heart failure? Circ Res 2003;93:896-906.

219. Small KM, Wagoner LE, Levin AM, et al: Synergistic polymorphisms of beta 1- and alpha 2C adrenergic receptors and the risk of congestive heart failure. N Engl J Med 2002;347:1135-1142.

220. Mialet Perez J, Rathz DA, Petrashevskaya NN, et al: Beta 1-adrenergic receptor polymorphisms confer differential function and predisposition to heart failure. Nat Med 2003;9:1300-1305.

221. Eisenach JH, McGuire AM, Schwingler RM, et al: The Arg 16/Gly beta 2-adrenergic receptor polymorphism is associated with altered cardiovascular responses to isometric exercise. Physiol Genomics 2004;16:323-328.

222. Terra SG, Pauly DF, Lee CR, et al: Beta-adrenergic receptor polymorphism and responses during titration of metoprolol controlled release/extended release in heart failure. Clin Pharmacol Ther 2005;77:127-137.

CHAPTER 34

Phosphodiesterase Inhibitors

Colin J. McMahon
Anthony C. Chang

In 1979, Alousi and colleagues[1] first showed that the bipyridine-derivative phosphodiesterase inhibitor (PDEI) amrinone possessed demonstrable increases in contractile force and vasodilatory effects without change in heart rate. Initial enthusiasm for this class of agents waned because early adult clinical trials showed an increase in mortality (see later sections). More recent investigations have shown the beneficial role of PDEIs, however, in the treatment of heart failure in adults and children.[2,3] The hemodynamic effects of PDEIs, increased inotropy and vasodilation with concomitant improved lusitropy (the property of diastolic relaxation), are unique as a class of cardiotonic drugs. Milrinone, with its shorter half-life, fewer side effects, and greater selectivity for the phosphodiesterase III isoenzyme, has become the PDEI of choice in the management of heart failure in the intensive care unit and the outpatient setting.

PHOSPHODIESTERASE INHIBITORS AND ADRENERGIC AGENTS

Mechanism of Action

In the 1970s, **cyclic AMP (cAMP)** was discovered as an important second messenger intimately involved in intracellular signaling.[4,5] cAMP, produced by enzyme cleavage of ATP, phosphorylates numerous cellular proteins through a cAMP-dependent protein kinase. It is broken down to the chemically inactive compound 5′AMP by the membrane-bound enzyme phosphodiesterase, which is associated with sarcoplasmic reticulum (SR) found in myocytes, vascular smooth muscle cells, and platelets (Fig. 34-1).

PDEIs selectively inhibit the isoenzyme phosphodiesterase III, increasing intracellular cAMP, which modulates cardiac contractile function and vascular tone.[6,7] Increased cAMP augments cardiac contractility by activating protein kinases, which increase activities of other essential intracellular cardiac proteins. More specifically, the PDEIs have a selective effect on the function of the SR because local increase in cAMP leads to activation of protein kinase A, which phosphorylates phospholamban. Because phospholamban normally inhibits the function of the SR by hindering its calcium pump, the phosphorylation of phospholamban by cAMP in effect "disinhibits" the SR and liberates cytosolic calcium.

This relatively isolated effect on the SR explains why highly type III–specific PDEIs increase the inotropic state without concomitant increase in heart rate.[8] cAMP also can promote improved contraction by another mechanism: activation of protein kinase (which catalyzes the transfer of phosphate groups from ATP), leading to faster calcium entry through the calcium channels.

All of this activity, as a result of increased cAMP, increases speed and force of not only cardiac contraction, but also relaxation. The relaxation of the myocardium is accelerated by reduction of cytosolic calcium (secondary to more efficient removal of calcium into the SR via the activated ATPase protein). Lastly, the vasodilatory effect of PDEIs is secondary to activation of protein kinase G by cAMP.[9]

Hemodynamic and Cardiac Effects of Phosphodiesterase Inhibitors

The main hemodynamic effects of PDEIs include increase in cardiac output, decrease in systemic and pulmonary vascular resistances, and decrease in filling pressures.[10] Similar to the systemic and pulmonary vasculature, the coronary circulation is dilated with the use of milrinone and undergoes a decrease in resistance.[11] These favorable changes occur usually without increase in myocardial oxygen consumption (as measured by heart rate–pressure product) to result in an increase in left ventricular external efficiency. Lastly, there is acceleration of isovolumic relaxation to indicate improved diastolic filling.[12] Other cardiac effects of PDEIs include dilation of epicardial coronary arteries and grafts,[13,14] anti-ischemic effects on myocardium,[15] and inhibition of proinflammatory cytokines.[16] All of these additional effects are particularly beneficial in the postoperative cardiac surgical patient.

Theoretical Advantages over Catecholamines

Although the PDEIs have longer times required for onset and termination of action compared with adrenergic agents, these agents have several advantages. One decided advantage for PDEIs is that these agents mediate their physiologic properties without interaction with myocardial β-receptors and are relatively independent from effects of receptor regulation. This ability is especially useful in heart failure because there is considerable down-regulation of β-receptors; there is

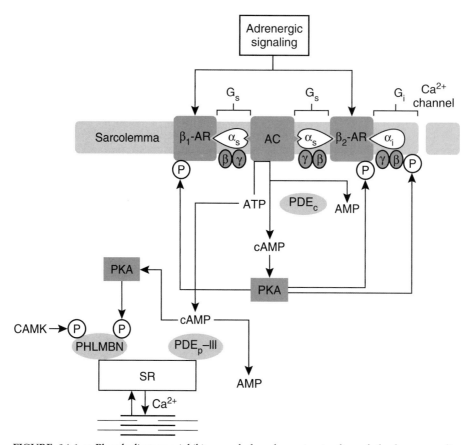

FIGURE 34-1 ■ **Phosphodiesterase inhibitors and the adrenergic signaling of the human cardiac myocyte.** Adrenergic receptor activation leads to increase in adenylate cyclase (AC) activity and subsequently cytosolic cyclic AMP (cAMP) formation. As a result, cAMP-dependent protein kinase A (PKA) is activated and increases the activities of intracellular cardiac proteins via phosphorylation. All of this activity results in increased force and speed of cardiac contraction and relaxation. One mechanism by which this activity is accomplished is via phosphorylation of the inhibitory actions of phospholamban (PHLMBN), which inhibits the calcium pump of the sarcoplasmic reticulum (SR). Phosphodiesterase inhibitors work via inhibition of the isoenzyme phosphodiesterase (PDE$_p$-III) related to the SR. The resultant increase in cAMP activates the cAMP-dependent PKA, which also disinhibits the SR via its phosphorylation of PHLMBN. All of these interactions lead to liberation of cytosolic calcium via the SR and to increase in the rate of calcium reuptake into the SR. The latter action increases the rate of relaxation. β$_1$-AR, β$_1$-adrenergic receptor; β$_2$-AR, β$_2$-adrenergic receptor; CAMK, calmodin-activated kinase; G$_i$, inhibitory G protein with α, β,and γ subunits; G$_s$, stimulatory G protein with α, β, and γ subunits; PDE$_c$, cytosolic phosphodiesterase; PDE$_p$, particulate SR-associated PDE III. (From Bristow MR, Port JD, Kelly RA: *Treatment of heart failure: Pharmacological methods.* In Braunwald E, Zipes DP, Libby P [eds]: *Heart Disease.* Philadelphia, WB Saunders, 2001, pp 579-581.)

blunting of the response to PDEIs, however, secondary to up-regulation of inhibitory G protein[17] and tachyphylaxis. PDEIs in the setting of acute heart failure may be beneficial in the case of increasing adrenergic support that fails to sustain adequate myocardial contractility and cardiac output. A reduction in the need for adrenergic support with the use of PDEIs also may allow up-regulation of α-receptors and β-receptors.

The PDEIs have other advantages over conventional catecholamines. First, higher doses of catecholamines can increase myocardial oxygen consumption; this is observed much less frequently with PDEIs because these agents increase inotropic state without concomitant increase in heart rate, resulting in a favorable myocardial oxygen supply-and-demand balance.[18]

This favorable balance is a considerable advantage in patients with decreased coronary flow reserve. Second, the propensity for dysrhythmias seen with prolonged use of catecholamines at higher doses usually is not associated with PDEIs in children. In addition to augmenting cardiac contractility, PDEIs result in cAMP-mediated vasodilation of arterial (systemic and pulmonary) and venous capacitance vessels. The vasodilating properties of PDEIs are superior to those of β-adrenergic agents, including isoproterenol.[19] Lastly, these agents also possess lusitropic properties, promoting diastolic ventricular relaxation as measured by micromanometer-derived time constant of left ventricular isovolumic relaxation τ.[20] PDEIs have an advantageous role when cardiac output is highly dependent on ventricular

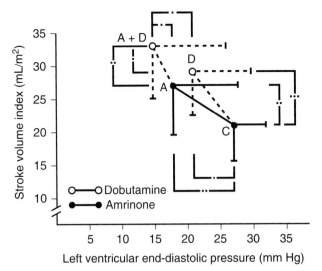

FIGURE 34-2 ■ Synergy between dobutamine (D) and amrinone (A). The hemodynamic effects of D, A, and both (A + D) are graphed with stroke volume index versus left ventricular end-diastolic pressure as parameters. As illustrated here, the additive effect of A + D resulted in a higher stroke volume index at a lower left ventricular end-diastolic pressure. (From Gage J, Rutman H, Lucido D, et al: *Additive effects of contractility and ventricular performance in patients with severe heart failure. Circulation* 1986;74:367-372.)

relaxation (e.g., patients after tetralogy of Fallot repair or after cavopulmonary anastomosis or Fontan operations).

Despite all of the aforementioned theoretical advantages of PDEIs over conventional adrenergic agents, there is evidence that a combined strategy is superior to single-drug regimen because there is synergy between these two classes of agents in treating the failing myocardium.[21] The addition of amrinone to any dose of dobutamine produced a higher cardiac index and lower systemic vascular resistance than either dobutamine or amrinone alone (Fig. 34-2).

PHOSPHODIESTERASE INHIBITOR USE IN ADULTS WITH HEART FAILURE

Amrinone

Amrinone (Inocor), the first PDEI used in clinical situations, is metabolized primarily by glucuronidation and acetylation, so the half-life can be unpredictable. Adults usually require a loading dose of 0.75 mg/kg and an infusion of 5 to 10 μg/kg/min. Major **side effects** include hypotension (which may be lessened with a slower infusion of the loading dose and concomitant infusion of volume), atrial or ventricular arrhythmias, and non-immune thrombocytopenia, which may be caused by the metabolite of amrinone, *N*-acetylamrinone.

Amrinone not only has the inotropic properties of catecholamines, but also the vasodilating properties of vasodilators. **Hemodynamic effects** of amrinone in adults include increase in cardiac index, increase in

pressure change over time, decrease in left ventricular end-diastolic pressure, and decreases in pulmonary capillary wedge pressure and right atrial pressure in patients with heart failure and in patients after cardiac surgery.[22,23]

Several studies have addressed the use of amrinone in patients after **cardiopulmonary bypass** (CPB). Hardy and Belisle,[24] reporting on the Montreal experience, suggested that type III PDEIs have a beneficial role in weaning failing hearts from CPB with specific beneficial effects on myocardial ischemia and reperfusion injury. In addition, a single intravenous dose of amrinone (1.5 mg/kg) improved velocity of circumferential fiber shortening and lowered systemic and pulmonary vascular resistances in adult patients after separation from CPB.[25] Patients undergoing elective surgery randomized to receive intravenous amrinone as prophylaxis had a significantly lower risk of failure to wean from CPB (7% versus 21%; *P* = .002), although this was statistically significant only in the group with left ventricular ejection fractions greater than 55%.[26] Hepatosplanchnic flow also has been shown to be improved with the use of PDEIs after cardiac surgery.[27]

Milrinone

Milrinone (Primacor), a more potent and more selective congener of amrinone, is designated chemically as 1,6-dihydro-2-methyl-6-oxo-(3,4′bipyridine)-5-carbonitrile lactate with an empirical formula of $C_{12}H_9N_{30}$. Milrinone is primarily bound to human plasma protein (70%) and excreted via the kidney as unchanged drug (83% of dose) and the rest of its glucuronide conjugate (12%). The usual dose in adults is 25 to 50 μg/kg bolus over 10 minutes followed by an infusion of 0.25 to 1 μg/kg/min. Milrinone exhibits a concentration-dependent response, and optimal effects are reported at 100 to 300 ng/mL.[28] Compared with amrinone, milrinone has the advantages of having a shorter half-life and a greater selectivity for the isoenzyme phosphodiesterase III.

Side effects include arrhythmias, which have been reported in 12.1% of adult patients with ventricular ectopy, nonsustained ventricular tachycardia, sustained ventricular tachycardia, and ventricular fibrillation. Milrinone also produces slight shortening of atrioventricular node conduction time, indicating the potential for increased ventricular response in patients with atrial flutter or fibrillation. Other side effects include hypotension (which can be stabilized with coadministration of low-dose dopamine at 4 μg/kg/min),[29] angina, headaches, hypokalemia, and tremor. The incidence of thrombocytopenia (0.4%) is significantly less than encountered with amrinone (2.4%).[30] There have been isolated reports of spontaneous bronchospasm and development of abnormal liver function tests.

Milrinone is termed an inodilator. For the equivalent increase in cardiac output, milrinone is superior to dobutamine in lowering systemic vascular resistance. Similarly, for the same decrease in mean arterial blood

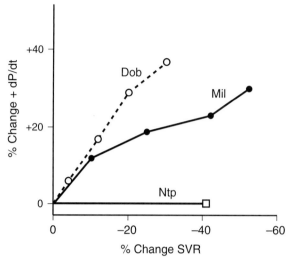

FIGURE 34-3 ■ Comparison of milrinone (Mil) with dobutamine (Dob) and nitroprusside (Ntp). The hemodynamic effects of Dob, Mil, and Ntp are shown with % change + pressure change over time (dP/dt) as a parameter of contractility and % change systemic vascular resistance (SVR). Mil, as an inodilator, for the equivalent increase in cardiac output, is superior to Dob in lowering SVR. Similarly, for the same decrease in mean arterial blood pressure, Mil is superior to Ntp in augmenting cardiac output. (From Colucci WS, Wright RF, Jaski BE, et al: *Milrinone and dobutamine in severe heart failure: Differing hemodynamic effects and individual patient responsiveness. Circulation* 1986;73:III-175-III-183.)

pressure, milrinone is superior to nitroprusside in augmenting cardiac output (Fig. 34-3).[31]

An early study reported significant hemodynamic benefits in a study of 20 patients with severe congestive heart failure (CHF),[32] including significant decreases in left ventricular end-diastolic pressure (27 ± 2 to 18 ± 2 mm Hg), pulmonary wedge pressure, systemic vascular resistance, and right atrial pressure and significant increases in cardiac index (1.9 ± 0.1 to 2.9 ± 0.2 L/min/ m²) and pressure change over time. Nineteen of these patients subsequently were transitioned to oral milrinone with continued improvement in symptoms. There were no reported complications during the study period.

The **Outcomes of a Prospective Trial of Intravenous Milrinone (Milrinone) for Exacerbation of Chronic Heart Failure (OPTIME-CHF)**[33] study investigated the interaction between the etiology of underlying CHF and the response to milrinone in patients with decompensated CHF. This was a prospective randomized trial with 949 patients with systolic dysfunction and decompensated CHF randomized to receive 48 to 72 hours of intravenous milrinone or placebo. The primary end point was days hospitalized from cardiac causes within 60 days of treatment. In this study, the primary end point was 13 days for ischemic patients and 11.7 days for nonischemic patients. Milrinone-treated patients with ischemic heart disease had a worse outcome than nonischemic patients in terms of the primary end point and composite of death or rehospitalization (42% versus 36% for placebo). In contrast, nonischemic patients treated with milrinone

improved in terms of primary end point and composite for death or rehospitalization (28% versus 35% placebo). This study showed bidirectional effect based on etiology of decompensated CHF in adults.

In the **postoperative setting**, a single loading dose of milrinone (50 μg/kg) was shown to facilitate weaning of adult patients from CPB with preexisting left ventricular dysfunction after coronary bypass graft surgery.[34] Studies have shown improvements in cardiac index and velocity of circumferential fiber shortening and left ventricular compliance in patients weaning from CPB treated with milrinone.[35,36] Recognized benefits of early PDEI administration after CPB include increased inotropy (left and right ventricles) and pulmonary vasodilation, possibly avoiding the need for mechanical assistance or placement on extracorporeal membrane oxygenation.[37,38] There is also good evidence for milrinone providing hemodynamic benefit and improving right ventricular diastolic function before[39] and after cardiac transplantation, even in the face of recipient chronic pulmonary hypertension.[40,41] Finally, milrinone increases cerebral blood flow after CPB.[42]

Oral milrinone clinical trials failed to show the same beneficial effects that the intravenous form had shown. The **Prospective Randomized Milrinone Survival Evaluation (PROMISE)**[43] study was one of the largest studies to date assessing the efficacy of oral milrinone in adults with severe chronic heart failure. This was a randomized prospective study assessing 1088 patients with severe CHF (New York Heart Association class III or IV) and advanced left ventricular dysfunction in which patients were allocated to a treatment group with oral milrinone, 40 mg daily (*n* = 561), or a placebo group (*n* = 527). In addition, all patients received conventional therapy with digoxin, diuretics, and angiotensin-converting enzyme inhibitor during the trial. The median follow-up duration was 6.1 months (range 1 day to 20 months). Compared with placebo, milrinone therapy was associated with a 28% increase in mortality from all causes (*P* = .038) and a 34% increase in mortality from cardiovascular causes (*P* = .016). Milrinone did not have a beneficial effect on survival in any treatment group. In addition, patients in the treatment group had more hospitalizations, were withdrawn from double-blinded therapy more frequently, and had more serious side effects, including hypotension and syncope. This study concluded that milrinone had deleterious side effects in treatment of adults with CHF, and the study was stopped before the proposed study end by the data and safety monitoring board.

Enoximone

Enoximone is a selective class III PDEI that is less potent than milrinone. It is available in oral form in Europe and the United States, but in intravenous form only in Europe. It is metabolized in the liver, but its metabolite is excreted in the kidney, so patients with renal or hepatic failure require dosage adjustments.

Prophylactic use of intravenous enoximone was found to be efficacious in older adults undergoing coronary artery graft surgery by decreasing the magnitude of post-CPB inflammation.[44] Enoximone initially was associated with an increased mortality rate and adverse effects when used in adults with CHF at doses of 4 to 5 mg/kg/day.[45] Follow-up studies on enoximone were more promising, however. Use of lower enoximone dosing (<3 mg/kg/day) regimens was successful in improving symptoms and medically bridging patients to cardiac transplantation.[46] In another investigation, Shakar and coworkers[47] combined low-dose enoximone with a β-blocker (metoprolol) in New York Heart Association class IV heart failure patients and showed significant improvements in functional classification and left ventricular ejection fraction in these patients. Lowes and associates[48] showed that low-dose enoximone improves exercise capacity after 12 weeks of therapy compared with placebo therapy in adults with New York Heart Association class II or III heart failure.

Vesnarinone

Vesnarinone is a quinolone-type PDEI that has hemodynamic benefits similar to the other PDEIs and class III antiarrhythmic properties, although the latter effect may not protect this drug from its proarrhythmic potential for ventricular arrhythmias.[49] Vesnarinone also is reported to be a potential cytokine inhibitor via inhibition of excessive cytotoxicity of natural killer cells.[50]

In the **Vesnarinone Survival Trial (VEST)**,[51] a short-term, placebo-controlled study, vesnarinone was shown to increase mortality in patients with severe heart failure when given at a dose of 60 mg/day. This study randomized 3833 patients with New York Heart Association class III or IV heart failure and a left ventricular ejection fraction of 30% or less despite optimal medical management to 60 mg/day of vesnarinone, 30 mg/day of vesnarinone, or placebo. There was a significant increase in mortality in the group receiving 60 mg/day, predominantly related to arrhythmic events. Quality of life improved significantly, however, in the vesnarinone group compared with the placebo group at 8 weeks (P < .001) and 16 weeks (P = .003). In a meta-analysis, Nony and colleagues[52] reported that patients with overt chronic CHF who took PDEIs compared with placebo were at increased risk of dying, but patients who took vesnarinone compared with placebo had a reduced risk of death. Despite the differences in these studies, vesnarinone has been discontinued in the United States.

ALTERNATIVE USES OF PHOSPHODIESTERASE INHIBITORS

Tsuchikane and associates[53] showed that cilostazol, a new PDEI that suppresses platelet aggregation and acts as a direct arterial vasodilator, significantly reduced restenosis after percutaneous coronary balloon angioplasty.

This beneficial effect may be secondary to increased synthesis of coronary vascular nitric oxide or cAMP-mediated inhibition of platelet aggregation, thrombus generation, and cytokine activation and smooth muscle proliferation.[54] PDEIs also have been shown to have beneficial effects in lung disease by improving right ventricular ejection fraction and oxygen delivery in canine oleic acid pulmonary injury[55] and ameliorating lung compliance in cardiogenic pulmonary edema.[56] In endotoxemic shock, endotoxin lipopolysaccharide previously was shown to be a trigger for systemic inflammatory response syndrome.[57] In an animal model, vesnarinone and amrinone were shown to prevent cytokine production and sepsis-related cardiac dysfunction.[58] Vesnarinone, when given in a rescue mode after endotoxemia, normalized sepsis-induced myocardial dysfunction and partially restored abnormal calcium cycling.[59] The authors concluded that although the underlying etiologies to these effects require further study, vesnarinone may be a useful agent in treating inflammatory-induced myocardial dysfunction. Lastly, amrinone has been shown to produce pulmonary vasodilation in an animal model of sepsis.[60]

The use of PDEIs can be extended to the microvasculature. In plastic surgery, amrinone improves survival of muscle flaps in reconstructive surgery via its microcirculation-enhancing effects.[61] Amrinone also has been used as a topical vasodilating agent.[62] Treatments for peripheral vascular disease usually include antiplatelet agents, and in more recent years PDEIs have been added to the treatment regimen.[63] New PDEIs with calcium-sensitizing activity, such as levosimendan[64] and pimobendan,[65] are discussed in Chapter 38.

PHOSPHODIESTERASE INHIBITOR USE IN CHILDREN

Because of the early data on the concentration-dependent negative inotropic effect of amrinone in a neonatal piglet model[66] and the unfavorable result of the adult milrinone clinical trial described previously, there were initial doubts about the use of PDEIs in children with heart failure. In contrast to amrinone, milrinone was shown to have a positive inotropic effect on the postischemic neonatal pig myocardium.[67] A subsequent study showed that the mechanism for milrinone to benefit the postischemic neonatal myocardium may be due to its potentiation of mitochondrial oxidative phosphorylation.[68] With increasing acceptance of milrinone as an inotropic agent with vasodilating properties in the treatment of heart failure in children, the broadest application of milrinone has been in children with low cardiac output syndrome after cardiac surgery.

Amrinone

Some authors report a larger bolus requirement of amrinone of 3 to 4 mg/kg in children.[69] Lawless and associates[70] recommended a lower infusion rate for neonates (3 to 5 μg/kg/min versus 10 μg/kg/min for infants). In a separate study, neonates were found to have a longer elimination half-life than infants.[71]

An early study on amrinone use in children with **pulmonary hypertension** showed that amrinone produced the greatest reduction in pulmonary vascular resistance in patients with increased pulmonary artery pressure and pulmonary vascular resistance.[72] Based on these data, amrinone should be avoided in patients with pulmonary hypertension and left-to-right shunt lesions because pulmonary overcirculation would be exacerbated. In patients with post- operative pulmonary hypertension without left-to-right shunting, amrinone would be beneficial because it is an efficacious pulmonary vasodilator.

Several studies, usually in small numbers of patients after cardiac surgery, examined the hemodynamic profile of amrinone. The use of amrinone in pediatric patients after **cardiac surgery** showed a decrease in systemic vascular resistance with or without concomitant increase in cardiac index.[73,74] Amrinone use was shown to be superior to a combined dopamine-nitroglycerin regimen in cardiac output after arterial switch operation and repair for complete atrioventricular septal defect.[75,76] Bailey and coworkers[77] compared the hemodynamic effects of amrinone versus sodium nitroprusside in 10 infants after cardiac surgery and showed that only amrinone resulted in a significant increase in cardiac index, but both agents resulted in decreases in mean blood pressure and systemic vascular resistance. Amrinone was found to have positive inotropic effects in infants after cardiac surgery by Teshima and colleagues,[78] who used echocardiographic indices such as velocity of circumferential fiber shortening corrected for heart rate and the stress-velocity index. A study examining the hemodynamic effects of amrinone after the Fontan operation also concluded that amrinone was effective in increasing cardiac output in these children.[79] Lastly, CPB may have significant effects on bioavailability of PDEIs such as amrinone. Williams and colleagues[80] found that after CPB approximately 20% of the drug becomes bound to the circuit, and after correcting for circuit uptake, serum amrinone levels were increased higher than predicted. CPB may result in significant perturbations in volume of distribution and the effects of PDEIs. In children with septic shock, a short-term dose-response study showed that amrinone improved cardiac index and oxygen delivery.[81]

Milrinone

For pediatric patients, a low-dose strategy for milrinone entails a bolus of 25 μg/kg followed by an infusion rate of 0.25 to 0.50 μg/kg/min, whereas a higher dose regimen includes a bolus of 50 to 75 μg/kg followed by an infusion of 0.50 to 1 μg/kg/min.[82] To avoid hypotension, the bolus dose can be administered over a longer period with concomitant volume infusion to minimize decrease in blood pressure.

To date, only a few studies have assessed the usefulness and efficacy of milrinone in children with low cardiac output state after **cardiac surgery**. Chang and associates[83] conducted the initial prospective study assessing intravenous milrinone use (bolus dose of 50 μg/kg over 10 minutes followed by an infusion of 0.50 μg/kg/min) in 10 neonates with low cardiac output syndrome after surgical repair of congenital heart defects. In their study, milrinone significantly improved the cardiac index from 2.1 ± 0.5 to 3 ± 0.8 L/min/m², reduced mean arterial pressure from 66 ± 12 to 57 ± 10 mm Hg, and decreased systemic and pulmonary vascular resistances by 37% and 27% (Fig. 34-4). The estimated myocardial oxygen consumption as indicated by pressure rate index remained unaffected, and there were no significant dysrhythmias. In addition, Bailey and coworkers[84] assessed the efficacy of milrinone in 20 children 3 to 22 months old with low cardiac output in the postoperative period. They reported a mean increase in cardiac index of 18% at a mean serum concentration of 235 ng/mL. The authors also recommended that children receive a bolus dose of 50 μg/kg before initiation of a 0.50 μg/kg/min maintenance infusion. Others have confirmed the increased volume of distribution and faster clearance with milrinone in children.[85]

The **Prophylactic Intravenous Use of Milrinone After Cardiac Operation in Pediatrics (PRIMACORP)** study was a large double-blinded, placebo-controlled trial with three parallel groups. More than 200 patients were treated with (1) a low-dose protocol, 25 μg/kg bolus over 1 hour followed by 0.25 μg/kg/min infusion for 35 hours; (2) a high-dose protocol, 75 μg/kg bolus followed by 0.75 μg/kg/min infusion over 35 hours; or (3) placebo. The clinical end point was a composite end point of death or development of low cardiac output state at 36 hours. The conclusion of this study was that a high-dose milrinone regimen significantly reduced the incidence of low cardiac output state with a relative risk reduction of 64% (Fig. 34-5). Experience with milrinone in complex single-ventricle neonates is small.[86]

A prospective double-blinded, placebo-controlled study assessed milrinone use in 12 children (age range 9 months to 15 years) with nonhyperdynamic **septic shock**.[87] This study showed significant increases in cardiac index, stroke volume index, right and left ventricular stroke work index, and oxygen delivery at 0.5, 1, and 2 hours after loading dosing in the treatment group without adverse events. A relatively high dose may be necessary in these septic shock pediatric patients for hemodynamic benefit.[88]

Enoximone

Pediatric experience with enoximone is limited, and the little experience principally comes from Europe. In an early study on infants after cardiac surgery, enoximone at a dose of 7.5 to 10 μg/kg/min (after a bolus dose

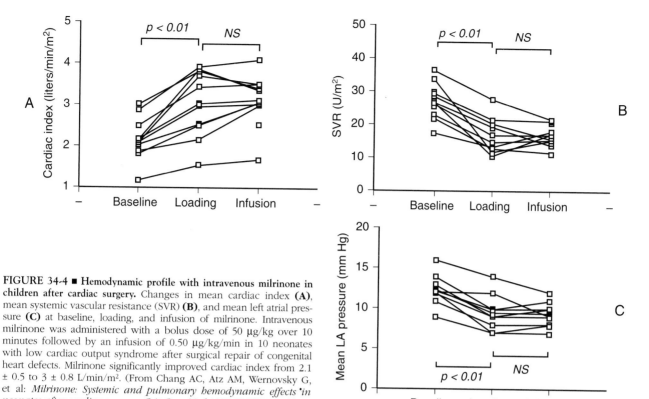

FIGURE 34-4 ■ **Hemodynamic profile with intravenous milrinone in children after cardiac surgery.** Changes in mean cardiac index **(A)**, mean systemic vascular resistance (SVR) **(B)**, and mean left atrial pressure **(C)** at baseline, loading, and infusion of milrinone. Intravenous milrinone was administered with a bolus dose of 50 μg/kg over 10 minutes followed by an infusion of 0.50 μg/kg/min in 10 neonates with low cardiac output syndrome after surgical repair of congenital heart defects. Milrinone significantly improved cardiac index from 2.1 ± 0.5 to 3 ± 0.8 L/min/m². (From Chang AC, Atz AM, Wernovsky G, et al: *Milrinone: Systemic and pulmonary hemodynamic effects in neonates after cardiac surgery. Crit Care Med* 1995;33:1907-1914.)

of 0.2 to 1 mg/kg) showed an increase in cardiac index by 28%,[89] and a more recent study showed a similar dosing range of 10 μg/kg/min infusion preceded by a bolus of 1 mg/kg.[90] In later studies on postoperative patients, various authors showed the expected hemodynamic improvements with enoximone in the presence

of low cardiac output syndrome.[91,92] Lastly, a study comparing enoximone (0.5 mg/kg bolus followed by an infusion of 10 μg/kg/min) with combination therapy of phenoxybenzamine and dobutamine showed that enoximone conferred no advantage in cardiac index or left ventricular stroke work index.[93]

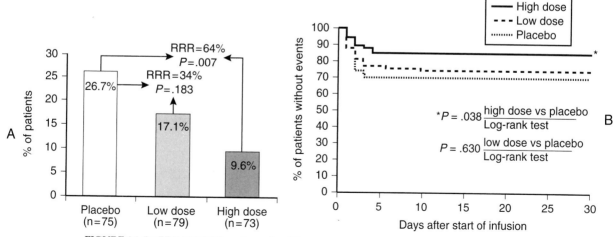

FIGURE 34-5 ■ **PRIMACORP study results. (A)** Primary end points of the PRIMACORP study: death or low cardiac output syndrome (LCOS) in the first 36 hours after study initiation (*n* = 227). There was a 64% relative risk reduction (RRR) in high-dose protocol patients compared with placebo patients. **(B)** Time to development of LCOS/death through final visit in patients treated with placebo, low-dose milrinone, and high-dose milrinone. Six additional patients developed LCOS after discontinuation of the drug infusion. (From Hoffman TM, Wernovsky G, Atz AM, et al: *Efficacy and safety of milrinone in preventing low cardiac output syndrome in infants and children after corrective surgery for congenital heart disease. Circulation* 2003;107:996-1002.)

CURRENT STATUS AND FUTURE TRENDS

PDEIs have become essential pharmacologic agents in the management of adults and children with CHF and low cardiac output syndrome. These agents augment myocardial contractility, increase venous and arterial dilation, and possess specific lusitropic effects with few side effects; PDEIs possess these properties without any increase in myocardial oxygen consumption. Milrinone has become a widely used PDEI in pediatric patients, especially in augmenting cardiac output after cardiac surgery and in septic shock, but also may include outpatient use in the near future. Additional studies could be directed toward more pharmacokinetic and pharmacodynamic profiles of milrinone and other new selective PDEIs in neonates and children. The PDEIs with calcium-sensitizing activity, such as levosimendan, may have a potential role in the pharmacologic support of the myocardium in the future.[94]

Key Points

■ The hemodynamic effects of PDEIs, increased inotropy and vasodilation with concomitant improved lusitropy, are unique as a class of cardiotonic drugs.

■ Milrinone, with its shorter half-life, fewer side effects, and greater selectivity for the phosphodiesterase III isoenzyme, has become the PDEI of choice in the management of heart failure in the intensive care unit and the outpatient setting.

■ PDEIs have a selective effect on the function of the SR because local increase in cAMP leads to activation of protein kinase A, which phosphorylates phospholamban. Because phospholamban normally inhibits the function of the SR by hindering its calcium pump, the phosphorylation of phospholamban by cAMP in effect disinhibits the SR and liberates cytosolic calcium. This relatively isolated effect on the SR explains why highly type III–specific PDEIs increase inotropic state without concomitant increase in heart rate.

■ The relaxation of the myocardium is accelerated by reduction of cytosolic calcium (secondary to more efficient removal of calcium into the SR via the activated ATPase protein), and the vasodilatory effect of PDEIs is secondary to activation of protein kinase G by cAMP.

■ The main hemodynamic effects of PDEIs include increase in cardiac output, decreases in systemic and pulmonary vascular resistances, and decrease in filling pressures. These favorable changes occur usually without increase in myocardial oxygen consumption (as measured by heart rate–pressure product) to result in an increase in left ventricular external efficiency. There is acceleration of isovolumic relaxation to indicate improved diastolic filling.

■ Other cardiac effects of PDEIs include dilation of epicardial coronary arteries and grafts, anti-ischemic effects on myocardium, and inhibition of proinflammatory cytokines. All of these additional effects are particularly beneficial in the postoperative cardiac surgical patient.

■ One decided advantage for PDEIs is that these agents mediate their physiologic properties without interaction with myocardial β-receptors and are relatively independent from effects of receptor regulation. This ability is especially useful in heart failure because there is considerable down-regulation of β-receptors; there is blunting of response to PDEIs, however, secondary to up-regulation of inhibitory G protein and tachyphylaxis.

■ There is evidence that a combined strategy is superior to single-drug therapy because there is synergy between these two classes of agents (adrenergic agents and PDEIs) in treating the failing myocardium.

■ Milrinone is considered an inodilator. For the equivalent increase in cardiac output, milrinone is superior to dobutamine in lowering systemic vascular resistance. Similarly, for the same decrease in mean arterial blood pressure, milrinone is superior to nitroprusside in augmenting cardiac output.

REFERENCES

1. Alousi AA, Farah AE, Lesher GY, et al: Cardiotonic activity of amrinone—Win 40680 (5-amino-3,4′-bipyridine-6(1H)-one). Circ Res 1979;45:666-667.
2. Feldman AM, McNamara DM: Reevaluating the role of phosphodiesterase inhibitors in the treatment of cardiovascular disease. Clin Cardiol 2002;25:256-262.
3. Hoffman TM, Wernovsky G, Atz AM, et al: Efficacy and safety of milrinone in preventing low cardiac output syndrome in infants and children after corrective surgery for congenital heart disease. Circulation 2003;107:996-1002.
4. Sutherland EW: On the biological role of cyclic AMP. JAMA 1970;214:1281-1288.
5. Robison GA, Butcher RW, Sutherland EW: Cyclic AMP. Annu Rev Biochem 1968;37:149-174.
6. Endoh M, Yamashita S, Taira N: Positive inotropic effect of amrinone in relation to cyclic nucleotide metabolism in the canine ventricular muscle. J Pharmacol Exp Ther 1982;221:775-783.
7. Colucci WS, Wright RF, Braunwald E: New positive inotropic agents in the treatment of congestive heart failure: Mechanisms of action and recent clinical developments. N Engl J Med 1986;314:290-299.
8. Bristow MR, Port JD, Kelly RA: Treatment of heart failure: Pharmacological methods. In Braunwald E, Zipes DP, Libby P (eds): Heart Disease, 6th ed. Philadelphia, WB Saunders, 2001, pp 579-581.
9. Jiang H, Colbran JL, Francis SH, et al: Direct evidence for cross-activation of cGMP-dependent protein kinase by cAMP in pig coronary arteries. J Biol Chem 1992;267:1015-1019.
10. Anderson JL, Baim DS, Fein SA, et al: Efficacy and safety of sustained intravenous infusions of milrinone in patients with severe congestive heart failure: A multicenter study. J Am Coll Cardiol 1987;9:711-722.
11. Monrad ES, Baim DS, Smith HS, et al: Effects of milrinone on coronary hemodynamics and myocardial energetics in patients with congestive heart failure. Circulation 1985;71:972-979.
12. Colucci WS: Cardiovascular effects of milrinone. Am Heart J 1991;121(6 Pt 2):1945-1947.

13. Cracowski JL, Stanke-Labesque F, Chavanon O, et al: Vasorelaxant actions of enoximone, dobutamine, and the combination on human arterial coronary bypass grafts. J Cardiovasc Pharmacol 1999;34:741-748.

14. Liu JJ, Doolan LA, Xie B, et al: Direct vasodilator effect of milrinone, an inotropic drug, on arterial coronary bypass grafts. FANZCA. J Thorac Cardiovasc Surg 1997;113:108-113.

15. Mitrovic V, Petrovic O, Bahavar H, et al: Antiischemic and hemodynamic effects of an oral single dose of 150 mg of the phosphodiesterase inhibitor enoximone in patients with coronary artery disease: Relation to plasma concentration. Cardiovasc Drugs Ther 1991;5:689-695.

16. Hayashida N, Tomoeda H, Oda T, et al: Inhibitory effect of milrinone on cytokine production after cardiopulmonary bypass. Ann Thorac Surg 1999;68:1661-1667.

17. Neumann J, Schmitz W, Scholz H, et al: Increase in myocardial Gi proteins in heart failure. Lancet 1988;2:936-937.

18. Baim DS: Effect of phosphodiesterase inhibition on myocardial oxygen consumption and coronary blood flow. Am J Cardiol 1989;63:23A-26A.

19. Firth BG, Ratner AV, Grassman ED, et al: Assessment of inotropic and vasodilator effects of amrinone versus isoproterenol. Am J Cardiol 1984;54:1331-1336.

20. Monrad ES, McKay RG, Baim DS, et al: Improvement in indexes of diastolic performance in patients with congestive heart failure treated with milrinone. Circulation 1984;70:1030-1037.

21. Gage J, Rutman H, Lucido D, et al: Additive effects of dobutamine and amrinone on myocardial contractility and ventricular performance in patients with severe heart failure. Circulation 1986;74:367-372.

22. LeJemtel T, Keung E, Sonnenblick EH: Amrinone: A new nonglycosidic, nonadrenergic cardiotonic agent effective in the treatment of intractable myocardial failure in man. Circulation 1979;59:1098-1104.

23. Goenen M, Pedermonte O, Baele P: Amrinone in the management of low cardiac output after open heart surgery. Am J Cardiol 1990;56:33B-38B.

24. Hardy JF, Belisle S: Inotropic support of the heart that fails to successfully wean from cardiopulmonary bypass: The Montreal Heart Institute experience. J Cardiothorac Vasc Anesth 1993;7:33-39.

25. Kikura M, Levy JH, Bailey JM, et al: A bolus of 1.5 mg/kg amrinone effectively improves low cardiac output state following separation from cardiopulmonary bypass in cardiac surgical patients. Acta Anaesthesiol Scand 1998;42:825-833.

26. Lewis KP, Appadurai IR, Pierce ET, et al: Prophylactic amrinone for weaning from cardiopulmonary bypass. Anaesthesia 2000;55:627-633.

27. Iribe G, Yamada H, Matsunaga A, et al: Effects of the phosphodiesterase III inhibitors, amrinone, milrinone, and olprinone on the hepatosplanchnic oxygen metabolism. Crit Care Med 2000;28:743-748.

28. Levy JH, Bailey JM, Deeb GM: Intravenous milrinone in cardiac surgery. Ann Thorac Surg 2002;73:325-330.

29. Karasawa F, Okuda T, Tsutsui M, et al: Dopamine stabilizes milrinone-induced changes in heart rate and arterial pressure during anesthesia with isoflurane. Eur Anaesthesiol 2003;20:120-123.

30. Kikura M, Lee MK, Safon RA: The effects of milrinone on platelets in patients undergoing cardiac surgery. Anesth Analg 1995;81:44-48.

31. Colucci WS, Wright RF, Jaski BE, et al: Milrinone and dobutamine in severe heart failure: Differing hemodynamic effects and individual patient responsiveness. Circulation 1986;73:III-175-III-183.

32. Baim DS, McDowell AV, Cherniles J, et al: Evolution of a new bipyridine inotropic agent—milrinone—in patients with severe congestive heart failure. N Engl J Med 1983;309:748-756.

33. Felker GM, Benza RL, Chandler AB, et al: Heart failure etiology and response to milrinone in decompensated heart failure: Results from the OPTIME-CHF study. J Am Coll Cardiol 2003;41:997-1003.

34. Lobato EB, Florete O Jr, Bingham HL: A single dose of milrinone facilitates separation from cardiopulmonary bypass in patients with pre-existing left ventricular dysfunction. Br J Anaesth 1998;81:782-784.

35. Kikura M, Levy JH, Michelsen LG, et al: The effect of milrinone on hemodynamics and left ventricular function after emergence from cardiopulmonary bypass. Anesth Analg 1997;85:16-22.

36. Lobato EB, Gravenstein N, Martin TD: Milrinone, not epinephrine, improves left ventricular compliance after cardiopulmonary bypass. J Cardiothorac Vasc Anesth 2000;14:374-377.

37. Doolan LA, Jones EF, Kalman J, et al: A placebo-controlled trial verifying the efficacy of milrinone in weaning high-risk patients from cardiopulmonary bypass. J Cardiothorac Vasc Anesth 1997;11:37-41.

38. Doyle AR, Dhir AK, Moors AH, et al: Treatment of perioperative low cardiac output syndrome. Ann Thorac Surg 1995;59:S3-S11.

39. Aranda JM, Schofield RS, Pauly DF, et al: Comparison of dobutamine versus milrinone therapy hospitalized patients awaiting cardiac transplantation: A prospective, randomized trial. Am Heart J 2003;145:324-329.

40. Chen EP, Bittner HB, David RD, et al: Hemodynamic and inotropic effects of milrinone after heart transplantation in the setting of recipient pulmonary hypertension. J Heart Lung Transplant 1998;17:669-678.

41. Chen EP, Craig DM, Bittner HB, et al: Pharmacological strategies for improving diastolic dysfunction in the setting of chronic pulmonary hypertension. Circulation 1998;97:1606-1612.

42. Sulek CA, Blas ML, Lobato EB: Milrinone increases middle cerebral artery blood flow velocity after cardiopulmonary bypass. J Cardiothorac Vasc Anesth 2002;16:64-69.

43. Packer M, Carver JR, Rodeheffer RJ, et al: Effect of oral milrinone on mortality in severe chronic heart failure. The PROMISE Study Research Group. N Engl J Med 1991;325:1468-1475.

44. Boldt J, Brosch C, Sutter S, et al: Prophylactic use of the phosphodiesterase III inhibitor enoximone in elderly cardiac surgery patients: Effect on hemodynamics, inflammation, and markers of organ function. Intensive Care Med 2002;28:1462-1469.

45. Uretsky BF, Jessup M, Konstam MA, et al, for the Enoximone Multicenter Trial Group: Multicenter trial of oral enoximone in patients with moderate to moderately severe congestive heart failure. Circulation 1990;82:774-780.

46. Narahara KA: Oral enoximone therapy in chronic heart failure: A placebo controlled randomized trial. The Western Enoximone Study Group. Am Heart J 1991;121:1471-1479.

47. Shakar SF, Abraham WT, Gilbert EM, et al: Combined oral positive inotropic and beta-blocker therapy for treatment of refractory class IV heart failure. J Am Coll Cardiol 1998;31:1336-1340.

48. Lowes BD, Higginbotham MB, Petrovich L, et al: Low-dose enoximone improves exercise capacity in chronic heart failure. J Am Coll Cardiol 2000;36:501-508.

49. Yoshimura A, Yoshioka K, Hino M, et al: Investigation on SCH00013, a novel cardiotonic agent with Ca+ sensitizing action: Influence on experimentally induced ventricular arrhythmias in dogs. Arzneimittelforschung 1999;49:420-426.

50. Sasayama S, Matsumori A: Vesnarinone: A potential cytokine inhibitor. J Card Fail 1996;2:251-258.

51. Cohn JN, Goldstein SO, Greenberg BH, et al: A dose-dependent increase in mortality with vesnarinone among patients with severe heart failure. Vesnarinone Trial Investigators. N Engl J Med 1998;339:1810-1816.

52. Nony P, Boissel JP, Lievre M, et al: Evaluation of the effect of phosphodiesterase inhibitors on mortality in chronic heart failure patients: A meta-analysis. Eur J Clin Pharmacol 1994;46:191-196.

53. Tsuchikane E, Fukuhara A, Kobayashi T, et al: Impact of cilostazol on restenosis after percutaneous coronary balloon angioplasty. Circulation 1999;100:21-26.

54. Ikeda U, Ikeda M, Kano S, et al: Effect of cilostazol, a cAMP phosphodiesterase inhibitor, on nitric oxide production by vascular smooth muscle cells. Eur J Pharmacol 1996;314:197-202.

55. Ishikawa S, Nakazawa K, Yokooyama K, et al: Amrinone improves right ventricular ejection fraction and oxygen delivery without deterioration of extravascular lung water in canine oleic acid pulmonary injury. Anaesth Intensive Care 1998;26:355-359.

56. Takeda S, Matsumura J, Ikezaki H, et al: Milrinone improves lung compliance in patients receiving mechanical ventilation for cardiogenic pulmonary edema. Acta Anaesthesiol Scand 2003;47: 714-719.

57. Muller-Werdan U, Reithman C, Werdan C: Cytokines and the Heart: Molecular Mechanisms of Septic Cardiomyopathy. Austin, Tex, RG Landes, 1996.

58. Takeuchi K, del Nido PJ, Ibrahim AE, et al: Vesnarinone and amrinone reduce the systemic inflammatory response syndrome. J Thorac Cardiovasc Surg 1999;117:375-382.

59. Takeuchi K, del Nido PJ, Poutias DN, et al: Vesnarinone restores contractility and calcium handling in early endotoxemia. Circulation 2000;102:III-365-III-369.

60. Allen EM, Rowin M, Pappas JB, et al: Hemodynamic effects of N-acetylamrinone in a porcine model of group B streptococcal sepsis. Drug Metab Dispos 1996;24:1028-1031.

61. Ichioka S, Nakatsuka T, Sato Y, et al: Amrinone, a selective phosphodiesterase inhibitor, improves microcirculation and flap survival: A comparative study with prostaglandin E1. J Surg Res 1998;75:42-48.

62. Ichioka S, Nakatsuka T, Ohura N, et al: Topical application of amrinone for relief of vasospasm. J Surg Res 2000;93:149-155.

63. Beebe HG, Dawson DL, Cutler BS, et al: A new pharmacological treatment for intermittent claudication: Results of a randomized, multicenter trial. Arch Intern Med 1999;159:2041-2050.

64. Poole-Wilson PA, Xue SR: New therapies for the management of acute heart failure. Curr Cardiol Rep 2003;5:229-236.

65. Chatterjee K, De Marco T: Role of nonglycosidic inotropic agents: Indications, ethics, and limitations. Med Clin North Am 2003;87: 391-418.

66. Ross-Ascuitto N, Ascuitto R, Chen V, et al: Negative inotropic effects of amrinone in the neonatal piglet. Circ Res 1987;61:847-852.

67. Ross-Ascuitto NT, Ascuitto RJ, Ramage D: Positive inotropic, vasodilatory, and chronotropic effects of milrinone on the post-ischemic neonatal pig heart. Am J Cardiol 1989;64:414-419.

68. Pridjian AK, Frohlich ED, VanMeter CH, et al: Pharmacologic support with high-energy phosphate preservation in the postischemic neonatal heart. Ann Thorac Surg 1995;59:1435-1438.

69. Allen-Webb EM, Ross MP, Pappas JB, et al: Age-related amrinone pharmacokinetics in a pediatric population. Crit Care Med 1994;22:1016-1024.

70. Lawless S, Burckart G, Diven W, et al: Amrinone in neonates and infants after cardiac surgery. Crit Care Med 1989;17:751-754.

71. Laitinen P, Ahonen J, Olkkola KT, et al: Pharmacokinetics of amrinone in neonates and infants. J Cardiothorac Vasc Anesth 2000;14:378-382.

72. Robinson BW, Gelband H, Mas MS, et al: Selective pulmonary and systemic vasodilator effects of amrinone in children: New therapeutic implications. J Am Coll Cardiol 1993;21: 1461-1465.

73. Skippen P, Taylor R, Bohn D: Amrinone in infants and children after cardiac surgery. Crit Care Med 1990;18(Suppl):268S.

74. Berner M, Jaccard C, Oberhansli I, et al: Hemodynamic effects of amrinone in children after cardiac surgery. Intensive Care Med 1990;16:85-88.

75. Laitinen P, Happonen JM, Sairanen H, et al: Amrinone versus dopamine and nitroglycerin in neonates after arterial switch operation for transposition of the great arteries. J Cardiothorac Vasc Anesth 1999;13:186-190.

76. Laitinen P, Happonen JM, Sairanen H, et al: Amrinone versus dopamine-nitroglycerin after reconstructive surgery for complete atrioventricular septal defect. J Cardiothorac Vasc Anesth 1997;11:870-874.

77. Bailey JM, Miller BE, Kanter KR, et al: A comparison of the hemodynamic effects of amrinone and sodium nitroprusside in infants after cardiac surgery. Anesth Analg 1997;84:294-298.

78. Teshima H, Tobita K, Yamamura H, et al: Cardiovascular effects of a phosphodiesterase III inhibitor, amrinone, in infants: Noninvasive echocardiographic evaluation. Pediatr Int 2002;44:259-263.

79. Sorensen GK, Ramamoorthy C, Lynn AM, et al: Hemodynamic effects of amrinone in children after Fontan surgery. Anesth Analg 1996;82:241-246.

80. Williams GD, Sorenson GK, Oakes R, et al: Amrinone loading during cardiopulmonary bypass in neonates, infants, and children. J Cardiothorac Vasc Anesth 1995;9:278-282.

81. Irazuzta JE, Pretzlaff RK, Rowin ME: Amrinone in pediatric refractory septic shock: An open label pharmacodynamic study. Pediatr Crit Care Med 2001;2:24-28.

82. Bailey JM, Miller BE, Lu W, et al: The pharmacokinetics of milrinone in pediatric patients after cardiac surgery. Anesthesiology 1999; 90:1012-1018.

83. Chang AC, Atz AM, Wernovsky G, et al: Milrinone: Systemic and pulmonary hemodynamic effects in neonates after cardiac surgery. Crit Care Med 1995;23:1907-1914.

84. Bailey JM, Miller BE, Lu W, et al: The pharmacokinetics of milrinone in pediatric patients after cardiac surgery. Anesthesiology 1999; 90:1012-1018.

85. Ramamoorthy C, Anderson GD, Williams GD, et al: Pharmacokinetics and side effects of milrinone in infants and children after open heart surgery. Anesth Aanlg 1998;86:283-289.

86. Reinoso-Barbero F, Garcia-Fernandez FJ, Diez-Labajo A, et al: Postoperative use of milrinone for Norwood procedure. Paediatr Anaesth 1996;6:342-343.

87. Barton P, Garcia J, Kouatli A, et al: Hemodynamic effects of i.v. milrinone lactate in pediatric patients with septic shock: A prospective, double-blinded, randomized, placebo-controlled, interventional study. Chest 1996;109:1302-1312.

88. Lindsay CA, Barton P, Lawless S, et al: Pharmacokinetics and pharmacodynamics of milrinone lactate in pediatric patients with septic shock. J Pediatr 1998;132:329-334.

89. Schranz D, Huth R, Dahm M, et al: Acute hemodynamic response to intravenous enoximone: An animal study and preliminary report in infants after cardiac surgery. J Cardiovasc Pharmacol 1989;14(Suppl I):S62-S68.

90. Booker PD, Gibbons S, Stewart JI, et al: Enoximone pharmacokinetics in infants. Br J Anaesth 2000;85:205-210.

91. Hausdorf G, Friedel N, Berdjis F, et al: Enoximone in newborns with refractory postoperative low output states. Eur J Cardiothorac Surg 1992;6:311-317.

92. Hausdorf G: Experience with phosphodiesterase inhibitor in pediatric cardiac surgery. Eur J Anesthesiol 1993;8(Suppl): 25-30.

93. Innes PA, Frazer RS, Booker PD, et al: Comparison of the hemodynamic effects of dobutamine with enoximone after open heart surgery in small children. Br J Anaesth 1994;72:77-81.

94. Amsallem E, Kasparian C, Haddour G, et al: Phosphodiesterase III inhibitors for heart failure. Cochrane Database Syst Rev 2005;1:CD062230.

CHAPTER 35

Use of Vasodilators in Heart Failure

Stephen A. Stayer

The hemodynamic descriptors of decompensated heart failure are elevated filling pressures with associated decreased cardiac output. Systemic vascular resistance (SVR) is increased in heart failure from activation of the neurohormonal axis and the renin-angiotensin and sympathetic nervous systems (see Chapters 5 and 6).[1] With these changes, blood flow to the kidney, skeletal muscle, and splanchnic beds is preferentially redistributed to the heart, lungs, and brain.

Heart failure induces changes in the sympathetic nervous system and the renin-angiotensin system such that the SVR usually is elevated as a result of vasoconstriction. This pathophysiology creates an unfavorable ventricular-vascular coupling because SVR is a major component of vascular elastance (see Chapters 7 and 8). Vasodilators decrease SVR, filling pressures, and myocardial work and increase perfusion to vascular beds of various organs; in short, these agents optimize ventricular-vascular coupling.

Vasodilators commonly are divided into medications that cause venodilation versus arterial vasodilation. A venodilator reduces preload, pulmonary and hepatic congestion, and diastolic wall stress, whereas an arteriodilator reduces SVR and myocardial work and preserves or improves cardiac output. Adult heart failure studies indicate that the increase in cardiac output from vasodilator therapy occurs primarily from a reduction in mitral regurgitation,[2,3] but long-term outcome after vasodilator therapy has shown varying results. Despite salutary effects on exercise tolerance, pure vasodilators alone do not alter the natural history of the disease. Drugs that affect the neurohormonal activation (drugs that block the adrenergic and renin-angiotensin systems) promote growth and prevent remodeling of the failing heart and have more beneficial effects compared with pure vasodilators (see later). The angiotensin II–mediated deleterious effects are ameliorated by agents such as angiotensin-converting enzyme (ACE) inhibitors; these effects surpass the vasodilating properties of these agents. Although phosphodiesterase inhibitors are considered vasodilators, these agents are discussed in Chapter 34.

Because of the limited population of pediatric heart failure patients and the diversity of etiologies, large-scale pediatric therapeutic trials on the various vasodilators have not been performed. Most of the data regarding vasodilator therapy for heart failure are derived from adult studies. This chapter reviews adult evidence of vasodilator treatment of heart failure and emphasizes the pediatric studies that exist.

NITROVASODILATORS AND HEART FAILURE

Nitric oxide activates guanylate cyclase, and increases the formation of cGMP in vascular smooth muscle cells. Nitrovasodilators produce vascular smooth muscle relaxation by mimicking the activity of nitric oxide, and the pharmacologic activity depends on biotransformation into nitrogen oxides within the blood and vascular tissue.[4] This class of drugs reduces filling pressures and symptoms, and in adult studies these drugs have been shown to decrease mitral regurgitation from a reduction in left ventricular volume and a decrease in annular distention.[3]

Nitroprusside

Nitroprusside is a potent, short-acting vasodilator that produces balanced effects on venous and arterial vasodilation that has a rapid onset and is quickly metabolized to nitric oxide and cyanide; these pharmacologic properties make it an excellent drug that can be titrated to effect in the treatment of acute congestive heart failure in the intensive care unit.[5] Cyanide is produced and metabolized to thiocyanate by the liver; cyanide toxicity may develop after prolonged use, especially in patients with hepatic and renal dysfunction or in patients with poor hepatic perfusion secondary to a low cardiac output state. When used for adults with acute decompensated heart failure, nitroprusside improves cardiac output, reduces filling pressures, reduces atrial volumes, and reduces regurgitation of mitral and tricuspid valves.[2,6]

Nitroprusside has been shown to improve the hemodynamic profile of children with low cardiac output from sepsis or acute respiratory distress syndrome.[7] In children with heart failure resulting from **left-to-right shunts**, nitroprusside should be used with caution. Beekman and colleagues[8] studied infants with a large ventricular septal defect undergoing cardiac catheterization. Although right atrial and pulmonary artery wedge pressures were decreased by 53%, the investigators observed a marked decrease in systemic blood flow with an increase in pulmonary-to-systemic shunting. Subramanyam and coworkers[9] also studied children (1.5 to 15 years old) with ventricular septal defects in the cardiac catheterization laboratory and found varying responses to nitroprusside depending on the underlying pathophysiology. Patients with elevated left ventricular filling pressures showed an improvement in systemic flow and a decrease in filling pressures, pulmonary artery pressures, and left-to-right shunting; most of the patients with normal left ventricular filling pressures had an increase in left-to-right shunt. These studies reveal that nitroprusside would have a varying effect on patients with left-to-right shunting depending on the hemodynamic profile. In patients who have a long-standing volume burden and who have developed significant elevations in left ventricular end-diastolic pressure, nitroprusside is likely to improve cardiac output by decreasing SVR, filling pressures, atrial dilation, and possibly atrioventricular valve regurgitation, whereas other patients are likely to develop a reduction in cardiac output from pulmonary vasodilation.

Nitroprusside generally improves the condition of patients with heart failure from **valvar regurgitation** or **stenosis**. In patients with aortic regurgitation, vasodilators significantly improve cardiac performance and decrease the regurgitant volume and left ventricular filling pressures.[10] Nitroprusside also has similar beneficial hemodynamic effects in patients with mitral regurgitation.[11-13] Vasodilators should be used with caution, however, in patients with heart failure from left-sided obstructive lesions, such as aortic stenosis or obstructive hypertrophic cardiomyopathy. These patients have a hypertrophied myocardium and may develop endocardial ischemia from a decrease in coronary artery perfusion pressure. Ikram[13a] studied the hemodynamic properties of nitroprusside in 35 patients with aortic stenosis and found limited benefit with modest effects on filling pressures and cardiac output in the group overall, but nitroprusside improved the hemodynamic status of a subgroup of patients with aortic stenosis who had high filling pressures and impaired left ventricular function. Khot and colleagues[14] determined the hemodynamic responses in 25 adult patients with severe aortic stenosis and decompensated heart failure and showed that nitroprusside produces a rapid and marked improvement in cardiac function in these patients without inducing hypotension (Fig. 35-1). Similar to the patients with impaired ventricular function in Ikram's study, patients in this study had decompensated heart failure. The traditional caveat that vasodilators should be avoided in fixed valvar stenosis may be an oversimplification of hemodynamics in this disease.

Nitroprusside is sometimes a first-line drug for patients with acute **congestive heart failure** or patients with chronic congestive heart failure experiencing acute decompensation. The recommended starting dose is 0.5 μg/kg/min and is titrated to a reduction in filling

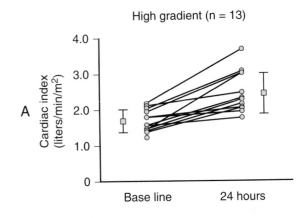

High gradient (n = 13)

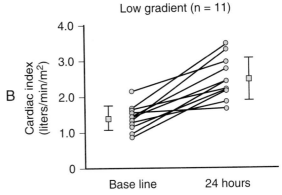

Low gradient (n = 11)

FIGURE 35-1 ■ Nitroprusside infusion in patients with aortic stenosis. Graphs illustrate the changes in cardiac indices in patients with high (>30 mm Hg) and low (<30 mm Hg) aortic stenosis gradients. There was no significant difference in cardiac indices between these two groups. The squares and error bars represent means ± SD. (From Khot UN, Novaro GM, Popovic ZB, et al: *Nitroprusside in critically ill patients with left ventricular dysfunction and aortic stenosis. N Engl J Med* 2003;348:1756-1763.)

pressures and a reduction in symptoms. As opposed to its use for the treatment of acute hypertension, nitroprusside does not need to be titrated to reduce blood pressure when treating acute heart failure. Adult patients usually are monitored with invasive hemodynamic monitoring during nitroprusside therapy,[15] but the use of nitroprusside alone is not an absolute indication for such monitoring in pediatric patients. The dose may be titrated to clinical signs and symptoms, such as hepatomegaly and resting respiratory rate, or to noninvasive blood pressure monitoring and periodic echocardiography to assess filling volumes and valve regurgitation. Vasodilators commonly are used with diuretics for the treatment of heart failure, and nitroprusside should be titrated carefully in a hypovolemic patient, who may experience an excessive decrease in blood pressure from vasodilation. In addition, most patients require transition to an oral vasodilating medication because the abrupt withdrawal of nitroprusside may produce recurrence of heart failure and rebound hypertension.[16]

Nitroglycerin

Nitroglycerin is metabolized in the liver and has a short plasma half-life; side effects include hypotension, tachycardia, and hypoxemia. Compared with nitroprusside, nitroglycerin is a more powerful venodilator and a mild arteriolar vasodilator and coronary vasodilator[5]; these properties make it useful as a vasodilator in patients with ischemic heart disease. Nitroglycerin reduces filling pressures by increasing venous capacitance.

There is limited information about the hemodynamics and pharmacokinetics of nitroglycerin use in children. Zeng and colleagues[17] studied the use of nitroglycerin in 26 children with left-to-right shunts lesions and found a reduction in filling pressures without a change in pulmonary-to-systemic flow ratio (Qp:Qs) measured echocardiographically. Tamura and Kawano[18] studied the hemodynamic effects of nitroglycerin in 20 neonates with heart failure of varying etiologies. Two patients had greater than 10% decrease in blood pressure at a dose of 2 μg/kg/min, but none of the remaining 18 patients exhibited significant blood pressure changes at doses of 4 μg/kg/min or greater. These neonatal patients had improved urine output, decreases in central venous pressure, and improved echocardiographic measurements of systolic function.[18] Transdermal nitroglycerin also has been studied in children; however, significantly lower plasma levels are produced from this method of administration, and the hemodynamic effects are limited.[19]

RENIN-ANGIOTENSIN SYSTEM INHIBITORS AND HEART FAILURE

Angiotensin Converting Enzyme (ACE) Inhibitors

ACE inhibitors are the mainstay in heart failure treatment in adults and commonly are used to treat pediatric heart failure patients. Numerous adult studies show consistent reductions in morbidity and mortality.[20-22] The renin-angiotensin-aldosterone and catecholamine systems are activated in adults and children with heart failure; studies of infants and children in heart failure find correlations between clinical heart failure scores and plasma renin and norepinephrine levels.[23,24]

Renin is secreted by the juxtaglomerular apparatus in response to decreased renal perfusion and protects glomerular perfusion pressure through angiotensin II–induced efferent arteriolar constriction. Angiotensin II produces many actions that contribute to the progression of heart failure. These compensatory mechanisms are responsible for heart failure symptoms and impact on morbidity and mortality in adults. Pharmacologic strategies to ameliorate the symptoms of heart failure are aimed at altering the sequence of renin production leading to increases in angiotensin II and aldosterone (Fig. 35-2).

ACE catalyzes the metabolic conversion of angiotensin I to angiotensin II, and the primary action of ACE inhibitors occurs from blocking this conversion (see Chapters 5 and 6). ACE also is responsible for the activation of bradykinin, which has vasodilatory and natriuretic properties that are in opposition to the vasoconstrictive and salt-retaining properties of angiotensin II.[25] Angiotensin II also stimulates growth factors that regulate endothelial, cardiomyocyte, and fibroblast growth, development, and function (Table 35-1). In animal and in vitro studies, these factors cause excessive growth and fibrosis of the myocardium through fibroblast and gene modulation. This maladaptive sequence results in hypertrophy, fibrosis, and apoptosis secondary to an excess deposition of extracellular matrix, a process called *left ventricular remodeling*. Remodeling produces alterations in ventricular mass, chamber size, and shape

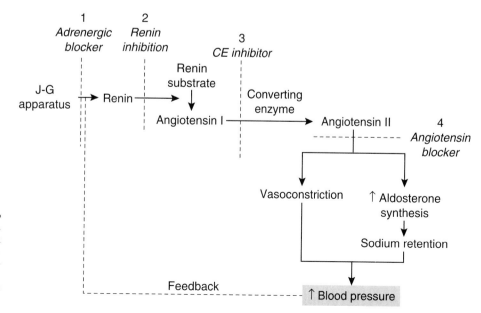

FIGURE 35-2 ■ Sites of action to inhibit the renin-angiotensin system. The activity of the renin-angiotensin system may be inhibited at four sites. CE, converting enzyme, J-G, juxtaglomerular. (From Kaplan NM: *Clinical Hypertension.* Baltimore, Williams & Wilkins, 1998, p 223.)

TABLE 35-1

Actions of Angiotensin II That Contribute to Heart Failure
Vasoconstriction
Sodium retention
Myocyte hypertrophy
Myocardial and vascular fibroproliferation
Myocyte apoptosis
Generation of oxygen-free radicals
Endothelial dysfunction
Sympathetic activation
Diminished thrombolysis

that develop from myocardial injury, pressure loading, or volume loading. It seems that local myocardial renin-angiotensin system is activated more in the failing heart.

ACE inhibitors have been shown to mitigate this process of angiotensin-mediated maladaptation to heart failure.[26,27] Angiotensin II is formed from angiotensin I via either the ACE or the protease chymase pathway. The former pathway is abundant in cardiac myocytes, fibroblasts, vascular smooth muscle cells, and endothelial tissue, whereas the latter is found in mast cells and other interstitial cells. Angiotensin II formation is only partially blocked by an ACE inhibitor in adult heart failure patients, but is almost completely inhibited by an inhibitor of chymase; ACE inhibitors achieve only partial inhibition of angiotensin II production.[28-30] ACE inhibitors block the degradation of bradykinin, a vasodilating hormone. ACE inhibitors also promote vasodilation by increasing prostaglandins and decreasing endothelins. Other effects of ACE inhibitors include reduction of renal vascular resistance, increase in renal blood flow, and decrease in glomerular capillary pressure.

Captopril undergoes hepatic and renal metabolism and produces a varying blood pressure response, particularly in neonates; the dosing of captopril should be age dependent. Enalapril, a newer class of ACE inhibitors, differs from captopril in that the molecular structure does not include the sulfhydryl group (believed to be responsible for some of the side effects observed with captopril), and the half-life is longer than that of captopril. Side effects of ACE inhibitor therapy include proteinuria, hyperkalemia (caused by reduction in aldosterone production), cough, and neutropenia. New ACE inhibitors include lisinopril (Fig. 35-3).

There has been much experience with captopril and enalapril in the treatment of adult heart failure (Fig. 35-4). Three large-scale, placebo-controlled studies of ACE inhibitors showed reductions in overall mortality, prolonged survival, and improved quality of life in adult patients with direct relation to the degree of severity of chronic heart failure.[20-22] Animal studies revealed that ACE inhibitors play a role in limiting cardiovascular remodeling, which is believed to be the primary mechanism by

which these drugs reduce cardiovascular morbidity and mortality. ACE inhibitors produce a regression of hypertrophy and normalization of glucose use in rats with pressure-loaded ventricles.[31] This effect has potential negative consequences in pediatric patients, however, by reducing hypertrophy of the developing myocardium, which is the primary mechanism of myocardial growth beyond 6 months of age.

Because there are many causes of heart failure in children, this section divides studies of ACE inhibitors by the etiologies of heart failure. In general, ACE inhibitors have been shown to decrease the Qp:Qs and improve weight gain in children with **left-to-right shunts**. It seems that the primary mechanism of action of ACE inhibitors is through a reduction of SVR with a minimal effect on pulmonary vascular resistance (PVR). In all of the following studies, either captopril or enalapril was added to conventional therapy with digoxin and diuretics. First, Scammell and colleagues[32] studied captopril therapy in 18 infants with heart failure from large left-to-right shunts. This study showed that weight gain improved, heart rate and respiratory rate decreased, and plasma sodium concentration increased.[32] Shaw and coworkers[33] also reported an increase in weight gain and decreases in heart and respiratory rates from captopril therapy in infants with poorly controlled heart failure. Studies from Shaddy and colleagues[34] and Montigny and associates[35] evaluated the acute hemodynamic effects of captopril in infants with large left-to-right shunts and found varying hemodynamic effects depending on the baseline SVR and PVR. Captopril decreased SVR and decreased Qp:Qs in most patients, especially patients with elevated SVR. In patients with normal SVR or with elevated PVR, there was a significant decrease in PVR, however, and an increase in left-to-right shunting.[34,35] A few infants in the studies by Shaddy and Shaw developed transient renal insufficiency, including one infant who developed renal failure. Webster and coworkers[36] measured the hemodynamic effects of intravenous enalaprilat in children with left-to-right shunts and showed that enalaprilat lowered systemic pressure and maintained systemic flow. Although patients without significantly elevated PVR had a decrease in left-to-right shunting, patients with elevated PVR had varying responses.[36] Lastly, Sluysmans and colleagues[37] studied the effects of enalaprilat followed by oral enalapril in eight infants with large VSD and congestive heart failure. Seven of the eight patients showed a favorable response with a decrease in Qp:Qs by 17%. One of the patients showed a paradoxical response, however, with a decrease in systemic cardiac output, an increase in systemic resistance, and poor feeding and weight loss.[37]

Patients with heart failure from **valvar regurgitation** improve as a result of vasodilator therapy, which reduces afterload, decreases ventricular end-diastolic pressure, and reduces pulmonary venous congestion.

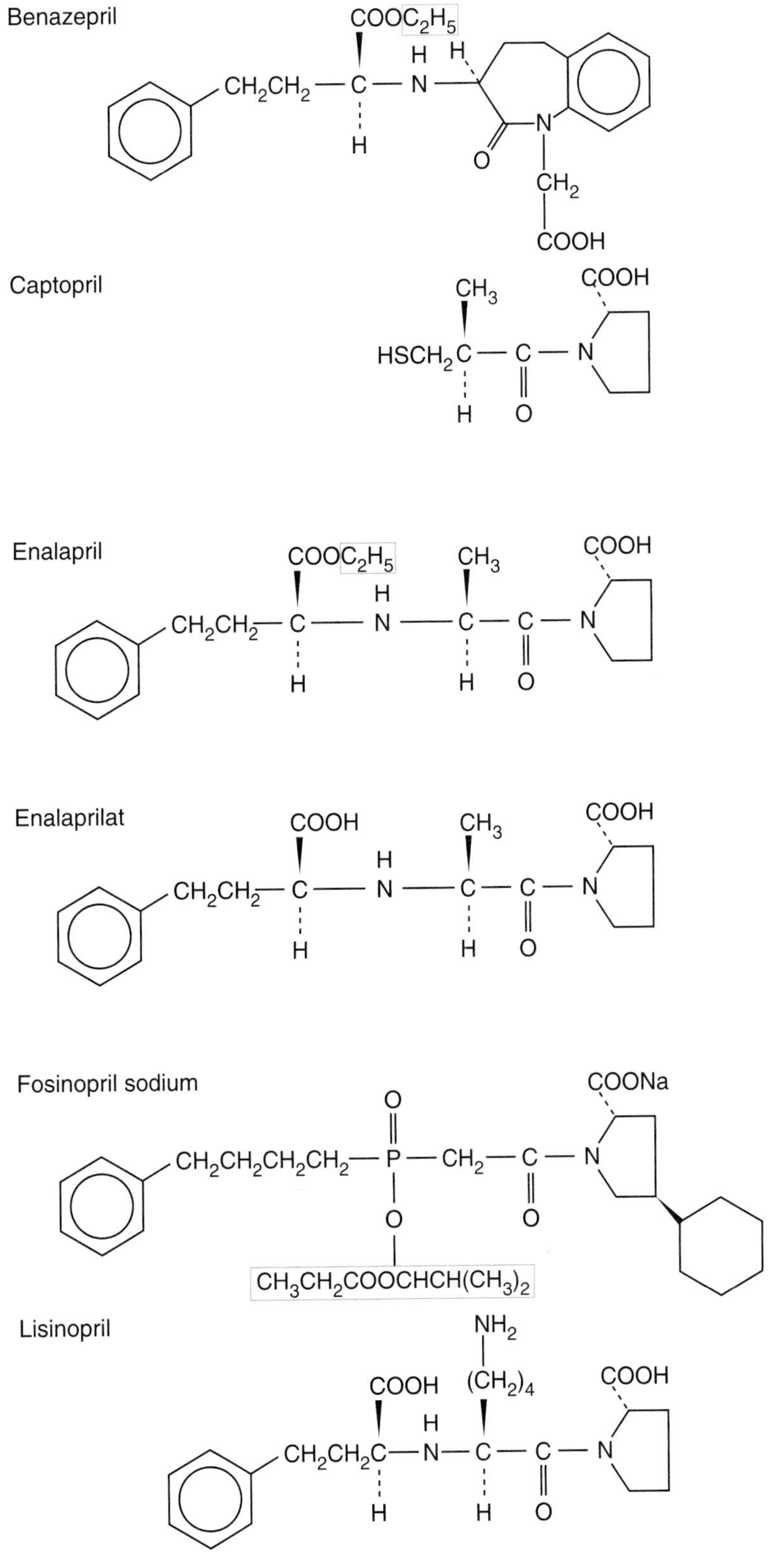

Benazepril

Captopril

Enalapril

Enalaprilat

Fosinopril sodium

Lisinopril

FIGURE 35-3 ■ **Angiotensin-converting enzyme inhibitors.** Only captopril, enalaprilat, and lisinopril are in their active forms. The rest of the angiotensin-converting enzyme inhibitors seen are inactive until esterases remove the structures enclosed in the box. (From Jackson EK: *Renin and angiotensin*. In Hardman JG, Limbird, LE (eds): Goodman and Gilman's *The Pharmacological Basis of Therapeutics*, 10th ed. New York, McGraw-Hill, p. 822, 2001.)

An adult study showed that enalapril therapy is superior to ·that of a direct vasodilator, hydralazine, because enalapril significantly reduces left ventricular mass index.[38] Some evidence also exists that ACE inhibitor therapy may have the same beneficial effect in children. Alehan and Ozkutlu[39] reported that long-term captopril therapy was shown to reduce left ventricular dilation and hypertrophy in children with aortic insufficiency. In addition, two other nonrandomized, noncontrolled studies of enalapril use in children with aortic or mitral regurgitation have been published. Although in one study all patients had a favorable response, the other study showed that only 7 of 12 children experienced clinical improvement.[40,41]

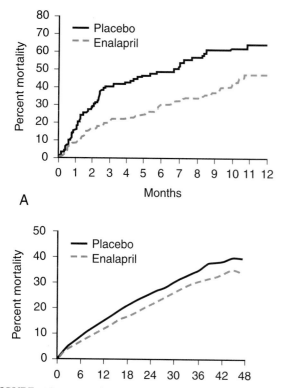

FIGURE 35-4 ■ **Enalapril therapy in adults with heart failure.** The Class IV Cooperative North Scandinavian Enalapril Survival Study (CONSENSUS) **(A)** and the Studies of the Left Ventricular Dysfunction Prevention Study (SOLVD) **(B)** show lower probability of death compared with placebo. (From Smith TW, Kelly RA, Stevenson LW, et al: *Management of heart failure.* In Braunwald E, Zipes D, Libby P, (eds): *Heart Disease,* 6th ed. Philadelphia, WB Saunders, p. 583, 1997.)

Significant increases in serum renin levels have been documented in patients with **coarctation of the aorta** compared with control patients and patients with essential hypertension.[42] Captopril has been used to treat heart failure unresponsive to conventional therapy associated with severe coarctation of the aorta.[43] Data from this study showed that clinical signs of heart failure improved, blood pressure was lowered, and left ventricular ejection fraction improved. Caution should be used in the infant with coarctation because there seems to be an association of acute renal failure with ACE inhibitor therapy.[44]

ACE inhibitor therapy theoretically would be beneficial to the **Fontan** patient because of evidence of high SVR after the Fontan procedure.[45] In addition, ventricular hypertrophy and the associated diastolic dysfunction have a more profoundly negative influence on Fontan hemodynamics. A randomized placebo-controlled study of ACE inhibitor therapy in Fontan patients show no change, however, in SVR, resting cardiac index, ventricular diastolic filling patterns, or exercise capacity after 10 weeks of therapy.[46]

Cardiomyopathy is a disease state that affects the ventricular myocardium and typically is divided into dilated, hypertrophic, and restrictive cardiomyopathies. Bengur and colleagues[47] studied the acute hemodynamic effects of captopril in 16 children with either dilated or restrictive cardiomyopathy who were treated with captopril. These authors found that 11 of the 12 patients with dilated cardiomyopathy had significant increases in cardiac index and stroke volume and decrease in SVR. Compared with adult studies, these authors did not observe a change in filling pressures. In addition, Stern and associates[48] measured echocardiographic changes associated with captopril use in 12 children with cardiomyopathy and found significant reductions in end-systolic and end-diastolic volumes. There is some evidence that ACE inhibitors may have beneficial effects on survival similar to that reported in adults. Lewis and Chabot[49] compared survival in patients with dilated cardiomyopathy: 27 patients were treated with ACE inhibitors, and 54 patients received conventional therapy. The groups were similar in age and in clinical and hemodynamic measures. These authors observed improved survival after 1 and 2 years of therapy with ACE inhibitors.[49]

There are no pediatric studies of ACE inhibitor application to hypertrophic cardiomyopathy. Available experimental and clinical data suggest that agents interfering with ACE, the angiotensin I receptor, or the mineralocorticoid receptor may have cardioprotective effects by inducing a reversal of the exaggerated growth of cardiac cell and regression of abnormalities in fibrillar collagen.[50] In addition, Bengur and colleagues[47] concluded that captopril therapy probably should be avoided in children with restrictive cardiomyopathy because of the observation of decreased aortic pressure without improvement in cardiac output in this group of patients. In this study, only four patients with restrictive cardiomyopathy were studied. Lastly, there are studies in patients with doxorubicin-related cardiomyopathy that reveal enalapril therapy reduces afterload and mitigates further deterioration of contractility. A 10-year follow-up study revealed that left ventricular mass, performance, and afterload improved over the first 6 years, but all of these parameters deteriorated between 7 and 10 years.[51]

Buchhorn and associates[52] compared the outcomes of infants with **left-to-right shunts** heart failure treated with captopril (1 mg/kg) versus propranolol (1.9 mg/kg) as a third drug after digoxin and diuretic therapy. Patients were not randomized: Patients treated from 1993 to 1995 received captopril, and patients treated from 1996 to 1998 received propranolol. Among the propranolol-treated patients, heart failure scores, plasma renin levels, and length of hospital stay were lower, and weight gain was higher. In patients who underwent cardiac catheterization, left atrial pressures and end-diastolic ventricular pressures were lower compared with the captopril group.

The safety of ACE inhibitors and the incidence of side effects seem to be similar to those of adults, with the most common side effects being hypotension and renal insufficiency. The decrease in blood pressure is not dose related. Children are likely to be symptomatic with either a low dose or high dose depending on the degree of ACE inhibition.[53] Blood pressure should be monitored regularly when starting therapy, especially in patients who are being treated concomitantly with diuretics. The incidence of renal failure is unknown, but it seems to be related to young age and the presence of left-to-right shunting.[41] Thirty percent to 60% of adults experience coughing when receiving ACE inhibitor therapy, requiring discontinuation of this class of medication in many patients.[54,55] The exact incidence of coughing from ACE inhibitors in children is unknown.

The use of ACE inhibitors has become an integral part of the management of heart failure in children. The beneficial effects for these agents are as follows: (1) ACE inhibitors prevent generation of angiotensin II effects of vasoconstriction, (2) ACE inhibitors decrease deactivation of bradykinin and kallidin (and promote vasodilation), and (3) ACE inhibitors result in slow ventricular remodeling (by decreasing fibrosis and hypertrophy).

Angiotensin Receptor Blockers

Angiotensin receptor blockers (ARBs) antagonize the effect of angiotensin II no matter which pathway of production (ACE or chymase). This class of drugs seems to be as effective as ACE inhibitors in improving symptoms, reducing mortality, reducing wedge pressures, and increasing cardiac output; there are, however, no pediatric studies of ARBs.

A multicenter study of an ARB, candesartan, divided the study population into three groups.[57] One group included heart failure patients with preserved ventricular function (i.e., left ventricular ejection fraction >40%). Candesartan had a moderate impact on preventing admissions for heart failure, but no impact on the cardiovascular death rate.[56] A second group of patients had heart failure and reduced left ventricular function and were being treated with ACE inhibitors. Of these patients, 55% also were treated with β-blockers and 17% with spironolactone. The addition of candesartan to ACE inhibitor and other treatments reduced the incidence of cardiovascular death and reduced the total number of hospital admissions for congestive heart failure. The greatest reduction in death and hospital admissions for congestive heart failure was in the last group of patients with heart failure and reduced left ventricular function who were intolerant to ACE inhibitor therapy.[58]

OTHER VASODILATORS AND HEART FAILURE

Arterial Vasodilators

Hydralazine is a direct-acting vasodilator that affects systemic and pulmonary vascular beds and increases renal and skeletal blood flow. It has a short half-life requiring dosing four times per day and is eliminated by acetylation in the liver. Side effects include a systemic reaction similar to lupus, flushing, headaches, and occasional salt and water retention. Although hydralazine reduces symptoms of heart failure and improves exercise tolerance, hydralazine and isosorbide dinitrate did not produce the same reduction in mortality compared with enalapril treatment of adults with chronic heart failure.[59]

Beekman and colleagues[60] studied the hemodynamic effects of hydralazine in seven children with large ventricular septal defect, all of whom had evidence of pulmonary hypertension. Hydralazine produced an effect within 5 minutes, and the peak effect was at 35 minutes, resulting in a significant increase in systemic blood flow and a decrease in left-to-right shunt.[60] Similar to other studies of vasodilator use in children with heart failure from **left-to-right shunts**, the effects of hydralazine on Qp:Qs vary depending on SVR before hydralazine administration. Patients who have high SVR show the greatest effect from hydralazine, which decreased SVR and Qp:Qs.[61,62]

Artman and colleagues[63] studied the effects of hydralazine in infants with heart failure from **dilated cardiomyopathy**. Hydralazine decreased filling pressures, decreased blood pressure, and increased cardiac output in these patients. Of the 13 patients studied, 10 patients continued with oral hydralazine after the initial catheterization study, and 8 of these 10 patients showed sustained clinical improvement. There is no reported experience with the vasodilator minoxidil as a treatment for heart failure in children.

Calcium Channel Antagonists

Adult studies of calcium channel antagonists indicate that this class of medications produces direct vasodilation and can be used successfully to reduce blood pressure. The use of these agents seems to have no effect on the natural history of heart failure. The oldest and most widely used classification of these drugs is based on their chemical structure: benzothiazepines, phenylalkylamines, and dihydropyridines, exemplified by diltiazem, verapamil, and nifedipine. Side effects of calcium channel blockers include hypotension. These drugs produce mainly arteriolar vasodilation by preventing vascular smooth muscle contraction through interference with calcium influx after depolarization.

This same mechanism produces myocardial depression and negative inotropic actions noted with the first generation of calcium channel antagonists, most notably verapamil. Although early studies of verapamil therapy for **hypertrophic cardiomyopathy** were promising, especially when combined with surgical therapy,[64] a more recently published cohort study of childhood hypertrophic cardiomyopathy found no benefit from verapamil.[65]

The dihydropyridine class of calcium channel antagonists includes nifedipine, felodipine, nicardipine, and amlodipine. These medications produce more significant vasodilation with less negative inotropic effects compared with the other classes of calcium channel blockers. Adult heart failure studies do not show benefit from these medications, but they may be used safely in patients with ischemic heart disease. Almost all pediatric studies of these medications are related to control of hypertension rather than to treatment of heart failure. Berisha and associates[66] studied pediatric patients with **left-to-right shunts** (ventricular septal defects) and found that 10 mg of sublingual nifedipine reduced SVR and increased heart rate. Among patients with pulmonary hypertension, nifedipine also reduced left-to-right shunting. Caution should be exercised with the administration of sublingual nifedipine because there are case reports of the development of profound hypotension when this drug has been used to treat hypertensive pediatric patients.[67-69] Intravenous nicardipine may have utility in the treatment of acute decompensated heart failure because the ability to titrate to effect is similar to nitroprusside. Nicardipine has a rapid onset of action, producing a 30% reduction in mean arterial pressure within 1 minute, and the duration of action is approximately 3 hours.[70]

Vasodilator Prostaglandins

Prostaglandins are biologically active eicosanoids that produce either vasodilation (prostaglandin E_1 prostacyclin), or vasoconstriction (thromboxane). Two clinical trials of intravenous prostacylin have been performed in adults with heart failure revealing improved outcomes in patients with right ventricular failure secondary to primary pulmonary hypertension,[71] but increased mortality in patients with biventricular failure.[72] The outcomes of these studies fit well with the current understanding of the pathophysiology of heart failure. Prostacyclin is a potent pulmonary and systemic vasodilator, and patients with right heart failure secondary to pulmonary hypertension benefit from the reduction in myocardial work from a reduction in afterload. Prostacyclin, similar to other direct vasodilators, has no effect on the ventricular remodeling associated with biventricular heart failure. Prostacyclin also is used in pediatric patients with pulmonary hypertension. Because it requires constant infusion, and discontinuation has been associated with rebound acute right heart decompensation, it is typically reserved for patients with pulmonary hypertension who have failed conventional medical therapy.

Prostaglandin E_1 also produces pulmonary vasodilation and has been used to treat pulmonary hypertension prophylactically after heart transplantation in children.[73] In addition, there is evidence in adults with refractory heart failure that prostaglandin E_1 is more effective than dobutamine or prostacyclin as a bridge to cardiac transplantation.[74,75]

α-Adrenergic Antagonists

Phentolamine and phenoxybenzamine are α-antagonists that sometimes are used as vasodilators in the cardiovascular intensive care unit. These drugs are not commonly used to treat heart failure. Nicergoline, an α-blocking vasodilator, has been studied in 10 children with heart failure from a large ventricular septal defect. Systemic and pulmonary arterial pressures were reduced by nicergoline, and the Qp:Qs decreased in 8 of the 10 patients.[76]

Dopamine Agonists

Fenoldopam is a direct-acting vasodilator that acts on the postsynaptic dopamine 1 receptor producing vasodilation in renal, coronary, cerebral, and splanchnic vasculature. Fenoldopam has been used to control blood pressure in children,[77] but there is no reported experience with the use of this drug for the treatment of heart failure in children. There is limited reported use of this drug for heart failure in adults, however, because the physiologic profile of this drug should be favorable for the treatment of acute heart failure with its ability to improve renal blood flow.[78,79]

Nitric Oxide

Inhaled nitric oxide is a direct pulmonary vasodilator that is devoid of effects on the systemic vasculature; it is used to treat heart failure with associated pulmonary hypertension and used in patients requiring a left ventricular assist device to optimize cardiac output.[80] Before the clinical use of nitric oxide, Konstam and associates[81] studied 10 adults with pulmonary hypertension, most of whom had biventricular failure. Nitroglycerin and nitroprusside reduced pulmonary arterial pressures, and these authors found a direct linear relationship between the vasodilator-induced decreases in pulmonary arterial end-systolic pressure and in right ventricular end-systolic volume. These agents also affect the systemic circulation, however, producing a significant decrease in systemic arterial pressure. Kieler-Jensen and coworkers[82] compared the hemodynamic effects of inhaled nitric oxide with intravenous prostacyclin, prostaglandin E_1, and sodium nitroprusside in patients after heart transplantation and showed that SVR and PVR were lowest with prostacyclin, which produced the highest cardiac output. In this study, inhaled nitric oxide was the only selective pulmonary vasodilator. Nitric oxide should be used with caution to treat pulmonary hypertension associated with left ventricular dysfunction because the decrease in PVR is associated with an increase in left ventricular filling pressure in many of these patients.[83-87]

Others

Vasodilators such as the α_1-adrenergic antagonist prazosin and the central α_2-adrenergic agonist clonidine are used as antihypertensive agents. There is virtually no reported experience with the use of these vasodilators for heart failure in children.

CURRENT STATUS AND FUTURE TRENDS

Vasodilators are a mainstay of heart failure treatment in adults and children. Patients with acute onset of heart failure and patients with decompensation from chronic heart failure benefit from use of short-acting vasodilators, most of which are administered as a continuous infusion. Although nitroprusside and nitroglycerin traditionally have been used in this setting, newer medications, such as fenoldopam and nesiritide, may have advantages secondary to improved preservation of renal perfusion. These potent vasodilators are not titrated to lower blood pressure, but to reduce cardiac filling pressure and heart failure symptoms.

ACE inhibitors are the mainstay of heart failure therapy for adults and children. New information about the complex interplay of the renin-angiotensin system continues to come forth from research, including recent revelation of the new ACE 2, which has direct effects on cardiac function.[88] Although long-term efficacy studies of ACE inhibitor therapy for pediatric heart failure are still lacking, this class of vasodilators will provide the foundation for large clinical trials and novel new treatments of chronic heart failure in children.[89,90] Future therapies in pediatric heart failure may be combined therapy with several agents that have vasodilating properties and inhibiting capabilities of the renin-angiotensin-aldosterone system.[91]

Key Concepts

■ Angiotensin II–mediated deleterious effects are ameliorated by ACE inhibitors; these effects surpass the vasodilating properties of these agents.

■ Nitric oxide activates guanylate cyclase and increases the formation of cGMP in vascular smooth muscle cells. Nitrovasodilators produce vascular smooth muscle relaxation by mimicking the activity of nitric oxide, and the pharmacologic activity depends on biotransformation into nitrogen oxides within the blood and vascular tissue.

■ Nitroprusside has been shown to improve the hemodynamic profiles of children with low cardiac output from sepsis or acute respiratory distress syndrome. In children with heart failure secondary to left-to-right shunting, nitroprusside should be used with caution.

■ Nitroprusside improved the hemodynamic status of a subgroup of patients with aortic stenosis who had high filling pressures and impaired left ventricular function. The traditional caveat that vasodilators should be avoided in fixed valvar stenosis may be an oversimplification of hemodynamics in this disease.

■ Compared with nitroprusside, nitroglycerin is a more powerful venodilator and a mild arteriolar vasodilator and coronary vasodilator; these properties make it useful as a vasodilator in patients with ischemic heart disease.

■ ACE catalyzes the metabolic conversion of angiotensin I to angiotensin II, and the primary action of ACE inhibitors occurs from blocking this conversion. ACE also is responsible for the activation of bradykinin, which has vasodilatory and natriuretic properties that are in opposition to the vasoconstrictive and salt-retaining properties of angiotensin II. Angiotensin II also stimulates growth factors that regulate endothelial, cardiomyocyte, and fibroblast growth, development, and function.

■ ACE inhibitors have been shown to mitigate the process of angiotensin-mediated maladaptation to heart failure. Angiotensin II is formed from angiotensin I via either the ACE or the protease chymase pathway. The former pathway is abundant in cardiac myocytes, fibroblasts, vascular smooth muscle cells, and endothelial tissue, whereas the latter is found in mast cells and other interstitial cells. Angiotensin II formation is only partially blocked by an ACE inhibitor in adult heart failure patients, but it is almost completely inhibited by an inhibitor of chymase; ACE inhibitors achieve only partial inhibition of angiotensin II production.

■ ACE inhibitors produce a regression of hypertrophy and normalization of glucose use in rats with pressure loaded ventricles. This effect has potential negative consequences in pediatric patients, however, by reducing hypertrophy of the developing myocardium, which is the primary mechanism of myocardial growth beyond 6 months of age.

■ In general, ACE inhibitors have been shown to decrease the Qp:Qs and improve weight gain in children with left-to-right shunts.

■ Patients with heart failure from valvar regurgitation improve as a result of vasodilator therapy, which reduces afterload, decreases ventricular end-diastolic pressure, and reduces pulmonary venous congestion.

■ The safety of ACE inhibitors and the incidence of side effects seem to be similar to those of adults, with the most common side effects being hypotension and renal insufficiency.

■ The use of ACE inhibitors has become an integral part of the management of heart failure in children. The beneficial effects for these agents are as follows: (1) ACE inhibitors prevent generation of angiotensin II effects of vasoconstriction, (2) ACE inhibitors decrease deactivation of bradykinin and kallidin (and promote vasodilation), and (3) ACE inhibitors result in slow ventricular remodeling (by decreasing fibrosis and hypertrophy).

■ Angiotensin receptor blockers antagonize the effect of angiotensin II no matter which pathway of production (ACE or chymase). This class of drugs seems to be as effective as ACE inhibitors in improving symptoms, reducing mortality, reducing wedge pressures, and increasing cardiac output.

■ Similar to other studies of vasodilator use in children with heart failure from left-to-right shunts, the effects of hydralazine on Qp:Qs vary depending on SVR before hydralazine administration. Patients who have high SVR show the greatest effect from hydralazine, which decreased SVR and Qp:Qs.

■ Although early studies of verapamil therapy for hypertrophic cardiomyopathy were promising, especially when combined with surgical therapy, a more recently published cohort study of childhood hypertrophic cardiomyopathy found no benefit from verapamil.

REFERENCES

1. Kaye DM, Lambert GW, Lefkovits J, et al: Neurochemical evidence of cardiac sympathetic activation and increased central nervous system norepinephrine turnover in severe congestive heart failure. J Am Coll Cardiol 1994;23:570-578.
2. Guiha NH, Cohn JN, Mikulic E, et al: Treatment of refractory heart failure with infusion of nitroprusside. N Engl J Med 1974;291:587-592.
3. Rosario LB, Stevenson LW, Solomon SD, et al: The mechanism of decrease in dynamic mitral regurgitation during heart failure treatment: Importance of reduction in the regurgitant orifice size. J Am Coll Cardiol 1998;32:1819-1824.
4. Harrison DG, Bates JN: The nitrovasodilators: New ideas about old drugs. Circulation 1993;87:1461-1467.
5. Leier CV, Bambach D, Thompson MJ, et al: Central and regional hemodynamic effects of intravenous isosorbide dinitrate, nitroglycerin and nitroprusside in patients with congestive heart failure. Am J Cardiol 1981;48:1115-1123.
6. Hamilton MA, Stevenson LW, Child JS, et al: Acute reduction of atrial overload during vasodilator and diuretic therapy in advanced congestive heart failure. Am J Cardiol 1990;65:1209-1212.
7. Apukhtina TE, Doletskii AS, Avdeeva ON, Timoshchenko OA: [The use of sodium nitroprusside in the treatment of heart failure in critically ill children]. Anesteziol Reanimatol 1991;50-53.
8. Beekman RH, Rocchini AP, Rosenthal A: Hemodynamic effects of nitroprusside in infants with a large ventricular septal defect. Circulation 1981;64:553-558.
9. Subramanyam R, Tandon R, Shrivastava S: Hemodynamic effects of sodium nitroprusside in patients with ventricular septal defect. Eur J Pediatr 1982;138:307-310.
10. Miller RR, Vismara LA, DeMaria AN, et al: Afterload reduction therapy with nitroprusside in severe aortic regurgitation: Improved cardiac performance and reduced regurgitant volume. Am J Cardiol 1976;38:564-567.
11. Goodman DJ, Rossen RM, Holloway EL, et al: Effect of nitroprusside on left ventricular dynamics in mitral regurgitation. Circulation 1974;50:1025-1032.
12. Chatterjee K, Parmley WW, Swan HJ, et al: Beneficial effects of vasodilator agents in severe mitral regurgitation due to dysfunction of subvalvar apparatus. Circulation 1973;48:684-690.
13. Grossman W, Harshaw CW, Munro AB, et al: Lowered aortic impedance as therapy for severe mitral regurgitation. JAMA 1974;230:1011-1013.
13a. Ikram H, Low CJ, Crozier IG: Hemodynamic effects of nitroprusside or valvular aortic stenosis. Am J Cardiol 1992;69:361-366.
14. Khot UN, Novaro GM, Popovic ZB, et al: Nitroprusside in critically ill patients with left ventricular dysfunction and aortic stenosis. N Engl J Med 2003;348:1756-1763.
15. Stevenson LW: Management of acute decompensation. In Mann DL (ed): Heart Failure. Philadelphia, WB Saunders, 2004, pp 595-601.
16. Packer M, Meller J, Medina N, et al: Rebound hemodynamic events after the abrupt withdrawal of nitroprusside in patients with severe chronic heart failure. N Engl J Med 1979;301:1193-1197.
17. Zeng H, Sun L, Li W, Du J: Effect of intravenous nitroglycerin on hemodynamics in infants and children with congestive heart failure. Chin Med J (Engl) 2000;113:328-331.
18. Tamura M, Kawano T: Effects of intravenous nitroglycerin on hemodynamics in neonates with refractory congestive heart failure or PFC. Acta Paediatr Jpn 1990;32:291-298.
19. Vaksmann G, Pariente-Khayat A, Godart F, et al: Effects of transdermal nitroglycerin in children with congestive heart failure: A Doppler echocardiographic study. Pediatr Cardiol 2001;22:11-13.
20. Effects of enalapril on mortality in severe congestive heart failure: Results of the Cooperative North Scandinavian Enalapril Survival Study (CONSENSUS). The CONSENSUS Trial Study Group. N Engl J Med 1987;316:1429-1435.
21. Effect of enalapril on survival in patients with reduced left ventricular ejection fractions and congestive heart failure. The SOLVD Investigators. N Engl J Med 1991;325:293-302.
22. Effect of enalapril on mortality and the development of heart failure in asymptomatic patients with reduced left ventricular ejection fractions. The SOLVD Investigators. N Engl J Med 1992;327:685-691.
23. Buchhorn R, Hammersen A, Bartmus D, Bursch J: The pathogenesis of heart failure in infants with congenital heart disease. Cardiol Young 2001;11:498-504.
24. Ross RD, Daniels SR, Schwartz DC, et al: Plasma norepinephrine levels in infants and children with congestive heart failure. Am J Cardiol 1987;59:911-914.
25. Linz W, Wiemer G, Gohlke P, et al: Contribution of kinins to the cardiovascular actions of angiotensin-converting enzyme inhibitors. Pharmacol Rev 1995;47:25-49.
26. McDonald KM, D'Aloia A, Parrish T, et al: Functional impact of an increase in ventricular mass after myocardial damage and its attenuation by converting enzyme inhibition. J Card Fail 1998;4:203-212.
27. McDonald KM: Anti-remodeling effects of ACE inhibitors. Coron Artery Dis 1995;6:295-301.
28. Urata H, Ganten D: Cardiac angiotensin II formation: The angiotensin-I converting enzyme and human chymase. Eur Heart J 1993;14(Suppl I):177-182.
29. Urata H, Nishimura H, Ganten D: Chymase-dependent angiotensin II forming systems in humans. Am J Hypertens 1996;9:277-284.
30. Urata H, Nishimura H, Ganten D, Arakawa K: Angiotensin-converting enzyme-independent pathways of angiotensin II formation in human tissues and cardiovascular diseases. Blood Press 1996;2(Suppl):22-28.
31. Wambolt RB, Henning SL, English DR, et al: Regression of cardiac hypertrophy normalizes glucose metabolism and left ventricular function during reperfusion. J Mol Cell Cardiol 1997;29:939-948.
32. Scammell AM, Arnold R, Wilkinson JL: Captopril in treatment of infant heart failure: A preliminary report. Int J Cardiol 1987;16:295-301.
33. Shaw NJ, Wilson N, Dickinson DF: Captopril in heart failure secondary to a left to right shunt. Arch Dis Child 1988;63:360-363.
34. Shaddy RE, Teitel DF, Brett C: Short-term hemodynamic effects of captopril in infants with congestive heart failure. Am J Dis Child 1988;142:100-105.
35. Montigny M, Davignon A, Fouron JC, et al: Captopril in infants for congestive heart failure secondary to a large ventricular left-to-right shunt. Am J Cardiol 1989;63:631-633.
36. Webster MW, Neutze JM, Calder AL: Acute hemodynamic effects of converting enzyme inhibition in children with intracardiac shunts. Pediatr Cardiol 1992;13:129-135.
37. Sluysmans T, Styns-Cailteux M, Tremouroux-Wattiez M, et al: Intravenous enalaprilat and oral enalapril in congestive heart failure secondary to ventricular septal defect in infancy. Am J Cardiol 1992;70:959-962.

38. Lin M, Chiang HT, Lin SL, et al: Vasodilator therapy in chronic asymptomatic aortic regurgitation: Enalapril versus hydralazine therapy. J Am Coll Cardiol 1994;24:1046-1053.

39. Alehan D, Ozkutlu S: Beneficial effects of 1-year captopril therapy in children with chronic aortic regurgitation who have no symptoms. Am Heart J 1998;135:598-603.

40. Seguchi M, Nakazawa M, Momma K: Effect of enalapril on infants and children with congestive heart failure. Cardiol Young 1992;2:14-19.

41. Leversha AM, Wilson NJ, Clarkson PM, et al: Efficacy and dosage of enalapril in congenital and acquired heart disease. Arch Dis Child 1994;70:35-39.

42. Fallo F, Maragno I, Mantero F: Resistance to captopril in hypertension of coarctation of the aorta. Int J Cardiol 1985;9:111-113.

43. Schneeweiss A: Cardiovascular drugs in children: Angiotensin-converting enzyme inhibitors. Pediatr Cardiol 1988;9:109-115.

44. Wood EG, Bunchman TE, Lynch RE: Captopril-induced reversible acute renal failure in an infant with coarctation of the aorta. Pediatrics 1991;88:816-818.

45. Akagi T, Benson LN, Green M, et al: Ventricular performance before and after Fontan repair for univentricular atrioventricular connection: Angiographic and radionuclide assessment. J Am Coll Cardiol 1992;20:920-926.

46. Kouatli AA, Garcia JA, Zellers TM, et al: Enalapril does not enhance exercise capacity in patients after Fontan procedure. Circulation 1997;96:1507-1512.

47. Bengur AR, Beekman RH, Rocchini AP, et al: Acute hemodynamic effects of captopril in children with a congestive or restrictive cardiomyopathy. Circulation 1991;83:523-527.

48. Stern H, Weil J, Genz T, et al: Captopril in children with dilated cardiomyopathy: Acute and long-term effects in a prospective study of hemodynamic and hormonal effects. Pediatr Cardiol 1990;11:22-28.

49. Lewis AB, Chabot M: The effect of treatment with angiotensin-converting enzyme inhibitors on survival of pediatric patients with dilated cardiomyopathy. Pediatr Cardiol 1993;14:9-12.

50. Gonzalez A, Lopez B, Diez J: Fibrosis in hypertensive heart disease: Role of the renin-angiotensin-aldosterone system. Med Clin North Am 2004;88:83-97.

51. Lipshultz SE, Lipsitz SR, Sallan SE, et al: Long-term enalapril therapy for left ventricular dysfunction in doxorubicin-treated survivors of childhood cancer. J Clin Oncol 2002;20:4517-4522.

52. Buchhorn R, Ross RD, Hulpke-Wette M, et al: Effectiveness of low dose captopril versus propranolol therapy in infants with severe congestive failure due to left-to-right shunts. Int J Cardiol 2000;76:227-233.

53. Grenier MA, Fioravanti J, Truesdell SC, et al: Angiotensin-converting enzyme inhibitor therapy for ventricular dysfunction in infants, children and adolescents: A review. Prog Pediatr Cardiol 2000;12:91-111.

54. Lacourciere Y: The incidence of cough: A comparison of lisinopril, placebo and telmisartan, a novel angiotensin II antagonist. Telmisartan Cough Study Group. Int J Clin Pract 1999;53:99-103.

55. Wu SC, Liu CP, Chiang HT, Lin SL: Prospective and randomized study of the antihypertensive effect and tolerability of three antihypertensive agents, losartan, amlodipine, and lisinopril, in hypertensive patients. Heart Vessels 2004;19:13-18.

56. Yusuf S, Pfeffer MA, Swedberg K, et al: Effects of candesartan in patients with chronic heart failure and preserved left-ventricular ejection fraction: The CHARM-Preserved Trial. Lancet 2003;362:777-781.

57. McMurray JJ, Ostergren J, Swedberg K, et al: Effects of candesartan in patients with chronic heart failure and reduced left-ventricular systolic function taking angiotensin-converting-enzyme inhibitors: The CHARM-Added trial. Lancet 2003;362:767-771.

58. Granger CB, McMurray JJ, Yusuf S, et al: Effects of candesartan in patients with chronic heart failure and reduced left-ventricular systolic function intolerant to angiotensin-converting-enzyme inhibitors: The CHARM-Alternative trial. Lancet 2003;362:772-776.

59. Cohn JN, Johnson G, Ziesche S, et al: A comparison of enalapril with hydralazine-isosorbide dinitrate in the treatment of chronic congestive heart failure. N Engl J Med 1991;325:303-310.

60. Beekman RH, Rocchini AP, Rosenthal A: Hemodynamic effects of hydralazine in infants with a large ventricular septal defect. Circulation 1982;65:523-528.

61. Nakazawa M, Takao A, Chon Y, et al: Significance of systemic vascular resistance in determining the hemodynamic effects of hydralazine on large ventricular septal defects. Circulation 1983;68:420-424.

62. Artman M, Parrish MD, Boerth RC, et al: Short-term hemodynamic effects of hydralazine in infants with complete atrioventricular canal defects. Circulation 1984;69:949-954.

63. Artman M, Parrish MD, Appleton S, et al: Hemodynamic effects of hydralazine in infants with idiopathic dilated cardiomyopathy and congestive heart failure. Am Heart J 1987;113:144-150.

64. Seiler C, Hess OM, Schoenbeck M, et al: Long-term follow-up of medical versus surgical therapy for hypertrophic cardiomyopathy: A retrospective study. J Am Coll Cardiol 1991;17:634-642.

65. Ostman-Smith I, Wettrell G, Riesenfeld T: A cohort study of childhood hypertrophic cardiomyopathy: Improved survival following high-dose beta-adrenoceptor antagonist treatment. J Am Coll Cardiol 1999;34:1813-1822.

66. Berisha S, Goda A, Kastrati A, et al: Acute haemodynamic effects of nifedipine in patients with ventricular septal defect. Br Heart J 1988;60:149-155.

67. Gauthier B, Trachtman H: Short-acting nifedipine. Pediatr Nephrol 1997;11:786-787.

68. Sasaki R, Hirota K, Masuda A: Nifedipine-induced transient cerebral ischemia in a child with Cockayne syndrome. Anaesthesia 1997;52:1236.

69. Truttmann AC, Zehnder-Schlapbach S, Bianchetti MG: A moratorium should be placed on the use of short-acting nifedipine for hypertensive crises. Pediatr Nephrol 1998;12:259.

70. Flynn JT, Pasko DA: Calcium channel blockers: Pharmacology and place in therapy of pediatric hypertension. Pediatr Nephrol 2000;15:302-316.

71. Shapiro SM, Oudiz RJ, Cao T, et al: Primary pulmonary hypertension: Improved long-term effects and survival with continuous intravenous epoprostenol infusion. J Am Coll Cardiol 1997;30:343-349.

72. Califf RM, Adams KF, McKenna WJ, et al: A randomized controlled trial of epoprostenol therapy for severe congestive heart failure: The Flolan International Randomized Survival Trial (FIRST). Am Heart J 1997;134:44-54.

73. Bauer J, Dapper F, Demirakca S, et al: Perioperative management of pulmonary hypertension after heart transplantation in childhood. J Heart Lung Transplant 1997;16:1238-1247.

74. Pacher R, Stanek B, Hulsmann M, et al: Prostaglandin E1 infusion compared with prostacyclin infusion in patients with refractory heart failure: Effects on hemodynamics and neurohumoral variables. J Heart Lung Transplant 1997;16:878-881.

75. Stanek B, Sturm B, Frey B, et al: Bridging to heart transplantation: Prostaglandin E1 versus prostacyclin versus dobutamine. J Heart Lung Transplant 1999;18:358-366.

76. Cloez JL, Isaaz K, Marchal C, et al: [Hemodynamic effects of an alpha-blocking vasodilator in cardiac insufficiency caused by left-right shunt in children]. Arch Mal Coeur Vaiss 1986;79:677-682.

77. Strauser LM, Pruitt RD, Tobias JD: Initial experience with fenoldopam in children. Am J Ther 1999;6:283-288.

78. Potluri S, Uber P, Mehra M: Difficult cases in heart failure: Expanding the therapeutic armamentarium in decompensated heart failure: Using intravenous fenoldopam. Congest Heart Fail 2001;7:51-52.

79. Nussmeier NA: Improving perioperative outcomes in patients with end-stage heart failure. Rev Cardiovasc Med 2003;4(Suppl 1): S29-S34.

80. Hare JM, Shernan SK, Body SC, et al: Influence of inhaled nitric oxide on systemic flow and ventricular filling pressure in patients receiving mechanical circulatory assistance. Circulation 1997;95: 2250-2253.

81. Konstam MA, Salem DN, Isner JM, et al: Vasodilator effect on right ventricular function in congestive heart failure and pulmonary hypertension: End-systolic pressure–volume relation. Am J Cardiol 1984;54:132-136.

82. Kieler-Jensen N, Lundin S, Ricksten SE: Vasodilator therapy after heart transplantation: Effects of inhaled nitric oxide and intravenous prostacyclin, prostaglandin E1, and sodium nitroprusside. J Heart Lung Transplant 1995;14:436-443.

83. Loh E, Stamler JS, Hare JM, et al: Cardiovascular effects of inhaled nitric oxide in patients with left ventricular dysfunction. Circulation 1994;90:2780-2785.

84. Hayward CS, Kalnins WV, Rogers P, et al: Left ventricular chamber function during inhaled nitric oxide in patients with dilated cardiomyopathy. J Cardiovasc Pharmacol 1999;34:749-754.

85. Hayward CS, Rogers P, Keogh AM, et al: Inhaled nitric oxide in cardiac failure: Vascular versus ventricular effects. J Cardiovasc Pharmacol 1996;27:80-85.

86. Natori S, Hasebe N, Jin Y, et al: Effect of inhaled nitric oxide on cardiovascular response to catecholamine in heart failure. J Cardiovasc Pharmacol 2000;36(Suppl 2):S55-S60.

87. Natori S, Hasebe N, Jin YT, et al: Inhaled nitric oxide modifies left ventricular diastolic stress in the presence of vasoactive agents in heart failure. Am J Respir Crit Care Med 2003;167:895-901.

88. Boehm M, Nabel EG: Angiotensin converting enzyme 2: A new cardiac regulator. N Engl J Med 2002;347:1795-1797.

89. Masoudi FA, Rathore SS, Wang Y, et al: National patterns of use and effectiveness of angiotensin converting enzyme inhibitors in older patients with heart failure and left ventricular systolic dysfunction. Circulation 2004;110:724-731.

90. Patten RD, Soman P: Prevention and reversal of LV remodeling with neurohormonal inhibitors. Curr Treat Options Cardiovasc Med 2004;6:313-625.

91. McMurray JJ, Pfeffer MA: Heart failure. Lancet 2005;365:1877-1889.

CHAPTER 36

β-Adrenergic Receptor Blockade

Robert E. Shaddy

Waagstein and colleagues[1] first reported the use of β-adrenergic receptor antagonists (β-blockers) in a small group of adults with heart failure in 1975, but most clinicians considered β-blockers to be contraindicated in heart failure. Since then, there have been enormous advances in the development and subsequent analysis of numerous β-blockers to determine the safety and efficacy of these medications in the treatment of heart failure in adults. β-Blockers now are considered to be standard of care for adults with heart failure. Pediatric studies are under way to determine whether equal efficacy and safety exist with their use in children. See Chapters 18, 20, and 24 for additional discussions of β-blockers in treating heart failure in dilated and hypertrophic cardiomyopathy and the role of β-blockers in arrhythmias and heart failure.

β-BLOCKER THERAPY IN HEART FAILURE

β-Adrenergic Receptors and Heart Failure

β-Adrenergic receptors in the adult myocardium consist of primarily β_1-receptors and β_2-receptors, with a much smaller contribution from β_3-receptors. The **β_1-adrenergic receptors** constitute 75% to 80% of the nonfailing adult myocardium and younger myocardium,[2] and norepinephrine has high affinity for these receptors. Overexpression of the β_1-receptor at relatively low levels (about fivefold) in mice causes myocyte hypertrophy, apoptosis, and a dilated cardiomyopathy.[3] In contrast, knockout of the β_1-receptor in a mouse model results in no change in basal heart rate or blood pressure, but a blunted response to catecholamines.

The **β_2-adrenergic receptor** has distinct properties from the β_1-receptor. It constitutes only 20% to 25% of the β-adrenergic receptors in the nonfailing adult myocardium and younger myocardium.[2] Epinephrine, rather than norepinephrine, has a high affinity for the β_2-receptor, and overexpression at extremely high levels (about 100-fold) in mice causes a dilated cardiomyopathy. In a mouse β_2-adrenergic receptor knockout model, it has a similar effect as the β_1-receptor knockout model in that there is essentially no change in basal heart rate or blood pressure, but a blunted response to catecholamines.[3]

There are many alterations in β-adrenergic receptors in the failing myocardium.[2,4] In this situation, the β_1-receptor-to-β_2-receptor ratio approximates 50:50. The β_1-receptors and β_2-receptors are uncoupled, and the β_1-receptors are down-regulated. There is up-regulation of the β-adrenergic receptor kinase and inhibitory G protein, both of which contribute to uncoupling of the receptor. There also is down-regulation of adenylate cyclase. Some experts consider these processes to be adaptive in that they provide a partial "shield" against the harmful effects of chronic adrenergic stimulation.

In the pediatric myocardium, investigators have found down-regulation of β-adrenergic receptor density in infants with large left-to-right shunts and children with severe cyanotic and acyanotic congenital heart disease.[5] This down-regulation is seen most in the β_1-adrenergic receptors, but also to a lesser extent in the β_2-receptors.[6] Buchhorn and colleagues[7] correlated this β-adrenergic receptor down-regulation to a worse postoperative outcome in children undergoing surgical repair of a congenital heart lesion.

Adrenergic Receptors and Genetic Polymorphism

The novel analysis of α-receptor and β-receptor polymorphisms in patients with heart failure has provided a new paradigm for approaching not only the mechanisms of heart failure, but also the approach to the treatment of heart failure with agents such as β-blockers. Small and coworkers[8] performed genotyping on 159 patients with heart failure and 189 controls. They found that in African American patients, the odds ratio for heart failure in individuals homozygous for the alpha2Cdel322-325 polymorphism compared with other α_{2C}-adrenergic receptor genotypes was 5.65. With regard to the β-adrenergic receptor, there was no increased risk of heart failure in individuals with the beta1Arg389 polymorphism alone. There was a markedly increased risk of heart failure, however, among individuals who were homozygous for both polymorphism variants (odds ratio 10.11; $P = .004$). The alpha2Cdel322-325 and beta1Arg389 receptors act synergistically to increase the risk of heart failure in African Americans. This new information ultimately may allow for a unique opportunity to tailor antiadrenergic therapy to patients who are most likely to respond and patients who may benefit most from it.[9]

Rationale for β-Blocker Use

The rationale for the use of β-blockers, developed from molecular, cellular, animal, and human studies, involves the prevention and reversal of adrenergically mediated intrinsic myocardial dysfunction and remodeling. There are many adverse effects on myocytes from prolonged adrenergic stimulation. There are alterations in gene expression that lead to myocyte dysfunction, including re-expression of fetal genes for myocyte hypertrophy and the development of increased sarcoplasmic reticulum Ca^{2+}-ATPase (SERCA2) and adult forms of myosin heavy chain and troponin.[10] Other alterations include cell loss via necrosis or apoptosis or both; cell and chamber remodeling; and alterations in the interstitial matrix, including depletion of fibrillar collagen and activation of matrix metalloproteinases.[2,10]

β-Blockers have many proved and hypothesized effects on the myocardium. β-Blockers may depress myocardial function acutely because of their effects on blocking the ongoing adrenergic stimulation. Long-term beneficial effects include prevention of deterioration in myocardial function, improved systolic myocardial function, and reversal of the detrimental remodeling process seen in heart failure. Some β-blockers also can reverse abnormalities of the β-adrenergic receptor signal transduction pathway that occurs with heart failure.

The exact **mechanism of action** of β-blockers in heart failure is still being defined. However, A large body of basic science and clinical investigation supports the concept that the major beneficial effect of β-blockers in heart failure is the prevention or reversal of myocardial dysfunction that occurs in heart failure secondary to sympathetic activation, primarily from norepinephrine.[2] These adverse effects of sympathetic activation include increased ventricular volumes and pressures as a result of peripheral vasoconstriction, cardiac hypertrophy and coronary vasoconstriction leading to ischemia, increased programmed cell death, and increased risk of arrhythmias. Other proposed beneficial effects of β-blockers may be their negative chronotropic effects, up-regulation of β-adrenergic receptors (although many β-blockers do not up-regulate receptors), coronary vasodilatory effects, and possibly antioxidant effects (in β-blockers such as carvedilol).

Lowes and associates[11] studied gene expression in adults with dilated cardiomyopathy who were treated with β-blockers. They showed an increase in SERCA mRNA and α-myosin heavy chain mRNA, and a decrease in β-myosin heavy chain mRNA in subjects who had improvement in left ventricular function compared with subjects who did not. This study showed that in idiopathic dilated cardiomyopathy, improvements in left ventricular function by β-blocking agents are associated specifically with favorable changes in the expression of genes encoding SERCA and α and β isoforms of myosin heavy chain, but not β-adrenergic receptors. This represents a type of molecular remodeling in the form of reversal of induction of the fetal gene program in patients who have a favorable myocardial response to treatment.[11]

β-Blocker Use in Heart Failure

The β-blockers are heterogeneous in pharmacologic characteristics and are classified by mechanism of action (Table 36-1). Differences between β-blockers used in heart failure are related primarily to their α-receptor and β-receptor selectivities, but also their non–receptor-mediated actions, such as antioxidant effects. First-generation β-blockers, such as propranolol, are non-selective. Although second-generation β-blockers, such as metoprolol and bisoprolol, are β_1-selective, the third-generation β-blockers, such as bucindolol and carvedilol, have a vasodilator capability, which can mitigate against the potential decreased systolic function observed with adrenergic blockade. Carvedilol even has antioxidant properties. Although there is a plethora of β-blockers in clinical use, only agents with large clinical experiences for heart failure are discussed.

The **general principle of use** of β-blockers in patients with heart failure is to start at a low dose (≤20% of target dose) and titrate upward very slowly over a course of weeks (with an incremental increase in drug dosage once every 1 to 2 weeks). Patients need to be under close supervision because exacerbation of heart failure can ensue as adrenergic blockade occurs.

TABLE 36-1

Differences Between Types of β-Adrenergic Receptor Antagonists					
β-Blocker	Generation	β-Blocking Activity	α-Blocking Activity	Antioxidant Activity	Pediatric Experience
Propranolol	First	β_1/β_2	No	No	Yes
Metoprolol	Second	β_1	No	No	Yes
Bisoprolol	Second	β_1	No	No	No
Bucindolol	Third	β_1/β_2	α_1	No	No
Carvedilol	Third	β_1/β_2	α_1	Yes	Yes

On initiation and escalation of therapy with β-blockers, serial measurements of ventricular function may show a temporary worsening of parameters before eventual improvement over months. Significant bradycardia usually requires reduction in β-blocker dose. If a patient receiving maintenance β blockade decompensates, use of a phosphodiesterase inhibitor should be considered to augment cardiac output because these agents are not antagonized by β blockade.[12]

Contraindications include asthma, second-degree or third-degree heart block, severe bradycardia, decompensated heart failure, cardiogenic shock, hepatic or renal impairment, and hypersensitivity to the drug. These agents also can mask manifestations of hypoglycemia or thyrotoxicosis. Adverse effects that involve the cardiovascular system include vasodilatory effects (particularly when using β-blockers with ancillary vasodilatory properties), exacerbation of heart failure, and bradycardia. Extracardiac side effects include bronchoconstriction, central nervous system effects such as depression or agitation, Raynaud phenomenon, and hypoglycemia (See also appendix on drugs).

β-BLOCKER THERAPY IN ADULTS WITH HEART FAILURE

There is a preponderance of clinical trials and clinical experience with the use of β-blockers in adults. The overall results show that β-blockers are associated with at least a 30% reduction in all-cause mortality and 40% reduction in hospitalizations.[13,14] In adults, current recommendations are that all patients with stable heart failure secondary to left ventricular systolic dysfunction should receive a β-blocker, unless they are unable to tolerate treatment with these drugs or have a contraindication to their use.[15] The usefulness of β-blocker therapy in asymptomatic left ventricular dysfunction has not been widely investigated.

Metoprolol

Metoprolol is a β_1-selective agent without ancillary properties and has its extended-release tablet form as metoprolol CR/XL. The first multicenter trial of β-blockers in adults with heart failure was the **Metoprolol in Dilated Cardiomyopathy (MDC)** trial.[16] In this study, 383 adults with nonischemic dilated cardiomyopathy and mild-to-moderate heart failure were randomized to receive placebo or metoprolol. The primary end point was a combined risk of death or transplantation listing; this study showed no effect on the primary end point. In the follow-up to the MDC trial, the **Metoprolol CR/XL Randomized Intervention Trial in Congestive Heart Failure (MERIT-HF)** (See appendix) trial was designed to see whether a long-acting form of metoprolol could improve survival in adults with heart failure.[17] This study randomized 3991 patients with stable heart failure to

placebo or metoprolol CR/XL. The study was stopped early because of a significant beneficial effect of metoprolol as shown by a 34% decrease in all-cause mortality, a 38% decrease in cardiovascular mortality, and a 41% reduction in sudden death.

Bisoprolol

Bisoprolol, similar to metoprolol, is a β_1-selective agent with a 120-fold higher affinity for β_1-receptors. The **Cardiac Insufficiency Bisoprolol Study (CIBIS-I)** randomized 641 adults with ischemic or nonischemic cardiomyopathy to placebo or bisoprolol (5 mg/day) with a primary end point of all-cause mortality.[18] Similar to the MDC trial, there was an insignificant (22%) reduction in mortality, although there was a significant reduction in hospitalizations because of heart failure. It is likely that both of these studies were statistically underpowered to show survival benefit in patients who received β blockade. The CIBIS-II trial randomized 2647 adults with heart failure to either placebo or bisoprolol at 10 mg/day (compared with 5 mg/day in CIBIS-I).[19] This trial also was stopped early because of a significant decrease in mortality in the β-blocker treatment arm: 11.8% versus 17.3%.

Bucindolol

Bucindolol is a nonselective β-blocking agent without intrinsic sympathomimetic activities, but with sympatholytic properties.[9] In the **Beta-blocker Evaluation of Survival (BEST)** trial, bucindolol was not shown to improve survival in adults with mild-to-moderate heart failure.[20] The authors speculated that the difference between the survival benefit found in other β-blocker trials and the BEST trial could be due to different patient populations or possibly the unique pharmacologic properties of bucindolol. The sympatholytic properties of bucindolol may diminish its potential benefit in the treatment of chronic heart failure. This sympatholytic property also has been found to be detrimental in studies examining the effect of moxonidine in heart failure. Moxonidine lowers norepinephrine through central imidazoline or α_2-adrenergic receptor activation plus possible presynaptic α_2-adrenergic receptor agonism.[9] This drug increased mortality by more than 50% in the **Moxonidine Congestive Heart Failure (MOXCON)** trial, with the study being stopped prematurely because of safety concerns.[21]

Carvedilol

Carvedilol is a third-generation nonselective β_1-adrenergic and β_2-adrenergic blocking agent with α_1-blocking properties, which results in vasodilating properties and offers an advantage in the treatment of heart failure. It also has ancillary properties of antagonism at prejunctional β-adrenoceptors and acts as an antioxidant. All of these properties contribute to its effect in reversing cardiac remodeling in animal models and patients with heart failure.[22]

In 1996, two studies finally showed a survival benefit from the use of β-blockers in adults with chronic heart failure. In the **Multicenter Oral Carvedilol Heart Failure Assessment (MOCHA)** trial, Bristow and colleagues[23] randomized 345 adults with ischemic or nonischemic cardiomyopathy to receive either placebo or carvedilol (12.5 mg to 50 mg daily). The primary end point was submaximal exercise; there was no benefit from carvedilol on the primary end point. There was a statistically significant dose-dependent reduction, however, in mortality and hospitalization. Mortality decreased from 14.3% in the placebo group to 4.8% in the carvedilol 12.5 mg daily group, to 3.4% in the carvedilol 25 mg daily, and to 1.1% in the carvedilol 50 mg daily group (Fig. 36-1). There was a similar dose-dependent increase seen in left ventricular ejection fraction. Packer and colleagues[24] also randomized 1094 adults with mild-to-moderate heart failure to placebo or carvedilol and found a 65% reduction in mortality in patients who received carvedilol and a 27% reduction in the risk of hospitalization for cardiovascular causes. Until more recently, β-blockers were recommended only for the treatment of mild-to-moderate heart failure in adults. The **Carvedilol Prospective Randomized Cumulative Survival Trial (COPERNICUS)** randomized 2389 adults with severe heart failure at 334 centers to either placebo or carvedilol and showed a 35% reduction in all-cause mortality (Fig. 36-2).[25]

Comparative Studies

Investigators have compared the safety and efficacy of different β-blockers in adults with heart failure. Metra and associates[26] randomized 150 adults with heart failure and left ventricular ejection fractions of less than 35% to receive either metoprolol or carvedilol. Compared with patients receiving metoprolol, patients receiving carvedilol showed larger increases in left ventricular ejection fraction (10.9% versus 7.2%) at rest, larger increases in left ventricular stroke volume and stroke work during exercise, and greater reductions in pulmonary artery and pulmonary capillary wedge pressures. The carvedilol group showed less improvement in maximal exercise tolerance, however, than the metoprolol group, but there were no differences between groups with regard to symptoms or submaximal exercise. Sanderson and coworkers[27] randomized 51 adults with heart failure and reduced left ventricular ejection fraction (26% ± 2%) to metoprolol (maximal dose 50 mg) or carvedilol (maximal dose 25 mg). In this study, there were no differences between groups with regard to changes in symptoms, left ventricular ejection fraction, or exercise capacity. Carvedilol had greater effects on blood pressure, left ventricular end-diastolic dimension, and mitral valve inflow. Carvedilol also has been shown to cause significant decreases in systemic and cardiac norepinephrine release, effects not seen with metoprolol.[28]

In a prospective crossover comparison of carvedilol and metoprolol, Maack and colleagues[29] studied 44 adult patients with ischemic or dilated cardiomyopathy who were stable on either carvedilol or metoprolol treatment. Before and 6 months after crossover of treatment, left ventricular ejection fractions had improved in both groups, although with dobutamine infusion, patients on crossover carvedilol had a lesser heart rate response during infusion and an increase in left ventricular ejection fraction after infusion that was not seen in the metoprolol crossover group. Bristow and colleagues[23] argued that this improved cardiac performance of carvedilol compared with metoprolol may represent the small but measurable incremental effect of adding β2-receptor and α1-receptor blockade, suggesting a potential advantage to a more comprehensive degree of β blockade.

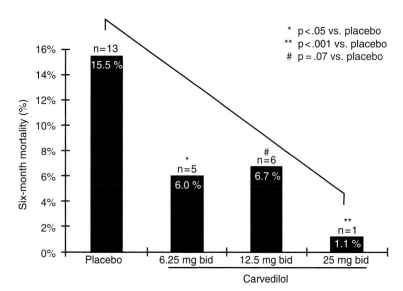

* p<.05 vs. placebo
** p<.001 vs. placebo
\# p = .07 vs. placebo

FIGURE 36-1 ■ Results of the Multicenter Oral Carvedilol Heart Failure Assessment (MOCHA) Trial. Six-month crude mortality as deaths per randomized patients × 100 in patients treated with placebo, carvedilol 6.25 mg orally twice daily, carvedilol 12.5 mg orally twice daily, and carvedilol 25 mg orally twice daily. *n* = number of deaths in each group. (From Bristow MR, Gilbert EM, Abraham WT, et al: *Carvedilol produces dose-related improvements in left ventricular function and survival in subjects with chronic heart failure.* MOCHA Investigators. *Circulation* 1996;94: 2807-2816.)

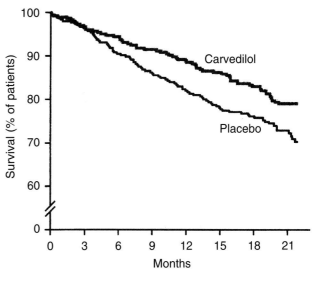

FIGURE 36-2 ■ Results of the Carvedilol Prospective Randomized Cumulative Survival (COPERNICUS) study. Kaplan-Meier analysis of time to death in the placebo group and the carvedilol group. The 35% lower risk in the carvedilol group was significant: $P = .00013$ (unadjusted) and $P = .0014$ (adjusted). (From Packer M, Fowler MB, Roecker EB, et al: *Effect of carvedilol on the morbidity of patients with severe chronic heart failure: Results of the carvedilol prospective randomized cumulative survival (COPERNICUS) study. Circulation* 2002;106:2194-2199.)

β-BLOCKER THERAPY IN CHILDREN WITH HEART FAILURE

Although there are profound differences in the etiology of heart failure between children and adults, the neurohormonal activation of heart failure in children is similar to adults. Current experience on the use of β-blockers in children with heart failure is limited to the small published case series described subsequently, and multicenter, randomized, controlled clinical trials to assess the efficacy of β-blockers in ameliorating heart failure are much needed in the pediatric population.

Propranolol

Propranolol is a nonselective β-blocker with equal affinity for β_1-receptors and β_2-receptors and does not block α-adrenergic receptors. It has negative inotropic and chronotropic actions on the heart. Its first-pass effect in the liver results in low bioavailability and marked differences in plasma concentrations in children.[30] Propranolol has been widely accepted as a pharmacologic therapy for myriad of clinical conditions in children, including hypercyanotic spells in tetralogy of Fallot, hypertrophic cardiomyopathy, hypertension, and tachydysrhythmias.

The experience with use of propranolol in heart failure in children is limited. Buchhorn and colleagues[31,32] reported the beneficial effects of propranolol in infants with congestive heart failure resulting from left-to-right intracardiac shunts. In these studies, treatment with propranolol resulted in lower respiratory rates and heart rates and improved weight gain. There also were significant changes in circulating neurohormonal parameters.

These effects of propranolol seem to be better than the effects seen with low-dose captopril.[33] These investigators also showed alterations in neurohormonal activation and receptor regulation in patients with heart failure and congenital heart disease. When comparing the patients treated with digoxin and diuretics with patients treated with these medications and β blockade, they showed that β-blockers partially prevent down-regulation of β_2-receptor and angiotensin II receptor genes and up-regulation of endothelin A receptor and connective tissue growth factor genes.[34] There is also evidence for β blockade to reverse depressed heart rate variability in infants with heart failure.[35] There may be some benefit of β-blockers in this clinical setting, although further study is indicated.

Metoprolol

Shaddy and coworkers[36] first reported experience with the use of β-blockers in children with heart failure in three teenagers who were referred for evaluation for heart transplantation because of congestive heart failure from left ventricular dysfunction secondary to anthracyclines used in the treatment of malignancies. All patients were receiving diuretics, digoxin, and angiotensin-converting enzyme inhibitors without significant improvements in left ventricular function or symptoms before starting metoprolol. Metoprolol was started at the low dose of 12.5 mg/day divided into two daily doses and gradually increased to approximately 100 mg/day. Two patients had long-term improvements in left ventricular function and symptoms and were no longer considered for transplantation. The third patient received minimal, if any, benefit from metoprolol and ultimately underwent heart transplantation 34 months after starting metoprolol.

Shaddy[37] subsequently reported experience with the beneficial effects of metoprolol in four young children with congestive heart failure with left ventricular dysfunction. Shaddy and coworkers[38] also reported a multi-institutional experience with metoprolol in the treatment of 15 children, age 8.6 ± 1.3 years (range 2.5 to 15 years), with congestive heart failure resulting from idiopathic dilated cardiomyopathy (9 patients), anthracycline cardiomyopathy (3 patients), Duchenne muscular dystrophy cardiomyopathy (1 patient), postmyocarditis cardiomyopathy (1 patient), and postsurgical cardiomyopathy (1 patient). All patients had been treated with conventional medications (digoxin, diuretics, and angiotensin-converting enzyme inhibitors) for 22.5 ± 9 months before starting metoprolol. Metoprolol was started at 0.1 to 0.2 mg/kg/dose given twice daily and slowly increased over a period of several weeks to a final dose of 1.1 ± 0.1 mg/kg/day (range 0.5 to 2.3 mg/kg/day). Between the time point of stabilization on conventional medications and the initiation of metoprolol therapy, there was no significant change in fractional shortening (13.1% ± 1.2% versus 15% ± 1.2%) or ejection fraction (25.6% ± 2.1% versus 27% ± 3.4%). After metoprolol therapy for 23.2 ± 7 months, there were significant increases in fractional shortening (23.3% ± 2.6%) and ejection fraction (41.1% ± 4.3%; $P < .05$) (Fig. 36-3). There were no significant adverse events noted with the exception of asymptomatic sinus bradycardia in one patient, who responded to outpatient reduction in metoprolol dose. From this study, it was concluded that metoprolol improves ventricular function in some children with dilated cardiomyopathy and congestive heart failure.

Carvedilol

Bruns and associates[39] reported a retrospective analysis of a multicenter experience of carvedilol for the treatment of chronic heart failure in a group of 46 children. At some time point (no primary end point was defined), two thirds of the patients reported improvement in symptoms, although adverse outcomes occurred in 30% of the patients. More than one half of the patients experienced side effects, including dizziness, hypotension, and headaches. The authors concluded that there might be some benefit to the use of β-blockers in children with heart failure, although prospective trials are necessary to determine this.

Laer and colleagues[40] also showed improvements in symptoms and left ventricular systolic performance in a small group of pediatric patients treated with carvedilol. In examining the pharmacokinetics of carvedilol in this group of children, they found that the elimination half-life of carvedilol was about 50% shorter in children with heart failure than in healthy adult volunteers. Gachara and associates[41] reported their experience with the use

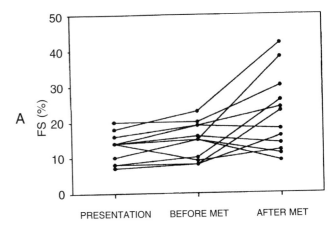

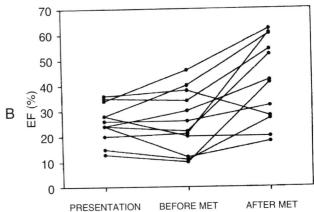

FIGURE 36-3 ■ Metoprolol treatment of dilated cardiomyopathy with congestive heart failure in children. Fractional shortening (FS) and ejection fraction (EF) in patients at three points in time: (1) presentation, which was the time the patient was first diagnosed with cardiomyopathy and after stabilization on conventional medications; (2) before metoprolol, just before starting metoprolol and after having been maintained on conventional medications for a mean period of 22.5 ± 9 months (range 0.5 to 119 months); and (3) after metoprolol, after receiving metoprolol for a mean period of 23.2 ± 7 months (range 1.2 to 102 months). MET, metoprolol. (From Shaddy RE, Tani LY, Gidding SS, et al: *Beta-blocker treatment of dilated cardiomyopathy with congestive heart failure in children: A multi-institutional experience.* J Heart Lung Transplant 1999;18:269-274.)

of open-label carvedilol in eight symptomatic infants with dilated cardiomyopathy. In their study, left ventricular ejection fraction and symptoms improved over 4.5 ± 2 months of carvedilol treatment. There were no significant adverse events or deaths in this group.

More recently, Azeka and coworkers[42] reported the results of a double-blinded, placebo-controlled study of 22 pediatric patients with severe left ventricular dysfunction who were randomized to placebo or carvedilol. In their study, there were four deaths and one heart transplantation in the carvedilol group and two deaths and two heart transplantations in the placebo group. In patients who survived and were not transplanted, left ventricular ejection fraction and fractional shortening improved only in patients treated with carvedilol. There is a high incidence of adverse effects in children who receive carvedilol for the treatment of heart failure.[39] Of note is the potential interaction of carvedilol with digoxin because oral clearance of digoxin is decreased by half with carvedilol.[43]

The only comparison of different types of β-blockers in children with heart failure failed to show any obvious differences in left ventricular systolic performance indices in a small group of children treated with either metoprolol or carvedilol.[44] There also have been case reports of β-blockers reversing pulmonary hypertension in children.[45,46] One possible mechanism would be the decrease in pulmonary arterial pressures secondary to improved left ventricular function, although there may be other direct mechanisms as well.

CURRENT STATUS AND FUTURE TRENDS

β-Blockers need to be used with extreme caution, and patients need to be monitored closely because there could be exacerbation of heart failure, particularly in patients with new-onset or more severe heart failure. Use of these medications is controversial in severe heart failure with decompensation. Compared with angiotensin-converting enzyme inhibitors, β-blockers provide less reduction in mortality in patients with worsening heart failure.[47] The reduction in mortality for patients with mild-to-moderate heart failure was greater for β-blockers compared with angiotensin-converting enzyme inhibitor.[48] Dosing in children has been extrapolated from adult data,[38,39] and the ideal dosing schedules for β-blockers in children with heart failure are unknown.

Although studies suggest a beneficial effect of β-blockers in certain pediatric patients with heart failure, all of the studies are too small to draw definitive conclusions about improvements in symptoms and mortality. There is an ongoing multicenter, placebo-controlled, double-blinded randomized trial of carvedilol in children with heart failure symptoms resulting from systemic ventricular dysfunction.[49] There is still little evidence as to whether β-blockers improve function in right or single ventricles.[50] It is hoped that the current multicenter carvedilol trial will provide some important information regarding this and other issues specific to children and β-blockers.[51]

Key Concepts
■ The rationale for the use of β-blockers, developed from molecular, cellular, animal, and human studies, involves the prevention and reversal of adrenergically mediated intrinsic myocardial dysfunction and remodeling.

■ β-Blockers may depress myocardial function acutely because of their effects on blocking the ongoing adrenergic stimulation. Long-term beneficial effects include prevention of deterioration in myocardial function, improved systolic myocardial function, and

reversal of the detrimental remodeling process seen in heart failure.

■ Differences between β-blockers used in heart failure are related primarily to their α-receptor and β-receptor selectivities, but also their non–receptor-mediated actions, such as antioxidant effects.

■ The general principle in the use of β-blockers in patients with heart failure is to start at a low dose (≤20% of target dose) and titrate upward very slowly over weeks (with incremental increase in drug dosage once every 1 to 2 weeks). Patients need to be under close supervision because exacerbation of heart failure can ensue as adrenergic blockade occurs.

■ There is a preponderance of clinical trials and clinical experience with the use of β-blockers in adults. The overall results show that β-blockers are associated with at least a 30% reduction in all-cause mortality and 40% reduction in hospitalizations.

■ Although there are profound differences in the etiologies of heart failure between children and adults, the neurohormonal activation of heart failure in children is similar to adults.

■ Current experience on the use of β-blockers in children with heart failure is limited to small published case series. Multicenter, randomized, controlled clinical trials to assess the efficacy of β-blockers in ameliorating heart failure are much needed in pediatric patients.

■ Compared with angiotensin-converting enzyme inhibitors, β-blockers have less reduction in mortality in patients with worsening heart failure. The reduction in mortality for patients with mild-to-moderate heart failure was greater for β-blockers compared with angiotensin-converting enzyme inhibitors.

REFERENCES

1. Waagstein F, Hjalmarson A, Varnauskas E, Wallentin I: Effect of chronic beta-adrenergic receptor blockade in congestive cardiomyopathy. Br Heart J 1975;37:1022-1036.
2. Bristow MR: Mechanism of action of beta-blocking agents in heart failure. Am J Cardiol 1997;80:26L-40L.
3. Rohrer DK, Chruscinski A, Schauble EH, et al: Cardiovascular and metabolic alterations in mice lacking both beta1- and beta2-adrenergic receptors. J Biol Chem 1999;274:16701-16708.
4. Port JD, Bristow MR: Altered beta-adrenergic receptor gene regulation and signaling in chronic heart failure. J Mol Cell Cardiol 2001;33:887-905.
5. Kozlik-Feldmann R, Kramer HH, Wicht H, et al: Distribution of myocardial beta-adrenoceptor subtypes and coupling to the adenylate cyclase in children with congenital heart disease and implications for treatment. J Clin Pharmacol 1993;33:588-595.
6. Brodde OE, Zerkowski HR, Borst HG, et al: Drug- and disease-induced changes of human cardiac beta 1- and beta 2-adrenoceptors. Eur Heart J 1989;10(Suppl B):38-44.
7. Buchhorn R, Hulpke-Wette M, Ruschewski W, et al: Beta-receptor downregulation in congenital heart disease: A risk factor for complications after surgical repair? Ann Thorac Surg 2002;73:610-613.
8. Small KM, Wagoner LE, Levin AM, et al: Synergistic polymorphisms of beta1- and alpha2C-adrenergic receptors and the risk of congestive heart failure. N Engl J Med 2002;347:1135-1142.

9. Bristow M: Antiadrenergic therapy of chronic heart failure: Surprises and new opportunities. Circulation 2003;107:1100-1102.

10. Colucci WS, Sawyer DB, Singh K, Communal C: Adrenergic overload and apoptosis in heart failure: Implications for therapy. J Card Fail 2000;6(2 Suppl 1):1-7.

11. Lowes BD, Gilbert EM, Abraham WT, et al: Myocardial gene expression in dilated cardiomyopathy treated with beta-blocking agents. N Engl J Med 2002;346:1357-1365.

12. Bohm M, Deutsch HJ, Hartmann D, et al: Improvement of postreceptor events by metoprolol treatment in patients with chronic heart failure. J Am Coll Cardiol 1997;30:992-996.

13. Foody JM, Farrell MH, Krumholz HM: Beta-Blocker therapy in heart failure: scientific review. JAMA 2002;287:883-889.

14. Tendera M, Ochala A: Overview of the results of recent beta blocker trials. Curr Opin Cardiol 2001;16:180-185.

15. Packer M, Cohn J: Consensus recommendations for the management of chronic heart failure. Am J Cardiol 1999;83:1A-38A.

16. Waagstein F, Bristow MR, Swedberg K, et al: Beneficial effects of metoprolol in idiopathic dilated cardiomyopathy: Metoprolol in Dilated Cardiomyopathy (MDC) Trial Study Group. Lancet 1993; 342:1441-1446.

17. Effect of metoprolol CR/XL in chronic heart failure: Metoprolol CR/XL Randomised Intervention Trial in Congestive Heart Failure (MERIT-HF). Lancet 1999;353:2001-2007.

18. A randomized trial of beta-blockade in heart failure: The Cardiac Insufficiency Bisoprolol Study (CIBIS). CIBIS Investigators and Committees. Circulation 1994;90:1765-1773.

19. The Cardiac Insufficiency Bisoprolol Study II (CIBIS-II): A randomised trial. Lancet 1999;353:9-13.

20. A trial of the beta-blocker bucindolol in patients with advanced chronic heart failure. N Engl J Med 2001;344:1659-1667.

21. Coats AJ: Heart Failure 99: The MOXCON story. Int J Cardiol 1999;71:109-111.

22. Moe G: Carvedilol in the treatment of chronic heart failure. Expert Opin Pharmacother 2001;2:831-843.

23. Bristow MR, Gilbert EM, Abraham WT, et al: Carvedilol produces dose-related improvements in left ventricular function and survival in subjects with chronic heart failure. MOCHA Investigators. Circulation 1996;94:2807-2816.

24. Packer M, Bristow MR, Cohn JN, et al: The effect of carvedilol on morbidity and mortality in patients with chronic heart failure. U.S. Carvedilol Heart Failure Study Group. N Engl J Med 1996; 334:1349-1355.

25. Packer M, Fowler MB, Roecker EB, et al: Effect of carvedilol on the morbidity of patients with severe chronic heart failure: Results of the carvedilol prospective randomized cumulative survival (COPERNICUS) study. Circulation 2002;106:2194-2199.

26. Metra M, Giubbini R, Nodari S, et al: Differential effects of beta-blockers in patients with heart failure: A prospective, randomized, double-blind comparison of the long-term effects of metoprolol versus carvedilol. Circulation 2000;102:546-551.

27. Sanderson JE, Chan SK, Yip G, et al: Beta-blockade in heart failure: A comparison of carvedilol with metoprolol. J Am Coll Cardiol 1999;34:1522-1528.

28. Azevedo ER, Kubo T, Mak S, et al: Nonselective versus selective beta-adrenergic receptor blockade in congestive heart failure: Differential effects on sympathetic activity. Circulation 2001;104: 2194-2199.

29. Maack C, Elter T, Nickenig G, et al: Prospective crossover comparison of carvedilol and metoprolol in patients with chronic heart failure. J Am Coll Cardiol 2001;38:939-946.

30. Gorodischer R, Koren G: Cardiac drugs. In Yaffe SJ, Aranda JV (eds): Pediatric Pharmacology. Philadelphia, WB Saunders, 345-354, 1992.

31. Buchhorn R, Bartmus D, Siekmeyer W, et al: Beta-blocker therapy of severe congestive heart failure in infants with left to right shunts. Am J Cardiol 1998;81:1366-1368.

32. Buchhorn R, Hulpke-Wette M, Hilgers R, et al: Propranolol treatment of congestive heart failure in infants with congenital heart disease: The CHF-PRO-INFANT Trial: Congestive Heart Failure in Infants Treated with Propanol. Int J Cardiol 2001;79:167-173.

33. Buchhorn R, Ross RD, Hulpke-Wette M, et al: Effectiveness of low dose captopril versus propranolol therapy in infants with severe congestive failure due to left-to-right shunts. Int J Cardiol 2000;76:227-233.

34. Buchhorn R, Hulpke-Wette M, Ruschewski W, et al: Effects of therapeutic beta blockade on myocardial function and cardiac remodelling in congenital cardiac disease. Cardiol Young 2003;13:36-43.

35. Buchhorn R, Hulpke-Wette M, Nothroff J, Paul T: Heart rate variability in infants with heart failure due to congenital heart disease: Reversal of depressed heart rate variability by propranolol. Med Sci Monit 2002;8:CR661-CR666.

36. Shaddy RE, Olsen SL, Bristow MR, et al: Efficacy and safety of metoprolol in the treatment of doxorubicin-induced cardiomyopathy in pediatric patients. Am Heart J 1995;129:197-199.

37. Shaddy RE: Beta-blocker therapy in young children with congestive heart failure under consideration for heart transplantation. Am Heart J 1998;136:19-21.

38. Shaddy RE, Tani LY, Gidding SS, et al: Beta-blocker treatment of dilated cardiomyopathy with congestive heart failure in children: A multi-institutional experience. J Heart Lung Transplant 1999;18:269-274.

39. Bruns LA, Chrisant MK, Lamour JM, et al: Carvedilol as therapy in pediatric heart failure: An initial multicenter experience. J Pediatr 2001;138:505-511.

40. Laer S, Mir TS, Behn F, et al: Carvedilol therapy in pediatric patients with congestive heart failure: A study investigating clinical and pharmacokinetic parameters. Am Heart J 2002;143:916-922.

41. Gachara N, Prabhakaran S, Srinivas S, et al: Efficacy and safety of carvedilol in infants with dilated cardiomyopathy: A preliminary report. Indian Heart J 2001;53:74-78.

42. Azeka E, Franchini Ramires JA, Valler C, Alcides Bocchi E: Delisting of infants and children from the heart transplantation waiting list after carvedilol treatment. J Am Coll Cardiol 2002;40:2034-2038.

43. Ratnapalan S, Griffiths K, Costei AM, et al: Digoxin-carvedilol interactions in children. J Pediatr 2003;142:572-574.

44. Williams RV, Tani LY, Shaddy RE: Intermediate effects of treatment with metoprolol or carvedilol in children with left ventricular systolic dysfunction. J Heart Lung Transplant 2002;21:906-909.

45. Buchhorn R, Hulpke-Wette M, Wessel A, Bursch J: Beta-blocker therapy in an infant with pulmonary hypertension. Eur J Pediatr 1999;158:1007-1008.

46. Horenstein MS, Ross RD, Singh TP, Epstein ML: Carvedilol reverses elevated pulmonary vascular resistance in a child with dilated cardiomyopathy. Pediatr Cardiol 2002;23:100-102.

47. Effects of enalapril on mortality in severe congestive heart failure: Results of the Cooperative North Scandinavian Enalapril Survival Study (CONSENSUS). The CONSENSUS Trial Study Group. N Engl J Med 1987;316:1429-1435.

48. Effect of enalapril on survival in patients with reduced left ventricular ejection fractions and congestive heart failure. The SOLVD Investigators. N Engl J Med 1991;325:293-302.

49. Shaddy RE, Curtin EL, Sower B, et al: The Pediatric Randomized Carvedilol Trial in Children with Heart Failure: Rationale and design. Am Heart J 2002;144:383-389.

50. Quaife RA, Christian PE, Gilbert EM, et al: Effects of carvedilol on right ventricular function in chronic heart failure. Am J Cardiol 1998;81:247-250.

51. Hoch M, Netz H: Heart failure in pediatric patients. Thorac Cardiovasc Surg 2005;53 Suppl 2: S129-134.

CHAPTER 37

Low Cardiac Output Syndrome in the Intensive Care Setting

Catherine L. Dent
David P. Nelson

Previous chapters have discussed medical therapeutic strategies for patients with various diagnoses, such as myocarditis, various types of cardiomyopathy, and valvular insufficiency and stenosis; this chapter focuses on the most common heart failure clinical scenario in the cardiac intensive care setting: the postoperative surgical patient with low cardiac output. In recent decades, significant advances in surgical techniques and pediatric cardiac intensive care have contributed to marked improvements in morbidity and mortality after pediatric cardiac surgery. Despite these improvements, patients remain at risk for low cardiac output and impaired systemic oxygen delivery, especially in the early postoperative period. The transient decrease in cardiac output after cardiac surgery has been referred to as low cardiac output syndrome (LCOS).

LCOS in the early postoperative period is due primarily to transient myocardial dysfunction, compounded by acute changes in myocardial loading conditions, including postoperative increases in systemic vascular resistance (SVR), pulmonary vascular resistance (PVR), or both. Residual cardiac abnormalities, even if minor, may aggravate further an underlying low cardiac output state. Surgical repair of cardiac malformations exposes the myocardium to periods of ischemia, resulting in transient myocardial stunning or damage. Cardiopulmonary bypass (CPB), which activates the complement and inflammatory cascades,[1,2] also contributes to myocardial injury, alterations in pulmonary and systemic vascular reactivity, and pulmonary dysfunction.[3-6] In addition, some repairs require ventriculotomy, which further exacerbates myocardial dysfunction. Although advances in myocardial protection, cardioplegia, and perfusion techniques have reduced perioperative cardiovascular injury dramatically, even relatively simple cardiac procedures still are associated with measurable myocardial dysfunction.[7]

Several studies have documented the predictable and reproducible decreases in cardiac output after surgery for congenital heart defects in neonates, infants, and young children.[8,9] In an early study of neonates undergoing arterial switch operation, the median decrease in cardiac index, which occurred typically 6 to 12 hours after CPB, was 32%. Nearly one fourth of these infants had a cardiac index nadir of less than 2 L/min/m² after surgery.[8] Figure 37-1 shows this decrease in output

occurs without significant changes in atrial filling pressure or inotropic support, suggesting the presence of contractile dysfunction or increased ventricular afterload because SVR increases during this same period. Wall stress analysis of a subgroup of these patients 1 to 2 weeks after surgery showed that myocardial function was normalized or augmented, indicating postoperative myocardial depression in these patients was a transient phenomenon.[10] Data from the multicenter PRIMACORP (PRophylactic Intravenous use of Milrinone After Cardiac Operations in Pediatrics) study indicate that the incidence of postoperative LCOS is significant, ranging from 10% in treated patients to 27% in control patients.[11]

Morbidity and mortality associated with LCOS are high. In the early days of infant cardiac surgery, surgical mortality approached 20%.[12] Although LCOS is associated with lower mortality in the current era, it results in increased hospital stay, increased resource use, and possible long-term cognitive dysfunction.[13] Prompt recognition, diagnosis, and management of LCOS are fundamental to optimal cardiac intensive care and essential for optimal patient outcome.

CLINICAL SIGNS OF LOW CARDIAC OUTPUT SYNDROME

The signs and symptoms of LCOS result from the combined effects of systemic and pulmonary venous congestion and inadequate systemic blood flow with poor end-organ perfusion. Respiratory compromise resulting from pulmonary venous congestion is one of the earliest signs of heart failure in children, but this may not be detected immediately in mechanically ventilated patients. Systemic venous congestion typically results in hepatomegaly, pleural effusions, ascites, and peripheral edema. Typical signs of inadequate end-organ perfusion or cardiogenic shock include tachycardia, poor peripheral perfusion, oliguria, and ultimately metabolic acidosis. Clinical assessment of systemic perfusion is an important, albeit nonquantitative, indicator of LCOS. In particular, assessment of capillary refill time or core toe temperature gradient or both may be helpful, although neither capillary refill time nor core toe temperature gradient has been carefully validated. Although postoperative LCOS may cause hypotension, systemic blood pressure

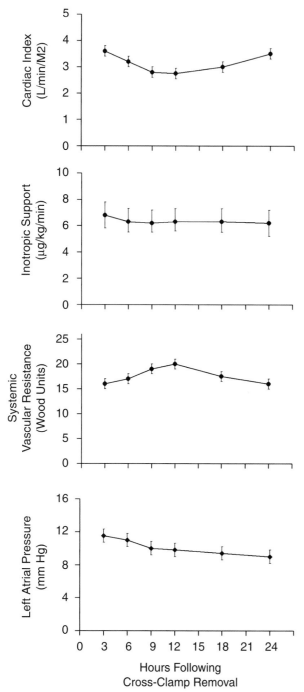

FIGURE 37-1 ■ Serial measurements of cardiac index, inotropic support, systemic vascular resistance, and left atrial pressure after arterial switch procedure. With stable inotropic support, cardiac index decreases during the first 12 postoperative hours, returning to normal at 24 hours after surgery. During this same period, systemic vascular resistance increases, returning to baseline at 24 hours. (From Wernovsky G, Wypij D, Jonas RA, et al: *Postoperative course and hemodynamic profile after the arterial switch operation in neonates and infants: A comparison of low-flow cardiopulmonary bypass and circulatory arrest. Circulation* 1995;92:2226-2235.)

is a particularly poor indicator of systemic perfusion in children, who can increase markedly their systemic vascular tone. Hypotension and bradycardia tend to be late consequences of LCOS, frequently occurring only minutes before cardiac arrest. Intractable cardiogenic shock results in unrelenting metabolic acidosis and ultimately multiorgan failure, including acute renal failure, gastrointestinal complications, and central nervous system compromise. Because LCOS is magnified in patients with palliated physiology or residual cardiac abnormalities, multiorgan system failure is more likely in such patients.

Respiratory insufficiency after congenital heart surgery can manifest as alterations in PVR, reduced pulmonary compliance, or defects in pulmonary gas exchange. Its time course mimics the predictable decrease in cardiac index,[14] and its intensity varies greatly among patients.[15] The fact that many pediatric patients are extubated early after cardiac surgery indicates that pulmonary dysfunction is often minimal, but patients with LCOS typically require increased levels and longer periods of ventilatory support after surgery.[16] Pleural effusions and ascites, which exacerbate pulmonary mechanical and gas exchange defects in patients with LCOS, may require attention and appropriate drainage.

Because the ability to maintain renal blood flow and glomerular filtration is lost during cardiogenic shock in infants, **oliguria** is one of the most important clinical indicators of LCOS. In patients with marginal renal perfusion, a period of prerenal azotemia usually precedes acute renal failure. Progression of the renal insult to acute tubular necrosis usually necessitates the support of pressure-dependent renal blood flow.[17] The incidence of acute renal failure after cardiac surgery ranges from 2.4% to 8%, but transient renal insufficiency with a reduced creatinine clearance is common.[8,18] Risk factors include perioperative ischemia, hypotension, and acidosis.[17] If supportive therapy with inotropes, fluids, and intravenous diuretics is ineffective, hemofiltration or peritoneal dialysis may be necessary. Peritoneal dialysis is usually the preferred method of renal replacement therapy, with fewer clinical complications. Studies evaluating the acute hemodynamic effects of peritoneal dialysis after surgical repair of congenital heart defects report that fluid shifts caused by dialysate instillation are well tolerated and hemodynamically beneficial.[18,19] Arteriovenous hemofiltration is often poorly tolerated in infants after cardiac surgery because of hemodynamic instability. Continuous venovenous hemofiltration may be beneficial in some patients, but its disadvantages include access difficulties and the need for systemic anticoagulation.[20]

Enteral feeding intolerance may be evident in patients with LCOS and central venous hypertension and may be compounded by high-dose inotropes and narcotic infusions. General attention should be paid to the nutritional needs of the postoperative patient, and patients with LCOS often require parenteral nutrition. Because bacteremia or sepsis may result from poor intestinal mucosal integrity, however, the early institution of trophic enteral feeding may be beneficial.[21] Hepatic hypoperfusion in patients with LCOS also may result in hepatic insufficiency. If the hepatic insult is severe, patients may develop coagulopathy as a result of reduced hepatic synthesis of coagulation factors. Coagulopathy in this setting may not be due exclusively to hepatic dysfunction. A component of disseminated intravascular coagulation is common after CPB. Quantitative measurements of factors VII and VIII may help differentiate between these two causes of coagulopathy. Severe gastrointestinal complications, such as bleeding, mesenteric ischemia, or necrotizing enterocolitis, can occur and be fatal.

Neurologic abnormalities also are relatively common after neonatal heart surgery. In children requiring hypothermic circulatory arrest or continuous low-flow bypass for vital organ support during cardiac repair, 20% experienced some form of neurologic dysfunction shortly after surgery.[13] Prolonged periods of circulatory arrest were associated with a higher incidence of clinical and subclinical seizures in the early postoperative period. In this same cohort, transient clinical seizures or ictal activity observed on electroencephalographic monitoring within 48 hours of surgery were associated with worsened neurodevelopmental outcomes at 1 and 2.5 years of age.[22] Although central nervous system injury is believed to result from intraoperative events,[23] postoperative LCOS with associated cerebral hypoperfusion may exacerbate central nervous system injury further.[13]

DIAGNOSIS OF LOW CARDIAC OUTPUT SYNDROME

Prompt diagnosis of LCOS are fundamental tenet of cardiac intensive care. Optimal postoperative management includes continuous monitoring of pulse oximetry, end-tidal carbon dioxide, atrial and arterial waveforms, and multiple ECG leads.[24] Pulmonary arterial pressure monitoring is useful in select patients.[25] At present, direct measurement of myocardial performance or cardiac output in children is primarily a research tool and not feasible for routine clinical monitoring of patients. Cardiac output and systemic perfusion usually are assessed indirectly by monitoring vital signs, peripheral perfusion, urine output, and acid-base status. The length of time spent in intensive care and the amount and duration of ventilatory and inotropic support probably reflect cardiac output indirectly.[16] Finally, limited data suggest that intensive care unit acuity scores may predict mortality accurately in pediatric cardiac surgery patients.[26]

Investigators have proposed **serum lactate** levels as a marker of diminished systemic perfusion and as a predictor of outcome after cardiac surgery. Elevated or rising lactate levels in the early postoperative period indicate inadequate oxygen delivery and suggest increased risks of morbidity and mortality.[27-29] Progressive increases in serum lactate levels may enhance the predictive value of monitoring lactate levels postoperatively.[30] Blood lactate levels may become elevated only with significant circulatory dysfunction, after the anaerobic threshold has been reached, below the point when oxygen consumption becomes dependent on oxygen delivery.[31] In addition, elevated blood lactate might not reflect the current state of well-being, but rather relate to prior (preoperative or intraoperative) periods of diminished tissue perfusion with end-organ injury and inability to metabolize existing lactate.

Mixed-venous oxygen saturation (SvO_2) and the arterial-venous oxygen saturation difference ($SaO_2 - SvO_2$) often are used to assess cardiac output and oxygen delivery. In patients with intracardiac shunts, superior vena cava (SVC) saturation is the best estimate of SvO_2[32]; many investigators have advocated continuous or intermittent monitoring of SVC saturation in postoperative patients.[15,33-35] Low SvO_2 and elevated $SaO_2 - SvO_2$ are sensitive predictors of low systemic blood flow and inadequate oxygen delivery; $SaO_2 - SvO_2$ difference greater than 40% suggests significant impairment in cardiac output and inadequate tissue delivery of oxygen.[36] Monitoring of SVC saturation is particularly useful after Norwood palliation because systemic output in these patients depends on myocardial performance and the balance of systemic and pulmonary blood flow. Figure 37-2 shows saturation (SaO_2 and SVC) and blood pressure data from a patient after the Norwood procedure during the first 4 hours after surgery. In the two episodes of low cardiac output (decreased SvO_2) shown, changes in SvO_2 are mirrored by only slight changes in blood pressure and SaO_2, showing that alterations in systemic output are poorly reflected by blood pressure and SaO_2. In patients after the Norwood procedure, anaerobic metabolism and metabolic acidosis are more common when the absolute SvO_2 decreases to less than 30%.[37] The oxygen extraction ratio (calculated as $[SaO_2 - SvO_2]/SaO_2$) reflects the relationship between oxygen delivery and oxygen demand. Excessive oxygen extraction reflects a limited supply of oxygen to the tissues, increasing the risk for tissue anaerobic metabolism, lactic acid production, and end-organ injury. An oxygen extraction ratio value greater than 0.5 corresponds to inadequate oxygen delivery and increased mortality.[33]

Combined analysis of serum lactate and SvO_2 improves the predictive accuracy of LCOS determination. Trittenwein and colleagues[36] analyzed postoperative hemodynamic and laboratory data from 218 pediatric patients in an effort to establish entry criteria for

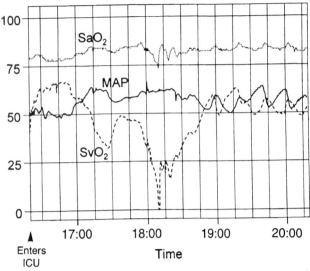

FIGURE 37-2 ■ Multichannel recording of arterial saturation (SaO2), mean arterial blood pressure (MAP), and superior vena cava saturation (SvO2) during the first 4 hours after the Norwood procedure in a patient with aortic atresia. The Y axis common to all three curves represents percent saturation and MAP mostly. The X axis indicates time, marked in 15-minute intervals. Two episodes of decreased SvO2 are shown. Changes in SvO2 are mirrored by only slight changes in MAP, and SaO2 remains within the acceptable range. These data show that SaO2 alone cannot be relied on to indicate a balanced circulation. (From Tweddell JS, Hoffman GM, Fedderly RT, et al: *Phenoxybenzamine improves systemic oxygen delivery after the Norwood procedure. Ann Thorac Surg* 1999;67:161-168.)

postoperative cardiac extracorporeal membrane oxygenation after pediatric open heart surgery. Multiple regression analyses revealed SvO2 and serum lactate levels as independent predictors of death, so inclusion of both variables in a predictive model improved the predictive accuracy of the model.[36]

Measurement of **mixed-cerebral oxygen saturation** by continuous near-infrared spectroscopy has been used to estimate the balance between cerebral oxygen delivery and consumption. Near-infrared spectroscopy has been applied to adults and children during CPB and in children during deep hypothermic circulatory arrest to assess adequacy of cerebral oxygen delivery.[38,39] It has been suggested that mixed-cerebral oxygen saturation values may correlate with SvO2 to provide a noninvasive measure of cardiac output, but confirmatory studies are necessary.

Although the techniques are challenging, cardiac output and myocardial performance have been measured directly in postoperative pediatric patients after congenital heart surgery. Measurement of cardiac output by **thermodilution method** can be done in the intensive care unit, but results may be unreliable in patients with low cardiac output, tricuspid regurgitation, or intracardiac shunts. Thermodilution measurements fail to reflect the interaction between oxygen delivery and tissue oxygen extraction[40] and may be misleading if tissue oxygen demand is not considered.[41] "Normal" cardiac output may be inadequate in times of increased

oxygen demand, whereas "reduced" cardiac output may be sufficient during times of lower oxygen demand. Measurement of SvO2 or the oxygen extraction ratio better assesses the relationship between oxygen supply and demand to identify patients at risk for LCOS.[33] An alternative is the **Fick method**, especially in patients with intracardiac shunts or low cardiac output.[40,42] Because the Fick method requires accurate measurement of systemic oxygen consumption, the presence of an endotracheal tube leak can seriously confound Fick cardiac output analysis.

Other methods of cardiac output assessment used in pediatric cardiac surgery patients include thoracic impedance measurements and detachable extravascular aortic Doppler ultrasound flow probes.[43] Considering all of these modalities, only Fick cardiac output measurements reflect the interaction between oxygen delivery and tissue oxygen extraction.[40]

Accurate measurement of myocardial performance in the postoperative pediatric cardiac surgical patient is extremely difficult and not well characterized. Poor echocardiographic windows, hemodynamic instability, and variable inotropic support have confounded noninvasive analyses of myocardial function in pediatric patients. Studies using **microconductance catheters** to record ventricular pressure-volume loops postoperatively showed depressed systolic function in patients undergoing uncomplicated corrective cardiac surgical procedures even with short CPB and aortic cross-clamp times.[7] Conductance catheters have been used to assess load-independent measures of left ventricular and right ventricular function in the early postoperative period after cardiac surgery.[7,44]

Although diastolic dysfunction is believed to play an important role in LCOS, accurate assessment of diastolic performance remains obscure. **Echocardiography** has been used to assess restrictive right ventricular physiology (right ventricular diastolic dysfunction) after corrective repair for tetralogy of Fallot, by determining the presence of antegrade flow into the pulmonary artery during ventricular diastole.[45]

CAUSES OF LOW CARDIAC OUTPUT AFTER CONGENITAL HEART SURGERY

Low cardiac output after congenital heart surgery is usually due to related and interacting factors. Although defects in myocardial systolic or diastolic contractile function usually accompany LCOS, myocardial contractile dysfunction always should be considered a diagnosis of exclusion, and other potential causes of LCOS, such as altered ventricular loading and residual cardiac lesions, should be ruled out before initiating therapy with inotropic or lusitropic agents. Changes in ventricular loading are integral to myocardial performance after congenital heart surgery. **Ventricular preload** is often inadequate because of blood loss, perioperative fluid shifts, changes in diastolic compliance, or physiologic changes resulting from the surgical procedure (e.g., Fontan or shunted single-ventricle physiology).[46] Also, cardiac tamponade, which impairs preload by altering diastolic compliance, always should be considered in patients showing signs of LCOS. Increases in intrathoracic pressure resulting from blood/fluid tamponade or pneumothorax limit venous return and impede ventricular filling. Myocardial tamponade can result from diffuse intrathoracic fluid accumulation or a localized collection of blood clot or fluid that preferentially limits venous return to one or more chambers of the heart in a local manner.

Ventricular afterload is often increased after CPB procedures, resulting from CPB-mediated vascular injury and the resultant altered vascular reactivity. Systemic and pulmonary endothelial dysfunctions have been observed after CPB with or without circulatory arrest, presumably resulting from ischemia-reperfusion injury to the endothelium.[47-51] Systemic vasoconstriction increases the afterload on the left or systemic ventricle, whereas pulmonary vasoconstriction increases afterload on the right or pulmonary ventricle. A pulmonary hypertensive crisis causes an acute increase in right ventricular afterload, which shifts the interventricular septum into the systemic ventricle, substantially decreasing the preload of the systemic ventricle. The acute increase in right ventricular afterload and decrease in left ventricular preload can diminish cardiac output dramatically. A pulmonary hypertensive crisis most often manifests with acute systemic hypotension and diminished perfusion. Arterial oxygen saturation decreases only when right-to-left intracardiac shunting can occur.

Residual anatomic or electrophysiologic abnormalities are likely to diminish cardiac output after congenital heart surgery. Uncorrected anatomic defects, such as outflow obstruction or valvar insufficiency, reduce the effective stroke volume, increasing myocardial demands. Similarly, persistence of a left-to-right intracardiac shunt yields excessive pulmonary blood flow and diminishes systemic blood flow. Low cardiac output could be exacerbated by arrhythmias, which limit ventricular filling or compromise atrioventricular synchrony or both. Arrhythmias are relatively common after congenital heart surgery.[52-54] It seems likely that a correlation exists between LCOS and certain rhythm disturbances, particularly junctional ectopic tachycardia (JET), although this has not been clearly shown. Careful evaluation for residual cardiac abnormalities is indicated in any patient with low cardiac output, especially when patients do not follow their expected postoperative course after heart surgery.

MOLECULAR MECHANISMS OF BYPASS-MEDIATED MYOCARDIAL INJURY

Repair or palliation of most forms of congenital heart disease requires use of CPB for circulatory support.

Despite advances in perfusion technology, patients undergoing CPB uniformly develop a systemic inflammatory response resulting in tissue injury with transient myocardial dysfunction, which contributes to postoperative morbidity and mortality.[2,8] The mechanism of bypass-mediated tissue injury is presumed to be multifactorial. Circulatory support with CPB involves obligate periods of myocardial and pulmonary ischemia with subsequent reperfusion. Neonatal cardiac surgery may use hypothermic circulatory arrest, which results in whole body ischemia-reperfusion. These planned periods of ischemia-reperfusion initiate tissue and vascular injury throughout the body.[8,55,56] Activation of blood components by the extracorporeal circuit may exacerbate this process.[17] The resultant post-CPB inflammatory response involves cytokine and endotoxin release[56-59]; initiation of the complement, coagulation, and fibrinolytic cascades[2,60]; and leukocyte-endothelial interactions.[61] This process ultimately leads to the development of edema, tissue injury, and organ damage, most notably in the heart and lungs.[1] Mechanisms of contractile dysfunction after cardiac surgery remain elusive, but evidence suggests that cardiomyocytes are injured by oxygen-derived free radicals and intracellular calcium overload during early reperfusion.[45,55,62] Other potential causes of myocardial contractile dysfunction after congenital heart surgery include cytokine-mediated negative inotropy,[63,64] cardiomyocyte apoptosis,[65] alterations in adrenergic receptor signaling,[66,67] and decreases in calcium responsiveness of the sarcomeric contractile apparatus as a result of troponin degradation.[68-72]

Various interventions have been proposed to decrease inflammatory injury after CPB. Although the efficacy of most of these strategies has not been evaluated rigorously, many are used routinely. Conventional and modified ultrafiltration has been shown to improve fluid balance and increase cardiac output in patients after CPB,[73,74] which suggests removal of inflammatory cytokines that may depress myocardial function. Peritoneal dialysis also has been shown to remove inflammatory mediators,[75] but its effect on cardiac output and performance has not been assessed. Heparin-coated bypass circuits may blunt leukocyte activation and decrease cytokine production by reducing the contact of blood with artificial circuit surfaces.[60,76,77] Although these modalities have been shown to reduce levels of circulating cytokines and inflammatory mediators, correlation with outcome has not been established.

Studies in animal bypass models suggest that treatment with agents directed against cytokines, adhesion molecules,[47,48,56,78,79] or activated complement[80] may diminish CPB-mediated inflammatory injury, but most of these agents have not been tested in humans. Perioperative glucocorticoid treatment has been shown to reduce the intensity of the postoperative inflammatory response by altering myocardial and circulating cytokine levels and has been associated with improved oxygen delivery in the immediate postoperative period.[81-84]

TREATMENT OF LOW CARDIAC OUTPUT SYNDROME

Management of postoperative LCOS includes optimization of preload and afterload; prompt diagnosis of residual cardiac lesions; prevention of hypoxia, anemia, and acidosis; and administration of pharmacologic agents to improve myocardial contractile function.[85] In addition, in low cardiac output associated with right heart failure, some children may benefit from the creation or enlargement of an atrial level shunt to allow right-to-left shunting.

Minimize Oxygen Requirements

Reduced cardiac output and increased systemic oxygen consumption can adversely alter the systemic oxygen balance after CPB. One study of children age 2 months to 15 years showed a significant increase in oxygen consumption after CPB.[41] Peak oxygen consumption correlated significantly with an increase in central temperature. Fever in the setting of LCOS should be treated aggressively with antipyretic medication or surface cooling. A cooling blanket may be useful, but shivering should be avoided because it may be associated with an increase in oxygen consumption. Total oxygen consumption can be decreased by the induction of heavy sedation, paralysis, or mild hypothermia that reduces the metabolic rate.[86] Case reports of moderate hypothermia induction for patients with refractory LCOS suggest this may be a potential therapy for LCOS.[87,88]

Ensure Adequate Preload

Inadequate preload is common in postoperative cardiac surgical patients. Potential causes of postoperative hypovolemia include bleeding, excessive ultrafiltration, and vasodilation from rewarming or afterload reduction.[46] Cardiac tamponade, which impairs preload by altering diastolic compliance, always should be considered in patients showing signs of LCOS. Increased mediastinal pressure, with fluid or extrapleural air, can lead to myocardial compression with LCOS and should be treated promptly. Myocardial swelling, which may limit myocardial filling and prevent adequate output, may necessitate sternal reopening.

Although true ventricular preload is the end-diastolic ventricular volume, preload assessment can be estimated from right and left atrial pressures. Continual reassessment of the optimal preload is essential because ventricular compliance and subsequent preload needs often change postoperatively. Figure 37-3A graphically shows how preload determination is predominantly a "trial-and-error" process. When atrial pressure is low, fluid administration augments end-diastolic volume and increases stroke volume. With successive fluid administration, however, increases in stroke volume become limited because of the nonlinear nature of the ventricular diastolic compliance. Preload augmentation also is limited by elevations in left ventricular end-diastolic pressure, which results

in clinically significant edema formation and potential impairment of myocardial perfusion. Hemodynamic pressure monitoring data always should be interpreted with an understanding of the patient's underlying physiology. A poorly compliant ventricle, such as with right ventricular dysfunction after tetralogy of Fallot repair, would be expected to have higher end-diastolic and right atrial pressures than a normal heart and may rely on higher filling pressures to generate adequate output. Patients with diastolic dysfunction may require more extensive postoperative volume administration to maintain preload and cardiac output. These patients also would benefit from lusitropic therapy intended to improve diastolic ventricular filling. Figure 37-3B illustrates how a change in ventricular diastolic compliance affects atrial pressure. Enhanced lusitropy should result in a greater stroke volume for a comparable atrial pressure.

Prompt Recognition of Arrhythmias

Early recognition of postoperative arrhythmias is imperative; a baseline postoperative surface ECG always should be obtained for comparison with preoperative and subsequent postoperative tracings. Continuous ECG monitoring during the postoperative period also is essential. Sinus bradycardia, bundle branch block, and atrioventricular block can occur after many cardiac surgical procedures; temporary atrial and ventricular pacing wires typically are placed to facilitate pacing, if necessary. Arrhythmias occur frequently in postoperative cardiac surgical patients and may require overdrive pacing, cardioversion, or pharmacologic intervention.[53] Hoffman and coworkers[53] reviewed the incidence of arrhythmias in postoperative cardiac surgical patients and observed the most common rhythm disturbances to be nonsustained ventricular and supraventricular tachycardia with incidences of 22% and 12%, respectively. Sustained ventricular, junctional, and supraventricular arrhythmias also were common with incidences of 6%, 5%, and 4%, respectively. Loss in atrioventricular synchrony can compromise preload, increase pulmonary congestion, and significantly diminish cardiac output; maintenance of atrioventricular synchrony is essential (via pacing, if necessary).

Junctional ectopic tachycardia (JET) is a common tachyarrhythmia that usually occurs in the first 48 hours after surgery, especially after procedures involving closure of a ventricular septal defect and in younger patients.[52] It is generally poorly tolerated, especially in patients with unstable hemodynamics. Early recognition of JET and other arrhythmias may be aided by careful surveillance of atrial pressure waveforms; loss of the distinct a and v waves, indicating loss of atrioventricular synchrony, is often the first indication of arrhythmia or atrioventricular dyssynchrony or both. Hypomagnesemia is a frequent occurrence after pediatric heart surgery and may contribute to the onset of JET. A study reported a reduction in the incidence of JET with administration

FIGURE 37-3 ■ Paired changes in pressure volume and Starling relationships with isolated manipulations in preload (A), lusitropy (B), contractility (C), and afterload (D). End-diastolic point A and stroke volume A (SV_A) for each pair of graphs represent the initial baseline hemodynamic condition. **A,** The effect of preload recruitment on the pressure-volume and Starling relationships. Fluid volume administration augments end-diastolic volume from points A to B, with the increase in stroke volume represented as the difference between SV_A and SV_B. Because diastolic compliance is nonlinear, increases in stroke volume are progressively less with further fluid administration (SV_C and SV_D). End-diastolic volumes A, B, C, and D define the diastolic compliance relationship. Preload augmentation is limited by elevations in left ventricular (LV) end-diastolic pressure, which can lead to impaired myocardial perfusion and elevations in atrial pressure, with resultant transcapillary leak and edema formation. **B,** The beneficial effects of positive lusitropy on the pressure-volume and Starling relationships. Enhanced ventricular compliance corresponds to an increased end-diastolic volume for the same end-diastolic pressure, augmenting stroke volume without increasing atrial pressure. Enhanced lusitropy results in a greater stroke volume for a comparable atrial pressure. **C,** The beneficial effects of positive inotropy on the pressure-volume and Starling relationships. Increases in contractility are shown as enhancement of the end-systolic pressure-volume relationship, shown by increases in the slopes of lines A through C on the left-hand graph. At constant preload, increased contractility enhances ejection during isovolumic contraction, decreasing the end-systolic volume and increasing stroke volume (from SV_A to SV_B to SV_C). Enhanced contractility results in a greater stroke volume for a comparable preload. **D,** The beneficial effects of afterload reduction on the pressure-volume and Starling relationships. From baseline conditions A or C, afterload reduction allows the heart to eject to a lower systolic pressure and volume (points B and D), enhancing ejection and augmenting stroke volume (SV_A to SV_B and SV_C to SV_D). At normal contractility (slope AB), the ventricle responds to altered afterload with only small changes in stroke volume (SV_A to SV_B). Neonatal and failing hearts are particularly sensitive to alterations in afterload. Benefits of afterload reduction are more pronounced in neonatal hearts and in the setting of poor contractility. With reduced contractility (as shown by the reduced slope of end-systolic pressure volume relationship CD), the increase in stroke volume is greater for a comparable change in afterload. Afterload reduction results in a greater stroke volume for a comparable preload.

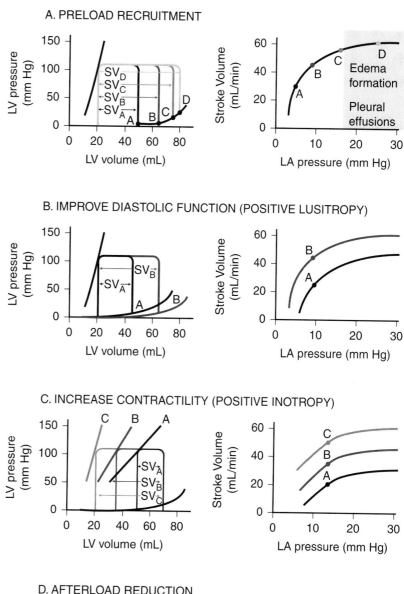

A. PRELOAD RECRUITMENT

B. IMPROVE DIASTOLIC FUNCTION (POSITIVE LUSITROPY)

C. INCREASE CONTRACTILITY (POSITIVE INOTROPY)

D. AFTERLOAD REDUCTION

of intravenous magnesium in the early postoperative period.[89] After JET is diagnosed, treatment is directed toward the re-establishment of atrioventricular synchrony. If the hemodynamics allow it, an effort should be made to discontinue adrenergic agents, which contribute to the onset of JET and increase the JET rate.[52] Pacing, either atrial (if atrioventricular conduction is preserved) or atrioventricular sequential, is the initial therapy of choice. If the junctional rate is too fast to allow pacing,

the goal of pharmacologic therapy is to provide rate control to allow institution of atrial or dual-chamber pacing. Although intravenous amiodarone generally is considered the drug of choice,[90] induction of hypothermia and procainamide administration also have been shown to be effective.[91] Finally, because common wisdom suggests that the risk of JET is greater in the presence of low output ("low cardiac output begets JET"), the diagnosis of JET should prompt the cardiac intensivist to search for other causes of LCOS, including other residual cardiac lesions.

Prompt Diagnosis of Residual Cardiac Lesions

Residual cardiac lesions in the postoperative patient can lead to LCOS and result in increased morbidity and mortality. Pressure and oximetry data from indwelling intracardiac catheters and transesophageal or surface echocardiography should be used to rule out residual structural lesions in patients with LCOS after CPB. Catheterization should be considered if LCOS persists and the etiology remains elusive. Careful evaluation for residual cardiac abnormalities is indicated, especially when patients do not follow their expected postoperative course after heart surgery. Prompt diagnosis of residual structural lesions can help direct medical management optimally or may prompt surgical or catheter-based intervention.

Treatment of Depressed Myocardial Contractility

Because low cardiac output after pediatric heart surgery often is associated with some level of contractile dysfunction, inotropic support in the early postoperative period is usually necessary. Figure 37-3C shows the beneficial effects of positive inotropy on the pressure-volume and Starling relationships. At constant preload, increased contractility should enhance ejection during isovolumic contraction to increase stroke volume. Because inotropic agents have unwanted side effects, it is important to assess the efficacy of these agents after initiation or dosage adjustment. Figure 37-3 illustrates the potential usefulness of Starling curves to assess the efficacy of most hemodynamic interventions. The Starling relationship specifies the therapeutic goal of all inotropic agents: Enhanced contractility should result in a greater stroke volume for a comparable preload. Measurement of stroke volume is not routine in postoperative patients, so an alternative to the true Starling relationship is illustrated in Figure 37-4. Because stroke volume is not monitored easily, indirect measures of cardiac output (e.g., SVC saturation) or measures of end-organ perfusion (e.g., urine output) may be plotted against atrial pressure to attain a "modified" Starling relationship. Points A through C of Figure 37-4 illustrate how preload recruitment is used to increase SVC saturation or urine output. Because preload recruitment is limited, however, inotropic agents are used to improve SVC saturation or urine output by shifting the Starling relationship leftward (point D in Fig. 37-4). Using the modified Starling relationship, the therapeutic goal of enhanced contractility is improvement in systemic blood flow for a comparable preload (reflected as improved SVC saturation and enhanced organ perfusion).

Inotropic agents are routinely used in pediatric cardiac surgical patients to help re-establish adequate myocardial function during and after surgery. Table 37-1 lists the agents most commonly used in pediatric

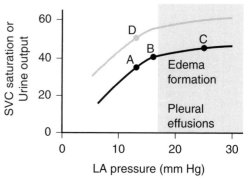

FIGURE 37-4 ■ Modified Starling relationship. Because stroke volume is not easily monitored, indirect measures of cardiac output (superior vena cava [SVC] saturation) or measures of end-organ perfusion (urine output) may be plotted against left atrial (LA) pressure to attain a "modified" Starling relationship. Fluid administration augments preload and leads to improvements in SVC saturation and end-organ perfusion (point A to point B). Preload augmentation is limited, however; progressive fluid administration is limited by increasing atrial pressures, until edema formation ensues (point C). Alternate ways to improve SVC saturation or urine output include afterload reduction and improvements in lusitropy or inotropy, which all shift the Starling relationship leftward (point D). The therapeutic goal of enhanced lusitropy, increased contractility, or afterload reduction is improvement in systemic blood flow for a comparable preload (reflected as improved SVC saturation and enhanced organ perfusion).

cardiac intensive care for LCOS. Support often is initiated with a low-dose infusion of dopamine (3 to 5 µg/kg/min). The infusion rate is titrated to produce the desired systemic blood pressure. High doses of dopamine rarely are used because of increasing vasoconstrictor and chronotropic effects with higher doses. Dobutamine generally produces less tachycardia than dopamine and may decrease systemic afterload. These effects may be particularly desirable when treating patients with dilated cardiomyopathies or volume-loaded ventricles with excessive pulmonary blood flow. Epinephrine is a more potent inotrope than dopamine or dobutamine because of its greater myocardial α1-adrenergic and β1-adrenergic effects and

TABLE 37-1

Common Inotropic Agents for the Treatment of Low Cardiac Output Syndrome		
Inotropic Agent	**Loading Dose**	**Infusion Dose Range**
Dopamine	None	3-10 µg/kg/min
Dobutamine	None	3-20 µg/kg/min
Milrinone	50-100 µg/kg over 60 min	0.5-1 µg/kg/min
Amrinone	0.75-1 mg/kg over 60 min	5-10 µg/kg/min
Calcium chloride	None	5-20 mg/kg/hr
Epinephrine	None	0.03-0.2 µg/kg/min
Arginine vasopressin	None	0.0003-0.006 U/kg/min

is preferred for treatment of severe ventricular dysfunction. High-dose epinephrine (>0.1 ug/kg/min) frequently results in tachycardia and systemic vasoconstriction. Epinephrine often is used in combination with intravenous vasodilators, such as milrinone, sodium nitroprusside, or phenoxybenzamine, to treat ventricular dysfunction and decrease systemic afterload (or at least attenuate the α1 effects of epinephrine). The use of high-dose catecholamines for inotropic support has disadvantages because they can increase afterload substantially, promote tachycardia and proarrhythmic effects, increase myocardial oxygen consumption, and depress the myocardial adrenergic response by downregulating β-adrenergic receptors. Prolonged use of high-dose catecholamines may amplify cardiomyocyte injury further, aggravating diastolic and systolic ventricular dysfunction.[92]

The use of **phosphodiesterase inhibitors**, which do not show many of the shortcomings common to catecholamine therapy, has increased considerably in recent years. Phosphodiesterase inhibitors improve cardiac index by enhancing systolic and diastolic functions and by reducing SVR and PVR. Phosphodiesterase inhibitors, including amrinone and its derivative milrinone, inhibit breakdown of cyclic AMP (cAMP) by the phosphodiesterase III isozyme.[93] By blocking the breakdown of intracellular cAMP, calcium transport into the cell is enhanced, and myocyte contractility is improved. In addition, reuptake of calcium is a cAMP-dependent process so that these agents may enhance diastolic relaxation of the myocardium by increasing the rate of calcium reuptake after systole. Phosphodiesterase inhibitors increase cardiac muscle contractility and vascular muscle relaxation without increasing myocardial oxygen consumption or ventricular afterload.[94] In pediatric patients, milrinone is used more frequently than amrinone because of its shorter half-life and lower incidence of thrombocytopenia.[11,95-98]

The ability to achieve a rapid hemodynamic response on initiation of milrinone is crucial after separation from CPB, when uncompensated LCOS can result quickly in the deterioration of hemodynamic status and subsequent secondary organ dysfunction. For patients at high risk for LCOS, some centers prefer to load with milrinone during CPB to avoid potential hypotension associated with loading in the ICU setting. The clinical usefulness of phosphodiesterase inhibitors in pediatric patients is similar to that of milrinone in adult heart failure patients.[99-101] Phosphodiesterase inhibitors have been shown to improve cardiac index effectively, while decreasing SVR and PVR.[94,95] The multicenter PRIMA-CORP study showed that the use of milrinone in children early after congenital heart surgery reduces the incidence of LCOS.[11] Because renal dysfunction results in delayed clearance of milrinone and amrinone, patients with renal insufficiency are at risk for toxicity secondary to excessive drug levels.[97,102] Continuous infusion rates should be adjusted based on creatinine clearance to avoid excessive and prolonged vasodilation, especially in neonates.

Calcium supplementation also warrants discussion. Cardiac contraction and relaxation are mediated by cyclic fluctuations in cytoplasmic calcium concentration. In the adult heart, calcium released from the sarcoplasmic reticulum accounts for most of the calcium that binds to troponin C. In the neonate, the sarcoplasmic reticular system is relatively sparse and undifferentiated so that the neonatal myocardium depends more on extracellular calcium stores for contractile function.[68] Maintenance of adequate extracellular calcium is essential for normal myocardial contractile function in all patients, but especially in neonates. Hypocalcemia occurs frequently in the postoperative period and may be pronounced in patients with 22q11 deletion syndrome and in neonates with transient hypoparathyroidism. Transfusion of citrate-treated blood, which chelates calcium, and administration of loop diuretics may exacerbate the hypocalcemia. Ionized calcium, the physiologically active form of calcium, should be monitored frequently in the postoperative period, and normal or supernormal levels should be maintained with supplementation. Many centers routinely use calcium infusions in neonates after CPB to augment and stabilize extracellular ionized calcium, especially in patients with 22q11 deletion syndrome.

A new class of drugs known as **calcium sensitizers** has been used in adults for the treatment of heart failure and low cardiac output states. These drugs act directly on the contractile protein system and are believed to increase cardiac contractility by sensitizing cardiac myofibrils to calcium without increasing intracellular calcium. They also may increase cAMP through phosphodiesterase inhibition, enhancing contractility and decreasing afterload. Levosimendan, one of the first calcium sensitizers, has been shown to be beneficial in adult patients in acute severe heart failure,[103,104] but its safety and efficacy in pediatric patients have not been established.

Although the mechanism is unclear, investigators have advocated **thyroid hormone** therapy as a potential treatment for LCOS.[105-107] During CPB, circulating levels of the thyroid hormones triiodothyronine and thyroxine are reduced; these deficiencies can persist for several days and may play a role in postoperative myocardial depression.[105] One small study showed hemodynamic improvement in infants with refractory LCOS when treated with triiodothyronine.[106] Another randomized study reported that children given postoperative triiodothyronine supplementation had significantly higher cardiac output after surgery than children given placebo.[107]

Arginine vasopressin has been advocated as a therapeutic option for pediatric patients with refractory hypotension after surgery, to improve systemic arterial blood pressure when conventional therapies fail.[108] Arginine vasopressin also has been shown to be effective for refractory hypotension in patients on mechanical circulatory support.[109,110]

Preoperative and postoperative patients can develop prolonged low cardiac output that requires escalating inotropic support and is refractory to other therapy. Data suggest that relative adrenal insufficiency contributes to morbidity in critically ill adult patients, and low-dose **corticosteroid** administration has been suggested as an option for patients with refractory LCOS. In a retrospective study of neonates receiving escalating, high-dose epinephrine, inotrope requirements were observed to decrease significantly within 24 hours of corticosteroid treatment.[111] The results of this study are shown in Figure 37-5. Some patients showed low random cortisol levels with a normal adrenocorticotropic hormone stimulation test, suggesting adrenal insufficiency. These data suggest stress-dose hydrocortisone (50 mg/m^2/day) may help reduce inotropic requirements in pediatric patients with LCOS refractory

to conventional therapy. The physiologic basis for the reduction in inotropic support after arginine vasopressin and corticosteroid therapy is obscure, but they may share a similar mechanism because arginine vasopressin serves as a potent stimulus for adrenocorticotropin.[112]

Afterload Reduction for Systemic Ventricular Failure

Elevated afterload is particularly detrimental to the neonatal heart, especially when compounded by postoperative myocardial dysfunction. Afterload reduction is often beneficial in postoperative patients showing signs of LCOS. If high-dose catecholamines cannot be avoided, afterload reduction and vasodilator therapy should be considered to counter catecholamine vasoconstrictor effects. Figure 37-3D shows beneficial effects of afterload reduction on pressure volume and Starling relationships. It also shows an important principle: Benefits of afterload reduction are particularly pronounced in neonatal hearts and in the setting of poor contractility. With neonatal hearts or impaired contractility, afterload reduction is particularly useful to augment stroke volume and overall cardiac output. As with inotropic agents, it is important to assess efficacy of these agents after initiation or dosage adjustment because vasodilator agents also have unwanted side effects. As shown in Figure 37-3, the therapeutic goal of afterload reduction should be a greater stroke volume for a comparable preload. As noted previously, however, because measurement of stroke volume is not routine in postoperative patients, the modified Starling relationship can be used to assess efficacy of most hemodynamic interventions, including afterload reduction (see Fig. 37-4). As shown in Figure 37-4, the therapeutic goal of afterload reduction is improvement in systemic blood flow for a comparable preload (reflected as improved SVC saturation and enhanced organ perfusion).

Some centers advocate use of the potent vasodilator **phenoxybenzamine**, an α–adrenergic blocking agent, in select pediatric patients after cardiac surgery.[35] Because phenoxybenzamine is a potent vasodilator with a long half-life (>24 hours), its use may be complicated by severe hypotension. For this reason, many centers prefer to use **sodium nitroprusside** for afterload reduction and vasodilator therapy in patients with congenital heart disease. Although nitroprusside may be a slightly less effective vasodilator than phenoxybenzamine, its therapeutic effects are easier to titrate because of its short half-life and rapid onset of action. Sodium nitroprusside also has been advocated in patients with excessive pulmonary blood flow after Norwood palliation.[34] In such patients, the dual effects of nitroprusside include afterload reduction for improvement of myocardial performance and reduction of systemic vascular resistance to improve the balance of pulmonary and systemic blood flow. **Phosphodiesterase inhibitors** also commonly are used for afterload reduction in pediatric patients with congenital heart disease. These agents are

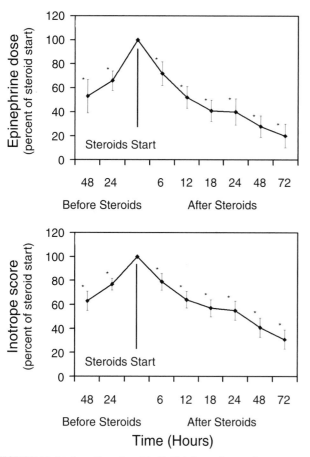

FIGURE 37-5 ■ Steroid use in critically ill infants after cardiac surgery. Epinephrine doses and inotropic scores in critically ill infants after heart surgery show significant decreases after administration of steroids. Values are plotted as a percentage of the baseline values at the time steroid administration was initiated. (From Shore S, Nelson DP, Pearl JM, et al: *Usefulness of corticosteroid therapy in decreasing epinephrine requirements in critically ill infants with congenital heart disease. Am J Cardiol* 2001;88:591-594.)

particularly useful in postoperative pediatric cardiac surgical patients because enhanced inotropic and lusitropic effects are combined with systemic and pulmonary vasodilation. In patients who require high doses of adrenergic agents, it is especially important to use one or more vasodilator agents simultaneously.

Management of Pulmonary Hypertension

Children with many forms of congenital heart disease, particularly children with elevated pulmonary pressure or blood flow preoperatively, are prone to develop postoperative elevations in PVR. Additionally, CPB-mediated inflammation results in alterations in pulmonary vascular reactivity, because of pulmonary vascular endothelial injury.[51] This endothelial injury may result in excess thromboxane production, decreased production of endogenous nitric oxide synthase, and pulmonary microemboli. A reduction in exhaled nitric oxide, endogenously produced by the pulmonary vascular endothelium, may be a marker of endothelial injury.[113,114] Increased endothelin-1 production by the pulmonary vascular endothelium occurs after deep hypothermic circulatory arrest.[6] Increases in PVR increase right ventricular afterload, aggravating right ventricular dysfunction and low cardiac output. In patients with elevated pulmonary arterial pressures, careful evaluation for anatomic causes of elevated PVR should be performed. In particular, anatomic or physiologic causes of pulmonary venous obstruction should be eliminated.

Management of postoperative pulmonary hypertension begins with prevention. Infants and children at risk should be identified preoperatively. Strategies to minimize stimuli known to induce pulmonary hypertension should be employed, including avoidance of hypoxia, hypercarbia, acidosis, agitation, pain, and tracheal stimulation. Therapy may include deep sedation and analgesia with a continuous opioid infusion (e.g., fentanyl) alone or in combination with a benzodiazepine. Neuromuscular blockade may allow more precise control of ventilation. Elevations in PVR can be managed by increasing arterial pH through the induction of alkalosis. Because hyperventilation may increase mean airway pressure and compromise venous return, administration of sodium bicarbonate may be a superior way to induce alkalosis. Induction of metabolic alkalosis with bicarbonate administration in postoperative neonates has been shown to reduce PVR and pulmonary arterial pressure, with a corresponding increase in cardiac index.[115] As discussed subsequently, ventilation strategies should aim to avoid atelectasis and maintain end-expiratory lung volume at functional residual capacity, while minimizing intrathoracic pressures. An appropriate tidal volume and inspiratory time and judicious use of positive end-expiratory pressure (PEEP) usually are required to attain these goals. Hyperventilation strategies have been employed, but careful attention

to mean airway pressure is needed. In particular, because high-frequency jet ventilation (HFJV) reduces mean airway pressure and PVR while maintaining a similar $Paco_2$, it may be ideally suited to patients with right ventricular dysfunction or pulmonary hypertension or both.

Pulmonary vasodilators are often necessary to lower pulmonary arterial pressure and pulmonary vascular resistance after congenital heart surgery.[116] In addition to their systemic vasodilator effects, milrinone and amrinone are effective pulmonary vasodilators. Isoproterenol also is an effective pulmonary vasodilator, but its suboptimal side-effect profile has limited its use significantly. Additionally, it may be less effective in the presence of endothelial dysfunction.[117] Use of nonspecific vasodilators may be limited by their deleterious systemic effects, including systemic hypotension and aggravation of existing defects in pulmonary gas exchange. Inhaled nitric oxide acts selectively on the pulmonary vasculature, however. Studies have shown that inhaled nitric oxide is an effective way to reduce PVR,[118] with fewer pulmonary hypertensive crises,[119] in postoperative neonates. Type III (milrinone, amrinone) and type V (sildenafil) phosphodiesterase inhibitors have been shown to enhance pulmonary vasodilatory effects of inhaled nitric oxide and reduce rebound pulmonary hypertension after discontinuation of nitric oxide therapy.[120] Studies evaluating the efficacy of sildenafil in postoperative pulmonary hypertension are ongoing. The endothelin receptor antagonist, bosentan, also acts to dilate the pulmonary vasculature, although pediatric data are limited.[121] Limited data with arginine and substance P suggest a benefit of these agents in restoring pulmonary endothelial function.[122]

Management of Right Ventricular Failure

Right heart failure is a common complication of congenital heart surgery and one of the common causes of LCOS. Factors contributing to postoperative right ventricular dysfunction include difficulties with right heart myocardial protection and right ventriculotomy, which is required for the surgical correction of many congenital heart lesions. Patients undergoing right heart procedures, including tetralogy of Fallot and Fontan procedures, often have restrictive physiology (diastolic right ventricular dysfunction), characterized by antegrade diastolic pulmonary arterial flow coinciding with atrial systole.[123,124]

Children with acute right ventricular restrictive physiology have a decreased cardiac index because the stiff right ventricle has impaired diastolic filling.[45] These patients typically have a slower postoperative recovery and a prolonged stay in the intensive care unit with longer periods of inotropic and ventilatory support. Alterations in left ventricular filling also may occur, because of the hypertensive right ventricle. Alterations in ventricular compliance make patients with right ventricular failure particularly sensitive to alterations in venous return caused by intrathoracic pressure changes. As discussed subsequently, these patients benefit from ventilation strategies that minimize intrathoracic pressure.[123-126] Patients with right ventricular failure may benefit from manipulation of PVR to minimize right ventricular afterload. Phosphodiesterase inhibitors are particularly beneficial in these patients because of the combined lusitropic and pulmonary vasodilatory effects.

The ability to maintain a right-to-left shunt at the atrial level is beneficial in patients with right ventricular dysfunction. In patients undergoing the modified Fontan procedure, fenestration between the Fontan pathway and atrium is associated with reduced pleural effusion and significantly shorter hospital stays.[127] In patients who undergo tetralogy of Fallot repair, a right-to-left atrial shunt similarly can be facilitated by maintaining the patency of the foramen ovale or by creating a small fenestration in the atrial septum.

Mechanical Support
Mechanical circulatory support should be considered in patients who have refractory (but potentially reversible) LCOS.[128] In pediatric patients, mechanical support is provided by extracorporeal membrane oxygenation or ventricular assist device. The choice may depend on the patient's weight or presence of pulmonary dysfunction. Extracorporeal membrane oxygenation can be used in patients with life-threatening pulmonary disease or postcardiotomy ventricular failure, whereas a ventricular assist device can be used in infants without pulmonary involvement. With both techniques, patients are sedated and usually paralyzed and receive minimal inotropic support. Early intervention and aggressive management are keys to the overall outcome with mechanical circulatory support. Mechanical support is discussed in greater detail in Section IV.

VENTILATION STRATEGIES AFTER PEDIATRIC CARDIAC SURGERY

Cardiopulmonary Interactions
Because the cardiorespiratory system functions as a unit, ventilation (spontaneous and mechanical) can have a profound effect on hemodynamics. These effects may be particularly pronounced in infants after cardiac surgery. An understanding of the complex interactions between the cardiovascular and respiratory systems is crucial to the management of these patients. Alterations in intrathoracic pressure and lung volume affect dynamic and loading conditions of the right ventricle and left ventricle differently, often having opposing effects. The right ventricle and left ventricle traditionally are considered separately in discussions of cardiopulmonary interactions. These effects highlight the central role of cardiopulmonary interactions in the management of patients with low cardiac output.

A transient increase in intrathoracic pressure decreases right ventricular preload and decreases left ventricular afterload, whereas spontaneous inspiration or negative intrathoracic pressure increases right ventricular preload and increases left ventricular afterload. Effects of ventilation on right ventricular afterload or PVR depend primarily on lung volume, with PVR lowest at functional residual capacity. Because the effects of intrathoracic pressure changes are opposite for the right ventricle and left ventricle, the ventilation strategy depends on whether right ventricular or left ventricular dysfunction predominates. In patients with systemic ventricular contractile dysfunction, positive intrathoracic pressure may be beneficial because the predominant effect is to reduce left ventricular afterload. Venous return effects of positive intrathoracic pressure are amplified in lesions with no right ventricle (Glenn and Fontan procedures) or in patients with right ventricular failure, especially patients with restrictive physiology after tetralogy of Fallot repair.[123-126]

Lung Recruitment in Patients with Congenital Heart Disease
Although lung recruitment is recognized to be an important principle for the ventilation of patients with respiratory failure, lung volume also is an important factor in the management of patients with congenital heart disease. A study observed that gas exchange defects in patients early after Norwood palliation were ameliorated by increasing PEEP, presumably resulting in alveolar recruitment.[15] In addition to the lung volume effects on PVR, adequate lung volume ensures optimal lung compliance and pulmonary gas exchange. Ventilation strategies for patients with congenital heart disease should strive to maintain an "open lung," striving for a normal functional residual capacity.

Ventilation Effects on Pulmonary Blood Flow
Manipulation of pulmonary blood flow is often necessary in patients with congenital heart disease, because of either excessive or diminished pulmonary blood flow. Manipulation of PVR in patients with congenital heart defects traditionally has emphasized the use of oxygen, carbon dioxide, and acid-base status.[129,130] Similar to management of patients with pulmonary hypertension, ventilation strategies for patients with diminished pulmonary blood flow entail lung recruitment, supplemental inspired oxygen, hyperventilation, and alkalosis. In patients with large left-to-right shunts, including infants with single-ventricle physiology, subatmospheric oxygen (fraction of inspired oxygen 0.17 to 0.19) or induction of respiratory acidosis can increase PVR, decrease SVR, and decrease pulmonary flow.[131] Subatmospheric oxygen should be used with caution because it may cause pulmonary venous desaturation, which may affect systemic oxygen delivery detrimentally, particularly in a postoperative patient.[15] Respiratory acidosis

can be induced either through alveolar hypoventilation or by altering inspired carbon dioxide concentrations in mechanically ventilated, paralyzed patients. Data from newborns with hypoplastic left heart syndrome suggest inhaled carbon dioxide may be more effective than subatmospheric oxygen to increase cerebral or systemic perfusion (or both) in ventilated, paralyzed patients, but these studies did not assess the effect of inspired carbon dioxide in spontaneously ventilated patients.[131-133] Increases in PVR also can be induced by PEEP, independent of SVR.[130] When lung compliance is normal, PEEP increases PVR by compressing interalveolar pulmonary arterioles. Increased levels of PEEP should be used with caution, however, because PEEP may reduce cardiac output by impeding venous return.

Effects of Positive-Pressure Ventilation on Left Ventricular Failure

As noted earlier, the ventilation strategy depends on whether right ventricular or left ventricular dysfunction predominates. Positive intrathoracic pressure is often beneficial in patients with systemic ventricular dysfunction resulting from diminished left ventricular afterload. In addition to optimal lung recruitment, higher levels of PEEP may be hemodynamically beneficial in these patients. Tidal volumes should be maintained in the range of 8 to 10 mL/kg to avoid overdistention, which could increase PVR and right ventricular afterload.[134] There is evidence that shorter inspiratory times may augment left ventricular filling in patients with systemic ventricular dysfunction.[135] Because alterations in thoracic pressure may have opposing hemodynamic effects, hemodynamic effects of all ventilatory maneuvers should be evaluated carefully with respect to systemic oxygen delivery.

Effects of Positive-Pressure Ventilation on Right Ventricular Failure

As noted earlier, alterations in ventricular compliance make patients with right ventricular failure particularly sensitive to changes in venous return caused by adjustments in intrathoracic pressure. Spontaneous inspiration enhances diastolic flow and overall cardiac output in these patients, so early extubation can be beneficial. Because of the detrimental effects of positive-pressure ventilation on right ventricular dynamics, alternative modes of ventilation, such as negative-pressure ventilation or HFJV, have been studied. Because HFJV reduces mean airway pressure and PVR while maintaining a similar $PaCO_2$, it may be ideally suited to patients with right ventricular dysfunction or pulmonary hypertension or both. In postoperative Fontan patients, HFJV decreased mean airway pressure, reduced PVR, and increased cardiac index.[136] Similarly, negative-pressure ventilation has been shown to augment cardiac output in patients with restrictive physiology after tetralogy of Fallot repair (Fig. 37-6).[123,124,126] Similar results were

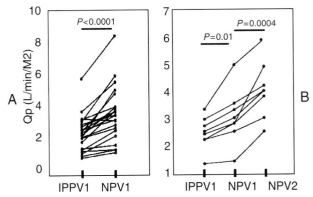

FIGURE 37-6 ■ Improvement in pulmonary blood flow (Qp) in acute postoperative tetralogy of Fallot patients after institution of negative-pressure ventilation (NPV). **A,** Qp for tetralogy of Fallot patients after conversion from conventional intermittent positive-pressure ventilation (IPPV) to NPV. **B,** Further improvement in Qp for a subgroup of patients in which NPV was extended for an additional period. (From Shekerdemian LS, Bush A, Shore DF, et al: *Cardiorespiratory responses to negative pressure ventilation after tetralogy of fallot repair: A hemodynamic tool for patients with a low-output state. J Am Coll Cardiol* 1999;33:549-555.)

observed in patients with Fontan physiology.[125] Although technical challenges associated with negative-pressure ventilation in postoperative cardiac surgery patients have prevented its widespread use, ventilation strategies used for patients with right ventricular failure should aim to minimize mean airway pressure, while maintaining lung volume at functional residual capacity, where lung function, PVR, and right ventricular afterload are optimal. To ensure minimal right ventricular afterload in patients with right ventricular dysfunction, the ventilation strategy should be tailored to avoid increases in PVR.

CURRENT STATUS AND FUTURE TRENDS

LCOS, one of the most significant complications of congenital heart surgery in children, results from the combined effects of transient myocardial dysfunction and alterations in ventricular loading conditions. Residual cardiac lesions and arrhythmias increase the risk for LCOS and aggravate further the underlying low output state. Recognition of LCOS after surgery is fundamental to cardiac intensive care and paramount to the prevention of associated morbidity and mortality. Monitoring of SvO_2 or SVC saturation and serum lactate is valuable for circulatory assessment. Treatment strategies may vary according to the underlying etiologic factors and clinical presentation. Prompt diagnosis of residual cardiac abnormalities is indicated especially when patients do not follow their predicted postoperative course. The mainstay of therapy, after the possibility of residual structural defects has been ruled out, is optimization of preload and afterload, improvements of tissue perfusion and oxygenation, and enhancement of myocardial function with the use of inotropic and vasodilator agents. The modified Starling relationship can be used to assess the efficacy of hemodynamic interventions aimed to treat LCOS. In the future, innovative methods of assessing myocardial performance and therapeutic measures will improve the management and evaluation of LCOS.[137,138]

Key Concepts

■ LCOS in the early postoperative period is due primarily to transient myocardial dysfunction, compounded by acute changes in myocardial loading conditions, including postoperative increases in SVR, PVR, or both.

■ At present, direct measure of myocardial performance or cardiac output or both in children is primarily a research tool and not feasible for routine clinical monitoring of patients. Cardiac output and systemic perfusion usually are assessed indirectly by monitoring vital signs, peripheral perfusion, urine output, and acid-base status.

■ Blood lactate levels may become elevated only with significant circulatory dysfunction, after the anaerobic threshold has been reached, below the point when oxygen consumption becomes dependent on oxygen delivery.

■ Conductance catheters have been used to assess load-independent measures of left ventricular and right ventricular function in the early postoperative period after cardiac surgery.

■ Mechanisms of contractile dysfunction after cardiac surgery are elusive, but evidence suggests that cardiomyocytes are injured by oxygen-derived free radicals and intracellular calcium overload during early reperfusion. Other potential causes of myocardial contractile dysfunction after congenital heart surgery include cytokine-mediated negative inotropy, cardiomyocyte apoptosis, alterations in adrenergic receptor signaling, and decreases in calcium responsiveness of the sarcomeric contractile apparatus as a result of troponin degradation.

■ When atrial pressure is low, fluid administration augments end-diastolic volume and increases stroke volume. With successive fluid administration, however, increases in stroke volume become limited because of the nonlinear nature of the ventricular diastolic compliance.

■ The use of high-dose catecholamines for inotropic support has disadvantages because they can increase afterload substantially, promote tachycardia and proarrhythmic effects, increase myocardial oxygen consumption, and depress the myocardial adrenergic response by down-regulating β–adrenergic receptors. Phosphodiesterase inhibitors increase cardiac muscle contractility and vascular muscle relaxation without increasing myocardial oxygen consumption or ventricular afterload.

■ In the neonate, the sarcoplasmic reticular system is relatively sparse and undifferentiated so that the neonatal myocardium depends more on extracellular calcium stores for contractile function.

■ Arginine vasopressin has been advocated as a therapeutic option for pediatric patients with refractory hypotension after surgery, to improve systemic arterial blood pressure when conventional therapies fail.

■ Data suggest that relative adrenal insufficiency contributes to morbidity in critically ill adult patients, and low-dose corticosteroid administration has been suggested as an option for patients with refractory LCOS.

■ A transient increase in intrathoracic pressure decreases right ventricular preload and decreases left ventricular afterload, whereas spontaneous inspiration or negative intrathoracic pressure increases right ventricular preload and increases left ventricular afterload. Effects of ventilation on right ventricular afterload or PVR depend primarily on lung volume, with PVR lowest at functional residual capacity.

REFERENCES

1. Boyle EM Jr, Pohlman TH, Johnson MC, Verrier ED: Endothelial cell injury in cardiovascular surgery: The systemic inflammatory response. Ann Thorac Surg 1997;63:277-284.
2. Hall RI, Smith MS, Rocker G: The systemic inflammatory response to cardiopulmonary bypass: Pathophysiological, therapeutic, and pharmacological considerations. Anesth Analg 1997;85:766-782.
3. Asimakopoulos G, Smith PL, Ratnatunga CP, Taylor KM: Lung injury and acute respiratory distress syndrome after cardiopulmonary bypass. Ann Thorac Surg 1999;68:1107-1115.
4. Burns SA, Newburger JW, Xiao M, et al: Induction of interleukin-8 messenger RNA in heart and skeletal muscle during pediatric cardiopulmonary bypass. Circulation 1995;92:II-315-II-321.
5. Chai PJ, Williamson JA, Lodge AJ, et al: Effects of ischemia on pulmonary dysfunction after cardiopulmonary bypass. Ann Thorac Surg 1999;67:731-735.
6. Kirshbom PM, Page SO, Jacobs MT, et al: Cardiopulmonary bypass and circulatory arrest increase endothelin-1 production and receptor expression in the lung. J Thorac Cardiovasc Surg 1997;113:777-783.
7. Chaturvedi RR, Lincoln C, Gothard JW, et al: Left ventricular dysfunction after open repair of simple congenital heart defects in infants and children: Quantitation with the use of a conductance catheter immediately after bypass. J Thorac Cardiovasc Surg 1998;115:77-83.
8. Wernovsky G, Wypij D, Jonas RA, et al: Postoperative course and hemodynamic profile after the arterial switch operation in neonates and infants: A comparison of low-flow cardiopulmonary bypass and circulatory arrest. Circulation 1995;92:2226-2235.
9. du Plessis AJ, Jonas RA, Wypij D, et al: Perioperative effects of alpha-stat versus pH-stat strategies for deep hypothermic cardiopulmonary bypass in infants. J Thorac Cardiovasc Surg 1997;114:991-1001.
10. Colan SD, Trowitzsch E, Wernovsky G, et al: Myocardial performance after arterial switch operation for transposition of the great arteries with intact ventricular septum. Circulation 1988;78:132-141.

11. Hoffman TM, Wernovsky G, Atz AM, et al: Efficacy and safety of milrinone in preventing low cardiac output syndrome in infants and children after corrective surgery for congenital heart disease. Circulation 2003;107:996-1002.

12. Parr GV, Blackstone EH, Kirklin JW: Cardiac performance and mortality early after intracardiac surgery in infants and young children. Circulation 1975;51:867-874.

13. Bellinger DC, Wypij D, Kuban KC, et al: Developmental and neurological status of children at 4 years of age after heart surgery with hypothermic circulatory arrest or low-flow cardiopulmonary bypass. Circulation 1999;100:526-532.

14. Nagashima M, Imai Y, Seo K, et al: Effect of hemofiltrated whole blood pump priming on hemodynamics and respiratory function after the arterial switch operation in neonates. Ann Thorac Surg 2000;70:1901-1906.

15. Taeed R, Schwartz SM, Pearl JM, et al: Unrecognized pulmonary venous desaturation early after Norwood palliation confounds Qp:Qs assessment and compromises oxygen delivery. Circulation 2001;103:2699-2704.

16. Cullen S, Shore D, Redington A: Characterization of right ventricular diastolic performance after complete repair of tetralogy of Fallot: Restrictive physiology predicts slow postoperative recovery. Circulation 1995;91:1782-1789.

17. Feltes T: Postoperative recovery from congenital heart disease. In Garson AJ, Bricker JT, Fisher DJ, Neish SR (eds): The Science and Practice of Pediatric Cardiology. Baltimore, Williams & Wilkins, 1997, pp 2387-2413.

18. Dittrich S, Dahnert I, Vogel M, et al: Peritoneal dialysis after infant open heart surgery: Observations in 27 patients. Ann Thorac Surg 1999;68:160-163.

19. Dittrich S, Vogel M, Dahnert I, et al: Acute hemodynamic effects of post cardiotomy peritoneal dialysis in neonates and infants. Intensive Care Med 2000;26:101-104.

20. Leyh RG, Notzold A, Kraatz EG, et al: Continuous venovenous haemofiltration in neonates with renal insufficiency resulting from low cardiac output syndrome after cardiac surgery. Cardiovasc Surg 1996;4:520-525.

21. Stechmiller JK, Treloar D, Allen N: Gut dysfunction in critically ill patients: A review of the literature. Am J Crit Care 1997;6:204-209.

22. Rappaport LA, Wypij D, Bellinger DC, et al: Relation of seizures after cardiac surgery in early infancy to neurodevelopmental outcome: Boston Circulatory Arrest Study Group. Circulation 1998;97:773-779.

23. du Plessis AJ: Neurologic disorders. In Chang AC, Hanley FL, Wernovsky G, Wessel DL (eds): Pediatric Cardiac Intensive Care. Baltimore, Williams & Wilkins, 1998, pp 369-386.

24. Perioperative care: Management of the infant and neonate with congenital heart disease. In Castaneda A, Jonas RA, Mayer JE, et al (eds): Cardiac Surgery of the Neonate and Infant. Philadelphia, WB Saunders, 1994, pp 65-87.

25. Gold JP, Jonas RA, Lang P, et al: Transthoracic intracardiac monitoring lines in pediatric surgical patients: A ten-year experience. Ann Thorac Surg 1986;42:185-191.

26. Zobel G, Rodl S, Rigler B, et al: Prospective evaluation of clinical scoring systems in infants and children with cardiopulmonary insufficiency after cardiac surgery. J Cardiovasc Surg (Torino) 1993;34:333-337.

27. Duke T, Butt W, South M, Karl TR: Early markers of major adverse events in children after cardiac operations. J Thorac Cardiovasc Surg 1997;114:1042-1052.

28. Siegel LB, Dalton HJ, Hertzog JH, et al: Initial postoperative serum lactate levels predict survival in children after open heart surgery. Intensive Care Med 1996;22:1418-1423.

29. Munoz R, Laussen PC, Palacio G, et al: Changes in whole blood lactate levels during cardiopulmonary bypass for surgery for congenital cardiac disease: An early indicator of morbidity and mortality. J Thorac Cardiovasc Surg 2000;119:155-162.

30. Charpie JR, Dekeon MK, Goldberg CS, et al: Serial blood lactate measurements predict early outcome after neonatal repair or palliation for complex congenital heart disease. J Thorac Cardiovasc Surg 2000;120:73-80.

31. Ronco JJ, Fenwick JC, Wiggs BR, et al: Oxygen consumption is independent of increases in oxygen delivery by dobutamine in septic patients who have normal or increased plasma lactate. Am Rev Respir Dis 1993;147:25-31.

32. Freed MD, Miettinen OS, Nadas AS: Oximetric detection of intracardiac left-to-right shunts. Br Heart J 1979;42:690-694.

33. Rossi AF, Seiden HS, Gross RP, Griepp RB: Oxygen transport in critically ill infants after congenital heart operations. Ann Thorac Surg 1999;67:739-744.

34. Rossi AF, Sommer RJ, Lotvin A, et al: Usefulness of intermittent monitoring of mixed venous oxygen saturation after stage I palliation for hypoplastic left heart syndrome. Am J Cardiol 1994;73:1118-1123.

35. Tweddell JS, Hoffman GM, Fedderly RT, et al: Phenoxybenzamine improves systemic oxygen delivery after the Norwood procedure. Ann Thorac Surg 1999;67:161-168.

36. Trittenwein G, Pansi H, Graf B, et al: Proposed entry criteria for postoperative cardiac extracorporeal membrane oxygenation after pediatric open heart surgery. Artif Organs 1999;23:1010-1014.

37. Hoffman GM, Ghanayem NS, Kampine JM, et al: Venous saturation and the anaerobic threshold in neonates after the Norwood procedure for hypoplastic left heart syndrome. Ann Thorac Surg 2000;70:1515-1521.

38. Kurth CD, Steven JM, Nicolson SC: Cerebral oxygenation during pediatric cardiac surgery using deep hypothermic circulatory arrest. Anesthesiology 1995;82:74-82.

39. Kurth CD, Steven JM, Nicolson SC, Jacobs ML: Cerebral oxygenation during cardiopulmonary bypass in children. J Thorac Cardiovasc Surg 1997;113:71-79.

40. Nunez S, Maisel A: Comparison between mixed venous oxygen saturation and thermodilution cardiac output in monitoring patients with severe heart failure treated with milrinone and dobutamine. Am Heart J 1998;135:383-388.

41. Li J, Schulze-Neick I, Lincoln C, et al: Oxygen consumption after cardiopulmonary bypass surgery in children: Determinants and implications. J Thorac Cardiovasc Surg 2000;119:525-533.

42. Wippermann CF, Huth RG, Schmidt FX, et al: Continuous measurement of cardiac output by the Fick principle in infants and children: Comparison with the thermodilution method. Intensive Care Med 1996;22:467-471.

43. Lequier LL, Leonard SR, Nikaidoh H, et al: Extravascular Doppler measurement of cardiac output in infants and children after operations for congenital heart disease. J Thorac Cardiovasc Surg 1999;117:1223-1225.

44. Brookes CI, White PA, Bishop AJ, et al: Validation of a new intraoperative technique to evaluate load-independent indices of right ventricular performance in patients undergoing cardiac operations. J Thorac Cardiovasc Surg 1998;116:468-476.

45. Chaturvedi RR, Shore DF, Lincoln C, et al: Acute right ventricular restrictive physiology after repair of tetralogy of Fallot: Association with myocardial injury and oxidative stress. Circulation 1999;100:1540-1547.

46. Burrows FA, Williams WG, Teoh KH, et al: Myocardial performance after repair of congenital cardiac defects in infants and children: Response to volume loading. J Thorac Cardiovasc Surg 1988;96:548-556.

47. Schermerhorn ML, Tofukuji M, Khoury PR, et al: Sialyl Lewis oligosaccharide preserves cardiopulmonary and endothelial function after hypothermic circulatory arrest in lambs. J Thorac Cardiovasc Surg 2000;120:230-237.

48. Schermerhorn ML, Nelson DP, Blume ED, et al: Sialyl Lewis oligosaccharide preserves myocardial and endothelial function during cardioplegic ischemia. Ann Thorac Surg 2000;70:890-894.

49. Sellke FW, Tofukuji M, Stamler A, et al: Beta-adrenergic regulation of the cerebral microcirculation after hypothermic cardiopulmonary bypass. Circulation 1997;96:II-304-II-310.

50. Stamler A, Wang SY, Aguirre DE, et al: Cardiopulmonary bypass alters vasomotor regulation of the skeletal muscle microcirculation. Ann Thorac Surg 1997;64:460-465.

51. Wessel DL, Adatia I, Giglia TM, et al: Use of inhaled nitric oxide and acetylcholine in the evaluation of pulmonary hypertension and endothelial function after cardiopulmonary bypass. Circulation 1993;88:2128-2138.

52. Hoffman TM, Bush DM, Wernovsky G, et al: Postoperative junctional ectopic tachycardia in children: Incidence, risk factors, and treatment. Ann Thorac Surg 2002;74:1607-1611.

53. Hoffman TM, Wernovsky G, Wieand TS, et al: The incidence of arrhythmias in a pediatric cardiac intensive care unit. Pediatr Cardiol 2002;23:598-604.

54. Rhodes LA, Wernovsky G, Keane JF, et al: Arrhythmias and intra-cardiac conduction after the arterial switch operation. J Thorac Cardiovasc Surg 1995;109:303-310.

55. Entman ML, Smith CW: Postreperfusion inflammation: A model for reaction to injury in cardiovascular disease. Cardiovasc Res 1994;28:1301-1311.

56. Dreyer WJ, Michael LH, Millman EE, et al: Neutrophil sequestration and pulmonary dysfunction in a canine model of open heart surgery with cardiopulmonary bypass: Evidence for a CD18-dependent mechanism. Circulation 1995;92:2276-2283.

57. Dreyer WJ, Burns AR, Phillips SC, et al: Intercellular adhesion molecule-1 regulation in the canine lung after cardiopulmonary bypass. J Thorac Cardiovasc Surg 1998;115:689-699.

58. Kilbridge PM, Mayer JE, Newburger JW, et al: Induction of inter-cellular adhesion molecule-1 and E-selectin mRNA in heart and skeletal muscle of pediatric patients undergoing cardiopulmonary bypass. J Thorac Cardiovasc Surg 1994;107:1183-1192.

59. Blume ED, Nelson DP, Gauvreau K, et al: Soluble adhesion molecules in infants and children undergoing cardiopulmonary bypass. Circulation 1997;96:II-352-II-357.

60. Grossi EA, Kallenbach K, Chau S, et al: Impact of heparin bonding on pediatric cardiopulmonary bypass: A prospective randomized study. Ann Thorac Surg 2000;70:191-196.

61. Hansen PR: Role of neutrophils in myocardial ischemia and reperfusion. Circulation 1995;91:1872-1885.

62. Bolli R, Marban E: Molecular and cellular mechanisms of myocardial stunning. Physiol Rev 1999;79:609-634.

63. Kan H, Finkel MS: Interactions between cytokines and neuro-hormonal systems in the failing heart. Heart Fail Rev 2001;6:119-127.

64. Stangl V, Baumann G, Stangl K, Felix SB: Negative inotropic mediators released from the heart after myocardial ischaemia-reperfusion. Cardiovasc Res 2002;53:12-30.

65. Pearl JM, Nelson DP, Schwartz SM, et al: Glucocorticoids reduce ischemia-reperfusion-induced myocardial apoptosis in immature hearts. Ann Thorac Surg 2002;74:830-837.

66. Buchhorn R, Hulpke-Wette M, Ruschewski W, et al: Beta-receptor downregulation in congenital heart disease: A risk factor for complications after surgical repair? Ann Thorac Surg 2002;73:610-613.

67. Schwinn DA, Leone BJ, Spahn DR, et al: Desensitization of myocardial beta-adrenergic receptors during cardiopulmonary bypass: Evidence for early uncoupling and late downregulation. Circulation 1991;84:2559-2567.

68. Schwartz SM, Duffy JY, Pearl JM, Nelson DP: Cellular and molecular aspects of myocardial dysfunction. Crit Care Med 2001;29:S214-S219.

69. Schwartz SM, Duffy JY, Pearl JM, et al: Glucocorticoids preserve calpastatin and troponin I during cardiopulmonary bypass in immature pigs. Pediatr Res 2003;54:91-97.

70. McDonough JL, Arrell DK, Van Eyk JE: Troponin I degradation and covalent complex formation accompanies myocardial ischemia/reperfusion injury. Circ Res 1999;84:9-20.

71. McDonough JL, Labugger R, Pickett W, et al: Cardiac troponin I is modified in the myocardium of bypass patients. Circulation 2001;103:58-64.

72. Gao WD, Atar D, Liu Y, et al: Role of troponin I proteolysis in the pathogenesis of stunned myocardium. Circ Res 1997;80:393-399.

73. Davies MJ, Nguyen K, Gaynor JW, Elliott MJ: Modified ultrafiltration improves left ventricular systolic function in infants after cardiopulmonary bypass. J Thorac Cardiovasc Surg 1998;115:361-370.

74. Chaturvedi RR, Shore DF, White PA, et al: Modified ultrafiltration improves global left ventricular systolic function after open-heart surgery in infants and children. Eur J Cardiothorac Surg 1999;15:742-746.

75. Bokesch PM, Kapural MB, Mossad EB, et al: Do peritoneal catheters remove pro-inflammatory cytokines after cardiopulmonary bypass in neonates? Ann Thorac Surg 2000;70:639-643.

76. Steinberg BM, Grossi EA, Schwartz DS, et al: Heparin bonding of bypass circuits reduces cytokine release during cardiopulmonary bypass. Ann Thorac Surg 1995;60:525-529.

77. Ozawa T, Yoshihara K, Koyama N, et al: Clinical efficacy of heparin-bonded bypass circuits related to cytokine responses in children. Ann Thorac Surg 2000;69:584-590.

78. Forbess JM, Ibla JC, Lidov HG, et al: University of Wisconsin cerebroplegia in a piglet survival model of circulatory arrest. Ann Thorac Surg 1995;60:S494-S500.

79. Weyrich AS, Ma XY, Lefer DJ, et al: In vivo neutralization of P-selectin protects feline heart and endothelium in myocardial ischemia and reperfusion injury. J Clin Invest 1993;91:2620-2629.

80. Chai PJ, Nassar R, Oakeley AE, et al: Soluble complement receptor-1 protects heart, lung, and cardiac myofilament function from cardiopulmonary bypass damage. Circulation 2000;101:541-546.

81. Lodge AJ, Chai PJ, Daggett CW, et al: Methylprednisolone reduces the inflammatory response to cardiopulmonary bypass in neonatal piglets: Timing of dose is important. J Thorac Cardiovasc Surg 1999;117:515-522.

82. Checchia PA, Backer CL, Bronicki RA, et al: Dexamethasone reduces postoperative troponin levels in children undergoing cardiopulmonary bypass. Crit Care Med 2003;31:1742-1745.

83. Schroeder VA, Pearl JM, Schwartz SM, et al: Combined steroid treatment for congenital heart surgery improves oxygen delivery and reduces postbypass inflammatory mediator expression. Circulation 2003;107:2823-2828.

84. Bronicki RA, Backer CL, Baden HP, et al: Dexamethasone reduces the inflammatory response to cardiopulmonary bypass in children. Ann Thorac Surg 2000;69:1490-1495.

85. Lowes BD, Simon MA, Tsvetkova TO, Bristow MR: Inotropes in the beta-blocker era. Clin Cardiol 2000;23:III-11-III-16.

86. Moat NE, Lamb RK, Edwards JC, et al: Induced hypothermia in the management of refractory low cardiac output states following cardiac surgery in infants and children. Eur J Cardiothorac Surg 1992;6:579-585.

87. Dalrymple-Hay MJ, Deakin CD, Knight H, et al: Induced hypothermia as salvage treatment for refractory cardiac failure following paediatric cardiac surgery. Eur J Cardiothorac Surg 1999;15:515-518.

88. Deakin CD, Knight H, Edwards JC, et al: Induced hypothermia in the postoperative management of refractory cardiac failure following paediatric cardiac surgery. Anaesthesia 1998;53:848-853.

89. Dorman BH, Sade RM, Burnette JS, et al: Magnesium supplementation in the prevention of arrhythmias in pediatric patients undergoing surgery for congenital heart defects. Am Heart J 2000;139:522-528.

90. Raja P, Hawker RE, Chaikitpinyo A, et al: Amiodarone management of junctional ectopic tachycardia after cardiac surgery in children. Br Heart J 1994;72:261-265.

91. Walsh EP, Saul JP, Sholler GF, et al: Evaluation of a staged treatment protocol for rapid automatic junctional tachycardia after operation for congenital heart disease. J Am Coll Cardiol 1997;29:1046-1053.

92. Singh K, Communal C, Sawyer DB, Colucci WS: Adrenergic regulation of myocardial apoptosis. Cardiovasc Res 2000;45: 713-719.

93. Bailey JM, Miller BE, Kanter KR, et al: A comparison of the hemodynamic effects of amrinone and sodium nitroprusside in infants after cardiac surgery. Anesth Analg 1997;84:294-298.

94. Chang AC, Atz AM, Wernovsky G, et al: Milrinone: Systemic and pulmonary hemodynamic effects in neonates after cardiac surgery. Crit Care Med 1995;23:1907-1914.

95. Bailey JM, Miller BE, Lu W, et al: The pharmacokinetics of milrinone in pediatric patients after cardiac surgery. Anesthesiology 1999; 90:1012-1018.

96. Latifi S, Lidsky K, Blumer JL: Pharmacology of inotropic agents in infants and children. Prog Pediatr Cardiol 2000;12:57-79.

97. Lindsay CA, Barton P, Lawless S, et al: Pharmacokinetics and pharmacodynamics of milrinone lactate in pediatric patients with septic shock. J Pediatr 1998;132:329-334.

98. Ramamoorthy C, Anderson GD, Williams GD, Lynn AM: Pharmacokinetics and side effects of milrinone in infants and children after open heart surgery. Anesth Analg 1998;86: 283-289.

99. Wright EM, Skoyles J, Sherry KM: Milrinone in the treatment of low output states following cardiac surgery. Eur J Anaesthesiol 1992;(Suppl 55):21-26.

100. Feneck RO: Intravenous milrinone following cardiac surgery: I. Effects of bolus infusion followed by variable dose maintenance infusion. The European Milrinone Multicentre Trial Group. J Cardiothorac Vasc Anesth 1992;6:554-562.

101. Monrad ES, Baim DS, Smith HS, et al: Effects of milrinone on coronary hemodynamics and myocardial energetics in patients with congestive heart failure. Circulation 1985;71:972-979.

102. Lebovitz DJ, Lawless ST, Weise KL: Fatal amrinone overdose in a pediatric patient. Crit Care Med 1995;23:977-980.

103. Slawsky MT, Colucci WS, Gottlieb SS, et al: Acute hemodynamic and clinical effects of levosimendan in patients with severe heart failure. Study investigators. Circulation 2000;102: 2222-2227.

104. Nawarskas JJ, Anderson JR: Levosimendan: A unique approach to the treatment of heart failure. Heart Dis 2002;4:265-271.

105. Portman MA, Fearneyhough C, Ning XH, et al: Triiodothyronine repletion in infants during cardiopulmonary bypass for congenital heart disease. J Thorac Cardiovasc Surg 2000;120:604-608.

106. Carrel T, Eckstein F, Englberger L, et al: Thyronin treatment in adult and pediatric heart surgery: Clinical experience and review of the literature. Eur J Heart Fail 2002;4:577-582.

107. Bettendorf M, Schmidt KG, Grulich-Henn J, et al: Tri-iodothyronine treatment in children after cardiac surgery: A double-blind, randomised, placebo-controlled study. Lancet 2000;356:529-534.

108. Rosenzweig EB, Starc TJ, Chen JM, et al: Intravenous arginine-vasopressin in children with vasodilatory shock after cardiac surgery. Circulation 1999;100:II-182-II-186.

109. Argenziano M, Choudhri AF, Oz MC, et al: A prospective randomized trial of arginine vasopressin in the treatment of vasodilatory shock after left ventricular assist device placement. Circulation 1997;96:II-286-II-290.

110. Morales DL, Gregg D, Helman DN, et al: Arginine vasopressin in the treatment of 50 patients with postcardiotomy vasodilatory shock. Ann Thorac Surg 2000;69:102-106.

111. Shore S, Nelson DP, Pearl JM, et al: Usefulness of corticosteroid therapy in decreasing epinephrine requirements in critically ill infants with congenital heart disease. Am J Cardiol 2001;88: 591-594.

112. Liu JP, Robinson PJ, Funder JW, Engler D: The biosynthesis and secretion of adrenocorticotropin by the ovine anterior pituitary is predominantly regulated by arginine vasopressin (AVP): Evidence that protein kinase C mediates the action of AVP. J Biol Chem 1990;265:14136-14142.

113. Pearl JM, Nelson DP, Wellmann SA, et al: Acute hypoxia and reoxygenation impairs exhaled nitric oxide release and pulmonary mechanics. J Thorac Cardiovasc Surg 2000;119:931-938.

114. Beghetti M, Silkoff PE, Caramori M, et al: Decreased exhaled nitric oxide may be a marker of cardiopulmonary bypass-induced injury. Ann Thorac Surg 1998;66:532-534.

115. Chang AC, Zucker HA, Hickey PR, Wessel DL: Pulmonary vascular resistance in infants after cardiac surgery: Role of carbon dioxide and hydrogen ion. Crit Care Med 1995;23:568-574.

116. Ivy D: Diagnosis and treatment of severe pediatric pulmonary hypertension. Cardiol Rev 2001;9:227-237.

117. Friedman M, Wang SY, Stahl GL, et al: Altered beta-adrenergic and cholinergic pulmonary vascular responses after total cardiopulmonary bypass. J Appl Physiol 1995;79:1998-2006.

118. Adatia I, Atz AM, Jonas RA, Wessel DL: Diagnostic use of inhaled nitric oxide after neonatal cardiac operations. J Thorac Cardiovasc Surg 1996;112:1403-1405.

119. Miller OI, Tang SF, Keech A, et al: Inhaled nitric oxide and prevention of pulmonary hypertension after congenital heart surgery: A randomised double-blind study. Lancet 2000;356: 1464-1469.

120. Ivy DD, Kinsella JP, Ziegler JW, Abman SH: Dipyridamole attenuates rebound pulmonary hypertension after inhaled nitric oxide withdrawal in postoperative congenital heart disease. J Thorac Cardiovasc Surg 1998;115:875-882.

121. Barst RJ, Ivy D, Dingemanse J, et al: Pharmacokinetics, safety, and efficacy of bosentan in pediatric patients with pulmonary arterial hypertension. Clin Pharmacol Ther 2003;73:372-382.

122. Schulze-Neick I, Penny DJ, Rigby ML, et al: L-arginine and substance P reverse the pulmonary endothelial dysfunction caused by congenital heart surgery. Circulation 1999;100:749-755.

123. Shekerdemian LS, Schulze-Neick I, Redington AN, et al: Negative pressure ventilation as haemodynamic rescue following surgery for congenital heart disease. Intensive Care Med 2000; 26:93-96.

124. Shekerdemian LS, Bush A, Shore DF, et al: Cardiorespiratory responses to negative pressure ventilation after tetralogy of Fallot repair: A hemodynamic tool for patients with a low-output state. J Am Coll Cardiol 1999;33:549-555.

125. Shekerdemian LS, Bush A, Shore DF, et al: Cardiopulmonary interactions after Fontan operations: Augmentation of cardiac output using negative pressure ventilation. Circulation 1997;96: 3934-3942.

126. Shekerdemian LS, Shore DF, Lincoln C, et al: Negative-pressure ventilation improves cardiac output after right heart surgery. Circulation 1996;94:II-49-II-55.

127. Bridges ND, Mayer JE Jr, Lock JE, et al: Effect of baffle fenestration on outcome of the modified Fontan operation. Circulation 1992;86:1762-1769.

128. del Nido PJ, Duncan BW, Mayer JE Jr, et al: Left ventricular assist device improves survival in children with left ventricular dysfunction after repair of anomalous origin of the left coronary artery from the pulmonary artery. Ann Thorac Surg 1999;67: 169-172.

129. Conte S, Hansen PB, Jensen T, et al: Early experience with the Norwood procedure. Cardiovasc Surg 1997;5:315-319.

130. Riordan CJ, Randsbeck F, Storey JH, et al: Effects of oxygen, positive end-expiratory pressure, and carbon dioxide on oxygen delivery in an animal model of the univentricular heart. J Thorac Cardiovasc Surg 1996;112:644-654.

131. Tabbutt S, Ramamoorthy C, Montenegro LM, et al: Impact of inspired gas mixtures on preoperative infants with hypoplastic left heart syndrome during controlled ventilation. Circulation 2001;104:I-159-I-164.

132. Ramamoorthy C, Tabbutt S, Kurth CD, et al: Effects of inspired hypoxic and hypercapnic gas mixtures on cerebral oxygen saturation in neonates with univentricular heart defects. Anesthesiology 2002;96:283-288.

133. Bradley SM, Simsic JM, Atz AM: Hemodynamic effects of inspired carbon dioxide after the Norwood procedure. Ann Thorac Surg 2001;72:2088-2094.

134. Cheifetz IM, Craig DM, Quick G, et al: Increasing tidal volumes and pulmonary overdistention adversely affect pulmonary vascular mechanics and cardiac output in a pediatric swine model. Crit Care Med 1998;26:710-716.

135. Meliones J, Kocis K, Bengur AR, Snider AR: Diastolic function in neonates after the arterial switch operation: Effects of positive pressure ventilation and inspiratory time. Intensive Care Med 2000;26:950-955.

136. Meliones JN, Bove EL, Dekeon MK, et al: High-frequency jet ventilation improves cardiac function after the Fontan procedure. Circulation 1991;84:III-364-III-368.

137. Duffy JY, Nelson DP, Schwartz SM, et al: Glucocorticoids reduce cardiac dysfunction after cardiopulmonary bypass and circulatory arrest in neonatal piglets. Pediatr Crit Care Med 2004;5:28-34.

138. Tortoriello T, Stayer SA, Mott AR, et al: A noninvasive estimation of mixed venous oxygen saturation using near-infrared spectroscopy by cerebral oximetry in pediatric cardiac surgery patients. Pediatr Anaesth 2005;15:495-503.

CHAPTER 38

New Drugs for Heart Failure

Brady S. Moffett

New agents for the treatment of heart failure are often the subject of careful scrutiny, heated debate, and intense interest. Development of these agents for children tends to be more difficult because of the smaller numbers of patients with heart failure and the relative lack of funding to conduct sizable clinical trials. It has been estimated that only 3% of the federal research and development budget is used for pediatric research.[1] As a result of the small amount of available data, approximately 75% of prescription medications have inadequate information regarding pediatric use.[2,3] A keen knowledge of pathophysiology and pharmacology is necessary to treat pediatric patients with heart failure adequately.

Rapid developmental changes occur in childhood that can create varying effects on drug pharmacokinetics and pharmacodynamics.[4] Absorptive profiles of oral medications are inconsistent with gastric pH, intestinal motility, and activity of drug-metabolizing enzymes altering with age. The volumes of distribution for certain medications also change as a child grows. Underdeveloped enzymes can be of great concern in the pharmacotherapy of children, as experience with chloramphenicol and "gray baby" syndrome has shown. Finally, the processes that allow excretion of medications in adult patients are still under development in infants, possibly resulting in supratherapeutic concentrations of drugs and unwanted side effects.

This chapter focuses on the new and emerging therapies for heart failure that have relevance in infants and children at present or in the near future. Many of the therapies reviewed have neither pediatric indications nor data to support use in children and may not be available currently. The latest medications for heart failure are being developed in adults, and the sound judgment and experience of the clinician are required to apply these medications safely and appropriately in pediatric patients with heart failure (See also other chapters in this section).

ANGIOTENSIN RECEPTOR BLOCKERS

Angiotensin receptor blockers (ARBs) are an emerging therapy in the treatment of heart failure. ARBs block the angiotensin I (AT-I) receptor, preventing the binding of angiotensin II (AT-II), a potent vasoconstrictor.[5] Blocking of this receptor also prevents activation of the later steps of the renin-angiotensin-aldosterone (RAA) hormonal cascade and inhibits the release of norepinephrine and aldosterone.

There are many potential benefits to blocking the AT-I receptor. There is a more complete AT-I receptor blockade with ARBs compared with angiotensin-converting enzyme (ACE) inhibitors because AT-II is formed by routes other than the RAA system. By virtue of blocking only the AT-I receptor, the AT-II receptor may be activated. The AT-II receptor, when stimulated, results in peripheral vasodilation, cell antiproliferative effects, cell differentiation, and tissue repair.[6] Because ARBs do not affect ACE and do not alter levels of bradykinin or substance P, the side effect of cough is eliminated. Bradykinin has cardioprotective and antihypertensive effects, however, which may be attenuated with ARB therapy.[6,7] ARBs also have been shown to reverse vascular hypertrophy, aortic constriction, and left ventricular hypertrophy in animal models. Target organ damage in animals with congestive heart failure (CHF) that have been treated with ARBs also has been minimized.[8-10]

In human subjects, ARBs promote reversal of left ventricular hypertrophy and have beneficial hemodynamic effects similar to those of ACE inhibitors.[11] The **ELITE (Evaluation of Losartan In The Elderly) trial** showed reduced left ventricular hypertrophy similar to that of ACE inhibitors.[12] In addition, the **ELITE II trial** showed that there was no difference in all-cause mortality, and that **losartan**, the ARB used in the trial, was tolerated better than captopril.[13] These studies were conducted with patients 60 years old or older with left ventricular ejection fractions of less than 40%. The **RESOLVD (Randomized Evaluation of Strategies for Left Ventricular Dysfunction) trial**, which enrolled 768 adult patients receiving **candesartan**, enalapril, or both, found that combination therapy increased left ventricular ejection fraction at the end of 43 weeks. This improvement was believed to be due to more complete neurohormonal blockade with the combination of an ACE inhibitor and an ARB.[14] **Val-HeFT (Valsartan–Heart Failure Trial)** enrolled 5010 adult patients with left ventricular ejection fractions of less than 40% and placed them on either placebo or **valsartan** in addition to standard heart failure therapy (which consisted of ACE inhibitors, digoxin, diuretics, and β-blockers). Patients who were receiving the ARB in addition to standard heart failure therapy had significant reductions in combined mortality and morbidity at 27 months.[15]

More recent trials, **CHARM (Candesartan in Heart Failure Reduction in Mortality and Morbidity)** and **VALIANT (Valsartan in Acute Myocardial Infarction)**, have shown that ARBs with and without ACE inhibitors improve morbidity and mortality in adult patients with heart failure.[16-19] A higher incidence of side effects was seen in the VALIANT trial, however, in patients who received valsartan and captopril. A more recent meta-analysis of randomized controlled trials with ARBs measured all-cause mortality and hospitalization resulting from heart failure.[20] No difference in mortality was noted in any subgroup of patients receiving ARBs. The combination of ARBs and ACE inhibitors significantly decreased hospitalizations, however. Because of the variety of ARBs used in the various trials and some differences in study outcomes, the authors of the meta-analysis warn of presuming that all ARBs are equal in their effects.

Although benefits have been seen in adults treated with ARBs, there is little literature regarding the use of ARBs in children with heart failure. The pharmacokinetic parameters of **irbesartan** have been described in 6-year-old patients.[21-23] Irbesartan has not been studied as widely as other ARBs, however, and, as mentioned earlier, the beneficial effects of ARBs may not be class-wide. Before ARBs can be implemented successfully in children, pharmacokinetic and appropriate dosing information must be available, along with a suitable oral formulation for the youngest patients.

β-BLOCKERS

Heart failure resulting from ventricular remodeling has been shown to be a complex process, encompassing many neurohormonal pathways. The continual stimulation by endogenous catecholamines (e.g., norepinephrine) alters myocardial contractility, function, and myocyte gene expression, leading to ventricular fibrosis and remodeling.[24-26] β-Blockers are theorized to decrease intrinsic myocyte remodeling by blocking excessive β-adrenergic stimulus.[24,25] In addition to preventing ventricular remodeling, β-blockers have been proposed to have antiarrhythmic effects, coronary artery vasodilatory effects, negative chronotropic effects, positive lusitropic effects, and beneficial myocyte metabolic effects.[27]

Most data concerning β-blocker use are in adult heart failure,[28] but there are convincing data concerning the benefits of **carvedilol** and **metoprolol** in pediatric heart failure. Pharmacokinetic studies currently are under way for carvedilol to determine more accurate dosing information for pediatric patients.[29] The data concerning these medications and other β-blockers are discussed in Chapter 36.

Newer β-blockers, including **nebivolol**, currently are in development outside of the United States. Nebivolol is a highly selective $β_1$-adrenergic blocker with endothelial relaxation and vasodilating effects. This vasorelaxant effect has not been documented with any other β-blocker. The mechanism for vasorelaxation is due to generation of endothelial nitric oxide, possibly through interactions with the estrogen receptor.[30] Production of nitric oxide also may result in lusitropic effects.[31] Nebivolol also has been shown to have antioxidant and antiproliferative properties.[32,33] With administration of nebivolol, blood pressure is lowered acutely, and peripheral vascular resistance is decreased.[34] These effects have been shown to be beneficial in adults with CHF, reducing left ventricular end-diastolic pressure and heart rate, while maintaining cardiac output.[35,36] Nebivolol also has been shown to improve exercise tolerance over atenolol and placebo.[37]

The effects of nebivolol also have been compared with other β-blockers in CHF. Nebivolol or atenolol was given for 6 months in 26 adult patients with hypertension and left ventricular diastolic dysfunction. Both agents showed similar reductions in heart rate, blood pressure, and left ventricular mass. Nebivolol showed a lower reduction in cardiac index and a greater increase in stroke volume.[38] Currently, nebivolol is not approved for use in the United States, and there is no pediatric dosing.

The pediatric use of β-blockers is expected to become more prevalent. The benefits of metoprolol and carvedilol in heart failure in infants and children are already recognized, and refinement of practices will ensue. Large randomized trials are necessary to determine the role and effectiveness of nebivolol in the treatment of heart failure in children.

ENDOTHELIN RECEPTOR ANTAGONISTS

The molecule plasma endothelin-1 (ET-1) acts on two main receptors in the vasculature: endothelin-A (ET_A) and endothelin-B (ET_B). The ET_A receptor has been noted for vasoconstriction, cell proliferation, and platelet aggregation effects, whereas the ET_B receptor has been shown to mediate smooth muscle relaxation through nitric oxide and prostacyclin release and is a major route of ET-1 clearance. The ET_B receptor also has been shown to prevent leukocyte adhesion to the vascular wall (Figs. 38-1 and 38-2).[39] The use of ET receptor antagonists in heart failure is currently not routine practice.

Selective and nonselective ET receptor antagonists have shown some benefit in adults with CHF. **Darusentan** and **sitaxsentan**, selective ET_A receptor antagonists, have been tested in adults with CHF. Sitaxsentan primarily has been studied in pulmonary hypertension secondary to heart failure in adults.[40,41]

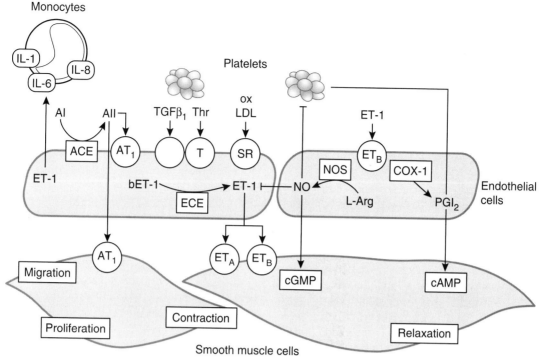

FIGURE 38-1 ■ Endothelin-1 (ET-1) and receptors. ET-1 exerts vasoconstriction and proliferation via ET_A receptors on smooth muscle cells. Endothelial ET_B receptors mediate vasodilation via release of nitric oxide (NO) and prostacyclin (PGI_2). ET_B receptors in the lung clear ET-1 from plasma. AI, AII, angiotensin I, II; AT, angiotensin receptor; COX, cyclooxygenase; ECE, endothelin-converting enzyme; IL, interleukin; L-Arg, L-arginine; NOS, nitric oxide synthase; oxLDL, oxidized low-density lipoprotein; SR, scavenger receptor; T, thrombin receptor; TGF, transforming growth factor; Thr, thrombin. (From Spieker LE, Noll G, Ruschitzka FT, Luscher TF: *Endothelin receptor antagonists in congestive heart failure: A new therapeutic principle for the future? J Am Coll Cardiol* 2001;37:1493-1505.)

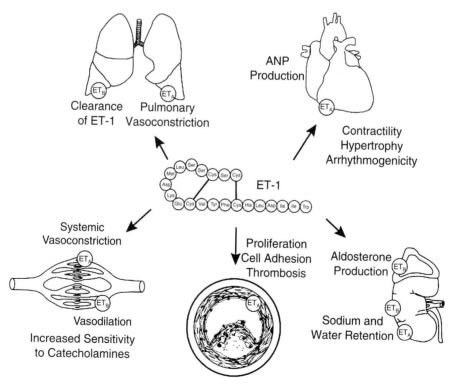

FIGURE 38-2 ■ Pathophysiologic role of endothelin-1 (ET-1) in congestive heart failure. In the heart, ET-1 contributes to contractility. In addition to its vasoconstrictive effects in the systemic and pulmonary circulation, ET-1 leads to hypertrophy of myocardial and smooth muscle cells. The pulmonary circulation is an important source of ET-1, but also is involved in the clearance of ET-1. In the kidney, ET-1 regulates sodium and water excretion. ANP, atrial natriuretic peptide. (From Spieker LE, Noll G, Ruschitzka FT, Luscher TF: *Endothelin receptor antagonists in congestive heart failure: A new therapeutic principle for the future? J Am Coll Cardiol* 2001;37:1493-1505.)

Darusentan has been studied in adults with CHF and shows not only vasodilatory activity, but also some neurohormonal modulation.[42] Darusentan also has been shown to improve cardiac index and other hemodynamic parameters in patients with heart failure.[43,44] Although darusentan has shown increased flow-mediated vasodilation in CHF patients,[45] increased heart failure symptoms were associated with darusentan treatment in studies where adverse events were reported.

Dual (ET_A and ET_B) ET receptor antagonism has been evaluated more thoroughly and may be more beneficial than selective receptor antagonism. **Bosentan**, currently approved by the U.S. Food and Drug Administration (FDA) for treatment of primary pulmonary hypertension, and **tezosentan**, an investigational agent, have been studied in patients with heart failure. Bosentan, given orally and intravenously, has shown acute vasodilatory activities in patients with CHF.[46-48] Bosentan has been reported to be hepatotoxic, however, at much lower doses than what was used in trials for treatment of CHF.[49] Long-term studies are needed to determine if this side effect is of concern. Tezosentan, given intravenously, has shown benefit in adult patients with CHF, primarily in the acute setting. Initially, tezosentan improved hemodynamic parameters during short-term infusions in patients with New York Heart Association (NYHA) class III or IV heart failure.[50-52] The **RITZ-4 (Randomized Intravenous Tezosentan Study) trial** concluded that short-term infusions of tezosentan did not offer significant benefit compared with placebo in acute decompensated CHF.[53] The **RITZ-5 (Randomized Intravenous Tezosentan for the Treatment of Pulmonary Edema) trial** also showed that tezosentan did not improve pulmonary edema in patients with CHF. Patients who received higher dosages of tezosentan had worse outcomes.[54] Further studies are warranted, possibly with lower doses of tezosentan.

Pediatric data for the ET receptor antagonists are sparse at best. Bosentan, in the oral formulation, has pharmacokinetic dosing for 2-year-old patients, but there are no safety or efficacy data.[55] In addition, bosentan has been noted to take 3 months before benefit is seen in primary pulmonary hypertension, which may lead one to believe that a patient may not see benefit for many months. The use of these agents in children should elicit a deep concern, particularly with bosentan's history of hepatotoxicity.[49] Treatment of CHF in children using ET receptor antagonists may become less relevant if further investigation into these agents reveals increased morbidity or mortality in adults.

PHOSPHODIESTERASE INHIBITORS

Enoximone is a highly selective type III phosphodiesterase inhibitor that is approved for oral and intravenous use in Europe. It is approximately one tenth as potent as milrinone and is renally eliminated. Dosage reductions in renal failure are similar to that of milrinone. In contrast to milrinone, enoximone is significantly hepatically metabolized and has an active metabolite, and dosage reductions are indicated in patients with hepatic failure.[56]

Patients with NYHA class IV CHF have shown improvement when treated with enoximone in many studies. Low-dose oral enoximone (25 mg) was shown to improve exercise tolerance in adult patients with NYHA class II or III CHF over a 12-week period.[57] Oral enoximone also has proved its use as a pharmacologic bridge to heart transplantation in adults with severe heart failure.[58] Combination therapy of enoximone and a β-blocker has shown benefit in patients with NYHA class IV heart failure.[59] Enoximone does not attenuate the effects of β-blockers, which was shown in a trial comparing enoximone and dobutamine.[60] Currently a phase III trial with oral enoximone in NYHA class III or IV heart failure is under way (ESSENTIAL trial), and this trial may facilitate FDA approval of enoximone in the United States.[61]

Several trials have shown that intravenous enoximone is beneficial in infants with low cardiac output states.[62-66] Enoximone has shown benefit in the postoperative setting, particularly when weaning patients from cardiopulmonary bypass after cardiac surgery. There is considerable debate whether these benefits are greater than the benefits of phenoxybenzamine and dobutamine. Enoximone may confer some benefit in this particular scenario because of the shorter half-life compared with phenoxybenzamine.[67,68] The similar pharmacokinetic parameters, which have been exhibited in adults and infants with enoximone, would enable initiation of this medication in children with heart failure.[69] If oral enoximone is approved for adult patients in the United States, extrapolated dosing for pediatric patients should be readily available. (Please see Chapter 34 for additional discussions on amrinone and milrinone.)

ALDOSTERONE ANTAGONISTS

Eplerenone (Inspra) is a selective aldosterone receptor antagonist that chemically differs from spironolactone by the presence of a 9α, 11α-epoxy bridge and a 17α carbomethoxy moiety in place of a thioacetyl group (Fig. 38-3).[70] Eplerenone is a competitive antagonist of aldosterone at mineralocorticoid receptors; it has been shown to antagonize the effects of aldosterone in the kidney, blood vessels, and heart.[71-75] In vivo studies have shown that eplerenone and spironolactone have similar potencies and mineralocorticoid effects, but eplerenone may have fewer endocrine disturbances because of its lower binding affinity for progesterone and androgen receptors.[76-79]

Eplerenone is approximately 100% orally bioavailable and reaches peak serum concentration level in

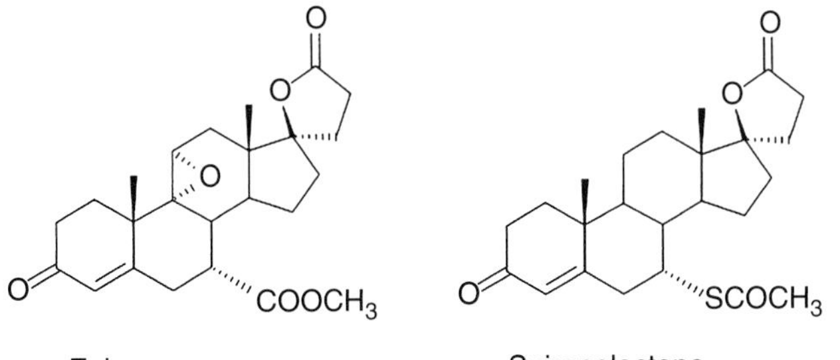

Eplerenone   Spironolactone

FIGURE 38-3 ■ **Eplerenone and spironolactone.** (From Moore TD, Nawarskas JJ, Anderson JR: Eplerenone: *A selective aldosterone receptor antagonist for hypertension and heart failure. Heart Dis* 2003;5:354-363.)

1 to 2 hours. It is significantly protein bound and metabolized hepatically by the cytochrome P-450 system, but significant drug interactions through this pathway with eplerenone are not yet known.[80,81] On treatment with eplerenone, increased serum aldosterone, plasma renin, and sodium excretion have been noted in phase I trials.[82,83] The pharmacokinetic parameters do not correlate with duration of action or other pharmacodynamic parameters.[83]

A dose-finding study with eplerenone was performed in patients with NYHA class II, III, or IV heart failure with an ejection fraction of less than 40% and maintained on an ACE inhibitor and a diuretic.[84] The patients were given eplerenone, 25 mg/day, 25 mg twice daily, 50 mg/day, or 100 mg/day; spironolactone, 25 mg/day; or placebo for 12 weeks. There were significant decreases in serum brain natriuretic peptide in the spironolactone and eplerenone groups, but no significant changes in NYHA class. Patients who received 100 mg/day of eplerenone had a higher incidence of hyperkalemia. It was concluded that a dose of 50 mg/day is safe and possibly effective for adult patients with heart failure.

Patients with mild-to-moderate hypertension and left ventricular hypertrophy were randomized to receive eplerenone, enalapril, or both.[85] Left ventricular hypertrophy was significantly reduced with the combination versus eplerenone alone, but not for enalapril alone or eplerenone alone. The authors stated that a low-dose combination of both agents may be more beneficial than monotherapy with either agent. Eplerenone also has been studied in patients with essential hypertension and left ventricular hypertrophy.[86] Patients ($n = 202$) were randomized to receive eplerenone, enalapril, or combined eplerenone and enalapril. The patients were evaluated at a 9-month end point. All treatments were shown to have reduced systolic and diastolic blood pressures. The combination of eplerenone and enalapril was shown to be the most effective in reducing left ventricular size, and eplerenone alone was as effective as enalapril alone in reducing left ventricular size. The side

effect of cough was more common in patients treated with enalapril, and hyperkalemia was more common in patients treated with eplerenone.

The largest trial in adult patients is **EPHESUS (Eplerenone Post-Acute Myocardial Infarction Heart Failure Efficacy and Survival Study).**[87] This double-blinded, placebo-controlled study enrolled 6632 patients with acute myocardial infarction complicated by left ventricular dysfunction and heart failure. Patients had an average ejection fraction of 33 ± 6 %, approximately 85% were receiving an ACE inhibitor, 75% were receiving a β-blocker, 60% were receiving a diuretic, 88% were on aspirin, and 47% were receiving a 3-hydroxy-3-methylglutaryl coenzyme A reductase inhibitor. The primary end points were death from any cause or cardiovascular causes and hospitalization from heart failure, acute myocardial infarction, stroke, or ventricular arrhythmia. Eplerenone was shown to reduce mortality at all end points. The incidence of hyperkalemia was slightly lower with eplerenone than with spironolactone.

The current recommended dose of eplerenone to treat hypertension in adults is 50 mg once daily, which may be increased to 50 mg twice a day.[88] A single-dose pharmacokinetic study enrolling 18 patients older than 2 years of age and younger than 16 years has been performed. There were no statistically significant differences in maximum concentration, area under the curve, and maximum threshold. The only covariate altering the pharmacokinetics of eplerenone was body weight. Eplerenone is one of the few new drugs on the horizon for treatment of heart failure in infants and children that has pediatric dosing.[89]

CALCIUM-SENSITIZING AGENTS

Calcium-sensitizing agents may be beneficial in heart failure by prolonging the effects of calcium in the myocardium. These agents do not affect the levels of calcium in the myocardium, and this benefit may lead to decreased incidences of arrhythmias from calcium overload.[90] Development of these agents has created considerable interest, which may be due partly to their unique mechanism of action.

Levosimendan (Simdax) is an inodilatory drug that was discovered by using troponin C as a target protein[91] and has shown positive chronotropy, positive inotropy, and vasodilatory effects.[92] Levosimendan binds to calcium-saturated troponin C complexes, and stabilizes the troponin C–calcium complex without affecting the initial calcium-binding capabilities of troponin C. This ability allows for a longer half-life and more effective use of calcium in the myocardium.[93] Myocardial levels of cyclic AMP may be increased by levosimendan through phosphodiesterase inhibition, but this is debatable.[94-96] Some data have shown that lower concentrations of levosimendan stimulate L-type calcium channels in human ventricular myocardium, which indicates phosphodiesterase inhibition activity.[97] Other studies have shown that the phosphodiesterase inhibition properties of levosimendan occur only at higher doses, which are not clinically relevant.[98,99] At this time, the phosphodiesterase inhibition activities of levosimendan seem to be a relatively minor mechanism for its beneficial effects.

In vitro data have suggested that an active metabolite of levosimendan, OR-1896, may be responsible for increased calcium ion concentration in the myocardium, at clinically relevant concentrations of the parent drug.[100,101] The vasodilatory effects of levosimendan have been attributed to the opening of ATP-sensitive potassium channels in vascular smooth muscle cells; this has been shown in animal models.[102-104] At higher concentrations, the potassium channel effects of levosimendan are attenuated.[105]

The pharmacokinetics of levosimendan have been published along with studies detailing possible interactions with other medications.[106-113] No difference has been shown in the pharmacokinetic parameters of levosimendan in healthy patients compared with patients with CHF.[114,115] The effects of levosimendan extend far beyond the discontinuation of the infusion in adults, owing to active metabolites with half-lives of nearly 80 hours after an infusion period of 24 hours.[111,114-116]

Levosimendan has shown benefit in adult patients with CHF. Continuous infusions of levosimendan at doses of 0.1 to 0.4 µg/kg/min have increased cardiac output and stroke volume, with only slight increases in heart rate. These infusions also resulted in decreased coronary, pulmonary, and peripheral vascular resistance.[117,118] Levosimendan also provides symptomatic relief without increasing myocardial oxygen consumption.[119] In patients with NYHA class III or IV heart failure secondary to an ischemic event, a bolus dose of levosimendan of 6 to 24 µg/kg over 10 minutes followed by an infusion of 0.05 to 0.2 µg/kg/min was well tolerated and led to favorable hemodynamic effects.[120] Oral levosimendan has been studied in patients with NYHA class III or IV heart failure secondary to coronary artery disease or dilated cardiomyopathy. Eight of these patients were being treated with a β-blocker, and five were being treated with a long-acting nitrate. Single doses of 1 mg and 4 mg of levosimendan resulted in significant decreases in pulmonary capillary wedge pressure and right atrial pressure; these one-time doses also resulted in significant increases in cardiac output. Because these were only one-time doses, the effect of continuous dosing could not be described.[121] Oral levosimendan also has shown benefit in weaning patients with severe heart failure (NYHA class IV) from inotropic therapy.[122]

Three large clinical trials with levosimendan have been performed. Slawsky and colleagues[123] enrolled 146 patients with NYHA class III or IV heart failure in a multicenter, double-blinded, placebo-controlled study with levosimendan. Patients who received the drug were given 0.1 to 0.4 µg/kg/min, up-titrated over 4 hours.

The authors noted a 28% increase in stroke volume and a 39% increase in cardiac index in the levosimendan group compared with placebo. There were moderate increases in heart rate at the higher end of the dose range. Patients also seemed to improve in regard to dyspnea and fatigue in the levosimendan group. The authors concluded that levosimendan may be beneficial in the short-term management of decompensated heart failure.[123] The **RUSSLAN trial** was a placebo-controlled, double-blind study that evaluated the safety and efficacy of levosimendan in patients with left ventricular failure complicating acute myocardial infarction. Levosimendan, 0.1 to 0.4 µg/kg/min, or placebo was given intravenously for 6 hours to 504 patients. The incidences of ischemia and hypotension were the same between all groups except for a higher incidence in patients receiving the highest dose of the drug. The patients receiving levosimendan at doses of 0.1 to 0.2 µg/kg/min did not have increased incidence of hypotension or ischemia, and the risk of worsening heart failure was reduced.[124] Dobutamine was compared with levosimendan in the **Levosimendan Infusion versus Dobutamine (LIDO) study**, which enrolled adult patients with low output heart failure. An initial loading dose of 24 µg/kg of levosimendan, followed by an infusion of 0.1 µg/kg/min, was administered to 103 patients. In 100 patients, dobutamine was infused at a dose of 5 µg/kg/min for 24 hours with no loading dose. Five patients in the levosimendan group and six patients in the dobutamine group had dose-limiting events leading to temporary discontinuation of the medications. Overall, 47% of the levosimendan patients had adverse events compared with 42% in the dobutamine group. The primary hemodynamic end point was achieved in 28% of the levosimendan patients and 15% of the dobutamine patients. At 180 days, 26% of the levosimendan patients had died compared with 38% of the dobutamine patients. These statistically significant percentages led the authors to conclude that levosimendan may be a better choice than dobutamine for severe low output heart failure.[125] A phase III study with levosimendan in adult patients with acute decompensated heart failure currently is being conducted in the United States.[126]

Pimobendan is another calcium-sensitizing agent that has a slightly separate mechanism of action compared with levosimendan. Pimobendan has a higher level of phosphodiesterase inhibition at clinically relevant serum levels and inhibits the production of inflammatory cytokines.[127,128] Higher intracellular calcium levels result, which have been shown to increase patient mortality.[129] Pimobendan also has been shown to prolong cardiac relaxation, which can impair diastolic function.[128]

Several small studies concerning the benefits of the use of pimobendan in heart failure, cor pulmonale, and dilated cardiomyopathy have been conducted.[129-131] One placebo-controlled trial that enrolled 317 patients with an ejection fraction of less than 45% showed some detrimental effects in the pimobendan group, however.

After 24 weeks, patients who had taken either 2.5 mg or 5 mg of pimobendan had improved exercise capacity, but the hazard of death was 1.8 times higher than the placebo group.[132] In another randomized, double-blind, placebo-controlled study, patients received pimobendan, 1.25 mg or 2.5 mg, or placebo for 52 weeks. The hospitalization rate for pimobendan was less than for placebo, but not significantly different. The incidence of cardiac events was 45% lower in the pimobendan group. The authors concluded that pimobendan lowers cardiac morbidity and increases physical activity levels in patients with heart failure.[133] Currently, pimobendan does not seem to have a role in the treatment of heart failure in infants and children, but this may change with further studies.

Two other agents, EMD 57033 and CGP 48506, that have pure calcium sensitization effects and no phosphodiesterase III inhibition have shown increased contractility in isolated myocytes with no change in energy consumption.[134] Another calcium-sensitizing agent known as MCC 135 is currently undergoing a phase III clinical trial in the United States and has shown some beneficial effect in animal studies.[126,135]

TUMOR NECROSIS FACTOR-α INHIBITORS

Tumor necrosis factor (TNF)-α, also known as myocardial depressant factor, is a proinflammatory cytokine that has been associated with cardiac dysfunction and poor outcomes in adults with CHF.[136,137] Elevated levels of TNF-α and other myocardial inflammatory factors have been associated with heart failure in children with congenital heart disease.[138] The primary mechanism for the detrimental effects of TNF-α is depression of nitric oxide endothelial relaxation, although the exact mechanism of TNF-α is complex and has not been elucidated completely (Fig. 38-4).[139] By inhibiting TNF-α, vasoreactivity can be restored.

Etanercept (Enbrel), a TNF-α inhibitor, has been tested in adult patients with NYHA class III or IV CHF. It was tolerated well and showed reductions in symptoms and improvement in left ventricular function.[140,141] It also was noted to improve endothelial vasoreactivity in adults with CHF.[142] Two large studies, the **RENAISSANCE (Randomized ENBREL North American Strategy to Study Antagonism of Cytokines) trial** and the **RECOVER (Research into ENBREL: Cytokine antagonism in Ventricular Dysfunction) trial** were performed to evaluate the effectiveness of etanercept in heart failure.[143] The **RENEWAL (Randomized Etanercept Worldwide Evaluation) trial** summarized the aforementioned studies and found no statistically significant differences between placebo and etanercept groups in effectiveness or in safety profiles. In one trial arm, there were indications of worsening heart failure in patients who received etanercept. More recently,

worsening of CHF and new-onset CHF have been identified in postmarketing reports with etanercept in patients treated for rheumatoid arthritis.[144,145] The mechanism for these adverse events is currently unclear and has halted the further development of etanercept as an agent in the treatment of heart failure.[144]

Infliximab (Remicade) is a monoclonal antibody against TNF-α that also was studied in adults with CHF.[146] The **Anti-TNF Therapy Against Congestive Heart Failure (ATTACH) trial** was a randomized, placebo-controlled trial with infliximab in 150 adults with NYHA class III or IV heart failure. Patients who received low to medium doses of infliximab showed no improvement, and patients who received high doses had increased mortality. There also have been postmarketing reports of new-onset and worsening heart failure in patients who received infliximab for treatment of rheumatoid arthritis or Crohn disease.[146,147] Although these particular agents may not be options for the treatment of heart failure at present, other agents that manipulate TNF-α may prove useful in the future.[147]

NEUTRAL ENDOPEPTIDASE INHIBITORS

When elevated, natriuretic peptides, such as atrial natriuretic peptide (ANP), result in increased natriuresis and decreased activation of the RAA system. Atrial wall stretch is believed to be the primary stimulus for production of ANP.[148] Neutral endopeptidase (NEP) is the major pathway for the enzymatic breakdown of these natriuretic peptides (Fig. 38-5). Increased natriuretic and vasodilatory properties can be expressed by preventing the breakdown of endogenous ANP via NEP inhibition (Fig. 38-6).[148] Varying forms of exogenously administered natriuretic peptides have shown benefit in patients with heart failure, but they must be given intravenously and have short half-lives.[149] Oral forms of NEP inhibitors have been developed and evaluated in patients with heart failure.

Candoxatril is an NEP inhibitor that has been noted to increase circulating plasma ET and natriuretic peptide levels in patients with chronic heart failure.[150] Candoxatril has been tested more recently against furosemide in adult patients with mild, stable, chronic heart failure.[151] Both agents induced natriuresis, diuresis, and similar changes in hemodynamic parameters. In contrast to furosemide, candoxatril did not induce any significant changes in neurohormonal factors, such as plasma renin or plasma aldosterone levels. Exercise capacity was increased in patients treated with candoxatril compared with a slight decrease in exercise capacity in patients treated with furosemide. Another study noted improved physical signs and symptoms with candoxatril compared with furosemide in patients with NYHA class I or II heart failure.[152] Finally, compared with captopril, candoxatril was equally tolerated and showed similar improvements in patients during treadmill exercise tests.

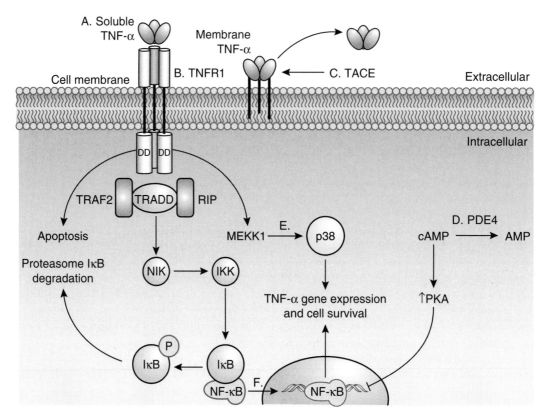

FIGURE 38-4 ■ **Potential targets for the inhibition of tumor necrosis factor (TNF)-α signaling pathways or protein expression.** Given the complexity of TNF-α signaling and the various mechanisms associated with the regulation of TNF expression, there are many potential targets for the inhibition of TNF-related activities. Some protein-based inhibitors target the TNF-α molecule or its receptor (**A** and **B**), which prevents the resultant signaling pathways. Additional targets include TNF-converting enzyme (TACE) (**C**), which processes the 26-κDa membrane form of TNF-α to the soluble 17-κDa form, preventing its release into the circulation. Molecules targeting intracellular TNF-related signaling pathways also have been identified, including inhibitors of phosphodiesterase 4 (PDE4) (**D**) and p38 (**E**). Additionally, nuclear factor-κB (NF-κB) inhibitors include molecules targeting the activities of upstream signaling events involved in the initial activation of NF-κB (NF-κB-inducing kinase [NIK], inhibitor of NF-κB [IB] kinase [IKK], IB degradation). Inhibition of the activation of NF-κB (**F**) prevents the synthesis of NF-κB inducible genes, which include many proinflammatory cytokines and other important inflammation-related proteins. NF-κB inhibition also can promote cell death in certain sensitive cell types, including cancers, suggesting the use of NF-κB inhibitors as potential cancer therapeutics. DD, death domain; MEKK1, mitogen-activated protein kinase 1; PKA, protein kinase A; RIP, receptor-interacting protein; TNFR1, TNF receptor 1; TRADD, TNFR1-associated death domain–containing protein; TRAF2, TNFR-associated factor 2. (See also Color Section) (From Palladino MA, Bahjat FR, Theodorakis EA, Moldawer LL: *Anti-TNF-alpha therapies: The next generation. Nat Rev Drug Discov* 2003;2:736-746.)

Sixty patients with NYHA class III or IV heart failure were randomized to receive candoxatril, captopril, or placebo for 12 weeks. The authors concluded that candoxatril may provide similar symptomatic benefits as ACE inhibitors in patients with CHF,[153] but most of the data with candoxatril are in patients with mild heart failure. It remains to be seen if patients with more severe heart failure would experience similar beneficial effects.

Ecadotril, another NEP inhibitor, also has been tested in adult patients with CHF. Initially, ecadotril had been shown to elevate plasma ANP levels, decrease plasma renin, and decrease pulmonary capillary wedge pressure in a few patients.[154] Larger trials have shown dramatically different results compared with patients

treated with candoxatril.[155] A dose escalation trial of ecadotril enrolled 50 ambulatory patients with an ejection fraction of less than 35%. At the end of the trial, no differences in neurohormonal levels were detected between ecadotril and placebo. The study was not designed to detect differences in NYHA class. This result was striking, considering that nearly all other trials with NEP inhibitors have shown some degree of change in ANP, aldosterone, or other neurohormonal levels. The dose of ecadotril used in this trial may not have been adequate, or in vivo activity may be absent.

Theoretically, NEP inhibitors could have a tremendous therapeutic advantage in the treatment of heart failure. There has been considerable controversy over the

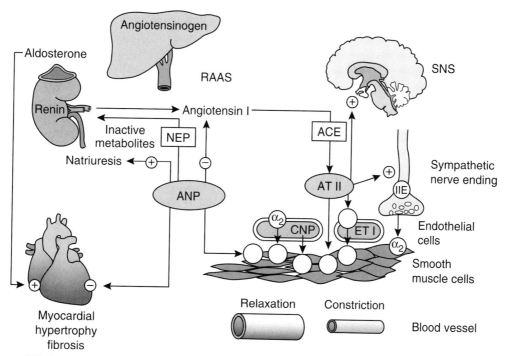

FIGURE 38-5 ■ Neutral endopeptidase (NEP) inhibition. The acute effect of NEP inhibitors on the cardiovascular system. Significant lowering of the blood pressure was documented in experimental models and in some clinical studies. Long-term treatment has shown only a moderate effect probably because of stimulation of the renin angiotensin aldosterone system (RAAS) or because of down-regulation of atrial natriuretic peptide (ANP) receptors. AT II, angiotensin II; ET-1, endothelin 1; CNP, C natriuretic peptide; ACE, angiotensin-converting enzyme; SNS, sympathetic nervous system. (From Worthley MI, Corti R, Worthley SG: *Vasopeptidase inhibitors: Will they have a role in clinical practice? Br J Clin Pharmacol* 2004;57:27-36.)

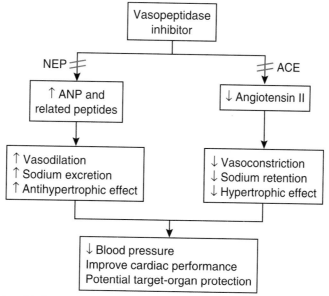

FIGURE 38-6 ■ Mechanism of action of vasopeptidase inhibitors. ACE, angiotensin-converting enzyme; ANP, atrial natriuretic peptide; NEP, neutral endopeptidase. (From Weber M: *Emerging treatments for hypertension: Potential role for vasopeptidase inhibition. Am J Hypertens* 1999;12: 139S-147S.)

effectiveness of these agents, however.[156] **Omapatrilat**, another NEP inhibitor that also inhibits ACE, has shown beneficial effects in patients with heart failure. It also has exhibited a higher rate of angioedema than ACE inhibitors.[157] Currently the effectiveness of NEP inhibitors in the treatment of heart failure is unclear. The significant difference in efficacy between the two studies previously mentioned highlights the traditional challenges of extrapolating drugs tested in adult trials to pediatric patients. As the neurohormonal mechanisms in heart failure are elucidated further, the role that NEP inhibitors play will be defined more clearly.

VASOPRESSIN ANTAGONISTS

Arginine vasopressin has been known to have many effects, based on the receptor that it stimulates (Table 38-1). Endogenous arginine vasopressin has been proved to be a potent vasoconstrictor in humans through V1a receptors, via an increase in cytosolic calcium.[158] Endogenous arginine vasopressin also causes water and sodium retention via V2 receptors and plays a fundamental role in proliferation of vascular endothelial growth factor.[159] Vasopressin antagonists are the newest agents designed to combat these effects in heart failure by blocking the V1a or V2 receptors. Many beneficial effects of vasopressin antagonists have been shown in animal models of CHF, and human trials are beginning to show similar results.[160-163]

Affinity for the V1a and V2 receptors has been noted in YM087, a vasopressin receptor antagonist currently known as **conivaptan**.[164-166] Although conivaptan is classified as a V1a/V2 receptor antagonist, it was shown to have a less pronounced action on the V1a receptor compared with the V2 receptor.[167] The diuretic effects of conivaptan have been shown in multiple animal studies in intravenous and oral dosage forms.[168,169] Ventricular remodeling mechanisms mediated by arginine vasopressin also have been attenuated by conivaptan.[159,170] A trial was performed with conivaptan in 142 patients with NYHA class III or IV heart failure. Patients received a single dose of 10 mg, 20 mg, or 40 mg of conivaptan. Patients were required to be on a diuretic or an ACE inhibitor and optionally could be receiving digoxin or a β-blocker. Many exclusion criteria were involved, including patients with congenital heart disease. The results noted that pulmonary capillary wedge pressure was significantly reduced and remained reduced for 8 hours after 20 mg and 40 mg of conivaptan with no other changes in hemodynamic parameters. Urine output also was increased in all dosage groups compared with placebo. The only significant adverse event correlated with conivaptan that was greater than placebo was headache.[171] Other V1a/V2 receptor antagonists, such as YM471, also have shown potent and long-acting V1a/V2 receptor blockade in animal and human cells, although less research has been published on YM471.[172-174]

Selective V1a receptor vasopressin antagonists, such as **relcovaptan** (SR49059), have been tested to determine their roles as treatment options in CHF.[175-178] In heart failure models, relcovaptan has shown beneficial effects by improving cardiac function via inhibition of the mitogenic effects of arginine vasopressin and decreasing cytosolic calcium concentrations.[179-181] The vasodilatory effect of relcovaptan on human arteries has been shown in several different trials, encompassing uterine arterioles, radial arteries, and arterial bypass grafts.[182-184] Phase I trials have shown that relcovaptan is safe in healthy adult volunteers.[185,186]

Finally, **tolvaptan** (OPC 41061) is an oral V2 receptor antagonist that has been studied in adults with CHF. Patients received tolvaptan or placebo for 25 days without fluid restriction. Compared with placebo, the tolvaptan group of patients had decreased edema and normalized serum sodium.[187] A trial currently is ongoing in the United States to test the acute and chronic effects of tolvaptan in adults with worsening CHF.[188]

Trials with vasopressin antagonists in humans have elucidated more clearly the role of these agents in heart failure. Further research is needed to determine their

TABLE 38-1

Location and Physiologic Actions of Arginine Vasopressin Receptor Subtypes		
Receptor Subtypes	**Site of Action**	**Arginine Vasopressin Activation Effects**
V$_{1a}$	Vascular smooth muscle cells Platelets Lymphocytes and monocytes Adrenal cortex	Vasoconstriction Platelet aggregation Coagulation factor release Glycogenolysis
V$_{1b}$	Anterior pituitary	ACTH and β-endorphin release
V$_2$	Renal collecting duct principal cells	Free water reabsorption

ACTH, adrenocorticotropin hormone.
From Lee CR, Watkins ML, Patterson JH, et al: Vasopressin: A new target for the treatment of heart failure. Am Heart J 2003;146:9–18.

place in the arsenal of medications used currently to treat heart failure. Pediatric use is expected to follow, pending FDA approval and pharmacokinetic studies.

CURRENT STATUS AND FUTURE TRENDS

Many of the new pharmacologic agents described in this chapter that are used for heart failure in adults eventually will be used in children with heart failure. As the trial with milrinone has shown, however, failure of a clinical trial with a drug in adults does not portend suboptimal results in pediatric patients with heart failure because mechanisms of heart failure differ. Finally, future pharmacologic strategies, such as dopamine–β-hydoxy-lase inhibition, apoptosis inhibition, G protein–coupled receptor modifiers, intracellular signal transduction pathway modifiers, and gene therapy, all will yield potential drugs for the treatment of heart failure in adults and children.

Pharmacogenomics, or the search for genetic polymorphisms that can influence drug therapy, will have a significant impact on the pharmacologic treatment of heart failure. Several targets have been identified for pharmacogenomic evaluation. Currently the matching of medications to a particular genotype to minimize side effects and maximize efficacy is not possible, but the progress that has been made shows great promise for the future of genomic medicine.

The RAA system is well known as a target in the treatment of heart failure. ACE inhibitors have proved that they are beneficial therapies by manipulating the RAA system. The response to ACE inhibitors often varies, however. African Americans do not respond as well to ACE inhibitors, with fewer reductions in morbidity and mortality than in other races.[189-191] These differences in response may be due to genetic polymorphisms for genes encoding ACE, angiotensinogen, and AT-II receptors.[192-195] Other studies have examined the influences of ACE genotypes on cardiovascular responses to ACE inhibitors and found significant differences in blood pressure reduction among various racial groups. Studies with left ventricular dysfunction have had conflicting results, however, in regard to RAA genetic polymorphisms.[196] An example of multiple genetic polymorphisms correlating with clinically significant results has been shown with two RAA genes and ACE inhibitor–induced cough.[197] Multiple polymorphisms are likely to be the pathway by which response to medications is likely deduced.

β-Blockers are an important treatment modality for patients with heart failure, and the level of β-receptor expression may determine the effectiveness of therapy. The genes that code for β_1-adrenergic and β_2-adrenergic receptors have shown different rates of expression between whites and African Americans. Studies currently are under way to determine if polymorphisms in the β_1-receptor gene influence the blood pressure response

to β-blockers. Response to β-blocker therapy in heart failure also has been correlated with ACE inhibitor genotype polymorphisms. Patients with dilated cardiomyopathy have shown increased transplant-free survival at 2 years for a particular ACE genotype.[198] In addition, pharmacogenetic factors influence expressions of CYP2D6 and metabolism of the β-blockers metoprolol, carvedilol, timolol, and propranolol.[199]

Digoxin, historically a mainstay in the treatment of heart failure, also can be affected by genetic polymorphisms. Digoxin is a substrate for P-glycoprotein, a drug efflux pump expressed in multiple sites in the body. P-glycoprotein is encoded by a multidrug resistance gene (*MDR-1*). It has been shown that healthy volunteers with particular genotypes for *MDR-1* can have varying excretion rates and serum levels of digoxin, possibly resulting in therapeutic failure.[200]

As with other directions in traditional drug development, pediatric experience with pharmacogenomics also has been limited. Case reports of adverse events from decreased metabolism of drugs are available, but offer little proactive insight into pediatric pharmacotherapy.[201] Investigation into this area of the interface between pharmacologic treatment and genetic polymorphisms undoubtedly would result in improved care for pediatric patients with heart failure.[202-204]

Key Concepts

■ ARBs block the AT-I receptor, preventing the binding of AT-II, a potent vasoconstrictor. Blocking of the AT-I receptor also prevents activation of the later steps of the RAA hormonal cascade and inhibits the release of norepinephrine and aldosterone.

■ The continual stimulation by endogenous catecholamines (e.g., norepinephrine) can alter myocardial contractility, function, and myocyte gene expression, leading to ventricular fibrosis and remodeling. β-Blockers are theorized to decrease intrinsic myocyte remodeling by blocking excessive β-adrenergic stimulus.

■ Nebivolol is a highly selective β_1-adrenergic blocker with endothelial relaxation and vasodilating effects. This vasorelaxant effect has not been documented with any other β-blocker. The mechanism for vasorelaxation is due to generation of endothelial nitric oxide, possibly through interactions with the estrogen receptor.

■ The molecule plasma ET-1 acts on two main receptors in the vasculature: ET_A and ET_B. The ET_A receptor has been noted for vasoconstriction, cell proliferation, and platelet aggregation effects, whereas the ET_B receptor has been shown to mediate smooth muscle relaxation through nitric oxide and prostacyclin release and is a major route of ET-1 clearance.

■ Eplerenone is a competitive antagonist of aldosterone at mineralocorticoid receptors; it has been shown to antagonize the effects of aldosterone in the kidney, blood vessels, and heart. In vivo studies have shown that eplerenone and spironolactone have similar potencies and mineralocorticoid effects, but eplerenone may have fewer endocrine disturbances because of its lower binding affinity for progesterone and androgen receptors.

■ The combination of eplerenone and enalapril was shown to be the most effective in reducing left ventricular size, and eplerenone alone was as effective as enalapril alone in reducing left ventricular size.

■ Levosimendan is an inodilatory drug discovered by using troponin C as a target protein and has shown positive chronotropy, positive inotropy, and vasodilatory effects. Levosimendan binds to calcium-saturated troponin C complexes, and stabilizes the troponin C–calcium complex without affecting the initial calcium-binding capabilities of troponin C.

■ Elevated levels of TNF-α and other myocardial inflammatory factors have been associated with heart failure in children with congenital heart disease. The primary mechanism for the detrimental effects of TNF-α is depression of nitric oxide endothelial relaxation, although the exact mechanism of TNF-α is complex and has not been elucidated completely.

■ NEP is the major pathway for the enzymatic breakdown of these natriuretic peptides. Increased natriuretic and vasodilatory properties can be expressed by preventing the breakdown of endogenous ANP via NEP inhibition.

■ Endogenous arginine vasopressin has been proved to be a potent vasoconstrictor in humans through V1a receptors, via an increase in cytosolic calcium. Endogenous arginine vasopressin also causes water and sodium retention via V2 receptors and plays a fundamental role in proliferation of vascular endothelial growth factor. Vasopressin antagonists are the newest agents designed to combat these effects in heart failure by blocking the V1a or V2 receptors.

■ Future pharmacologic strategies, such as dopamine–β-hydoxylase inhibition, apoptosis inhibition, G protein–coupled receptor modifiers, intracellular signal transduction pathway modifiers, and gene therapy, all will yield potential drugs for the treatment of heart failure in adults and children.

■ Pharmacogenomics, or the search for genetic polymorphisms that can influence drug therapy, will have a significant impact on the pharmacologic treatment of heart failure.

REFERENCES

1. Roberston WO: Chemicals, children, and research $'s. Vet Hum Toxicol 1998;40:308-309.
2. Smyth RL, Weindling AM: Research in children: Ethical and scientific aspects. Lancet 1999;354(Suppl 2):SII-21-SII-24.
3. Campbell H, Surry SAM, Royle EM: A review of randomized controlled trial published in the *Archives of Disease in Childhood* from 1982-96. Arch Dis Child 1998;79:192-197.
4. Kearns GL: Impact of developmental pharmacology on pediatric study design: Overcoming the challenges. J Allergy Clin Immunol 2000;106:S128-S138.
5. Burnier M: Angiotensin II type 1 receptor blockers. Circulation 2001;103:904-912.
6. de Gasparo M, Levens N: Does blockade of angiotensin II receptors offer clinical benefits over inhibition of angiotensin-converting enzyme? Pharmacol Toxicol 1998;82:257-271.
7. Willienheimer R, Dahlof B, Rydberg E, Erhardt L: AT1-receptor blockers in hypertension and heart failure: Clinical experience and future directions. Eur Heart J. 1999;20:997-1008.
8. Kim S, Ohta K, Hamaguchi A, et al: Angiotensin II type 1 receptor antagonist inhibits gene expression of transforming growth factor-β1 and extracellular matrix in cardiac and vascular tissue of hypertensive rats. J Pharmacol Exp Ther 1995;273:509-515.
9. Obayashi M, Yano M, Kohno M, et al: Dose-dependent effect of ANG II-receptor antagonist on myocyte remodeling in rat cardiac hypertrophy. Am J Physiol 1997;273(4 Pt 2):H1824-H1831.
10. Rockman HA, Wachorst SP, Mao L, Ross J Jr: ANG II receptor blockade prevents ventricular hypertrophy and ANF gene expression with pressure overload in mice. Am J Physiol 1994;226(6 Pt 2):H2468-H2475.
11. Crozier I, Ikram H, Awan N, et al: Losartan in heart failure: Hemodynamic effects and tolerability. Circulation 1995;91:691-697.
12. Pitt B, Segal R, Martinez FA, et al: Randomised trial of losartan versus captopril in patients greater than 65 with heart failure (Evaluation of Losartan In The Elderly study, ELITE). Lancet 1997;349:747-752.
13. Pitt B, Poole-Wilson PA, Segal R, et al: Effect of losartan compared with captopril on mortality in patients with symptomatic heart failure: Randomized trial—the losartan heart failure survival study ELITE II. Lancet 2000;355:1582-1587.
14. McKelvie RS, Yusuf S, Pericak D, et al, RESOLVED Pilot study investigators: Comparison of candesartan, enalapril, and their combination in congestive heart failure: Randomized Evaluation of Strategies for Left Ventricular Dysfunction (RESOLVD) pilot study. Circulation 1999;100:1056-1064.
15. Maggioni AP, Anand I, Gottlieb SO, et al, Val-HeFT investigators: Effects of valsartan on morbidity and mortality in patients with heart failure not receiving angiotensin-converting enzyme inhibitors. J Am Coll Cardiol 2002;40:1414-1421.
16. Yusuf S, Pfeffer MA, Swedberg K, et al, CHARM Investigators and Committees: Effects of candesartan in patients with chronic heart failure and reduced left-ventricular systolic function taking angiotensin-converting-enzyme inhibitors: The CHARM-Added trial. Lancet 2003;362:767-771.
17. McMurray JJ, Ostergren J, Swedberg K, et al, CHARM Investigators and Committees: Effects of candesartan in patients with chronic heart failure and reduced left-ventricular systolic function intolerant to angiotensin-converting-enzyme inhibitors: The CHARM-Alternative trial. Lancet 2003;362:772-776.
18. Granger CB, McMurray JJ, Yusuf S, et al, CHARM Investigators and Committees: Effects of candesartan in patients with chronic heart failure and preserved left-ventricular ejection fraction: The CHARM-Preserved trial. Lancet 2003;362:777-781.
19. Winkelmann BR: American Heart Association scientific sessions. Expert Opin Investig Drugs 2004;13:435-445.
20. Jong P, Demers C, McKelvie RS, Liu PP: Angiotensin receptor blockers in heart failure: Meta-analysis of randomized controlled trials. J Am Coll Cardiol 2002;39:463-470.
21. Marino MR, Vachharajani NN: Pharmacokinetics of irbesartan are not altered in special populations. J Cardiovasc Pharmacol 2002;40:112-122.
22. Sakarcan A, Tenney F, Wilson JT, et al: The pharmacokinetics of irbesartan in hypertensive children and adolescents. J Clin Pharmacol 2001;41:742-749.
23. Vachharajani NN, Shyu WC, Smith RA, Greene DS: The effects of age and gender on the pharmacokinetics of irbesartan. Br J Clin Pharmacol 1998;46:611-613.

24. Kaye DM, Lefkovits J, Jennings GL, et al: Adverse consequences of high sympathetic nervous activity in the failing human heart. J Am Coll Cardiol 1995;26:1257-1263.

25. Bristow MR: Mechanism of action of beta-blocking agents in heart failure. Am J Cardiol 1997;80:26L-40L.

26. Ross RD, Daniels SR, Schwartz DC, et al: Plasma norepinephrine levels in infants and children with congestive heart failure. Am J Cardiol 1987;59:911-914.

27. Shaddy R: Beta-adrenergic blockers in the treatment of pediatric heart failure. Prog Pediatr Cardiol 2000;12:113-118.

28. Patterson JH, Rodgers JE: Expanding role of beta-blockade in the management of chronic heart failure. Pharmacotherapy 2003;23: 451-459.

29. National Institutes of Health: National Institutes of Health Clinical Trials webpage. Available at: www.clinicaltrials.gov. Accessed April 30, 2004.

30. Garban HJ, Buga GM, Ignarro LJ: Estrogen receptor-mediated vascular responsiveness to nebivolol: A novel endothelium-related mechanism of therapeutic vasorelaxation. J Cardiovasc Pharmacol 2004;43:638-644.

31. Paulus WJ, Shah AM: NO and cardiac diastolic function. Cardiovasc Res 1999;43:595-606.

32. Brehm BR, Wolf SC, Bertsch D, et al: Effects of nebivolol on proliferation and apoptosis on human coronary artery smooth muscle and endothelial cells. Cardiovasc Res 2001;49:430-439.

33. Janssen PM, Zeitz O, Hasenfuss G: Transient and sustained impacts of hydroxy radicals on sarcoplasmic reticulum function: The protective effects of nebivolol. Eur J Pharmacol 1999;366:223-232.

34. McLay JS, Irvine N, McDevitt DG: Clinical pharmacology of nebivolol. Drug Invest 1991;3(Suppl 1):31-32.

35. Wisenbaugh T, Katz I, Davis J, et al: Long-term (3 month) effects of a new beta-blocker (nebivolol) on cardiac performance in dilated cardiomyopathy. J Am Coll Cardiol 1993;21:1094-1110.

36. Brehm BR, Wolf SC, Gorner S, et al: Effect of nebivolol on left ventricular function in patients with chronic heart failure: A pilot study. Eur J Heart Fail 2002;4(6):757-763.

37. Uhlir O, Dvorak I, Gregor P, et al: Nebivolol in the treatment of cardiac failure: A double-blind controlled clinical trial. J Card Fail 1997;3:271-276.

38. Nodari S, Meatra M, Dei Cas L: Beta-blocker treatment of patients with diastolic heart failure and arterial hypertension: A prospective, randomized, comparison of the long-term effects of atenolol vs. nebivolol. Eur J Heart Fail 2003;5:621-627.

39. Spieker LE, Noll G, Ruschitzka FT, Luscher TF: Endothelin receptor antagonists in congestive heart failure: A new therapeutic principle for the future? J Am Coll Cardiol 2001;37:1493-1505.

40. Ooi H, Colucci WS, Givertz MM: Endothelin mediates increased pulmonary vascular tone in patients with heart failure. Circulation 2002;106:1618-1621.

41. Givertz MM, Colucci WS, LeJemtel TH, et al: Acute endothelin A receptor blockade causes selective pulmonary vasodilation in patients with chronic heart failure. Circulation 2000;101:2922-2927.

42. Philipp S, Monti J, Pagel I, et al: Treatment with darusentan over 21 days improved cGMP generation in patients with chronic heart failure. Clin Sci 2002;103:2495-2535.

43. Luscher TF, Enseleit F, Pacher R, et al: Hemodynamic and neurohormonal effects of selective endothelin A (ETA) receptor blockade in chronic heart failure. Circulation 2002;106:2666-2672.

44. Speiker LE, Mitrovic V, Noll G, et al: Acute hemodynamic and neurohormonal effects of selective ETA receptor blockade in patients with congestive heart failure. J Am Coll Cardiol 2000;35: 1745-1752.

45. Berger R, Stanek B, Hulsmann M, et al: Effects of endothelin A receptor blockade on endothelin function in patients with chronic heart failure. Circulation 2001;103:981-986.

46. Sutsch G, Kiowski W, Yan XW, et al: Short-term oral endothelin-receptor antagonist therapy in conventionally treated patients with symptomatic severe chronic heart failure. Circulation 1998;98:2262-2268.

47. Sutsch G, Bertel O, Kiowski W: Acute and short-term effects of the nonpeptide endothelin-1 receptor antagonist bosentan in humans. Cardiovasc Drug Ther 1997;10:717-725.

48. Kiowski W, Sutsch G, Hunziker P, et al: Evidence for endothelin-1-mediated vasoconstriction in severe chronic heart failure. Lancet 1995;346:732-736.

49. Bosentan package insert. South San Francisco, Calif, Actelion Pharmaceuticals US Inc, 2003.

50. Schalcher C, Cotter G, Reisin L, et al: The dual endothelin receptor antagonist tezosentan acutely improves hemodynamic parameters in patients with advanced heart failure. Am Heart J 2001;142:340-349.

51. Torre-Amione G: A pilot safety trial of prolonged (48 hour) infusion of the dual endothelin receptor antagonist tezosentan in patients with advanced heart failure. Chest 2001;120:460-466.

52. Torre-Amione G, Young JB, Durand JB, et al: Hemodynamic effects of tezosentan, an intravenous dual endothelin receptor antagonist, in patients with Class III to Class IV congestive heart failure. Circulation 2001;103:973-980.

53. O'Conner CM, Gattis WA, Adams KF, et al: Tezosentan in patients with acute heart failure and acute coronary syndromes: Results of the Randomized Intravenous Tezosentan Study (RITZ-4). J Am Coll Cardiol 2003;41:1452-1457.

54. Kaluski E, Kobrin I, Zimlichman R, et al: RITZ-5: Randomized Intravenous TeZosentan (an endothelin A/B antagonist) for the treatment of pulmonary edema. J Am Coll Cardiol 2003;41:204-210.

55. Data on file: Bosentan use in pediatrics. South San Francisco, Calif, Actelion Pharmaceuticals, Inc., 2003.

56. Vernon MW, Heel RC, Brogden RN: Enoximone: A review of its pharmacological properties and therapeutic potential. Drugs 1991;42:997-1017.

57. Lowes BD, Higginbotham M, Petrovich L, et al: Low-dose enoximone improves exercise capacity in chronic heart failure. Enoximone Study Group. J Am Coll Cardiol 2000;36:501-508.

58. Friedel N, Teebken M, Lemme A, et al: Enoximone as pharmacologic "bridging" to heart transplantation. Z Kardiol 1991;80 (Suppl):27-33.

59. Shakar SF, Abraham WT, Gilbert EM, et al: Combined oral positive inotropic and beta-blocker therapy for treatment of refractory class IV heart failure. J Am Coll Cardiol 1998;31:1336-1340.

60. Metra M, Nodari S, D'Aloia A, et al: Beta-blocker therapy influences the hemodynamic response to inotropic agents in patients with heart failure. J Am Coll Cardiol 2002;40:1248-1258.

61. National Institutes of Health: National Institutes of Health Clinical Trials webpage. Available at: www.clinicaltrials.gov. Accessed February 21, 2004.

62. Hausdorf G, Friedel N, Berdjis F, et al: Enoximone in newborns with refractory low cardiac output states (LOS). Eur J Cardiothorac Surg 1992;6:311-317.

63. Hausdorf G: Experience with phosphodiesterase inhibitors in paediatric cardiac surgery. Eur J Anaesthesiol 1993;8(Suppl):25-30.

64. Schranz D, Bauer J, Wiemann J, et al: Treatment of low cardiac output syndrome after surgery of congenital heart defects: Value of enoximone. Z Kardiol 1994;83:83-89.

65. Hausdorf G, Loebe M: Treatment of low cardiac output syndrome in newborn infants and children. Z Kardiol 1994;83(Suppl 2): 91-100.

66. Cossilini M, Ferri F, Giupponi A, et al: Enoximone in the treatment of postoperative low cardiac output syndrome in pediatric heart surgery: Open study in tetralogy of Fallot. Minerva Anestesiol 1997;63:213-219.

67. Innes PA, Frazer RS, Booker PD, et al: Comparison of the hemodynamic effects of dobutamine with enoximone after open heart surgery in small children. Br J Anaesth 1994;72:77-81.

68. Bevilacqua S, Del Sarto P, Tommasini G, et al: Enoximone weaning from mechanical circulation support in pediatric patients. Minerva Anestesiol 1997;63:9-16.

69. Booker PD, Gibbons S, Stewart JI, et al: Enoximone pharmacokinetics in infants. Br J Anaesth 2000;85:205-210.

70. Delyani JA, Rocha R, Cook CS, et al: Eplerenone: A selective aldosterone receptor antagonist (SARA). Cardiovasc Drug Rev 2001;19:185-200.

71. Takeda T, Miyamori I, Yoneda T, et al: Production of aldosterone in isolated rat blood vessels. Hypertension 1995;25:170-173.

72. Takeda T, Miyamori I, Yoneda T, et al: Regulation of aldosterone synthase in human vascular endothelial cells by angiotensin II and adrenocorticotropin. J Clin Endocrinol Metab 1996;81: 2797-2800.

73. Ullian ME, Islam MM, Robinson CJ, et al: Resistance to mineralcorticoids in Wistar-Furth rats. Am J Physiol 1997;272(3 Pt 2):H1454-H1461.

74. Rocha R, Chander PN, Zuckerman A, et al: Role of aldosterone in renal vascular injury in stroke-prone hypertensive rats. Hypertension 1999;33(1 Pt 2):232-237.

75. Horiuchi M, Nishiyana H, Hama J, et al: Characterization of renal aldosterone receptors in genetically hypertensive rats. Am J Physiol 1993;264(2 Pt 2):F286-F291.

76. Quashning T, Ruschitzka F, Shaw S, et al: Aldosterone receptor antagonism normalizes vascular function in liquorice-induced hypertension. Hypertension 2001;37(2 Pt 2):801-805.

77. Rocha R, Stier CT, Kifor I, et al: Aldosterone: A mediator of myocardial necrosis and renal arteriopathy. Endocrinology 2000; 141:3871-3878.

78. Ward MR, Kanellakis P, Ramsey D, et al: Eplerenone suppresses constrictive remodeling and collagen accumulation after angioplasty in porcine coronary arteries. Circulation 2001;104:467-472.

79. Delyani JA, Robinson EL, Rudolph AE: Effect of a selective aldosterone receptor antagonist in myocardial infarction. Am J Physiol Heart Circ Physiol 2001;281:H647-H654.

80. Delyani JA, Myles K, Funder J: Eplerenone (SC 66110), a highly selective aldosterone antagonist (Abstract). Am J Hypertens 1998;11:94A.

81. Micromedex: Spironolactone—drug evaluation. Online healthcare series. Available at: URL:http://www.micromedex.com/products/ hcsonline/. Cited October 12, 2003.

82. Roniker B: Eplerenone, a selective antagonist of the aldosterone receptor (Abstract). Hypertension 1997;30:995.

83. Martin J, Krum H: Eplerenone (GD Searle & Co.). Curr Opin Invest Drugs 2001;12:521-524.

84. Pitt B, Roniker B: Eplerenone, a novel selective aldosterone receptor antagonist (SARA) dose finding study in patients with heart failure (Abstract). J Am Coll Cardiol 1999;33:S188A-S189A.

85. Pitt B, Reichek N, Metscher B, et al: Efficacy and safety of eplerenone, enalapril, and eplerenone/enalapril combination therapy in patients with left ventricular hypertrophy (Abstract). Am J Hypertens 2002;15(Pt 2):23A.

86. Pitt B, Reicheck N, Willnebrock R, et al: Effects of eplerenone, enalapril, and eplerenone/enalapril in patients with essential hypertension and left ventricular hypertrophy: The 4E-left ventricular hypertrophy study. Circulation 2003;108:1831-1838.

87. Pitt B, Remme W, Zannad F, et al, for the EPHESUS study group: Eplerenone, a selective aldosterone blocker, in patients with left ventricular dysfunction after myocardial infarction. N Engl J Med 2003;348:1309-1321.

88. Eplerenone Package insert. Kalamazoo, Mich, Pfizer Pharmaceuticals Group, October 2003.

89. Data on file: Use in pediatrics. Kalamazoo, Mich, Pfizer Pharmaceuticals Group, October 2003.

90. Haikala H, Linden I-B: Mechanisms of action of calcium-sensitizing drugs. J Cardiovasc Pharmacol 1995;26(Suppl 1):S10-S19.

91. Levijoki J, Piero P, Kaivola J, et al: Further evidence for the cardiac troponin C mediated calcium sensitization by levosimedan: Structure-response and binding analysis with analogs of levosimendan. J Mol Cell Cardiol 2000;32:479-491.

92. Tassani P, Schad H, Heimisch W, et al: Effect of the calcium sensitizer levosimendan on the performance of ischaemic myocardium in anaesthetized pigs. Cardiovasc Drugs Ther 2002;16:435-441.

93. Edes I, Kiss E, Kitada Y, et al: Effects of levosimendan, a cardiotonic agent targeted to troponin C, on cardiac function and on phosphorylation and Ca2+ sensitivity of cardiac myofibrils and sarcoplasmic reticulum in guinea pig heart. Circ Res 1995;77:107-113.

94. Sato S, Hassan Talukder M, Sugawara H, et al: Effects of levosimendan on myocardial contractility and Ca++ transients in aequorin-loaded right ventricular papillary muscles and indo-1-loaded single ventricular cardiomyocytes of the rabbit. J Mol Cell Cardiol 1998;30:1115-1128.

95. Virag L, Hala O, Marton A, et al: Cardiac electrophysiologic effects of levosimendan, a new calcium sensitizer. Gen Pharmacol 1996;27:551-556.

96. Kleerekoper Q, Putkey JA: Drug binding to cardiac troponin C. J Biol Chem 1999;274:23932-23939.

97. Zimmermann N, Boknik P, Gams E, et al: Calcium sensitization as a new principle of inotropic therapy in end-stage heart failure? Eur J Cardiothorac Surg 1998;14:70-75.

98. Hasenfuss G, Pieske B, Kretschmann B, et al: Effects of calcium sensitizers on intracellular calcium handling and myocardial energetics. J Cardiovasc Pharmacol 1995;26(Suppl 1):S45-S51.

99. Varro A, Papp JG: Classification of positive inotropic actions based on electrophysiologic characteristics: Where should calcium sensitizers be placed? J Cardiovasc Pharmacol 1995;26 (Suppl 1):S32-S44.

100. Takahashi R, Talukder MAH, Endoh M: Effects of OR-1896, and active metabolite of levosimendan, on contractile force and aequorin light transients in intact rabbit ventricular myocardium. J Cardiovasc Pharmacol 2000;36:118-125.

101. Takahashi R, Hassan Talukder M, Endoh M: Inotropic effects of OR-1896, an active metabolite of levosimendan, on canine ventricular myocardium. Eur J Pharm 2000;400:103-112.

102. Yokoshiki H, Katsube Y, Sunagawa M, Sperelakis N: Levosimendan, a novel Ca2+ sensitizer, activates the glibenclamide-sensitive K+ channel in rat arterial myocytes. Eur J Pharmacol 1997;333:249-259.

103. Kopustinskiene D, Pollesello P, Saris N: Levosimendan is a mitochondrial KATP channel opener. Eur J Pharmacol 2001;428:311-314.

104. Lepran I, Papp J: Effect of long-term oral pretreatment with levosimendan on cardiac arrhythmias during coronary artery occlusion in conscious rats. Eur J Pharmacol 2003;464:171-176.

105. Katsube Y, Hagiwara N, Kasanuki H, et al: Effects of levosimendan: A novel Ca2+ sensitizer, on ionic currents of human cardiac cells (Abstract). Eur Heart J 1999;20:610.

106. Antila S, Honkanen T, Lehtonen L, Neuvonen PJ: The CYP3A4 inhibitor intraconazole does not affect the pharmacokinetics of a new calcium-sensitizing drug levosimendan. Int J Clin Pharmacol Ther 1998;36:446-449.

107. Sundberg S, Lehtonen L: Haemodynamic interactions between the novel calcium sensitizer levosimendan and isosorbide-5-mononitrate in healthy subjects. Eur J Clin Pharmacol 2000; 55:793-799.

108. Antila S, Jarvinen A, Akkila J, et al: Studies on psychomotoric effects and pharmacokinetic drug interactions of the new calcium sensitizing drug levosimendan and ethanol. Arnzneimittelforschung 1997;47:816-820.

109. Antila S, Eha J, Heinpalu M, et al: Haemodynamic interactions of a new calcium sensitizing drug levosimendan and captopril. Eur J Clin Pharmacol 1996;49:451-458.

110. Antila S, Asko J, Honkanen T, Lehtonen L: Pharmacokinetic and pharmacodynamic interactions between the novel calcium sensitizer levosimendan and warfarin. Eur J Clin Pharmacol 2000; 56:705-710.

111. Lilleberg J, Antila S, Karlsson M, et al: Pharmacokinetics and pharmacodynamics of simendan, a novel calcium sensitizer, in healthy volunteers. Clin Pharmacol Ther 1994;56:554-563.

112. Antila S, Huuskonen H, Nevalainen T, et al: Site dependent bioavailability and metabolism of levosimendan in dogs. Eur J Pharm Sci 1999;9:85-91.

113. Valjakka-Koskela R, Hirvonen J, Monkkonen J, et al: Transdermal delivery of levosimendan. Eur J Pharm Sci 2000;11:343-350.

114. Kivikko M, Antila S, Eha J, et al: Pharmacodynamics and safety of a new calcium sensitizer, levosimendan, and its metabolites during an extended infusion in patients with severe heart failure. J Clin Pharmacol 2002;42:43-51.

115. Kivikko M, Antila S, Eha J, et al: Pharmacokinetics of levosimendan and its metabolites during and after a 24-hour continuous infusion in patients with severe heart failure. Int J Clin Pharmacol Ther 2002;40:465-471.

116. Kivikko M, Lehtonen L, Colucci W, et al: Sustained hemodynamic effects of intravenous levosimendan. Circulation 2003;107:81-86.

117. Lilleberg J, Nieminen S, Akkila J, et al: Effects of a new calcium sensitizer, levosimendan, on haemodynamics, coronary blood flow and myocardial substrate utilization early after coronary artery bypass grafting. Eur Heart J 1998;19:660-668.

118. Nijwahan N, Nicolosi A, Montgomery M, et al: Levosimendan enhances cardiac performance after cardiopulmonary bypass: A prospective, randomized placebo-controlled trial. J Cardiovasc Pharmacol 1999;34:219-228.

119. Ukkonen H, Saraste M, Akkila J, et al: Myocardial efficiency during levosimendan infusion in congestive heart failure. Clin Pharmacol Ther 2000;68:522-531.

120. Nieminen M, Akkila J, Hasenfuss G, et al: Hemodynamic and neurohormonal effects of continuous infusion of levosimendan in patients with congestive heart failure. J Am Coll Cardiol 2000;36:1903-1912.

121. Harjola V, Peuhkurinen K, Nieminen M, et al: Oral levosimendan improves cardiac function and hemodynamics in patients with severe congestive heart failure. Am J Cardiol 1999;83:4(I)-8(I).

122. Hosenpud J: Levosimendan, a novel myofilament calcium sensitizer, allows weaning of parenteral inotropic therapy in patients with severe congestive heart failure. Am J Cardiol 1999;83:9(I)-11(I).

123. Slawsky M, Colucci W, Gottlieb S, et al: Acute hemodynamic and clinical effects of levosimendan in patients with severe heart failure. Circulation 2000;102:2222-2227.

124. Moiseyev V, Poder P, Andrejevs N, et al: Safety and efficacy of a novel calcium sensitizer, levosimendan, in patients with left ventricular failure due to an acute myocardial infarction: A randomized, placebo-controlled, double-blind study (RUSSLAN). Eur Heart J 2002;23:1422-1432.

125. Follath F, Cleland JGF, Just H, et al: Efficacy and safety of intravenous levosimendan compared with dobutamine in severe low-output heart failure (the LIDO study): A randomized double-blind trial. Lancet 2002;360:196-202.

126. National Institutes of Health: National Institutes of Health Clinical Trials webpage. Available at: www.clinicaltrials.gov. Accessed April 30, 2004.

127. Matsumori A, Nunokawa Y, Sasayama S: Pimobendan inhibits the activation of the transcription factor NF-kappaB: A mechanism which explains its inhibition of cytokine production and inducible nitric oxide synthetase. Life Sci 2000;67:2513-2519.

128. Bohm M, Morano I, Pieske B, et al: Contribution of cAMP-phosphodiesterase inhibition and sensitization of the contractile proteins for calcium to the inotropic effect of pimobendan in the failing human myocardium. Circ Res 1991;68:689-701.

129. Nakatani M, Shirotani T, Kobayashi K, et al: Effects of low dose pimobendan in patients with cor pulmonale. J Cardiol 1999;34:79-83.

130. Shiga T, Wakaumi M, Yajima T, et al: Beta-blocker therapy combined with low-dose pimobendan in patients with idiopathic dilated cardiomyopathy and chronic obstructive heart disease: Report on two cases. Cardiovasc Drugs Ther 2002;16:259-263.

131. Sasaki T, Kubo T, Komamura K, et al: Effects of long-term treatment with pimobendan on neurohormonal factors in patients with non-ischemic chronic moderate heart failure. J Cardiol 1999;33:317-325.

132. Lubsen J, Just H, Hjalmarsson AC, et al: Effect of pimobendan on exercise capacity in patients with heart failure: Main results from the Pimobendan in Congestive Heart Failure (PICO) trial. Heart 1996;76:223-231.

133. Effects of pimobendan on adverse cardiac events and physical activities in patients with mild to moderate chronic heart failure: The Effects of Pimobendan on Chronic Heart Failure study (EPOCH study). Circ J 2002;66:149-157.

134. Brixius K, Reicke S, Reuter H, Schwinger R: Effects of the Ca2+ sensitizers EMD 57033 and CGP 48506 on myocardial contractility and Ca2+ transients in human ventricular and atrial myocardium. Z Kardiol 2002;91:312-318.

135. Satoh N, Sato T, Shimada M, et al: Lusitropic effect of MCC-135 is associated with improvement of sarcoplasmic reticulum function in ventricular muscles of rats with diabetic cardiomyopathy. J Pharmacol Exp Ther 2001;298:1161-1166.

136. Levine B, Kalman J, Mayer L, et al: Elevated circulating levels of tumor necrosis factor in severe chronic heart failure. N Engl J Med 1990;323:236-241.

137. Torre-Amione G, Kapadia S, Benedict C, et al: Proinflammatory cytokine levels in depressed left ventricular ejection fraction: A report from the Studies of Ventricular Dysfunction (SOLVD). J Am Coll Cardiol 1996;27:1201-1206.

138. Mou S, Haudek S, Lequier L, et al: Myocardial inflammatory activation in children with congenital heart disease. Crit Care Med 2002;30:827-832.

139. Wang P, Ba ZF, Chaudry IH: Administration of tumor necrosis factor alpha in vivo depresses endothelium-dependent relaxation. Am J Physiol 1994;266:H2535-H2541.

140. Deswal A, Bozkurt B, Seta Y, et al: Safety and efficacy of a soluble P75 tumor necrosis factor receptor (Enbrel, Entanercept) in patients with advanced heart failure. Circulation 1999;99:3224-3226.

141. Bozkurt B, Torre-Amione G, Warren M, et al: Results of targeted anti-tumor necrosis factor therapy with Etanercept (ENBREL) inpatients with advanced heart failure. Circulation 2001;103:1044-1047.

142. Fichtlscherer S, Rossig L, Breuer S, et al: Tumor necrosis factor antagonism with Etanercept improves systemic endothelial vasoreactivity in patients with advanced heart failure. Circulation 2001;104:3023-3025.

143. Etanercept (Enbrel): Data on file. Seattle, Wash, Amgen Corporation, 2002.

144. Etanercept (Enbrel) package insert. Seattle, Wash, Amgen Corporation, 2002.

145. Anker SD, Coats AJ. How to RECOVER from RENAISSANCE? The significance of the results of RECOVER, RENAISSANCE, RENEWAL and ATTACH. Int J Cardiol 2002;86:123-130.

146. Infliximab (Remicade) package insert. Malvern, Penn, Centocor, Inc, 2003.

147. Feldman AM, McTiernan C: Is there any future for tumor necrosis factor antagonists in chronic heart failure? Am J Cardiovasc Drugs 2004;4:11-19.

148. Edwards BS, Zimmerman RS, Schwab TR, et al: Atrial stretch, not pressure, is the prinicipal determinant controlling the release of atrial natriuretic factor. Circ Res 1988;62:191-195.

149. Seymour AA, Swerdel JN, Abboa-Offei B: Antihypertensive activity during inhibition of neutral endopeptidase and angiotensin converting enzyme. J Cardiovasc Pharmacol 1991;17:456-465.

150. Mcdowell G, Coutie W, Shaw C, et al: The effect of the neutral endopeptidase inhibitor drug, candoxatril, on circulating levels of two of the most potent vasoactive peptides. Br J Clin Pharmacol 1997;43:329-332.

151. Westheim AS, Bostrom P, Christensen CC, et al: Hemodynamic and neuroendocrine effects for candoxatril and frusemide in mild stable chronic heart failure. J Am Coll Cardiol 1999;34:1794-1801.

152. Northridge DB, Newby DE, Rooney E, et al: Comparison of the short-term effects of candoxatril, an orally active neutral endopeptidase inhibitor, and furosemide in the treatment of

patients with chronic heart failure. Am Heart J 1999;138:1149-1157.

153. Northridge DB, Currie PF, Newby DE, et al: Placebo-controlled comparison of candoxatril, an orally active neutral endopeptidase inhibitor, and captopril in patients with chronic heart failure. Eur J Heart Fail 1999;1:67-72.

154. Kahn JC, Patey M, Dubois-Rande JL, et al: Effect of sinorphan on plasma atrial natriuretic factor in congestive heart failure. Lancet 1990;335:118-119.

155. O'Conner CM, Gattis WA, Gheorghiade M, et al: A randomized trial of ecadotril versus placebo in patients with mild to moderate heart failure: The U.S. ecadotril pilot safety study. Am Heart J 1999;138:1140-1148.

156. Francis GS: Is there still a future for neutral endopeptidase inhibitors? Am Heart J 1999;138:1007-1008.

157. Rouleau JL, Pfeffer MA, Stewart DJ, et al: Comparison of vasopeptidase inhibitor, omapatrilat, and lisinopril on exercise tolerance and morbidity in patients with heart failure: IMPRESS randomized trial. Lancet 2000;356:615-620.

158. Segarra G, Medina P, Vila JM, et al: Increased contraction to noradrenaline by vasopressin in human renal arteries. J Hypertension 2002;20:1373-1379.

159. Tahara A, Saito M, Tsukada J, et al: Vasopressin increases vascular endothelial growth factor secretion from human vascular smooth muscle cells. Eur J Pharmacol 1999;368:89-94.

160. Yatsu T, Tomura Y, Tahara A, et al: Pharmacology of conivaptan hydrochloride (YM087), a novel vasopressin V1A/V2 receptor antagonist. Nippon Yakurigaku Zasshi 1999;114(Suppl 1):113P-117P.

161. Yatsu T, Tomura Y, Tahara A, et al: Cardiovascular and renal effects of conivaptan hydrochloride (YM087), a vasopressin V1A and V2 receptor antagonist, in dogs with pacing-induced congestive heart failure. Eur J Pharmacol 1999;376:239-246.

162. Yatsu, T, Kusayama T, Tomura Y, et al: Effect of conivaptan, a combined vasopressin V1A and V2 receptor antagonist, on vasopressin-induced cardiac and haemodynamic changes in anaesthetized dogs. Pharmacol Res 2002;46:375-381.

163. Wada K, Tahara A, Arai Y, et al: Effect of the vasopressin receptor antagonist conivaptan in rats with heart failure following myocardial infarction. Eur J Pharmacol 2002;450:169-177.

164. Tahara A, Tomura Y, Wada K, et al: Effect of YM087, a potent non-peptide vasopressin antagonist, on vasopressin-induced hyperplasia and hypertrophy of cultured smooth-muscle cells. J Cardiovasc Pharmacol 1997;30:759-766.

165. Tahara A, Saito M, Sugimoto T, et al: Pharmacological characterization of YM087, a potent, nonpeptide human vasopressin V_{1A} and V_2 receptor antagonist. Naunyn Schmeidebergs Arch Pharmacol 1998;357:63-69.

166. Tahara A, Tomura Y, Wada K, et al: Pharmacological a profile of YM087, a novel potent nonpeptide vasopressin V_{1A} and V_2 receptor antagonist, in vitro and in vivo. J Pharmacol Exp Ther 1997;282:301-308.

167. Burnier M, Fricker AF, Hayoz D, et al: Pharmacokinetic and pharmacodynamic effects of YM087, a combined V1/V2 vasopressin receptor antagonist in normal subjects. Eur J Clin Pharmacol 1999;55:633-637.

168. Tomura Y, Tahara A, Tsukada J, et al: Pharmacologic profile of orally administered YM087, a vasopressin antagonist, in conscious rats. Clin Exp Pharmacol Physiol 1999;26:399-403.

169. Yatsu T, Tomura Y, Tahara A, et al: Pharmacologic profile of YM087, a novel nonpeptide dual vasopressin V1A and V2 receptor antagonist, in dogs. Eur J Pharmacol 1997;321:225-230.

170. Tahara A, Tomura Y, Wada K, et al: Effect of YM087, a potent nonpeptide vasopressin antagonist, on vasopressin-induced protein synthesis in neonatal rat cardiomyocyte. Cardiovasc Res 1998;38:198-205.

171. Udleson JE, Smith WB, Hendrix GH, et al: Acute hemodynamic effects of conivaptan, a dual V1A and V2 vasopressin receptor antagonist, in patients with advanced heart failure. Circulation 2001;104:2417-2423.

172. Tsukada J, Tahara A, Tomura Y, et al: Effects of YM471, a non-peptide AVP V(1A) and V(2) receptor antagonist, on human AVP receptor subtypes expressed in CHO cells and oxytocin receptors in human uterine smooth muscle cells. Br J Pharmacol 2001;133:746-754.

173. Tsukada J, Tahara A, Tomura Y, et al: Effect of YM471, an orally active non-peptide arginine vasopressin receptor antagonist, on human vascular smooth muscle cells. J Hypertension 2002;20:1807-1814.

174. Tsukada J, Tahara A, Tomura Y, et al: Pharmacological characterization of YM471, a novel potent vasopressin V(1A) and V(2) receptor antagonist. Eur J Pharmacol 2002;446:129-138.

175. Loichot C, Cazaubon C, De Jong W, et al: Nitric oxide, but not vasopressin V2 receptor-mediated vasodilation, modulates vasopressin-induced renal vasoconstriction in rats. Naunyn Schmeidebergs Arch Pharmacol 2000;361:319-326.

176. Serradeil-Le Gal C, Wagnon J, Garcia C, et al: Biochemical and pharmacological properties of SR 49059, a new, potent, nonpeptide antagonist of rat and human vasopressin V1a receptors. J Clin Invest 1993;92:224-231.

177. Heinemann A, Horina G, Stauber RE, et al: Lack of effect of a selective vasopressin V1a receptor anatagonist SR 49059, on potentiation by vasopressin of adrenoceptor-mediated pressor responses in the rat mesenteric arterial bed. Br J Pharmacol 1998;125:1120-1127.

178. Serradeil-Le Gal C, Villanova G, Boutin M, et al: Effects of SR 49059, a non-peptide antagonist of vasopressin-induced coronary vasoconstriction in conscious rabbits. Fundam Clin Pharmacol 1995;9:17-24.

179. Van Kerckhoven R, Lankhuizen I, van Veghel R, et al: Chronic vasopressin V(1a) but not V(2) receptor antagonism prevents heart failure in chronically infarcted rats. Eur J Pharmacol 2002;449:135-141.

180. Serradeil Le-Gal C, Bourrie B, Raufaste D, et al: Effect of a new, potent, non-peptide V1a vasopressin antagonist, SR 49059, on the binding and mitogenic activity of vasopressin on Swiss 3T3 cells. Biochem Pharmacol 1994;47:633-641.

181. Serradeil Le-Gal C, Herbert JM, Delisse C, et al: Effect of SR-49059, a vasopressin V1a antagonist, on human vascular smooth muscle cells. Am J Physiol 1995;268(1 Pt 2):H404-H410.

182. Kostrzewska A, Laudanski T, Steinwall M, et al: Effects of the vasopressin V1a receptor antagonist, SR 49059, on the response of human uterine arteries to vasopressin and other vasoactive substances. Acta Obstet Gynecol Scand 1998;77:3-7.

183. Weber R, Pechere-Bertschi A, Hayoz D, et al: Effects of SR 49059, a new orally active and specific vasopressin V1 receptor antagonist, on vasopressin-induced vasoconstriction in humans. Hypertension 1997;30:1121-1127.

184. Liu JJ, Chen JR, Buxton BB, et al: Potent inhibitory effect of SR 49059, an orally active non-peptide vasopressin Via receptor antagonist, on human arterial coronary bypass graft. Clin Sci (Lond) 1995;89:481-485.

185. Brouard R, Laporte V, Serradeil-Le Gal C, et al: Safety, tolerability, and pharmacokinetics of SR 49059, a V1a vasopressin receptor antagonist, after repeated oral administration in healthy volunteers. Adv Exp Med Biol 1998;449:455-465.

186. Thibonnier M, Kilani A, Rahmann M, et al: Effects of the non-peptide V1 vasopressin receptor antagonist SR49059 in hypertensive patients. Hypertension 1999;341:293-1300.

187. Gheorghiade M, Niazi I, Ouyang J: Vasopressin V2-receptor blockade with tolvaptan in patients with chronic heart failure: Results from a double-blind, randomized trial. Circulation 2003;107:2690-2696.

188. Gheorghiade M, Gattis WA, Barbagelata A: Rationale and study design for a multicenter, randomized, double-blind, placebo-controlled study of the effects of tolvaptan on the acute and

chronic outcomes of patients hospitalized with worsening congestive heart failure. Am Heart J 2003;145(2 Suppl):S51-S54.

189. Materson BJ, Reda DJ, Cushman WC: Department of Veteran's Affairs single drug therapy of hypertension study: Revised figures and new data. Department of Veteran's Affairs Cooperative Study Group on Antihypertensive agents. Am J Hypertens 1995;8: 189-192.

190. Carson P, Ziesche S, Johnson G, et al: Racial differences in response to therapy for heart failure: Analysis of the vasodilator heart failure trials. Vasodilator-Heart Failure Trial Study group. J Card Fail 1999;5:178-187.

191. Exner DV, Dries DL, Domanski MJ, et al: Lesser response to angiotensin-converting enzyme inhibitor therapy in black as compared with white patients with left ventricular dysfunction. N Engl J Med 2001;344:1351-1357.

192. Dieaguez-Lucena JL, Aranda-Lara P, Ruiz-Galdon M, et al: Angiotensin I-converting enzyme genotypes and angiotensin II receptors: Response to therapy. Hypertension 1996;28:98-103.

193. Danser AH, Schalekamp MA, Bax WA, et al: Angiotensin converting enzyme in the human heart: Effect of the deletion/insertion polymorphism. Circulation 1995;92:1387-1388.

194. Winkelman BR, Russ AP, Nauck M, et al: Angiotensin M235T polymorphism is associated with plasma angiotensinogen and cardiovascular disease. Am Heart J 1999;137:698-705.

195. Van Geel PP, Pinto YM, Voors AA, et al: Angiotensin II type 1 receptor A1166C gene polymorphism is associated with an increased response to angiotensin II in human arteries. Hypertension 2000;35:717-721.

196. Sasaki M, Oki T, Iuchi A, et al: Relationship between the angiotensin converting enzyme gene polymorphism and the effects of enalapril on left ventricular hypertrophy and impaired diastolic filling in essential: M-mode hypertension and pulsed Doppler echocardiographic studies. J Hypertens 1996;14: 1403-1408.

197. Takahashi T, Yamaguchi E, Furuya K, et al: The ACE gene polymorphism and cough threshold for capsaicin after cilazapril usage. Respir Med 2001;95:130-135.

198. McNamara DM, Holubkov R, Janosko K, et al: Pharmacogenetic interactions between beta-blocker therapy and the angiotensin converting enzyme deletion polymorphism in patients with congestive heart failure. Circulation 2001;103:1644-1648.

199. Marez D, Legrand M, Sabbagh N, et al: Polymorphism of the cytochrome P450 CYP2D6 gene in a European population: Characterization of 48 mutations and 53 alleles, their frequencies and evolution. Pharmacogenetics 1997;7:193-202.

200. Cascorbi I, Gerloff T, Johne A, et al: Frequency of single nucleotide polymorphisms in the P-glycoprotein drug transporter MDR1 gene in white subjects. Clin Pharmacol Ther 2001;69:169-174.

201. Kearns GL: Pharmacogenetics and development: Are infants and children at increased risk for adverse outcomes? Curr Opin Pediatr 1995;7:220-233.

202. Leeder JS, Kearns GL: Pharmacogenetics in pediatrics: Implications for practice. Pediatr Clin North Am 1997;44:55-77.

203. Jain KK: Role of pharmacoproteomics in the development of personalized medicine. Pharmacogenomics 2004;5:331-336.

204. Muszkat M, Stein CM: Pharmacogenetics and response to beta-adrenergic receptor antagonists in heart failure. Clin Pharmacol Ther 2005;77:123-126.

CHAPTER 39

Cardiac Resynchronization Therapy and Heart Failure

Gaurav Arora
Richard Friedman

Cardiac pacing was first developed as a tool to treat patients with bradyarrhythmias. With advances in pacing, it became clear that pacing not only could maintain a baseline heart rate, but also could affect the hemodynamic profile. With this revelation came attempts to augment cardiac output with the use of pacing in patients with severe heart failure. Initial attempts focused on dual-chamber pacing using the right atrium and right ventricle. Ultimately, this approach was found to be inconsistent in increasing cardiac output in patients with heart failure.

In 1994, the first report of biventricular pacing appeared. Subsequently, there have been numerous reports of biventricular and left ventricular pacing resulting in improved hemodynamic profiles, specifically in regard to increasing cardiac output in patients with depressed systolic function who did not have the traditional bradycardia indication for pacing. These approaches more recently have evolved into the concept now commonly referred to as cardiac resynchronization therapy (CRT), a pacing therapy that attempts to re-establish the synchronous contraction between the left ventricular free wall and the interventricular septum so that left ventricular efficiency is maximized (Fig. 39-1). In 2001, the first resynchronization device became available in the United States, and in the year that followed, devices that combine biventricular pacing capability with implantable cardioverter defibrillators were approved for use.

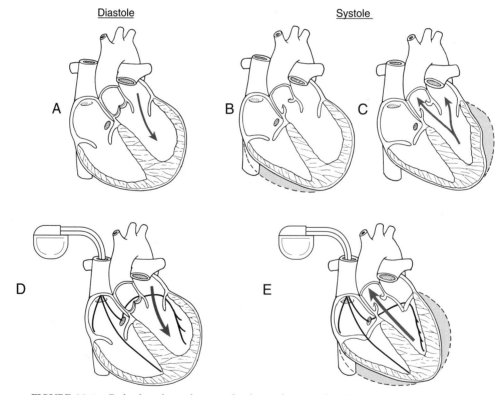

FIGURE 39-1 ■ **Pathophysiology of ventricular dyssynchrony and mechanisms of action for cardiac resynchronization therapy (CRT).** Heart failure. **A,** Atrioventricular dyssynchrony results in extended isovolumic contraction time and reduction in diastolic filling time. Contribution of atrial systole also is suboptimal. **B,** Interventricular and intraventricular dyssynchrony results in earlier activation of the right ventricle and septum compared with the left ventricular free wall and prestretch of the left ventricular free wall. There is disorganization of the ventricular contraction, decrease of pumping efficiency, and abnormal local wall strain and wall motion. **C,** Delayed contraction of the left ventricular free wall results in reduced diastolic filling time, inefficient contraction, and mitral regurgitation, all of which lead to diminished stroke volume. CRT. **D,** CRT increases diastolic filling time via optimization of the time delay between atrial sensed and ventricular pacing events. **E,** CRT to resynchronize interventricular and intraventricular contraction reduces mitral regurgitation and increases stroke volume.

RATIONALE FOR CARDIAC RESYNCHRONIZATION THERAPY

Pacing Site

Despite advances in medical therapy, patients with severe congestive heart failure (CHF) resulting from ischemic and nonischemic cardiomyopathy continue to have high morbidity and mortality. Adult patients with advanced CHF often have evidence of conduction delay on the ECG, most often left bundle-branch block (LBBB). With increasing QRS duration, mortality increases.[1] Significant interventricular conduction delay results in uneven activation of the ventricular myocardium, with regions of early and late activation. Dyskinetic activation of the ventricle increases ventricular wall stress, decreases pressure measured over time (dP/dt), increases left ventricular end-diastolic pressure, and impairs systolic function. In addition, there is dyssynchrony between the right and left ventricles and septal dyskinesis.[2]

In the early 1990s, several studies proposed the use of right-sided dual-chamber pacing to augment cardiac output.[3] Traditional dual-chamber pacing (DDD) and atrial sensing, ventricular pacing (VDD) with short atrioventricular (AV) delays were attempted. Despite initial enthusiasm, subsequent studies were unable to show reliably an improvement in ventricular function.[4] Other investigators proposed that pacing the right ventricular outflow tract rather than the traditional location in the right ventricular apex would improve cardiac output. The theory was that the more normal superoinferior activation sequence would approximate the normal activation sequence seen in sinus rhythm. Randomized studies to address this theory failed to show any substantial, reproducible benefits in ejection fraction, cardiac output, or symptoms.[5]

In the initial report of biventricular pacing, the patient was a 54-year-old man with New York Heart Association (NYHA) class IV heart failure and significant conduction disturbances. Standard transvenous leads were placed in the right atrium and right ventricle. A transvenous lead placed in the coronary sinus (CS) was used to pace the left atrium, and an epicardial lead was placed to stimulate the left ventricle. After 6 weeks of pacing, the patient showed marked improvement in clinical status, with a weight loss of 17 kg as a result of disappearance of peripheral edema and improvement to NYHA class II.[6]

Subsequent attempts have focused on biventricular and left ventricular stimulation in an attempt to increase cardiac output. Initially, left ventricular pacing was accomplished with the use of traditional transvenous right atrial and right ventricular leads and an epicardial left ventricular lead implanted via thoracotomy. Another option is to perform a transseptal procedure for endocardial placement of the left ventricular lead, but this technique introduces a significant risk of thromboembolic events. Subsequent successful design efforts were concentrated on the development of transvenous leads that could be placed into the CS and lodged in a distal cardiac vein, allowing pacing of the left ventricular free wall. Currently, most CRT is accomplished via the transvenous route with a CS left ventricular lead, obviating the need for general anesthesia or a thoracotomy.

CRT has several proposed mechanisms of benefit, including increased left ventricular filling time (longer diastolic filling interval), reduced mitral regurgitation, and decreased septal dyskinesis (improved ventricular synchrony).[2] In addition, numerous studies have shown the significant benefits of CRT, in terms of hemodynamics (ejection fraction, cardiac output, and blood pressure) and symptoms (quality-of-life scores, NYHA class, and exercise tolerance [frequently measured in the 6-minute walk test]). These benefits are independent of whether the left ventricular lead is placed via an epicardial or a transvenous approach. Largely as a result of these studies, biventricular pacing devices were approved by the U.S. Food and Drug Administration in 2001.[7]

Lead Placement

As mentioned previously, with the first biventricular devices, the left ventricular lead was placed via an epicardial approach through a limited thoracotomy. This approach is usually successful in establishing a well-functioning left ventricular lead, but there are added morbidity and mortality concerns with the procedure. In addition, there are concerns about post-thoracotomy pain.[8] Also, avoidance of the use of general anesthesia in patients with severe CHF would be beneficial.

Later, specially developed transvenous leads were made available for implantation via the CS (Figs. 39-2 and 39-3). The technique has been facilitated with the development of a steerable sheath that is placed in the CS with the assistance of a guidewire. Often, angiography of the coronary venous system is performed to obtain a visual "roadmap." The lead is implanted over the guidewire, with the goal of inserting it as distally as possible, avoiding diaphragmatic stimulation. The transvenous approach has the advantage of a limited surgical procedure, but requires technical expertise with a certain learning curve required to master the procedure. Studies have reported a 3.6% to 13% incidence of failure to place a transvenous CS lead successfully,[9-11] with a complication rate (including need for lead repositioning) of 3.9% to 9.3%.[10-13]

Another transvenous approach involves performing a transseptal procedure and placing the left ventricular lead endocardially. One series reported improved left ventricular shortening fraction and left ventricular tissue Doppler imaging (TDI) with the left ventricular endocardial approach as opposed to the traditional epicardial CS approach. With the placement of a left ventricular endocardial lead, anticoagulation is necessary to prevent a cerebrovascular accident. The endocardial approach is reserved for patients in whom a standard transvenous

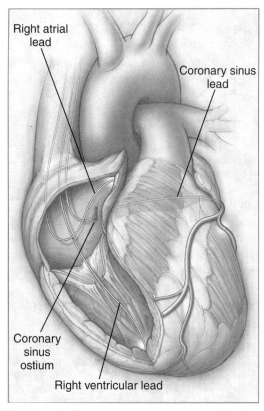

FIGURE 39-2 ■ Cardiac resynchronization therapy with leads in place.
The three leads of cardiac resynchronization therapy are seen in the
right atrium, right ventricle, and coronary sinus (to function as the left
ventricle pacing lead). (See also Color Section) (Courtesy of Guidant,
Indianapolis, IN.)

CS lead could not be placed.[14] Complications of this
procedure include complete heart block; CS dissection
or perforation; need to replace, reposition, or remove
pacing leads; and death.

The specific location of where on the left ventricular
surface the lead should be positioned has been studied.
Ansalone and colleagues[15] evaluated 31 patients who
were undergoing biventricular pacing using the standard
transvenous CS approach. Before pacing, TDI was used
to measure conduction delay in the interventricular
septum and inferior, posterior, lateral, and anterior walls
of the left ventricle before the procedure. Hemodynamics
were measured at baseline and after implantation. One
day after implantation, all patients showed improvements
in left ventricular ejection fraction (LVEF), NYHA class,
and left ventricular end-diastolic volume (LVEDV). The
subset of patients whose lead placement was at the most
delayed site of ventricular activation by TDI showed the
greatest degree of hemodynamic improvement at the time
of follow-up measurement.[15] Butter and associates[16]
compared pacing the left ventricular free wall with
pacing the left ventricular anterior wall. Each patient
underwent temporary pacing at both locations and had
aortic pulse pressure and left ventricular dP/dt measured
using pressure-tipped catheters. All patients in biventricular and left ventricular pacing arms showed improvements
in pulse pressure and left ventricular dP/dt. Pacing at
the left ventricular free wall was superior, however, to

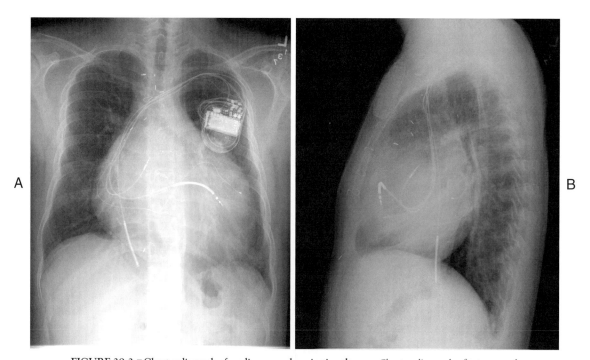

FIGURE 39-3 ■ Chest radiograph of cardiac resynchronization therapy. Chest radiograph of a teenaged
patient with complex congenital heart disease with left ventricular dysfunction and heart failure.
Posteroanterior (A) and lateral (B) radiographs show cardiomegaly with a biventricular pacing system
and an implantable cardioverter defibrillator. The three leads seen are positioned in the right atrium,
in the right ventricular apex, and along the coronary sinus and into the posterolateral coronary vein
(which serves as the left ventricle lead). An additional defibrillation coil is seen in the inferior vena cava.

pacing at the left ventricular anterior wall. In addition, in approximately one third of patients tested, pacing in the anterior wall worsened hemodynamics, whereas free wall pacing improved the measurements. The opposite situation never occurred. The study also assessed conduction delay, as measured by the difference between initial sensed atrial activity on the atrial pacing catheter compared with the site of ventricular activation. In 28 of 30 patients, intrinsic conduction delays were longer to the free wall.[16]

To maximize benefit from CRT, it seems prudent to assess the maximal site of conduction delay in the ventricle during sinus rhythm and to implant a lead that would pace from this site. Pacing may be via a transvenous CS or epicardial or endocardial left ventricular lead, all of which offer similar benefits. Baker and coworkers[12] showed that patients with existing dual-chamber right ventricular pacemakers feasibly could be upgraded to a biventricular system with a low rate of complications.

Timing of Pacing

In the initial studies of biventricular pacing, left ventricular stimulation and right ventricular stimulation were simultaneous. Eventually, devices were developed that could be programmed to provide a short delay between left ventricular activation and right ventricular activation. O'Cochlain and colleagues[17] reported the results of varying interventricular activation times on QRS duration. They studied 26 patients with severe CHF and LBBB who had biventricular devices implanted. The left ventricular-to-right ventricular activation time was varied by ± 50 msec and the QRS duration was measured on the surface ECG. These authors found that the narrowest QRS duration was found most often with a left ventricular-to-right ventricular delay of −30 msec (left ventricular preceding right ventricular). Overall, the narrowest QRS was found at −30 msec and −25 msec in most patients, although there were patients for whom the maximum QRS narrowing was derived at 0 to +30 msec. This finding suggested that each individual patient has an optimal interventricular (and presumably AV) delay.[17]

Sogaard and coworkers[18] used TDI with tissue tracking and three-dimensional echocardiography to evaluate LVEF in patients with biventricular pacing and varying intraventricular pacing delays. Patients ($n = 21$) with severe CHF, LBBB, and biventricular pacing were studied, and the results showed that sequential ventricular activation was superior to simultaneous pacing in terms of improved LVEF. In their study, the intraventricular activation times varied ± 20 msec. Approximately half of the patients improved with left ventricular preactivation, whereas the other half had maximal benefit with right ventricular preactivation. Sequential ventricular activation is often superior to simultaneous activation, and pacing delays should be individualized for maximal benefit.[18]

Initial studies proposed that AV synchrony and optimization of AV times were the primary mechanisms responsible for improvement with CRT. Although optimization of AV delay and improved left ventricular filling may be partially responsible for hemodynamic improvement, data suggest that intraventricular synchrony is more likely to be the major mechanism responsible. Leon and associates[19] studied 20 patients with severe CHF, LBBB, and atrial fibrillation with biventricular pacing. The patients showed significant improvements in LVEF, NYHA class, quality-of-life score, left ventricular end-diastolic dimension, and QRS duration and decreased hospitalizations. Because these patients did not have AV synchrony, the results suggest that the primary mode of improvement with biventricular pacing is ventricular resynchronization.[19] In short, CRT is based on correction of conduction disturbances that are associated with heart failure, which include delayed ventricular activation and ventricular dyssynchrony.

BENEFITS OF CARDIAC RESYNCHRONIZATION THERAPY IN HEART FAILURE

After initial case reports showed short-term benefit of biventricular pacing, several large trials were completed to evaluate the safety, efficacy, and long-term effects of CRT (Table 39-1 and Fig. 39-4). For most clinical trials, enrollment criteria included patients with moderate-to-severe CHF (NYHA class III or IV) regardless of cause (ischemic or nonischemic), LVEF of less than 35%, and evidence of conduction delay (QRS duration >130 msec). Patients had stable medical regimens and had no recent cardiovascular events (myocardial infarction or cerebrovascular accident). The target patient was one with severe CHF on maximal medical therapy, with evidence of conduction delay and no significant recent changes in medical regimen or clinical status.

In most studies, patients served as their own controls, with crossover designs used to test the effects of pacing. Generally, biventricular pacing was compared with no pacing, although several studies also included separate right ventricular pacing arms, left ventricular pacing arms, or both. Numerous end points were used to measure improvement, including quality-of-life score, NYHA class, exercise tolerance (measured by 6-minute walk distance), number of hospital admissions, LVEF, cardiac output, dP/dt, pulmonary capillary wedge pressure, degree of mitral regurgitation, left ventricular end-diastolic dimension, LVEDV, and QRS duration.

Quality of Life

The Minnesota Living with Heart Failure questionnaire was used in several trials to assess patients' quality of life. CRT showed consistent improvements in patients' quality of life scores in all instances where it was measured,

TABLE 39-1

Summary of Cardiac Resynchronization Therapy Trials

Study	Design	Patients	Results
COMPANION[30]	Multicenter, prospective, randomized, controlled	1600 patients (terminated early) with DCM, NYHA classes III/IV, IVCD with 3 arms: drug therapy only, drug + CRT, drug + CRT/ICD	Combined all-cause mortality and hospitalizations decreased 20% in device arms; 40% reduction in total mortality with combined CRT/ICD
PATH-CHF[8]	Single-blinded, randomized, crossover, controlled	42 patients with DCM, NYHA classes III/IV, IVCD	Improved exercise tolerance (6-min walk), QOL, and NYHA class
MIRACLE[9]	Prospective, randomized, double-blinded, parallel, controlled	453 patients with DCM, NYHA classes III/IV, IVCD	Improved exercise capacity, NYHA class, QOL, LVEF, and LVEDD; decreased hospitalizations
MUSTIC[20]	Randomized, crossover	131 patients with DCM, NYHA class III, IVCD, with sinus rhythm and atrial fibrillation	Improved exercise capacity, NYHA class, and QOL; decreased hospitalizations. Improvement slightly less in atrial fibrillation group
InSync[10]	Prospective, multicenter	117 patients with DCM, NYHA classes III/IV, IVCD	Improved exercise capacity, QOL, NYHA class, QRS duration, LVEF, and LVEDD
Ventak CHF[29]	Prospective, blinded, randomized	32 patients with DCM, NYHA classes II/III/IV, IVCD with indications for ICD placement	Significant decrease in appropriate therapy for ventricular arrhythmias with CRT versus no CRT

CRT, cardiac resynchronization therapy; DCM, dilated cardiomyopathy; ICD, implantable cardioverter defibrillator; IVCD, intraventricular conduction delay; LVEDD, left ventricular end-diastolic dimension; LVEF, left ventricular ejection fraction; NYHA, New York Heart Association; QOL, quality of life.

from 12 weeks to 2 years after implantation.[8-11,13,19-21] Although quality of life is a subjective measure, the consistent improvement across large trials with CRT represents solid evidence for patient improvement.

New York Heart Association Class
Numerous studies have shown consistently an improvement in NYHA class with CRT. This benefit was observed

12 weeks after implantation through 2 years of follow-up.[8-11,13,19-22] In most trials, most patients improved by at least one NYHA class.

Exercise Tolerance
The 6-minute walk test commonly was used as a surrogate marker for overall exercise tolerance. In this test, patients are asked to use maximum effort to walk for

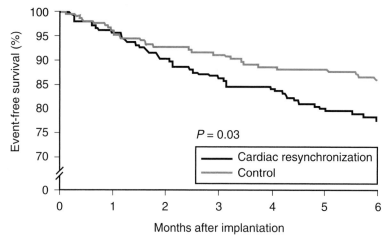

FIGURE 39-4 ■ Multicenter In Sync Randomized Clinical Evaluation (MIRACLE) Trial. The Kaplan-Meier estimates of the time to death or hospitalization for exacerbation of heart failure in the control and resynchronization groups in the MIRACLE trial. A total of 453 patients were enrolled. The trial showed that the risk of an event was 40% lower in the treated group. (From Abraham WT, Fisher WG, Smith AL, et al: *Cardiac resynchronization in chronic heart failure. N Engl J Med* 2002;346:1845-1853.)

6 minutes, and the distance traveled is measured. When measured 12 weeks to 2 years postimplantation, the 6-minute walk test was shown to improve significantly and consistently in patients receiving CRT.[8-11,13,20,21]

Hospitalizations

In all trials in which hospitalizations were assessed, the use of CRT consistently was associated with a decrease in number of hospital days or admission per patient 2 years after initiation of CRT.[9,13,19-21]

Left Ventricular Ejection Fraction

LVEF was consistently improved in patients receiving CRT, from early postimplantation to 2 years.[9-11,13,15,19,20,23] Critics of CRT have argued that most markers for improvement are subjective and may not be clinically significant (quality of life, NYHA class, 6-minute walk), but the consistent and significant improvement in LVEF would argue that patient improvement is real. In addition, the improvement in ejection fraction correlates with improved NYHA class, exercise tolerance, and decreased chamber size.

Chamber Size

In addition to improving function, there is continuing evidence that CRT results in reverse remodeling of the ventricle. Sogaard and colleagues[22] used three-dimensional echocardiography and TDI to measure left ventricular dimensions and function in 25 patients with biventricular pacing. They showed persistent improvement in LVEF over time and a decrease in LVEDV and left ventricular end-systolic volume. This study suggests that in addition to improved mechanical function, these patients had evidence of favorable reverse remodeling.[22] Ansalone and colleagues[15] confirmed similar benefits in patients with biventricular pacing and improved LVEDV and left ventricular end-systolic volume. At least one study showed that patients deemed to be non-responders to CRT had higher baseline LVEDVs, perhaps suggesting that there is a "point of no return" past which reverse remodeling may be unobtainable.[23] Other studies have shown consistent benefits of reducing left ventricular end-diastolic dimension with CRT.[9,10,19,23] Patients who respond to CRT show results similar to patients who have received other proven therapies for CHF, such as afterload reduction with angiotensin-converting enzyme inhibitors.

QRS Duration

Several studies have shown a benefit in terms of shortening QRS duration from immediately after implantation to 2 years postimplantation.[9,13,19] Although often used as a surrogate marker of success of resynchronization, narrowing of the QRS may not provide the entire benefit. Kass and coworkers[24] studied 18 patients with severe CHF and interventricular conduction delay. Left ventricular and biventricular pacing was found to be superior to right ventricular pacing alone with respect to measurement of dP/dt. Narrowing of QRS duration did not predict percent improvement in dP/dt, although baseline QRS duration did correlate with percent improvement. This finding suggests that the re-establishment of mechanical ventricular synchrony is necessary for CRT to be efficacious and that QRS narrowing alone is not a sufficient surrogate for hemodynamic improvement to be seen.[24]

In a canine model of CHF with LBBB, Leclercq and associates[25] compared biventricular pacing with left ventricular pacing, measuring chamber hemodynamics (dP/dt and aortic pulse pressure). Biventricular and left ventricular pacing improved hemodynamics, but only biventricular pacing improved electrical synchrony. Both modes of pacing had similar improvements in ejection fraction (23% at baseline compared with 28% with pacing), but left ventricular pacing increased electrical activation time (98 to 122 msec), whereas biventricular pacing shortened it (98 to 85 msec). Mechanical synchrony and electrical synchrony are not synonymous, and mechanical synchrony is the more critical of the two for hemodynamic improvement.[25] Extrapolation of this study would strengthen further the belief that QRS duration as a marker for improvement may not be adequate.

Decreased Sympathetic Activation

Sundell and associates[26] studied 10 patients with dilated cardiomyopathy and biventricular pacing. They performed echocardiography and positron emission tomography to evaluate LVEF and myocardial oxygen consumption with biventricular pacing and dobutamine infusion. They noted that CRT improved left ventricular function and myocardial efficiency (stroke volume) with no associated changes in myocardial perfusion or oxygen consumption. In addition, there was a significant increase in the serum brain natriuretic peptide level with CRT off versus activated. This study suggests that CRT improves myocardial function without the added expense (and risk) of increasing myocardial oxygen demand, in contrast to standard inotropic therapy, which does increase myocardial oxygen demand.[26]

Nelson and colleagues[27] measured arterial pulse pressure, which correlates with cardiac output and dP/dt as measures of systolic function and mixed venous oxygen saturation and arterial-CS oxygen difference as measures of myocardial oxygen consumption. These investigators showed improvements in the systolic parameters with biventricular or left ventricular pacing with decreased myocardial oxygen consumption. In contrast, with dobutamine, there were similar increases in systolic function, but a concomitant increase in myocardial oxygen consumption.[27]

Other studies also have shown a reduction in the average heart rate, which suggests decreased chronic sympathetic activation.[20] Hamdan and coworkers[28] used microneurography to measure sympathetic nerve activity, which was significantly decreased in patients with left ventricular pacing compared with pacing with right ventricular pacing, regardless of QRS duration. Increased myocardial oxygen demand may worsen supply-demand mismatch, which may provide the substrate for arrhythmias. Trials such as **Ventak-CHF** have shown the decreased need for the use of implantable cardioverter defibrillators in patients with biventricular pacing.[29] With CRT, there are decreased sympathetic activation and decreased myocardial oxygen consumption.

Mortality

Even in the largest single trials to date, it has been difficult to show a statistic difference in all-cause mortality between patients receiving standard therapy and patients receiving standard therapy and biventricular pacing. After considering the results of the **Comparison of Medical Therapy, Pacing, and Defibrillation in Chronic Heart Failure (COMPANION) trial**,[30] however, a meta-analysis analyzed the major studies for evidence of mortality benefit. With inclusion of the COMPANION data, there seems to be a significant reduction in all-cause mortality, with an odds ratio of 0.74 and a 95% confidence interval of 0.56 to 0.97. This study supports the notion that CRT not only improves patients' symptoms and hemodynamics, but also prolongs their lives.

CARDIAC RESYNCHRONIZATION THERAPY IN CHILDREN AND YOUNG ADULTS WITH CONGENITAL HEART DISEASE

To date, there is no large-scale randomized study in pediatric patients to evaluate the benefits of CRT. Several case reports and small case series have detailed the use of CRT in children and adults with congenital heart disease. Rodriguez-Cruz and colleagues[31] first reported the use of CRT in a 22-year-old man with congenitally corrected transposition of the great arteries, pulmonary atresia, and ventricular septal defect. He underwent a palliative shunt in the first weeks of life followed by placement of a right ventricle–to–pulmonary artery conduit at approximately 4 years of age. He also underwent placement of an epicardial pacemaker caused by surgical AV block. At age 22 years, he presented with symptoms of CHF and was found to have severe biventricular systolic dysfunction. Exercise testing showed his workload to be 64 W with an oxygen consumption of 19.6 mL/kg/min. His fractional area of change by echocardiography was 8%, and his left ventricular end-diastolic pressure measured at catheterization was 22 mm Hg. After optimization of his medical regimen, the patient underwent placement of a biventricular pacing system with a transvenous CS lead. One month after implantation, he was found to have marked

hemodynamic improvement. His workload increased 45% to 93 W, and his oxygen consumption improved by 17% to 23 mL/kg/min. His fractional area of change had increased 125% to 18%, and his left ventricular end-diastolic pressure decreased by 27% to 16 mm Hg.[31]

Blom and colleagues[32] reported the case of a 6-year-old boy with an initial diagnosis of multiple ventricular septal defects and severe mitral regurgitation. The patient underwent placement of a pulmonary artery band in the first year of life. At age 2 years, he had corrective surgery that involved takedown of the pulmonary artery band, closure of the ventricular septal defects, and mitral valve replacement. Six months later, he underwent repeat operation for closure of a residual ventricular septal defect via left ventriculotomy. After the last procedure, he had significant ventricular dysfunction that was attributed to inherent myocardial abnormalities and early age at mitral valve replacement and left ventriculotomy. The patient's LVEF was 27%. He also was noted to have failure to thrive, frequent hospital admissions for pulmonary infections, and reduced exercise tolerance. He had evidence of conduction delay, with first-degree AV block (PR interval 170 msec) and LBBB (QRS duration 160 msec). TDI was used to show intraventricular dyssynchrony by measuring the difference between the peak systolic velocities in the interventricular septum and the left ventricular lateral wall (at baseline the delay was 80 msec). He underwent implantation of a transvenous biventricular pacemaker. TDI after implantation revealed that ventricular synchrony had improved markedly with a septal-to-lateral delay of only 10 msec. After 1 year, the LVEF had improved to 38%, he had not been hospitalized for pulmonary infections, and he showed improved exercise tolerance.[32]

Roofthooft and associates[33] reported the use of epicardial biventricular pacing in a female infant with congenital heart disease. The underlying diagnosis was coarctation of the aorta with hypoplastic transverse aortic arch, subvalvar aortic stenosis, and large ventricular septal defect. She underwent aortic arch repair, resection of subvalvar aortic stenosis, and closure of the ventricular septal defect as a neonate. Postoperatively, she developed complete AV block, and a standard epicardial dual-chamber pacing system was implanted. She presented 3 weeks later with biventricular dysfunction. Cardiac catheterization revealed mild subaortic stenosis with a moderate recoarctation. She underwent balloon dilation of the coarctation with good hemodynamic result, but had no improvement in left ventricular function, with a LVEF of 25%. The ECG showed a PR interval of 100 msec and a QRS duration of 100 msec with a LBBB pattern. M-mode echocardiography was used to quantify the delay between septal motion and motion of the left ventricular posterior wall, which was 110 msec. The patient underwent placement of a left ventricular epicardial lead and change in her generator to a biventricular pacemaker. Six months later, measurement of the LVEF was 44%, and she had improved ventricular synchrony, with a septal-to-posterior wall delay of 55 msec.[33]

Janousek and colleagues[34] published the first case series of the use of CRT in pediatric patients. They studied the acute effects of epicardial CRT in 20 patients after congenital heart disease surgery. The requirements were evidence of AV or intraventricular conduction delay and need for inotropic support. The investigators used temporary epicardial pacing wires on the right atrium, right ventricle, and left ventricle. Resynchronization (AV or intraventricular or both) resulted in improved arterial systolic, mean, and pulse pressures. This result correlated well with initial QRS duration and degree of QRS shortening. Janousek and colleagues[34] proposed that temporary epicardial CRT could be used as an adjunct in the immediate postoperative period in patients with congenital heart disease.

Zimmerman and associates[35] studied 29 postoperative congenital heart disease patients using epicardial CRT, with temporary pacing leads placed at surgery. The patient population consisted of patients with single-ventricle and biventricular anatomy. They showed a significant increase in systolic blood pressure and cardiac index and shortening of the QRS duration in all patients. In their study, CRT facilitated weaning from cardiopulmonary bypass in two patients. Zimmerman and associates[35] also proposed that epicardial CRT could be used as an adjunct postoperative therapy.

Dubin and associates[36] studied seven patients with failing right ventricles and right ventricular conduction delay (right bundle-branch block [RBBB]) in an acute hemodynamic study. Patients who were to have clinically-indicated cardiac catheterizations performed underwent placement of pacing catheters in the right atrium and various sites in the right ventricle. A pressure-tip catheter was used to measure intraventricular pressures. Pacing was tested in three separate right ventricular sites: apex, outflow tract, and septum. AV pacing showed an improvement in cardiac index and narrowing of the QRS duration (Fig. 39-5). The site that produced the narrowest QRS duration was associated with the greatest increase in cardiac index in six of the seven patients. Although this study involved a small number of patients, it suggests that RV synchronization may be feasible in patients with congenital heart disease.

OTHER CONSIDERATIONS WITH CARDIAC RESYNCHRONIZATION THERAPY

Cost Implications

Although CRT has been shown to be clinically beneficial, the cost implications preclude widespread use at this time. In contrast to pharmacologic therapy, which is more readily available and cost-efficient, CRT requires a center of expertise and substantial cost. Currently in the United States, device costs alone range from $25,000 to $40,000, with total per-patient charges of $100,000 in some cases.[7] CRT has shown benefit in reducing hospitalizations per patient, which would reduce the cost of heart failure therapy.[20] From a cost perspective, the

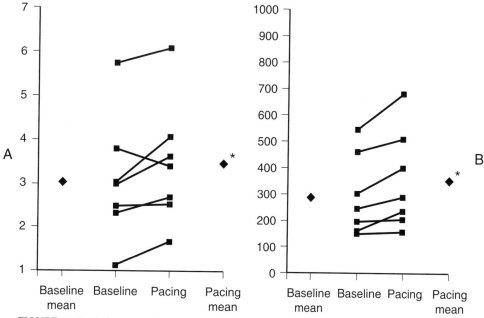

FIGURE 39-5 ■ **Right ventricular (RV) resynchronization.** Changes in cardiac index (CI) in L/min/m² **(A)** and RV pressure measured over time (dP/dt) in mm Hg/sec **(B)** are plotted at baseline and with resynchronization. The individual subjects are plotted with boxes, and the mean is plotted diamonds. CI and RV dP/dt increased with RV synchronization. (From Dubin AM, Feinstein JA, Reddy VM, et al: *Electrical resynchronization: A novel therapy for the failing right ventricle. Circulation* 2003;107:2287-2289.)

benefit of reduced hospitalizations would have to be weighed against the cost of implantation of devices. To date, a good economic analysis comparing the impact of CRT with the cost of heart failure therapy overall has not been published.

Left Ventricular Pacing

Most studies performed compared standard therapy with biventricular pacing versus standard medical therapy alone. Numerous studies included an arm with left ventricular pacing alone, however. In all studies performed, left ventricular pacing alone compared favorably with biventricular pacing and was shown consistently to be superior to right ventricular pacing alone or no pacing in all parameters measured.[24,25,37-39] At this time, left ventricular pacing alone is not recommended as primary therapy, although if for any reason it is not feasible to place a simultaneous right ventricular lead, left ventricular pacing alone likely would provide ventricular resynchronization in patients with predominant left ventricular conduction delay.

Right Ventricular Resynchronization

Most data regarding CRT involve patients with severe CHF and conduction delay, most frequently LBBB. Pediatric patients and adults with congenital heart disease rarely have LBBB. Most commonly, they have underlying RBBB. Although there have been no large-scale trials with patients with predominantly RBBB, several smaller case series have suggested that they may benefit from CRT as well.

As elucidated earlier, Dubin and coworkers[36] showed efficacy of CRT in patients with congenital heart disease and RBBB in a small case series. In addition, Garrigue and colleagues[40] studied 12 adults with RBBB and biventricular pacing. In their study, 9 of 12 patients, with regard to NYHA class, left ventricular end-diastolic dimension, treadmill performance, and narrowed QRS duration, improved with biventricular pacing. The three patients who did not improve did not have evidence of concomitant left ventricular delay as measured by TDI of the right ventricular free wall and left ventricular septal wall. This study suggests that a subset of patients with RBBB is still eligible for CRT if TDI shows substantial left ventricular dyssynchrony.[40]

CURRENT STATUS AND FUTURE TRENDS

Patients with severe CHF often have associated conduction delay, but it is uncertain whether this is cause or effect. CRT, in the form of left ventricular or biventricular pacing, has been shown to be beneficial, improving patients' symptoms and hemodynamics. In adult studies, the maximum benefit was obtained with pacing from the site of maximal ventricular delay, regardless of whether the route of pacing was epicardial or endocardial.

In addition, left ventricular and biventricular pacing had similar benefits, although at this time most CRT is performed with biventricular pacing. The technology of CRT is still evolving, with improving catheter and lead designs to minimize morbidity and maximize successful implantation.

Noninvasive parameters, such as TDI, can be used to assist with measurement of ventricular delay and efficacy of resynchronization. There is evidence that discoordinately contracting myocardium can lead to regional molecular alterations in the myocyte.[41] Studies of long-term benefit and of economic cost analysis of CRT remain to be performed, however.

Although there are no large studies in children and young adults with congenital heart disease, there is preliminary evidence to suggest that selected patients with congenital heart disease may benefit from CRT, perhaps with right ventricular pacing or alternative site pacing. Children with dilated cardiomyopathy also may benefit from this mode of innovative pacing.[42] The heterogeneous nature of pediatric patients with congenital heart disease continually will pose a special challenge in assessing the short-term and long-term clinical efficacy of CRT.

Key Concepts

- CRT is a pacing therapy that attempts to re-establish the synchronous contraction between the left ventricular free wall and the interventricular septum so that the left ventricular efficiency is maximized.

- In 2001, the first resynchronization device became available in the United States, and in the year that followed, devices that combine biventricular pacing capability with implantable cardioverter defibrillators were approved for use.

- Adult patients with advanced CHF often have evidence of conduction delay on ECG, most often LBBB.

- Significant interventricular conduction delay results in uneven activation of the ventricular myocardium, with regions of early and late activation. Dyskinetic activation of the ventricle increases ventricular wall stress, decreases dP/dt, increases left ventricular end-diastolic pressure, and impairs systolic function. In addition, there is dyssynchrony between the right and left ventricles and septal dyskinesis.

- Currently, most CRT is accomplished via the transvenous route with a CS left ventricular lead, obviating the need for general anesthesia or a thoracotomy.

- CRT has several proposed mechanisms of benefit, including increased left ventricular filling time (longer diastolic filling interval), reduced mitral regurgitation, and decreased septal dyskinesis (improved ventricular synchrony).

- With the placement of a left ventricular endocardial lead, anticoagulation is necessary to prevent a cerebrovascular accident. The endocardial approach is reserved for patients in whom a standard transvenous CS lead could not be placed.

- To maximize benefit from CRT, it seems prudent to assess the maximal site of conduction delay in the ventricle during sinus rhythm and implant a lead that would pace from this site.
- Sequential ventricular activation is often superior to simultaneous activation, and pacing delays should be individualized for maximal benefit.
- Although optimization of AV delay and improved left ventricular filling may be partially responsible for hemodynamic improvement, data suggest that intraventricular synchrony is more likely to be the major mechanism responsible.
- Critics of CRT have argued that most markers for improvement are subjective and may not be clinically significant (quality of life, NYHA class, 6-minute walk), but the consistent and significant improvement in LVEF would argue that patient improvement is real. In addition, the improvement in ejection fraction correlates with improved NYHA class, exercise tolerance, and decreased chamber size.
- Although often used as a surrogate marker of success of resynchronization, narrowing of the QRS may not provide the entire benefit. Mechanical synchrony and electrical synchrony are not synonymous, and mechanical synchrony is the more critical of the two for hemodynamic improvement.
- With CRT, there is decreased sympathetic activation and decreased myocardial oxygen consumption.
- To date, a good economic analysis comparing the impact of CRT with the cost of heart failure therapy overall has not been published.
- Most data regarding CRT involve patients with severe CHF and conduction delay, most frequently LBBB. Children and adults with congenital heart disease rarely have LBBB.
- Although there are no large studies in children and young adults with congenital heart disease, there is preliminary evidence to suggest that selected patients with congenital heart disease may benefit from CRT, perhaps right ventricular pacing or alternative site pacing.
- The heterogeneous nature of pediatric patients with congenital heart disease will continually pose a special challenge in assessing the short-term and long-term clinical efficacy of CRT.

REFERENCES

1. Iuliano S, Fisher SG, Karasik PE, et al, Department of Veterans Affairs Survival Trial of Antiarrhythmic Therapy in Congestive Heart Failure: QRS duration and mortality in patients with congestive heart failure. Am Heart J 2002;143:1085-1091.
2. Gerber TC, Nishimura RA, Holmes DR Jr, et al: Left ventricular and biventricular pacing in congestive heart failure. Mayo Clin Proc 2001;76:803-812.
3. Hoechleitner M, Hortnagl H, Ng CK, et al: Usefulness of physiologic dual-chamber pacing in drug-resistant idiopathic dilated cardiomyopathy. Am J Cardiol 1990;66:198-202.
4. Gold MR, Feliciano Z, Gottlieb SS, Fisher ML: Dual-chamber pacing with a short atrioventricular delay in congestive heart failure: A randomized study. J Am Coll Cardiol 1995;26:967-973.
5. Victor F, Leclercq C, Philippe M, et al: Optimal right ventricular pacing site in chronically implanted patients. J Am Coll Cardiol 1999;33:311-316.
6. Cazeau S, Ritter P, Bakdach S, et al: Four chamber pacing in dilated cardiomyopathy. Pacing Clin Electrophysiol 1994;17:1974-1979.
7. Leclercq C, Hare JM: Ventricular resynchronization. Circulation 2004;109:296-299.
8. Auricchio A, Stellbrink C, Sack S, et al, Pacing Therapies in Congestive Heart Failure (PATH-CHF) Study Group: Long-term clinical effect of hemodynamically optimized cardiac resynchronization therapy in patients with heart failure and ventricular conduction delay. J Am Coll Cardiol 2002;39:2026-2033.
9. Abraham WT, Fisher WG, Smith AL, et al, MIRACLE Study Group: Cardiac resynchronization in chronic heart failure. N Engl J Med 2002;346:1845-1853.
10. Kuhlkamp V, InSync 7272 ICD World Wide Investigators: Initial experience with an implantable cardioverter-defibrillator incorporating cardiac resynchronization therapy. J Am Coll Cardiol 2002;39:790-797.
11. Reuter S, Garrigue S, Barold SS, et al: Comparison of characteristics in responders versus nonresponders with biventricular pacing for drug-resistant congestive heart failure. Am J Cardiol 2002;89:346-350.
12. Baker CM, Christopher TJ, Smith PF, et al: Addition of a left ventricular lead to conventional pacing systems in patients with congestive heart failure. Pacing Clin Electrophysiol 2002;25:1166-1171.
13. Molhoek SG, Bax JJ, van Erven L, et al: Effectiveness of resynchronization therapy in patients with end-stage heart failure. Am J Cardiol 2002;90:379-383.
14. Garrigue S, Jais P, Espil G, et al: Comparison of chronic biventricular pacing between epicardial and endocardial left ventricular stimulation using Doppler tissue imaging in patients with heart failure. Am J Cardiol 2001;88:858-862.
15. Ansalone G, Giannantoni P, Riccci R, et al: Doppler myocardial imaging to evaluate the effectiveness of pacing sites in patients receiving biventricular pacing. J Am Coll Cardiol 2002;39:489-499.
16. Butter C, Auricchio A, Stellbrink C, et al, Pacing Therapy for Chronic Heart Failure (PATH-CHF-II) Study Group: Effect of resynchronization therapy stimulation site on the systolic function of heart failure patients. Circulation 2001;104:3026-3029.
17. O'Cochlain B, Delurgio D, Leon A, Langberg J:. The effect of variation in the interval between right and left ventricular activation on paced QRS duration. Pacing Clin Electrophysiol 2001;24:1780-1782.
18. Sogaard P, Egeblad H, Pedersen AK, et al: Sequential versus simultaneous biventricular resynchronization for severe heart failure. Circulation 2002;106:2078-2084.
19. Leon AR, Greenberg JM, Kanuru N, et al: Cardiac resynchronization in patients with congestive heart failure and chronic atrial fibrillation. J Am Coll Cardiol 2002;39:1258-1263.
20. Linde C, Leclercq C, Rex S, et al, Multisite Stimulation In Cardiomyopathies (MUSTIC) Study Group: Long-term benefits of biventricular pacing in congestive heart failure: Results from the Multisite Stimulation In Cardiomyopathy (MUSTIC) study. J Am Coll Cardiol 2002;40:111-118.
21. Cazeau S, Leclercq C, Lavergne T, et al, Multisite Stimulation in Cardiomyopathies (MUSTIC) Study Investigators: Effects of multisite biventricular pacing in patients with heart failure and intraventricular conduction delay. N Engl J Med 2001;344:873-880.
22. Sogaard P, Egeblad H, Kim WY, et al: Tissue Doppler imaging predicts improved systolic performance and reversed left ventricular remodeling during long-term cardiac resynchronization therapy. J Am Coll Cardiol 2002;40:723-730.

23. Stellbrink C, Breithardt OA, Franke A, et al, PATH-CHF Investigators; Pochet T, Salo R, Kramer A, Spinelli J, CPI Guidant Congestive Heart Failure Research Group: Impact of cardiac resynchronization therapy using hemodynamically optimized pacing on left ventricular remodeling in patients with congestive heart failure and ventricular conduction disturbances. J Am Coll Cardiol 2001;38:1957-1965.

24. Kass DA, Chen CH, Curry C, et al: Improved left ventricular mechanics from acute VDD pacing in patients with dilated cardiomyopathy and ventricular conduction delay. Circulation 1999;99:1567-1573.

25. Leclercq C, Faris O, Tunin R, et al: Systolic improvement and mechanical resynchronization does not require electrical synchrony in the dilated failing heart with left bundle-branch block. Circulation 2002;106:1760-1763.

26. Sundell J, Engblom E, Koistinen J, et al: The effects of cardiac resynchronization therapy on left ventricular function, myocardial energetics, and metabolic reserve in patients with dilated cardiomyopathy and heart failure. J Am Coll Cardiol 2004;43:1027-1033.

27. Nelson GS, Berger RD, Fetics BJ, et al: Left ventricular or biventricular pacing improves cardiac function at diminished energy costs in patients with dilated cardiomyopathy and left bundle-branch block. Circulation 2000;102:3053-3059.

28. Hamdan MH, Zagrodzky JD, Joglar JA, et al: Biventricular pacing decreases sympathetic activity compared with right ventricular pacing in patients with depressed ejection fraction. Circulation 2000;102:1027-1032.

29. Higgins SL, Yong P, Scheck D, et al, Ventak CHF Investigators: Biventricular pacing diminishes the need for implantable cardioverter defibrillator therapy. J Am Coll Cardiol 2000;36:824-827.

30. Bristow MR, Saxon LA, Boehmer J, et al, Comparison of Medical Therapy, Pacing and Defibrillation in Heart Failure (COMPANION) Investigators: Cardiac-resynchronization therapy with or without an implantable defibrillator in advanced chronic heart failure. N Engl J Med 2004;350:2140-2150.

31. Rodriguez-Cruz E, Karpawich PP, Lieberman RA, Tantengco MV: Biventricular pacing as alternative therapy for dilated cardiomyopathy associated with congenital heart disease. Pacing Clin Electrophysiol 2001;24:235-237.

32. Blom NA, Bax JJ, Ottenkamp J, Schalij MJ: Transvenous biventricular pacing in a child after congenital heart surgery as an alternative therapy for congestive heart failure. J Cardiovasc Electrophysiol 2003;14:1110-1112.

33. Roofthooft MTR, Blom NA, Rijlaarsdam MEB, et al: Resynchronization therapy after congenital heart surgery to improve left ventricular function. Pacing Clin Electrophysiol 2003;26:2042-2044.

34. Janousek J, Vojtovic P, Hucin B, et al: Resynchronization pacing is a useful adjunct to the management of acute heart failure after surgery for congenital heart defects. Am J Cardiol 2001;88:145-152.

35. Zimmerman FJ, Starr JP, Koenig PR, et al: Acute hemodynamic benefit of multisite ventricular pacing after congenital heart surgery. Ann Thorac Surg 2003;75:1775-1780.

36. Dubin AM, Feinstein JA, Reddy VM, et al: Electrical resynchronization: A novel therapy for the failing right ventricle. Circulation 2003;107:2287-2289.

37. Leclercq C, Kass DA: Retiming the failing heart: Principles and current clinical status of cardiac resynchronization. J Am Coll Cardiol 2002;39:194-201.

38. Auricchio A, Stellbrink C, Block M, et al, Guidant Congestive Heart Failure Research Group: Effect of pacing chamber and atrioventricular delay on acute systolic function of paced patients with congestive heart failure. Circulation 1999;99:2993-3001.

39. Blanc JJ, Etienne Y, Gilard M, et al: Evaluation of different ventricular pacing sites in patients with severe heart failure. Circulation 1997;96:3273-3277.

40. Garrigue S, Reuter S, Labeque JN, et al: Usefulness of biventricular pacing in patients with congestive heart failure and right bundle branch block. Am J Cardiol 2001;88:1436-1441.

41. Spragg DD, Leclercq C, Loghmani M, et al: Regional alterations in protein expression in the dyssynchronous failing heart. Circulation 2003;108:929-932.

42. Nurnberg JH, Butter C, Abdul-Kahliq H, et al: Successful cardiac resynchronization therapy in a 9-year-old boy with dilated cardiomyopathy. Z Kardiol 2005;94:44-48.

CHAPTER 40

Catheter Device Therapy for Heart Failure

Vivian Dimas
Anthony C. Chang

Orthotopic heart transplantation remains the only definitive therapy for children who develop end-stage heart failure.[1] In the adult population, lack of adequate supply of organ donors has led to the development of implantable and paracorporeal types of mechanical assist devices as bridges to transplantation or destination therapy (see Chapters 45 to 50). Most of these devices are designed solely for adults and are not suited for children. Although attempts have been made at downsizing various devices, these devices remain oversized for most pediatric patients.

The National Heart, Lung and Blood Institute convened with a task force in January 2001 to identify the most important research priorities associated with pediatric cardiovascular disease.[1] Specific focus was placed on improving surgical and transcatheter therapies for the treatment of heart failure in children, including the creation of materials for cardiovascular bioprostheses, development of cardiovascular cell therapies, and development of minimally invasive surgical and transcatheter therapies. Although there is virtually no pediatric experience with most of the transcatheter therapies discussed in this chapter, these support modalities are likely to be part of the future strategy in the acute management of heart failure in children.

INTRA-AORTIC BALLOON PUMP

The intra-aortic balloon pump (IABP), first introduced by Kantrowitz and colleagues in 1968, is the most common method for myocardial support in adults because of its ease of implantation and removal.[2-9] Use has been limited in children, however, because of size constraints and other anatomic considerations (e.g., the compliance of the aorta). Although extracorporeal membrane oxygenation (ECMO) (see Chapter 46) commonly has been employed as a means of circulatory support in pediatric patients, centers that do not have ECMO capabilities have used alternative therapies such as the IABP and have shown that IABPs can be used safely and effectively in pediatric patients.[3,10,11]

Under normal conditions, coronary blood flow depends on total coronary vascular resistance, resulting from changes in coronary arteriolar tone. Changes in coronary arteriolar tone are controlled by multiple mechanisms, including metabolic, neurohormonal, endothelial-mediated, α-adrenergic, and myogenic effects. Adjustments to coronary arteriolar tone are made in response to various physiologic effects, which are necessary to augment coronary flow. Because coronary venous oxygen tension is normally very low at less than 20 mm Hg, increased oxygen demand is achieved predominantly by improvement in myocardial oxygen delivery rather than increased extraction.[3] Regulatory mechanisms do not act uniformly throughout the coronary vasculature. When coronary artery pressures decrease to levels such that autoregulatory mechanisms cannot increase oxygen delivery to the myocardium, mechanical factors become the principal determinants of coronary flow. These forces include, but are not limited to, aortic root pressure, ventricular wall stress, and intraventricular pressure. IABP provides support to the failing myocardium by improving mechanical factors to augment coronary artery flow and myocardial oxygen delivery.

IABP uses a counterpulsation technique to improve diastolic pressure in the aorta and reduce afterload, reducing myocardial oxygen consumption and improving cardiac output. Counterpulsation works by inflating the balloon during diastole, just after aortic valve closure, and deflating the balloon during systole, just before the opening of the aortic valve leaflets.[4-7,9,12-15] The catheter is connected to a pneumatic pump, which inflates and deflates the balloon in time with the cardiac cycle and timed with either the R wave of the ECG or the arterial waveform. Helium gas is used to inflate the balloon due to its low viscosity, which allows for rapid inflation and deflation. This low viscosity is especially crucial when using the IABP in children, in whom relatively rapid inflation and deflation times are necessary because of more rapid heart rates in children. Patient selection and timing are crucial in the successful deployment of IABP because the main role of IABP is to prevent left ventricular deterioration, and the IABP must be instituted before ventricular failure when the ventricle no longer can sustain cardiac output.

Several sizes of pediatric balloon catheters are available, ranging from 2.5-cc to 20-cc balloons on 4.0F to 7.0F catheters, and a new pediatric console capable of tracking heart rates to 210 beats/min (Datascope Corporation, Parasmus, NJ) is available (Fig. 40-1). The diameter of

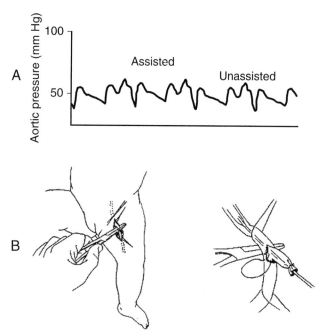

FIGURE 40-1 ■ Intraaortic balloon pumping (IABP) in infants and children. A, The arterial pressure waveform illustrates IABP support at a 1:2 ratio and demonstrates the assisted beat with afterload reduction and diastolic augmentation. B, Schematic diagrams show insertion of a small balloon into the femoral artery for IABP. The common femoral artery is isolated via a vertical groin incision. The balloon catheter is inserted through a sidearm graft of polytetrafluoroethylene, which is sewn to a longitudinal arteriotomy in the femoral artery. (From Pinkney KA, Minich LL, Tani LY, et al: *Current results with intraaortic balloon pumping in infants and children. Ann Thorac Surg* 2002;73:887-891.)

the inflated balloons is 6 to 12 mm with a nominal length of 12.8 to 19.5 cm, depending on the size of balloon catheter used. Previous studies recommended using a balloon volume of 50% to 60% of the patient's stroke volume. Balloon length is often the major determinant for the size of balloon catheter used. Ideally the tip of the balloon should not extend past the first lumbar vertebra and should be no higher than the angle of the manubrium. In smaller children, however, even the smallest balloons may extend past the origins of the renal arteries.[3,16] In children weighing less than 4 kg, surgical placement directly into the ascending aorta may be the preferred approach.[2,3,5,9,10] In larger children, access via the femoral artery can be obtained either by direct visualization or through a percutaneous approach (see Fig. 40-1). Pediatric IABP catheters do not contain a central lumen for pressure monitoring as do adult catheters, so efficacy is determined mainly by systemic arterial pressure and improvement in end-organ function.

Difficulties in performing counterpulsation in children have been attributed to multiple factors, including patient size limitations, potential increased distensibility of the aorta that may result in less effective augmentation, and difficulty tracking and timing the IABP to faster heart rates. In several studies, adequate diastolic augmentation was obtained, however, despite the increased compliance of the aorta, and effective tracking

and device timing were accomplished successfully even at heart rates of 210 beats/min with newer techniques for timing.[2,10,11,17,18] In addition, timing from the radial artery waveform in children resulted in substantial timing errors and decreased effectiveness of the IABP, highlighting the need for better timing methods in these smaller patients.[17] Minich and colleagues[10] proposed using M-mode echocardiography for the timing of discharge because this method allows balloon inflation and deflation to be timed more accurately to aortic valve opening and closure, resulting in fewer timing errors and better device efficacy.[10,11,17]

In pediatric patients, IABPs have been used in a myriad of left ventricular failure disease states as acute support, a bridge to transplantation, or bridge-to-bridge (to a long-term support device).[20-22] The IABP was used in a 2-kg infant who had significant left ventricular dysfunction of unknown etiology.[18] The IABP has also been used successfully in the treatment of primarily right ventricular failure secondary to elevated pulmonary vascular resistance.[19]

Multiple complications have been reported in children, including limb ischemia, mesenteric ischemia, bleeding, thromboembolic phenomena, and complications resulting from inappropriate device placement. Overall, the complication rates for IABP have continued to improve, reported from 7% to 22%, with limb ischemia being the most commonly reported complication in children.[2,12,23]

Survival has continued to increase with the advent of improved technology with survival rates ranging from 57% to 66%.[2,10,11] In comparison, the survival rate for ECMO reported by the Extracorporeal Life Support Organization (ELSO) registry was 38% and 43% for neonatal and pediatric cardiac patients.[24] Although use remains limited in the pediatric population, IABPs can be employed successfully for acute myocardial rescue and should be considered an essential transcatheter support modality in the treatment of refractory cardiogenic shock in children.[5,8,11,18,20,21,25]

PERCUTANEOUS VENTRICULAR ASSIST DEVICES

Although much emphasis has been placed on surgically placed acute or chronic mechanical support devices, more recent technologic advances have led to the development of percutaneously placed ventricular assist devices (VADs). Several percutaneous devices currently are approved for placement in humans, including the Hemopump, the Impella Recover LV, the A-Med Percutaneous Ventricular Assist Device, the TandemHeart PTVA System, and the Cancion CRS (see atlas on devices for additional details and literature).

The **Hemopump** (Johnson & Johnson Interventional Systems, Rancho Cordova, CA), first successfully used in 1988, is an intra-aortic axial flow pump used to provide 1 week of ventricular support. It consists of an axial

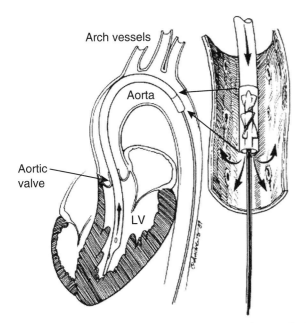

FIGURE 40-2 ■ The Hemopump percutaneous ventricular assist device. The diagram illustrates the Hemopump device that pumps blood from the left ventricle (LV) to the descending thoracic aorta. The details of the pump impeller are seen on the right. (From Duncan JM, Frazier OH, Radovancevic B, et al: *Implantation techniques for the Hemopump. Ann Thorac Surg* 1989;48:733-735)

flow pump enclosed within a silicone cannula, along with a drive cable and a purge fluid system (Fig. 40-2). There are two types of Hemopump. One has a 21F cannula, designed for introduction through a peripheral vessel, and a maximum pump rate of 3.5 L/min; this type is suitable only as a partial assist device. The other type has a 31F cannula and was designed for the transthoracic approach with a flow rate of 6 L/min. This pump permits complete unloading of the left ventricle, but requires sternotomy for insertion. When the pump rotates, blood is drawn from the ventricle and pumped into the thoracic aorta. The Hemopump unloads the ventricle directly and has the ability to reduce the end-diastolic or intraventricular cavitary pressure. Power is provided through a percutaneous drive-line connected to an external electromechanical console. There is very limited experience in children with the Hemopump.

The **Impella LP 2.5** (CardioSystems AG, Aachen, Germany), from a line of devices produced since 1991, is a 12F catheter system that is inserted percutaneously via the femoral artery and can deliver 2.5 L/min of blood flow. The tip of the cannula is placed in the left ventricle over a guidewire using either fluoroscopy or transesophageal imaging for guidance. Blood is drawn into the device through the cannula tip in the left ventricle and is discharged upstream from the impeller via several side ports in the ascending aorta. This pump is currently under clinical investigation in the United States, but already is approved for use in Europe with a large cumulative experience.

The **A-Med Percutaneous Ventricular Assist Device** (A-Med Systems, Inc, West Sacramento, CA), first used in 1999, is a percutaneously placed intravascular pump and cannula system designed to provide temporary left ventricular and circulatory support for patients with acute heart failure. It includes two pump-catheter systems that employ a small, externally mounted centrifugal pump connected to coaxial catheter systems. The total circuit volume of each system is approximately 30 mL. The left ventricular system is inserted percutaneously in the femoral artery into the left ventricle, and the right ventricular system is inserted via the internal jugular vein and placed so that the take-up ports are in the right atrium and the distal delivery port is in the main pulmonary artery. Although this device was designed to be used as a VAD for 3 days, currently it is used only to augment the heart's pumping capability during coronary artery bypass.

The **TandemHeart pVAD** (CardiacAssist, Inc, Pittsburgh, PA) is a centrifugal pump capable of delivering a cardiac output of 4 L/min. The upper housing provides a conduit for inflow and outflow of blood; the lower housing assembly allows communication with the controller, the means for rotating the impeller of the percutaneous VAD, and the infusion line for anticoagulation and cooling for the bearing. The controller is a microprocessor-based electromechanical drive and infusion system and generates the signals to drive the percutaneous VAD. The device requires a low pump prime volume of only about 10 mL and is placed percutaneously via the femoral vessels. This device uses a hydrodynamic fluid bearing that supports a spinning rotor, which rotates between 3000 and 7500 rpm with little hemolysis. The left atrial cannula (21F) is placed via a standard transseptal procedure from the femoral vein, and the aortic outflow cannula (14F to 19F) is placed retrograde into the lower abdominal aorta via the femoral artery.

This device was designed for the stabilization of patients in acute heart failure with poor systemic perfusion, off-loading the left ventricle to decrease workload and to allow recovery. The device has been available since May 2000 and has been used for short-term stabilization of patients with cardiogenic shock until recovery of the myocardium or definitive supportive or replacement therapy can be achieved; it is currently approved for support for 14 days.[26] In addition, it can be placed during high-risk revascularization procedures to provide a means of cardiac support should ventricular function deteriorate. In experienced hands, it can be placed in approximately 30 minutes, allowing for rapid and easy institution of ventricular assist.

The **Cancion Cardiac Recovery System (CRS)** (Orqis Medical Corp, Lake Forest, CA), first used in 2003, has an inflow cannula that is placed directly into the peripheral vessel using a sheathless technique. The inflow cannula is connected to the bearingless

Cancion pump, which contains an internal rotor, or impeller; the pump fits on top of the bearingless Cancion motor, which drives the pump magnetically. The system also consists of two arterial access conduits, a small centrifugal pump and motor, and the control system. The blood is returned back to the descending aorta via the pigtail outflow cannula, which is placed in the femoral artery using standard techniques. This device currently is undergoing feasibility trials in the United States.

Percutaneously placed VADs can be implanted rapidly either in the catheterization laboratory or in the intensive care setting. Initial results of the aforementioned devices from feasibility studies in adult patients with heart failure are promising. Continued efforts to improve and even miniaturize these devices will provide additional resuscitative tools for the pediatric cardiologist to initiate lifesaving support for critically ill children in a timely manner.

TRANSCATHETER VALVE REPLACEMENT

Pulmonary regurgitation after repair of right ventricular outflow tract obstruction is tolerated for many years, but ultimately leads to right ventricular dilation and eventual dysfunction (see Chapter 21). If the pulmonary insufficiency is left untreated, progressive right ventricular failure develops.[27-29] As right ventricular failure progresses, patients are at increased risk of developing ventricular arrhythmias, which may lead to sudden cardiac death. Timing of pulmonary valve placement in these patients is debated. Ideally, placement of the pulmonary valve should occur before right ventricular failure, when remodeling and contractile recovery of the ventricle may not be possible. Several articles have described attempts to define the appropriate timing of valve placement and whether or not placement of the valve actually results in clinical and hemodynamic improvement.[27-29]

Traditionally, pulmonary valve placement has been performed surgically on cardiopulmonary bypass. Bonhoeffer and associates[30] have shown successful implantation of stent-mounted pulmonary valves initially in animal studies and more recently in patients who had successful implantation of a pulmonary valve in the right ventricular outflow tract (Fig. 40-3). Theoretical advantages of the percutaneous valve implantation technique include a less invasive procedure with shorter recovery time and possible further right ventricular preservation by not subjecting an already failing right ventricle to cardiopulmonary bypass.

Patients who have had a valveless repair of the right ventricular outflow tract tend to develop significant right ventricular outflow tract dilation as pulmonary insufficiency worsens. Bovine venous valves come in a variety of sizes (range 8 to 24 mm). In Bonhoeffer's initial lamb experiment, an 18-mm bovine valve harvested from

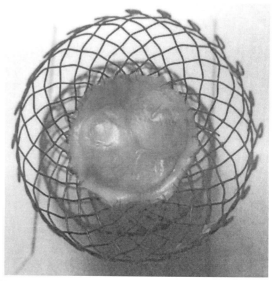

FIGURE 40-3 ■ Pulmonary valve implantation. The front view of the stent used for pulmonary valve implantation, showing the valve in the closed position as seen from the ventricular side. (From Boudjemline Y, Agnoletti G, Bonner D, et al: *Percutaneous pulmonary valve replacement in a large right ventricular outflow tract: An experimental study. J Am Coll Cardiol* 2004;43:1082-1087.)

bovine jugular vein was sutured to a balloon expandable platinum stent. The valved stent was hand-crimped onto the inflatable portion of either an 18-mm, 20-mm, or 22-mm balloon catheter. The size of balloon catheter chosen was based on the size of the pulmonary artery as measured by angiography. When the stent was placed on the balloon catheter, assembly was front-loaded onto a 16F Mullins long sheath. The valved stent was placed using fluoroscopic guidance. Of the seven lambs in which successful implantation was accomplished, six were angiographically competent after implantation, with the remaining stent only mildly regurgitant after placement. No complications were noted immediately after valve placement, although one valve was mildly stenotic with a 15 mm Hg pressure gradient between the right ventricle and pulmonary artery. Two months after implantation, the valved stents were able to be easily removed.[30]

In a more recent study, Boudjemline and colleagues[31] implanted a pulmonary valve and downsized the pulmonary artery from 30 mm to 18 mm. This technique would make it feasible to decrease the diameter of the pulmonary artery, which tends to be dilated in these patients, to the diameter of available valves (22 mm). The self-expandable stent in this study was created from nitinol in the shape of a conduit with a central restriction. The extremities of the stent were 30 mm in diameter with a central restriction 15 mm long and 18 mm in diameter. The stent was covered with polytetrafluoroethylene membrane, and a naturally valved segment of bovine jugular vein was mounted to the restricted portion of the stent.

Two types of implantation were performed in ewes. The first implantation method involved deployment of the valved stent in a single procedure. The second implantation method was stepwise, with implantation of the nonvalved stent followed by valve implantation 6 to 10 weeks later. After implantation, successful reduction in pulmonary artery diameter was achieved, and all pulmonary valves implanted (either in a single or stepwise fashion) were competent after placement.

Thrombus formation between the stent and pulmonary artery wall secondary to blood entrapment was a concern. Although no thromboembolism was noted on postmortem examination, the risk exists especially in patients in whom an adequate seal does not develop between the pulmonary artery wall and the covered stent.[31] Longevity of implanted valves varies from 1 to 15 years.[28,32-36] Bovine jugular vein conduits have been used as a right ventricle-to-pulmonary conduit in pediatric congenital heart surgery. Long-term follow-up is not yet available, but early results are promising.[37-39]

TRANSCATHETER DELIVERY OF BIOMATERIALS

Research efforts have been focused on improving the subset of patients who do not improve because of residual left ventricular dysfunction, patients with genetic disorders of the myocardium, and patients with diffuse or distal coronary artery disease.[40-60] Initial results have shown regenerative capabilities of hematopoietic stem cells and skeletal myoblasts when directly injected into damaged, but viable myocardium.[44,55,61-76] In addition, angiogenic growth factors are being evaluated for their ability to generate new vessels in the ischemic myocardium.[77] Lastly, effectiveness of gene therapy is determined by a combination of the effects of gene delivery into the target tissue, the entry of the new genetic material into cells, and the expression of the transfected gene in the target tissue.[78] Currently, multiple delivery routes exist for the aforementioned biologic materials, including retrograde coronary venous delivery, transvenous intramyocardial delivery, direct endocardial delivery, and video thoracoscopic epicardial or intrapericardial delivery.[60,72,77,79-85]

Transvenous coronary access is accomplished by placing a catheter in the right atrium and engaging the coronary sinus. When the catheter is placed successfully in the coronary sinus, a wire is placed in either the great cardiac vein or the middle cardiac vein. A balloon-tipped Swan-Ganz catheter is placed over the wire, and the wire is withdrawn. The balloon is inflated to occlude the vein completely, and the injection is performed.[60] Intravascular administration (intravenous or intracoronary) is relatively safe and easy to perform, but it delivers a relatively low percentage of total treatment dose to the heart. In addition, it results in exposure of nontarget organs.[82] Transthoracic transepicardial injection and direct myocardial injection, although providing

excellent localization, are limited because of the additional risk of a required thoracotomy.[82] Intrapericardial delivery offers the theoretical advantage of prolonged exposure of the coronary arteries and myocardium to the injectate, but it too requires a more invasive means of delivery. Direct endocardial delivery seems to have much promise as a delivery mechanism because it allows for direct localization and injection without significant exposure of nontarget organs.[56,57,72,78,86,87]

There are essentially two categories for delivery of cells intramyocardially: needle or non-needle injection systems. All needle-based systems are coaxial systems, with an outer shaft and inner core injecting lumen. The core has a hypodermic needle at its distal tip for injection, and is able to be advanced and withdrawn independently of the outer shaft. All needle-based catheter injection systems are designed for percutaneous placement in the femoral artery and the left ventricle using fluoroscopic guidance (Fig. 40-4).[88]

The first catheter used in humans was the **Biosense-Webster Myostar** (Waterloo, Belgium). Its core lumen is attached to a 27-gauge needle. The handle of the catheter contains controls for tip deflection, needle advancement, and lumen injection. It uses nonfluoroscopic techniques for endocardial contact, in particular the **NOGA** (Biosense-Webster, Waterloo, Belgium) system. Localization of the catheter tip within the left ventricle can be accomplished by various methods. The NOGA catheter system uses electromechanical mapping as its primary imaging method, using a specialized transmission probe positioned at the distal tip of the catheter connected to a central imaging console. It is able to locate areas of damaged or hibernating myocardium via electropotentials.[89,90] In addition, the **Bioheart MyoCath** (Bioheart, Inc, Santa Rosa, CA) has a 25-gauge needle for injection and uses radiographic imaging for guidance.

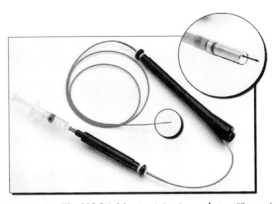

FIGURE 40-4 ■ **The NOGA Myostar injection catheter.** The catheter is seen with the needle in the extended position *(inset)*. The catheter is advanced into the left ventricle, and the catheter tip is placed against the endocardial surface with the needle extended into the myocardium to deliver the cells. (See also Color Section) (From Perin EC, Dohmann HF, Borojevic R, et al: *Transendocardial autologous bone marrow cell transplantation in severe, chronic ischemic heart failure.* Circulation 2003;107:2294-2302.)

Finally, the **Stiletto** (Boston Scientific SciMed, Inc, Natick, MA) has three separate components, which move independently of one another. It contains two steerable guiding catheters (9F and 7F) and an inner spring-loaded needle for injection. This system has the added benefit of being able to be advanced into the left ventricle over a guidewire.[88]

Non-needle–based catheter systems include catheters designed to access the coronary venous system or catheters designed to deliver the injectate by injecting through the coronary arteries. Intracoronary injection may result in less uptake of the injectate during its first pass, allowing the injectate to be taken up by other tissues rather than the target tissue itself. Ease of use, accuracy of delivery of injectate, and tissue retention of the injectate using each of these methods are being evaluated. Additionally, methods for tagging injected cells to determine their location and degree of tissue retention are being evaluated because none of the previously described injection techniques can confirm that the injectate has entered the myocardium.[84,88,91,92]

Animal and human studies have documented cellular differentiation capabilities of stem cells and skeletal myoblasts. Several studies have been performed that suggest a strong association between smooth muscle proliferation, lesion instability, and the expression of **basic fibroblast growth factor** in human atherosclerotic plaques obtained by coronary atherectomy.[82] Inoue and coworkers[93] described expression of vascular endothelial growth factor and its receptors in atherosclerotic lesions of the human coronary artery, with the presence of inflammatory mononuclear cells within the plaques. These data suggest that there may be proatherogenic effects as a consequence of intracoronary or intravenous administration of angiogenic growth factors. Whether this potential is only theoretical remains to be determined.[82]

Laham and colleagues[77] performed a randomized, double-blind, placebo-controlled study of basic fibroblast growth factor comparing 10 μg or 100 μg with placebo in patients with ungraftable myocardial territories who were undergoing coronary artery bypass graft surgery for the treatment of ischemic coronary artery disease. After completion of all coronary bypasses to portions of the myocardium that could be revascularized, multiple linear incisions were made in the epicardial fat surrounding the target vessel, which could not be revascularized. Heparin-alginate pellets containing either basic fibroblast growth factor or placebo were inserted into the epicardial fat and secured with polypropylene (Prolene) suture. Two to three pellets were placed in each incision, with a total of 10 pellets used in each patient. The mean clinical follow-up period was 16 months, and there were no recurrences of angina in the 100-μg basic fibroblast growth factor group. There was significant improvement in defect size by nuclear perfusion imaging in the 100-μg group and a trend, although not significant, toward reduction in the target ischemic area in the 100-μg group. This study showed the feasibility of using this mode of drug delivery in patients with viable myocardium that is not able to be adequately revascularized.[77]

The FIRST trial (FGF Initiating RevaScularization Trial) was a multicenter, randomized, double-blind, placebo-controlled trial to evaluate the efficacy and safety of **recombinant fibroblast growth factor** at 0 μg/kg, 0.3 μg/kg, 3 μg/kg, or 30 μg/kg dosing via single intracoronary infusion. Efficacy was evaluated at 90 and 180 days postinjection by exercise tolerance test, myocardial nuclear perfusion imaging, Seattle Angina Questionnaire, and Short-Form 36 questionnaire. The investigators found exercise tolerance was improved at 90 days in all groups, but the angina score as measured by the Seattle Angina Questionnaire and physical component summary scale of the Short-Form 36 were significantly reduced in patients who received the recombinant fibroblast growth factor compared with the placebo group. At 180 days, there were no significant differences among the groups. Adverse events were similar between the two groups except for hypotension, which occurred with higher frequency in the 30-μg/kg recombinant fibroblast growth factor group.[94]

Perin and colleagues[57] performed a prospective, nonrandomized, open-label study injecting **bone marrow mononuclear cells** for treatment of severe heart failure secondary to ischemic heart disease to determine its feasibility and utility for the treatment of severe congestive heart failure. Electromechanical mapping was used to identify viable myocardium (unipolar voltage ≥6.9 mV). The bone marrow–derived stem cells were injected intramyocardially into these areas. Perin and colleagues[57] found a significant reduction in total reversible defect and improvement in global left ventricular function within the treatment group. At 4 months, there was a significant improvement in ejection fraction from baseline and significant improvement in mechanical function of the injected segments as documented by electromechanical mapping. There were no significant adverse effects noted. Perin and Willerson (personal communication) currently are performing the first U.S. Food and Drug Administration–approved randomized, double-blind study of cardiac stem cell therapy in the United States at the Texas Heart Institute in patients with heart failure and severe coronary disease.

Many questions concerning stem cell therapy remain unanswered: What is the optimal number of stem cells to implant? Is there a threshold number of stem cells needed? When is the ideal time for injection after the ischemic injury? In addition, the ideal delivery strategy has yet to be determined, and the long-term functioning of the stem cells is unknown. The potential for stem cells to regenerate contracting myocardium and improve ventricular remodeling seems promising in the short-term, but long-term efficacy has not been evaluated. As with any new therapy, there are negative aspects to

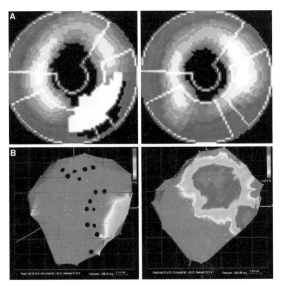

FIGURE 40-5 ■ **Single-photon emission computed tomography (SPECT) polar maps and electromechanical maps. A,** SPECT polar map at baseline shows an inferolateral ischemic area in white and nonreversible stress defect in black *(left)*. Follow-up SPECT at 2 months *(right)* after autologous bone marrow cell transplantation shows complete resolution of ischemic defect. **B,** Electromechanical map from the inferior position. Mechanical map at the time of the injection procedure *(left)*. shows the 15 injection sites in black. Follow-up mechanical map at 4 months *(right)* shows marked improvement in contractile function in the injected area. (See also Color Section) (From Perin EC, Dohmann HF, Borojevic R, et al: *Transendocardial autologous bone marrow cell transplantation in severe, chronic ischemic heart failure. Circulation* 2003;107:2294-2302.)

therapy as well. One such concern is the possible arrhythmogenic potential that stem cells exhibit intrinsically[95] or owing to secondary effects, such as fibroblast formation with enhancement of scar formation.[96] Additionally, if injected stem cells are not completely incorporated into the myocardium, they may adversely affect the electrical conduction system of the heart.[97] The primary application for stem cell therapy is treatment of ischemic heart failure (Fig. 40-5). If this technology could be applied to the treatment of nonischemic congestive heart failure, particularly patients with primary cardiac muscle disease, perhaps its benefit could be realized in pediatric patients as well.

CURRENT STATUS AND FUTURE TRENDS

In the current era, transplantation remains the only definitive therapy for the treatment of refractory heart failure; however, it cannot meet the growing demands of the rapidly expanding population of patients with severe congestive heart failure. The future seems to be in the creation of devices that can assist a failing myocardium, rather than transplantation. Percutaneous strategies for the treatment of heart failure have improved considerably the treatment options available in adult patients. We currently are awaiting larger scale human trials to determine the efficacy and safety of these

new strategies, including percutaneous assist devices and valve replacement. Financial support and intellectual investment for the development of treatment strategies in children should improve significantly the likelihood that these treatment options will be available to pediatric patients in the future. One of the promising devices is the CentriMag® Left Ventricular Assist system (Levitronic LLC, Waltham, MA).

Stem cell therapy has shown the potential to improve cardiovascular function in patients with ischemia, but the mechanisms by which stem cells improve tissue repair are not clearly understood. Additionally, there is a risk that stem cells may exacerbate tissue injury by mobilization of inflammatory mediators, if given at the wrong time.[98] There is evidence from human and animal studies that tissue regeneration can occur, but which progenitor cells are most successful in regenerating myocardium needs to be elucidated further.[54] Another shortfall is the ability to follow patient progress and confirm the short-term and long-term successes of stem cell therapy by observing their distribution and functional effect via noninvasive imaging. Currently, noninvasive imaging techniques have not reached the cellular level; advances in imaging, particularly nuclear imaging, are being designed that may help detect even small changes in regional blood flow distribution and function, further assisting in documenting differential effect of stem cell therapy.[99] Evidence currently suggests further definitive clinical trials are necessary, specifically randomized, controlled clinical trials. The risk-to-benefit ratio is not in favor of the patient and should be evaluated before future clinical studies.[54,98,100,101]

Key Concepts

■ When coronary artery pressures decrease to levels such that autoregulatory mechanisms cannot increase oxygen delivery to the myocardium, mechanical factors become the principal determinants of coronary flow. These forces include, but are not limited to, aortic root pressure, ventricular wall stress, and intraventricular pressure. The IABP provides support to the failing myocardium by improving mechanical factors to augment coronary artery flow and myocardial oxygen delivery.

■ Patient selection and timing are crucial in the successful deployment of the IABP because the main role of the IABP is to prevent left ventricular deterioration, and it must be instituted before ventricular failure when the ventricle no longer can sustain cardiac output.

■ Difficulties in performing counterpulsation in children have been attributed to multiple factors, including patient size limitations, potential increased distensibility of the aorta that may result in less effective augmentation, and difficulty tracking and timing the IABP to faster heart rates.

■ Multiple complications have been reported in children, including limb ischemia, mesenteric ischemia, bleeding, thromboembolic phenomena, and complications resulting from inappropriate device placement. Overall the complication rates for IABP have continued to improve, reported from 7% to 22%, with limb ischemia being the most commonly reported complication in children.

■ Although use remains limited in pediatric patients, IABPs can be employed successfully for acute myocardial rescue and should be considered an essential transcatheter support modality in the treatment of refractory cardiogenic shock in children.

■ Although much emphasis has been placed on surgically placed acute or chronic mechanical support devices, more recent technologic advances have led to the development of percutaneously placed VADs. Several percutaneous devices currently are approved for placement in humans, including the Hemopump, the Impella Recover LV, the A-Med Percutaneous Ventricular Assist Device, the TandemHeart PTVA System, and the Cancion CRS.

■ Percutaneously placed VADs can be implanted rapidly either in the catheterization laboratory or in the intensive care setting. Initial results of these devices from feasibility studies in adult patients with heart failure are promising.

■ Theoretical advantages of the percutaneous valve implantation technique include a less invasive procedure with shorter recovery time and possible further right ventricular preservation by not subjecting an already failing right ventricle to cardiopulmonary bypass.

■ Currently, multiple delivery routes exist for the biologic materials, including retrograde coronary venous delivery, transvenous intramyocardial delivery, direct endocardial delivery, and video thoracoscopic epicardial or intrapericardial delivery.

■ There are essentially two categories for delivery of cells intramyocardially: needle or non-needle injection systems. All needle-based systems are coaxial systems, with an outer shaft and inner core injecting lumen. Non–needle-based catheter systems include catheters designed to access the coronary venous system and catheters designed to deliver the injectate by injecting through the coronary arteries.

■ Many questions concerning stem cell therapy remain unanswered: What is the optimal number of stem cells to implant? Is there a threshold number of stem cells needed? When is the ideal time for injection after the ischemic injury? In addition, the ideal delivery strategy has yet to be determined, and the long-term functioning of the stem cells is unknown.

REFERENCES

1. Clark EGJ: National Heart, Lung, and Blood Institute report of the Task Force on Research in Pediatric Cardiovascular Disease. Washington, DC, 2002.

2. Akomea-Agyin C, et al: Intraaortic balloon pumping in children. Ann Thorac Surg 1999;67:1415-1420.

3. Booker PD: Intra-aortic balloon pumping in young children. Paediatr Anaesth 1997;7:501-507.

4. Cohen M, Urban P, Christenson JT, et al: Intra-aortic balloon counterpulsation in US and non-US centres: Results of the Benchmark Registry. Eur Heart J 2003;24:1763-1770.

5. Fukumasu H, Blaylock R, Veasy LG, et al: Intra-aortic balloon pumping device for infants. Clin Cardiol 1979;2:348-353.

6. Mehlhorn U, Kroner A, de Vivie ER: 30 years clinical intra-aortic balloon pumping: Facts and figures. Thorac Cardiovasc Surg 1999;47(Suppl 2):298-303.

7. Schmid C, Wilhelm M, Reimann A, et al: Use of an intraaortic balloon pump in patients with impaired left ventricular function. Scand Cardiovasc J 1999;33:194-198.

8. Veasy LG, Blalock RC, Orth JL, et al: Intra-aortic balloon pumping in infants and children. Circulation 1983;68:1095-1100.

9. Veasy LG, Webster HF, McGough EC: Intra-aortic balloon pumping: Adaptation for pediatric use. Crit Care Clin 1986;2:237-249.

10. Minich LLT, McGough LY, Shaddy EC, et al: A novel approach to pediatric intraaortic balloon pump timing using M-mode echocardiography. Am J Cardiol 1997;80:170-181.

11. Pinkney KA, Minich LL, Tani LY, et al: Current results with intra-aortic balloon pumping in infants and children. Ann Thorac Surg 2002;73:887-891.

12. Ferguson J III, Cohen M: The current practice of intra-aortic balloon counterpulsation: Results from the Benchmark Registry. J Am Coll Cardiol 2001;38:1456-1462.

13. Ferrari G, Gorczynska K, Minno R, et al: IABP assistance: A test bench for the analysis of its effects on ventricular energetics and hemodynamics. Int J Artif Organs 2001;24:274-280.

14. Jeevanandam V, Jayakar D, Anderson AS, et al: Circulatory assistance with a permanent implantable IABP: Initial human experience. Circulation 2002;106(12 Suppl 1):I-183-I-188.

15. Kern MJ, Aguirre FV, Caracciolo EA, et al: Hemodynamic effects of new intra-aortic balloon counterpulsation timing methods in patients: A multicenter evaluation. Am Heart J 1999;137:1129-1136.

16. Pollock JC, Williams MC, Edmonds WG, et al: Intraaortic balloon pumping in children. Ann Thorac Surg 1980;29:522-528.

17. Pantalos GM, Minich LL, Tani LY, et al: Estimation of timing errors for the intraaortic balloon pump use in pediatric patients. ASAIO J 1999;45:166-171.

18. del Nido PJ, Swan PR, Benson LN, et al: Successful use of intraaortic balloon pumping in a 2-kilogram infant. Ann Thorac Surg 1988;46:574-576.

19. Arafa OE, Geiran OR, Andersen K, et al: Intraaortic balloon pumping for predominantly right ventricular failure after heart transplantation. Ann Thorac Surg 2000;70:1587-1593.

20. Inoue YK, Kaneko H, Yoshizawa H, Morikawa Y: Rescue of a child with fulminant myocarditis using percutaneous cardiopulmonary support. Pediatr Cardiol 2000;21:158-160.

21. Minich LL, Tani LY, Hawkins JA, et al: Intra-aortic balloon pumping in children with dilated cardiomyopathy as a bridge to transplantation. J Heart Lung Transplant 2001;20:750-754.

22. Scheinin SR, Parnis B, Ott SM, et al: Mechanical circulatory support in children. Eur J Cardiothorac Surg 1994;8:537-540.

23. Van de Wal HJ, Bennink GB, Benatar AA: Complication of intra-aortic balloon pumping in a pediatric patient. Eur J Cardiothorac Surg 1995;9:602-603.

24. Conrad SA, Rycus PT, Dalton H: Extracorporeal Life Support Registry Report 2004; ASAIO J 2005;51:4-10.

25. Park JH, Gersony DT: Intraaortic balloon pump management of refractory congestive heart failure in children. Pediatr Cardiol 1993;14:19-22.

26. Holger TL, Hambrecht B, Boudriot R, et al: Reversal of cardiogenic shock by percutaneous left atrial-to-femoral arterial bypass assistance. Circ J 2001;104:2917-2922.

27. Bove EK, Bryrum RE, Sondheimer CJ, et al: Improved right ventricular function following late pulmonary valve replacement for

residual pulmonary insufficiency or stenosis. J Thorac Cardiovasc Surg 1985;90:50-55.

28. Discigil BD, Puga JA, Schaff FJ, et al: Late pulmonary valve replacement after repair of tetralogy of Fallot. J Thorac Cardiovasc Surg 2001;121:344-351.

29. Thierren JS, McLaughlin SC, Liu PR, et al: Pulmonary valve replacement in adults late after repair of tetralogy of Fallot: Are we operating too late? J Am Coll Cardiol 2000;36:1670-1675.

30. Bonhoeffer P, Boudjemline Y, Saliba Z, et al: Transcatheter implantation of a bovine valve in pulmonary position: A lamb study. Circulation 2000;102:813-816.

31. Boudjemline Y, Agnoletti G, Bonner D, et al: Percutaneous pulmonary valve replacement in a large right ventricular outflow tract: An experimental study. J Am Coll Cardiol 2004;43:1082-1087.

32. Conte SR, Benedict J, Gewillig E, et al: Homograft valve insertion for pulmonary regurgitation late after valveless repair of right ventricular outflow tract obstruction. Eur J Cardiothorac Surg 1999;15:143-149.

33. Kirklin JB, Maehara EH, Pacifico T, et al: Intermediate-term fate of cryopreserved allograft and xenograft valved conduits. Ann Thorac Surg 1987;44:598-606.

34. Meldrum-Hanna WC, Cartmill T, Johnson T, et al: Late results of right ventricular outflow tract reconstruction with Bjork-Shiley valved conduits. Br Heart J 1986;55:371-375.

35. Schlichter AK, Mayorquim C, Simon RC, et al: Five-to fifteen-year follow-up of fresh autologous pericardial valved conduits. J Thorac Cardiovasc Surg 2000;119:869-879.

36. Schlichter AK, Mayorquim C, Simon RC, et al: Long-term follow-up of autologous pericardial valved conduits. Ann Thorac Surg 1996;62:155-160.

37. Chatzis AG, Bobos NM, Kirvassilis D, et al: New xenograft valved conduit (Contegra) for right ventricular outflow tract reconstruction. Heart Surg Forum 2003;6:396-398.

38. Bove TD, Wauthy H, Goldstein P, et al: Early results of valved bovine jugular vein conduit versus bicuspid homograft for right ventricular outflow tract reconstruction. Ann Thorac Surg 2002;74:536-541.

39. Breymann TT, Boethig WR, Blanz D, et al: Bovine valved venous xenografts for RVOT reconstruction: Results after 71 implantations. Eur J Cardiothorac Surg 2002;21:703-710.

40. Abbott JD, Giordano FJ: Stem cells and cardiovascular disease. J Nucl Cardiol 2003;10:403-412.

41. Al-Radi OO, Rao V, Li RK, et al: Cardiac cell transplantation: Closer to bedside. Ann Thorac Surg 2003;75:S674-S677.

42. Amrani DL, Port S: Cardiovascular disease: Potential impact of stem cell therapy. Exp Rev Cardiovasc Ther 2003;1:453-461.

43. Blatt A, Robinson D, Cotter G, et al: Improved regional left ventricular function after successful satellite cell grafting in rabbits with myocardial infarction. Eur J Heart Fail 2003;5:751-757.

44. Chiu RC: Bone-marrow stem cells as a source for cell therapy. Heart Fail Rev 2003;8:247-251.

45. Chiu RC: Adult stem cell therapy for heart failure. Exp Opin Biol Ther 2003;3:215-225.

46. Dowell JD, Rubart M, Pasumarthi KB, et al: Myocyte and myogenic stem cell transplantation in the heart. Cardiovasc Res 2003;58:336-350.

47. Forrester JS, Price MJ, Makkar RR: Stem cell repair of infarcted myocardium: An overview for clinicians. Circulation 2003;108:1139-1145.

48. Fraser JK, Schreiber RE, Zuk PA, et al: Adult stem cell therapy for the heart. Int J Biochem Cell Biol 2004;36:658-666.

49. Folkman J: Angiogenic therapy of the human heart. Circulation 1998;97:628-629.

50. Haider H, Tan AC, Aziz S, et al: Myoblast transplantation for cardiac repair: A clinical perspective. Mol Ther 2004;9:14-23.

51. Hassink RJ, Brutel de la Riviere A, Mummery CL, et al: Transplantation of cells for cardiac repair. J Am Coll Cardiol 2003;41:711-717.

52. Itescu S, Schuster MD, Kocher AA: New directions in strategies using cell therapy for heart disease. J Mol Med 2003;81:288-296.

53. Kovacic JC, Graham RM: Stem-cell therapy for myocardial diseases. Lancet 2004;363:1735-1736.

54. Mathur A, Martin JF: Stem cells and repair of the heart. Lancet 2004;364:183-192.

55. Nir SG, David R, Zaruba M, et al: Human embryonic stem cells for cardiovascular repair. Cardiovasc Res 2003;58:313-323.

56. Perin EC, Geng YJ, Willerson JT: Adult stem cell therapy in perspective. Circulation 2003;107:935-938.

57. Perin EC, Dohmann HF, Borojevic R, et al: Transendocardial, autologous bone marrow cell transplantation for severe, chronic ischemic heart failure. Circulation 2003;107:2294-2302.

58. Schwartz Y, Kornowski R: Autologous stem cells for functional myocardial repair. Heart Fail Rev 2003;8:237-245.

59. Strauer BE, Kornowski R: Stem cell therapy in perspective. Circulation 2003;107:929-934.

60. Herity NA, Lo ST, Oei F, et al: Selective regional myocardial infiltration by the percutaneous coronary venous route: A novel technique for local drug delivery. Cathet Cardiovasc Interv 2000;51:358-363.

61. Tomita S, Li RK, Wiesel RD, et al: Autologous transplantation of bone marrow cells improves damaged heart function. Circulation 1999;100(19 Suppl):II-247-II-256.

62. Thompson RB, Emani SM, Davis BH, et al: Comparison of intracardiac cell transplantation: Autologous skeletal myoblasts versus bone marrow cells. Circulation 2003;108(Suppl 1):II-264-II-271.

63. Soukiasian HJ, Czer LS, Avital I, et al: A novel sub-population of bone marrow-derived myocardial stem cells: Potential autologous cell therapy in myocardial infarction. J Heart Lung Transplant 2004;23:873-880.

64. Sim EK, Jiang S, Ye L, et al: Skeletal myoblast transplant in heart failure. J Card Surg 2003;18:319-327.

65. Schuster MD, Kocher AA, Seki T, et al: Myocardial neovascularization by bone marrow angioblasts results in cardiomyocyte regeneration. Am J Physiol Heart Circ Physiol 2004;287:H525-H532.

66. Schumacher B, Pecher P, von Specht BU, et al: Induction of neoangiogenesis in ischemic myocardium by human growth factors: First clinical results of a new treatment of coronary heart disease. Circulation 1998;97:645-650.

67. Reffelmann T, Kloner RA: Cellular cardiomyoplasty—cardiomyocytes, skeletal myoblasts, or stem cells for regenerating myocardium and treatment of heart failure? Cardiovasc Res 2003;58:358-368.

68. Orlic D, Kajstura J, Chimenti S, et al: Bone marrow stem cells regenerate infarcted myocardium. Pediatr Transplant 2003;7(Suppl 3):86-88.

69. Menasche P: Skeletal myoblast transplantation for cardiac repair. Exp Rev Cardiovasc Ther 2004;2:21-28.

70. Menasche P: Myoblast-based cell transplantation. Heart Fail Rev 2003;8:221-227.

71. Kehat I, Kenyagin-Karsenti D, Snir M, et al: Human embryonic stem cells can differentiate into myocytes with structural and functional properties of cardiomyocytes. J Clin Invest 2001;108:407-414.

72. Herreros J, Prosper F, Perez A, et al: Autologous intramyocardial injection of cultured skeletal muscle-derived stem cells in patients with non-acute myocardial infarction. Eur Heart J 2003;24:2012-2020.

73. Heng BC, Haider HKh, Sim EK, et al: Strategies for directing the differentiation of stem cells into the cardiomyogenic lineage in vitro. Cardiovasc Res 2004;62:34-42.

74. Hagege AA, Carrion C, Menasche P, et al: Viability and differentiation of autologous skeletal myoblast grafts in ischaemic cardiomyopathy. Lancet 2003;361:491-492.

75. Boheler KR, Czyz J, Tweedie D, et al: Differentiation of pluripotent embryonic stem cells into cardiomyocytes. Circ Res 2002;91:189-201.

76. Agbulut O, Vandervelde S, Al Attor N, et al: Comparison of human skeletal myoblasts and bone marrow-derived CD133+ progenitors for the repair of infarcted myocardium. J Am Coll Cardiol 2004;44:458-463.

77. Laham RJ, Sellke FW, Edelman ER, et al: Local perivascular delivery of basic fibroblast growth factor in patients undergoing coronary bypass surgery: Results of a phase I randomized, double-blind, placebo-controlled trial. Circulation 1999;100:1865-1871.

78. Yla-Herttuala S, Martin JF: Cardiovascular gene therapy. Lancet 2000;355:213-222.

79. Barbash IM, Leor J, Feinberg MS, et al: Interventional magnetic resonance imaging for guiding gene and cell transfer in the heart. Heart 2004;90:87-91.

80. Kang HJ, Kim HS, Zhang SY, et al: Effects of intracoronary infusion of peripheral blood stem-cells mobilised with granulocyte-colony stimulating factor on left ventricular systolic function and restenosis after coronary stenting in myocardial infarction: The MAGIC cell randomised clinical trial. Lancet 2004;363:751-756.

81. Kornowski R, Fuchs S: Catheter-based transendocardial gene delivery for therapeutic myocardial angiogenesis. Int J Cardiovasc Interv 2000;3:67-70.

82. Kornowski R, Fuchs S, Leon MB, et al: Delivery strategies to achieve therapeutic myocardial angiogenesis. Circulation 2000;101:454-458.

83. Laham RJ, Post M, Sellke FW, et al: Therapeutic angiogenesis using local perivascular and pericardial delivery. Curr Interv Cardiol Rep 2000;2:213-217.

84. Laham RJ, Rezaee M, Post M, et al: Intrapericardial administration of basic fibroblast growth factor: Myocardial and tissue distribution and comparison with intracoronary and intravenous administration. Catheter Cardiovasc Interv 2003;58:375-381.

85. Yla-Herttuala S: Percutaneous transcoronary venous access for cellular cardiomyoplasty. Lancet 2003;362:1252.

86. Henry TD: Therapeutic angiogenesis. BMJ 1999;318:1536-1539.

87. Perin EC, et al: Improved exercise capacity and ischemia 6 and 12 months after transendocardial injection of autologous bone marrow mononuclear cells for ischemic cardiomyopathy. Circulation 2004;110(11 Suppl 1):II-213-II-218.

88. Sherman W: Cellular therapy for chronic myocardial disease: Nonsurgical approaches. Basic Appl Myol 2003;13:11-14.

89. Kornowski R, Fuchs S, Leon MB: Detection of myocardial viability in the catheterization laboratory using the Biosense-guided electromechanical mapping system. Int J Cardiovasc Interv 1999;2:125-128.

90. Sarmento-Leite R, Silva GV, Dohmann HF, et al: Comparison of left ventricular electromechanical mapping and left ventricular angiography: Defining practical standards for analysis of NOGA maps. Tex Heart Inst J 2003;30:19-26.

91. Hill JM, Dick AJ, Raman VK, et al: Serial cardiac magnetic resonance imaging of injected mesenchymal stem cells. Circulation 2003;108:1009-1014.

92. Rickers C, Gallegos R, Seethamraju ZJ, et al: Applications of magnetic resonance imaging for cardiac stem cell therapy. J Interv Cardiol 2004;17:37-46.

93. Inoue MI, Ueda H, Naruko M, et al: Vascular endothelial growth factor (VGEF) expression in human coronary athetrosclerotic lesions: Possible pathophysiological signficance of VEGF in progression of atherosclerosis. Circ J 1998;98:2108-2116.

94. Simons M, Annex BH, Laham RJ, et al: Pharmacological treatment of coronary artery disease with recombinant fibroblast growth factor-2: Double-blind, randomized, controlled clinical trial. Circulation 2002;105:788-793.

95. Raman SV, Cooke GE, Binkley PF: Stem cell-derived cardiomyocytes demonstrate arrhythmic potential. Circ J 2002;106:1294.

96. Lee MS, Makkar RR: Stem-cell transplantation in myocardial infarction: A status report. Ann Intern Med 2004;140:729-737.

97. Dengler TK, Katus HA: Stem cell therapy for the infarcted heart. Herz 2002;27:598-610.

98. Lew WY: Mobilizing cells to the injured myocardium: A novel rescue strategy or an unwelcome intrusion? J Am Coll Cardiol 2004;44:1521-1522.

99. Marzullo P: Nuclear imaging after cell implantation. Int J Cardiol 2004;95(Suppl 1):S53-S54.

100. Smits AM, van Vleit P, Hassink RJ, et al: The role of stem cells in cardiac regeneration. J Cell Mol Med 2005;9:25-36.

101. Yoon YS, Lee N, Scadova H: Myocardial regeneration with bone-marrow-derived stem cells. Biol Cell 2005;97:253-263.

CHAPTER 41

Pediatric Heart Transplantation

William J. Dreyer
Steven A. Webber

The first pediatric cardiac transplantation was performed in December 1967 a few days after the first adult cardiac transplantation was performed.[1] Although the transplant was an historic event, the patient survived only a few hours. Additional procedures were attempted in the ensuing years; however, long-term survival was not achieved, primarily because of a lack of effective immunosuppressive medications. Interest in cardiac transplantation waned in the 1970s, and it was not until the introduction of cyclosporine-based immunosuppressive regimens in 1979 that long-term survival became feasible. Cooley performed the first successful orthotopic cardiac transplantation in 1984 while Bailey performed the first successful neonatal orthotopic cardiac transplantation in 1985.

In the 1980s and 1990s, a resurgence in interest and dramatic strides in adult and pediatric cardiac transplantation occurred. Advances including improved donor and recipient selection, improvement in the preservation of donor hearts, refinements in surgical technique, and the ability to detect and treat allograft rejection have contributed to the length of patient survival and improved quality of life. Significant limitations still exist, however, including the lifelong need for immunosuppressive medications and the potential toxicities associated with the continued use of these drugs, the development of post-transplant lymphoproliferative disease, and chronic rejection or transplant coronary vascular disease. This chapter updates the clinician regarding the current status of pediatric cardiac transplantation, highlights advances in the field, identifies ongoing controversies and problematic areas of management, and introduces potential new prospects for the future management of these challenging patients. Additional information can be obtained from several other recent reviews.[2-4]

INDICATIONS FOR CARDIAC TRANSPLANTATION

At our institution, cardiac transplantation is considered an alternative therapy when no other form of long-term palliation is considered possible. **Dilated cardiomyopathy** is the principal diagnosis for most of these patients. Heart failure refractory to appropriate medical therapy is the primary indication for cardiac transplantation in our patient population. Defining "refractory to appropriate medical therapy" is not always easy, however. Patients with heart failure symptoms who cannot be weaned from intravenous inotropic support fall into this category. Patients managed on diuretics, angiotensin-converting enzyme inhibitors, and β-blockers with or without digoxin who have persistent New York Heart Association class III or IV heart failure symptoms, ongoing failure to thrive, or severely depressed ventricular function after 6 months of appropriate therapy should be considered candidates for cardiac transplantation.

Patients with **surgically palliated congenital heart disease** no longer amenable to additional surgery who have ongoing heart failure symptoms or a degree of cyanosis that severely limits their day-to-day living constitute a second major group of patients undergoing cardiac transplantation. Occasionally, patients have what is otherwise considered inoperable congenital heart disease (e.g., hypoplastic left heart syndrome with severe tricuspid valve insufficiency or depressed right ventricular function or both, certain severe cases of Ebstein anomaly), and cardiac transplantation should be considered as a primary therapeutic option. More controversial is cardiac transplantation as primary therapy of patients with uncomplicated hypoplastic left heart syndrome. Most centers today perform staged reconstruction with some modification of the Norwood approach with excellent short-term results. Other lesions with a high risk for sudden death without cardiac transplantation (i.e., restrictive cardiomyopathy, intractable ventricular arrhythmias, Kawasaki disease with giant coronary artery aneurysms) constitute a small but important group in which cardiac transplantation should be considered.

The appropriate indications for cardiac transplantation in children were the focus of a consensus statement from the Pediatric Committee of the American Society of Transplantation.[5] The committee also identified other areas of continuing controversy. Survivors of childhood **malignancy** previously treated with anthracyclines, with or without mediastinal radiation, who go on to develop intractable heart failure represent a difficult management dilemma. The risk of recurrent disease or new-onset malignancy in the face of long-term immunosuppression after transplantation is poorly defined.

Much less experience exists with concurrent or recently treated malignancy, especially primary cardiac tumors. Our experience has included one patient with a left atrial rhabdomyosarcoma who had primary resection, chemotherapy, and cardiac transplantation. He died from metastatic disease refractory to further chemotherapy. Similar experience has been documented in the literature.[6-8] Similarly, cardiac transplantation in children with chronic infection with hepatitis B, hepatitis C, or human immunodeficiency virus (HIV) is controversial, in part because so little experience in this area has been documented. Most data have been extrapolated from adults, or from transplantation of other organs.

Data from the Seventh Official Pediatric Report of the Registry for the International Society of Heart and Lung Transplantation (ISHLT) show that the indications for cardiac transplantation vary as a function of age. For the period of January 1996 through June 2003, among infants younger than 1 year old, 30% had cardiomyopathy, and 66% had congenital heart disease. Among children 1 to 10 years old, 52% had cardiomyopathy, and among adolescents 11 to 17 years old, 62% had cardiomyopathy. Congenital heart disease was the indication for transplantation in 37% and 28% of patients in these two groups, respectively.[9]

EVALUATION AND MANAGEMENT OF THE RECIPIENT

At our institution, a team of specialists, including cardiologists, infectious disease specialists, immunologists, nutritionists, social and financial counselors, and child life specialists, evaluates every prospective recipient. Pretransplant evaluation includes a detailed history, physical examination, hemodynamic assessment by cardiac catheterization, and complete anatomic evaluation of the heart and pulmonary vasculature. Estimation of indexed pulmonary vascular resistance (PVR) (see later) is a vital component in determining suitability for transplantation. Determination of ABO type, determination of the presence of antibodies against human HLA, and screening for serologic evidence of prior exposure to several infectious agents (Toxoplasma, cytomegalovirus, Epstein-Barr virus (EBV), varicella zoster, herpes simplex, hepatitis A through D, and HIV) are performed. Evaluations of other organ system functions by standard biochemical and imaging techniques are essential for determining suitability for and risk of transplantation and for planning immediate postoperative care. Contraindications to transplantation are elevated PVR index, active infection or malignancy, and noncardiac conditions that limit life expectancy. Poor social support and medical noncompliance also can be contraindications to cardiac transplantation.

Management of a pretransplant patient poses many challenges. A high percentage of patients require intravenous inotropic support and await cardiac transplantation while hospitalized. Patients managed on an outpatient basis return to the clinic at least once every 4 weeks. Optimizing nutrition and maintaining overall conditioning can be difficult in this end-stage population, but are paramount to the overall success of the patient's perioperative course. Malnutrition and growth failure are common secondary to anorexia and vomiting associated with high venous pressures and low cardiac output and are worsened by malabsorption and the hypermetabolic state of heart failure. Comorbid disorders, such as protein-losing enteropathy and chronic liver and renal disease, may contribute to ongoing nutritional disorders. Before transplantation, immunizations should be given according to current recommendations, unless the probability of transplantation within the next month is high. Waiting times for heart transplant patients vary greatly and at our institution have ranged from 1 day to more than 2 years. Waiting times are based on the patient's severity of illness, blood type, and size. The highest priority is given to the sickest patients.

Pulmonary vascular resistance is a crucial issue in the evaluation of any candidate for cardiac transplantation. If the PVR is excessive and fixed, the thin-walled right ventricle of the donor heart, especially after an imposed ischemic time, acutely fails, and the patient cannot be weaned from cardiopulmonary bypass. The absolute upper limit of PVR index that is acceptable is uncertain, and institutional practices vary. In adults, a PVR greater than 5 Wood units, or a transpulmonary gradient greater than 15 mm Hg, correlates with increased perioperative mortality.[10] Children may be able to undergo successful transplantation with higher PVR indices than their adult counterparts, however.[11] At our institution, patients with a PVR index greater than 4 Wood units at cardiac catheterization undergo additional testing for reactivity of the pulmonary vascular bed in response to 100% oxygen and, if necessary, with the subsequent administration of inhaled nitric oxide up to 80 ppm. A fixed PVR index greater than 10 Wood units is considered a contraindication to cardiac transplantation.

SURGICAL CONSIDERATIONS IN HEART TRANSPLANTATION

Technique of Implantation

For patients with straightforward anatomy, two basic surgical techniques have been employed (Figs. 41-1 and 41-2). For years, **biatrial anastomoses** were performed, avoiding individual systemic and pulmonary venous connections. Patients were left with capacious atrial chambers, however, comprising donor and recipient components, contracting asynchronously. Since 1999, our surgeons have removed the entire right atrium and have left only a small cuff of left atrial tissue incorporating

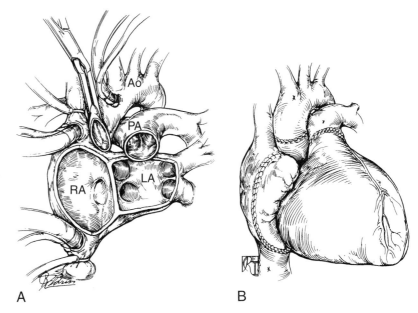

FIGURE 41-1 ■ Cardiac transplantation with biatrial anastomosis. A, The recipient cardiectomy has been completed via a median sternotomy after institution of cardiopulmonary bypass with aortic and bicaval cannulation. The four anastomoses were performed in the following sequence: (1) left atrial (LA), (2) aortic (Ao), (3) right atrial (RA), and (4) pulmonary artery (PA). B, The completed anastomoses are seen. (From Backer CL, Mavroudis C: *Pediatric transplantation.* In Stuart FP, Abecassis MM, Kaufman DB [eds]: *Organ Transplantation.* Georgetown, Tex, Landes Bioscience, 2000.)

the pulmonary veins. The donor left atrium is sewn into place, and **bicaval anastomoses** are performed, creating a more normal anatomic result. Theoretically, this technique is believed to improve sinus node function, invoke less tricuspid regurgitation, and improve cardiac output.[12,13] Only preliminary data are available in children, however, to show that outcomes are improved by this implantation technique.[14]

Transplantation for Complex Congenital Heart Disease

Children with complex congenital heart disease represent approximately one half of all referrals for consideration for transplantation. Other than newborns with hypoplastic

left heart syndrome, most of these children have undergone multiple prior surgical palliative or corrective procedures.[15] Frequently, there are stenoses, hypoplastic segments, or even discontinuities of the branch pulmonary arteries. Anomalies of systemic and pulmonary venous return, particularly in the context of **atrial isomerism** or mirror-imaged atrial arrangement, pose additional challenges for the surgeon. A series of reports described specialized surgical techniques for dealing with these complex anomalies of the heart and great vessels, including abnormalities of atrial arrangement.[15-19] In experienced centers, survival has been comparable with patients transplanted for cardiomyopathy, although the

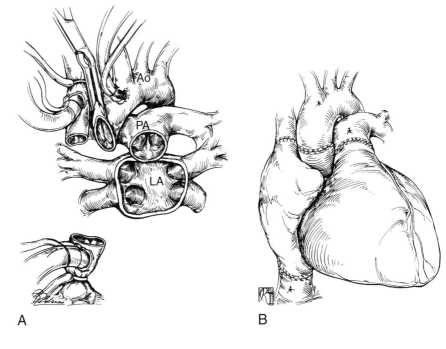

FIGURE 41-2 ■ Cardiac transplantation with bicaval anastomosis. A, The recipient cardiectomy has been completed via a median sternotomy after institution of cardiopulmonary bypass with aortic and bicaval cannulation. The recipient right atrium has been removed. The anastomoses were performed in the following sequence: (1) left atrial (LA), (2) aortic (Ao), (3) inferior vena cava, (4) pulmonary artery (PA), and (5) superior vena cava. B, The completed anastomoses are seen. (From Backer CL, Mavroudis C: *Pediatric transplantation.* In Stuart FP, Abecassis MM, Kaufman DB [eds]: *Organ Transplantation.* Georgetown, Tex, Landes Bioscience, 2000.)

donor ischemic times, postoperative stays in the intensive care unit, and length of hospitalization are prolonged compared with patients with cardiomyopathy.[15,16] Failure to recognize the presence of significant aortopulmonary collateral circulation in patients with cyanotic heart disease may contribute to high output failure occurring soon after transplantation.[20] This situation emphasizes the importance of comprehensive preoperative anatomic evaluation and planning in this difficult group of patients.

A patient with a **failed Fontan** procedure poses additional challenges related to premorbid states, such as protein-losing enteropathy, chronic liver disease, and pulmonary arteriovenous malformations. The last-mentioned are most common in patients with a previous classic Glenn anastomosis and when hepatic venous return is excluded from the cavopulmonary repair, especially in the setting of left isomerism. Resolution of small pulmonary arteriovenous malformations may occur after transplantation,[21] although it would seem unlikely that large lesions would regress rapidly. In the latter setting, the patient may remain severely cyanotic after transplantation, potentially leading to primary failure of the transplanted heart from hypoxemia. Increasing numbers of patients with complex palliated congenital heart disease are being referred for consideration of transplantation in adult life. Results from children cannot be readily extrapolated to adults. In general, the results of transplantation for congenital heart disease in adults are poor compared with the results in children, although the precise reasons for this are unclear.[22,23]

Mechanical Circulatory Support

Mechanical circulatory support has been used to bridge infants and children to cardiac transplantation for many years.[24] Extracorporeal membrane oxygenation or the use of a centrifugal pump head without an inline oxygenator for left ventricular support only are the techniques most widely used in infants and small children because pulsatile ventricular assist devices generally are not available for use in this population. In general, it is hard to support children more than 2 weeks using this technology, because of escalating problems with bleeding, sepsis, and secondary end-organ dysfunction. Pretransplant mortality is high, and the postoperative course is often difficult. The overall chance of achieving hospital discharge after listing for transplantation is around 50%.[24]

Older children can be successfully bridged to transplantation using ventricular assist devices originally designed for use in adults.[25,26] At our institution, we have successfully bridged seven children to transplantation using left heart or biventricular support with a Thoratec (Thoratec Laboratories, Berkeley, CA) assist device (see Chapter 48). The Thoratec system has been employed successfully in children weighing as little as 17 kg. In Europe, more effort has been extended to produce pneumatically driven paracorporeal devices for children.

The greatest experience is with the pediatric version of the Berlin Heart (Mediport Kardiotechnik, Berlin, Germany). A second, similar, system also has been developed in Germany (Medos HIA VAD, Stolberg, Germany). Both systems have been used successfully to bridge small children, including neonates, to transplantation.[27,28] Major obstacles to further development of such devices for children in the United States have been the small market, prolonged time to develop and test new systems, and the extremely high costs of such development. A push by clinicians and renewed interest by industry have resulted, however, in several new systems appropriate to pediatric use now in development.

IMMUNOSUPPRESSIVE THERAPY FOR HEART TRANSPLANTATION

The recipient of a transplanted heart invariably mounts an immune response to foreign antigens contained within the graft. All recipients, even neonates, require potent immunosuppressive therapy. This immune response is most vigorous in the early weeks and months after transplant, but is believed to persist for the life of the graft. In contrast to the case with some liver transplant patients, there is no evidence that recipients of cardiac transplants can be withdrawn from immunosuppressive therapy, even late after transplantation. Clinical immunosuppression aims to prevent or minimize the immune response of the host to donor antigens, while avoiding complications of immunodeficiency, such as infections and malignancy (Fig. 41-3 and Table 41-1). It is also important to minimize non-immune toxicities, including diabetes, nephrotoxicity, neurotoxicity, hyperlipidemia, bone marrow suppression, and Cushingoid side effects. Immunosuppressive therapy can be broken down into induction therapy, maintenance therapy, and rescue therapy in cases of acute rejection.

Induction Therapy

Induction therapy is used to produce an immunosuppressed state rapidly in the host patient immediately after transplantation. Drugs available for this purpose include **monoclonal** or **polyclonal antibody** preparations directed against T cells, such as OKT3 or antithymocyte globulin. More recently available are two monoclonal antibodies directed against the alpha chain of the interleukin-2 receptor, basiliximab and daclizumab. The use of induction therapy is controversial. Data reported in the Seventh Official Pediatric Report of the Registry for the ISHLT suggest that the percentage of patients receiving induction therapy of any form has increased in U.S. centers to almost 45%.[9] Despite an increased use of induction immunosuppressive therapy in pediatric recipients, a review of frequency-of-rejection and survival data has failed to show a significant beneficial effect from this treatment.

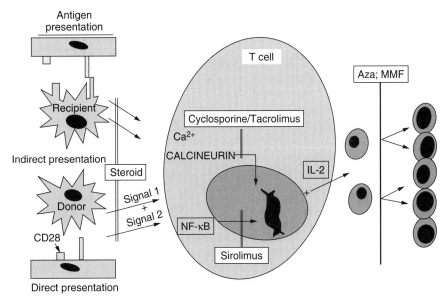

FIGURE 41-3 ■ Sites of action of immuno-suppressive agents. Schematic diagram shows the essential steps in immune recognition of allografts. Antigen presentation first involves either recipient (indirect presentation) or donor (direct presentation) antigen presenting cells. The HLA antigens and CD28 (costimu-latory ligands) are required to signal the T cells. The signaling process involves either a calcineurin or nuclear factor (NF)-κB pathway to increase nuclear transcription of cytokines such as interleukin (IL)-2. This increased nuclear transcription leads to expansion of T cell clones exhibiting graft-specific reactivity. The sites of action for steroids, cyclosporine, tacrolimus, sirolimus, azathioprine (Aza), and mycophenolate mofetil (MMF) are shown. (From Boucek RJ, Boucek MM: *Pediatric heart transplantation. Curr Opin Pediatr* 2002;14:611-619.)

Maintenance Immunosuppression

Maintenance immunosuppression regimens used in pediatric heart transplant recipients tend to be individual-specific and institution-specific. The strategies take advantage of the selectivity of immunosuppressive agents for critical pathways in graft rejection. Virtually all immunosuppressive regimens in children are based on the use of a calcineurin inhibitor, either **cyclosporine** or **tacrolimus**. Before 2000, nearly four fifths of all recipients received cyclosporine, with the remainder receiving tacrolimus.[29] The proportion of pediatric patients receiving tacrolimus has increased markedly, however. Now more than 40% of all patients receive tacrolimus-based immunosuppression,[9] although the

two agents have not been compared in randomized trials in children after thoracic organ transplantation. Usual doses of cyclosporine range from 5 to 10 mg/kg/day, and trough levels are usually maintained in the range of 100 to 300 ng/mL. The usual oral dose range for tacrolimus is 0.05 to 0.3 mg/kg/day, with trough levels maintained in the range of 5 to 15 ng/mL.

Most centers also use a second or third agent in the immunosuppression therapy.[29] Antiproliferative agents and corticosteroids are the most commonly used adjunctive therapies. **Azathioprine** has been the most commonly used antiproliferative agent, although now there is increasing use of **mycophenolate mofetil** (MMF). MMF is believed to be a more specific

TABLE 41-1

U.S. Food and Drug Administration–Approved Immunosuppressive Agents			
Generic Name	**Proprietary Name/Manufacturer**	**Type of Agent**	**Clinical Use**
Tacrolimus	Prograf/Fujisawa	Calcineurin inhibitor	Maintenance therapy
Microemulsion cyclosporines	Neoral/Novartis and other generic preparations	Calcineurin inhibitor	Maintenance therapy
Mycophenolate mofetil	CellCept/Roche	Inhibitor of de novo pathway of purine biosynthesis	Adjunctive therapy in lieu of azathioprine
Sirolimus (rapamycin)	Rapamune/Wyeth-Ayerst	TOR inhibitor	Adjunctive therapy in lieu of azathioprine or mycophenolate mofetil
Basiliximab	Simulect/Novartis	Antibody to IL-2 receptor	Induction therapy
Daclizumab	Zenapax/Roche	Antibody to IL-2 receptor	Induction therapy
Rabbit ATG	Thymoglobulin/SangStat	Rabbit polyclonal antibody	Induction therapy or treatment of severe rejection

ATG, antithymocyte globulin; IL-2, interleukin-2; TOR, target of rapamycin.
From Webber SA: The current state of and future prospects for cardiac transplantation in children. Cardiol Young 2003;13:64–83.

antilymphocyte agent. Azathioprine usually is administered in the range of 1 to 3 mg/kg/day. Absorption and metabolism of MMF vary with age, other drugs in the regimen, and time after transplantation. Doses of MMF vary widely, ranging from 30 to 50 mg/kg/day. At our institution, the starting dose of MMF is 20 mg/kg/dose given twice daily. The dosing of both agents should be adjusted based on the serial white blood cell count. More recently, serum mycophenolic acid levels have become available, with a recommended serum trough level of 2 to 4 considered efficacious.

There have been no randomized trials of MMF in children, but there was one large multicenter trial in adults after cardiac transplantation.[30] This was a randomized, blinded study from 28 centers in Australia, Europe, and North America comparing therapy consisting of cyclosporine, corticosteroids, and azathioprine with therapy with cyclosporine, corticosteroids, and MMF. There was a high withdrawal rate from the study—approximately two fifths of each group. Survival and rejection were similar in the two randomized groups. In patients who received mycophenolate, there was a statistically significant reduction in mortality at 1 year (6.2% versus 11.4% for patients receiving azathioprine). Survival at 3 years was 88% in patients treated with mycophenolate and 82% in patients receiving azathioprine. There was also a reduction in the requirement for treatment of rejection at 1 year.

Rapamycin, or **sirolimus**, is a newly introduced antiproliferative agent with a novel mechanism of immunosuppression with potent immunosuppressive properties.[31] Sirolimus blocks the costimulatory signal mediated by nuclear factor-κB, and there is increasing evidence that this agent can be used safely with cyclosporine and tacrolimus, despite the fact that it targets the same binding protein as tacrolimus. Sirolimus seems to act synergistically with the calcineurin inhibitors, blocking interleukin-2 signaling. Case reports support its efficacy in treating refractory rejection.[32] Indications for use of sirolimus after pediatric heart transplantation remain to be defined. Based on extrapolation from indications in other solid-organ transplantation, however, sirolimus could be useful to withdraw or reduce the dose of the calcineurin inhibitors for toxicity (e.g., renal dysfunction) or EBV-mediated lymphoproliferative disease after transplantation.[31] Trials also are under way to determine if therapeutic levels of sirolimus can reduce the proliferative component of accelerated graft coronary vascular disease (see later).

Similarly, **everolimus** is a new drug being developed for the prevention of acute and chronic rejection in solid-organ transplants. Everolimus is a proliferation inhibitor that acts synergistically with cyclosporine and has been effective in preclinical models of kidney, heart, and lung transplantation.[33] A single multicenter clinical trial in adult cardiac transplant patients performed in Europe comparing everolimus with azathioprine showed less coronary intimal thickening in the everolimus group over a 12-month interval.[34] Pediatric experience is limited to a few renal transplant patients in Europe,[35] but this drug is believed to hold significant promise as a future therapeutic agent in children and adults. U.S. Food and Drug Administration approval for clinical trials in the United States is currently pending.

Approximately three quarters of pediatric heart transplant recipients receive **corticosteroids** at the time of hospital discharge; however, by 3 years from transplantation, this has fallen to one half.[29] There are no randomized trials of routine use of corticosteroids versus their avoidance in children after heart transplantation. Long-term corticosteroid use in pediatric patients has been linked in some centers to several undesirable risks, such as higher risks for opportunistic infections, diabetes, and bone demineralization. Some centers have reported the withdrawal of corticosteroids in the medium term of 6 months to 2 years after transplantation[36,37] or even the avoidance of maintenance corticosteroids in the immunosuppressive regimen after transplantation.[38,39] It currently is speculated that the use of antibody induction therapy, tacrolimus as primary immunosuppressant, and newer adjunctive agents such as MMF and sirolimus may enhance the ability to achieve complete avoidance or early withdrawal of corticosteroids.

All of the currently available immunosuppressive medications have known side effects or toxicities. Side effects of cyclosporine include nephrotoxicity, hypertension, neurotoxicity, electrolyte imbalance, hirsutism, and gingival hyperplasia. Tacrolimus has similar side effects excluding the hirsutism and gingival hyperplasia, but has the added risk of causing hyperglycemia. The use of sirolimus is associated with hyperlipidemia and bone marrow suppression. Azathioprine can cause significant myelosuppression. MMF is less myelosuppressive than azathioprine, but has worse gastrointestinal side effects. The side effects of corticosteroids are well known and include Cushingoid habitus, increased appetite, hypertension, diabetes, gastritis and gastric ulceration, growth retardation, and osteoporosis. The associated side effects of these medications may dictate to some extent the specific regimen used in individual patients.

COMPLICATIONS AFTER HEART TRANSPLANTATION

Acute Cellular Rejection

Acute failure of the transplanted heart is the most common cause of death in the first 30 days after transplantation and occurs with greater frequency in infant recipients.[9,29] From 1 to 5 years after transplantation, acute cellular rejection and infection are the most common causes of death. Beyond 5 years, chronic rejection becomes the dominant cause of loss of either the heart or the patient. Understanding the timing of and risk factors for acute rejection is vital for designing logical strategies for surveillance and prevention. There is an important distinction between acute rejection and acute dysfunction of the heart. The two terms are not synonymous. Most acute rejection in the heart is not associated with overt dysfunction, although subtle subclinical abnormalities of diastolic function are common. When cardiac failure does occur in the first few years after transplantation, acute cellular rejection is the most likely diagnosis, although other pathologies must be entertained, such as humoral (antibody mediated) rejection,[40] acute presentation of chronic rejection secondary to post-transplant coronary artery disease, and viral myocarditis. An intriguing group of patients remains in whom acute dysfunction, sometimes reversible with augmentation of immunosuppression, occurs without evidence of significant cellular, humoral, or chronic rejection.[41] The pathophysiology of this phenomenon remains an enigma, making it hard to develop logical strategies for treatment.

Most recipients in childhood experience at least one episode of moderate or severe acute cellular rejection. Data from the Pediatric Heart Transplant Study, a research study group of 28 North American centers undertaking transplantation in children, shows that approximately two thirds of recipients are free from rejection by 1 month after transplantation, but this decreases to less than one third by 1 year.[2] The peak hazard, or instantaneous risk, for rejection after heart transplantation is around 1 to 2 months after transplantation. Late episodes of acute rejection (i.e., after >1 year post-transplantation) also have been studied more recently within the consortium.[42]

Episodes of acute rejection occurring late after transplantation were diagnosed in one quarter of recipients, with a probability of freedom from late rejection of 82% at 2 years and 73% at 3 years after transplantation. In contrast to the first episodes of rejection occurring early after transplantation, the hazard for late rejection is more constant, with an ongoing risk for as long as the cohort has been followed. This ongoing risk for acute rejection correlates with the clinical observation that recipients do not tolerate discontinuation of immunosuppression, which at this time must be considered a lifelong therapy.

Risk factors for rejection in children include older age at transplant, African American race, cytomegalovirus, gender mismatch, and a previous episode of rejection.[42-46] Hemodynamically significant rejection episodes predict a particularly poor outcome, with approximately 50% mortality in the year after the episode.[45,46]

There has been significant interest in the investigation of genetic risk factors of the recipient for outcomes regarding the transplanted organ and the well-being of the patient. Most attention has focused on genetic polymorphisms for cytokines, and other genes involved in immune responses. Awad and colleagues[47] have observed that high producers of the proinflammatory cytokine tumor necrosis factor-α and low producers of the anti-inflammatory cytokine interleukin-10 are more likely to experience recurrent cardiac rejection in the first year after transplantation. They also investigated polymorphisms of other genes that may influence outcome. Of particular interest are genes that influence individual responses to various immunosuppressive drugs, such as the multidrug resistance gene *MDR1*. The same group more recently has noted that certain polymorphisms of this gene, at exons 21 and 26, correlate with an increased chance of weaning children from corticosteroids within the first year after transplantation.[48] Most African Americans carry pharmacogenomic polymorphisms at loci that are associated with decreased immunosuppressive efficacy, perhaps explaining the observation that African Americans have poorer outcomes after transplantation, with worse profiles for rejection. These kinds of genetic studies hold promise that clinicians will be able to predict the risk of an individual patient for acute rejection and tailor immunosuppressive therapy to the needs of the individual.

Rejection in pediatric heart transplant recipients often is not associated with symptoms. However, recipients with rejection (especially infants) may present with a history of poor feeding, irritability, malaise, fever, nausea, and abdominal pain. Accompanying physical findings may include tachycardia, a gallop rhythm, rales, hepatomegaly, and new-onset arrhythmias. Although ECG evidence of low QRS voltages is a common finding, the specificity and sensitivity are poor. Numerous noninvasive tools have been used to diagnose cellular rejection with conflicting results. Although echocardiography has been widely used to diagnose cellular rejection,[49] in our experience, moderate acute cellular rejection frequently is associated with a normal or stable echocardiogram.

For this reason, most centers, including ours, still use rejection surveillance programs based on **endomyocardial biopsy**. The utility and safety of endomyocardial biopsy are well established.[50,51] An adequate biopsy sample should contain four to six pieces of endomyocardium. These samples are stained with hematoxylin and eosin, and a standard biopsy grading system developed by the ISHLT is used for grading the severity of the rejection and guiding treatment.[52] The biopsy sample also is useful in assessing the presence of viral genome by polymerase chain reaction, a marker for myocarditis and a predictor of poor outcome in some patients.[53-55] Episodes of moderate-to-severe acute cellular rejection are treated with intravenous methylprednisolone at 10 to 20 mg/kg for three to four doses, whereas episodes that are refractory to corticosteroids are treated with anti–T cell antibody preparations (e.g., OKT3 or antithymocyte globulin).

Humoral Rejection

Humoral rejection is much less common than cellular rejection and generally occurs when a patient with preformed anti-HLA antibodies receives an organ containing antigens to which the recipient has been sensitized previously. This allosensitization is usually due to prior blood product transfusion or homograft materials used during previous surgical palliations for congenital heart defects or associated with mechanical ventricular support. Most centers screen serum from each prospective transplant recipient for the presence of preformed anti-HLA, **panel reactive antibodies**. These antibodies are detected by testing the recipient's serum against a panel of lymphocytes from numerous donors selected to represent all of the common HLA antigens. The management of an ambulatory candidate with an elevated panel reactive antibodies screen is controversial. Prospective crossmatching of the candidate serum against lymphocytes from a prospective donor may be attempted, but often is not feasible because most donor hearts for children are procured from distant sites where recipient serum is not available. Attempts can be made to reduce the level of recipient anti-HLA antibodies.

Strategies that have been used to achieve this reduction of anti-HLA antibodies include the use of intravenous pooled immunoglobulin,[56] plasmapheresis,[57] and agents that may inhibit production of antibodies by B cells.[58,59] The newest agent in this regard is the anti–B cell monoclonal antibody, rituximab (Rituxan; Genentech Inc/IDEC Pharmaceuticals, South San Francisco, CA); this is a human/mouse chimeric monoclonal antibody directed against the CD20 antigen carried on almost all B cells.[60]

In a critically ill child, a negative prospective crossmatch is unlikely to be achieved before the death of the patient. A decision must be made as to whether the first ABO compatible donor of suitable size will be used, regardless of the potential result of crossmatching. These candidates can be managed with a similar protocol of plasmapheresis pretransplantation, which can be continued intraoperatively and postoperatively. This protocol should minimize the risk of hyperacute rejection with immediate vascular thrombosis and graft failure. Ongoing problems related to humoral sensitization may occur, including severe acute rejection often associated with graft dysfunction. The endomyocardial biopsy sample frequently shows marked edema and endothelial activation, but with little cellular infiltrate.

Few experimental studies are available to guide the treatment of humoral rejection beyond plasmapheresis[61]; however, in our own experience, a protocol of intravenous immunoglobulin and rituximab has been successful. Induction cytolytic therapy with anti–T cell antibodies is a consideration because humoral responses may up-regulate cellular immune responses. Triple-drug therapy is indicated, and MMF and rapamycin are logical choices for adjunctive therapy because they may suppress production of antibodies with greater efficiency than azathioprine. There is increasing evidence that antibodies play a role in the development of chronic rejection.[62] Although an aggressive approach to the management of the sensitized patient may allow for short-term and medium-term survival, the long-term consequences of transplanting sensitized children, especially with a positive crossmatch, are unknown.

Chronic Rejection or Post-transplantation Coronary Artery Disease

Coronary artery disease subsequent to transplantation is an accelerated vasculopathy that is the leading cause of death in late survivors of heart transplantation.[29] The pathology differs from that of ischemic heart disease in the normal adult population.[63] Typical allograft coronary artery disease consists of myointimal proliferation that is concentric and involves the entire length of the vessel, including intramyocardial branches with eventual luminal occlusion.

One third to one half of adult recipients have angiographic or autopsy evidence of coronary vascular disease by 5 years after transplantation. Moderate-to-severe disease occurred in 15% of patients registered in the multicenter adult Cardiac Transplant Research database maintained at the University of Alabama, Birmingham.[64] Using the same method of diagnosis, the incidence at 5 years after transplantation was 6% among recipients in the Pediatric Heart Transplant Study.[65] Overall, the incidence of any angiographic evidence of coronary disease was 3%, 12%, and 20% at 1, 3, and 5 years after transplantation of children in this dataset. The incidence of this serious complication depends on the method of survey. Most studies have relied on angiography for diagnosis, which tends to underestimate mild disease that may be present in the microvasculature.

Although immune and nonimmune mechanisms are likely to contribute to the development of coronary artery disease, immune mechanisms are probably of central importance in children. Even neonates, with no traditional risk factors, now are recognized to be at risk for the development of coronary artery disease. The immunobiology of chronic rejection is discussed in detail elsewhere.[66] Identification of specific risk factors for development of disease in children has been investigated more recently. Among 1032 recipients at 18 centers in the Pediatric Heart Transplant Study, older recipient age, older donor age (especially >30 years old), and greater number of episodes of rejection in the first year were the main risk factors for the development of coronary artery disease.[65] Donor age older than 30 years tripled the risk of disease at 5 years after transplantation.

The diagnosis of coronary vasculopathy is difficult. Patients are often asymptomatic until they present with sudden death. As the heart is denervated, patients usually do not experience typical ischemic chest pain. A symptom complex of atypical chest or abdominal pain coupled with other gastrointestinal complaints, heart failure, or syncope often may be the initial presentation.[67] Standard treadmill and nuclear scans for the detection of coronary artery disease generally are not adequate in this population. Myocardial perfusion scanning, dobutamine stress echocardiography, and MRI techniques are under investigation as more definitive noninvasive diagnostic techniques. Only limited experience has been reported at this time in children.[68,69]

Angiography traditionally has been the gold standard for detection of coronary artery disease in children and adults. Angiography has serious limitations, however, beyond the obvious facts that it is invasive and expensive as a screening tool. Angiography is a relatively insensitive marker of mild coronary artery disease secondary to the diffuse nature of the disease process and the propensity to affect small vessels, although severe epicardial disease that portends a poor prognosis is readily apparent. It has proved difficult to predict prognosis for patients with mild-to-moderate disease, many of whom may do well for several years after diagnosis. Some pediatric centers advocate listing for retransplantation at the time of diagnosis of any angiographic abnormality because of the progressive nature of the disease and the tendency for angiography to underestimate the degree of vessel involvement. Despite its limitations, in our institution, we continue to perform coronary angiography annually to assess risk. Intravascular coronary ultrasound has a greater sensitivity for detection of graft vasculopathy than angiography.

Studies in adults have reported the frequent occurrence of abnormalities on **intravascular ultrasound**, despite angiographically normal appearances of the coronary arteries.[70] Several studies from large programs involving children also have shown discrepancies between findings from coronary angiography and intravascular ultrasound, abnormalities commonly being predicted by ultrasound when angiography is deemed normal.[71-74] At present, however, correlation between intravascular coronary ultrasound findings and clinical outcome is lacking in pediatrics. Although intravascular ultrasound can be performed safely in children, its use in pediatric recipients may be limited because of the potential risks associated with the manipulation of these imaging catheters in small coronary vessels. As technology improves, and greater experience is gained, the long-term safety and prognostic value of these studies in children should be forthcoming. Prospective, multicenter studies are needed, however, to study the role of intravascular ultrasound in this patient population.

Beyond retransplantation, no effective treatment exists for established coronary artery disease because bypass grafting and coronary angioplasty have limited utility as a result of the diffuse nature of the disease. Similarly, stenting is of limited use because of intimal proliferation through the stent and because of progression of the

disease in other areas. Rapamycin-coated stents have shown great promise for preventing restenosis in ischemic heart disease,[75] but are relatively untested in this patient population. Even retransplantation represents a limited option. As a result of the re-do nature of the procedure, many patients experience greater perioperative morbidity. Existing end-organ toxicities from the first transplant also can render immunosuppression more difficult. Patients may be at risk for accelerated development of coronary vascular disease in the second organ, and a shortage of donors exist, especially for an older child, who will be competing with adults for donor organs.

Several pharmacologic approaches have been used for prevention of coronary artery disease after transplantation. Anecdotal reports, small clinical trials in adults, and experimental models in animals suggest that many agents may be potentially useful in the prevention of graft vasculopathy and coronary arterial events, including calcium antagonists, angiotensin-converting enzyme inhibitors, antioxidants such as vitamin E, statins, aspirin, and antiproliferative agents such as MMF and rapamycin. Rapamycin is of particular interest because it has been shown to prevent the development and progression of graft vasculopathy in numerous animal transplantation models, including primates.[76] It will take many years before it is known whether this or any other agent, can reduce the incidence and severity of chronic rejection in human recipients of transplanted hearts. A major side effect of this agent is hyperlipidemia, widely considered to be a risk factor for graft coronary artery disease. Because adherence to complex medical regimens is a significant challenge for many patients and families, it is hard to justify routine use of all of these agents in the absence of proof of efficacy. Large-scale multicenter trials of most of these therapies are unlikely ever to be performed, especially in children.

Infectious Complications

The spectrum of infections after transplantation in children and their prevention and treatment have been the focus of a recent review.[77] An increased prevalence of all forms of infection is seen. Most infections are caused by pathogens that also cause infection in nonimmunocompromised children. Common examples include respiratory viruses, *Streptococcus pneumoniae,* and varicella-zoster virus. All infections that may be seen in nonimmunocompromised patients can cause greater disease severity in the recipient of a transplanted heart, and strategies to achieve prevention and early treatment are imperative. Of particular note in this respect are infections caused by cytomegalovirus and EBV, which only rarely cause severe disease in the immunocompetent host. More rarely, opportunistic infections are seen, such as those due to *Pneumocystis carinii.* Although most infections are well tolerated, infection ranks comparable with early graft failure and rejection as main causes of death after heart transplantation in children.

Relatively few major advances in the prevention and management of infection after transplantation have been realized in recent years. Two important exceptions are infections with cytomegalovirus and EBV (see later). **Cytomegalovirus** is an important cause of morbidity after solid-organ transplantation, but symptomatic disease in children is relatively unusual.[78] Some groups have suggested that cytomegalovirus infection is a risk factor for development of coronary artery disease.[79] It is unknown whether this is true in children, but in an intravascular ultrasound study from Loma Linda, California, increases in maximal intimal thickness and intimal index correlated with cytomegalovirus seropositivity.[71] Since the 1990s, advances in diagnosis, prevention, and treatment of cytomegalovirus have been realized, including widespread availability of ganciclovir as an intravenous and oral antiviral agent, the development of cytomegalovirus immunoglobulin preparations, and assays for rapid diagnosis of active infection from peripheral blood samples (e.g., pp65 antigenemia test and polymerase chain reaction detection of viral genome). The optimal strategies for preventing infection with cytomegalovirus remain to be determined in children.

Recent years have seen major advances in understanding the nature of **Epstein-Barr virus** infection in the immunocompromised host. The immunobiology, nomenclature, management, and possibilities for prevention of symptomatic EBV disease and **post-transplant lymphoproliferative disorders** (PTLD) have been the topics of several recent reviews.[80-85] A review of the Pediatric Heart Transplant Study database identified 56 cases among 1184 primary transplants (4.7%) at 19 North American centers.[86] Greater than 80% were driven by EBV. There is a bimodal presentation of PTLD disease with the early-onset disease usually possessing a less aggressive polymorphic histology and an almost invariable association with primary infection by EBV. Late-onset PTLD, usually presenting beyond 3 years, can have highly varying histology and may be polymorphic, but is often monomorphic with histology resembling aggressive B cell lymphoma.

The clinical manifestations of PTLD are protean.[80] Fever, malaise, weight loss, abdominal pain, and vomiting and diarrhea are common presenting clinical features. In contrast to other transplanted solid organs, disease rarely is seen within the allograft. Most children who develop these disorders are diagnosed with lung nodules, mediastinal or abdominal adenopathy, or both. Gastrointestinal involvement is common, and bleeding, obstruction, or perforation may occur. Central nervous system involvement is rare. Monitoring of EBV viral load in peripheral blood of post-transplant patients by serial quantitative polymerase chain reaction shows promise for detecting early EBV disease and allows for the possibility of early therapeutic intervention.[81]

The development of very high viral loads should alert the physician to look for signs or symptoms of disease, even in an asymptomatic patient. We routinely monitor patients at transplantation who are at risk by monthly polymerase chain reaction for the first 6 to 12 months after transplantation and at the time of development of symptoms suggesting the disease. Studies at other institutions are under way to determine if a preemptive decrease in immunosuppression, use of immunoglobulin preparations with high titers of anti-EBV antibodies, or both can reduce safely the risk of lymphoproliferative disease when high viral loads are detected in an otherwise healthy child.

The mainstay of treatment of PTLD in children is reduction or temporary discontinuation of immunosuppression. In some institutions, this course of action has been associated with cure in approximately four fifths of cases with polymorphic histology. Rebound rejection is common and must be sought by increased echocardiographic and endomyocardial biopsy surveillance. PTLD rarely recurs, even if treatment with pulsed corticosteroid therapy for rebound rejection is required. The monomorphic forms are less likely to respond to a reduction in immunosuppression, but this typically is attempted as first-line therapy because complete remissions have been observed. Monomorphic disease may require treatment with conventional chemotherapeutic agents, as do overtly malignant lymphomas, such as Burkitt lymphoma.

Several other therapies have been proposed. Two therapies are of particular interest because they may treat the condition effectively without requiring global immunocompetence to be re-established. In this way, rebound rejection may be avoided. The first therapy is use of monoclonal antibodies directed against B cell antigens. More than nine tenths of lymphoproliferative disorders are of recipient B cell origin after heart transplantation. In the United States, rituximab is approved for the treatment of certain types of adult B cell non-Hodgkin lymphomas; most lesions express this antigen. Several reports now have suggested that this agent may be a useful therapy for B cell PTLD.[87-89] A trial of this agent in children with refractory disease is in progress. A second novel approach is cellular immunotherapy, whereby the patient is given an infusion of cytotoxic T lymphocytes directed against EBV-specific antigens. This infusion should result in control of the proliferation of the B cells infected with EBV, but without the risk of rejection. EBV-specific cytotoxic T cell therapy already has been developed and applied successfully for the management of PTLD in recipients of transplanted bone marrow.[90] Efforts to achieve this management in recipients of transplanted solid organs are under way in several centers, and preliminary data suggest this should be feasible.[91]

The safety and efficacy of many of the currently available vaccines have not been evaluated thoroughly in the solid-organ transplant recipient. In general, it is believed that immunization can help prevent infectious complications. Although pediatric heart transplant recipients generally are responsive to environmental pathogens after the immediate post-transplant period, immunizations with inactivated preparations against diphtheria, pertussis, tetanus, hepatitis B virus, *Haemophilus influenzae,* pneumococcus, and polio (Salk) are recommended.[92] We withhold these immunizations for the first 12 months post-transplant.

Live viral vaccines should be avoided, despite the apparent ability of pediatric heart recipients to overcome viral infections effectively. Although increasing experience suggests that varicella-naive recipients can acquire varicella immunity in response to wild-type infections, the varicella vaccine has not been studied adequately in heart transplant recipients. We routinely give varicella immunoglobulin for children exposed to varicella after heart transplantation. Also, antiviral therapy is employed when evidence of varicella infection is seen.

Nonimmune Complications

Our focus on rejection, infection, and malignancy emphasize the careful balance that must be achieved between overimmunosuppression and underimmunosuppression. In addition to these complications, recipients experience a wide array of other complications that are unrelated to their immune status; most of these complications reflect end-organ toxicities of immunosuppressive therapies.[93]

As stated earlier, **systemic hypertension** is a common complication, especially in patients receiving cyclosporine and steroid-based immunosuppression. Hypertension generally responds to standard antihypertensive agents, but occasionally can be quite resistant to treatment. At 5 years, 60% of pediatric heart transplant patients require at least one antihypertensive agent for blood pressure control.[29] The addition of an angiotensin-converting enzyme inhibitor or diltiazem has been shown to have some renal protective effects. For hypertensive patients with a history of congenital heart disease, hemodynamic assessment is recommended to rule out persistent structural heart disease, such as residual coarctation.

Hyperlipidemia also is common in children after heart transplantation.[94,95] Data show that children treated with cyclosporine experience more adverse lipid profiles compared with children treated with tacrolimus, and this effect occurs independent of the effects of corticosteroids.[96] Treatment with statins is generally quite effective, although rare cases of rhabdomyolysis indicate the need for careful monitoring during therapy.

Dose-related and idiosyncratic neurologic complications of current immunosuppressive regimens include seizures, tremors, paresthesias, and encephalopathies.[97] Common metabolic complications include hyperkalemia, hyperuricemia, hypomagnesemia, and, most

importantly, **diabetes mellitus**.[98] The relative diabetogenic effect of cyclosporine and tacrolimus is the subject of considerable controversy,[99] but the development of diabetes is rare after transplantation in preadolescents.[100] Adolescent age, obesity, and the need for high doses of corticosteroids have been identified as major risk factors. The diabetes reflects high peripheral insulin resistance and pancreatic insufficiency. This complication is likely to become less frequent with newer immunosuppressive regimens that allow for lower doses of calcineurin inhibitors and corticosteroids.

One of the most worrisome end-organ toxicities is that of progressive **renal dysfunction** resulting from calcineurin inhibitor renal toxicity. Most centers have observed no significant difference in renal function between cyclosporine and tacrolimus-based immunosuppressive regimens 7 years after transplantation.[101] With increasing numbers of patients surviving into the second decade after transplantation, the number of patients developing end-stage renal failure inevitably will increase. Also, estimates of creatinine clearance based on serum creatinine levels significantly underestimate the extent of renal dysfunction compared with nuclear medicine measurements of glomerular filtration rate.[101] In this study, nearly two fifths of patients during long-term follow-up had glomerular filtration rates greater than 2 SDs below the mean for normals. Increased use of adjunctive therapies without renal toxicity (e.g., rapamycin and MMF) should allow for reduced dosing of tacrolimus and cyclosporine. It is hoped that this approach will reduce the extent of chronic nephropathy associated with these agents. Some groups have attempted calcineurin-free immunosuppressive regimens, although this has not yet been attempted in cardiac recipients. Use of multiple immunosuppressive agents with differing end-organ toxicities, each at low dosage, represents a logical approach to minimizing side effects, while maintaining immunosuppressive efficacy. Such complex regimens are suitable only for the most motivated and compliant of patients, however, as most centers struggle with compliance using even the simplest of immunosuppressive regimens in adolescents. Studies also are under way on a new generation of potent calcineurin inhibitors that seem to exhibit minimal renal toxicity.[102]

SURVIVAL AND QUALITY OF LIFE

More recent data from the ISHLT show that survival for pediatric heart transplant recipients continues to improve over the 20-year interval followed by the Registry (Fig. 41-4).[9] In the period between 1982 and 1988, survival at 1 year post-transplant was approximately 75%; this survival has increased to almost 90% in the most recent period of 1999 to 2002. An analysis of the era effect on survival stratified by age of the recipient

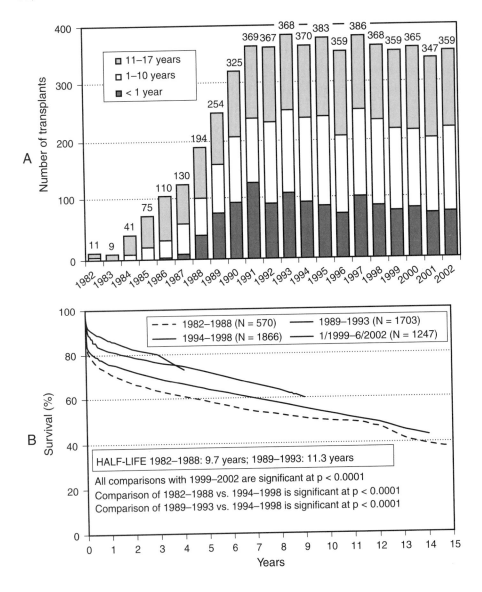

FIGURE 41-4 ■ Age distribution and survival of pediatric cardiac transplantation. **A,** Age distribution of pediatric heart recipients by year of transplantation up to 2003. The number has remained relatively constant since 1991. **B,** Kaplan-Meier survival curve is seen for pediatric heart transplantation by era. The 1-year and 3-year survivals have improved significantly since the early era. (From Boucek MM, Edwards LB, Keck BM, et al: *Registry for the International Society for Heart and Lung Transplantation: Seventh official pediatric report—2004. J Heart Lung Transplant* 2004;23:933-947.)

revealed that in infants younger than 1 year old, a great improvement in survival was noted in the period of 1994 to 1998. The 1-year survival of infants undergoing transplantation in the most recent era was approximately 85%; the 1-year survival of children and adolescents has not improved since the early 1990s and remains at approximately 90%. It is not obvious from the data that there has been any real improvement in late-decrement survival for any of the pediatric age groups, and overall 5-year survival remains at approximately 70%.

Causes of death and risk factors for survival have been analyzed in the Pediatric Heart Transplant Study.[103] The major causes of death are early graft failure, infection, and acute rejection. Together, these account for almost one half of all deaths after transplantation. Age at transplantation was not a significant risk factor for survival in the analysis of the data from 1993 to 2000 analyzed from the consortium of centers in the United States,

although a slight trend to lower survival was seen for infants. This difference was no longer apparent by 3 years from transplantation. Beyond the first 6 months of life, survival was almost identical in patients hospitalized versus patients cared for at home at the time of transplantation. Survival after transplantation was not influenced by prolonged ischemic time greater than 300 minutes. This observation has led some programs to procure organs from distances greater than 2000 miles. Diagnosis of hypoplastic left heart syndrome or other congenital heart disease was significantly associated with worse outcome in the first few years after transplantation. As noted previously, comparable outcomes among patients with and without congenital heart disease have been observed in several experienced centers.[15,16]

Most recipients are well rehabilitated and are in New York Heart Association class I. Full-time attendance at school is achieved in almost all patients within a few months of transplantation. Because the transplanted heart is denervated, heart transplant patients rely on catecholamine stimulation to increase heart rate and cardiac output. It has been reported that the maximum capacity for physical work and peak heart rate are only approximately two thirds of predicted, and that maximum volume of oxygen use is just 50% of normal controls.[104,105] The reasons for these changes are complex and include chronotropic incompetence and diastolic dysfunction of the allograft.

Although pediatric heart transplant survivors generally are reported to return to a good quality of life,[105-110] many recipients experience difficulties in psychosocial adjustment, with adolescents being most vulnerable.[106,107] Few studies have addressed the magnitude of this problem, and even fewer have sought solutions. In one of the few longitudinal studies conducted in children after heart or heart-lung transplantation, academic cognitive functioning was in the normal range and did not change as a function of time since transplant.[111] School performance was at a significantly lower level than healthy children, however, and the prevalence of behavior problems increased from 8% at 6 months to 29% at 3 and 5 years post-transplantation. In a longitudinal study in a small group of patients from Boston Children's Hospital, most (73.3%) patients still surviving almost a decade after heart transplantation showed psychological functioning within the normal range. The patients showed significant improvement over their emotional functioning before transplantation and maintained the same level of functioning that was described when the group averaged 2 years after transplantation.[108] Post-transplant medical severity did not correlate with post-transplant functioning. These results correspond to other studies in which illness severity was less important to a child's adaptation than other factors.[105-110,112] Most children and adolescents have the capacity for healthy psychological functioning after heart transplantation. The need for ongoing psychological assessment and intervention exists for patients and their families, however, because more than 25% likely will present with emotional adjustment difficulties. The factors that may facilitate or hinder coping with pediatric heart transplantation have not been well defined and should be the topic of further research.

Nonadherence to complicated and life-sustaining therapy is even less well studied. Normal adolescent development, combined with the complex psychological issues surrounding heart transplantation, create a large population of recipients at risk. Nonadherence has been linked to late rejection,[113,114] and high mortality rates in the adolescent age group associated with noncompliance have been a source of immense frustration for all who care for these individuals. Coordinated efforts between pediatricians, psychologists, and transplant teams are necessary to help identify patients at risk and design interventions that work to prevent unnecessary morbidity and mortality in this challenging group of patients.

CURRENT STATUS AND FUTURE TRENDS

Current studies are under way to (1) look at therapies that would obviate the need for cardiac transplantation, (2) extend preservation of the donor heart, and (3) induce a state of immune tolerance in heart transplant recipients. Bone marrow–derived stem cells have been injected successfully into the human myocardium and improved cardiac function in adult heart failure patients with ischemic cardiomyopathy.[115] Refinements in this type of cellular myoplasty someday could obviate the need for cardiac transplantation in most adult and pediatric cardiomyopathy patients. Because transplant coronary vascular disease represents the number one reason for late organ loss in cardiac transplant recipients, studies to understand and eliminate this pathologic process are paramount to graft preservation.

Immune tolerance remains the true holy grail of the transplant physician. Donor-specific tolerance after transplantation can be defined as a state in which the recipient permanently accepts the allograft without the need for long-term anti-rejection therapy, yet retains normal host immune responses to antigens other than those of the donor. The side effects of immunosuppressive medications and the risks of infection, lymphoproliferative disorders, and malignancy are avoided. Tremendous effort has been expended to understand how tolerance can be achieved.[116-118] Many experiments in small animals, particularly rodents, have been extended to subhuman primates. It is necessary that this tolerance be robust and long lasting.

Perturbations of the immune system of the recipient, such as immunologic responses to everyday infections, cannot result in loss of tolerance, or else rapid rejection of the transplanted organ would ensue. It has become apparent that, as one advances up the evolutionary tree, it becomes more difficult to achieve stable tolerance. We are likely many years away from this goal in humans. Nonetheless, the complex molecular and cellular events involved in induction of tolerance are becoming better elucidated, and this will enhance greatly the ability to achieve this goal. The current state of knowledge in this field and the potential huge benefits to patients from induction of tolerance have led many groups to suggest that the time is right to begin human trials. Initial emphasis has been placed on studies in transplantation of kidneys and pancreas in adults, in part because these are not life-supporting organs, and return to dialysis is possible if the strategies fail.

Children also offer some special opportunities. First, induction may be most readily achieved in the neonate, and transplantation in the neonatal and early infancy period is extremely rare for organs other than the heart.

In addition, the median sternotomy required for heart transplantation exposes the thymus gland, allowing for potential manipulation of this organ for induction of tolerance. In many small animal models, intrathymic inoculation of donor antigens, particularly bone marrow, results in development of donor-specific tolerance.[119] A trial of thymic tolerance by inoculation of the thymus gland with donor bone marrow concomitant with heart transplantation in children is currently under way at Children's Hospital of Pittsburgh. Other strategies for inducing transplantation tolerance are summarized elsewhere.[116-118]

Great improvements in outcomes after cardiac transplantation in children have occurred in the 1980s and 1990s. Surgeons have risen to the challenge of transplanting the heart in recipients having the most complex anatomy and have achieved great success in reducing early mortality. Mechanical support as a bridge to transplantation remains in its infancy, with few devices currently available for use in children, but new devices are now in development. Major advances also have occurred in recent years in understanding of the immune response to solid-organ allografts. Improved patient care is the result of these advances. New immunosuppressive agents now can be designed to target molecules and receptors that are known to be of central importance in the immune response to the allograft. There will be an explosion in the number of new drugs available for clinical use in the near future.

Understanding of risk factors for individual outcomes also is improving, including new knowledge about genetic factors. Improved understanding of the immune response to infection with EBV, combined with new strategies for monitoring and treatment, suggest that lymphoproliferative disorders may be prevented after transplantation or more satisfactorily treated in the years to come. It is becoming increasingly apparent that successful induction of tolerance and ABO-incompatible heart transplantation in infants may become a clinical reality within the next decade, potentially transforming transplantation from a palliative to a curative therapy, with expectations for indefinite survival of the transplanted organs.[120-122]

Key Concepts

■ Patients with a PVR index greater than 4 Wood units at cardiac catheterization undergo additional testing for reactivity of the pulmonary vascular bed in response to 100% oxygen and, if necessary, with the subsequent administration of inhaled nitric oxide up to 80 ppm. A fixed PVR index greater than 10 Wood units is considered a contraindication to cardiac transplantation.

■ Children with complex congenital heart disease now represent approximately one half of all referrals for consideration for transplantation. Other than newborns with hypoplastic left heart syndrome, most of these children have undergone multiple prior surgical palliative or corrective procedures. Frequently, there are stenoses, hypoplastic segments, or even discontinuities of the branch pulmonary arteries. Anomalies of systemic and pulmonary venous return, particularly in the context of isomerism or mirror-imaged atrial arrangement, pose additional challenges for the surgeon.

■ Despite an increased use of induction immunosuppressive therapy in pediatric recipients, a review of frequency-of-rejection and survival data failed to show a significant beneficial effect from this treatment.

■ Maintenance immunosuppression regimens used in pediatric heart transplant recipients tend to be individual-specific and institution-specific. The strategies take advantage of the selectivity of immunosuppressive agents for critical pathways in graft rejection. Virtually all immunosuppressive regimens in children are based on the use of a calcineurin inhibitor, either cyclosporine or tacrolimus.

■ Long-term corticosteroid usage in pediatric patients has been linked in some centers to several undesirable risks, such as higher risks for opportunistic infections, diabetes, and bone demineralization. Some centers have reported the withdrawal of corticosteroids in the medium term of 6 months to 2 years after transplantation or even the avoidance of maintenance corticosteroids in the immunosuppressive regimen after transplant.

■ Acute failure of the transplanted heart is the most common cause of death in the first 30 days after transplantation and occurs with greater frequency in infant recipients.

■ When cardiac failure does occur in the first few years after transplantation, acute cellular rejection is the most likely diagnosis, although other pathologies must be entertained, including humoral (antibody-mediated) rejection, acute presentation of chronic rejection secondary to post-transplant coronary artery disease, and viral myocarditis.

■ Risk factors for rejection in children include older age at transplant, African American race, cytomegalovirus, gender mismatch, and a previous episode of rejection. Hemodynamically significant rejection episodes predict a particularly poor outcome, with approximately 50% mortality in the year after the episode.

■ Most African Americans carry pharmacogenomic polymorphisms at loci that are associated with decreased immunosuppressive efficacy, perhaps explaining the observation that African Americans have poorer outcomes after transplantation, with worse profiles for rejection.

■ Humoral rejection is much less common than cellular rejection and generally occurs when a patient with preformed anti-HLA antibodies receives an organ containing antigens to which the recipient has been previously sensitized. This allosensitization is usually due to prior blood product transfusion or homograft materials used during previous surgical palliations for congenital heart defects or associated with mechanical ventricular support.

■ Coronary artery disease subsequent to transplantation is an accelerated vasculopathy that is the leading cause of death in late survivors of heart transplantation. The pathology differs from that of ischemic heart disease in the normal adult population. Typical allograft coronary artery disease consists of myointimal proliferation that is concentric and involves the entire length of the vessel, including intramyocardial branches with eventual luminal occlusion.

■ Older recipient age, older donor age (especially >30 years), and greater number of episodes of rejection in the first year were the main risk factors for the development of coronary artery disease.

■ Angiography is a relatively insensitive marker of mild coronary artery disease secondary to the diffuse nature of the disease process and the propensity to affect small vessels, although severe epicardial disease that portends a poor prognosis is readily apparent.

■ Beyond retransplantation, no effective treatment exists for established coronary artery disease because bypass grafting and coronary angioplasty have limited usefulness as a result of the diffuse nature of the disease.

■ There is a bimodal presentation of PTLD with early-onset disease usually possessing a less aggressive polymorphic histology and almost invariably being associated with primary infection by EBV. Late-onset PTLD, usually presenting beyond 3 years, can have highly varying histology and may be polymorphic, but is often monomorphic with histology resembling aggressive B cell lymphoma.

■ The 1-year survival of infants undergoing transplantation in the most recent era was approximately 85%; the 1-year survival of children and adolescents has not improved since the early 1990s and remains at approximately 90%.

REFERENCES

1. Kantrowitz A, Haller JD, Joos H, et al: Transplantation of the heart in an infant and an adult. Am J Cardiol 1968;22:782-790.
2. Webber SA: The current state of, and future prospects for, cardiac transplantation in children. Cardiol Young 2003;13:64-83.
3. Boucek RJ, Boucek MM: Pediatric heart transplantation. Curr Opin Pediatr 2002;14:611-619.
4. Blume ED: Current status of heart transplantation in children: Update 2003. Pediatr Clin North Am 2003;50:1375-1391.
5. Fricker FJ, Addonizio L, Bernstein D, et al: Heart transplantation in children: Indications. Pediatr Transplant 1999;3:333-342.
6. Ward KM, Canter CE, Webber SA, et al: Anthracycline cardiomyopathy and pediatric heart transplantation (Abstract). J Heart Lung Transplant 2002;21:64.
7. Morgan E, Pahl E: Early heart transplantation in a child with advanced lymphoma. Pediatr Transplant 2002;6:509-512.
8. Armitage JM, Fricker FJ, del Nido P, et al: A decade (1982-1992) of pediatric cardiac transplantation and the impact of FK506 immunosuppression. J Thorac Cardiovasc Surg 1993;105:464-472.
9. Boucek MM, Edwards LB, Keck BM, et al: Registry for the International Society for Heart and Lung Transplantation: Seventh official pediatric report—2004. J Heart Lung Transplant 2004;23:933-947.
10. Murali S, Kormos R, Uretsky B, et al: Preoperative pulmonary hemodynamics and early mortality after orthotopic cardiac transplantation: The Pittsburgh experience. Am Heart J 1993;126:896-904.
11. Gajarski R, Towbin J, Bricker J, et al: Intermediate follow-up of pediatric heart transplant recipients with elevated pulmonary vascular resistance index. J Am Coll Cardiol 1994;23:1682-1687.
12. El Gamel A, Yonan NA, Grant S, et al: Orthotopic cardiac transplantation: Comparison of standard and bicaval Wythenshawe techniques. J Thorac Cardiovasc Surg 1995;109:721-730.
13. Trento A, Czer LSC, Blanche C: Surgical techniques for cardiac transplantation. Semin Thorac Cardiovasc Surg 1996;8:126-132.
14. Pigula F, Ghandi S, Cipriani L, et al: Bicaval anastomosis for pediatric heart transplantation (Abstract).Transplantation 1999;67: S642.
15. Webber SA, Fricker FJ, Michael M, et al: Orthotopic heart transplantation in children with congenital heart disease. Ann Thorac Surg 1994;58:1664-1669.
16. Hsu DT, Quaegebeur JM, Michler RE, et al: Heart transplantation in children with congenital heart disease. J Am Coll Cardiol 1995;26:743-749.
17. Vricella LA, Razzouk AJ, Gundry SR, et al: Heart transplantation in infants and children with situs inversus. J Thorac Cardiovasc Surg 1998;116:82-89.
18. Vricella LA, Razzouk AJ, del Rio M, et al: Heart transplant for hypoplastic left heart syndrome: Modified technique for reducing circulatory arrest time. J Heart Lung Transplant 1998;17:1167-1171.
19. Cooper M, Fuzesi L, Addonizio L, et al: Pediatric heart transplantation after operations involving the pulmonary arteries. J Thorac Cardiovasc Surg 1991;102:386-394.
20. Kirshman US, Hsu DT, Donnelly CM, et al: Management of aortopulmonary collaterals in children following heart transplantation for complex congenital heart disease (Abstract). J Heart Lung Transplant 1997;16:71.
21. Lamour JM, Hsu DT, Kichuk MR, et al: Regression of pulmonary arteriovenous malformations following heart transplantation. Pediatr Transplant 2000;4:280-284.
22. Webber SA, Pigula FA: Heart and lung transplantation in adult congenital heart disease. In Gatzoulis M, Webb G, Daubeney P (eds): Diagnosis and Management of Adult Congenital Heart Disease. London, Harcourt Publishers Limited, 2003, pp. 93-98.
23. Pigula FA, Gandhi S, Ristich J, et al: Cardiopulmonary transplantation for congenital heart disease in the adult. J Heart Lung Transplant 2001;20:297-303.
24. Del Nido PJ, Armitage JM, Fricker FJ, et al: Extracorporeal membrane oxygenation support as a bridge to pediatric heart transplantation. Circulation 1994;90(Pt II):II-66-II-69.
25. Helman DN, Addonizio LJ, Morales DLS, et al: Implantable left ventricular ventricular assist devices can successfully bridge adolescent patients to transplant. J Heart Lung Transplant 2000;16:121-126.
26. Reinhartz O, Keith FM, El-Banayosy A, et al: Multi-center experience with the Thoratec ventricular assist device in children and adolescents. J Heart Lung Transplant 2001;20:439-448.
27. Hetzer R, Loebe M, Potapov EV, et al: Circulatory support with pneumatic paracorporeal ventricular assist device in infants and children. Ann Thorac Surg 1998;66:1498-1506.
28. Weyand M, Kececioglu D, Kehl HG: Neonatal mechanical bridging to total orthotopic heart transplantation. Ann Thorac Surg 1998;66:519-522.

29. Boucek MM, Edwards LB, Keck BM, et al: The Registry of the International Society for Heart and Lung Transplantation: Fifth official pediatric report—2001 to 2002. J Heart Lung Transplant 2002;21:826-938.

30. Kobashigawa J, Miller L, Renlund D, et al: A randomized active-controlled trial of mycophenolate mofetil in heart transplant recipients. Transplantation 1998;66:507-515.

31. Sindhi R, Webber SA, Venkataramanan R, et al: Sirolimus for rescue and primary immunosuppression in transplanted children receiving tacrolimus. Transplantation 2001;72:851-855.

32. Straatman LP, Coles JG: Pediatric utilization of rapamycin for severe cardiac allograft rejection. Transplantation 2000;70:541-543.

33. Nashan B: Review of the proliferation inhibitor everolimus. Exp Opin Invest Drugs 2002;11:1845-1857.

34. Eisen HJ, Tuzcu EM, Dorent R, et al, RAD B253 Study Group: Everolimus for the prevention of allograft rejection and vasculopathy in cardiac transplant recipients. N Engl J Med 2003;349:847-858.

35. Hoyer PF, Ettenger R, Kovarik JM, et al, Everolimus Pediatric Study Group. Everolimus in pediatric de nova renal transplant patients. Transplantation 2003;75:2082-2085.

36. Webber SA: Fifteen Years of pediatric heart transplantation at the University of Pittsburgh: Lessons learned and future prospects. Pediatr Transplant 1997;1:8-21.

37. Canter CE, Moorhead S, Saffitz JE, et al: Steroid withdrawal in the pediatric heart transplant recipient initially treated with triple immunosuppression. J Heart Lung Transplant 1994;13:74-80.

38. Bailey L, Assaad A, Trimm R, et al: Orthotopic transplantation during early infancy as therapy for incurable congenital heart disease. Ann Surg 1988;208:279-286.

39. Leonard HCO, Sullivan JJ, Darj HH: Long term follow-up of pediatric cardiac transplant recipients on a steroid-free regime: The role of endomyocardial biopsy. J Heart Lung Transplant 2000;19:469-472.

40. Schuurman HJ, Jambroes G, Borleffs JC, et al: Acute humoral rejection after heart transplantation. Transplantation 1988;46:603-605.

41. Mills RM, Naftel DC, Kirklin JK, et al: Heart transplant rejection with hemodynamic compromise: A multi-institutional study of the role of endomyocardial infiltrate. J Heart Lung Transplant 1997;16:813-821.

42. Webber SA, Naftel DC, Parker J, et al, the Pediatric Heart Transplant Study: Late rejection episodes greater than 1 year after pediatric heart transplantation: Risk factors and outcomes. J Heart Lung Transplant 2003;22:869-875.

43. Rotondo K, Naftel DC, Boucek R, et al: Allograft rejection following cardiac transplantation in infants and children: A multi-institutional study. J Heart Lung Transplant 1996;15:S80.

44. Kawauchi M, Gundry SR, de Begona JA, et al: Male donor into female heart increases the risk of pediatric heart allograft rejection. Ann Thorac Surg 1993;55:716-718.

45. Mills RM, Naftel DC, Kirklin JK, et al: Heart transplant rejection with hemodynamic compromise: A multi-institutional study of the role of endomyocardial infiltrate. J Heart Lung Transplant 1997;16:813-821.

46. Pahl E, Naftel DC, Canter CE, et al, The Pediatric Heart Transplant Study: Death after rejection with severe hemodynamic compromise in pediatric heart transplant recipients: A multi-institutional study. J Heart Lung Transplant 2001;20:279-287.

47. Awad MR, Webber SA, Boyle GJ, et al: The effect of cytokine gene polymorphism on pediatric heart allograft outcome. J Heart Lung Transplant 2001;20:625-630.

48. Zheng HX, Webber SA, Zeevi A, et al: MDR1 polymorphisms at exons 21 and 26 predict steroid weaning in pediatric heart transplant patients. Hum Immunol 2002;63:765-770.

49. Webber SA:Cardiac transplantation. In Tejani AH, Harmon WE, Fine RN (eds): Pediatric Solid Organ Transplantation. Copenhagen, Munksgaard, 2000, pp 404-411.

50. Wagner K, Oliver MC, Boyle GJ, et al: Endomyocardial biopsy in pediatric heart transplant recipients: A useful exercise? (Analysis of 1169 biopsies.) Pediatr Transplant 2000;4:186-192.

51. Pophal SG, Sigfusson G, Booth KL, et al: Complications of endomyocardial biopsy in children. J Am Coll Cardiol 1999;34: 105-110.

52. Billingham ME, Cary NR, Hammond ME, et al: A working formulation for the standardization of nomenclature in the diagnosis of heart and lung rejection: Heart Rejection Study Group. J Heart Transplant 1990;9:587-593.

53. Bowles NE, Ni J, Kearney DL, et al: Detection of viruses in myocardial tissues by polymerase chain reaction: Evidence of adenovirus as a common cause of myocarditis in children and adults. J Am Coll Cardiol 2003;42:466-472.

54. Shirali GS, Ni J, Chinnock RE, et al: Association of viral genome with graft loss in children after cardiac transplantation. N Engl J Med 2001;344:1498-1503.

55. Bowles NE, Shirali GS, Chinnock RE, et al: Association of viral genome with transplant coronary arteriopathy and graft loss in children following cardiac transplantation. J Heart Lung Transplant 2001;20:198.

56. Glotz D, Haymann JP, Sansonetti N, et al: Suppression of HLA-specific alloantibodies by high dose intravenous immunoglobulin (IVIg): A potential tool for transplantation of immunized patients. Transplantation 1993;56:335-337.

57. John R, Lietz K, Burke E, et al: Intravenous immunoglobulin reduces anti-HLA alloreactivity and shortens time to cardiac transplantation in highly sensitized left ventricular assist device recipients. Circulation 1999;100:229-235.

58. Anderson C, Sicard G, Etheredge E: Pretreatment of renal allograft recipients with azathioprine and donor specific blood products. Surgery 1982;92:315-321.

59. Jordan SC: Management of the highly HLA-sensitized patient: A novel role for intravenous gammaglobulin. Am J Transplant 2002;2:691-692.

60. Sawada T, Fuchinoue S, Kawase T, et al: Preconditioning regimen consisting of anti-CD20 monoclonal antibody infusions, splenectomy and DFPP-enabled non-responders to undergo ABO-incompatible kidney transplantation. Clin Transplant 2004;18:254-260.

61. Grauhan O, Muller J, v Baeyer H, et al: Treatment of humoral rejection after heart transplantation. J Heart Lung Transplant 1998;17:1184-1194.

62. Suciu-Foca N, Reed E, Marboe C, et al: The role of anti-HLA antibodies in heart transplantation. Transplantation 1991;51:716-724.

63. Billingham ME: Histopathology of graft coronary disease. J Heart Lung Transplant 1990;119;3:538-544.

64. Costanzo MR, Naftel DC, Pritzker MR, et al: Heart transplant coronary artery disease detected by coronary angiography: A multi-institutional study of preoperative donor and recipient risk factors. Cardiac Transplant Research Database. J Heart Lung Transplant 1998;17:744-753.

65. Pahl E, Naftel D, Kuhn M, et al: The incidence and impact of transplant coronary disease pediatric recipients: A 9 year multi-institutional study (Abstract). Circulation 2002;106(Suppl): II-396.

66. Shirwan H: Chronic allograft rejection. Transplantation 1999;68: 715-726.

67. Pahl E, Zales VR, Fricker FJ, et al: Posttransplant coronary artery disease in children: A multicenter national survey. Circulation 1994;90(Pt 2):II-56-II-60.

68. Larsen RL, Applegate PM, Dyar DA, et al: Dobutamine stress echocardiography for assessing coronary artery disease after transplantation in children. J Am Coll Cardiol 1998;32:515-520.

69. Pahl E, Crawford SE, Swenson JM, et al: Dobutamine stress echocardiography: Experience in pediatric heart transplant recipients. J Heart Lung Transplant 1999;18:725-732.

70. St Goar FG, Pinto FJ, Alderman EL, et al: Intracoronary ultrasound in cardiac transplant recipients: in vivo evidence of "angiographically silent" intimal thickening. Circulation 1992;85:979-987.

71. Kuhn MA, Jutzy KR, Deming DD, et al: The medium-term findings in coronary arteries by intravascular ultrasound in infants and children after heart transplantation. J Am Coll Cardiol 2000;36:250-254.

72. Dent CL, Canter CE, Hirsch R, Balzer DT: Transplant coronary artery disease in pediatric heart transplant recipients. J Heart Lung Transplant 2000;19:240-248.

73. Schratz LM, Meyer RA, Schwartz DC: Serial intracoronary ultrasound in children: Feasibility, reproducibility, limitations, and safety. J Am Soc Echocardiogr 2002;15:782-790.

74. Costello JM, Wax DF, Binns HJ, et al: A comparison of intravascular ultrasound with coronary angiography for evaluation of transplant coronary disease in pediatric heart transplant recipients. J Heart Lung Transplant 2003;22:44-49.

75. Morice MC, Serruys PW, Sousa JE, et al, RAVEL Study Group: A randomized comparison of a sirolimus-eluting stent with a standard stent for coronary revascularization. N Engl J Med 2002;346:1773-1780.

76. Ikonen TS, Gummert JF, Serkova N, et al: Efficacies of sirolimus (rapamycin) and cyclosporine in allograft vascular disease in non-human primates: Trough levels of sirolimus correlate with inhibition of progression of arterial intimal thickening. Transpl Int 2000;13(Suppl 1):S314-S320.

77. Michaels MG: Infectious complications. In Tejani AH, Harmon WE, Fine RN (eds): Pediatric Solid Organ Transplantation. Copenhagen, Munksgaard, 2000, pp 404-410.

78. Kanter K, Pahl E, Naftel DC, et al, Pediatric Heart Transplant Study Group: Preventing CMV infection in pediatric heart transplant recipients: Does prophylaxis work? (Abstract). J Heart Lung Transplant 1998;17:59-60.

79. Koskinen PK, Nieminen MS, Krogerus LA, et al: Cytomegalovirus infection and accelerated cardiac allograft vasculopathy in human cardiac allografts. J Heart Lung Transplant 1993;12:724-729.

80. Webber SA, Green M: Post-transplantation lymphoproliferative disorders: Advances in diagnosis, prevention and management. Prog Pediatr Cardiol 2000;11:145-157.

81. Green M, Reyes J, Webber SA, et al: The role of viral load in the diagnosis, management and possible prevention of Epstein-Barr virus-associated posttransplant lymphoproliferative disease following solid organ transplantation. Curr Opin Organ Transplant 1999;4:292-296.

82. Rowe DT, Qu L, Reyes J, et al: Use of quantitative competitive PCR to measure Epstein-Barr virus genome load in the peripheral blood of pediatric transplant recipients with lymphoproliferative disorders. J Clin Microbiol 1997;35:1612-1615.

83. Qu L, Green M, Webber SA, et al: Epstein-Barr virus gene expression in the peripheral blood of transplant recipients with persistent circulating viral loads. J Infect Dis 2000;182:1013-1021.

84. Boyle GJ, Michaels MG, Webber SA, et al: Post transplant lymphoproliferative disorders in pediatric thoracic organ recipients. J Pediatr 1997;131:309-313.

85. Nalesnik MA: The diverse pathology of post-transplant lymphoproliferative disorders: The importance of a standardized approach. Transplant Infect Dis 2001;3:88-96.

86. Webber SA, Bowman P, Naftel D, et al: Post-transplant lymphoproliferative disorders: Experience with 56 cases at 19 pediatric heart transplant centers (Abstract). Circulation 2002;106(Suppl):II-718.

87. Webber SA, Fine RN, McGhee W, et al: Anti-CD20 monoclonal antibody (Rituximab) for pediatric post-transplant lymphoproliferative disorders: A preliminary multicenter experience (Abstract). Am J Transplant 2001;1(Suppl 1):469.

88. Grillo-López AJ, Lynch J, Coiffier B, et al: Rituximab therapy of lymphoproliferative disorders in immunosuppressed patients. Ann Oncol 1999;10(Suppl 3):179.

89. Milpied N, Vasseur B, Parquet N, et al: Humanized anti-CD20 monoclonal antibody (Rituximab) in posttransplant B-lymphoproliferative disorders: A retrospective analysis on 32 patients. Ann Oncol 2000;11(Suppl 1):113-116.

90. Rooney CM, Smith CA, Ng CY, et al: Use of gene-modified virus-specific T lymphocytes to control Epstein-Barr virus related lymphoproliferation. Lancet 1995;345:9-13.

91. Khanna R, Bell S, Sherritt M, et al: Activation and adoptive transfer of Epstein-Barr virus-specific cytotoxic T cells in solid organ transplant patients with posttransplant lymphoproliferative disease. Proc Natl Acad Sci U S A 1999;96:10391-10396.

92. Neu AM, Fivush BA: Recommended immunization practices for pediatric renal transplant recipients. Pediatr Transplant 1998;2:263-269.

93. Boyle GJ: Other complications. In Tejani AH, Harmon WE, Fine RN (eds): Pediatric Solid Organ Transplantation. Copenhagen, Munksgaard, 2000, pp 411-416.

94. Chin C, Rosenthal D, Bernstein D: Lipoprotein abnormalities are highly prevalent in pediatric heart transplant recipients. Pediatr Transplant 2000;4:193-199.

95. Penson MG, Winter WE, Fricker FJ, et al: Tacrolimus-based triple drug immunosuppression minimizes serum lipid elevations in pediatric cardiac transplant recipients. J Heart Lung Transplant 1999;18:707-713.

96. Law YM, Yim R, Agatista PK, et al: Lipid profiles in pediatric thoracic recipients are determined by the immunosuppressive regimens (Abstract). J Heart Lung Transplant 2002;21:172.

97. Walker R, Brochstein J: Neurologic complications of immunosuppressive agents. Neurol Clin 1988;6:261-277.

98. Asante-Korang A, Boyle GJ, Webber SA, et al: Experience of FK 506 immunosuppression in pediatric heart transplantation: A study of long-term adverse effects. J Heart Lung Transplant 1996;15:415-422.

99. First MR, Gerber DA, Hariharan S, et al: Posttransplant diabetes mellitus in kidney allograft recipients: Incidence, risk factors, and management. Transplantation 2002;73:379-386.

100. Wagner K, Webber SA, Kurland G, et al: New onset diabetes mellitus in pediatric thoracic organ recipients under tacrolimus based immunosuppression. J Heart Lung Transplant 1997;16:275-282.

101. English RF, Pophal SA, Bacanu S, et al: Long-term comparison of tacrolimus and cyclosporine induced nephrotoxicity in pediatric heart transplant recipients. Am J Transplant 2002;2:769-773.

102. Abel MD, Aspeslet LJ, Broski AP, et al: Phase II trial of ISATX247, a novel calcineurin inhibitor, in renal transplantation. Am J Transplant 2002;2(Suppl 3):379.

103. Shaddy RE, Naftel DC, Kirklin JK, et al: Outcome of cardiac transplantation in children: Survival in a contemporary multiinstitutional experience. Pediatric Heart Transplant Study. Circulation 1996;94(9 Suppl):II-69-II-73.

104. Nixon PA, Fricker FJ, Noyes BE, et al: Exercise testing in pediatric heart and/or lung transplant recipients. Chest 1995;107:1328-1335.

105. Hsu DT, Garofano RP, Douglas JM, et al: Exercise performance after pediatric heart transplantation. Circulation 1993;88(Pt II):238-242.

106. Uzark KC, Sauer SN, Lawrence KS, et al: The psychosocial impact of pediatric heart transplantation. J Heart Lung Transplant 1992;11:1160-1167.

107. Wray J, Pot-Mees C, Zeitlin H, et al: Cognitive function and behavioural status in pediatric heart and heart-lung transplant recipients: The Harefield experience. BMJ 1994;309:837-841.

108. Slater JA: Psychiatric aspects of organ transplantation in children and adolescents. Child Adolesc Psychiatr Clin N Am 1994;3:557-598.

109. DeMaso DR, Twente AW, Spratt EG, O'Brien P: The impact of psychological functioning, medical severity, and family functioning in pediatric heart transplantation. J Heart Lung Transplant 1995;14:1102-1108.

110. Wray J, Yacoub MH: Psychological evaluation of children after heart and heart-lung transplantation. In Kapoor AS, Laks H, Schroeder JS, Yacoub MH (eds): Cardiomyopathies and Heart-Lung Transplantation. New York, McGraw-Hill, 1991, pp 447-460.

111. Nixon PA, Morris KA: Quality of life in pediatric heart, heart-lung, and lung transplant recipients. Int J Sports Med 2000;2(Suppl):S109-S111.

112. Wray J, Radley-Smith R, Yacuob M: Effect of cardiac or heart-lung transplantation on the quality of life of the paediatric patient. Qual Life Res 1992;1:41-46.

113. Serrano-Ikkos E, Lask B, Whitehead B, Eisler I: Unsatisfactory adherence after pediatric heart and heart-lung transplantation. J Heart Lung Transplant 1998;17:1177-1183.

114. Ringewald JM, Gidding SS, Crawford SE, et al: Nonadherence is associated with late rejection in pediatric heart transplant recipients. J Pediatr 2001;139:75-78.

115. Perin EC, Dohmann HF, Borojevic R, et al: Transendocardial, autologous bone marrow cell transplantation for severe, chronic ischemic heart failure. Circulation 2003;107:2294-2302.

116. Kurtz J, Sykes M: Tolerance: A review of its mechanisms in the transplant setting. In Tejani AH, Harmon WE, Fine RN (eds): Pediatric Solid Organ Transplantation. Copenhagen, Munksgaard, 2000, pp 74-87.

117. Turka LA: Transplantation tolerance. Medscape Transplantation, 2000. Available at: www.medscape.com/Medscape/transplantation/ClinicalMgmt/CM.v05/public/index-CM.v05.html.

118. Kirk A: Immunosuppression without immunosuppression? How to be a tolerant individual in a dangerous world. Transplant Infect Dis 1999;1:65-75.

119. Remuzzi G, Perico N, Carpenter CB, Sayegh M: The thymic way to transplantation tolerance. J Am Soc Nephrol 1995;5:1639-1646.

120. Foreman C, Gruenwald C, West L: ABO-incompatible heart transplantation: A perfusion strategy. Perfusion 2004;19:69-72.

121. Rao JN, Hasan A, Hamilton JR, et al: ABO-incompatible heart transplantation in infants: The Freeman Hospital experience. Transplantation 2004;77:1389-1394.

122. West LJ: Targeting antibody-mediated rejection in the setting of ABO-incompatible infant heart transplantation: Graft accommodation vs B cell tolerance. Curr Drug Targets Cardiovasc Haematol Discord 2005;5:223-232.

CHAPTER 42

Surgical Strategies for the Failing Systemic Ventricle

David L. S. Morales
Charles D. Fraser, Jr.

In contrast to the earlier years of congenital heart surgery, when the effort was more on achieving better survival in neonatal palliative or corrective repairs of complex lesions, the focus currently has come to include the longevity and performance of the systemic ventricle. In other words, because operative mortality rates of less than 1% for arterial switch operations (ASOs) and Fontan procedures has been achieved at many large institutions, this outcome has led cardiac surgeons and cardiologists to be held even more accountable for the long-term outcomes of present surgeries and surgeries performed in the past (i.e., atrial switch operations and atriopulmonary Fontan procedures).[1] Another significant group of patients includes children who have two adequate ventricles, but the systemic ventricle is the morphologic right ventricle (mRV), and the pulmonary ventricle is the morphologic left ventricle (mLV). The mRV may fail in time, and the mLV may become deconditioned and unable to reclaim its function as the systemic ventricle. This situation is encountered in patients with congenitally corrected transposition of the great arteries (ccTGA) and in patients who present late with transposition of the great arteries (TGA).

The mRV generally is accepted not to be as effective or as reliable as a systemic ventricle in the long-term as the mLV. Depending on the congenital anomaly or operation, the incidence of significant mRV failure at 10 years ranges from 10% to 33%.[2,3] Surgeries relying on the mRV as the systemic ventricle can result in a mortality rate of 50% by 20 years, almost all secondary to mRV dysfunction, with reoperation rates of 60% during those years.[4] This survival rate translates into 50% of these children dying before age 20. Some studies show good systemic mRV function in patients after atrial switch operations at 10 to 15 years with excellent resting mRV systolic function.[5,6] Most authors agree, however, that the mRV response to even submaximal exercise can be abnormal.[7]

The mRV does not seem well suited to be the systemic ventricle for several reasons (see Chapter 16). First, the myocardial **fiber arrangement** in the mRV is different than that of the mLV, as are the fibers themselves. These differences do not allow the mRV to respond to afterload stress acutely or chronically similar to the mLV; this has been shown by a deficient increase

in minute work index and, more grossly, by an inadequate increase in ejection fraction when the mRV is exposed to afterload stress (i.e., exercise).[8]

Second, the **coronary blood supply** of the mRV contributes to its inability to function as the systemic ventricle. The mRV has only one coronary artery to supply its ever-growing muscle mass, so the supply of blood to that increasing mRV systemic ventricular muscle mass is established mainly by coronary collaterals and neovascularization. The coronary supply during exercise and stress for a systemic mRV may not always be adequate, leading to chronic subclinical ischemia. These repeated episodes of ischemia eventually can lead to chronic systolic and diastolic dysfunction. All 22 patients studied 15 years after atrial switch operations had fixed or reversible perfusion defects in the mRV.[9]

Third, the mRV was arranged to be efficient in its usual crescent shape, but not the spherical one it is transformed to by the stresses associated with functioning as the systemic ventricle; this has serious pathophysiologic implications on the **atrioventricular valve** (AVV). In contrast to the two well-balanced papillary muscles of the mLV, the mRV has an AVV with multiple papillary muscles that are septophilic. As the mRV changes its **geometry** to that of a sphere, the interventricular septum (IVS) changes its position and bows toward the mLV. This shift in the IVS commonly causes distortion of the subvalvular apparatus and subsequently systemic AVV regurgitation. This effect leads to volume loading of the mRV with a steady increase in end-diastolic volume over time, resulting in more dilation and increasing tricuspid regurgitation with eventual decline in ventricular function.[10] The spherical form of the mRV also causes the tricuspid annulus to become more circular in shape, which also leads to leaflet malcoaptation and insufficiency.

Fourth, another geometrical disadvantage for the mRV is that the **free wall** of the mRV has a bellows-like action during systole and is not as well coordinated with the septum in regard to vector forces and temporal relations. Finally, the reduction in the septal contribution to contraction also may be attributable to the differences in the **conduction systems** of the mRV and mLV. The mRV has two distinct conduction pathways, in contrast to the array of pathways seen on the left. The mRV is not as well suited to ensure maximum coordination of the multiple muscular components of ventricular contraction. This asynchrony of the muscular components causes a diminution of the efficiency and the effective output of the mRV. Tricuspid regurgitation leading to atrial enlargement and eventually atrial arrhythmias further adds to this discord. The loss of atrioventricular synchrony is one of the most significant contributing factors to heart failure in these patients because it does not allow for efficient ventricular filling or function.[11]

Aside from valve repairs or replacements, there are several procedures available for improving the failing systemic ventricle in the palliated or corrected congenital heart patient. These procedures involve either making the mLV function as the systemic ventricle or making the mRV function more efficiently and can be quite complex and associated with significant morbidity and mortality. The only other alternative for these children is often orthotopic heart transplantation, with the disadvantages of a 30% attrition rate while on the transplant waiting list and a limited life expectancy even after a successful transplantation.[12] Procedures that could palliate these children for a significant time interval at a good functional level should be considered alongside orthotopic heart transplantation in treating systemic ventricular failure.

Four strategies for patients with failing or failed ventricles are discussed in this chapter: (1) Fontan conversion for the failed Fontan, (2) double-switch operation for patients with ccTGA, (3) ASO for failed atrial switch operation, and (4) late ASO for dextraposed transposition of the great arteries (D-TGA). The application of these surgical strategies in regard to timing, candidacy, and expected outcomes is delineated. Additional procedures and simple devices that are on the horizon for the failing systemic ventricle that do not involve mechanical support or assist devices also are introduced.

FONTAN CONVERSION FOR THE FAILED FONTAN

In 1971, Fontan was the first to place the pulmonary and systemic circulations in series with one ventricle.[13] Although this surgery was a significant contribution to the care of patients with tricuspid atresia, it soon was recognized that Fontan's original procedure and its modifications could be of benefit to many other patients with single-ventricle physiology. The Fontan circulation has become the accepted final arrangement for most patients with a single-ventricle physiology.

Exclusion of a ventricle from the pulmonary circulation has resulted in several physiologic and anatomic sequelae. First, there can be turbulence and energy loss in the flow of the Fontan circulation, which can lead to stasis, thrombosis, and eventually partial obstruction. This entire process contributes to a significant **increase in systemic venous pressures**. One effect of this

increase in venous pressure is an increase in hydrostatic pressure, which results in an increase in production of lymph followed by a loss of albumin, antibodies, and lymphocytes with a significant decrease in oncotic pressure. These hydrodynamic changes (decreased oncotic pressure and increased hydrostatic pressure) contribute to the **generalized edema** with recurrent **effusions** and **protein-losing enteropathy (PLE)** sometimes seen in older Fontan patients. These complications in particular can be devastating to quality of life and can be associated with late mortality.[14,15] The loss of entropy of the systemic venous inflow in a Fontan circulation, especially in an atriopulmonary type of Fontan, allows for stasis and baffle **thrombus**. On close inspection, 20% of Fontan patients have some degree of thrombus in their connection.[16] Baffle thrombi not only promote increased systemic venous pressure secondary to partial obstruction, but also can lead to repeated subclinical pulmonary emboli. Chronically, this situation can lead to increasing pulmonary vascular hypertension, which further begets baffle stasis and obstruction.[15] Chronic pulmonary emboli seem to be an underappreciated cause contributing to Fontan failure. The chronically elevated right atrial pressure often leads to significant **right atrial dilation**. A dilated right atrium not only causes inefficient flow dynamics, but also can cause direct compression of the right pulmonary veins, further contributing to increasing pulmonary resistance. There also is a subset of Fontan patients with classic Glenn procedures who get a significant right-to-left shunt and cyanosis secondary to **pulmonary arteriovenous fistulas**. All of these changes are a detriment to Fontan circulation and contribute to cyanosis, systemic venous stasis, and an overall weakened state of health.

One of the most devastating late complications for the Fontan patient is **systemic ventricular failure**, with only cardiac transplantation or death as its end point. The etiology for ventricular failure after a Fontan operation may be multifactorial. First, right atrial enlargement seen in late Fontan circulations perpetuates atrial arrhythmias, and the loss of atrioventricular coordination and inefficient ventricular preloading could contribute to suboptimal myocardial performance. Second, the increased right atrial pressure in the Fontan patient causes coronary sinus hypertension, which decreases myocardial perfusion and propagates ventricular diastolic dysfunction. This chronic low-level ischemia coupled with the loss of atrioventricular synchrony over time may lead to systemic ventricular dilation and failure. Finally, there could be long-term effects of cyanosis on single ventricular performance.

Present forms of the Fontan operation, such as the lateral tunnel or the extracardiac conduit, do not have the same rate of Fontan failure as the earlier atriopulmonary version of the procedure. Both of the current types of Fontan operations have shown better flow hydrodynamics, and the extracardiac conduit has the theoretical advantage of fewer atrial suture lines,[17,18] which may contribute to less atrial arrhythmias.[19] As mentioned earlier, patients who have a failed Fontan circulation sometimes are provided the opportunity to have the original Fontan operation converted to the more current Fontan.

The indications and timing of such a Fontan conversion surgery are uncertain. Most larger series have a few lateral tunnel Fontan patients presenting for Fontan conversion secondary to the dilation of the right atrial wall[11]; this dilated portion of the lateral tunnel can serve as a substrate for arrhythmias or a nidus for thrombus and an obstruction to the right pulmonary venous return. At first, the Fontan conversions focused on changing the Fontan connection from atriopulmonary connections or Bjork right atrial–to–right ventricular connections to the total cavopulmonary connections. The earlier series showed that surgeons could perform these procedures safely with low operative mortality (0% to 6.5%) and excellent survival (90% at median follow-up durations of 18 to 25 months). These earlier results showed significant improvement in hemodynamics after conversion, and greater than 87% of patients had significant improvement in their symptoms. More than 75% of the surviving patients in the two largest series were in New York Heart Association (NYHA) class I at medium-term follow-up.[14,15,20,21]

These series on Fontan conversion patients all revealed important lessons learned in regard to (1) fenestration, (2) PLE, (3) atrial arrhythmias, and (4) timing.[14,15,20,21] First, most of the authors thought it was unnecessary to include a **fenestration** during these Fontan conversions because these patients are a much different cohort from primary Fontan patients. The patients with failing Fontans already are accustomed to Fontan physiology with elevated venous pressures; the Fontan conversion should encourage more efficient Fontan flow by decreasing the resistance in the Fontan circulation, allowing more flow and decreased venous pressure. The only exception to this nonfenestration practice is patients with PLE. If one believes that decreased cardiac output is a significant causative factor for PLE, fenestrating these patients may be beneficial because a fenestration should help to maintain a minimal cardiac output.

Second, some of these reports also concluded that patients with **protein-losing enteropathy** are not good candidates for conversion and can have a high short-term mortality (>50%). Although the literature did not support PLE being an absolute contraindication, it should be recognized as a significant risk factor for a poor outcome and in and of itself should not be a reason for Fontan conversion.

Third, although clinical and hemodynamic improvements were consistently reported with Fontan conversion, these results were tempered by the high rate of either new or recurrent **atrial arrhythmias** after the surgery.[11] Because the atrial arrhythmias negatively affected the hemodynamic profile, more recent series of Fontan conversion have treated atrial arrhythmias aggressively with intraoperative ablative therapy. Most protocols consist of a right modified atrial maze procedure for atrial reentrant tachycardia or atrial flutter and a modified left atrial maze for atrial fibrillation. Although a variety of energy sources have been used to create these ablations, cryoablation has been the most favored for its good results, reliability, and ease of use. Using this or similar arrhythmia management protocols, freedom from atrial dysrhythmias of 70% to 90% at mid-term (approximately 1.5 to 3 years) follow-up has been reported.[11,22] Because the restoration of sinus rhythm is a goal of most groups performing Fontan conversions, the practice of placing permanent pacemakers in patients has become more routine.[11,22] This practice ensures rate-responsive sinus rhythm regardless of the high postoperative incidence of sinus node dysfunction or recurrent atrial arrhythmias in these patients. Postoperative rhythm disturbances not only would be a hemodynamic insult, but also would require repeat sternotomy or thoracotomy for pacemaker placement because of lack of venous access for a transvenous pacing system. As underscored by more recent data, the ability to re-establish atrioventricular synchrony is probably one of the most important elements of the Fontan conversion.

Lastly, groups that advocate performing Fontan conversions have deduced that the best candidates are patients who have specific problems related to their Fontan circulation. Some authors even purport a direct correlation between hemodynamic and symptomatic results with the number of preoperative Fontan-related issues (i.e., baffle obstruction, arrhythmia, subclinical pulmonary emboli). Although patients with isolated decreased systemic ventricular function may improve with the decompression of the coronary sinus, the response in these patients to conversion is inconsistent. In addition, Fontan patients in NYHA class IV heart failure may not benefit from a Fontan conversion, leading more often to their transition to orthotopic heart transplantation. The largest series to date reported that 60% of NYHA class IV patients required orthotopic heart transplant after Fontan conversion.[11] Timing of intervention seems to be crucial in improving on these patients' results. Earlier intervention for the atriopulmonary Fontan seems to be desirable because the sequence of right atrial dilation to atrial reentry tachycardia to atrial fibrillation in these patients is clearly detrimental. There seems to be a benefit to interrupting this sequence at its earlier stages, as shown by the more favorable results in patients with less systemic ventricular failure and without atrial arrhythmias. The improved results from early Fontan conversion also may be attributable to the avoidance of worsening heart failure secondary to multiple antiarrhythmic drugs with cardiodepressive effects and chronic loss of atrioventricular synchrony.

Following is a suggested management protocol for these difficult patients that incorporates the more recent literature on Fontan conversion and our own practice. At the first signs of atrial arrhythmias, conduit obstruction, significant atrial enlargement, or valvular dysfunction, the concept of Fontan conversion and the option of transplantation should be introduced. Although exact timing of conversion is specific for each patient depending on their constellation of symptoms, we advocate intervening during the early stages of the failing Fontan. To consider converting these patients only when they have become marginal transplantation candidates would yield poor outcomes. Although PLE is not a contraindication per se, most clinicians think that the expectations for Fontan conversion for these patients should be guarded. When a candidate has been selected, the procedure should consist of the takedown of the old Fontan connection and creation of a total cavopulmonary connection, which could be an extracardiac conduit or a lateral tunnel Fontan. There seems to be consensus that in the presence of preexisting atrial arrhythmias, intraoperative ablation surgery should be performed, probably with cryoablation. If atrial reentry tachycardia or atrial flutter exists, we perform a modified right atrial maze specific for the patient's cardiac lesion, and if atrial fibrillation exists, a standard transseptal modified left atrial maze is performed (Fig. 42-1). Permanent pacemakers should be placed in all patients who undergo ablation surgery. Prophylactic arrhythmia ablation surgery has not been shown to be helpful in primary Fontan patients, and there are no data at this time to show its place in Fontan conversion patients. Atrial debulking for significant atrial dilation also is performed if necessary, especially if clot, atrial arrhythmia, or pulmonary venous compression is a complicating factor. One also should perform any concomitant repairs to the heart (i.e., systemic AVV repair)

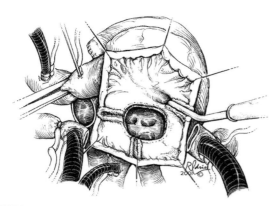

FIGURE 42-1 ■ **The maze procedure.** A right atrial modified maze procedure in a patient with tricuspid atresia. This intraoperative electrophysiologic procedure reduces the likelihood of postoperative intra-atrial reentrant tachycardia and is an essential part of the Fontan conversion operation. (From Mavroudis C, Backer CL, Deal BJ: *Total cavopulmonary conversion and maze procedure for patients with failure for the Fontan operation. J Thorac Cardiovasc Surg* 2001; 122:863-871.)

to increase further the likelihood of recovery of ventricular function. Patients who required orthotopic heart transplants (0% to 7%) all were in NYHA class IV heart failure or had long-standing malignant atrial arrhythmias preoperatively. These patients perhaps could have been more successful conversions had intervention occurred sooner, underscoring the importance of early and aggressive surgical intervention in this patient cohort.

A retrospective review of our experience with 30 Fontan conversions comparing extracardiac conduit with lateral tunnel patients showed that there were no differences between these patients in duration of intubation, inotropic support, intensive care unit stay, hospital stay, or postoperative rhythm disturbances. NYHA class, mortality, and late arrhythmias also did not differ at mid-term follow-up (3 years). Extracardiac conduit provides the surgeon the advantages of not arresting the heart, decreasing the sutures needed in the atrium (possible arrhythmogenic foci), and excluding all atrial tissue so that atrial dilation is theoretically no longer a possibility. To date, no studies have shown a difference between these two methods of total cavopulmonary connection for Fontan conversion. This general protocol has resulted in no hospital deaths and only one late death at our institution. These excellent mid-term results have been seen in other programs as well, with hospital mortalities of 0% to 5% with almost uniform improvements (>90%) in NYHA class and exercise endurance.[11,22] The late recurrence of atrial arrhythmia can be expected to be between 10% and 30% with almost all recurrent arrhythmias being able to be medically controlled.

There is a growing body of data to support the notion that Fontan conversion can be accomplished safely and with high expectations for significant hemodynamic and symptomatic improvement. Whether the long-term result of this therapy will be as a destination therapy or as a bridge to transplantation or permanent mechanical support is unknown, but present results advocate Fontan conversion as an effective primary therapy for the failing Fontan patient.

DOUBLE-SWITCH OPERATION FOR CONGENITALLY CORRECTED TRANSPOSITION OF THE GREAT ARTERIES

Congenitally-correction transposition of the great arteries (ccTGA) is an uncommon form of congenital heart disease with atrioventricular and ventriculoarterial discordance (S, L, L or I, D, D); in this lesion, the mRV is associated with the systemic circulation. Although the small fraction of patients with ccTGA who do not have any associated anomalies (1%) theoretically could have a normal physiology and no symptoms,[23,24] the natural history of these patients is that of significant lifetime risks of systemic mRV failure and AVV insufficiency.[25-28]

Most patients with ccTGA have a combination of the following associated anomalies: ventricular septal defect (VSD) (80%), pulmonary stenosis/atresia (50%), systemic AVV regurgitation, or congenital heart block.

The classic surgical approach to this lesion was to treat the associated anomalies, leaving the mRV as the ventricle in the systemic circulation. These operations usually consisted of closing the VSD through the right atrium and addressing the subpulmonic/pulmonary stenosis with muscle resection or a spiral outflow tract patch or bypassing it with an mLV to pulmonary artery conduit. **Complete heart block** is often seen either preoperatively in its congenital form or postoperatively and treated with implantation of a permanent pacemaker. The estimated incidence of complete heart block without surgery is 2% per year and increases to 20% to 30% postoperatively.[25] The systemic AVV usually was addressed at the time of initial repair or subsequently when regurgitation became severe. Progression of **AVV regurgitation** requiring intervention after classic repair ranged from 40% to 80% in long-term follow-up and was the major reason for repeat intervention in all the large series.[26,27] Because repair of the tricuspid valve was rarely successful in ccTGA when the mRV was left in the systemic circulation, valve replacement often was required with all of its drawbacks.[27] Besides a high incidence of dysplastic systemic AVV that results in insufficiency of the valve, the mRV with its septophilic systemic AVV also becomes incompetent as the interventricular septum bows left into the low-pressured mLV. The frequently seen improvement in systemic AVV regurgitation with pulmonary artery banding (PAB) and shifting of the interventricular septum toward the mRV attests to this hypothesis.

The classic approach to ccTGA produced acceptable short-term results with operative mortalities usually around 10% to 15%. The mid-term and long-term results were disappointing, however, in many regards. Long-term survival at 10 years ranged from 50% to 60%, and in one larger series, 70% to 100% of these late deaths were attributable to **systemic mRV failure**.[26-28] Of the patients who survived, 40% to 60% required a reoperation, with most being attempts to salvage the failing right ventricle (by addressing systemic AVV regurgitation or complete heart block or both).[27-29] These poor long-term results brought into question the conceptual approach of leaving the mRV in the systemic circulation in patients with ccTGA.

Placing the mLV into the systemic circulation was first accomplished by Mee and Yamagishi in the same year (1989) with the technique of an anatomic correction for ccTGA.[30,31] These initial reports were followed by several later series purporting the favorable results of this dramatic change in surgical approach. The anatomic surgical corrections of ccTGA are (1) a double-switch operation (atrial with ASOs) for ccTGA patients without pulmonary stenosis or (2) a Rastelli repair with an atrial switch operation for ccTGA patients with pulmonary stenosis or atresia (Fig. 42-2). This approach, although technically complex, was adopted by several groups in the early 1990s, whose results proved that the procedures could be done with low hospital mortality (5% to 10%) and good functional outcomes (NYHA class I) for greater than 90% of survivors in early follow-up.[31-33] Since the 1990s, these results have continued to improve secondary to myriad of factors, including better cardiopulmonary bypass, anesthesia, postoperative care, and surgical technique. The most essential improvement has been the cumulative experience gained in the timing of and the preparation for definitive surgical intervention in this heterogeneous group of patients.

The following can be a general surgical management scheme for ccTGA patients.

(1) Patients with ccTGA, a nonrestrictive VSD, and no pulmonary stenosis usually have unrestricted pulmonary blood flow and require PAB early in infancy. Repair should be undertaken when cyanosis becomes significant with a double-switch operation and VSD closure.

(2) Patients with ccTGA, VSD, and pulmonary stenosis/pulmonary atresia can have a well-balanced circulation or inadequate pulmonary blood flow. The latter situation warrants a systemic-to-pulmonary artery shunt. Patients who are well balanced and clinically asymptomatic can be a controversial group because despite their high functional status, serial echocardiography may show declining systemic ventricular function or abnormal exercise testing or both. The low hospital mortality reported by most recent studies raises the issue of how early these patients should go for anatomic correction.[34-36] Presently, most authors still think that clinically asymptomatic patients should be followed closely and treated aggressively when symptoms manifest. The patients in this category require a combined Rastelli/atrial switch repair, which should be delayed until they outgrow their pulmonary blood flow with the expectation that more time, it is hoped, would allow for a larger conduit.

(3) Patients with ccTGA, intact IVS, or a restrictive VSD have balanced circulations, but a high incidence of systemic AVV regurgitation, which contributes to an often relentless and progressive systemic ventricular dysfunction. The physiology of this cohort is a spectrum differentiated according to the amount of mRV dysfunction and mLV preparedness. Patients who present with no or mild mRV dysfunction and a prepared left ventricle secondary to early presentation or mild pulmonary stenosis can proceed to double-switch operation. Patients who present later with an unprepared mLV (mLV-to-mRV ratio <0.7 or IVS bowing into a crescent-shaped mLV) and moderate or less mRV dysfunction can undergo mLV retraining by PAB.[10] The science and art of mLV retraining via PAB are discussed in greater detail later. In brief, the PAB is placed to increase the

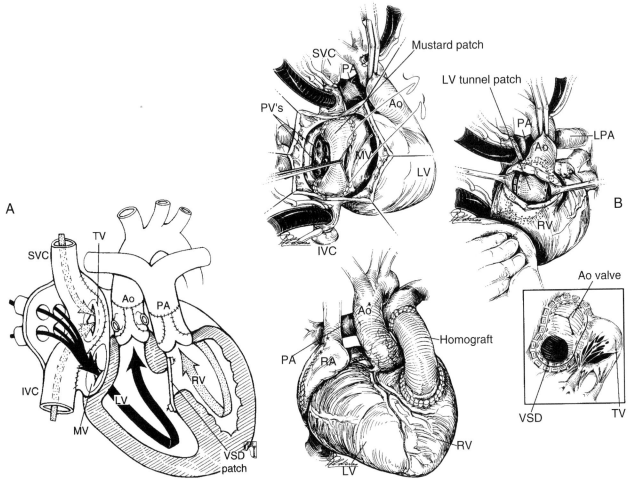

FIGURE 42-2 ■ The double-switch operation. A, The Senning plus arterial switch operations are illustrated. **B,** The Mustard plus Rastelli operations are illustrated in sequence. The atrial reconstruction is performed and followed by the Rastelli operation with the right ventricular incision used to baffle the left ventricular blood through the ventricular septal defect (VSD) to the aorta (Ao). The right ventricle (RV)–to–pulmonary artery (PA) continuity is established with a valved homograft conduit. After both of these complex surgeries, concordant atrioventricular and ventriculoarterial connections are established. IVC, inferior vena cava; LPA, left pulmonary artery; LV, left ventricle; MV, mitral valve; PVs, pulmonary veins; RA, right atrium; SVC, superior vena cava; TV, tricuspid valve. (From Karl T, Cochrane AD: *Congenitally corrected transposition of the great arteries.* In Mavroudis C, Backer C [eds]: *Pediatric Cardiac Surgery*, p. 488 (**A**), p. 491 (**B**), Philadelphia, Mosby, 2003.)

mLV pressure to 80% systemic pressure, tolerating only mild mLV dysfunction and shifting the IVS toward the mRV. This increase in afterload helps the mLV gain mass via hypertrophy and maybe hyperplasia. The shift in the IVS often causes an improvement in mRV function by allowing better systemic AVV coaptation. The mLV is considered prepared in most series when the mLV-to-mRV ratio is greater than 70% with near-normal mLV function and when notable thickening of the mLV wall has occurred. The time for retraining of the mLV for ccTGA differed among groups from medians of 2 months to 12 months.[25,35,36] This disparity in the length of training among the different series seemed to indicate that older patient cohorts required longer training periods.

After satisfactory mLV training, these patients would proceed to the double-switch operation.

(4) Patients with ccTGA, IVS, and moderate-to-severe mRV dysfunction are difficult in terms of devising a surgical strategy. The declining systemic function complicates the training of the mLV because these patients often do not tolerate PAB. The increase in competence of the systemic AVV with PAB only worsens the systemic ventricular function because the mRV no longer would be able to decompress via the AVV, causing some degree of acute failure and hemodynamic embarrassment or even death. The limited options for these patients are to do a double-switch operation with an untrained left ventricle and support the patients postoperatively with

a ventricular assist device or perform an orthotopic heart transplant. The former option is suitable only for prepubescent patients because mLV retraining on mechanical assistance in young adults is rarely successful. The therapeutic options and outcomes for this cohort are the least favorable of all the ccTGA patients.[25,34]

Certain anatomic and clinical issues should be considered before choosing to do an anatomic repair over the classic repair. First, although a moderate degree of mLV or AVV hypoplasia is a relative contraindication to anatomic repair, moderate hypoplasia of the systemic mRV or AVV is not. One may need to create a pulsatile Glenn shunt or tolerate cyanosis from an atrial fenestration to do an anatomic repair.[34] Second, if the systemic AVV straddles the VSD, biventricular repair is probably not an option. Third, older patients (>15 years old) with an unprepared mLV (no pulmonary stenosis) do not seem to tolerate training well because the ventricular response to an increased afterload usually is limited to maladaptive hypertrophy causing diastolic dysfunction and endocardial ischemia.[10,25,34,36] Fourth, certain characteristics of the VSD (small orifice or noncommittable or both) in patients with pulmonary stenosis can make an anatomic repair exceedingly difficult, if not impossible. Although posterior and inferior enlargement of these VSDs is possible, this surgical modification potentially can compromise the conduction system and the septal perfusion.[37] Lastly, although certain groups have listed coronary anatomy as a possible contraindication to the double-switch, our institutional preference is to perform the double-switch operation regardless of the coronary artery pattern (as with ASO for D-TGA).[38]

The evolution of the anatomic repair for ccTGA in the 1990s has yielded impressive results with zero or very low hospital mortality[25,30,34-36]; overall, these series report on 114 patients with only 4 deaths. The mid-term clinical results have been encouraging, with all series reporting greater than 90% of patients being in NYHA class I with follow-up periods of 3 to 7 years. Groups that have investigated exercise function have found that these anatomically corrected patients had normal exercise tolerance. All reports also comment on the significant improvement in AVV regurgitation in most patients, often going from severe to mild insufficiency. The freedom of intervention at 5 years is about 85% and at 7 years is about 78%. Although the double-switch results are improvements over the classic repair, late complications, such as neo–aortic insufficiency and atrial baffle obstruction, are beginning to be reported and need to be followed closely. Another frequent complication is complete heart block requiring a permanent pacemaker, with most recent series reporting an incidence of 0% to 14%.[25,35]

Although creating a circulation in which the mLV is the systemic ventricle is the ideal arrangement, the risk and success for such a complex anatomic repair for

patients with ccTGA were in doubt. In the 1990s, several groups clearly showed the safety and effectiveness of such a therapeutic strategy. Anatomic correction is presently the preferred therapy for most symptomatic ccTGA patients with favorable anatomy, although cautious enthusiasm should be exercised. These patients need continued surveillance to determine the long-term results of the retrained mLV and its semilunar valve and the atrial baffle.

ARTERIAL SWITCH OPERATION ("RE-SWITCH") FOR FAILED ATRIAL SWITCH OPERATION

A challenging but relatively uncommon form of systemic mRV failure occurs in patients who had a prior atrial switch procedure (Senning or Mustard) for D-TGA. With the success and adoption of the ASO in the 1980s and 1990s, the scope of this problem seems to be finite. There is a relatively large population of patients who have undergone Mustard or Senning procedures in the prior decades, however, who are now adults and probably will present over the next decade with a clinical syndrome of systemic mRV failure, tricuspid regurgitation, or atrial arrhythmias. Many authors have estimated the incidence for systemic ventricular failure in patients after atrial switch operations to be 7% to 10% per 10 years in simple D-TGA with higher rates (15%) for patients with D-TGA and VSD.[39-41]

The therapeutic options for atrial switch patients with a failing systemic ventricle are limited to tricuspid valve repair or replacement, orthotopic heart transplantation, or ASO. The results of **tricuspid repair/replacement** in these patients have been disappointing because even if successful, the failing right ventricle does not seem to improve with this intervention. The 10-year survival for patients with a failing systemic mRV with an ejection fraction of less than 45% after tricuspid valve replacement has been shown to be less than 25%.[27,42] **Transplantation** for congenital heart disease in children and adolescents has been documented clearly to be less satisfying than adult data. Transplantation also continues to be plagued with the problems of donor paucity (with a 30% mortality while awaiting orthotopic heart transplant), rejection, coronary artery disease, immunosuppressive therapy, compliance with medications, and the need for repeat transplantation. The **arterial switch operation** is usually a two-stage therapeutic strategy:[43] The first stage is to retrain the underloaded and underdeveloped mLV through a single or multiple periods of PAB until the mLV-to-mRV ratio is greater than 80% (Fig. 42-3), and this preparatory stage is followed by the ASO, which includes takedown of the atrial baffle. There is, however, a small cohort of patients in almost all series that has significant subpulmonic obstruction and mLV hypertrophy; these patients also have adequate substrates

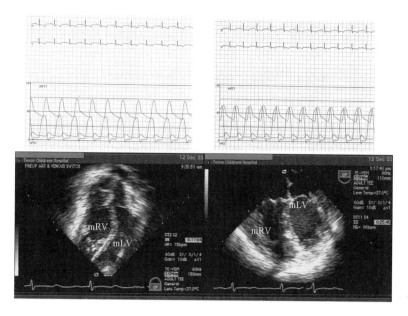

FIGURE 42-3 ■ **Intraoperative assessment of switch candidate during pulmonary artery banding.** Arterial tracing and echocardiography of morphologic right ventricle (mRV) and morphologic left ventricle (mLV) before *(left)* and after *(right)* pulmonary artery banding tightening (see text for details).

for a single-stage ASO that omits the mLV retraining stage.[44-46]

In addition to Mee's experience, which has cumulatively reported on 29 patients who underwent this surgical strategy, other series have been reported, albeit with limited number of patients.[45,46] A comparison between patients who were retrained and patients who failed that stage is essential to delineate which patients are appropriate candidates for this therapeutic strategy. Of the patients who enter the retraining stage, 50% to 75% become suitable substrates for the anatomic ASO, and the remaining patients proceed to orthotopic heart transplant or death despite maximal medical therapy.

A third cohort of patients results from the mLV retraining—patients who symptomatically improved after the PAB. This improvement is secondary to the intraventricular septal shift that allows improved systemic AVV function and a decrease in systemic mRV volume overload. Some of these patients improve sufficiently to obviate the need to become candidates for ASO. The PAB served as a prolonged bridge to transplantation. The mortality from mLV retraining ranges from 0% to 15%, but all series document that the postoperative course of these patients after PAB is often protracted and challenging.

Although the mean time required for successful mLV retraining ranged from 13 to 26 months,[42,45] this number is not useful information because the training of these patients needs to be quite individualized depending on several factors.[44-46] The issues for determination of the mLV training period include the following: (1) The particular anatomy of the patient (i.e., subpulmonary stenosis) may have caused some degree of elevated mLV pressures and hypertrophy (i.e., the period of mLV training can be shortened or in some cases omitted); (2) the starting mLV-to-mRV pressure ratio is important

because if this pressure ratio is low (<0.3), one usually can expect a prolonged retraining period with more than one banding procedure (and patients undergoing successful ASO had statistically higher ratios at the end of mLV retraining)[45]; and (3) the age of the patient is important because prepubescent patients often can be switched with less than ideal hemodynamics even if a ventricular assist device is required postoperatively.

Some investigators have documented that postpubescent patients cannot be expected to respond as well to this surgical strategy even with ideal hemodynamics because they seem to have a higher mortality rate.[10] Although there are isolated reports of patients being converted to ASO late into their 20s or 30s, the larger experiences have shown that patients older than 12 years of age have a significantly higher failure rate (80%) compared with patients younger than 12 years of age (40%).[45] This is an extremely important aspect for the ASO in this setting because most patients who will present as candidates for this procedure are growing older.[45] At our institution, consideration of these factors along with careful clinical observation and hemodynamic assessment determine the need and length of mLV retraining.

Several methods have been proposed to assess the mLV readiness during the retraining period: pressure volume loops, mLV wall thickness, pressure ratios, myocardial biopsies, and ventricular geometry.[10,44-47] The one common criterion for all series has been an mLV-to-mRV ratio of greater than 0.7 to 0.8 with good mLV function. The mLV wall thickness of greater than 7 to 8 mm also has been purported by some series to be an absolute criterion, but the accurate assessment of the true muscle thickness of the mLV wall has been difficult. Using MRI, clinicians have reported that 40% of mLV thickness was actually fibrosis on pathologic examination. In addition, edema of the tissues after banding has made the measurement of LV wall thickness difficult.[48] Some investigators began using MRI with T2-weighted images to distinguish myocardial edema from mass acquisition with the caveat, however, that the edema represents cellular damage that leads to undesired fibrosis/scarring.[45]

Most series come from experienced surgeons who use the constellation of pressure data, patient clinical status, and left ventricle geometry and function to determine which patients are adequate substrates for the ASO. This strategy still results in a 16% to 35% mortality for all the patients who undergo PAB and a short-term mortality of 25% to 45% for patients who undergo the ASO.[44-46] Almost all of the short-term mortalities consist of postoperative, in-hospital deaths. These results highlight that even if criteria are met, it is difficult to be certain that the mLV is truly prepared, especially in these patients, who tend to present in the postpubescent period.

The inability to predict successful ASO in these patients is due to factors that are still unclear. It has been suggested in at least one study that the chronically involuted mLV has abnormal underdevelopment of the native coronary circulation, which with increasing age is less likely to be revitalized during and after load retraining. This underdevelopment is a result of a declining coronary reserve caused by a decrease in capillary density, large-caliber coronary arteries, and intramural coronary perfusion.[45,47,49] The neovascularization that does develop under the duress of mLV retraining is a functionally inferior circulation unable to support the requirements of a systemic ventricle long-term. This may be one of the factors to help explain the unpredictable results of the strategy. Patients who do survive the perioperative period enjoy excellent long-term functional results with greater than 90% being in NYHA class I.[44,45]

The increasing experience at some centers with this strategy to convert a failed atrial switch operation to the ASO has allowed these centers to start identifying some morbidities, including neo–aortic insufficiency and persistent atrial arrhythmias. **Neo aortic insufficiency** requiring valve replacement ranges from 10% to 20%, whereas mild neo–aortic valvular insufficiency requiring close observation is 40% after mLV retraining and ASO.[42,49] In addition, the hopes of **atrial arrhythmias** resolving as atrial pressures decreased have not been realized. This observation is perhaps not surprising when considering the additional suturing and manipulation of the atria during the second stage involving takedown of the atrial switch before the ASO. The largest and most recent series showed that preoperative arrhythmias were the only variable to be a risk factor for failing PAB retraining and ASO.[45] Mavroudis[46] and others have become aggressive with the treatment of both of these morbidities by performing neo–aortic valve reconstruction during the ASO and modified atrial maze procedures in patients with atrial tachyarrhythmias.

The patient with a failing systemic ventricle and heart failure after atrial switch palliation for TGA presents a therapeutic dilemma. The arterial re-switch strategy has become an alternative to orthotopic heart transplantation for these patients. Enthusiasm for this strategy is constrained by the retraining process through serial PABs, which can be hazardous and unpredictable, and by the challenging postoperative course after the ASO. In the face of severe mRV failure and atrial arrhythmias in a postpubescent patient with a prior atrial switch operation, many authors believe transplantation still should be the preferred treatment modality. The ASO can be a successful management strategy, however, in a carefully select cohort of patients with the opportunity for excellent functional and long-term results. The future role of mechanical assist devices in these patients remains to be elucidated.

LATE ARTERIAL SWITCH

The performance of an ASO in the first 3 weeks of life to achieve anatomic correction of D-TGA is the present standard of care. A small cohort of these TGA patients with an intact ventricular septum or restrictive VSD presents late secondary to low birth weight, delayed referral, or perinatal complications. Their late presentation raises the issue of the adequacy of the deconditioned mLV to assume the work of the systemic ventricle.

Late ASO in most series has been defined loosely as performing the ASO in children older than 3 weeks old; there have been case reports and even a few small series, however, of older infants (3 weeks to 2 months of age) with TGA and IVS in whom a primary ASO was performed with good results.[50,51] A series from Foran and colleagues[50] reported 37 infants with minimal mortality (1 of 37) and minimal postoperative mechanical support (1 of 37). The same group showed no significant difference in mortality or mechanical support when the older infant group was compared with a group of patients who had ASO at younger than 21 days of age.[50] This strategy correlates with a postmortem study of 61 infants with uncorrected TGA and IVS that showed normal or near-normal left ventricular wall thickness in infants 2 months of age.[52] It is also possible that patients with TGA and IVS presenting for the first time at older than 3 weeks may have persistence of the ductus arteriosus or a delayed decline in the pulmonary artery resistance, both of which would allow the left ventricular mass to be maintained.

The assumption that the crescent shape geometry of the mLV correlates to an mLV that is unfit to serve as a systemic ventricle for life is yet unproved. Although most authors agree that pressure unloading the mLV eventually begins to change its physiologic and molecular structure, this time course is relatively uncertain. In contrast, other authors believe that age alone should not be the determining factor for the management strategy for TGA, but rather left ventricular mass should be the deciding factor (lower limits defined to be <20 g/m²). Lacour-Gayet and associates[53] used the criteria that patients with a left ventricular mass of less than 35 g/m² necessitated retraining, which led to an age distribution of patients who got mLV retraining of 9 days to 8 months; the authors submitted that further studies are needed to determine a more accurate lower limit of mLV mass.

There are several management strategies for patients with TGA and IVS who present late with a potentially failing mLV. The **primary ASO** is performed with the expectation that a certain percentage of these patients will require ventricular support, usually extracorporeal membrane oxygenation (ECMO) or ventricular assist device, while their mLV retrains (see Chapters 45-47).[54] The period of mLV retraining on mechanical support can be expected usually to be less than 10 days and to be required only in about 10% of patients when ASO is performed on patients 3 weeks to 3 months old.[50] A criticism of this management strategy is that ECMO not only exposes these patients to its well-documented morbidities, but also that ECMO places a large strain on personnel and financial resources. Other groups argue that the aforementioned burdens are relatively less for institutions that regularly use ECMO. These groups also think that retraining the mLV after correction, with an oxygenated state, proves better for long-term systemic ventricular function than retraining the mLV in a cyanotic milieu.[50,51] The required length of retraining on mechanical support and the percentage of patients needing support seem to be age dependent, with increasing age requiring support more often and for longer periods. Performing primary ASO in patients older than 2 months old with TGA and IVS has been reported only in case reports or as outliers in several series. Most authors believe that primary ASO in patients older than 2 months would carry a much higher mechanical support and mortality burden than the rapid two-stage ASO. We believe using age as a cutoff is too broad a criterion, and that any infant with no obvious involution of the mLV should undergo catheterization to determine if the mLV-to-mRV pressure ratio is greater than 80%. If this value is met and is in congruence with our overall perception of the patient, we believe it is reasonable to proceed with primary ASO.

The **rapid two-stage arterial switch operation** is a management protocol that contains three principal steps: choosing a suitable candidate, PAB to pressure train the mLV (with a concomitant aortopulmonary shunt), and performing the ASO. The criteria (e.g., age, left ventricle geometry, mLV-to-mRV pressure ratio, myocardial mass) to determine which mLVs are unprepared to assume the work of the systemic ventricle have been discussed in detail in prior sections. After determining that the mLV of the late-presenting D-TGA/IVS patient is involuted, PAB should be placed. Not only is the mLV pressure loaded, but also the systemic mRV is

volume loaded, explaining the often challenging postoperative management of these patients.

A tight PAB leading to quicker retraining is not better because rapid increases in mLV mass and hypertrophy has been linked to a significant reduction in late mLV function.[55] Many surgeons place a conservative PAB, realizing that they may have to reoperate in the early postoperative period to tighten the band. Most series have training periods of 7 to 15 days. Longer periods of mLV retraining, employed in other cohorts of patients (i.e., arterial switch for failed atrial switch operation), are not beneficial in this group. Prolonged training in late ASO patients has been documented to increase mLV dysfunction, arrhythmias, aortic insufficiency, and subaortic stenosis.[56]

When the patient's mLV has met the particular institutional criteria for preparedness, an ASO should be performed in a timely manner. Many institutions use this management strategy with a hospital mortality of less than 5%, a late cardiac mortality of less than 5%, and excellent clinical results, with almost all patients being in NYHA class I.[53,56-58] There are, however, several concerns with this management scheme. First, the significant afterload burden from a tight band and the volume burden from a systemic-to-pulmonary shunt can lead to significant ventricular dysfunction, which some patients do not tolerate. Their bands are either loosened or taken off altogether, with the latter maneuver representing a failure of this strategy (10%).[53,56-58] Second, the acute stress caused by significant pressure and volume loads probably induces subendocardial ischemia, which may explain the late mLV dysfunction seen in patients retrained too quickly.[55] This late dysfunction has not been documented in patients undergoing primary ASO, unless coronary complications have ensued. Third, there has been concern that the rapid two-stage ASO would produce a higher incidence of aortic insufficiency. Lastly, the fundamental question of the two-stage strategy, as with all mLV-PAB retraining strategies, is the type of muscle being stimulated (hyperplasia versus hypertrophy). The mitotic function of the myocyte is lost in the first weeks of life, leaving only hypertrophy as an adaptive response to stress. This latter response is not predictable and may be maladaptive, possibly contributing to late mLV dysfunction.[10,59] Despite these concerns, one cannot deny the almost uniform success of the major centers with this management strategy in this difficult cohort. The rapid two-stage ASO is the standard of care for TGA/IVS patients with a significantly deconditioned mLV.

The **atrial switch operation** is a third management strategy for these patients, but is usually invoked when ASO is not possible because of an mLV that does not tolerate retraining or because of an associated cardiac anomaly that precludes an ASO. The well-documented early and late morbidities of baffle obstruction, systemic mRV failure, atrial arrhythmias, and systemic

AVV insufficiency render this a less attractive option than ASO. Greater than 80% of atrial switch patients survive more than 10 years and even longer with good-to-excellent functional status and quality of life.[60] When right ventricular and tricuspid valve function are favorable, the atrial switch operation can still be an acceptable option, especially as an extended bridge to transplantation or even as a destination therapy, for patients unable to undergo ASO.

(4) **Orthotopic heart transplantation** is the last option. Orthotopic heart transplant is usually reserved as the fourth option in the care of these patients.

The management of patients with TGA/IVS who present late has been a success as a result of an understanding of retraining the involuted mLV. The results for these patients clinically in regard to morbidity and mortality and their functional status are considered almost the same as those for patients who underwent primary ASO.

SURGICAL STRATEGIES FOR VENTRICULAR RESHAPING

Congestive heart failure is characterized by a progressive loss of cardiac function that stimulates compensatory mechanisms at the molecular, cellular, and genetic levels that eventually become maladaptive. The macroscopic manifestation of this complex remodeling process are the changes in shape and size of the systemic ventricle. The increases in sphericity and dilation of the ventricle cause a decrease in myocardial perfusion and an increase in myocardial stretching, which lead to further biochemical and cellular maladaptations. This self-perpetuating decline in function eventually leads to end-stage heart failure. Some authors believe that this cycle can be interrupted by surgical interventions that restore the normal shape and size of the systemic ventricle. The law of LaPlace (wall tension = [intraventricular pressure × ventricular radius]/2 × wall thickness) is the basis for this rationale of reducing the size of the left ventricle: If the ventricular radius is reduced by surgical means, the wall tension also is lessened.

This cellular and geometric reverse remodeling phenomenon has been achieved in varying degrees via medications, such as angiotensin-converting enzyme and β blockade; ventricular mechanical support; and left ventricular volume reduction surgeries, such as the Batista operation and the Dor procedure.[61,62] **The Batista operation** (Fig. 42-4), also called partial left ventriculectomy, initially was used to treat patients with cardiomyopathy related to Chagas disease. In this operation, the normal ventricular tissue between the anterior and posterior papillary muscles is resected with mitral valve repair or replacement. **The Dor procedure** (Fig. 42-5), also called endoventricular circular patch plasty repair of the left ventricle with associated coronary grafting or surgical ventricular restoration, has been applied to patients with left ventricular dysfunction after an infarction with either akinesis or dyskinesis. Lastly, **mitral valve reconstructive surgery** has been shown to aid in reshaping the left ventricle and reducing its size, improving hemodynamics.[63]

In some countries where ventricular assist devices and transplantation are not options, left ventricular volume reduction surgery has been performed in children with dilated cardiomyopathy without congenital anatomic defects. These series have been small but promising with some significant initial improvements in

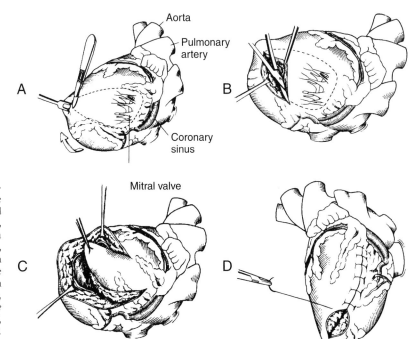

FIGURE 42-4 ■ **The Batista operation.** In this operation, the normal ventricular tissue between the anterior and posterior papillary muscles is resected along with mitral valve repair or replacement. **A,** The extent of the myocardial resection is in the area of the circumflex marginal coronary artery. **B** and **C,** The excision of the inferolateral myocardium between the papillary muscles is seen. **D,** The restoration of the left ventricular cavity is seen with placement of a continuous suture. (From Westaby S, Katsumata T, Frazier OH: *Surgical restoration of the failing left ventricle.* In Narula J, Virmani R, Ballester M, et al [eds]: *Heart Failure: Pathogenesis and Treatment.* p. 627, London, Martin Kunitz, 2002.)

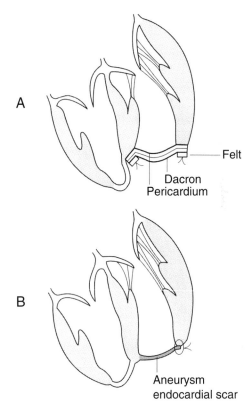

FIGURE 42-5 ■ The Dor procedure. The procedure includes a looped stitch around the aneurysm to shrink the area. An endoventricular Dacron patch is used to exclude the areas that are akinetic or dyskinetic. The operation transforms the failing ventricle from a spherical to its original elliptical shape. **A,** A pericardial covered Dacron patch is used. **B,** An autogenous endocardium from septal scar is seen. (See also Color Section) (From Westaby S, Katsumata T, Frazier OH: *Surgical restoration of the failing left ventricle.* In Narula J, Virmani R, Ballester M, et al, [eds]: *Heart Failure: Pathogenesis and Treatment,* p. 625. London, Martin Kunitz, 2002.)

LV function and clinical status.[64] The adult data have shown that the initial promising results of volume restorative surgery wane quickly and that the initial improvements do not truly represent an increase in contractility (end-diastolic volume decreases after volume reduction surgery, but stroke volume remains the same). The increase in ejection fraction often noted in these studies did not represent any change in contractility.[65]

Another concept to restore left ventricular function is to provide a support girdle for the failed ventricle. One such procedure experimentally and clinically tested for aiding a failing ventricle is **dynamic cardiomyoplasty**, which entails the training of skeletal muscle to contract in concert with ventricular muscle and assist or boost its function. In this procedure, the latissimus dorsi muscle is wrapped around the heart muscle and is electrically paced in synchrony with ventricular systole. The true benefit of cardiomyoplasty is not the pumping action of the skeletal muscle, but rather its containment of the ventricle—the so-called girdling effect.[66] This finding, coupled with the current enthusiasm toward surgical therapies of remodeling and reshaping strategies, resulted in the development of the current generation of passive mechanical cardiac support devices.

Of the passive ventricular constraint support devices, the **CorCap** (Acorn Cardiovascular, Inc, St. Paul, MN) (Fig. 42-6) has been among the most extensively used. The CorCap is a netlike device that is positioned around the cardiac ventricles and is anchored to the atrioventricular groove; it is designed to reduce ventricular volume acutely.[67] The CorCap has a unique polyester knit with multiple filaments that create compliance characteristics so that compliance in the apical-to-base vector is greater than that in the circumferential vectors.[67,69] This arrangement allows the heart to change from the maladaptive spherical shape to its more functional elliptical shape. In experimental investigations, the CorCap not only prevented progressive left ventricular dilation, but also caused the left ventricle to reshape without inducing a restrictive physiology.[68,69] This reshaping helped to reduce functional mitral regurgitation and did not disturb epicardial and myocardial surface vessels, as shown by angiography and cellular studies.[67] The changes induced by CorCap seemed to improve diastolic function, as shown by decreased end-diastolic volumes and pressures and by more sophisticated measurements with conductance catheters, which exhibited a leftward shift of the end-systolic pressure volume relationship. At a cellular and biochemical level, this reshaping correlated with improved adrenergic signaling and calcium cycling and decreased myocardial oxygen consumption. These multiple adaptive changes at all levels to passive restraint and reshaping argue that the CorCap can lead to reverse remodeling of the failing ventricle.[67,69]

Initial clinical studies of the CorCap focused on safety to ensure that a constrictive physiology was not present. Hemodynamic studies were done on 15 patients and showed pressure volume loops and coronary artery flow measurements with no physiologic or hemodynamic embarrassment. At 1-year follow-up, cardiac size was reduced (left ventricular end-diastolic diameter, left ventricular end-systolic diameter), ejection fraction was improved, and functional and clinical status was improved. Concomitant coronary artery bypass grafts done at the time of CorCap implant all were patent by angiography. In the 10 patients undergoing only the CorCap procedure, the hemodynamic, functional, and quality-of-life results were similar to the entire cohort of CorCap patients.[70] The application of this device in small children with congenital heart defects would be limited by somatic outgrowth.

CorCap, or a similar device such as the **Myosplint** (Myocor, Maple Grove, MN) (Fig. 42-7), may be applicable during interstage management or as an adjunct to valvular repair for regurgitation.[71] An even more promising application for these devices is in older adolescents who present with a failing systemic ventricle (i.e., classically corrected ccTGA, patients after failed atrial switch operations), who cannot tolerate mLV retraining. The mechanical restraining device possibly

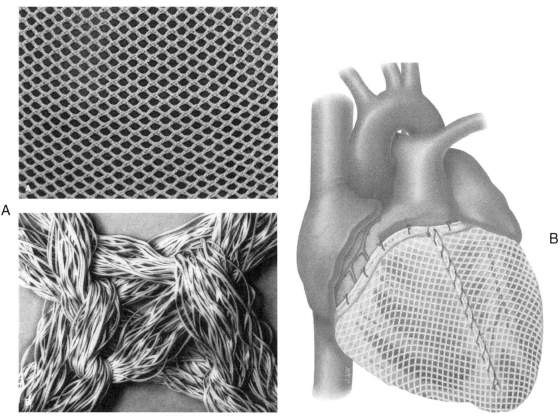

FIGURE 42-6 ■ The CorCap device. This fabric mesh implant device is designed to reduce wall stress by passive support to reverse the progression of ventricular dilation. Several sizes are available. **A,** Scanning electron microscopy shows the area of the open-weave construction. **B,** The device is seen wrapped around the ventricles to arrest progressive dilation of the ventricles. (See also Color Section for part B). (From Westaby S, Katsumata T, Frazier OH: *Surgical restoration of the failing left ventricle.* In Narula J, Virmani R, Ballester M, et al [eds]: *Heart Failure: Pathogenesis and Treatment,* p. 643. London, Martin Kunitz, 2002.)

could serve to extend the pre–orthotopic heart transplant time period.

The investigations with these passive restraint devices have focused on the safety of the devices, but the preliminary hemodynamic and functional results are encouraging. A passive restraint device (e.g., the Acorn cardiac support device or the Myosplint device) does not cure the failing systemic ventricle, but it is possible through reshaping the ventricle and improving AVV and diastolic function that a significant bridge to a destination therapy can be achieved with a good functional status. This is one of the many exciting new surgical therapies being developed for congestive heart failure that may become a useful surgical tool for congenital heart surgeons treating children with heart failure.

CURRENT STATUS AND FUTURE TRENDS

The increasing success of palliating patients with congenital cardiac malformations in the 1980s and 1990s has led to a new cohort of late survivors. This cohort is

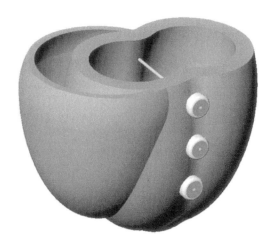

FIGURE 42-7 ■ The Myosplint device. This transcavitary tensioning device consists of three rods with wide buttons at either end. The pads at either end of the rod are made of high-strength polymer with polyester velour to encourage tissue incorporation. The rods are inserted in such a way as to change the left ventricle shape from globular to bilobular, reducing the radius of the left ventricular dimension. (See also Color Section). (From Westaby S, Katsumata T, Frazier OH: *Surgical restoration of the failing left ventricle.* In Narula J, Virmani R, Ballester M, et al [eds]: *Heart Failure: Pathogenesis and Treatment,* p. 645. London, Martin Kunitz, 2002.)

the one of the fastest growing populations of patients undergoing congenital heart surgery. The earlier interventional successes of these patients sometimes are accompanied by the burden of the ever-growing population of these patients who have cardiac dysfunction late after repair. This patient population provides the congenital heart surgeon with new challenges in the treatment of a unique form of heart failure. As in the adult patient population, assist devices and cardiac transplantation are likely to play essential roles in the treatment of these pediatric and adolescent patients with heart failure, but they have significant limitations. There are opportunities for innovative palliative surgical strategies and simple devices that would benefit these patients.[72,73] In the near future, tissue engineering may even yield a strategy that incorporates the patient's own cardiomyocytes into ventricular scar tissue.[74]

Key Concepts

■ Aside from valve repairs or replacements, there are several procedures available for improving the failing systemic ventricle in the palliated or corrected congenital heart patient. These procedures involve either making the mLV function as the systemic ventricle or making the mRV function more efficiently and can be quite complex and associated with significant morbidity and mortality.

■ The etiology for ventricular failure after a Fontan operation may be multifactorial. First, right atrial enlargement seen in late Fontan circulations perpetuates atrial arrhythmias, and the loss of atrioventricular coordination and inefficient ventricular preloading could contribute to suboptimal myocardial performance. Second, the increased right atrial pressure in the Fontan patient causes coronary sinus hypertension, which decreases myocardial perfusion and propagates ventricular diastolic dysfunction.

■ Because the atrial arrhythmias negatively affected the hemodynamic profile, more recent series of Fontan conversion have treated atrial arrhythmias aggressively with intraoperative ablative therapy. Most protocols consist of a right modified atrial maze procedure for atrial reentrant tachycardia or atrial flutter and a modified left atrial maze for atrial fibrillation.

■ At the first signs of atrial arrhythmias, conduit obstruction, significant atrial enlargement, or valvular dysfunction, the concept of Fontan conversion and the option of transplantation should be introduced.

■ There is a growing body of data to support the notion that Fontan conversion can be accomplished safely and with high expectations for significant hemodynamic and symptomatic improvements. Whether the long-term result of this therapy will be as a destination therapy or as a bridge to transplantation or permanent mechanical support is unknown, but present results advocate Fontan conversion as an effective primary therapy for the failing Fontan patient.

■ Besides a high incidence of dysplastic systemic AVV that results in insufficiency of the valve, the mRV with its septophilic systemic AVV also becomes incompetent as the interventricular septum bows left into the low-pressured mLV. The frequently seen improvement in systemic AVV regurgitation with PAB and shifting of the interventricular septum toward the mRV attests to this hypothesis.

■ The anatomic surgical corrections of ccTGA include a double-switch operation (atrial with ASO) for ccTGA patients without pulmonary stenosis and a Rastelli repair with an atrial switch operation for ccTGA patients with pulmonary stenosis or atresia.

■ Although the double-switch results are improvements over the classic repair, late complications, such as neo–aortic insufficiency and atrial baffle obstruction, are beginning to be reported and need to be followed closely.

■ Anatomic correction is presently the preferred therapy for most symptomatic ccTGA patients with favorable anatomy, although cautious enthusiasm should be exercised. These patients need continued surveillance to determine the long-term results of the retrained mLV and its semilunar valve and the atrial baffle.

■ The therapeutic options for atrial switch patients with a failing systemic ventricle are limited to tricuspid valve repair or replacement, orthotopic heart transplantation, or ASO.

■ The ASO is usually a two-stage therapeutic strategy: The first stage is to retrain the underloaded and underdeveloped mLV through a single or multiple periods of PAB until the mLV-to-mRV ratio is greater than 80%, and this preparatory stage is followed by the ASO, which includes takedown of the atrial baffle.

■ A third cohort of patients results from the mLV retraining—patients who symptomatically improved after the PAB. This improvement is secondary to the intraventricular septal shift that allows improved systemic AVV function and a decrease in systemic mRV volume overload.

■ Several methods have been proposed to assess the mLV readiness during the retraining period: pressure volume loops, mLV wall thickness, pressure ratios, myocardial biopsies, and ventricular geometry.

■ Neo–aortic insufficiency requiring valve replacement ranges from 10% to 20%, whereas mild neo–aortic valvular insufficiency requiring close observation is 40% after mLV retraining and ASO.[42,49] In addition, the hopes of atrial arrhythmias resolving as atrial pressures decreased have not been realized.

■ The law of LaPlace (wall tension = [intraventricular pressure × ventricular radius]/2 × wall thickness) is the basis for this rationale of reducing the size of the left ventricle: If the ventricular radius is reduced by surgical means, the wall tension also is lessened.

■ The Batista operation, also called partial left ventriculectomy, initially was used to treat patients with cardiomyopathy related to Chagas disease. The Dor procedure, also called endoventricular circular patch plasty repair of the left ventricle with associated coronary grafting, has been applied to patients with left ventricular dysfunction after an infarction with either akinesis or dyskinesis. Mitral valve reconstructive surgery also has been shown to aid in reshaping the left ventricle and reducing its size, improving hemodynamics.

■ A passive restraint device (e.g., the Acorn cardiac support device or the Myosplint device) does not cure the failing systemic ventricle, but it is possible through reshaping the ventricle and improving AVV and diastolic function that a significant bridge to a destination therapy can be achieved with a good functional status.

REFERENCES

1. DiBardino DJ, Allison AE, Vaughn WK, et al: Current expectations for newborns undergoing the arterial switch operation. Ann Surg 2004;239:588-598.

2. Williams WG, Trusler GA, Kirklin JW, et al: Early and late results for a protocol for simple transposition leading to an atrial switch (Mustard) repair. J Thorac Cardiovasc Surg 1998;95:717-726.

3. Turina MI, Siebermann R, VonSegesser L, et al: Late function deterioration after atrial correction for transposition of the great arteries. Circulation 1989;80(Suppl):I-162-I-167.

4. Mee RBB: Arterial switch or right ventricular failure following Mustard or Senning operations. In Stark J, Pacifico A (eds): Reoperations in Cardiac Surgery. New York, Springer, 1989, pp 217-232.

5. Moons P, De Bleser L, Budts W, et al: Health status, functional abilities, and quality of life after the Mustard or Senning operation. Ann Thorac Surg 2004;77:1359-1365.

6. Graham TP, Burger J, Bender HW, et al: Improved right ventricular function after intra-atrial repair of transposition of the great arteries. Circulation 1985;72(Suppl):II-45-II-51.

7. Page E, Perrault H, Flore P, et al: Cardiac output response to dynamic exercise after arterial switch repair for transposition of the great arteries. Am J Cardiol 1996;77:892-897.

8. Borow KM, Keane JF, Castaneda AR, et al: Systemic ventricular function in patients with tetrology of Fallot, ventricular septal defect, and transposition of the great arteries repaired during infancy. Circulation 1981;64:878-882.

9. Millane T, Bernard EJ, Jaeggi E, et al: Role of ischemia and infarction in late right ventricular dysfunction after atrial repair of transposition of the great arteries. J Am Coll Cardiol 2000;35:1661-1668.

10. Poirier NC, Mee RBB: Left ventricular reconditioning and anatomical correction for systemic right ventricular dysfunction. J Thorac Cardiovasc Surg (Pediatr Card Surg Seminar) 2000;3:198-215.

11. Mavroudis C, Backer CL, Deal BJ: Total cavopulmonary conversion and maze procedure for patients with failure for the Fontan operation. J Thorac Cardiovasc Surg 2001;122:863-871.

12. Boucek MM, Edwards LB, Keck BM, et al: Registry for the International Society for Heart and Lung Transplantation: Seventh official pediatric report—2004. J Heart Lung Transplant 2004;23:933-947.

13. Fontan F, Mounicot FB, Bauder E, et al: "Correction" de L'Atresia Tricuspidienne: rappot de deux cas "corriqes" par l'utilisation d'une technique chirurqicale nouvelle. Ann Chir Thorac Cardiovasc 1971;10:39-47.

14. Mavroudis C, Backer CL: Arterial switch after failed atrial baffle procedures for transposition of the great arteries. Ann Thorac Surg 2000;69:851-857.

15. Van Son JAM, Mohr FW, Hamnsch J, et al: Conversion of atriopulmonary or lateral atrial tunnel cavopulmonary anastomosis to extracardiac conduit Fontan modification. Eur J Cardiothorac Surg 1999;15:150-158.

16. Jahangiri M, Ross DB, Redington AN, et al: Thromboembolism after the Fontan procedure and its modifications. Ann Thorac Surg 1994;58:1510-1514.

17. DeLeval MR, Dubini G, Migliavacca F, et al: Use of computational fluid dynamics in the design of surgical procedures: Application to the study of competitive flows in cavopulmonary connections. J Thorac Cardiovas Surg 1996;111:502-511.

18. DeLeval MR, Kilner P, Gewillig M, Bull C: Total cavopulmonary connection: A logical alternative to atriopulmonary connection for complex Fontan operations: Experimental studies and early clinical experience. J Thorac Cardiovasc Surg 1988;96:682-695.

19. Gandhi SK, Bromberg BI, Rodefeld MD, et al: Lateral tunnel suture line variation reduces atrial flutter after modified Fontan operation. Ann Thorac Surg 1996;61:1299-1309.

20. Marcellentti CF, Hanley FL, Mavroudis C, et al: Revision of previous Fontan connections to total extracardiac cavopulmonary anastamosis: A multicenter experience. J Thorac Cardiovasc Surg 2000;119:340-346.

21. Conte S, Gewillig M, Eyskens B, et al: Management of late complications after classic Fontan procedure by conversion to total cavopulmonary connection. Cardiovasc Surg 1999;7:651-655.

22. Weinstein S, Cua C, Chan D, Davis JT: Outcome of symptomatic patients undergoing extracardiac Fontan conversion and cryoablation. J Thorac Cardiovasc Surg 2003;126:529-536.

23. Anselmi G, Munoz S, Machado I, et al: Complex cardiovascular malformations associated with the corrected type of transposition of the great vessels. Am Heart J 1963;66:14.

24. Allwork SP, Bentall HH, Becker AE, et al: Congenitally corrected transposition of the great arteries: Morphological study of 32 cases. Am J Cardiol 1976;38:910-913.

25. Langley SM, Winlaw DS, Stumper O, et al: Midterm results after restoration of the morphological left ventricle to the systemic circulation in patients with congenitally corrected transposition of the great arteries. J Thorac Cardiovasc Surg 2003;125:500-507.

26. Termignon JL, Leca F, Vouhe PR, et al: "Classic" repair of congenitally corrected transposition and ventricular septal defect. Ann Thorac Surg 1996;62:199-206.

27. Van Son JA, Danielson GK, Huhta JC, et al: Late results of systemic atrioventricular valve replacement in corrected transposition. J Thorac Cardiovasc Surg 1995;109:642-653.

28. McGarth LB, Kirklin JW, Blackstone EH, et al: Death and other events after cardiac repair in discordant atrioventricular connection. J Thorac Cardiovasc Surg 1985;90:711-728.

29. Sano T, Riesenfeld T, Karl TR, et al: Intermediate-term outcome after intracardiac repair of associated cardiac defects in patients with atrioventricular and ventriculoarterial discordance. Circulation 1995;92(Suppl 9):II-272-II-278.

30. Karl TR, Weintraub RG, Brizard CP, et al: Senning plus arterial switch operation for discordant (congenitally corrected) transposition. Ann Thorac Surg 1997;64:495-502.

31. Yamagishi M, Imai Y, Hoshino S, et al: Anatomic correction of atrioventricular discordance. J Thorac Cardiovasc Surg 1993;105:1067-1076.

32. Yagihara T, Kishimoto H, Isobe F, et al: Double switch operation in cardiac anomalies with atrioventricular and ventriculoarterial discordance. J Thorac Cardiovasc Surg 1994;107:351-358.

33. Ilbawi MN, DeLeaon SY, Backer CL, et al: An alternative approach to the surgical management of physiologically corrected transposition with ventricular septal defect and pulmonary stenosis or atresia. J Thorac Cardiovasc Surg 1990;100:410-415.

34. Ilbawi MN, Ocampo CB, Allen BS, et al: Intermediate results of the anatomic repair for congenitally corrected transposition. Ann Thorac Surg 2002;73:594-600.

35. Devaney EJ, Charpie JR, Ohye RG, Bove EL: Combined arterial switch and Senning operation for congenitally corrected transposition of the great arteries: Patient selection and intermediate results. J Thorac Cardiovasc Surg 2003;125:500-507.

36. Imamura M, Drumond-Webb JJ, Murphy DJ, et al: Results of the double switch operation in the current era. Ann Thorac Surg 2000;70:100-105.

37. Reddy VM, McElhinney D, Silverman N, et al: Double switch procedure for anatomical repair of congenitally corrected transposition of the great arteries in infants and children. Eur Heart J 1997;18:1470-1477.

38. McKay R, Anderson R, Smith A: The coronary arteries in hearts with discordant atrioventricular connections. J Thorac Cardiovasc Surg 1996;111:988-997.

39. Williams WG, Trusler GA, Kirklin JW, et al: Early and late results for a protocol for simple transposition leading to an atrial switch (Mustard) repair. J Thorac Cardiovasc Surg 1988;95:717-726.

40. Turina MI, Siebenmann R, von Segesser L, et al: Late functional deterioration after atrial correction for transposition. Circulation 1989;80(Suppl):I-162-I-167.

41. Carrel T, Pfammatter JP: Complete transposition of the great arteries: Surgical concepts for patients with systemic right ventricular failure following intraarterial repair. Thorac Cardiovasc Surg 2000;48:224-227.

42. Cochrane AD, Karl TR, Mee RBB: Staged conversion to arterial switch for later failure of the systemic right ventricle. Ann Thorac Surg 1993;56:854-862.

43. Mee RBB: Severe right ventricular failure after Mustard or Senning operations: Two staged repair: Pulmonary artery banding and switch. J Thorac Cardiovasc Surg 1986;92:385-390.

44. Daebritz SH, Tiete AR, Sachweh JS, et al: Systemic right ventricular failure after atrial switch operation: Midterm results of conversion into an arterial switch. Ann Thorac Surg 2001;71:1255-1259.

45. Poirier NC, Yu JH, Brizard CP, Mee RBB: Long-term results of left ventricular reconditioning and anatomic correction for systemic right ventricular dysfunction after atrial switch procedures. J Thorac Cardiovasc Surg 2004;127:975-981.

46. Marvroudis C, Backer CL: Arterial switch after failed atrial baffle procedures for transposition of the great arteries. Ann Thorac Surg 2000;69:851-857.

47. DeGiovanni JV: Left ventricular retraining in preparation for a late arterial switch in patients with a failing atrial repair for transposition: Proceedings of the International Workshop on Left Ventricular Retraining. Bergamo, Italy, International Heart School, 1996, pp 95-105.

48. Helvind MH, McCarthy JF, Imamura M, et al: Ventriculo-arterial discordance: Switching the morphologically left ventricle into the systemic circulation after 3 months of age. Eur J Cardiothorac Surg 1998;14:173-178.

49. Chang AC, Wernovsky G, Wessel DL, et al: Surgical management of late right ventricular failure after Mustard or Senning repair. Circulation 1992;86(Suppl 2):140-149.

50. Foran JP, Sullivan ID, Elliott MJ, de Leval MR: Primary arterial switch operation for transposition of the great arteries with intact ventricular septum in infants older than 21 days. J Am Coll Cardiol 1998;31:883-889.

51. Davis AM, Wilkinson JL, Karl TR, Mee RBB: Transposition of the great arteries with intact ventricular septum arterial switch repair in patients 21 days of age or older. J Thorac Cardiovasc Surg 1993;106:111-115.

52. Lev M, Rimoldi H, Paiva R, Arcilla R: The quantitative anatomy of simple complex transposition. Am J Cardiol 1969;23:409-416.

53. Lacour-Gayet F, Piot D, Zoghibi J, et al: Surgical management and indication of left ventricular retraining in arterial switch for transposition of the great arteries with intact ventricular septum. Eur J Cardiothoracic Surg 2001;20:824-829.

54. Naughton P, Mossad E: Retraining the LV after ASO: Emerging uses for the left ventricular assist device in pediatric cardiac surgery. J Cardiothorac Vasc Anesth 2000;14:454-456.

55. Boutin C, Wernovsky G, Sanders SP, et al: Rapid two-stage arterial switch operation: Evaluation of the left ventricular systolic mechanics late after an acute pressure overload stimulus in infancy. Circulation 1994;90:1294-1303.

56. Al Qethamy HO, Aizaz K, Aboelnazar SA, et al: Two-stage arterial switch operation: Is late ever too late? Asian Cardiovasc Thorac Ann 2002;10:235-239.

57. Jonas RA, Giglia TM, Sanders SP, et al: Rapid, two-stage arterial switch for transposition of the great arteries and intact ventricular septum beyond the neonatal period. Circulation 1989;80(3 Pt 1):I-203-I-208.

58. Corn AE, Hurni M, Payot M, et al: Adequate left ventricular preparation allows for arterial switch despite late referral. Cardiol Young 2003;13:49-52.

59. Boutin C, Wernovsky G, Sanders SP, et al: Rapid two-stage arterial switch operation: Acquisition of left ventricular mass after pulmonary artery banding in infants with transposition of the great arteries. Circulation 1994;90:1304-1309.

60. Moons P, DeBessler L, Budts W, et al: Health status, functional abilities, and quality of life after the Mustard or Senning operation. Ann Thorac Surg 2004;77:1359-1365.

61. Goldstein S, Sabbah N: Ventricular remodeling and angiotensin converting enzyme inhibitors. J Cardiovasc Pharmacol 1994;24: S27-S31.

62. Frazier OH, Benedict CR, Radovancevic B, et al: Improved left ventricular function after chronic left ventricular unloading. Ann Thorac Surg 1996;62:675-681.

63. Chen FY, Cohn LH: The surgical treatment of heart failure: A new frontier: Nontransplant surgical alternatives to heart failure. Cardiol Rev 2002;10:326-333.

64. Park P, Jun T, Sung K, et al: Midterm results of left ventricular volume reduction surgery in children with dilated cardiomyopathy. STS 40th annual meeting. San Antonio, Tx 2004, Abstract 63.

65. Abe T, Fukada J, Morishita K: The Batista procedure: Fact, fiction and its role in the management of heart failure. Heart Fail Rev 2001;6:195-199.

66. Kass DA, Baughman KL, Pak PH, et al: Reverse remodeling from cardiomyoplasty in human heart failure: External constraint versus active assist. Circulation 1995;91:2314-2318.

67. Oz MC, Konertz WF, Kleber FX, et al: Global surgical experience with the Acorn cardiac support device. J Thorac Cardiovasc Surg 2003;126:983-991.

68. Pilla JJ, Blom AS, Brockman DJ, et al: Ventricular constraint using the Acorn cardiac support device reduces myocardial akinetic area in an ovine model of acute infarction. Circulation 2002;106 (12 Suppl):I207-I211.

69. Chaudhry PA, Anagnostopoulos PV, Mishima T, et al: Acute ventricular reduction with the acorn cardiac support device: Effect on progressive left ventricular dysfunction and dilation in dogs with chronic heart failure. J Card Surg 2001;16:118-126.

70. Kleber FX, Sonntang S, Krebs H, et al: Follow-up on passive cardiomyoplasty in congestive heart failure: Influence of the Acorn cardiac support device on left ventricular function. J Am Coll Cardiol 2001;37(Suppl A):143A.

71. Sabbah HN: The cardiac support device and the myosplint: Treating heart failure by targeting left ventricular size and shape. Ann Thorac Surg 2003;756:s13-s19.

72. Popovic ZB, Saracino G, Deserranno D, et al: Echocardiographic assessment of regional ventricular function after device-based change of left ventricular shape. J Am Soc Echocardiogr 2004;17:411-417.

73. Oz MC, Konertz WF, Raman J, et al: Reverse remodeling of the failing ventricle: Surgical intervention with the Acorn cardiac support device. Congest Heart Fail 2004;10:96-104.

74. Kofidis T, deBruin JL, Hoyt G, et al: Myocardial restoration with embryonic stem cell bioartificial tissue transplantation. J Heart Lung Transplant 2005;24:737-744.

CHAPTER 43

Sudden Death and Implantable Cardioverter Defibrillators in Heart Failure

Naomi J. Kertesz
Bryan C. Cannon

Supraventricular and ventricular arrhythmias are common in adults with cardiomyopathy and heart failure, but are relatively uncommon in children. Regardless, arrhythmias can cause symptoms, a worsening of heart failure, or sudden cardiac death. This chapter addresses the evaluation and management of children and young adults with heart failure and arrhythmias who may be at risk for sudden death and may require treatment with an implantable cardioverter defibrillator (ICD).

SUPRAVENTRICULAR TACHYARRYTHMIAS

Atrial arrhythmias, including atrial fibrillation, atrial flutter, and reentrant supraventricular arrhythmias, have been reported in 10% to 20% of children with **dilated cardiomyopathy** (DCM).[1-7] The most recent report of arrhythmias in children with DCM is from 1998,[5] and the largest series included only 81 patients.[2] Supraventricular arrhythmias are common in adults with **hypertrophic cardiomyopathy** (HCM). Paroxysmal supraventricular tachycardia and atrial fibrillation can be detected on 24-hour Holter monitoring in 30% of adults[9] and 10% of children.[8] Sustained or symptomatic episodes are much less common, but warrant therapy. Established atrial fibrillation is uncommon in children, whereas it can occur in 30% of adults. In addition, although there is an association between HCM and Wolff-Parkinson-White syndrome, the incidence of a true accessory pathway is an uncommon finding.[9]

In patients presenting with sustained atrial fibrillation or flutter, sinus rhythm with improved atrial contribution to cardiac output is preferred. At least one attempt to terminate the tachyarrhythmia is warranted. This strategy also provides an opportunity to determine if an underlying atrial tachycardia or sick sinus syndrome is inducing the flutter or fibrillation. Treatment with a β-blocker or pacing may be necessary (see also Chapter 20). Anticoagulation is an important part of managing a patient with atrial fibrillation or flutter. The American Heart Association guidelines are clear on the necessity of anticoagulation before and after cardioversion in a patient with an unclear time of onset of the arrhythmia.[10] Based on numerous clinical trials in adults, the current standard of care is to anticoagulate patients with warfarin and maintain their international normalized ratio at 2.5 (range 2 to 3).[11-14] In patients with HCM in whom no underlying trigger for the arrhythmia can be found, treatment with amiodarone has been advocated by McKenna and others[9,15] because atrial fibrillation can cause significant morbidity and mortality. In patients in whom sinus rhythm cannot be maintained, ventricular rate control is important and can be attempted with the combination of digoxin and a β-blocker. Other potential therapies include radiofrequency ablation and, as a last resort, atrioventricular node ablation.

Restrictive cardiomyopathy (RCM) accounts for 3% to 5%[16,17] of pediatric cardiomyopathy. Atrial flutter, atrial tachycardia, Wolff-Parkinson-White syndrome with supraventricular tachycardia, first-degree atrioventricular block, and complete atrioventricular block all have been reported in patients with RCM.[18-20] Patients with RCM are particularly vulnerable because sinus tachycardia in this population can result in significant ST-segment changes consistent with ischemia and may be the inciting factor for lethal ventricular arrhythmias (see Chapter 19). These patients may require β blockade, but they are such a fragile group that they are likely to require initiation of such therapy in the hospital and possibly hospitalization until transplantation.

VENTRICULAR TACHYARRHYTHMIAS

Most cases of DCM and HCM are idiopathic; 42% are caused by inborn errors of metabolism, malformation syndromes, neuromuscular disorders, myocarditis, and familial isolated cardiomyopathy.[16] Forty-one percent of patients receive the diagnosis of cardiomyopathy within the first 12 months of life. Given the large spectrum of etiologies and age range at diagnosis, making specific recommendations regarding the incidence of arrhythmias and their management is difficult.

Sudden Death and Implantable Cardioverter Defibrillators

Since first being reported by Mirowski,[20a] ICDs have played an increasing role in the treatment of ventricular arrhythmias and prevention of sudden death. ICDs initially were used for secondary prevention (survivors of cardiac arrest or sustained ventricular tachycardia or fibrillation);

however, many studies are now focusing on the impact of using these devices for primary prevention (patients who are believed to be at high risk for sudden death). As further research progresses, the indications for these devices are constantly evolving. Similar to pacemakers, ICDs typically are implanted transvenously and consist of a generator and one or more leads (Fig. 43-1). Currently available ICDs all have bradycardia pacing capabilities, and many have rate-responsive pacing ability. In addition, many have the ability to burst pace or overdrive pace terminate atrial arrhythmias in addition to the ability to identify, pace terminate, or defibrillate ventricular arrhythmias (Fig. 43-2). In addition to its sensing and pacing capabilities, the ventricular lead has one or two coils used for defibrillation. The most recent generation of ICDs also includes the ability to use a coronary sinus lead for biventricular pacing. Initially designed only to treat ventricular arrhythmias, newer devices include algorithms to detect and treat atrial arrhythmias.

Children and patients with congenital heart disease pose unique and difficult challenges to the use of ICDs. Specifically the size of the device and the leads have provided the greatest hurdles. The first generation of ICDs consisted of patches placed epicardially with epicardial sensing leads, and the generator was placed in the abdomen (Fig. 43-3). As the technology has evolved, the devices now are placed entirely transvenously (Fig. 43-4). Small children, patients with left-to-right shunts, and patients with no vascular access cannot have transvenous systems, however. Alternatives have included the use of subcutaneous arrays and subcutaneous coils[21] (Fig. 43-5) and the placement of transvenous leads in the operating

room via direct access to the right atrium (Fig. 43-6). Children and young adults also pose unique challenges from a programming perspective. Thirty percent of patients can experience inappropriate ICD discharges because of atrial arrhythmias and sinus tachycardia (Fig. 43-7).[22,23] The use of dual-chamber defibrillators should reduce the incidence of inappropriate shocks. Children with congenital heart disease and cardiomyopathy may experience sudden death from atrial arrhythmias with rapid atrioventricular conduction and from ventricular arrhythmias.[24] In addition, attempts at termination of these arrhythmias may result in their acceleration and pose a risk of sudden death if no defibrillation is available.

Lastly, the indications for the use of ICDs in children are based largely on retrospective studies in children. In the remainder of this chapter, we review many of the adult trials that have shaped the current indications for ICD therapy in adults and the pediatric data that are available in patients with cardiomyopathy and heart failure.

Dilated Cardiomyopathy

The mortality in children with DCM varies with the underlying diagnosis; the mortality rate in the cardiomyopathy registry at 2 years after diagnosis was 13.6% with an additional 12.7% receiving a transplant within 2 years of diagnosis.[16] Reports of sudden death in children with DCM range from 5% to 15%,[1-7] but the latest report is from 1998, and there are no large studies reviewing the incidence of sudden death in children. In addition, no large pediatric studies reviewing the appropriateness or effectiveness of amiodarone or ICD therapy in this population have been done.

In the Framingham Heart Study, the 5-year mortality was 62% in men and 42% in women,[25,26] and the mortality rate was related to the severity of heart failure. A significant number of deaths in adults with heart failure are sudden (30% to 50%), and most are attributed to a ventricular tachyarrhythmia (although determining a nonarrhythmic cause can be difficult). In addition, despite an increasing frequency of ventricular arrhythmias as heart failure and left ventricular dysfunction worsen in adults, the percentage of sudden death actually declines as heart failure severity increases (Fig. 43-8).[27] In adults with New York Heart Association class III or IV heart failure, especially patients awaiting cardiac transplantation, a greater number die suddenly from a bradyarrhythmia rather than a tachyarrhythmia.[28]

In adults, the severity of left ventricular dysfunction is the most powerful predictor of mortality in patients with idiopathic DCM and heart failure. A reduced left ventricular ejection fraction (LVEF) has been shown to correlate strongly with poor survival. In one study, 84% of patients with ischemic DCM and LVEF of less than 35% died over a mean of 39 months compared with 46% of patients with LVEF of greater than 35%. Other indices of left ventricular and right ventricular function also have been shown to predict mortality in patients with cardiomyopathy. Other clinical predictors of poor

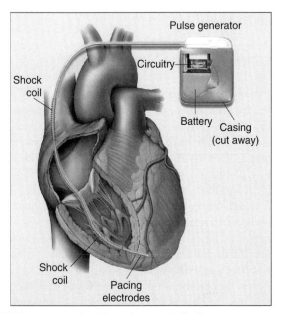

FIGURE 43-1 ■ Implantable cardioverter defibrillator. The implantable cardioverter defibrillator system is shown with the pulse generator and the lead that is used for pacing and defibrillation. (See also Color Section) (From DiMarco JP: Implantable cardioverter-defibrillators. N Engl J Med 2003;349:1836-1847.)

ID#	Date/Time	Type	V. Cycle	Last Rx	Success	Duration
1	Jul 09 16:18:46	VF	260 ms	VF Rx 1	Yes	11 sec

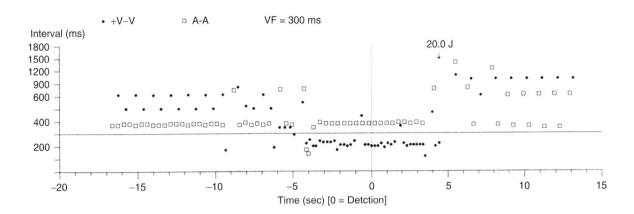

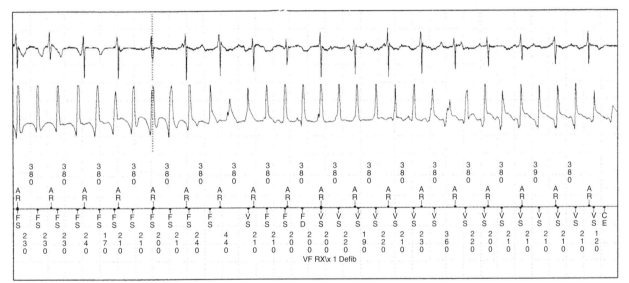

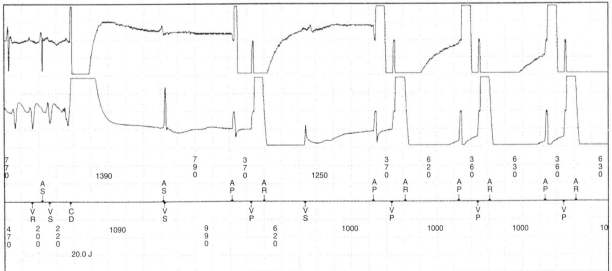

FIGURE 43-2 ■ **Appropriate shock delivered by implantable cardioverter defibrillator.** This tracing represents the information that is obtained when interrogating an implantable cardioverter defibrillator after an appropriate discharge. From *top* to *bottom*, the graph plots the atrial and ventricular rates prior to, during, and after defibrillation. The tracings represent the electrograms from the atrial, and ventricular leads and from an annotated marker channel. At the beginning of the tracing the ventricular rate is in the ventricular fibrillation zone as noted by FS on the ventricular marker channel. The criteria for treatment has been met as noted by FD (fibrillation detect) on the ventricular marker channel. The device then charges and delivers a 20-J shock as noted by CD (charge delivered) on the marker channel. The ventricular fibrillation is terminated and the ventricular pacing begins.

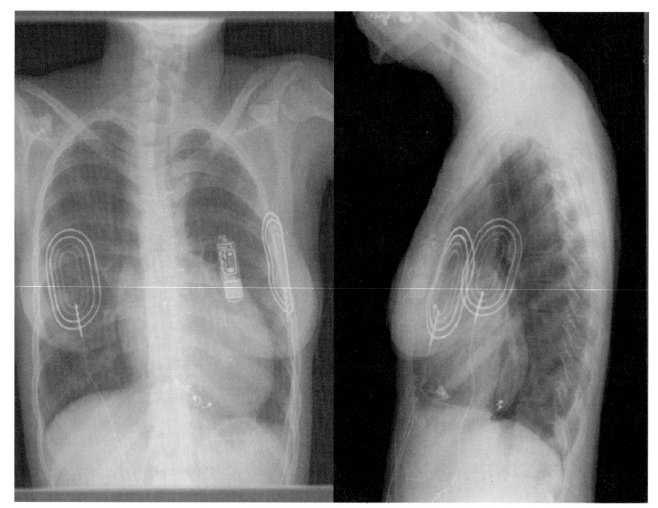

FIGURE 43-3 ■ **Epicardial implantable cardioverter defibrillator.** Epicardial implantable cardioverter defibrillator. These x-rays show the patches placed subcutaneously with the implantable cardioverter defibrillator generator in the abdomen. The first generation of these devices required the patches to be placed directly on the heart. With advances in technology, the patches could be placed subcutaneously, but the ventricular sensing and pacing lead still needed to be placed epicardially.

outcome in adults with heart failure include left bundle branch block and first-degree and second-degree atrioventricular blocks.[29] Finally, the incidence of sudden death is significantly greater in patients with syncope; this population may have a 1-year sudden death rate of 45%.[30-32] Knight and colleagues[33] prospectively evaluated patients with nonischemic DCM, unexplained syncope, and a negative electrophysiology study and compared them with patients with nonischemic DCM and cardiac arrest who were treated with a defibrillator. Both groups received a similar number of appropriate defibrillator shocks, reinforcing the importance of syncope as a predictor of sudden death.

Multiform premature ventricular contractions, ventricular couplets, and nonsustained ventricular tachycardia are present in 80% to 90% of patients with DCM. In patients with congestive heart failure, ventricular arrhythmias often become more frequent and complex as left ventricular function deteriorates.[29] Ventricular arrhythmias have been reported as independent predictors of total

cardiac mortality or sudden cardiac death or both by some investigators, but not by others. Arrhythmic complexity was a major predictor of survival in 218 patients studied by DeMaria and associates,[34] although not as strong as LVEF or stroke work index. In contrast, Romero and coworkers[35] found Lown grade 4 or greater ventricular arrhythmias to be independent predictors of sudden death in patients with ischemic DCM.

Programmed electrical stimulation has been found to be predictive of sustained ventricular arrhythmias and sudden death in patients with ischemic cardiomyopathy. The results in nonischemic DCM have not been as encouraging, however. Grimm and colleagues[36] evaluated the role of programmed ventricular stimulation for arrhythmia risk prediction in patients with nonischemic DCM (LVEF ≤35%) and spontaneous nonsustained ventricular tachycardia. All patients underwent programmed ventricular stimulation and were divided into patients with and without inducible sustained ventricular tachycardia or fibrillation. Arrhythmic events during

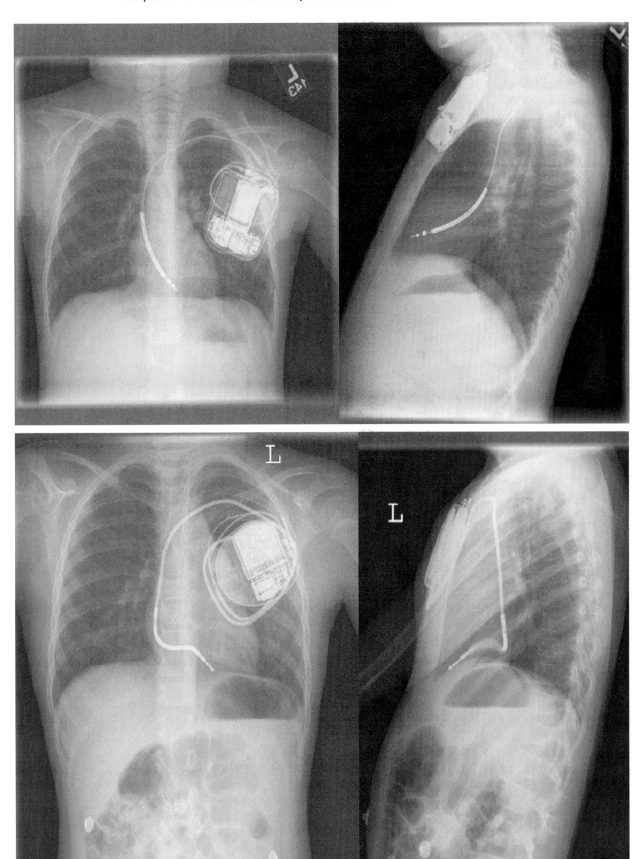

FIGURE 43-4 ■ Transvenous implantable cardioverter defibrillators in children. These two sets of X-rays show transvenous single-chamber implantable cardioverter defibrillators in small children. Despite the newer, relatively smaller devices, they are still quite large for children. In addition, note the amount of extra lead that is coiled around the device.

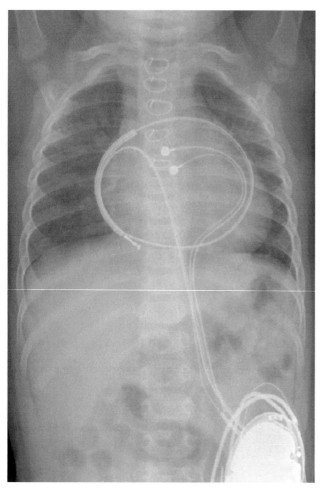

FIGURE 43-5 ■ Epicardial implantable cardioverter defibrillator. In this infant, a subcutaneous coil was placed around the heart, a pacing lead was placed epicardially, and the generator was placed in the abdomen.

follow-up occurred in 4 of 13 patients with inducible ventricular arrhythmias compared with 5 of 21 patients without inducible ventricular arrhythmias, 1 of whom died suddenly after discharge from the hospital without an ICD. The authors subsequently reviewed all studies of programmed ventricular stimulation in patients with nonischemic DCM without a history of sustained ventricular arrhythmias. In the patients with no inducible monomorphic ventricular tachycardia, there were high rates of arrhythmia recurrence and sudden death, although lower than in patients with inducible ventricular tachycardia. These and other studies have concluded that a negative electrophysiology study should not be the sole reason for not providing prophylactic therapy.[29]

β-Blocker therapy not only has been shown to be useful in the treatment of heart failure, but also is believed to be beneficial in preventing ventricular arrhythmias. This strategy has not been advocated as sole therapy, however. Since the CAST (Cardiac Arrhythmia Suppression Trial) study, most research has focused on the use of amiodarone in the prevention of sustained ventricular arrhythmias and sudden death. The randomized trial of low-dose amiodarone in severe congestive heart failure, **GESICA** (Grupo de Estudio de la Sobrevida en la Insuficiencia Cardiaca en Argentina),[37] sought to evaluate prospectively the effect of low-dose amiodarone on 2-year mortality in patients with severe heart failure. The investigators randomized 516 patients with advanced heart failure (New York Heart Association classes II through IV with LVEF <35%) primarily resulting from nonischemic cardiomyopathy and nonsustained ventricular tachycardia to amiodarone versus standard therapy. Amiodarone resulted in a 28% reduction in total mortality and a 27% reduction in sudden death.

CHF-STAT (Survival Trial of Antiarrhythmic Therapy in Congestive Heart Failure)[38] randomly assigned 674 patients with symptoms of congestive heart failure, cardiac enlargement, 10 or more premature ventricular contractions per hour, and LVEF of less than or equal to 40% to receive amiodarone or placebo. The primary end point was mortality. There was no significant difference in overall mortality or sudden death between the two groups. In the 196 patients with nonischemic DCM, however, there was a trend toward reduction in overall mortality in patients who received amiodarone (P = .07). In addition, in the entire group, there was no difference in mortality between the patients in whom episodes of ventricular tachycardia were eliminated by amiodarone at 2 weeks and the patients in whom such episodes continued to occur.

Given the current state of flux in regard to the use of ICDs for primary prevention in adults with cardiomyopathy, **MADIT II** (Multicenter Automatic Defibrillator Implantation Trial)[39] clarified the use of ICD implantation for primary prevention in patients with ischemic cardiomyopathy. Patients with LVEF of less than 30% and a prior myocardial infarction were randomized to receive an ICD or conventional medical therapy. Both groups also received appropriate therapy with angiotensin-converting enzyme (ACE) inhibitors, β-blockers, and diuretics. During an average follow-up of 20 months, defibrillator therapy was associated with a 31% reduction in total mortality. Electrophysiologic testing and the presence of ventricular arrhythmias were not eligibility criteria.

Given these data, the **Marburg Cardiomyopathy Study**[40] attempted to determine a method of noninvasive risk stratification in adults with idiopathic DCM. This group prospectively evaluated 343 patients who were between 16 and 70 years old, had LVEF of less than 45%, and left ventricular end-diastolic diameter of greater than 56 mm. This study investigated the predictability of major arrhythmic events on the basis of echocardiography, 12-lead ECG, signal averaged ECG, arrhythmias, and heart rate variability on digital 24-hour Holter ECG, baroreflex sensitivity, and microvolt T wave alternans. During 52 months of follow-up, major arrhythmic events (sustained ventricular tachycardia, ventricular fibrillation, or sudden death) occurred in 46 patients (13%). By multivariate

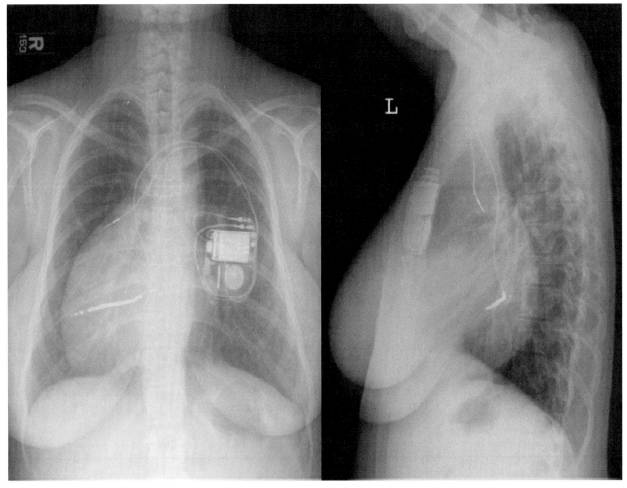

FIGURE 43-6 ■ **Transvenous implantable cardioverter defibrillator placement via sternotomy.** Because of the patient's complex anatomy, a transvenous system could not be placed via a subclavian puncture. The patient was taken to the operating room, and her leads were placed transvenously via an opening in the superior vena cava/right atrium junction.

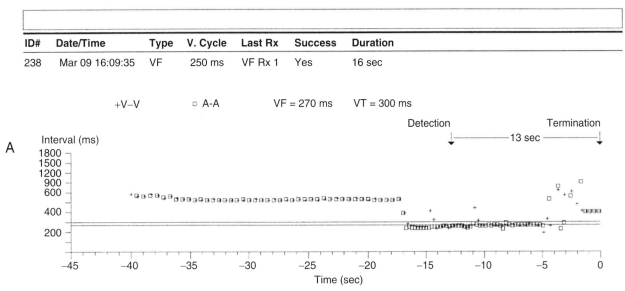

FIGURE 43-7 ■ **Inappropriate shock delivered by implantable cardioverter defibrillator for rapidly conducting atrial flutter.** These tracings show how a rapidly conducting atrial arrhythmia can lead to an implantable cardioverter defibrillator delivering a shock for what it identifies as ventricular fibrillation. **A,** The relationship of the atrial and ventricular cycle lengths during sinus rhythm and atrial flutter.

Continued

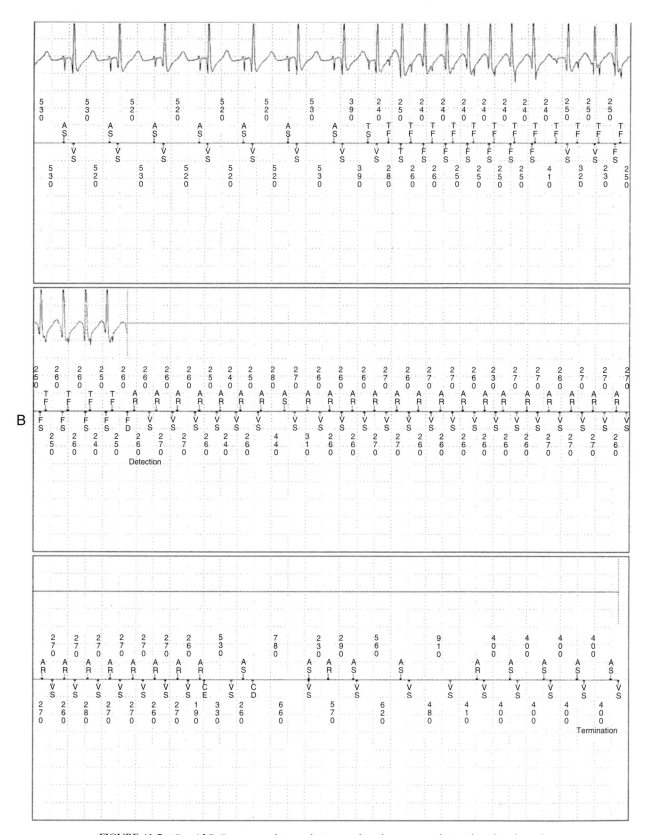

FIGURE 43-7 ■ Cont'd B, From *top* to *bottom,* the intracardiac electrograms, the atrial marker channel, and the ventricular marker channel. Initially the patient is in sinus rhythm. The atrial flutter then begins and is briefly not conducted 1:1. After a few beats, there is 1:1 atrioventricular conduction, and the ventricular rate is in the ventricular fibrillation zone as noted by *FS* on the ventricular marker channel. At *FD,* the device has determined that this is ventricular fibrillation, and at *CD* it delivers a 30-J shock that terminates the atrial flutter.

FIGURE 43-8 ■ Sudden death and total mortality. Annual mortality and sudden death in trials in heart failure. The various trials are listed by severity of heart failure from class I to IV. (From Stevenson WG, Stevenson LW: Prevention of sudden death in heart failure. J Cardiovasc Electrophysiol 2001;12:112-114.)

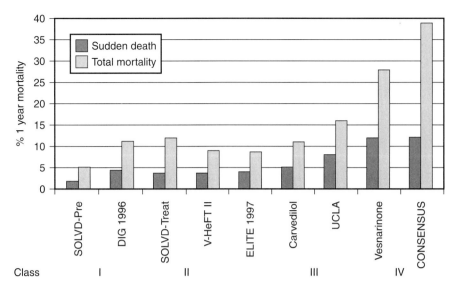

analysis, LVEF was the only significant arrhythmia risk predictor in this patient population. Lack of β-blocker use and presence of nonsustained ventricular tachycardia on Holter monitoring were significant univariate predictors of major arrhythmic events. The combination of LVEF of less than 30% and nonsustained ventricular tachycardia showed an eightfold arrhythmia risk compared with patients with LVEF of greater than 30% without nonsustained ventricular tachycardia. The authors admit, however, that the potential clinical usefulness of the combination of LVEF of less than 30% and nonsustained ventricular tachycardia for selection of patients for prophylactic ICD therapy is limited by a positive predictive value for arrhythmic events of less than 50% during 72 months of follow-up (according to the Kaplan-Meier estimate).

Given the success of ICD as primary prevention in patients with ischemic cardiomyopathy and the data that seem to suggest a decreased ejection fraction could be predictive of sudden death, three prospective trials in patients with idiopathic DCM were performed to determine the usefulness of ICD therapy as primary prevention.

First, **CAT** (Cardiomyopathy Trial)[41] enrolled 104 patients between ages 18 and 70 years with DCM and impaired left ventricular function (LVEF <30%) who were symptomatic for less than 9 months and were in New York Heart Association class II or III. Patients with a history of prior myocardial infarction or myocarditis were excluded. Patients with a history of symptomatic ventricular tachycardia were excluded. The primary end point was all-cause mortality at 1 year. Patients were assigned randomly to ICD treatment versus control. The mean follow-up was 22.8 months. After 1 year, six patients were dead (four in the ICD group and two in the control group), but no sudden deaths occurred during the first and second years of follow-up. After a mean follow-up of 5.5 years, 30 deaths had occurred (13 in

the ICD group and 17 in the control group). Cumulative survival was not significantly different between the two groups, and the study was terminated because of the overall low mortality rate. The authors speculate that this in part was because of the high use of ACE inhibitors in the study participants. This trial did not provide evidence in favor of prophylactic ICD implantation in patients with DCM of recent onset and impaired LVEF.

AMIOVIRT (Amiodarone Versus Implantable Cardioverter-Defibrillator Randomized Trial)[42] studied patients with nonischemic DCM and asymptomatic nonsustained ventricular tachycardia. This trial compared the total mortality during therapy with amiodarone or an ICD in patients with nonischemic DCM and nonsustained ventricular tachycardia. A total of 103 patients with nonischemic DCM with LVEF of less than 35% and asymptomatic nonsustained ventricular tachycardia were randomized to either amiodarone or ICD therapy. Patients with new-onset DCM were excluded, in contrast to the CAT study. Optimal medical therapy with ACE inhibitors, β-blockers, and potassium-sparing diuretics was attempted throughout the duration of the study. At the first interim analysis, the study enrollment was stopped because the prospective stopping rule for the inability to achieve statistical significance was reached. The 1- and 3-year survival rates in the patients treated with amiodarone were not statistically different from patients who received an ICD. The distribution of sudden versus nonsudden deaths was similar in both groups. In addition, 16 of 51 patients who received an ICD received an appropriate ICD discharge, whereas 25 of 52 patients initially treated with amiodarone had the drug discontinued because of adverse side effects. An ICD was inserted in eight patients initially treated with amiodarone (four because of amiodarone intolerance). The 3-year survival rate in this cohort was 89%. The authors concluded that the study seemed to represent a departure from the usual interpretation of superiority of the ICD over amiodarone shown in previous studies. Not only was the total mortality found not to be statistically different with amiodarone versus ICD in patients with nonischemic DCM and nonsustained ventricular tachycardia, but there also was a trend toward amiodarone being more effective than the ICD in preventing symptomatic ventricular tachycardia. The lack of statistically different survival rates and the trend toward a substantial cost savings with amiodarone provide an argument favoring amiodarone as the initial therapy to prevent death in patients with nonischemic DCM and nonsustained ventricular tachycardia.

Finally, the **DEFINITE** (Defibrillators in Non-Ischemic Cardiomyopathy Treatment Evaluation) trial[43] sought to determine whether the prophylactic implantation of an ICD would reduce the incidence of sudden death compared with standard medical therapy consisting of ACE inhibitors and β-blockers. In this study, 438 patients with nonischemic DCM, LVEF of less than 36%, and at least ten premature ventricular contractions per hour or nonsustained ventricular tachycardia were assigned randomly to receive standard medical therapy versus standard medical therapy and a single-chamber ICD. The standard medical therapy consisted of an ACE inhibitor and β-blockers. The primary end point was death from any cause; sudden death from arrhythmia was a secondary end point. Therapy with an ICD significantly reduced the risk of sudden death from arrhythmia ($p = .006$) and resulted in a risk of death from any cause that approached but did not reach statistical significance. The authors concluded that the routine implantation of an ICD could not be recommended for all patients with nonischemic DCM and severe left ventricular dysfunction. The reduction in sudden death from arrhythmia and an apparent benefit of ICDs in subgroup analyses suggest, however, that the use of these devices should be considered on a case-by-case basis.

Most studies involving survivors of sudden cardiac death or patients with sustained ventricular tachycardia primarily have involved patients with coronary artery disease. Of the prospective randomized trials of ICD therapy, only AVID (Antiarrhythmic versus Implantable Defibrillator), CIDS (Canadian Implantable Defibrillator Study), and CASH (Cardiac Arrest Survival Hamburg) included patients with nonischemic DCM. Because only AVID[44] has data on the nonischemic subgroup, only this study is reviewed here. This study sought to determine whether amiodarone or ICD was superior in treating patients who had been resuscitated from near-fatal ventricular fibrillation or who had undergone cardioversion from sustained ventricular tachycardia. One group of patients was treated with implantation of ICD, and the other received class III antiarrhythmic drugs, primarily amiodarone. There were 1,013 patients in whom follow-up was complete. The authors concluded that among survivors of ventricular fibrillation or sustained ventricular tachycardia causing severe symptoms, the ICD was superior to antiarrhythmic drugs for

increasing overall survival. Steinberg and colleagues[45] evaluated the 106 patients without coronary artery disease (not all of whom had DCM). One half of the patients were randomized to conventional drug therapy and one half to ICD implant; the overall mortality rates were less in patients randomized to ICD therapy.

In light of this review of the adult literature, some important points need to be addressed before attempting to apply what has been learned in adults to children. First, the underlying etiology of DCM is more varied in children, and includes neuromuscular, infectious, familial, and idiopathic etiologies. The prognosis of children in different centers has varied not only based on the etiology, but also depending on the age at diagnosis.[7] The prognosis of idiopathic DCM diagnosed in childhood may differ significantly from that diagnosed in adults. Specifically, the incidence of sudden death and nonsustained ventricular tachycardia based on previous studies and research being done at our institution is much lower in children than in their adult counterparts. The use of ICDs or amiodarone for primary prevention must be evaluated on a case-by-case basis. The use of ICDs has been well documented in children to be effective, and ICDs can and should be used for secondary prevention.[46,47]

Hypertrophic Cardiomyopathy
The issues regarding the treatment of ventricular arrhythmias in patients with heart failure and HCM have similar difficulties as mentioned previously with patients with DCM. Heart failure is uncommon in patients with HCM, but can be a relatively late manifestation. The mechanisms contributing to arrhythmogenesis include adaptations in the electrical, contractile, metabolic, and structural properties of the heart, which all have been shown in animal models of heart failure. This ventricular remodeling process has been associated with increased risks for ventricular tachyarrhythmias and sudden cardiac death.[48] Because there are no specific guidelines for this subgroup of pediatric patients, a review of the literature regarding therapy for ventricular arrhythmias in adults with HCM is warranted.

As in DCM, much of the research in HCM has focused on risk stratification and prevention of sudden death. Sudden death occurs with a frequency of about 1% or less per year in adults with HCM and 2% to 4% in children.[15] These data have been revised as more community-based studies have shown a lower sudden death risk in relation to the tertiary referral center data. As in nonischemic DCM, programmed stimulation has a low positive predictive accuracy in patients with HCM, and many cardiologists now use noninvasive criteria for risk stratification. In a review of ICD use in patients with HCM, 4 of 12 (33%) patients without an inducible ventricular tachycardia had an appropriate ICD discharge compared with 19 of 79 (24%) with inducible ventricular tachycardia.[49]

Elliott and associates[50] sought to identify which patients with HCM are at high risk of sudden death in a cohort of 368 patients followed at a tertiary referral center. The five clinical risk factors for patients with HCM that were assessed were a family history of sudden cardiac death, unexplained syncope, nonsustained ventricular tachycardia on 48-hour cardioscan, abnormal blood pressure response during upright exercise testing, and maximal left ventricular wall thickness. An abnormal blood pressure response was defined as a failure of blood pressure to increase, or a decrease in blood pressure during exercise. The most predictive cutoff values were less than a 25 mm Hg increase or greater than a 15 mm Hg decrease in blood pressure. Of the 368 patients, 36 died; 22 (61%) deaths were sudden. Family histories of sudden death and unexplained syncope were combined into a single risk factor because of evidence of interaction in statistical analysis. Patients with HCM who had two or more risk factors had a significantly lower estimate of 6-year survival from sudden death compared with patients with one or no risk factors (72% versus 94% with a risk ratio of 5.6), but nonsustained ventricular tachycardia was not significantly associated with sudden death. The authors concluded that the presence of two or more risk factors was associated with a 4% to 5% estimated annual sudden death risk, which may be high enough to justify prophylactic antiarrhythmic therapy.

Given that community-based studies have shown a 1% annual mortality, significantly lower than what is reported in tertiary referral centers, Kofflard and coworkers[51] evaluated the clinical course and risk factors for sudden cardiac death in HCM in a large community-based population. In a cohort of 225 patients, there were 20 sudden deaths. Episodes of nonsustained and sustained ventricular tachycardia were present in 73 of 149 patients, but there was no significant difference in sudden cardiac death in patients with ventricular tachycardia on 24-hour cardioscan. With multivariate statistical analysis, only syncope was an independent predictor for sudden cardiac death.

In contrast to the adult DCM population, no prospective randomized trials have been performed to compare the prevention of sudden death in high-risk HCM patients with the use of amiodarone versus ICDs. As in patients with DCM, it is accepted practice to treat patients with HCM who have experienced cardiac arrest or sustained ventricular arrhythmias, or both, aggressively with an ICD. As discussed earlier, primary prevention should be considered in patients with HCM with two or more risk factors, and these patients should be offered prophylaxis with an ICD or amiodarone.

Maron and coworkers[49] conducted a retrospective multicenter study on the efficacy of ICDs in preventing sudden death in 128 patients (including 69 who were <41 years old) who were judged to be at high risk. In 43 patients, ICDs were implanted for secondary prevention. In the remaining 85 patients, the devices were implanted prophylactically for the following indications (alone or in combination): syncope, family history of sudden death, nonsustained ventricular tachycardia, and left ventricular wall thickness of at least 30 mm. In this patient population, 56 patients had inducible ventricular tachycardia or ventricular fibrillation during electrophysiology testing. Of the group, 25% had one or more episodes of inappropriate discharges. Twenty-nine patients, or 23%, had an appropriate discharge, and of these patients, 19 were in the group of 43 patients who received the ICD for secondary prevention, and 10 were in the group of 85 who had received the ICD for primary prevention. The age at which the first appropriate discharge occurred ranged from 11 to 83 years, and patients with appropriate discharges were most likely to be younger than 31 years or older than 55 years (Fig. 43-9).

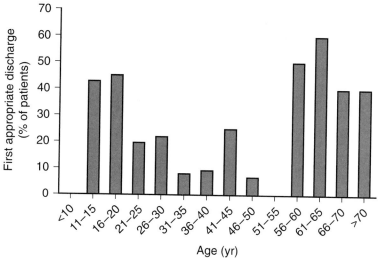

FIGURE 43-9 ■ Age at the time of the first appropriate defibrillator discharge in 29 patients. The bar for each age category shows the number of patients with appropriate discharges expressed as a proportion of the patients who were in the same age category at the time that the defibrillator was implanted. (Reproduced with permission from Maron BJ, Shen WK, Link MS, et al: Efficacy of implantable cardioverter-defibrillators for the prevention of sudden death in patients with hypertrophic cardiomyopathy. N Engl J Med 2000;342:365-373.)

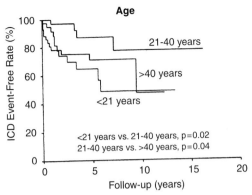

FIGURE 43-10 ■ Implantable cardioverter defibrillator intervention-free rates and risk factors. Young age (<21 years old) had a significantly lower implantable cardioverter defibrillator event-free rate. (From Begley DA, Mohiddin SA, Tripodi D, et al: Efficacy of implantable cardioverter-defibrillator therapy for primary and secondary prevention of sudden cardiac death in hypertrophic cardiomyopathy. Pacing Clin Electrophysiol 2003;26:1887.)

Begley and colleagues[52] reviewed 132 patients with HCM who received ICDs, including 47 patients for secondary prevention. There were 24 patients younger than 21 years who received an ICD for primary prevention and 20 patients younger than 21 years who received an ICD for secondary prevention. Twenty-seven patients received appropriate ICD shocks. Young patients (<21 years old) and older patients (>40 years old) had higher rates of therapeutic ICD discharges (Fig. 43-10). Serious complications occurred in 38 (29%) patients. The incidence of therapeutic shocks was related to age, but not to other reported risk factors, including severity of cardiac hypertrophy, nonsustained ventricular tachycardia during Holter monitoring, and abnormal blood pressure response to exercise. The authors concluded that risk stratification in HCM remains a major challenge. Given these data, ICDs should be regarded as the best current treatment for patients with a history of cardiac arrest or sustained ventricular arrhythmia and patients with a high-risk clinical profile on noninvasive clinical examination.[15]

Children with HCM are considered to represent a unique subset of patients with HCM. The etiologies of HCM in children are much more varied than in adults and include familial autosomal dominant HCM, genetic syndromes, and metabolic etiologies. In contrast to DCM, specific risk factors for young adults with HCM have been identified. As cited earlier, it seems that patients who receive an ICD before 20 years of age are more likely to have an ICD discharge. In addition, although the presence of nonsustained ventricular tachycardia is a known risk factor in adults with HCM, its presence in children also may be an independent marker of sudden death. Monserrat and associates[53] studied a group of 104 patients with nonsustained ventricular tachycardia and HCM who were 14 to 75 years old; 54 were younger than 20 years. The relative risk of sudden death in patients with nonsustained ventricular tachycardia varied with age, being highest in patients younger

than 30 years. Nonsustained ventricular tachycardia is associated with a substantial increase in all-cause mortality and sudden death risk in young patients with HCM. It seems that in children with familial autosomal dominant HCM, the noninvasive criteria to identify high-risk patients can be used, but the risk associated with the presence of nonsustained ventricular tachycardia is likely higher. In other forms of HCM, it is unclear how to risk stratify this population, and a case-by-case decision-making process should ensue.

Restrictive Cardiomyopathy

There is very little literature regarding the treatment of ventricular arrhythmias in pediatric patients with RCM. The incidence of sudden death in children with RCM as reported by Rivenes and colleagues[18] is 28%. These patients often had signs or symptoms of ischemia prior to sudden death. Although these authors advocate that β-blockers may be beneficial, ICD placement should be considered in patients with clinical evidence of ischemia, particularly in patients with documented ventricular arrhythmias.[18]

CURRENT STATUS AND FUTURE TRENDS

The use of ICDs is expanding rapidly in the United States and Europe. The impact of ICDs, more aggressive medical management, and biventricular pacing is being scrutinized not only for patients with heart failure, but also for patients with other disease processes. The expanding indications for ICD therapy have important medical and economic implications. The fact that pediatric patients constitute less than 1% of all ICD implantations does not diminish the need for clear indications for their use. In addition, special consideration must be given to the unique challenges that children and patients with congenital heart disease pose to the implanter and programmer of these devices. Given these issues, the Pediatric Electrophysiology Society is currently in the process of creating an ICD registry to address some of these issues.

Key Concepts
- Atrial arrhythmias, including atrial fibrillation, atrial flutter, and reentrant supraventricular arrhythmias, have been reported in 10% to 20% of children with DCM.
- Patients with RCM are particularly vulnerable because sinus tachycardia in this population can result in significant ST-segment changes consistent with ischemia and may be the inciting factor for lethal ventricular arrhythmias.
- Currently available ICDs all have bradycardia pacing capabilities, and many have rate-responsive pacing ability. In addition, many have the ability to burst pace or overdrive pace terminate atrial arrhythmias in addition to the ability to identify, pace terminate, or defibrillate ventricular arrhythmias.

■ The use of ICDs has been well documented in children to be effective and can and should be used for secondary prevention.

■ Thirty percent of patients can experience inappropriate ICD discharges because of atrial arrhythmias and sinus tachycardia.

■ In patients with congestive heart failure, ventricular arrhythmias often become more frequent and complex as left ventricular function deteriorates. Ventricular arrhythmias have been reported as independent predictors of total cardiac mortality or sudden cardiac death or both by some investigators, but not by others.

■ As in nonischemic DCM, programmed stimulation had a low positive predictive accuracy in patients with HCM; many cardiologists now use noninvasive criteria for risk stratification.

■ Primary prevention should be considered in patients with HCM with two or more risk factors, and these patients should be offered prophylaxis with an ICD or amiodarone.

■ Although the presence of nonsustained ventricular tachycardia is a known risk factor in adults with HCM, its presence in children also may be an independent marker of sudden death.

■ The fact that pediatric patients constitute less than 1% of all ICD implantations does not diminish the need for clear indications for their use.

REFERENCES

1. Muller G, Ulmer HE, Hage KJ, Wolf D: Cardiac dysrhythmias in children with idiopathic dilated or hypertrophic cardiomyopathy. Pediatr Cardiol 1995;16:56.

2. Lewis AB, Chabot M: Outcome of infants and children with dilated cardiomyopathy. Am J Cardiol 1991;68:365.

3. Ciszewski A, Bilinska ZT, Bubiszewska B, et al: Dilated cardiomyopathy in children: Clinical course and prognosis. Pediatr Cardiol 1994;15:121.

4. Wiles HB, McArthur PD, Taylor AB, et al: Prognostic features of children with idiopathic dilated cardiomyopathy. Am J Cardiol 1991;68:1372.

5. Arola A, Tuominen J, Ruuskanen O, Jokinen E: Idiopathic dilated cardiomyopathy in children: Prognostic indicators and outcome. Pediatrics 1998;101:369.

6. Friedman RA, Moak JP, Garson A Jr: Clinical course of idiopathic dilated cardiomyopathy in children. J Am Coll Cardiol 1991;18:152.

7. Griffin ML, Hernandez A, Martin TC, et al: Dilated cardiomyopathy in infants and children. J Am Coll Cardiol 1988;11:13944.

8. McKenna WJ, Franklin RCG, Nihoyannopoulos P, et al: Arrhythmia and prognosis in infants, children and adolescents with hypertrophic cardiomyopathy. J Am Coll Cardiol 1988;11:147.

9. McKenna WJ, Behr ER: Hypertrophic cardiomyopathy: management, risk stratification, and prevention of sudden death. Heart 2002;87:169.

10. Fuster V, Ryden LE, Asinger RW, et al; American College of Cardiology/American Heart Association Task Force on Practice Guidelines; European Society of Cardiology Committee for Practice Guidelines and Policy Conferences (Committee to Develop Guidelines for the Management of Patients with Atrial Fibrillation); North American Society of Pacing and Electrophysiology: ACC/AHA/ESC guidelines for the management of patients with atrial fibrillation: Executive summary: A report of the American College of Cardiology/American Heart Association Task Force on Practice Guidelines and the European Society of Cardiology Committee for Practice Guidelines and Policy Conferences (Committee to Develop Guidelines for the Management of Patients with Atrial Fibrillation) developed in collaboration with the North American Society of Pacing and Electrophysiology. Circulation 2001;104:2118.

11. Ezekowitz MD, Bridgers SL, James KE, et al: Warfarin in the prevention of stroke associated with nonrheumatic atrial fibrillation. N Engl J Med 1992;327:1406.

12. Atrial fibrillation investigators: Risk factors for stroke and efficacy of antithrombotic therapy in atrial fibrillation: Analysis of pooled data from five randomized controlled trials. Arch Intern Med 1994;154:1449.

13. Hyleck EM, Go AS, Chang Y, et al: Effect of intensity of oral anticoagulation on stroke severity and mortality in atrial fibrillation. N Engl J Med 2003;349:1019.

14. Podrid PJ: Management of arrhythmias in heart failure and cardiomyopathy. In Mann D (ed): Heart Failure: A Companion to Braunwald's Heart Disease. Philadelphia, WB Saunders, 2004, pp 683-704.

15. Elliott P, McKenna WJ: Hypertrophic cardiomyopathy. Lancet 2004;363:1881.

16. Lipshultz SE, Sleeper LA, Towbin JA, et al: The incidence of pediatric cardiomyopathy in two regions of the United States. N Engl J Med 2003;348:1647.

17. Nugent AW, Daubeney PEF, Chondros P, et al: The epidemiology of childhood cardiomyopathy in Australia. N Engl J Med 2003;348:1639.

18. Rivenes SM, Kearney DL, Smith O, et al: Sudden death and cardiovascular collapse in children with restrictive cardiomyopathy. Circulation 2000;102:876.

19. Weller RJ, Weintraub R, Addonizio LJ, et al: Outcome of idiopathic restrictive cardiomyopathy in children. Am J Cardiol 2002;90:501.

20. Lewis AB: Clinical profile and outcome of restrictive cardiomyopathy in children. Am Heart J 1992;123:1589.

20a. Mirowski M, Mower MM: Transvenous automatic defibrillator as an approach to prevention of sudden death from ventricular fibrillation. Heart Lung 1973;2:867-869.

21. Cannon BC, Friedman RA, Fenrich AL, et al: Innovative new techniques for placement of implantable cardioverter-defibrillator leads in patients with limited venous access to the heart. Heart Rhythm 2004;1:S51.

22. Love BA, Barrett KS, Alexander ME, et al: Supraventricular arrhythmias in children and young adults with implantable cardioverter defibrillators. J Cardiovasc Electrophysiol 2001;12:1097.

23. Chatrath R, Porter CJ, Ackerman MJ: Role of transvenous implantable cardioverter defibrillators in preventing sudden cardiac death in children, adolescents, and young adults. Mayo Clin Proc 2002;77:226.

24. Kammeraad JA, van Deurzen CH, Sreeram N, et al: Predictors of sudden cardiac death after Mustard or Senning repair for transposition of the great arteries. J Am Coll Cardiol 2004;44:1095.

25. Kannel WB, Plehn JF, Cupples LA: Cardiac failure and sudden death in the Framingham study. Am Heart J 1988;115:869.

26. McKee PA, Castelli WP, McNamara M, Kannel WB: The natural history of congestive heart failure: The Framingham study. N Engl J Med 1971;285:1141.

27. Stevenson WG, Stevenson LW: Prevention of sudden death in heart failure. J Cardiovasc Electrophysiol 2001;12:112.

28. Luu M, Stevenson WG, Stevenson LW, et al: Diverse mechanisms of unexpected cardiac arrest in advanced heart failure. Circulation 1989;80:1675.

29. Galvin JM, Ruskin JN: Ventricular tachycardia in patients with dilated cardiomyopathy. In Zipes DP, Jalife J (eds): Cardiac Electrophysiology: From Cell to Bedside, 4th ed. Philadelphia, WB Saunders, 2004, pp 575-587.

30. Fruhwald FM, Eber B, Schumacher M, et al: Syncope in dilated cardiomyopathy is a predictor of sudden cardiac death. Cardiology 1996;87:177.

31. Komajda M, Jais JP, Reeves F, et al: Factors predicting mortality in idiopathic dilated cardiomyopathy. Eur Heart J 1990; 11:824.

32. Middlekauff HR, Stevenson WG, Stevenson LW, Saxon LA: Syncope in advanced heart failure: High risk of sudden death regardless of origin of syncope. J Am Coll Cardiol 1993;21:110.

33. Knight BP, Goyal R, Pelosi F, et al: Outcome of patients with non-ischemic dilated cardiomyopathy and unexplained syncope treated with an implantable defibrillator. J Am Coll Cardiol 1999;33:1964.

34. DeMaria R, Gavazzi A, Caroli A, et al: Ventricular arrhythmias in dilated cardiomyopathy as an independent prognostic hallmark. Am J Cardiol 1992;69:1451.

35. Romero F, Pelliccia F, Cianfrocca C, et al: Predictors of sudden death in idiopathic dilated cardiomyopathy. Am J Cardiol 1989; 63:138.

36. Grimm W, Hoffman J, Menz V, et al: Programmed ventricular stimulation for arrhythmia risk prediction in patients with idiopathic dilated cardiomyopathy and nonsustained ventricular tachycardia. J Am Coll Cardiol 1998;32:739.

37. Doval HC, Nul DR, Grancelli HO, et al: Randomised trial of low-dose amiodarone in severe congestive heart failure. Grupo de Estudio de la Sobrevida en la Insuficiencia Cardiaca en Argentina (GESICA). Lancet 1994;344:493.

38. Singh SN, Fletcher RD, Fisher SG, et al; the Survival Trial of Antiarrhythmic Therapy in Congestive Heart Failure: Amiodarone in patients with congestive heart failure and asymptomatic ventricular arrhythmia. N Engl J Med 1995;333:77.

39. Moss AJ, Zareba W, Hall WJ, et al; the Multicenter Automatic Defibrillator Implantation Trial II investigators: Prophylactic implantation of a defibrillator in patients with myocardial infarction and reduced ejection fraction. N Engl J Med 2002;346:877.

40. Grimm W, Christ M, Bach J, et al: Noninvasive arrhythmia risk stratification in idiopathic dilated cardiomyopathy: Results of the Marburg Cardiomyopathy Study. Circulation 2003;108:2883.

41. Bansch D, Antz M, Boczor S, et al; the CAT investigators: Primary prevention of sudden cardiac death in idiopathic dilated cardiomyopathy. The Cardiomyopathy Trial (CAT). Circulation 2002;105:1453.

42. Strickberger SA, Hummel JD, Bartlett TG, et al; the AMIOVIRT investigators: Amiodarone versus implantable cardioverter-defibrillator: Randomized trial in patients with nonischemic dilated cardiomyopathy and asymptomatic nonsustained ventricular tachycardia—AMIOVIRT. J Am Coll Cardiol 2003;41:1707.

43. Kadish A, Dyer A, Daubert JP, et al; the Defibrillators in Non-Ischemic Cardiomyopathy Treatment Evaluation (DEFINITE) investigators: Prophylactic defibrillator implantation in patients with nonischemic dilated cardiomyopathy. N Engl J Med 2004; 350:2151.

44. The Antiarrhythmics Versus Implantable Defibrillators (AVID) investigators: A comparison of antiarrhythmic-drug therapy with implantable defibrillators in patients resuscitated from near-fatal ventricular arrhythmias. N Engl J Med 1997;337:1576.

45. Steinberg JS, Ehlert FA, Cannon DS, et al: Dilated cardiomyopathy vs. coronary artery disease in patients with VT/VF: Differences in presentation and outcome in the Antiarrhythmics Versus Implantable Defibrillators (AVID) registry. Circulation 1997;96:1.

46. Silka MJ, Kron J, Dunnigan A, Dick M 2nd: Sudden cardiac death and the use of implantable cardioverter-defibrillators in pediatric patients. The Pediatric Electrophysiology Society. Circulation 1993; 87:800.

47. Dubin AM, Berul CI, Bevilacqua LM, et al: The use of implantable cardioverter-defibrillators in pediatric patients awaiting heart transplantation. J Card Fail 2003;9:375.

48. Vos MA, Crijns HJ: Ventricular tachycardia in patients with hypertrophy and heart failure. In Zipes DP, Jalife J (eds): Cardiac Electrophysiology: From Cell to Bedside, 4th ed. Philadelphia, WB Saunders, 2004, pp 608-617.

49. Maron BJ, Shen W, Link MS, et al: Efficacy of implantable cardioverter-defibrillators for the prevention of sudden death in patients with hypertrophic cardiomyopathy. N Engl J Med 2000; 3442:365.

50. Elliott PM, Poloniecki J, Dickie S, et al: Sudden death in hypertrophic cardiomyopathy: Identification of high risk patients. J Am Coll Cardiol 2000;36:2212.

51. Kofflard MJM, Ten Cate FJ, van der Lee C, van Domburg RT: Hypertrophic cardiomyopathy in a large community-based population: Clinical outcome and identification of risk factors for sudden cardiac death and clinical deterioration. J Am Coll Cardiol 2003;41:987.

52. Begley DA, Mohiddin SA, Tripodi D, et al: Efficacy of implantable cardioverter defibrillator therapy for primary and secondary prevention of sudden cardiac death in hypertrophic cardiomyopathy. Pacing Clin Electrophysiol 2003;26:1887.

53. Monserrat L, Elliott PM, Gimeno JR, et al: Non-sustained ventricular tachycardia in hypertrophic cardiomyopathy: An independent marker of sudden death risk in young patients. J Am Coll Cardiol 2003;42:873.

CHAPTER 44
Surgical Valve Intervention for Valve Failure

Jeffrey S. Heinle

Intervention for valvular heart disease is frequently an important aspect of care of children and young adults with congenital heart disease. Previous chapters in this text have discussed the anatomy and pathophysiology of valvar stenosis and insufficiency and indications for valvar interventions and nonoperative strategies for valve lesions. This chapter discusses the surgical aspects of valve repair and replacement and reviews surgical outcomes in this group of often challenging patients.

Surgical interventions can be in the form of repair or replacement. Given the unique needs of active and growing children, valve repair should be considered whenever possible. Although valve replacement is an option for a failing valve, there is currently no ideal valve substitute, and selection of a valve must be individualized to each patient.

Improved survival in patients with congenital heart disease has resulted in a large population of adults with congenital heart disease.[1] In 2001, for the first time, the number of adults with congenital heart disease matched that of children.[2] With approximately 85% of infants with congenital heart disease surviving to adulthood, it is estimated that there are now more than 1 million adults in the United States with congenital heart disease.[2] Many of these patients require interventions or repeat interventions for their cardiac lesions, frequently in the form of valve interventions.

HISTORICAL ASPECTS OF VALVE INTERVENTION

The first attempts at surgical repair of valvular heart disease were closed procedures for the repair of mitral stenosis in the 1920s.[3,4] The first surgically implanted valve prosthesis was performed by Hufnagel in 1952[5]; a ball-valve prosthesis was implanted into the descending aorta for the treatment of aortic insufficiency. With the advent of successful cardiopulmonary bypass in 1953,[6] open heart surgery became a reality, and by the early 1960s, successful mechanical valve replacement was being reported for aortic and mitral valves,[7,8] ushering in the era of prosthetic cardiac valve replacement. In 1962, Ross[9] in England and Barratt-Boyes[10] in New Zealand first reported the use of homografts (allografts) for aortic valve replacement. In 1964, Rastelli performed the first

operation with the use of a right ventricle–to–pulmonary artery conduit in a patient with pulmonary atresia[11]; the use of an extracardiac conduit rendered repair of complex forms of congenital heart lesions possible. Ross[12] introduced the use of the pulmonary autograft in 1967, creating for the first time a viable valve with growth potential. Finally, in the late 1970s and 1980s, the importance and feasibility of valve reparative techniques to reproduce normal valve function were recognized and were championed by Carpentier in France.[13,14]

Valvuloplasty procedures also began initially in the surgical arena, with Brock[15] performing the first successful pulmonary valvuloplasty with a pulmonary valvulotome inserted via the right ventricle in 1948. The first successful percutaneous pulmonary valvuloplasty was performed by Kan in 1982[16]; this has become standard therapy in some congenital valvular heart lesions. More recently, percutaneous techniques for valve replacement have been described by Bonhoeffer and colleagues[17,18] (pulmonary valve) and Cribier and colleagues[19] (aortic valve).

VALVE REPAIR IN CHILDREN

Surgical intervention for valvular disease can be particularly difficult in children given the patient size and the need for somatic growth. Valve repair offers the possibility of growth in pediatric patients and avoids the risk of thromboembolism and need for long-term anticoagulation with its accompanying risk of bleeding and need for lifestyle alterations. As emphasized by Fraser,[20] growing children require a longitudinal management strategy not usually necessary in adult patients, and this strategy incorporates valve repair when possible. Restoring normal valve function while preserving the valve and valvar apparatus can have a profound effect on ventricular function. Because there is no ideal valve prosthesis that allows for growth and freedom from anticoagulation, thromboembolism, or repeat intervention, techniques for valve repair have become an important component in the surgical management of children with congenital heart disease.

Pulmonary Valve Repair
Since the first reported percutaneous pulmonary balloon valvuloplasty for **pulmonary stenosis** in 1982,[16]

percutaneous techniques have become relatively routine and have replaced surgical valvotomy as the initial therapy for this lesion. Surgery is considered in patients with persistent or recurrent stenosis after percutaneous attempts. These patients often have commissural fusion,[20] which can be relieved with open commissurotomy under direct vision with the use of cardiopulmonary bypass. If there is associated annular hypoplasia, this is addressed with an incision across the pulmonary annulus and placement of a transannular patch.

Pulmonary insufficiency is uncommon as a primary lesion, but is encountered frequently in patients after interventions involving the pulmonary valve (including repair of tetralogy of Fallot, pulmonary valvotomy, and transannular incisions). Although pulmonary insufficiency is often well tolerated for a long time, most patients eventually require intervention.

Aortic Valve Repair

Aortic stenosis is present in approximately 5% of patients with congenital heart disease,[21] with valvar aortic stenosis being the most common cause of left ventricular outflow tract obstruction. Complete or partial fusion of the leaflet commissures is usually present in patients with severe congenital aortic stenosis. Aortic valvuloplasty, using either percutaneous or open techniques, provides good palliation, allows the opportunity for growth, and delays the need for valve replacement[20-22] in patients with symptomatic aortic stenosis. Balloon valvuloplasty often is the initial therapy for patients with critical neonatal aortic stenosis.[20,23] For patients requiring surgical intervention, a variety of repair techniques have been described, including commissurotomy, shaving and thinning of the valve leaflets, mobilization of the valve mechanism, and leaflet extension.[24-26]

In patients who require surgical intervention, open aortic valvuloplasty is a safe and effective procedure for the relief of aortic stenosis.[21,22,24] The morbidity and mortality in neonates are higher than those in older infants and children. Postoperative hospital mortality in this critically ill group of neonates has been shown to be 33% to 52%,[21,27] whereas in older infants and children, hospital mortality is 1% or less.[21,22] In the same studies, actuarial 20-year survival rates ranged from 88% to 94%. Most neonates undergoing intervention required repeat intervention within 10 years. In older patients, 20-year freedom from reoperation was higher at 62% to 63%, with 90% of patients in New York Heart Association (NYHA) class I after valvuloplasty.

Aortic insufficiency may manifest as a result of an abnormal bicuspid aortic valve or may be associated with other cardiac lesions (e.g., ventricular septal defect [VSD], subaortic membrane). The problem of aortic insufficiency associated with a VSD is well recognized. In these patients, there is prolapse of the aortic valve cusp (usually the right) into the defect leading to elongation and poor coaptation of the leaflet edge, resulting in an insufficient valve. In less severe cases of aortic insufficiency, closure of the VSD alone may be adequate to prevent the progression of aortic insufficiency.[20] More severe cases of aortic insufficiency require valvuloplasty in addition to VSD repair. Trusler and coworkers[28] have described shortening on the free border of the redundant leaflet with resuspension of the commissure to address aortic insufficiency in these patients. Operative mortality is negligible, and long-term (10-year) freedom from repeat intervention is better than 80%.[29,30]

Surgical repair of insufficient bicuspid aortic valves has been well described by Fraser and associates.[31] In these patients, there is typically fusion of two leaflets of the valve. Excessive cusp tissue and inadequate commissural support lead to prolapse of the conjoined cusp and valvular insufficiency. Surgical repair involves resection of redundant leaflet tissue to create two equivalent-sized leaflets and subaortic annular plication to establish a larger zone of coaptation between the cusps. Using this technique[31] on 79 patients with a mean age of 39 years, there were no operative or postoperative deaths and a freedom from reoperation of 94% at 2 years. There was no need for anticoagulation and no reports of thromboembolic events; degree of aortic insufficiency at last follow-up was graded as 0.9 on a scale of 0 to 4. Repair of insufficient bicuspid aortic valves was believed to be safe and associated with a low incidence of recurrent aortic insufficiency. Similar results have been obtained in other adult studies.[32,33]

Mitral Valve Repair

Some of the earliest surgical valve interventions were directed at the mitral valve. Even after the development of a suitable mitral valve prosthesis for valve replacement, the morbidity and mortality associated with mitral valve replacement led to a renewed interest in mitral valve reparative techniques. In children, issues related to growth, risks of long-term anticoagulation therapy, thromboembolism, and prosthetic valve malfunction make mitral valve repair a particularly attractive alternative to valve replacement.[34] In the 1960s, Kay and Egerton[35] and Wooler and colleagues[36] described techniques for valve repair, but mitral valve repair gained wider acceptance in the 1980s after Carpentier's classification of mitral valve pathology and descriptions of effective repair techniques.[13,14]

Congenital **mitral stenosis** is a relatively rare isolated lesion that often is associated with other left-sided cardiac lesions[37] or annular hypoplasia. In symptomatic patients with congenital mitral stenosis requiring intervention in infancy, options for repair are limited, and mortality and repeat intervention rates are high.[38] For patients with parachute mitral valves, the subvalvular apparatus is narrowed, and attempts to split the chordae and papillary muscles can be challenging.[20] Isolated congenital mitral stenosis resulting from a supravalvar mitral ring can be addressed effectively with surgical resection of the ring.

Surgical intervention is performed more commonly for congenital **mitral regurgitation**[39] than for mitral stenosis, and the results for repair in children are good. Left ventricular function has been shown to normalize in children with chronic mitral regurgitation after valve repair.[40] Mitral regurgitation in children may be caused by anomalies of any component of the mitral apparatus: the leaflet itself, chordae, papillary muscle, or annulus.[41] Repair techniques can address all of these components and include annuloplasty, cleft repair, leaflet resection or enlargement, chordal shortening or transposition, and papillary muscle splitting.[39,42] Multiple studies[39,41-43] have shown the operative mortality for mitral valve repair in children to be less than 5%, with 5- and 10-year survival rates exceeding 80% and with more than 80% of patients in NYHA class I or II at late follow-up. The long-term (8 to 15 years) freedom from reoperation ranged from 70% to 90% in these studies. Mitral valve repair can be performed with low mortality and excellent results in terms of symptomatic improvement, long-term durability, and low incidences of reoperation and valve replacement.

Tricuspid Valve Repair

Tricuspid stenosis usually is associated with annular and right ventricular hypoplasia,[44] limiting the options for surgical repair.[20] **Tricuspid regurgitation** is more common and is amenable to surgical repair in most cases. Tricuspid regurgitation often is related to other underlying cardiac pathologies leading to annular dilation and poor coaptation of valve leaflets. In these cases, repair techniques must address the underlying pathology and the annular dilation. For tricuspid regurgitation, various annuloplasty techniques have been used to improve leaflet coaptation,[20] including posterior leaflet annuloplasty with obliteration of the posterior leaflet and anterior (DeVega) annuloplasty. Annuloplasty rings have been employed, but given the need for growth in children, probably should be reserved for use in older children with large annulus size. Kanter and associates[45] reviewed their use of DeVega annuloplasty for moderate-to-severe tricuspid regurgitation in 41 children at a mean age of 9.9 years. There were no early or late deaths, and postoperative tricuspid regurgitation was none or mild in 81% of patients early and 70% of patients late (mean follow-up 3.4 years). There was a 4.5% incidence of reoperation, and no patients had tricuspid stenosis.

Ebstein's anomaly is a variant of tricuspid regurgitation in which there are displacements of the septal and posterior leaflets of the tricuspid valve into the right ventricle, malformation of the anterior leaflet, atrialization of a portion of the right ventricle, dilation of the tricuspid annulus, and malformation of the right ventricle. Surgical techniques[46,47] to address this anomaly are aimed at restoring competency of the tricuspid valve, reducing annular dilation, plicating the atrialized ventricle, and

restoring right ventricular volume. Results for surgery in this lesion from two large series[48,49] have shown that repair is possible in most patients with excellent results. Operative mortality is less than 10%, and there is a low incidence of reoperation (6% to 10%) with greater than 90% of patients in NYHA class I or II postoperatively.

Valve repair offers an attractive option for children with valvular heart disease and avoids the problems associated with valve replacement in these active and growing patients. Results for valve repair in many lesions have been good, and children should be considered for repair when a good result can be anticipated. In children in whom valve repair either is not advisable or has failed, valve replacement is required.

TYPES OF VALVE REPLACEMENT

In patients requiring valve replacement, selection of prosthesis type must take into account many factors related to the prosthesis itself and factors related to patient status and lifestyle. Table 44-1 summarizes the characteristics of the ideal heart valve replacement for children. Despite the progress made in heart valve prostheses and the many options that have become available, the ideal valve for children that combines growth potential, durability, and low morbidity does not exist yet. Although mechanical valves have a long life span and excellent hemodynamics, these benefits are offset by the need for anticoagulation and the risk of thromboembolism. Although the tissue valves avoid the need for anticoagulation, these valves exhibit accelerated degeneration in children. This section reviews the options available for valve replacement in children and discusses the features and results associated with each valve type. Although there are many different models available for each valve type with similar characteristics among different manufacturers, references are made only to specific valves. Options for valve replacement fall into

TABLE 44-1

Characteristics of an Ideal Valve Replacement for Children
Excellent hemodynamics
Durable
No risk of thromboembolism
No anticoagulation required
Nonimmunogenic
Growth potential
Readily available
Silent
Affordable
Easy to implant/low operative risk

two major types: mechanical and tissue (biologic) valves, which include bioprosthetic (xenograft), allograft (homograft), and autograft valves.

Low-profile Mechanical Valves

Table 44-2 summarizes the advantages and disadvantages of available mechanical valve prostheses. In general, these valves are known for their excellent hemodynamics and durability, but have no potential for growth and generally require lifestyle alterations because of the need for anticoagulation. Although there are many types and brands of mechanical valves, the most commonly used type in children is the bileaflet valve because of the availability of small sizes, favorable hemodynamics, and low-profile. The most commonly used of these valves are the **St. Jude Medical mechanical valve** (St Jude Medical, Inc, St. Paul, MN) and the **Carbomedics bileaflet prosthesis** (CarboMedics, Inc, Austin, TX). Both of these valves are made from pyrolitic carbon because of the indestructible nature, thromboresistance, and biocompatibility.[50] In adult studies, there have been little differences in the hemodynamics, durability, and morbidity between these two valves.[51]

The St. Jude valve (Fig. 44-1) was introduced in 1977, and since then more than 1.5 million valves have been implanted worldwide. This valve is available in small sizes for pediatric use. A long-term follow-up study of the St. Jude valve documented excellent results in pediatric patients.[52] A typical postoperative echocardiogram after valve replacement is shown in Figure 44-2.

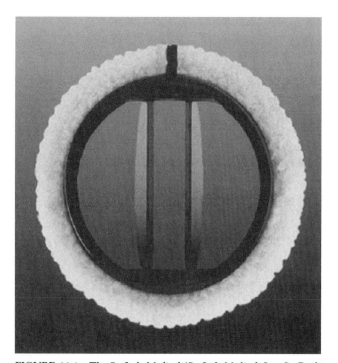

FIGURE 44-1 ■ The St. Jude Medical (St. Jude Medical, Inc, St. Paul, MN) bileaflet mechanical heart valve prosthesis. (Courtesy of St Jude Medical, Inc, St. Paul, MN.)

TABLE 44-2

Mechanical Valves	
Advantages	Disadvantages
Durable	Anticoagulation
Excellent hemodynamics	Thromboembolism
Small sizes available	Lifestyle constraints
Availability	No growth potential
	Noise

Because of reports of higher incidences of thrombosis and complications with mechanical valves implanted on the right side of the heart, their use in the pulmonary and tricuspid positions[53-55] usually is avoided, and tissue valves are favored instead in these positions. Although the avoidance of anticoagulation in children with mechanical valves has been suggested,[53,56] there are data showing an increased incidence of thromboembolic complications in children not receiving warfarin anticoagulation.[57,58] For this reason, more clinicians typically have used warfarin anticoagulation in all children receiving mechanical valves unless there are strong contraindications to its use. One strategy is to follow the American College of Cardiology/American Heart Association guidelines[59] for international normalized ratio (2 to 3 for aortic valves and 2.5 to 3.5 for mitral valves).

Bioprosthetic (Xenograft) Valves

Bioprosthetic valves are obtained or crafted from tissues from other species (typically porcine or bovine); these valves also are called *heterografts* or *xenografts*. They typically are treated with glutaraldehyde to stabilize the collagen cross-linking and improve durability and may be stented or unstented prostheses. Newer generations of these valves have incorporated various anticalcification techniques in an attempt to avoid early degeneration and valve failure. The advantages and disadvantages of these valves are summarized in Table 44-3. The major advantages of these types of valves are the low thromboembolic rates and lack of warfarin anticoagulation.

The phenomena of accelerated calcification and early degeneration of bioprosthesis in children and young adults are well recognized,[60,61] are believed to be related to accelerated calcium metabolism in children, and have limited the durability and use of these valves in pediatric patients. Because of the poorer hemodynamics in the smaller sizes and short life span of left-sided implants, most of these valves have been used for right-sided valve replacements, particularly for pulmonary valve replacement and right ventricular outflow tract (RVOT) reconstructions.

Many companies offer a wide variety of bioprosthetic devices, for RVOT reconstruction including the **Hancock bioprosthetic valved conduit**, a stented porcine valve

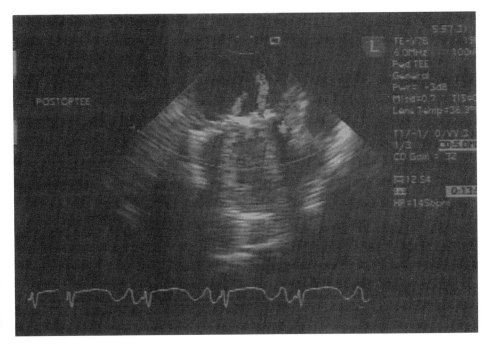

FIGURE 44-2 ■ Echocardiogram of the St. Jude Medical (St. Jude Medical, Inc, St. Paul, MN) mechanical prosthesis. The prosthesis is seen in the mitral position showing "physiologic" regurgitation along the hinge points. (Courtesy of Wanda Miller-Hance, MD, Texas Children's Hospital, Houston, TX.)

incorporated into a Dacron conduit (Fig. 44-3); the **PERIMOUNT pericardial bioprosthesis**, a stented valve with leaflets crafted from bovine pericardium (Fig. 44-4); and the **Contegra pulmonary valved conduit**, an unstented, valved, bovine jugular vein (Fig. 44-5). Results with the use of these devices are discussed subsequently in the section on pulmonary valve replacement.

Allograft Valves

Allografts (homografts) are human valves acquired from donor hearts, and the most commonly used of these valves are the aortic and pulmonary allografts (Fig. 44-6). The use of allograft valves was introduced in the early 1960s for aortic valve replacement[9,10]; allograft valves were used in RVOT reconstruction shortly thereafter.[62] In the 1980s, cryopreserved allografts were introduced, which greatly aided the storage and availability of these prostheses. In 1984, CryoLife (CryoLife, Inc, Kennesaw, GA) made commercially available cryopreserved human heart valves; more than 44,000 cryopreserved allograft heart tissue implants have been reported worldwide

(CryoValve Human Heart Valve Clinical Experience 2003 report).

Because allografts are human valves, they naturally have excellent hemodynamics, do not require anticoagulation, have extremely low thromboembolic event rates, and are potentially available in all sizes. From a surgical perspective, they have excellent handling

TABLE 44-3

Bioprosthetic Valves	
Advantages	Disadvantages
No anticoagulation	Tissue deterioration
No thromboembolism	Accelerated calcification
Silent	Hemodynamics
Availability	No growth potential

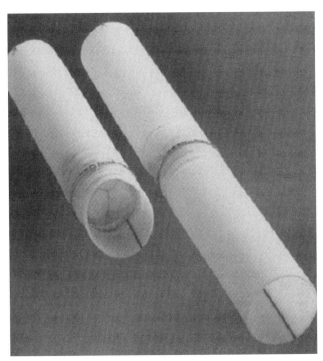

FIGURE 44-3 ■ The Hancock bioprosthetic valved conduit (Medtronic, Inc, Minneapolis, MN). (Courtesy of Medtronic, Inc, Minneapolis, MN.)

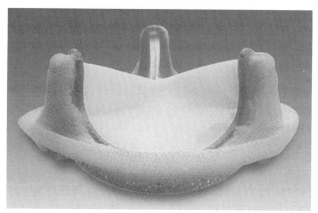

FIGURE 44-4 ■ The Carpentier-Edwards PERIMOUNT pericardial bioprosthesis (Edwards Lifesciences Corporation, Irvine, CA). (Courtesy of Edwards Lifesciences Corporation, Irvine, CA.)

characteristics, making implantation feasible even in small patients. The main disadvantages of these prostheses are accelerated degeneration in children as with bioprostheses, unpredictable durability, and limited donor availability (Table 44-4).[63,64] When used in RVOT reconstruction, the risk factors for earlier allograft degeneration include younger recipient age, longer donor ischemic time, allograft size mismatch, smaller allograft size, and use of an aortic allograft.[64-68] There are conflicting results regarding their durability versus bioprosthetic valve conduits for use in RVOT reconstructions,[69,70] and both options seem to be reasonable alternatives.

More recently, there have been concerns regarding the immunologic response elicited by these allografts

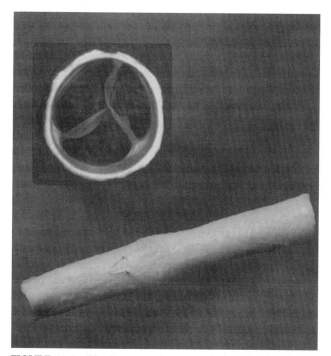

FIGURE 44-5 ■ The Contegra pulmonary valved conduit (Medtronic, Inc, Minneapolis, MN). (Courtesy of Medtronic, Inc, Minneapolis, MN.)

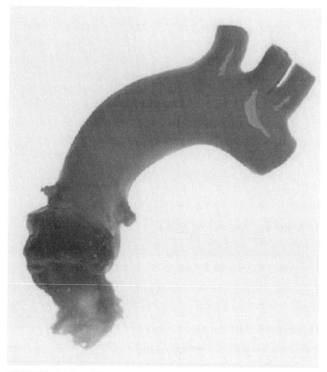

FIGURE 44-6 ■ The cryopreserved aortic allograft. (Courtesy of CryoLife, Inc, Kennesaw, GA.)

in terms of graft durability[71,72] and the development of high plasma reactive antibody levels after allograft implantation.[73,74] As pointed out by Shaddy and colleagues,[75] this HLA sensitization has the potential not only for causing deleterious effects on allograft function, but also for limiting the future opportunity of heart transplantation in patients who receive cryopreserved valve allografts. This situation has led to attempts at decellularizing allografts in the hopes of reducing immunogenicity while maintaining structural integrity and allowing for repopulation of the graft with functional host cells.[76] Early results with these decellularized allografts have shown a significantly lower level of antibody formation versus standard cryopreserved allografts,[77] although improvements in long-term durability are not yet proven.

TABLE 44-4

Allograft Valves	
Advantages	**Disadvantages**
Excellent hemodynamics	Tissue deterioration
No anticoagulation	Accelerated calcification
No thromboembolism	Availability
All sizes	Immunogenic
Silent	Cost
	No growth potential

Autograft Valves

The pulmonary autograft (Ross) procedure involves harvesting of the patient's pulmonary valve for auto-transplantation into the aortic position and recon-struction of the RVOT, typically with allograft tissue (Fig. 44-7). This procedure was described first by Ross in 1967[12] and offers an excellent hemodynamic result with no thromboembolic risk and no need for antico-agulation.[78-80] In addition, because it is a viable graft, its potential for growth makes it an attractive alternative for use in children and young adults.[78,81-83] This opera-tion requires reimplantation of the coronary arteries and has the disadvantage of substituting two-valve disease for single-valve disease (Table 44-5). Use of the auto-graft concept has been extended to reconstruction of small left ventricular outflow tract (the so-called Ross-Konno procedure) in infants and young children with good results.[84,85]

Late dilation of the neoaortic root after the Ross oper-ation has been observed,[86] and the fate of the pulmonary allograft is still an issue in children. Contraindications to the use of the pulmonary autograft in children include an abnormal pulmonary valve (preoperative pul-monary insufficiency, bicuspid valve, or significant leaflet fenestrations), aortic valve disease secondary to immune complex disease, Marfan syndrome, and ascending aorta or aortic root dilation (relative con-traindication).[78] More recent evidence suggests that primary aortic insufficiency as the indication for valve replacement may be a contraindication to the Ross

TABLE 44-5

Autograft Valves	
Advantages	**Disadvantages**
Excellent hemodynamics	Create two-valve disease
No anticoagulation	Conduit deterioration
No thromboembolism	Complex operations
Growth potential	
Silent	

procedure, given the higher incidence of late neoaortic insufficiency in this group of patients.[78,87]

In a review of the literature by Brown and cowork-ers,[21] early mortality after the Ross procedure ranged from 0% to 25% (although most centers now report an early mortality of <5%) with a late mortality of 0% to 5%. Freedom from autograft replacement was greater than 90% at 12 years in the series by Elkins and colleagues.[78] Given these excellent results, the potential for growth, and the low associated valve morbidity, the pulmonary auto-graft is considered by many surgeons to be the treatment of choice for children and young adults with congenital aortic stenosis.[79,80,82] It may be the closest option to the "ideal" valve currently available.

VALVE REPLACEMENT IN CHILDREN

Pulmonary Valve Replacement and Right Ventricular Outflow Tract Reconstruction

Placement of a right ventricle–to–pulmonary artery extra-cardiac conduit has made repair of complex forms of congenital heart disease possible.[11,62] The use of a right ventricle–to–pulmonary artery conduit is indicated in a wide variety of lesions involving the RVOT, including tetralogy of Fallot, pulmonary atresia (with or without VSD), truncus arteriosus, transposition of the great arter-ies with VSD and pulmonary stenosis, double-outlet right ventricle, RVOT reconstruction in the Ross proce-dure, and pulmonary insufficiency after previous RVOT interventions (Fig. 44-8). Although early results with these conduits are good, there was always the potential for conduit stenosis and insufficiency and the eventual need for conduit replacement. RVOT/pulmonary valve replace-ment is a common indication for valve replacement. There is at present no "perfect option" for restoring pul-monary valve competency, as is reflected by the wide variety of conduits and valves used in this location.

Progressive pulmonary insufficiency after RVOT inter-ventions (e.g., tetralogy of Fallot repair with transannular incisions) increases the risks of arrhythmia, sudden death, and progressive right ventricular dysfunction.[88-90] This increased risk has altered the initial management of patients to avoid right ventriculotomy when possible and to limit the length of transannular incisions in the hopes

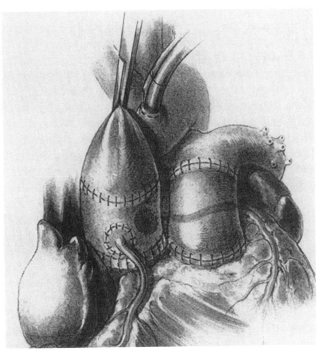

FIGURE 44-7 ■ The completed Ross procedure: Root replacement technique. (From Oury JH, Maxwell M: An appraisal of the Ross procedure: *Goals and technical guidelines. Oper Tech Card Thorac Surg* 1997;2:289-301.)

of minimizing postoperative pulmonary insufficiency.[91] In patients who do develop symptomatic or progressive pulmonary insufficiency, restoring pulmonary competency has been shown to significantly improve right ventricular function, functional class, exercise capacity, and atrial arrhythmias.[92,93] Indications for surgical intervention are not well established, and there is no clear consensus regarding timing of repeat intervention. Suggested indications for intervention include decreased exercise tolerance, right heart dysfunction, progressive right ventricular dilation, arrhythmia, progressive tricuspid regurgitation, and right ventricular hypertension.[69,92] Using these criteria, patients are often referred too late, however, and the effects of chronic pulmonary insufficiency may be irreversible. Because of this possibility and the fact that the mortality of RVOT interventions is extremely low (<2%[94,95]), several centers have suggested

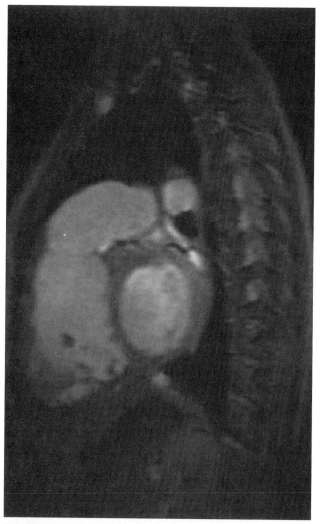

FIGURE 44-8 ■ MRI (sagittal section) of the right ventricle and right ventricular outflow tract. Image is from a patient after repair of tetralogy of Fallot with a transannular right ventricular outflow tract patch. Note the right ventricular dilation and dilation of the outflow tract patch. This study also showed severe pulmonary insufficiency and right ventricular dysfunction. (Courtesy of Wesley Vick, MD, Texas Children's Hospital, Houston, TX.)

a more aggressive approach to restoring pulmonary competency.[92,96-98] It could be argued that asymptomatic right ventricular dilation and asymptomatic pulmonary insufficiency that is moderate or severe may be adequate indications for intervention. MRI (see Fig. 44-8) has aided greatly in the assessment of right ventricular function (global and regional) and pulmonary regurgitant fraction[99] and probably should be an integral part of the follow-up for these patients.

Several large studies[65,69,95,100] have reviewed the results of extracardiac conduit placement in children for the repair of complex congenital heart defects in terms of survival and need for late repeat interventions. The Mayo Clinic[69] reviewed the results of 1,095 patients undergoing pulmonary ventricle–to–pulmonary artery reconstructions for complex lesions before 1992. The mean age at operation was 9.6 years, and mean follow-up was 10.9 years. Early mortality after repair was 3.7% for the latest decade with an actuarial survival of 77% at 10 years. Freedom from reoperation for conduit failure was 56% at 10 years, and risk of death for conduit replacement was 1.7%. In this study, heterograft Dacron conduits were more durable than allograft conduits. Baskett and associates[65] reviewed the results of 83 children receiving 96 allograft conduits at a mean age of 5.1 years. Operative mortality was 7%, and actuarial survival at 10 years was 92%. Freedom from reoperation was 71% at 9 years with a mean time to reoperation of 43 months. There were no deaths related to reoperation. Use of an aortic homograft and younger age at operation were risk factors for reoperation. Finally, Homann and colleagues[100] reported 505 patients over a 25-year period who underwent allograft or xenograft reconstruction of the RVOT at a median age of 4 years. After 10 years, 30% of the allografts and 70% of the xenografts had been replaced. Allografts in this study showed significantly better long-term durability than xenografts regardless of the age of the patient and size of the conduit at implantation.

Although xenograft conduits are a potential alternative for RVOT reconstruction, some studies have indicated that they may not be as durable as allograft conduits.[101-103] Others have noted that the presence of a pseudointimal peel within the Dacron portion of heterograft conduits limits their long-term durability.[60,104] Studies of homograft durability in children have shown varying results for freedom from allograft failure depending on the age at implantation and type of allograft used. Overall freedom from allograft failure was 82% at 8 years in Niwaya's study[64] and 74% at 5 years and 54% at 10 years in Tweddell's study.[66] Bando[67a] showed a 94% freedom from failure at 5 years with pulmonary allografts versus 70% for aortic allografts. Forbess and colleagues[68] noted a 5-year freedom of allograft failure of only 25% for patients younger than 1 year old compared with 81% for patients older than 10 years.

These results for conduit failure have led to the development and investigation of other alternatives for pulmonary valve replacement. Several reports have shown excellent short-term results with an unstented, porcine aortic root for RVOT reconstruction.[105-107] The U.S. Food and Drug Administration has granted a humanitarian device exemption for use of the Contegra pulmonary valved conduit (Medtronic, Inc, Minneapolis, MN) for its use in patients younger than 18 years old for correction or reconstruction of the RVOT in the following congenital heart malformations: pulmonary stenosis, tetralogy of Fallot, truncus arteriosus, transposition with VSD, and pulmonary atresia. In addition, this valve is indicated for the replacement of previously implanted but dysfunctional pulmonary homografts or valved conduits. It is not approved for use in primary RVOT reconstruction in the Ross procedure. This prosthesis is a valved, bovine jugular venous conduit with excellent handling characteristics that is available in diameters ranging from 12 to 22 mm. Several studies have shown good results in short-term and mid-term follow-up,[108-112] and it seems that it may be a satisfactory alternative to homograft conduit for RVOT reconstruction.[108] Concerns with this conduit include reports of thrombosis of the valve sinuses, distal anastomotic fibrosis and stenosis, and approximately a 20% incidence of moderate or greater regurgitation at 1-year follow-up.[108,109,113-115]

Aortic Valve Replacement

Mechanical, homograft, and autograft valves all have been employed in aortic valve replacement in children, but bioprosthetic (heterograft) valves generally have been avoided because of the early degeneration and structural failure in pediatric patients.[79] Although mechanical valves are readily available and easy to insert, they have the risk of thromboembolic complications, require anticoagulation, and do not have the potential for growth. Although homografts have excellent hemodynamics and are available in a wide range of sizes, they also do not have the potential for growth, and their durability varies. The pulmonary autograft may represent the ideal prosthesis for aortic valve replacement, given its excellent hemodynamics, durability, and growth potential.[79] The procedure possesses all of the issues described earlier for RVOT reconstruction, however.

In a review of the literature by Brown and colleagues,[21] early mortality for mechanical valve replacement in children ranged from 0% to 13% with most studies reporting a mortality of less than 5%; late mortality ranged from 0% to 5%. Intermediate-term results from Lupinetti and associates[116] showed no statistical difference in operative deaths between children receiving mechanical valves compared with human valves. Four-year freedom from valve-related complications was 61% in the mechanical valve group versus 88% in the human valve group. As opposed to the mechanical valves, there were no late deaths or thromboembolic events in the human valve group. Based on these results, Lupinetti and associates[116] concluded that human valves in children requiring aortic valve replacement are superior to mechanical valves in intermediate follow-up.

In the largest reported series of autograft operations in children in the United States, Elkins and coworkers[78] reported an operative mortality of 4.5%. At 12 years, the actuarial survival was 92%, the freedom from autograft replacement was excellent at 93%, and the freedom from RVOT homograft replacement was 90%. Similar results were shown by Al Halees and associates.[82] Survival and freedom from autograft replacement of the aortic valve are excellent in children, but the late function of the RVOT conduit remains a concern.

Mitral Valve Replacement

Mechanical valves are used almost exclusively for mitral valve replacement in children. Mitral valve replacement in the first several years of life carries a high operative mortality (17% to 37%) and repeat intervention rate.[117-119] Predictors of death in this age group included a diagnosis of atrioventricular septal defect or Shone syndrome and an increased ratio of prosthesis size to patient weight.

Two studies[120,121] have shown improved survival in the current era. In the study by Alexiou and colleagues,[121] operative mortality after 1990 was 3.6%, and 10-year survival was 86%; 16% of patients had valve-related or anticoagulation-related events, and 18% required repeat mitral valve replacement. In the study by Kojori and associates[120] of 137 mitral valve replacements in 104 children, the 6-month survival was 83%, and mortality 15 years after initial replacement was 19%. Bleeding related to anticoagulation was present in 5% of patients, whereas throm-boembolic events occurred in 4%. By 15 years, 19% of patients had died, and 71% of the valves had been replaced, leaving only 10% of patients surviving without the need for repeat mitral valve replacement.

Tricuspid Valve Replacement

Tricuspid valve replacement in children is a rare procedure, with the most common indications being endocarditis and Ebstein's anomaly not amenable to surgical repair. Use of bioprosthetic (xenograft) valves for tricuspid valve replacement usually is preferred over mechanical valves. In a series from the Mayo Clinic[122] of primary tricuspid valve replacement for Ebstein's anomaly in children (median age 14 years), the early mortality was 5.7%, and late mortality was 6%. Survival was worse in patients younger than 14 years old. Freedom from reoperation for valve replacement was 98% at 5 years and 82% at 10 years; this may reflect the fact that large valves (median size 33 mm) were able to be implanted in these patients. The authors concluded that tricuspid valve replacement with a bioprosthesis is a reasonable alternative in patients who are not suitable candidates for a good repair.

Percutaneous Valve Implantation

Percutaneous valve implantation offers the potential advantage of avoiding the potential deleterious effects of cardiopulmonary bypass and the risks of multiple

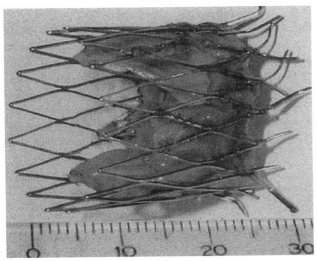

FIGURE 44-9 ■ **Percutaneous valve implantation.** A biologic valve sutured to an expandable stent for percutaneous implantation. (From the American Association for Thoracic Surgery.)

sternotomies. The valve used for these procedures is a xenograft sutured to an expandable stent (Fig. 44-9). Extensive work in the animal laboratory[123] led to the first successful percutaneous pulmonary valve implantation in humans by Bonhoeffer and colleagues in 2000[17] (Fig. 44-10). These investigators subsequently reported on eight children and adolescents with failing right ventricle-to-pulmonary conduits who underwent percutaneous implantation of a Contegra conduit mounted into an expandable stent.[18] All valves were successfully

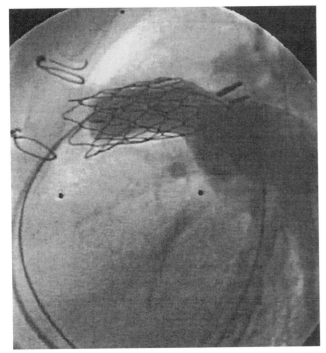

FIGURE 44-10 ■ **Pulmonary angiogram of percutaneous valve implantation.** Angiogram shows valvular competence of a percutaneously implanted pulmonary valve. (From Bonhoeffer P, Boudjemline Y, Qureshi A, et al: *Percutaneous insertion of the pulmonary valve. J Am Coll Cardiol* 2002;39:1664-1669.)

implanted, and six of the eight were competent immediately after implantation. Short-term follow-up revealed all patients to be improved clinically, and in all patients the valve was competent; four of the patients had residual RVOT obstruction. A cumulative experience of 56 patients with short-term follow-up (mean 4 months) showed a 98% freedom from regurgitation, a low rate (5%) of procedural complication, and no deaths.[123]

In 2002, the first percutaneous aortic valve implantation in a human was performed as a "last resort" in a patient with severe calcific aortic stenosis.[19] The early experience of percutaneous aortic valve implantations in adult patients was presented in 2004.[124] In five of the six patients, the valve could be positioned successfully, but in one patient the valve was ejected into the ascending aorta, and the patient died. On early follow-up, three of the five surviving patients have mild aortic insufficiency whereas the other two have severe insufficiency secondary to paravalvular leaks. Currently, this technique is a potential option only in patients who are not surgical candidates for valve replacement.

CURRENT STATUS AND FUTURE TRENDS

Valve repair and replacement constitute a significant proportion of operations for children with congenital heart lesions.[125] Surgical repair should be attempted when feasible because it offers the potential for growth of the valve and eliminates prosthetic valve-related morbidity. There is no "ideal" valve prosthesis available that provides the possibility of growth and long-term freedom from repeat intervention. Early postoperative results for repair and replacement in the current era are excellent, but late need for repeat intervention is frequent.

Additional bioengineering research can improve further the existing mechanical and biologic valves.[126] Although percutaneous valve replacement offers theoretical advantages over standard surgical techniques, medium-term and long-term results are lacking. State-of-the-art replacement of cardiac valves is far less than ideal, but the potential availability of tissue-engineered valves in the future may address some of these issues. Advances in this area include the development of different potential cell sources and cell-seeding techniques, matrix and scaffold development, polymer chemistry fabrication, and the advent of tissue-engineered neotissue in vitro.[127,128]

Key Concepts

■ With approximately 85% of infants with congenital heart disease surviving to adulthood, it is estimated that there are now more than 1 million adults in the United States with congenital heart disease. Many of these patients require interventions or repeat interventions for their cardiac lesions, frequently in the form of valve interventions.

- Valve repair offers the possibility of growth in pediatric patients and avoids the risk of thromboembolism and need for long-term anticoagulation with its accompanying risk of bleeding and need for lifestyle alterations.

- In patients who require surgical intervention, open aortic valvuloplasty is a safe and effective procedure for the relief of aortic stenosis. The morbidity and mortality in neonates are higher than those in older infants and children.

- In children, issues related to growth, risks of long-term anticoagulation therapy, thromboembolism, and prosthetic valve malfunction make mitral valve repair a particularly attractive alternative to valve replacement.

- Although there are many types and brands of mechanical valves, the most commonly used type in children is the bileaflet valve because of the availability of small sizes, favorable hemodynamics, and low-profile.

- Because of reports of higher incidences of thrombosis and complications with mechanical valves implanted on the right side of the heart, their use in the pulmonary and tricuspid positions usually is avoided, and tissue valves are favored instead in these positions.

- Bioprosthetic valves are obtained or crafted from tissues from other species (typically porcine or bovine); these valves also are called heterografts or xenografts.

- The phenomena of accelerated calcification and early degeneration of bioprosthesis in children and young adults are well recognized, are believed to be related to accelerated calcium metabolism in children, and have limited the durability and use of these valves in pediatric patients.

- Allografts (homografts) are human valves acquired from donor hearts, and the most commonly used of these valves are the aortic and pulmonary allografts.

- Because allografts are human valves, they naturally have excellent hemodynamics, do not require anticoagulation, have extremely low thromboembolic event rates, and are potentially available in all sizes. From a surgical perspective, they have excellent handling characteristics, making implantation feasible even in small patients. The main disadvantages of these prostheses are accelerated degeneration in children as with bioprostheses, unpredictable durability, and limited donor availability.

- There have been concerns regarding the immunologic response elicited by these allografts in terms of graft durability and the development of high plasma reactive antibody levels after allograft implantation.

- The pulmonary autograft (Ross) procedure involves harvesting of the patient's pulmonary valve for autotransplantation into the aortic position and reconstruction of the RVOT, typically with allograft tissue.

- Use of the autograft concept has been extended to reconstruction of small left ventricular outflow tract (the so-called Ross-Konno procedure) in infants and young children with good results.

- Contraindications to the use of the pulmonary autograft in children include an abnormal pulmonary valve (preoperative pulmonary insufficiency, bicuspid valve, or significant leaflet fenestrations), aortic valve disease secondary to immune complex disease, Marfan syndrome, and ascending aorta or aortic root dilation (relative contraindication).

- Given the excellent results, the potential for growth, and the low associated valve morbidity, the pulmonary autograft is considered by many surgeons to be the treatment of choice for children and young adults with congenital aortic stenosis.

- It could be argued that asymptomatic right ventricular dilation and asymptomatic pulmonary insufficiency that is moderate or severe may be adequate indications for intervention. MRI has aided greatly in the assessment of right ventricular function (global and regional) and pulmonary regurgitant fraction and probably should be an integral part of the follow-up for these patients.

- Mechanical, homograft, and autograft valves all have been employed in aortic valve replacement in children, but bioprosthetic (heterograft) valves generally have been avoided because of the early degeneration and structural failure in pediatric patients.

- Survival and freedom from autograft replacement of the aortic valve are excellent in children, but the late function of the RVOT conduit remains a concern.

- Percutaneous valve implantation offers the potential advantage of avoiding the potential deleterious effects of cardiopulmonary bypass and risks of multiple sternotomies. The valve used for these procedures is a xenograft sutured to an expandable stent.

REFERENCES

1. Marelli A, Rhame E, Pilote L: Congenital heart disease: Prevalence rates in a population of 5,363,695 adults (Abstract). J Am Coll Cardiol 2003;41(Suppl A):490A.
2. Warnes CA, Liberthson R, Danielson GK, et al: 32nd Bethesda Conference: Care of the adult with congenital heart disease. Task Force 1: The changing profile of congenital heart disease in adult life. J Am Coll Cardiol 2001;37:1171-1175.
3. Cutler EC, Levine SA: Cardiotomy and valvulotomy for mitral stenosis: Experimental observations and clinical notes concerning an operated case with recovery. Boston Med Surg J 1923;188:1023-1027.
4. Souttar HS: The surgical treatment of mitral stenosis. BMJ 1925; Oct 3:603-606.
5. Hufnagel C, Harvey WP, Rabil PJ, et al: Surgical correction of aortic insufficiency. Surgery 1954;35:673-680.
6. Gibbon J Jr: Application of a mechanical heart and lung apparatus to cardiac surgery. Minn Med 1954;37:171-180.
7. Starr A, Edwards M: Mitral replacement: Clinical experience with a ball valve prosthesis. Ann Surg 1961;154:726-740.
8. Gott VL, Alejo DE, Cameron DE: Mechanical heart valves: 50 years of evolution. Ann Thorac Surg 2003;76:S2230-S2239.
9. Ross DN: Homograft replacement of the aortic valve. Lancet 1962;2:487-492.
10. Barratt-Boyes BG: Homograft aortic valve replacement in aortic incompetence and stenosis. Thorax 1964;19:131-135.

11. Rastelli GC, Ongley PA, Davis GD, et al: Surgical repair for pulmonary valve atresia with coronary-pulmonary artery fistula: Report of a case. Mayo Clin Proc 1965;40:521-527.

12. Ross DN: Replacement of aortic and mitral valves with a pulmonary autograft. Lancet 1967;2:956-958.

13. Carpentier A, Deloche A, Dauptain I, et al: A new reconstructive operation for correction of mitral and tricuspid insufficiency. J Thorac Cardiovasc Surg 1971;61:1-13.

14. Carpentier A: Cardiac valve surgery: The "French Correction." J Thorac Cardiovasc Surg 1983;86:323-337.

15. Brock RC: Pulmonary valvulotomy for the relief of congenital pulmonary stenosis. BMJ 1948;Jun 12:1121-1126.

16. Kan J, White RJ, Mitchell S, Gardner T: Percutaneous balloon valvuloplasty: A new method for treating congenital pulmonary-valve stenosis. N Engl J Med 1982;307:540-542.

17. Bonhoeffer P, Boudjemline Y, Saliba Z, et al: Percutaneous replacement of pulmonary valve in a right-ventricle to pulmonary-artery prosthetic conduit with valve dysfunction. Lancet 2000;356: 1403-1405.

18. Bonhoeffer P, Boudjemline Y, Qureshi A, et al: Percutaneous insertion of the pulmonary valve. J Am Coll Cardiol 2002;39: 1664-1669.

19. Cribier A, Eltchaninoff H, Bash A, et al: Percutaneous transcatheter implantation of an aortic valve prosthesis for calcific aortic stenosis: First human case description. Circulation 2002; 106:3006-3008.

20. Fraser CD Jr: Technical considerations for valve repair in patients with congenital heart lesions. Curr Opin Cardiol 1998;13:96-104.

21. Brown JW, Ruzmetov M, Vijay P, et al: Surgery for aortic stenosis in children: A 40-year experience. Ann Thorac Surg 2003;76: 1398-1411.

22. Chartrand CC, Saro-Servando E, Vobecky JS: Long-term results of surgical valvuloplasty for congenital valvar aortic stenosis in children. Ann Thorac Surg 1999;68:1356-1359.

23. Gatzoulis MA, Rigby ML, Shinebourne EA, Redington AN: Contemporary results of balloon valvuloplasty and surgical valvotomy for congenital aortic stenosis. Arch Dis Child 1995;73:66-69.

24. Caspi J, Ilbawi MN, Roberson DA, et al: Extended aortic valvuloplasty for recurrent valvular stenosis and regurgitation in children. J Thorac Cardiovasc Surg 1994;107:1114-1120.

25. Grinda J, Latremouille C, Berrebi A, et al: Aortic cusp extension valvuloplasty for rheumatic aortic valve disease: Midterm results. Ann Thorac Surg 2002;74:438-443.

26. Ilbawi MN, DeLeon SY, Wilson WR, et al: Extended aortic valvuloplasty: A new approach for the management of congenital valvar aortic stenosis. Ann Thorac Surg 1991;52:663-668.

27. Gaynor JW, Bull C, Sullivan ID, et al: Late outcome of survivors of intervention for neonatal aortic valve stenosis. Ann Thorac Surg 1995;60:122-125.

28. Trusler GA, Moes CF, Kidd VS: Repair of ventricular septal defect with aortic insufficiency. J Thorac Cardiovasc Surg 1973;66:394.

29. Trusler GA, Williams WG, Smallhorn JF, Freedom RM: Late results after repair of aortic insufficiency with ventricular septal defect. J Thorac Cardiovasc Surg 1992;103:276-281.

30. Elgamal MA, Hakimi M, Lyons JM, Walters HL: Risk factors for failure of aortic valvuloplasty in aortic insufficiency with ventricualr septal defect. Ann Thorac Surg 1999;68:1350-1355.

31. Fraser CD Jr, Wang N, Mee RB, et al: Repair of insufficient bicuspid aortic valves. Ann Thorac Surg 1994;58:386-390.

32. Kasimir M, Simon P, Seebacher G, et al: Reconstructed bicuspid aortic valve after 10 years: Clinical and echocardiographic follow-up. Heart Surg Forum 2004;7:319-323.

33. Minakata K, Schaff HV, Zehr KJ, et al: Is repair of aortic valve regurgitation a safe alternative to valve replacement? J Thorac Cardiovasc Surg 2004;127:645-653.

34. Lamberti JJ, Mainwaring RD, George L, Oury JH: Management of systemic atrioventricular valve regurgitation in infants and children. J Card Surg 1993;8:612-621.

35. Kay JH, Egerton WS: The repair of mitral insufficiency associated with ruptured chordae tendinae. Ann Surg 1963;157:351-360.

36. Wooler GH, Nixon PG, Grimshaw VA, et al: Experiences with the repair of the mitral valve in mitral incompetence. Thorax 1962;17: 49-57.

37. Serraf A, Zoghbi J, Belli E, et al: Congenital mitral stenosis with or without associated defects: An evolving surgical strategy. Circulation 2000;102(19 Suppl 3):III-166-III-171.

38. Moore P, Adatia I, Spevak PJ, et al: Severe congenital mitral stenosis in infants. Circulation 1994;89:2099-2106.

39. Aharon AS, Laks H, Drinkwater DC, et al: Early and late results of mitral valve repair in children. J Thorac Cardiovasc Surg 1994; 107:1262-1270.

40. Krishnan US, Gersony WM, Berman-Rosenzweig E, Apfel HD: Late left ventricular function after surgery for children with chronic symptomatic mitral regurgitation. Circulation 1997;96:4280-4285.

41. Sugita T, Ueda Y, Matsumoto M, et al: Early and late results of partial plication annuloplasty for congenital mitral insufficiency. J Thorac Cardiovasc Surg 2001;122:229-233.

42. Chauvaud S, Fuzellier JF, Houel R, et al: Reconstructive surgery in congenital mitral valve insufficiency (Carpentier's techniques): Long-term results. J Thorac Cardiovasc Surg 1998;115:84-93.

43. Zias EA, Mavroudis C, Backer CL, et al: Surgical repair of the congenitally malformed mitral valve in infants and children. Ann Thorac Surg 1998;66:1551-1559.

44. Lewis DA, Tweddell JS: Valve repair and replacement in children. Curr Opin Cardiol 1997;12:63-69.

45. Kanter KR, Doelling NR, Fyfe DA, et al: De Vega tricuspid annuloplasty for tricuspid regurgitation in children. Ann Thorac Surg 2001;72:1344-1348.

46. Carpentier A, Chauvaud S, Mace L, et al: A new reconstructive operation for Ebstein's anomaly of the tricuspid valve. J Thorac Cardiovasc Surg 1988;96:92-101.

47. Danielson GK, Fuster V: Surgical repair of Ebstein's anomaly. Ann Surg 1982;196:499-504.

48. Chauvaud SM, Mihaileanu SA, Gaer JA, Carpentier AC: Surgical treatment of Ebstein's malformation: The Hopital Broussais' experience. Cardiol Young 1995;6:4-11.

49. Danielson GK, Driscoll DJ, Mair DD, et al: Operative treatment of Ebstein's anomaly. J Thorac Cardiovasc Surg 1992;104:1195-1202.

50. Bokros JC: Carbon in prosthetic heart valves. Ann Thorac Surg 1989;48:S49-S50.

51. Lim KH, Caputo M, Ascione R, et al: Prospective randomized comparison of CarboMedics and St Jude Medical bileaflet mechanical heart valve prostheses: An interim report. J Thorac Cardiovasc Surg 2002;123:21-32.

52. Cabalka AK, Emery RW, Petersen RJ, et al: Long-term follow-up of the St. Jude Medical prosthesis in pediatric patients. Ann Thorac Surg 1995;60(6 Suppl):S618-S623.

53. Ilbawi MN, Lockhart CG, Idriss FS, et al: Experience with St. Jude Medical valve prosthesis in children: A word of caution regarding right-sided placement. J Thorac Cardiovasc Surg 1987;93:73-79.

54. Kawachi Y, Masuda M, Tominaga R, Tokunaga K: Comparative study between St. Jude Medical and bioprosthetic valves in the right side of the heart. Jpn Circ J 1991;55:553-562.

55. Miyamura H, Kanazawa H, Hayashi J, Eguchi S: Thrombosed St. Jude Medical valve prosthesis in the right side of the heart in patients with tetralogy of Fallot. J Thorac Cardiovasc Surg 1987; 94:148-150.

56. Pass HI, Sade RM, Crawford FA, Hohn AR: Cardiac valve prosthesis in children without anticoagulation. J Thorac Cardiovasc Surg 1984; 87:832-835.

57. Serra AJ, McNicholas KW, Olivier HF Jr, et al: The choice of anticoagulation in pediatric patients with the St. Jude Medical valve prostheses. J Cardiovasc Surg (Torino) 1987;28:588-591.

58. McGrath LB, Gonzalez-Lavin L, Eldredge WJ, et al: Thromboembolic and other events following valve replacement in a pediatric population treated with antiplatelet agents. Ann Thorac Surg 1987;43:285-287.

59. Bonow RO, Carabello B, de Leon AC, et al: ACC/AHA guidelines for the management of patients with valvular heart disease: A report of the American College of Cardiology/American Heart Association Task Force on Practice Guidelines (Committee on Management of Patients with Valvular Heart Disease). J Am Coll Cardiol 1998;32:1486-1488.

60. Jonas RA, Freed MD, Mayer JE, Castaneda AR: Long-term follow-up of patients with synthetic right heart conduits. Circulation 1985;72(Suppl 2):II-77.

61. Castaneda AR, Jonas RA, Mayer JE, Hanley FL: Clinical and experimental aspects. In Castaneda AR, Jonas RA, Mayer JE, Hanley FL (eds): Cardiac Surgery of the Neonate and Infant. Philadelphia: WB Saunders, 1994, pp 109-122.

62. Ross DN, Somerville J: Correction of pulmonary atresia with a homograft aortic valve. Lancet 1966;2:1146-1147.

63. Clarke DR, Campbell DN, Hayward AR, Bishop DA: Degeneration of aortic valve allografts in young recipients. J Thorac Cardiovasc Surg 1993;105:934-942.

64. Niwaya K, Knott-Craig CJ, Lane MM, et al: Cryopreserved homograft valves in the pulmonary position: Risk analysis for intermediate-term failure. J Thorac Cardiovasc Surg 1999;117:141-146.

65. Baskett RJ, Ross DB, Nanton MA, Murphy DA: Factors in the early failure of cryopreserved homograft pulmonary valves in children: Preserved immunogenicity? J Thorac Cardiovasc Surg 1996;112:1170-1178.

66. Tweddell JS, Pelech AN, Frommelt PC, et al: Factors affecting longevity of homograft valves used in right ventricular outflow tract reconstruction for congenital heart disease. Circulation 2000;102(Suppl 3):III-130-III-135.

67. Bull C, Macartney FJ, Horvath P, et al: Evaluation of long-term results of homograft and heterograft valves in extracardiac conduits. J Thorac Cardiovasc Surg 1987;94:12-19.

67a. Bando K, Danielson GK, Schaff HV, et al: Outcome of pulmonary and aortic hemografts for right ventricular outflow tract reconstruction. J Thorac Cardiovasc Surg 1995;109:509-518.

68. Forbess JM, Shah AS, St Louis JD, et al: Cryopreserved homografts in the pulmonary position: Determinants of durability. Ann Thorac Surg 2001;71:54-59.

69. Dearani JA, Danielson GK, Puga FJ, et al: Late follow-up of 1095 patients undergoing operation for complex congenital heart disease utilizing pulmonary ventricle to pulmonary artery conduits. Ann Thorac Surg 2003;75:399-410.

70. Clarke DR, Bishop DA: Ten year experience with pulmonary allografts in children. J Heart Valve Dis 1995;4:384-391.

71. Hogan PG, O'Brien MF: Improving the allograft valve: Does the immune response matter? (Editorial). J Thorac Cardiovasc Surg 2003;126:1251-1253.

72. Baskett RJ, Nanton MA, Warren AE, Ross DB: Human leukocyte antigen-DR and ABO mismatch are associated with accelerated homograft valve failure in children: Implications for therapeutic interventions. J Thorac Cardiovasc Surg 2003;126:232-238.

73. Breinholt JP, Hawkins JA, Lambert LM, et al: A prospective analysis of the immunogenicity of cryopreserved nonvalved allografts used in pediatric heart surgery. Circulation 2000;102(Suppl III):III-179-III-182.

74. Hawkins JA, Breinholt J, Lambert L, et al: Class I and class II anti-HLA antibodies after implantation of cryopreserved allograft material in pediatric patients. J Thorac Cardiovasc Surg 2000;119:324-330.

75. Shaddy RE, Hunter D, Osborn KA, et al: Prospective analysis of HLA immunogenicity of cryopreserved valved allografts used in pediatric heart surgery. Circulation 1996;94:1063-1067.

76. Elkins RC, Dawson PE, Goldstein S, et al: Decellularized human valve allografts. Ann Thorac Surg 2001;71:S428-S432.

77. Hawkins JA, Hillman ND, Lambert LM, Shaddy RE: Immunogenicity of decellularized cryopreserved allografts in pediatric cardiac surgery: Comparison with standard cryopreserved allografts. J Thorac Cardiovasc Surg 2003;126:247-253.

78. Elkins RC, Lane MM, McCue C: Ross operation in children: Late results. J Heart Valve Dis 2001;10:736-741.

79. Turrentine MW, Ruzmetov M, Vijay P, et al: Biological versus mechanical aortic valve replacement in children. Ann Thorac Surg 2001;71(5 Suppl):S356-S360.

80. Lupinetti FM, Duncan BW, Lewin M, et al: Comparison of autograft and allograft aortic valve replacement in children. J Thorac Cardiovasc Surg 2003;126:240-246.

81. Elkins RC, Knott-Craig CJ, Ward KE, et al: Pulmonary autograft in children: Realized growth potential. Ann Thorac Surg 1994;57:1387-1394.

82. Al Halees Z, Pieters F, Qadoura F, et al: The Ross procedure is the procedure of choice for congenital aortic valve disease. J Thorac Cardiovasc Surg 2002;123:437-441.

83. Ross D: Replacement of the aortic valve with a pulmonary autograft: the "switch" operation. Ann Thorac Surg 1991;52:1346-1350.

84. Hraska V, Krajci M, Haun C, et al: Ross and Ross-Konno procedure in children and adolescents: Mid-term results. Eur J Cardiothorac Surg 2004;25:742-747.

85. Reddy VM, Rajasinghe HA, McElhinney DB, et al: Extending the limits of the Ross procedure. Ann Thorac Surg 1995;60(6 Suppl):S600-S603.

86. David TE, Omran A, Ivanov J, et al: Dilation of the pulmonary autograft after the Ross procedure. J Thorac Cardiovasc Surg 2000;119:210-220.

87. Laudito A, Brook MM, Suleman S, et al: The Ross procedure in children and young adults: A word of caution. J Thorac Cardiovasc Surg 2001;122:147-153.

88. Dietl C, Cazzaniga M, Dubner S, et al: Life-threatening arrhythmias and RV dysfunction after surgical repair of tetralogy of Fallot: Comparison between transventricular and transatrial approaches. Circulation 1994;90:II-7-II-12.

89. Bove E, Byrum C, Thomas F, et al: The influence of pulmonary insufficiency on ventricular function following repair of tetralogy of Fallot: Evaluation using radionuclide ventriculography. J Thorac Cardiovasc Surg 1983;85:691-696.

90. Nollert GD, Daebritz SH, Schmoeckel M, et al: Risk factors for sudden death after repair of tetralogy of Fallot. Ann Thorac Surg 2003;76:1901-1905.

91. Fraser CD Jr, McKenzie ED, Cooley DA: Tetralogy of Fallot: Surgical management individualized to the patient. Ann Thorac Surg 2001;71:1556-1563.

92. Discigil B, Dearani JA, Puga FJ, et al: Late pulmonary valve replacement after repair of tetralogy of Fallot. J Thorac Cardiovasc Surg 2001;121:344-351.

93. Eyskens B, Reybrouck T, Bogaert J, et al: Homograft insertion for pulmonary regurgitation after repair of tetralogy of Fallot improves cardiorespiratory exercise performance. Am J Cardiol 2000;85:221-225.

94. LeBlanc JG, Russell JL, Sett SS, Potts JE: Intermediate follow-up of right ventricular outflow tract reconstruction with allograft conduits. Ann Thorac Surg 1998;66:S174-S178.

95. Kanter KR, Budde JM, Parks WJ, et al: One hundred pulmonary valve replacements in children after relief of right ventricular outflow tract obstruction. Ann Thorac Surg 2002;73:1801-1806.

96. Warner KG, O'Brien PK, Rhodes J, et al: Expanding the indications for pulmonary valve replacement after repair of tetralogy of Fallot. Ann Thorac Surg 2003;76:1066-1071.

97. Bove EL, Kavey R, Byrum C, et al: Improved right ventricular function following late pulmonary valve replacementr for residual pulmonary insufficiency or stenosis. J Thorac Cardiovasc Surg 1985;90:50-55.

98. Therrien J, Siu SC, McLaughlin PR, et al: Pulmonary valve replacement in adults late after repair of tetralogy of Fallot: Are we operating too late? J Am Coll Cardiol 2000;36:1670-1675.

99. Sahn DJ, Vick GW: Review of new techniques in echocardiography and magnetic resonance imaging as applied to patients with congenital heart disease. Heart 2001;86(Suppl 2):II-41-II-53.

100. Homann M, Haehnel JC, Mendler N, et al: Reconstruction of the RVOT with valved biologic conduits: 25 years of experience with allografts and xenografts. Eur J Cardiothorac Surg 2000; 17:624-630.

101. Dittrich S, Alexi-Meskishvili VV, Yankah AC, et al: Comparison of porcine xenografts and homografts for pulmonary valve replacement in children. Ann Thorac Surg 2000;70:717-722.

102. Lange R, Weipert J, Homann M, et al: Performance of allografts and xenografts for right ventricular outflow tract reconstruction. Ann Thorac Surg 2001;71:S365-S367.

103. Schmid FX, Keyser A, Wiesenack C, et al: Stentless xenografts and homografts for right ventricular outflow tract reconstruction during the Ross operation. Ann Thorac Surg 2002;74:684-688.

104. Razzouk AJ, Williams WG, Cleveland DO, et al: Surgical connections from ventricle to pulmonary artery: Comparison of four types of valved implants. Circulation 1992;86(Suppl 2):II-154.

105. Kanter KR, Fyfe DA, Mahle WT, et al: Results with the freestyle porcine aortic root for right ventricular outflow tract reconstruction in children. Ann Thorac Surg 2003;76:1889-1894.

106. Chard RB, Kang N, Andrews DR, Nunn GR: Use of the Medtronic Freestyle valve as a right ventricular to pulmonary artery conduit. Ann Thorac Surg 2001;71:S361-S364.

107. Hartz RS, DeLeon SY, Lane J, et al: Medtronic freestyle valves in right ventricular outflow tract reconstruction. Ann Thorac Surg 2003;76:1896-1900.

108. Breymann T, Thies W, Boethig D, et al: Bovine valved venous xenografts for RVOT reconstruction: Results after 71 implants. Eur J Cardiothorac Surg 2002;21:703-710.

109. Boudjemline Y, Bonnet D, Massih TA: Use of bovine jugular vein to reconstruct the right ventricular outflow tract: Early results. J Thorac Cardiovasc Surg 2003;126:490-497.

110. Corno AF, Hurni M, Griffin H, et al: Bovine jugular vein as right ventricle-to-pulmonary artery valved conduit. J Heart Valve Dis 2002;11:242-247.

111. Bove T, Demanete H, Wauthy P, et al: Early results of valved bovine jugular vein conduits versus bicuspid homograft for right ventricular outflow tract reconstruction. Ann Thorac Surg 2002; 74:536-541.

112. Boethig D, Thies W, Hecker H, Breymann T: Mid term course after pediatric right ventricular outflow tract reconstruction: A comparison of homografts, porcine xenografts and Contegras. Eur J Cardiothorac Surg 2004;27:58-66.

113. Tiete AR, Sachweh JS, Roemer U, et al: Right ventricular outflow tract reconstruction with the Contegra bovine jugular vein conduit: A word of caution. Ann Thorac Surg 2004;77:2151-2156.

114. Kadner A, Dave H, Stallmach T, et al: Formation of a stenotic membrane at the distal anastomosis of bovine jugular vein grafts (Contegra) after right ventricular outflow tract reconstruction. J Thorac Cardiovasc Surg 2004;127:285-286.

115. Meyns B, Van Garsse L, Boshoff D, et al: The Contegra conduit in the right ventricular outflow tract induces supravalvular stenosis. J Thorac Cardiovasc Surg 2004;128:834-840.

116. Lupinetti FM, Duncan BW, Scifres AM, et al: Intermediate-term results in pediatric aortic valve replacement. Ann Thorac Surg 1999;68:521-525.

117. Zweng TN, Bluett MK, Mosca R, et al: Mitral valve replacement in the first 5 years of life. Ann Thorac Surg 1989;47:720-724.

118. Caldarone CA, Raghuveer G, Hills CB, et al: Long-term survival after mitral valve replacement in children aged <5 years: A multi-institutional study. Circulation 2001;104(12 Suppl 1):I-143-I-147.

119. Gunther T, Mazzitelli D, Schreiber C, et al: Mitral-valve replacement in children under 6 years of age. Eur J Cardiothorac Surg 2000;17:426-430.

120. Kojori AF, Chen R, Caldarone CA, et al: Outcomes of mitral valve replacement in children: A competing-risks analysis. J Thorac Cardiovasc Surg 2004;128:703-709.

121. Alexiou C, Galogavrou M, Chen Q, et al: Mitral valve replacement with mechanical prostheses in children: Improved operative risk and survival. Eur J Cardiothorac Surg 2001;20:105-113.

122. Kiziltan HT, Theodoro DA, Warnes CA, et al: Late results of bioprosthetic tricuspid valve replacement in Ebstein's anomaly. Ann Thorac Surg 1998;66:1539-1545.

123. Lutter G, Ardehali R, Cremer J, Bonhoeffer P: Percutaneous valve replacement: Current state and future prospects. Ann Thorac Surg 2004;78:2199-2206.

124. Cribier A, Eltchaninoff H, Tronc F, et al: Early experience with percutaneous transcatheter implantation of heart valve prosthesis for the treatment of end-stage inoperable patients with calcific aortic stenosis. J Am Coll Cardiol 2004;43:698-703.

125. Oury JH, Maxwell M: An appraisal of the Ross procedure: Goals and technical guidelines. Oper Tech Card Thorac Surg 1997;2:289-301.

126. Redaelli A, Bothorel H, Votta E, et al: 3-D simulation of the St. Jude Medical bileaflet valve opening process: Fluid-structure interaction study and experimental validation. J Heart Valve Dis 2004;13:804-813.

127. Breuer CK, Mettler BA, Anthony T, et al: Application of tissue-engineering principles toward the development of a semilunar heart valve substitute. Tissue Eng 2004;10:1725-1736.

128. Ketchedjian A, Kreuger P, Lukoff H, et al: Ovine panel reactive antibody assay of HLA responsivity to allograft bioengineered vascular scaffolds. J Thorac Cardiovasc Surg 2005;129:159-166.

CHAPTER 45

General Principles of Mechanical Cardiopulmonary Support

Anthony C. Chang
E. Dean McKenzie

The failing myocardium producing low cardiac output syndrome is a common clinical pathophysiologic state in the pediatric cardiac intensive care setting. Although the mainstay of therapy for the failing heart includes conventional catecholamines and new pharmacologic agents such as milrinone,[1,2] there are limitations in this form of therapy, especially in neonates because of age differences in sympathetic neurohumoral activity and adrenergic receptor agonism.[3] With improved technology in cardiopulmonary bypass and mechanical support equipment, results with mechanical cardiopulmonary support in infants, children, and young adults have steadily improved since the 1990s (Tables 45-1 and 45-2).[4-6] Use of mechanical cardiopulmonary support in children remains in its nascent stages, however, and is limited mainly to extracorporeal membrane oxygenation (ECMO).[7-25] Currently, use of pediatric mechanical circulatory support is an essential aspect of state-of-the-art pediatric cardiac intensive care,[26,27] and additional innovative modalities and extended indications for mechanical cardiopulmonary support are being explored.[28]

In children and adults, myocardial failure can be divided into (1) intrinsic failure of the myocardium from general pathophysiologic processes, such as myocardial ischemia, myocarditis/cardiomyopathy, graft rejection after transplantation, or injury from prolonged intraoperative course (prolonged cross-clamp time, insufficient myocardial protection, or coronary ischemia), and (2) extrinsic factors, such as sepsis or metabolic causes (e.g., acidosis or hypoxia). There are important differences, however, between pediatric and adult patients with cardiac failure. Pediatric patients with failing hearts usually have concomitant issues, such as right ventricular failure, pulmonary hypertension, profound hypoxemia, and anatomic variations that would provide daunting challenges to surgical cannulation and support strategy. In addition, mechanical support for pediatric patients with heart disease, particularly patients with congenital heart disease, demands even more forethought and individualization than for pediatric patients needing mechanical support for respiratory disease with normal intracardiac anatomy. See also Chapters 46 to 48.

CARDIAC INTENSIVE CARE BEFORE MECHANICAL SUPPORT: GENERAL PRINCIPLES

The present strategy of mechanical cardiopulmonary support is to use it as a bridge to either myocardial recovery or heart transplantation, although the concept for the failing heart requiring rest to recover is not entirely novel.[29] As with pediatric cardiac intensive care in general, the care of these critically ill patients should be delivered and coordinated by a multidisciplinary team involving a cardiologist; cardiac surgeon; cardiac anesthesiologist; intensivist or neonatologist; support personnel in perfusion, respiratory therapy, pharmacology, and nursing; and other relevant subspecialists, such as pulmonologists, nephrologists, hematologists, neurologists, and infectious disease specialists.

For all patients being considered for mechanical cardiopulmonary support, it is essential to make an accurate diagnosis of the cardiac anatomy and physiology before instituting support. One lesion that occasionally is misdiagnosed is anomalous left coronary artery from the pulmonary artery because these infants often have clinical presentations that mimic myocarditis and are amenable to surgical correction. In addition, total anomalous pulmonary venous connection previously was misdiagnosed often as pulmonary disease before the widespread use of color Doppler. Lastly, venous and aortic arch anatomy need close scrutiny before cannulation (especially the possibilities of an interrupted aortic arch or coarctation because these are difficult diagnoses to exclude in the presence of a patent ductus arteriosus).[30]

Before planned cardiac surgery, it is strategically beneficial to improve any significant preoperative ventricular dysfunction with pharmacologic means before surgery to lessen the likelihood of need for postoperative support. Cardiopulmonary bypass induces myocardial inflammation, which sometimes can lead to subsequent dysfunction, so increased myocardial wall stress (as seen in patients with deteriorating myocardial function) before surgery may decrease the necessary safety margin for successful separation from bypass after surgery. A 3-year-old child with severe mitral regurgitation and a shortening fraction of 22% (when the shortening fraction should be

TABLE 45-1

Extracorporeal Membrane Oxygenation for Children with Heart Disease

Author	Year	No. Patients/Age	Types of Patients	Support Duration Range	Weaned from Support (%)	Survival to Discharge (%)
Kanter et al[7]	1987 (1982-1985)	13/9 days-17.6 yr (mean 3.8 yr)	Postoperative (100%)	12 hr-9 days (mean 3.4 days)	54	46
Rogers et al[10]	1989 (1981-1987)	10/2 days-5 yr (NA)	Postoperative (100%)	15 hr-6 days (mean 3.8 days)	80	70
Weinhaus et al[9]	1989 (1985-1988)	13/2 days-7.4 yr (mean 1.4 yr)	Postoperative (93%)	6 hr-11.2 days (mean 3.8 days)	64	36
Anderson et al[11]	1990 (1971-1989)	16/NA	Postoperative (69%)	NA	NA	25
Klein et al[12]	1990 (1984-1989)	39/1 day-7 yr (mean 13.6 mo)	Postoperative (92%)	6 hr-9 days (mean 4.4 days)	61	58
Meliones et al[17]	1991 (1981-1990)	189/1 day-16.8 yr (median 7 mo)	Postoperative (93%)	NA (mean 4.8 days)	NA	43
Delius et al[14]	1992 (1981-1990)	25/1 day-8 yr (median 7 mo)	Postoperative (80%)	8 hr-15.8 days (mean 6.1 days)	52	40
Raithel et al[15]	1992 (1982-1991)	65/1 day-14 yr (mean 2.4 yr)	Postoperative (100%)	12.5 hr-17.6 days (mean 5.2 days)	68	35
Ziomek et al[16]	1992 (1989-1991)	24/14 hr-6 yr (mean 12.5 mo)	Postoperative (100%)	17 hr-8.3 days (mean 4 days)	75	54
Dalton et al[18]	1993 (1981-1990)	29/2 wk-7 yr (mean 1.4 yr)	Cardiac arrest (59%); postoperative (93%)	15 hr-9.2 days (NA)	62	45
Black et al[121]	1995 (1990-1994)	31/NA (mean 1.2 yr)	Postoperative (81%); myocarditis (19%)	NA (mean 5 days)	45	41
Walters et al[122]	1995 (1984-1994)	73/NA (median 7.2 mo)	Preoperative (10%); failure to wean (26%); postoperative (74%)	NA (mean 4.8 days)	67	58
del Nido[20]	1996 (1981-1994)	68/1 day-18 yr	NA	NA	NA	38
Mehta et al[23]	2000 (1995-1999)	34/1 day-17.5 yr (median 7 mo)	Postoperative (53%)	1 day-58 days (median 6.4 days)	50	35
Aharon et al[24]	2001 (1997-2000)	50/1 day-11 yr (median 40 days)	Postoperative (100%)	1 hr-15 days (mean 4 days)	60	50

NA, not available.

TABLE 45-2

ELSO Registry*

Category	Total	% Survived
Neonate		
Respiratory	19,061	77
Cardiac	2,215	38
Pediatric		
Respiratory	2,762	56
Cardiac	2,936	43
Adult		
Respiratory	972	53
Cardiac	474	33
Total	28,985	66

*Data up to July 2004.
ELSO, Extracorporeal Life Support Organization.

supranormal, or >30%) may benefit from 24 to 48 hours of inotropic support before surgery to decrease the end-diastolic and end-systolic dimensions and wall stress. In addition, certain congenital heart defects, such as anomalous left coronary artery from the pulmonary artery or transposition of the great arteries in an older infant, have an expected higher risk for postoperative ventricular dysfunction, and the awareness for possible use of mechanical support should be heightened.

After cardiac surgery, the decision for mechanical support should be anticipatory; indications include poor hemodynamic profile, metabolic acidosis, oliguria, poor perfusion, and increasing serum lactate level (>0.75 mmol/L/hr)[31] despite escalating inotropic support. Before placing a postoperative patient on support, it is prudent to rule out significant postoperative residua (e.g., residual atrioventricular valve regurgitation/stenosis or left-to-right shunt) or coronary insufficiency as a result of surgical manipulation (e.g., ostial stenosis or compression from conduit). Such an evaluation may require diagnostic and interventional cardiac catheterization. If the patient's condition is extremely unstable and warrants immediate support, it is technically feasible to obtain hemodynamic and angiographic data at a later time while on mechanical support by introducing brief periods of circuit interruptions. The presence of postoperative residua is not a contraindication for support, but rather a situation that warrants surgical or catheter intervention to improve the likelihood of eventual survival. In the absence of interventions for significant postoperative residua, the likelihood of survival even with mechanical cardiopulmonary support is low.[32]

In general, an anticipatory strategy for earlier institution of mechanical support is preferable to a forced resuscitative situation. For a 6-week-old infant with transposition of the great arteries after an arterial switch operation with left ventricular dysfunction and a left atrial pressure of 22 mm Hg, who is on inotropic support consisting of epinephrine at 0.4 μg/kg/min, mechanical support should be discussed before reaching the nadir period of cardiac output at 6 to 12 hours postoperatively.[33] Optimal timing of support implantation is subjective, but crucial to minimize end-organ ischemia and to maximize opportunity for multiorgan recovery. The use of ECMO for postcardiotomy support ranges from 1.5% to 8.3% in the literature, but it can be even less as observed at our institution (currently at <1%). Although entry criteria for postoperative cardiac ECMO support based on serum lactate levels have been proposed,[34] a concern about having such an approach is that it may simplify a very complex decision that should be made on a case-by-case basis. Such criteria can create intellectual limitations that discourage management flexibility, which is vital in perioperative cardiac intensive care.

Overall, the decision for institution of mechanical support should be individualized with consideration for hemodynamic instability (incessant tachycardia and hypotension with concomitant increased ventricular filling pressures), low (<1 mL/kg/hr) urine output, metabolic acidosis, poor perfusion with decreased capillary refill, and high level of inotropic support. As a guide, inotropic support with 0.2 μg/kg/min or more of epinephrine (without evidence for vasodilatory shock, such as seen in sepsis, in which case norepinephrine or vasopressin would be indicated) usually indicates sufficiently severe low cardiac output syndrome and may warrant mechanical support. This proactive approach of early use of mechanical support is particularly important because there may be irreversible damage in the neonatal myocardium at these excessive epinephrine dosages for sustained periods. Before a final decision for mechanical support is made, a thorough echocardiographic examination should be performed to rule out any

reversible mechanical problem (e.g., pericardial tamponade). Acute sternal opening in the intensive care unit is an acceptable strategy as a maneuver to improve oxygenation delivery[35] before mechanical support.

Preparation for mechanical support includes acquisition of packed red blood cells (2 U that are cytomegalovirus-negative irradiated and leukocyte reduced in case the patient becomes a transplantation candidate) and fresh frozen plasma. Baseline hematologic studies, such as complete blood cell count, prothrombin time and partial thromboplastin time, platelet count, activated clotting time, plasma hemoglobin, antithrombin III, fibrinogen, and thromboelastogram, also should be obtained. Lastly, arterial and venous lines and the endotracheal tube should be secured and be accessible during the cannulation process.

INDICATIONS AND CONTRAINDICATIONS FOR MECHANICAL SUPPORT

Appropriate patient selection and stabilization for mechanical support are paramount to maximize survival and outcome. The indications for mechanical cardiopulmonary support in children are discussed in this section.

Myocardial Dysfunction—Bridge to Recovery

Mechanical support in children with potentially reversible myocardial dysfunction, including postcardiotomy myocardial dysfunction (especially after surgery for lesions such as anomalous left coronary artery from the pulmonary artery[36,37] or for transposition of the great arteries and left ventricular dysfunction[38]), acute myocarditis, and other causes such as exacerbation in cardiomyopathy or acute post-transplantation rejection,[39] entails a clinical strategy to create a bridge to eventual myocardial recovery. Perioperative patients with postcardiotomy syndrome can be divided further into patients who fail to separate from cardiopulmonary bypass ("early" postcardiotomy cardiac failure) and patients who require mechanical support in the ensuing postoperative period (hours or days) as a result of myocardial dysfunction and low cardiac output syndrome ("late" postcardiotomy cardiac failure). Experiences in these patients show that there is a higher likelihood of survival if cannulation occurs after an initial period of stability versus immediately after cardiopulmonary bypass (except for children with anomalous left coronary artery from the pulmonary artery).

Children with acute fulminant myocarditis often die as a result of low cardiac output syndrome despite escalating inotropic support and can benefit greatly from mechanical support with eventual myocardial recovery.[40,41] In adult patients with fulminant myocarditis, aggressive hemodynamic support with assist technology has yielded excellent long-term survival.[42] Mechanical support probably is underused in children with this diagnosis; a child should not die of myocarditis without an attempt for myocardial recovery on mechanical support because survival in these patients is excellent.[43] In the absence of a severity of illness score for myocarditis, escalating inotropic support (particularly use of epinephrine) associated with relentless metabolic acidosis and elevated serum lactate should provide a clinical guideline for institution of mechanical support. Children with myocarditis on mechanical support usually require a relatively longer duration of support (>72 hours) compared with children with myocardial dysfunction after cardiac surgery.

Myocardial Dysfunction—Bridge to Transplantation

Children who are critically ill with primary myocardial failure secondary to dilated cardiomyopathy, end-stage congenital heart disease, or prolonged graft rejection after heart transplantation should be considered for mechanical cardiopulmonary support as a bridge to transplantation.[44,45] Although these children are less likely to recover myocardial function compared with patients in the previous category, there is nevertheless a continuum of recovery and reversibility of myocardial dysfunction. In addition, although ECMO has been the mainstay of therapy for this group of patients with survival of about 50%,[46-48] there is a growing need for more longer term (>2 weeks) mechanical support alternatives for these patients[49-51] because complications can develop during ECMO that would preclude transplantation before a donor heart is available.[52] Although extracorporeal life support can be used as a bridge to pediatric cardiac transplantation for at least 2 weeks with acceptable survival,[53] mortality while waiting for heart transplantation in patients on inotropic support, especially infants, is greater than 50% at 6 months.[54]

Cardiopulmonary Resuscitation

The use of mechanical support as a rescue device after failed conventional resuscitation initially was described by del Nido and colleagues[55] in pediatric cardiac patients and has been described in adults with acceptable results.[56,57] The capability for rapid deployment of a mechanical support system is essential for any cardiac intensive care unit and demands an organized team effort. It is essential for such a maneuver to be instituted within 20 minutes, and a crystalloid primed circuit is essential as the initial setup to obviate the need for blood products. The current survival results for such rescue therapy are 50% or greater as long as resuscitation is effective, and cannulation is performed in a timely manner.[58-60]

Preoperative Stabilization

Cardiopulmonary support can be applied in theory to any neonate who presents with profound hypoxemia or cardiovascular collapse or both before intervention is possible.[61] Clinical situations that demand such support in preoperative patients include patients with hypercyanotic spells[62]; pulmonary hypertensive crises[63]; or certain diagnoses, such as total anomalous pulmonary venous connection,[64,65] common pulmonary vein atresia,[66] or tetralogy of Fallot with absent pulmonary valve.[67] Timely surgical or catheter palliation or repair for these lesions remains an essential part of management, however.

Acute Respiratory Distress Syndrome

Parenchymal lung disease is the most common indication in neonates for use of ECMO, but good results have been observed with non-neonatal respiratory failure as well.[68] A patient with congenital heart disease could develop parenchymal lung disease before or after cardiac surgery and fail conventional therapy, such as high-frequency ventilation, surfactant administration, or inhaled nitric oxide. The highest risk patients include children with respiratory syncytial virus[69,70] or bronchopulmonary dysplasia[71] and unusual associated respiratory diseases, such as plastic bronchitis.[72] Duration of necessary support may be weeks rather than days because patients with lung parenchymal disease tend to recover over a longer period. Venovenous ECMO also has been used for respiratory disease in children with cardiac diagnoses, including a neonate after a Norwood operation.[73]

Severe Pulmonary Hypertension

In a few select patients, pulmonary hypertension with hemodynamic instability that is unresponsive to inhaled nitric oxide therapy or other therapy can benefit from mechanical support, especially in the postoperative period, during which pulmonary vascular resistance (PVR) may be transiently elevated.[74] Mechanical support is controversial, however, for any patient with irreversible pulmonary hypertension. For postoperative patients with pulmonary hypertension who are selected for mechanical support, any anatomic postoperative residua (e.g., residual shunt or pulmonary venous obstruction) must be ruled out by noninvasive imaging or cardiac catheterization while the patient is on mechanical support. The advent of inhaled nitric oxide has reduced the need for mechanical support for this indication.[75-77] Elevated right atrial pressure in a Fontan patient, indicating elevated PVR, also has been treated with ECMO.[78] Although mechanical support provides stability of hemodynamic profile and minimizes PVR (as a result of less aggressive mechanical ventilation), its use potentially can recreate the inflammatory milieu that leads to pulmonary vasoreactivity.

Malignant Dysrhythmias

Malignant dysrhythmias as an indication for mechanical support is a relatively infrequent clinical scenario. In a select few patients who failed conventional aggressive medical therapy for incessant tachydysrhythmias, a short trial on mechanical support may be warranted to avoid further deterioration secondary to potentially myocardial depressant effects of medical treatment, especially β blockade.

Patients who have benefited from mechanical support include patients with lethal arrhythmias associated with myocardial disease,[79] supraventricular tachycardia,[80] or junctional ectopic tachycardia or ventricular tachycardia after cardiac surgery.[81-83] It is imperative, however, that the presence of lethal tachydysrhythmias should promulgate the caretaker to seek etiologic factors, such as postoperative residua or coronary ischemia or both. The use of ECMO also has been reported for malignant ventricular tachydysrhythmias[84] and quinidine toxicity with refractory bradydysrhythmias and profound hypotension.[85]

Profound Cyanosis

In patients with severe cyanosis, the inherent anatomic or physiologic etiology for cyanosis needs to be diagnosed and palliated or corrected; the use of mechanical support for this reason should be decided on a case-by-case basis. An infant who is profoundly cyanotic after a bidirectional cavopulmonary anastomosis without an anatomic cause may benefit from inhaled nitric oxide and sternal opening; if these maneuvers fail, however, mechanical support could be justified to stabilize and resuscitate a patient, while diagnostic and possibly interventional catheterization is performed to delineate the etiologic factors for cyanosis.

Proactive Support

Proactive support is controversial, but may be valid in certain extremely high-risk clinical situations. High-risk interventional catheterizations, such as balloon valvotomy in a critically ill neonate with aortic stenosis, may warrant support on ECMO.[86,87] Certain electrophysiologic procedures also may be performed while on ECMO support to minimize end-organ ischemia in the event of a cardiac arrest.[88] Lastly, use of mechanical support in a proactive fashion for children after the Norwood palliative repair has been discussed.[89]

Miscellaneous Indications

There are numerous reported uses for ECMO for cardiopulmonary support for indications not listed here. Tracheal reconstruction[90] and heart/lung or lung transplantation[91] are examples of clinical situations that benefit from mechanical cardiopulmonary support during the perioperative period. Transport of a critically ill patient on ECMO also has been performed for certain situations.[92] Cardiac dysfunction from myocardial infarction,[93] tricyclic antidepressant overdose,[94] and even trauma or hypothermia are possible indications and require the caregiver to be flexible with its use. In addition, coexisting congenital diaphragmatic hernia and congenital heart disease has an acceptable survival after repair and support on ECMO.[95] Lastly, sepsis and meningococcal infection with cardiac dysfunction and intractable shock were reported to have a 67% survival.[96]

Near-absolute contraindications for support include very low weight (<1.5 kg), preexisting severe neurologic or intra-abdominal bleeding, Eisenmenger syndrome, and advanced multisystem organ failure or multiple congenital anomalies and/or chromosomal aberrations. Other conditions can be elusive contraindications. Results of mechanical support in the presence of pulmonary hemorrhage have been acceptable.[97] Sepsis is no longer an absolute contraindication to mechanical support, and survival has been good even with meningococcal disease.[98] Although single-ventricle patients have had a significantly lower survival after mechanical support, there is no reason to preclude any child with a single ventricle from support solely based on this anatomic diagnosis category because survival results have been acceptable.[99] If an anatomic diagnosis is deemed to be inoperable, mechanical support can be used only as a bridge to heart or heart/lung transplantation. Finally, ethical discussions should accompany the use of these support devices because some parents, laypeople, and physicians consider these therapies as heroic measures in select situations and patients and would not advocate this therapy.[100]

MECHANICAL DEVICE SELECTION

Present device selection for short-term support is a relatively limited choice between ECMO in its various technologic forms or centrifugal ventricular assist device (VAD) (Figs. 45-1 and 45-2 and Table 45-3). Longer term support options are virtually nonexistent for pediatric patients, especially for neonates and infants. Advantages of ECMO include its relative ease of implantation, rapid potential for stabilization, peripheral cannulation, capability for biventricular support, accommodation of neonatal size limitations, effective oxygenation, and large international neonatal and pediatric experience (see Table 45-3). Disadvantages are its requirement for blood prime, extensive anticoagulation, carotid artery ligation, nonpulsatile flow, decreased pulmonary blood flow, occasional inadequate left atrial decompression, relatively complex circuit that requires higher level of expertise, lack of durability, bleeding tendencies in postoperative patients, and relatively high incidences of neurologic complications.

Advantages of the VAD include its relative ease of use compared with ECMO, ease of implantation, fast setup time, low priming volume, and low-level anticoagulation because it usually does not have an oxygenator or a heat exchanger. There also is purported evidence that myocardial recovery may be superior to ECMO (although this is controversial if the left atrium is decompressed in ECMO support). Disadvantages include its shorter duration of usage and occasional thrombus formation in the circuit and its nonpulsatile flow nature. In addition, the right ventricle needs to be adequate in its function because it supplies preload to the left ventricle supported

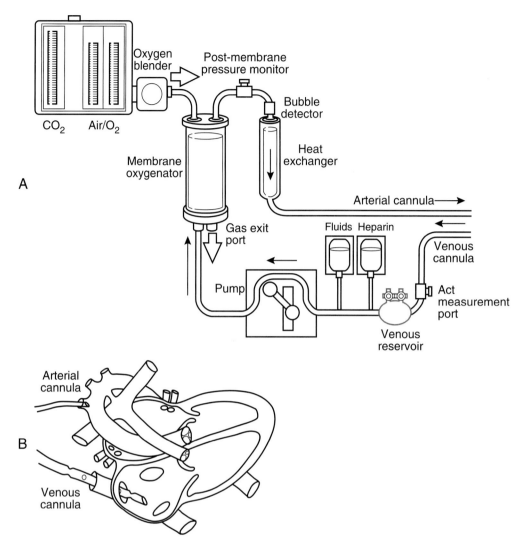

FIGURE 45-1 ■ Venoarterial extracorporeal membrane oxygenation (ECMO) circuit and cannulation for venoarterial ECMO. A, The setup for venoarterial ECMO via neck cannulation. This modality of support uses a roller pump system with a servo-regulatory mechanism for controlling circuit flow. The blood is drained into a compliant bladder and goes through the circuit above at rates of 100 to 150 $cm^3/kg/min$ in neonates and 75 to 100 $cm^3/kg/min$ in older infants. The servo-regulating bladder turns off the pump if venous return is inadequate. The ECMO circuit consists of the pump that pushes blood to a membrane or hollow fiber oxygenator followed by a heat exchanger. The blood gases can be adjusted by altering the sweep rate and composition of the gases passing across the membrane. The oxygenated blood is returned to the patient via the arterial cannula. A hemofilter may be attached via a circuit parallel to the oxygenator. **B,** Close-up view of the cannulation via the neck vessels for support with venoarterial ECMO. Cannulation can be peripheral via the right internal jugular vein and the common carotid artery, but also can be trans-sternal via the right atrial appendage and the aorta in the postcardiotomy cardiac surgical patient (although mediastinal bleeding and infection are potential complications). Patients with venous anomalies and patients who had a cavopulmonary anastomosis warrant special considerations for venous cannulation strategies. (**A** from Walker LK: *Myocardial assist devices.* In Nichols DG, Cameron DE, Greeley WJ, et al [eds]: *Critical Heart Disease in Infants and Children.* Philadelphia, Mosby, 1995, p 534; **B** from del Nido PJ: *Extracorporeal membrane oxygenation for cardiac support in children. Ann Thorac Surg* 1996;61:336-339.)

by the VAD. There is also a size limitation if biventricular support is needed.

At present, ECMO remains the mainstay support device in all neonates, unless there is isolated right or left ventricular dysfunction. In addition, pediatric support for biventricular dysfunction or hypoxemia is limited to ECMO because VADs for both ventricles are difficult to use because of size limitations in smaller patients. In the future, the decision for specific devices will become more complex as factors such as anticipated duration of support, patient size and age, necessity for biventricular support, and acceptable device complications all will enter into the decision-making process.

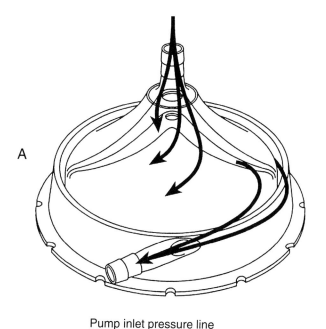

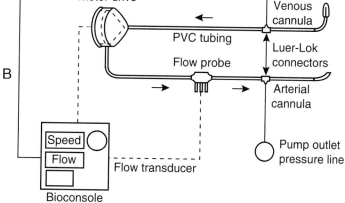

FIGURE 45-2 ■ **BioMedicus centrifugal pump and setup. A** and **B,** The blood enters the cones via the apex of the cone, and the kinetic energy of the spinning cones is transferred to the blood leaving the side-port. With this ventricular assist device, an extracorporeal centrifugal pump with acrylic rotator cones produces a vortex continuous flow, which creates a negative pressure that enables blood to move. The pump is magnetically coupled to a driver that controls the revolutions per minute (rpm). The BP-80 and BP-50 models have volumes of 80 mL and 50 mL, with the former capable of a maximal flow of 10 L/min. Heparin-bonded tubing can be used to minimize the need for aggressive anticoagulation. A flow probe is necessary with the centrifugal pump because the pump is afterload dependent and rpm in and of itself may not correlate accurately with flow. Mean arterial pressure is maintained by varying intravascular volume and rpm on the ventricular assist device console. An oxygenator also can be placed in cases of coexisting pulmonary failure. Cannulation is performed via the left atrium and aorta (left ventricular assist) or right atrium and pulmonary artery (right ventricular assist). (From Karl TR, Horton SB: *Centrifugal pump ventricular assist device in pediatric cardiac surgery.* In Duncan BW [ed]: *Mechanical Support for Cardiac and Respiratory Failure in Pediatric Patients.* New York, Marcel Dekker, 2001, pp 24, 25.)

CARDIAC INTENSIVE CARE DURING SUPPORT: GENERAL PRINCIPLES

Extracorporeal Membrane Oxygenation

It is imperative that the team understands not only the pathophysiology of the failing myocardium, but also the circulatory physiology of mechanical support.[101]

In addition, there are many more confounding issues with specifically cardiac patients that would be relevant during mechanical support (e.g., presence of atrial and ventricular septal defects, patent ductus arteriosus).

The heart during support has decreased work, oxygen consumption, and wall stress (if appropriately decompressed). The alterations in preload and afterload

TABLE 45-3

Extracorporeal Membrane Oxygenation (ECMO) Versus Centrifugal Ventricular Assist Device (VAD) for Children with Heart Disease		
	ECMO	Centrifugal VAD
Pediatric experience	Large (>4000 since 1989)	Growing (NA)
Ease of use	No	Yes
Membrane oxygenator	Yes	Possible
Peripheral cannulation	Yes	No
Ventricular cannulation	No	No
Anticoagulation	Yes	Yes (but less than ECMO)
Univentricular support	Yes	Yes
Biventricular support	Yes	Possible (but difficult in infants)
Need for left atrial decompression	Occasional	No
Duration of support	Days to weeks	Days to weeks
Patient mobility	No	No
Cost	High	Low
Complications	Moderate	Low

NA, not available.

on initiation of support and clinical significance of nonpulsatile flow are important concepts for the intensive care clinician. Central venous pressure usually is lowered as a result of adequate venous drainage and should be maintained low to minimize sequelae from elevated central venous pressure, such as pleural effusions, ascites, and deleterious effects on the cerebral, gastrointestinal, hepatic, and renal blood flows. Left atrial pressure (which can be estimated noninvasively by echocardiographic examinations of the position of the atrial septum) should be monitored carefully; inadequate unloading of the left atrium and ventricle with resultant distention can lead to mitral regurgitation and pulmonary edema and hemorrhage and minimize the likelihood of myocardial recovery. One strategy to decrease the left atrial pressure is to increase the ECMO flow to 150 cc/kg/min. If the left atrium continues to be distended, however, this may necessitate mechanical decompression via either surgical left atrial venting (with an additional cannula and a Y connector to the venous tubing of the ECMO circuit)[102] or balloon/blade atrial septostomy/septectomy with transseptal puncture.[103-105] The presence of aortopulmonary collaterals or patent ductus arteriosus and insufficiency of the aortic valve (occasionally as a result of flow of the arterial cannula directed at the aortic valve) can create a persistently elevated left atrial pressure. If an adequate atrial septal defect is present, as in some patients with congenital heart disease, no intervention should be necessary to decompress the left atrium.

Systolic hypertension and increased systemic vascular resistance[106] associated with ECMO are believed to be related to high plasma renin activity or due to higher ECMO flows and should be treated aggressively with vasodilators, such as nitroprusside, nitroglycerin, phenoxybenzamine, or milrinone. Adequate afterload

reduction decreases the likelihood of elevated left ventricular wall stress,[107,108] surgical bleeding, or intracranial hemorrhage.[109] Mean pressure should be maintained at what is appropriate for body weight (approximately 30 to 40 mm Hg in neonates and approximately 50 to 75 mm Hg in older children depending on size). Other etiologic factors for elevated systemic resistance include hypothermia, seizures, pain, and acidosis. Occasionally, intermittent doses of intravenous hydralazine may be necessary for more rapid treatment of elevated systolic blood pressure, although this therapy does not improve cardiac performance.[110]

Ideally, ventricular ejection manifested by arterial pulsations should be observed from the arterial line because this may be an indication of ventricular recovery. **Myocardial stun** can be observed in 5% of neonates on ECMO, even in infants without prior myocardial injury, and can be manifested by a lack of adequate arterial pulsations.[111] This stun phenomenon, which can manifest itself by even electromechanical dissociation, usually occurs within the first 6 hours after initiation of flow and can last 64 hours.[112] One theory for this lack of myocardial function is that it is due to the inability of the heart to eject antegrade against an excessively augmented afterload. Maneuvers to reduce afterload (either reduction in ECMO flow or institution of pharmacologic afterload reduction) and inotropic support potentially can improve this situation. In addition, coronary blood flow usually is perfused with blood ejected from the left ventricle except during very high bypass flows (>80% flow) or when the aortic valve is rendered incompetent.[113]

The myocardium on mechanical support should be in a more favorable milieu with decreased oxygen consumption (less tachycardia and wall stress if the ventricle is adequately unloaded) and increased myocardial perfusion (with augmentation of the coronary diastolic pressure and concomitant diminution of the end-diastolic filling pressure). Low-dose inotropic support can be used to maintain baseline inotropy and renal perfusion. Continuous monitoring of mixed venous saturation is used to maintain vigilance of overall cardiac output. In addition, elevated serum lactate levels and altered acid-base status should normalize after initiation of support to show adequate oxygen delivery. Overall, the right and left ventricular outputs decrease proportionally to the amount of bypass flow provided.[114]

Basic troubleshooting for patients on ECMO involves monitoring and interpretation of right and left atrial pressures and the mean arterial pressure. If the arterial pressure is low and the filling pressures are also low, one should consider (1) hypovolemia, and administer volume; (2) excessive bleeding (including occult bleeding), and correct coagulopathy; (3) vasodilation, and decrease vasodilators/initiate vasopressors; (4) excessive runoff into pulmonary circulation (shunts or collaterals, such as a large patent ductus arteriosus), and discuss with the cardiovascular surgeon the possibility of obliterating such a runoff; and (5) unfavorable venous cannula positions, and correct as needed with the surgical team. If the arterial pressure is low, but the filling pressures are elevated, one should consider (1) inadequate venous drainage from cannulae, and adjust as necessary; (2) tamponade, and perform echocardiography and consider an effort to re-explore the mediastinum[115]; (3) left atrial distention (see earlier); and (4) other issues, such as tension pneumothorax or hemothorax.[116] Patients with arrhythmias need special consideration while on mechanical support. If there are readily reversible issues, such as lowered mean perfusion pressure or metabolic derangements leading to arrhythmias, it is preferable to reverse these conditions (rather than performing cardiopulmonary resuscitation or countershock). Any resuscitation has potential deleterious sequelae, and chest compressions are contraindicated because this maneuver can easily dislodge the cannulae or injure the myocardium.

Although mechanical support gives a temporary reprieve from the constant threat of cardiac arrest, it remains a good strategy to continue to pursue aggressively any postoperative residua that may be amenable to interventional catheterization. Although transthoracic echocardiography can be limited because of suboptimal acoustic windows, it can be useful in delineating cannula position, intracardiac thrombi, or certain intracardiac anatomic residua.[117] Even transesophageal echocardiography can have inherent limitations for accurate diagnosis given that the loading conditions while on mechanical support make it less likely that residual defects can be assessed hemodynamically with Doppler studies.

Cardiac catheterizations can be performed safely while on extracorporeal membrane oxygenation and can aid in the diagnosis of potential residual lesions and in interventional therapy (balloon dilations, stent implantations, and coil placements).[118-120] Not correcting postoperative residua in patients on mechanical support contributes to poor survival.[121,122] Leaving a large interventricular communication after a corrective surgery reduces the effectiveness of ECMO because right atrial drainage is usually inadequate to decompress the left atrium. In addition, a patent ductus arteriosus may need to be closed because it can create a large amount of runoff.[123] Transport of these critically ill patients to the catheterization laboratory requires meticulous care during the entire process; potential complications can be avoided with support equipment that is attached directly to the bed (which may reduce the risk of dislodging cannulae).

In patients with **single ventricle** and shunts, the management of the shunt during the period of support (open, partially ligated, or totally ligated) is controversial, including the option of support without an oxygenator and relying on the aortopulmonary shunt as the sole source of pulmonary blood flow.[124,125] One report indicated a higher survival in 10 patients if the shunt remained open.[126] If the shunt is left totally open, adequate alveolar ventilation should be made sufficient to prevent pulmonary interstitial edema from excessive pulmonary blood. In addition, flow from the ECMO circuit may need to be increased to maintain pulmonary blood flow and adequate systemic perfusion. In certain patients with particularly low PVR, such as low-birth-weight neonates, leaving the shunt open may not be a feasible option because the pulmonary blood flow may be excessive. In addition, there is evidence that there are deleterious effects on cerebral oxygenation and hemodynamics when there is an aortopulmonary communication, such as the ductus arteriosus.[127] Totally occluding the shunt may lead to extensive pulmonary ischemia and infarction because bronchial flow alone may not be adequate to supply the pulmonary parenchyma. ECMO support for single-ventricle patients requires even more forethought and flexibility than for biventricular patients, but the general philosophical construct of single-ventricle physiology still applies (pulmonary blood flow and systemic blood flow balance as much as possible).[128]

In patients with single ventricle and bidirectional cavopulmonary anastomosis, this clinical scenario is particularly challenging. Cannulation would need to be in the superior vena cava and the right atrium because jugular venous cannulation alone may not supply sufficient venous return, and right atrial cannulation alone may not decompress the cerebral venous system adequately; cannulation of the common iliac vein may be needed. In Fontan patients, similar considerations may be needed to ensure adequate venous drainage.[129]

Progressive multisystem dysfunction on mechanical support is associated with decreased survival, and meticulous care and continual vigilance must be part of the care for these patients. For the respiratory system, the optimal ventilator management strategy during extracorporeal support is controversial. Animal studies show that pulmonary sequelae from prolonged venoarterial bypass are significant and include pulmonary edema with parenchymal necrosis and intra-alveolar hemorrhage.[130] Ventilatory support may be necessary to minimize atelectasis and to maximize oxygenation of blood returning to the left atrium (with the theoretical advantage that the coronary blood flow from the left ventricle can have the highest oxygen tension possible),[131] although the myocardium has relatively low oxygen consumption while on support and is an extremely efficient organ in extracting oxygen.

One ventilatory support approach is to maintain (1) 10 to 12 mL/kg of tidal volume and 5 to 10 cm H_2O of end-expiratory pressure (higher levels of PEEP may be efficacious in cases of mediastinal bleeding or excessive pulmonary blood flow); (2) relatively low rates of intermittent mechanical ventilation (10 to 15 per minute); and (3) inspired oxygen of 0.60 or less to minimize atelectasis, while not incurring barotrauma or oxygen toxicity. Adequate alveolar ventilation is even more essential in patients with single-ventricle physiology with an open aortopulmonary shunt (Blalock-Taussig shunt or patent ductus arteriosus). Another consideration is possible use of surfactant for lungs with unfavorable parenchymal changes because relative ischemia to the lungs during mechanical support can result in endothelial dysfunction and surfactant deficiency (similar to that observed with cardiopulmonary bypass).[132] Surfactant therapy may decrease pulmonary dysfunction and duration of ECMO.[133] Excessive fluid overload, evidenced by interstitial edema on chest radiograph, also can be addressed by use of hemofiltration via the extracorporeal circuits to remove excessive fluid and to improve gas exchange.[134]

There are occasional issues regarding gas exchange during support. Hypoxemia can result from malfunction of the membrane oxygenator (which routinely should be changed every 7 to 10 days), but a rare cause for low oxygen tension also can be pulmonary embolism.[135] If there is no malfunction of the oxygenator, the ECMO flow can be increased or the membrane size can be increased to improve oxygen tension. In situations of excessive carbon dioxide, the sweep gas flow rate can be increased to remove carbon dioxide. If the carbon dioxide is low, carbon dioxide can be added to the sweep gas (carbogen, which is a combination of 5% carbon dioxide and 95% oxygen, is used).

After successful resuscitation and cannulation for support, the neurologic system needs to be assessed, but this is limited because of neuromuscular blockade and narcotic analgesia. Fentanyl can be administered at a dose of 3 to 10 μg/kg/hr to maintain adequate analgesia, and benzodiazepines (e.g., midazolam or lorezepam) can be given intermittently or as a continuous infusion as adjunctive therapy. Chemical paralysis can be maintained with cisatracurium (0.2 to 0.4 mg/kg/hr) because it is

eliminated via Hoffman degradation and is less subject to accumulation in the face of renal and hepatic dysfunction.

Neurologic complications remain a major source of morbidity with neonates and children on mechanical support. Daily head ultrasound examinations should be performed, especially in the first few days because this is the highest risk period,[136] and cerebral blood flow velocities are found to be lower in neonates who had an intracranial hemorrhage while on ECMO.[137] Cerebrovascular accidents and hemorrhages can occur during any resuscitation and during the support period, so other investigative procedures, such as CT, may be necessary when feasible. In one study, serial head ultrasound combined with electroencephalography increased the predictive value of normal post-ECMO neuroimaging studies.[138] Seizures while on support also are common (manifested occasionally with tachycardia, elevated blood pressure, and pupillary changes), but often go undetected, and a study showed that intermittent-discontinuous electroencephalograms did not indicate poor prognosis if normalization of electroencephalogram occurred within 7 days.[139] Other useful indicators for early neuronal injury include measurements of serum neuron-specific enolase, S-100 protein,[140] or brain-type creatinine kinase.[141] There also may be benefit in maintaining children at cooler temperatures after cardiopulmonary arrest for higher likelihood of neurologic recovery.[142] An unfavorable imaging result can be useful to dictate timing of decannulation or to determine feasibility as a transplantation candidate. Longer term neurologic complications include acquired hydrocephalus associated with superior vena cava syndrome.[143]

Optimal renal perfusion during mechanical support is vital because **renal failure** with an elevated creatinine is a poor prognostic factor in the overall survival of pediatric patients on mechanical support. Low-dose dopamine and new drugs such as the dopamine-agonist fenoldopam[144] may have a role in the maintenance of renal perfusion while patients are on mechanical support with nonpulsatile flow. Peritoneal dialysis also can be used as a strategy to remove fluid in appropriate patients and may be beneficial for minimizing capillary leak syndrome by removing unwanted inflammatory mediators.[145]

There are reports of significant complications of the gastrointestinal system with patients on mechanical support, so nutrition probably should be parenteral rather than enteral, especially in the immediate postcannulation period.[146] Because some cardiac diagnoses (e.g., hypoplastic left heart syndrome and truncus arteriosus) are at higher risks for necrotizing enterocolitis, enteral feeding may need to be avoided in these patients, especially in the presence of low cardiac output. There is evidence for gastric tonometry pH as a predictor of survival in children on ECMO.[147] In addition, hepatic function should be monitored closely.

The hematologic system is a vital part of mechanical support management; an appropriate level of anticoagulation needs to be maintained, and hematologic abnormalities have correlations with morbidity. This is a particularly challenging aspect in the early postoperative period. Hematocrit is maintained about 40% to 50% for most cardiac patients with leukocyte-reduced cytomegalovirus-negative and irradiated packed red blood cells. The mainstay of anticoagulation therapy has been continuous intravenous infusion of heparin sodium (10 to 50 U/kg/hr) to maintain whole blood activated clotting time of 180 to 220 seconds, but more recent modification of circuits to include heparin-bonded tubing and silicone membrane oxygenator have decreased the need for aggressive anticoagulation. Vigilance is needed for device-related or mediastinal bleeding and bleeding in the central nervous system. There is an increased risk of hemorrhage and intracranial bleeding associated with low platelet counts, so appropriate platelet transfusion (given postmembrane with a 50% increase in heparin infusion during the transfusion to avoid thrombosis) to maintain a count greater than 100,000/μL is important to minimize bleeding complications.[148,149] In addition, routine echocardiography should be performed to survey for intracavitary thrombi (especially prevalent in patients on mechanical support with preexisting prosthetic valves) or pericardial fluid and blood collections.

In the presence of persistent significant **bleeding** (>10 mL/kg/hr), other blood products, including cryoprecipitate, fresh frozen plasma, aminocaproic acid (Amicar) at 30 mg/kg/hr for 72 hours (with a loading dose of 100 mg/kg over 5 to 10 minutes), and the kinin-inhibitor aprotinin at an infusion dose of 10,000 IU/kg/hr for 6 hours after a bolus of 30,000 IU/kg,[150,151] can be administered. Serum fibrinogen usually is maintained at greater than 100 mg/dL. Thromboelastography[152] has been useful in the more precise delineation of the bleeding and product profile. Normal maintenance issues during the support period involve clearing the mediastinum and surveillance of tubing for thrombi. In addition, hemolysis is monitored by plasma-free hemoglobin (should be <60 mg/dL). If plasma-free hemoglobin increases, and there is change in pressure gradient across the oxygenator, one should suspect thrombus formation and consider changing the pump head or even the circuit. A difference between ECMO and VAD is that the patients on VADs can have activated clotting times lower than patients on conventional ECMO (approximately 140 to 180 seconds).

An important complication during mechanical support is **infection**, such as sepsis or mediastinitis, which is especially prevalent in children on ECMO after the initial week of support; an open chest was shown to be an added risk factor.[153] Routine administration of antibiotics includes vancomycin, ceftazidime, and nystatin for *Candida* coverage. The risk for life-threatening infection in these patients is compounded by the usual intensive care unit–related infections of ventilated patients with central lines and prolonged usage of parenteral nutrition and antibiotics and is increased further by support device–related access, such as the mediastinum and cannulae, not to mention possible immunosuppression from prolonged ECMO support. Antibiotic coverage should be broadened appropriately, especially if transsternal cannulation was necessary, but dosages of antibiotics should be adjusted carefully for mechanical support to minimize toxicities.

Fluid and electrolyte issues include electrolyte disturbances, such as hypercalcemia/hypocalcemia[154,155] or hyperkalemia.[156] Diuresis can be encouraged with intermittent or continuous furosemide infusion. In addition, continuous hemofiltration via a circuit parallel to the oxygenator[157] can be used to maintain optimal fluid balance because these patients usually have capillary leak and fluid retention secondary to elevated levels of inflammatory mediators, but may be limited by flow rates.[158,159] Fluid administration in the form of albumin or lipids should be performed postmembrane to avoid thrombosis.

The use of drugs should be monitored carefully because pharmacokinetic profiles of various drugs are likely to be altered dramatically during mechanical support secondary to increased distribution volumes, drug absorption by circuit materials, impaired drug elimination, decreased renal clearance, and altered cerebral perfusion and blood-brain barrier function. Significant uptakes of drugs with losses of 40% to 98% have been noted with commonly used sedative drugs such as midazolam and diazepam.[160] Although occasionally pediatric patients are on mechanical support as a consequence of rejection after heart transplantation, there is virtually no information on the pharmacokinetic profiles of immunosuppressive agents in children on mechanical support.

Ventricular Assist Devices

Most of the aforementioned principles that pertain to ECMO apply to VADs with a few key differences. Although children with myocarditis, acute rejection, and end-stage congenital heart disease have some degree of biventricular dysfunction, left ventricular unloading with the VAD with concomitant physiologic assist of the right ventricle generally has made the use of biventricular VAD unnecessary. For left VADs, it is essential to appreciate its major inherent difference from ECMO: Cardiac output that is generated from the assist device depends entirely on right ventricular output; the right ventricular output is the preload to the left VAD. Inadequate filling of the left ventricular VAD can result from low intravascular volume, tamponade, improper cannula positioning, right ventricular dysfunction, elevated PVR, or dysrhythmias. Monitoring of central venous pressure is even more critical compared with ECMO, and frequent echocardiographic assessment of right ventricular function and estimation of right ventricular pressure are mandatory. An elevated central venous pressure indicates right ventricular dysfunction or elevated PVR or both, and these issues need to be treated in a timely fashion.

As in the management of patients on ECMO, overall management of the VAD is dictated by monitoring the filling and the systemic blood pressures. Low systemic blood pressures with a low left atrial pressure indicate hypovolemia/bleeding, sepsis, or right ventricular failure and should be treated with volume resuscitation or appropriate inotropic agents. A low inlet pressure may be secondary to collapse of the atrial wall around the cannula and can be managed by decreasing the revolutions per minute temporarily to allow the tissue to be freed from the cannula. Low systemic blood pressure with a high left atrial pressure may indicate tamponade or cannula malposition, and both of these possible situations can be checked by noninvasive imaging.

High systemic blood pressure with an elevated left atrial pressure can indicate fluid overload and should be treated with diuresis and afterload reduction. High systemic blood pressure with a low left atrial pressure requires special understanding. A constrained vortex system such as those of the centrifugal pumps used for VADs potentially increases sensitivity to peripheral vascular resistance. A low inlet pressure with a high outlet pressure could be due to change in cannula position, thrombus, or flow being too high for the cannula. All of the aforementioned situations also could lead to increased hemolysis.

The presence of an atrial septal defect should be evaluated before placement of the VAD to avoid the clinical situation of cyanosis (if left atrial pressure falls below the right atrial pressure). Other troubleshooting issues for the VAD involve (1) air in the system, which needs immediate attention (patient can be placed in the Trendelenburg position) and revision of the system if necessary, and (2) thrombus in the pump head, which requires more aggressive anticoagulation and possible exchange for a new component.

CONSIDERATIONS DURING THE WEANING PROCESS

Before the actual weaning process, cardiac and pulmonary support should be escalated to accommodate the weaning process to maintain adequate perfusion and oxygenation, normocarbia, and normal acid-base status. Parameters need to be established on a case-by-case basis because patients with congenital heart disease differ considerably in anatomy and physiology and oxygenation saturation and delivery.

During the usual weaning process over a 6- to 24-hour period, flow is slowly reduced in 5% to 10% decrements to 25% flow with unclamping of the bridge between the arterial and venous systems; anticoagulation strategy may need to be modified during this period, and ECMO flow probably should not be reduced to less than 100 to 200 cc/min to avoid thrombosis. If the bridge is used, cannulae should be flushed frequently (every 4 hours or so) to maintain patency. A trial period of 2 to 4 hours

off support can be used to ensure a higher likelihood of a successful decannulation. Some surgeons may prefer a shorter weaning period because any significant decrease in flow, particularly in infants, may be conducive to oxygenator failure. If the patient tolerates the weaning process, the arterial and venous cannulae are clamped.

Although it is useful to incorporate use of echocardiography[161] and even newer noninvasive methodology with ultrasound[162] to assess myocardial function, interpretation of such studies must take into account the general observation of decreased circumferential shortening and myocardial performance in the face of decreased preload and increased afterload with patients on mechanical support. Occasionally a patient fails to meet criteria for decannulation, yet survives after removal of support. One reason may be due to the relative large size of the venous cannula impeding sufficient venous return (especially in a neonate) to achieve adequate cardiac output.

The Extracorporeal Life Support Organization neonatal registry reports that the patients who had failure after decannulation the first time had an acceptable survival, but had a higher incidence of complications, especially neurologic and infectious.[163] There is no information on pediatric cardiac patients who required recannulation.

DECISION TO WITHDRAW FROM MECHANICAL SUPPORT

There is some evidence that prolonged support beyond 72 hours or longer is unfavorable for survival for certain indications (e.g., postcardiotomy syndrome), and every effort should be made to wean from support within this time period. Beyond this period, there should be serious consideration for either heart transplantation or termination of support if appropriate. In addition, other medical conditions, such as intracranial bleeding or intractable hemorrhage, should be considered potential reasons for termination of support. It is important to appreciate the differences in time of myocardial recovery in children with various indications for support. The expected myocardial recovery for postcardiotomy syndrome in the absence of postoperative residua or coronary insufficiency is usually not more than 72 hours and is considerably shorter than those for other disease states, such as fulminant myocarditis or acute respiratory distress syndrome.

CARDIAC INTENSIVE CARE AFTER SUPPORT: GENERAL PRINCIPLES

Low cardiac output syndrome can ensue even after initial success from weaning off mechanical support. Intensive care monitoring for bleeding and thromboses for vessels entered for cannulation during support should be complete, and vigilance for any potential neurologic injury should continue. Myocardial dysfunction and subsequent recovery are manifested by altered genetic expression of membrane receptors, extracellular matrix proteins, calcium cycling proteins, and contractile proteins. Whether reverse remodeling occurs as a result of signal transduction or changes in ultrastructural and extracellular matrix contents in patients after ventricular assist device implantation has been investigated only more recently.[164,165] In addition, there is evidence for reduction of β-receptor antibodies while on long-term mechanical support.[166] Clinical affirmation of this recovery has been reported in adult patients after extended bridge to cardiac transplantation.[167] Dystrophin, a protein responsible for structural integrity of the myocardium, is disrupted in the process of myocarditis; recovery of the myocardium during support in adults has been shown to be associated with recovery of this dystrophin complex. Work by Matta and colleagues[168] showed a molecular basis for the failing myocardium on mechanical support to effect eventual myocardial recovery. There also is evidence that early decrease in brain natriuretic peptide may indicate recovery of ventricular function during VAD support.[169] It remains to be seen whether this phenomenon is present in infants and children on mechanical support.[170]

CURRENT STATUS AND FUTURE TRENDS

Principles of use of mechanical circulatory support emphasize the need for an individualized approach. Indications should broaden to include pediatric patients with myocarditis and septic shock. Short-term use of mechanical devices has been limited to ECMO, but pediatric experience with VADs is growing. The pediatric experience with long-term devices is lacking, but the advent of small axial-type devices holds great promise as long-term devices in children.[171] Long-term biventricular support in neonates and infants remains a daunting challenge. With better clinical management, improved technology, and broader use of mechanical support devices and attention to economic restraints, survival for children with severe heart failure will continue to improve.

Key Concepts

■ Pediatric patients with failing hearts usually have concomitant issues, such as right ventricular failure, pulmonary hypertension, profound hypoxemia, and anatomic variations, that would provide daunting challenges to surgical cannulation and support strategy.

■ Before planned cardiac surgery, it is strategically beneficial to improve any significant preoperative ventricular dysfunction with pharmacologic means before surgery to lessen the likelihood of need for postoperative support. In addition, certain congenital heart defects, such as anomalous left coronary artery

from the pulmonary artery or transposition of the great arteries in an older infant, have an expected higher risk for postoperative ventricular dysfunction, and the awareness for possible use of mechanical support should be heightened.

■ Overall, the decision for institution of mechanical support should be individualized with consideration for hemodynamic instability (incessant tachycardia and hypotension with concomitant increased ventricular filling pressures), low (<1 mL/kg/hr) urine output, metabolic acidosis, poor perfusion with decreased capillary refill, and high level of inotropic support.

■ Children with acute fulminant myocarditis often die as a result of low cardiac output syndrome despite escalating inotropic support and can benefit greatly from mechanical support with eventual myocardial recovery.

■ In ECMO, left atrial pressure (which can be estimated noninvasively by echocardiographic examinations of the position of the atrial septum) should be monitored carefully; inadequate unloading of the left atrium and ventricle with resultant distention can lead to mitral regurgitation and pulmonary edema and hemorrhage and minimize the likelihood of myocardial recovery.

■ For left VADs, it is essential to appreciate its major inherent difference from ECMO: Cardiac output that is generated from the assist device depends entirely on right ventricular output; the right ventricular output is the preload to the left VAD. Inadequate filling of the left ventricular VAD can result from low intravascular volume, tamponade, improper cannula positioning, right ventricular dysfunction, elevated PVR, or dysrhythmias.

■ It is important to appreciate the differences in time of myocardial recovery in children with various indications for support. The expected myocardial recovery for postcardiotomy syndrome in the absence of postoperative residua or coronary insufficiency is usually not more than 72 hours and is considerably shorter than those for other disease states, such as fulminant myocarditis or acute respiratory distress syndrome.

REFERENCES

1. Chang AC, Atz A, Burke RP, et al: Milrinone: Systemic and pulmonary hemodynamic effects in neonates after cardiac surgery. Crit Care Med 1995;23:1907-1914.
2. Hoffman TM, Wernovsky G, Atz AM, et al: Prophylactic Intravenous Use of Milrinone after Cardiac Operation in Pediatrics (PRIMACORP) study. Am Heart J 2002;143:15-21.
3. Booker PD: Pharmacological support for children with myocardial dysfunction. Pediatr Anesth 2002;12:5-25.
4. Beghetti M, Rimensberger PC: Mechanical circulatory support in pediatric patients. Intensive Care Med 2000;26:350-352.
5. Duncan BW: Mechanical circulatory support for infants and children with cardiac disease. Ann Thorac Surg 2002;73:1670-1677.

6. Dalton HJ, Rycus PT, Conrad SA: Update on extracorporeal life support 2004. Semin Perinatol 2005;29:24-33.

7. Kanter KR, Pennington DG, Weber TR, et al: Extracorporeal membrane oxygenation for postoperative cardiac support in children. J Thorac Cardiovasc Surg 1987;93:27-35.

8. Redmond CR, Graves ED, Falterman KW, et al: Extracorporeal membrane oxygenation for respiratory and cardiac failure in infants and children. J Thorac Cardiovasc Surg 1987;93:199-204.

9. Weinhaus L, Canter C, Noetzel M, et al: Extracorporeal membrane oxygenation for circulatory support after repair of congenital heart defects. Ann Thorac Surg 1989;48:206-212.

10. Rogers AJ, Trento A, Siewers RD, et al: Extracorporeal membrane oxygenation for postoperative cardiogenic shock in children. Ann Thorac Surg 1989;47:903-906.

11. Anderson HL, Attorri RJ, Custer JR, et al: Extracorporeal membrane oxygenation for pediatric cardiopulmonary failure. J Thorac Cardiovasc Surg 1990;99:1011-1021.

12. Klein MD, Shaheen KW, Whittlesey GC, et al: Extracorporeal membrane oxygenation for circulatory support of children after repair of congenital heart disease. J Thorac Cardiovasc Surg 1990;100:498-505.

13. Ferrazzi P, Glauber M, DiDomenico A, et al: Assisted circulation for myocardial recovery after repair of congenital heart disease. Eur J Cardiothorac Surg 1991;5:419-423.

14. Delius RE, Bove EL, Meliones JN, et al: Use of extracorporeal life support in patients with congenital heart disease. Crit Care Med 1992;20:1216-1222.

15. Raithel SC, Pennington DG, Boegner E, et al: Extracorporeal membrane oxygenation in children after cardiac surgery. Circulation 1992;86(Suppl 2):305-310.

16. Ziomek S, Harrell JE, Fasules JW, et al: Extracorporeal membrane oxygenation for cardiac failure after congenital heart operation. Ann Thorac Surg 1992;54:861-868.

17. Meliones JN, Custer JR, Snedecor S, et al: Extracorporeal life support for cardiac assist in pediatric patients: Review of ELSO Registry data. Circulation 1991;84(5 Suppl):III-168-III-172.

18. Dalton HJ, Siewers RD, Fuhrman BP, et al: Extracorporeal membrane oxygenation for cardiac rescue in children with severe myocardial dysfunction. Crit Care Med 1993;21:1020-1028.

19. Pennington DG, Swartz MT: Circulatory support in infants and children. Ann Thorac Surg 1993;55:233-237.

20. del Nido PJ: Extracorporeal membrane oxygenation for cardiac support in children. Ann Thorac Surg 1996;61:336-339.

21. Walters HL, Hakimi M, Rice MD, et al: Pediatric cardiac surgical ECMO: Multivariate analysis of risk factors for hospital death. Ann Thorac Surg 1995;60:329-336.

22. Montgomery VL, Strotman JM, Ross MP: Impact of multiple organ system dysfunction and nosocomial infections on survival of children treated with extracorporeal membrane oxygenation after heart surgery. Crit Care Med 2000;28:526-531.

23. Mehta U, Laks H, Sadeghi A, et al: Extracorporeal membrane oxygenation for cardiac support in pediatric patients. Am Surg 2000;66:879-886.

24. Aharon AS, Drinkwater DC, Churchwell KB, et al: Extracorporeal membrane oxygenation in children after repair of congenital cardiac lesions. Ann Thorac Surg 2001;72:2095-2101.

25. ECMO Registry Report. Ann Arbor, Mich, Extracorporeal Life Support Organization, 2001.

26. Chang AC, Hanley FL, Wernovsky G, Wessel DL: Pediatric Cardiac Intensive Care. Baltimore, Williams & Wilkins, 1998.

27. Chang AC: Pediatric cardiac intensive care: Current state of the art and beyond the millennium. Curr Opin Pediatr 2000;12:238-246.

28. Pennington DG, Swartz MT: Circulatory support in infants and children. Ann Thorac Surg 1993;55:233-237.

29. Burch GE: On resting the human heart. Am Heart J 1966;71:422-428.

30. Kahwaji I, Ramaciotti C, Nikaidoh H, et al: Images in cardiovascular medicine: Echocardiographic diagnosis of anomalous drainage of the superior vena cava into the left atrium. Circulation 2003;107:1560-1561.

31. Charpie JR, Dekeon MK, Goldberg CS, et al: Serial blood lactate measurements predict early outcome after neonatal repair or palliation for complex congenital heart disease. J Thorac Cardiovasc Surg 2000;120:73-80.

32. Langley SM, Sheppard SB, Tsang VT, et al: When is extracorporeal life support worthwhile following repair of congenital heart disease in children? Eur J Cardiothorac Surg 1998;13:520-525.

33. Wernovsky G, Chang AC, Wessel DL: Intensive care. In Emmannouilides GC, Riemenschneider TA, Allen HD, et al (eds): Heart Disease in Infants, Children, and Adolescents. Baltimore, Williams & Wilkins, 2000, pp 398-439.

34. Trittenwein G, Pansi H, Graf B, et al: Proposed entry criteria for postoperative cardiac extracorporeal membrane oxygenation after pediatric open heart surgery. Artif Organs 1999;23:1010-1014.

35. Hakami M, Walters HL, Pinsky WW, et al: Delayed sternal closure after neonatal cardiac operations. J Thorac Cardiovasc Surg 1994;107:925-933.

36. Alexi-Meskishvili V, Hetzer R, Weng Y, et al: Successful extracorporeal circulatory support after aortic reimplantation of anomalous left coronary artery. Eur J Cardiothorac Surg 1994;8:533-536.

37. del Nido PJ, Duncan BW, Mayer Jr JE, et al: Left ventricular assist device improves survival in children with left ventricular dysfunction after repair of anomalous origin of the left coronary artery from the pulmonary artery. Ann Thorac Surg 1999;67:169-172.

38. Mee RB, Harada Y: Retraining of the left ventricle with a left ventricular assist device (BioMedicus) after the arterial switch operation. J Thorac Cardiovasc Surg 1991;101:171-173.

39. Mitchell MB, Campbell DN, Bielefeld MR, et al: Utility of extracorporeal membrane oxygenation for early graft failure following heart transplantation in infancy. J Heart Lung Transplant 2000;19:834-839.

40. Grundl PD, Miller SA, del Nido PJ, et al: Successful treatment of myocarditis using extracorporeal membrane oxygenation. Crit Care Med 1993;21:302-304.

41. Duncan BW, Bohn DJ, Atz AM, et al: Mechanical circulatory support for the treatment of children with acute fulminant myocarditis. J Thorac Cardiovasc Surg 2001;122:440-448.

42. Acker MA: Mechanical circulatory support for patients with acute-fulminant myocarditis. Ann Thorac Surg 2001;71(3 Suppl):S73-S76.

43. Lee KJ, McCrindle BW, Bohn DJ, et al: Clinical outcomes of acute myocarditis in childhood. Heart 1999;82:226-233.

44. Bohn D: Extracorporeal life support in heart and lung transplantation. Semin Thorac Cardiovasc Surg Pediatr Card Surg Annu 2001;4:94-102.

45. Levi D, Marelli D, Plunkett M, et al: Use of assist devices and ECMO to bridge pediatric patients with cardiomyopathy to transplantation. J Heart Lung Transplant 2002;21:760-770.

46. del Nido PJ, Armitage JM, Fricker FJ, et al: Extracorporeal membrane oxygenation support as a bridge to pediatric heart transplantation. Circulation 1994;90(5 Pt 2):II-66-II-69.

47. Hopper AO, Pageau J, Job L, et al: Extracorporeal membrane oxygenation for perioperative support in neonatal and pediatric cardiac transplantation. Artif Organs 1999;23:1006-1009.

48. Ishino K, Weng Y, Alexi-Meskishvili V, et al: Extracorporeal membrane oxygenation as a bridge to cardiac transplantation in children. Artif Organs 1996;20:728-732.

49. Farrar DJ, Hill JD: Univentricular and biventricular Thoratec VAD support as a bridge to transplantation. Ann Thorac Surg 1991;55:276-282.

50. Warnecke H, Berdjis F, Hennig E, et al: Mechanical left ventricular support as a bridge to cardiac transplantation in childhood. Eur J Cardiothorac Surg 1991;5:330-333.

51. Hetzer R, Loebe M, Weng Y, et al: Pulsatile pediatric ventricular assist device: Current results for bridge to transplantation. Semin Thorac Cardiovasc Surg Pediatr Card Surg Annu 1999;2:157-176.

52. Delius RE, Zwischenberger JB, Cilley R, et al: Prolonged extracorporeal life support of pediatric and adolescent cardiac transplant patients. Ann Thorac Surg 1990;50:791-795.

53. Gajarski RJ, Mosca RS, Ohye RG, et al: Use of extracorporeal life support as a bridge to pediatric cardiac transplantation. J Heart Lung Transplant 2003;22:28-34.

54. Morrow WR, Naftel D, Chinnock R, et al: Outcome of listing for heart transplantation in infants younger than six months: Predictors of death and interval to transplantation. The Pediatric Heart Transplantation Study Group. J Heart Lung Transplant 1997;16:1255-1266.

55. del Nido PJ, Dalton HJ, Thompson AE, et al: Extracorporeal membrane oxygenation for cardiac rescue in children with severe myocardial dysfunction. Crit Care Med 1993;21:1020-1028.

56. Kurose M, Okamoto K, Sato T, et al: Extracorporeal life support for patients undergoing prolonged external cardiac massage. Resuscitation 1993;25:35-40.

57. Chen YS, Chao A, Yu HY, et al: Analysis and results of prolonged resuscitation in cardiac arrest patients rescued by extracorporeal membrane oxygenation. J Am Coll Cardiol 2003;41:197-203.

58. Parra DA, Totapally BR, Zahn E, et al: Outcome of cardiopulmonary resuscitation in a pediatric cardiac intensive care unit. Crit Care Med 2000;28:3296-3300.

59. Dembitsky WP, Moreno-Cabral RJ, Adamson RM, et al: Emergency resuscitation using portable extracorporeal membrane oxygenation. Ann Thorac Surg 1993;55:304-309.

60. Duncan BW, Ibrahim AE, Hraska V, et al: Use of rapid deployment extracorporeal membrane oxygenation for the resuscitation of pediatric patients with heart disease after cardiac arrest. J Thorac Cardiovasc Surg 1998;116:305-311.

61. Salzer-Muhar UE, Marx M, Wimmer M: Pediatric cardiac extracorporeal membrane oxygenation in congenital heart disease: The cardiologist's view. Artif Organs 1999;23:995-1000.

62. Hunkeler NM, Canter CE, Donze A, et al: Extracorporeal life support in cyanotic congenital heart disease before cardiovascular operation. Am J Cardiol 1992;69:790-793.

63. McKay VJ, Stewart DL, Robinson TW, et al: Preoperative versus postoperative extracorporeal life support in neonatal cardiac patients. Perfusion 1997;12:179-186.

64. Lupinetti FM, Kulik TJ, Beekman RH, et al: Correction of total anomalous pulmonary venous connection in infancy. J Thorac Cardiovasc Surg 1993;106:880-885.

65. Stewart DL, Mendoza JC, Winston S, et al: Use of extracorporeal life support in total anomalous pulmonary venous drainage. J Perinatol 1996;16(2 Pt 1):186-190.

66. Dudell GG, Evans ML, Krous HF, et al: Common pulmonary vein atresia: The role of extracorporeal membrane oxygenation. Pediatrics 1993;91:403-410.

67. McDonnell BE, Raff GW, Gaynor JW, et al: Outcome after repair of tetralogy of Fallot with absent pulmonary valve. Ann Thorac Surg 1999;67:1391-1396.

68. Adolph V, Heaton J, Steiner R, et al: Extracorporeal membrane oxygenation for nonneonatal respiratory failure. J Pediatr Surg 1991;26:326-330.

69. Khongphatthanayothin A, Wong P, Samara Y, et al: Impact of respiratory syncytial virus infection on surgery for congenital heart disease: postoperative course and outcome. Crit Care Med 1999;27:1974-1981.

70. Moler FW, Palmisano JM, Green TP, et al: Predictors of outcome of severe respiratory syncytial virus-associated respiratory failure treated with extracorporeal membrane oxygenation. J Pediatr 1993;23:46-52.

71. Hibbs A, Evans JR, Gerdes M, et al: Outcome of infants with bronchopulmonary dysplasia who receive extracorporeal membrane oxygenation therapy. J Pediatr Surg 2001;36:1479-1484.

72. Brogan TV, Finn LS, Pyskaty DJ, et al: Plastic bronchitis in children: A case series and review of the medical literature. Pediatr Pulmonol 2002;34:482-487.

73. Boigner H, Trittenwein G, Marx M, et al: Pulmonary failure after Norwood procedure: Indication for extracorporeal membrane oxygenation? A case report. Artif Organs 1999;23:1036-1037.

74. Dhillon R, Pearson GA, Firmin RK, et al: Extracorporeal membrane oxygenation and the treatment of critical pulmonary hypertension in congenital heart disease. Eur J Cardiothorac Surg 1995;9:553-556.

75. Chang AC, Wernovsky G, Kulik T, et al: Management of the neonate with transposition of the great arteries and persistent pulmonary hypertension. Am J Cardiol 1991;68:1253-1255.

76. Cullen M, Splittgerber F, Sweezer W, et al: Pulmonary hypertension postventricular septal defect repair treated by extracorporeal membrane oxygenation. J Pediatr Surg 1986;21:675-677.

77. Goldman AP, Delius RE, Deanfield JE, et al: Nitric oxide might reduce the need for extracorporeal membrane support in children with critical postoperative pulmonary hypertension. Ann Thorac Surg 1996;62:750-755.

78. Saito A, Miyamura H, Kanazawa H, et al: Extracorporeal membrane oxygenation for severe heart failure after Fontan operation. Ann Thorac Surg 1993;55:153-155.

79. Thomas JA, Raroque S, Scott WA, et al: Successful treatment of severe dysrhythmias in infants with respiratory syncytial virus infections: Two cases and a literature review. Crit Care Med 1997;25:880-886.

80. Walker GM, McLeod K, Brown KL, et al: Extracorporeal life support as a treatment of supraventricular tachycardia in infants. Pediatr Crit Care Med 2003;4:52-54.

81. Azzam FJ, Fiore AC: Postoperative junctional ectopic tachycardia. Can J Anesth 1998;45:898-902.

82. Marino BS, Wernovsky G, Rychik J, et al: Early results of the Ross procedure in simple and complex left heart disease. Circulation 1999;100(19 Suppl):II-62-II-66.

83. Chen RJ, Ko WJ, Lin FY: Successful rescue of sustained ventricular tachycardia/ventricular fibrillation after coronary artery bypass grafting by extracorporeal membrane oxygenation. J Formos Med Assoc 2002;101:283-286.

84. Cohen MI, Gaynor JW, Ramesh V, et al: Extracorporeal membrane oxygenation for patients with refractory ventricular arrhythmias. J Thorac Cardiovasc Surg 1999;118:961-963.

85. Tecklenburg FW, Thomas NJ, Webb SA, et al: Pediatric ECMO for severe quinidine cardiotoxicity. Pediatr Emerg Care 1997;13:111-113.

86. Butler TJ, Yoder BA, Seib P, et al: ECMO for left ventricular assist in a newborn with critical aortic stenosis. Pediatr Cardiol 1994;15:38-40.

87. Ward CJ, Mullins CE, Barron LJ, et al: Use of extracorporeal membrane oxygenation to maintain oxygenation during pediatric interventional cardiac catheterization. Am Heart J 1995;130(3 Pt 1):619-620.

88. Carmichael TB, Walsh EP, Roth SJ: Anticipatory use of venoarterial extracorporeal membrane oxygenation for a high risk interventional high-risk cardiac procedure. Respir Care 2002;47:1002-1006.

89. Ungerleider R: Personal communcation, May, 2005.

90. Goldman AP, Macrae DJ, Tasker RC, et al: Extracorporeal membrane oxygenation as a bridge to definitive tracheal surgery in children. J Pediatr 1996;128:386-388.

91. Whyte RI, Deeb GM, McCurry KR, et al: Extracorporeal life support after heart or lung transplantation. Ann Thorac Surg 1994;58:754-758.

92. Wilson BJ, Heiman HS, Butler TJ, et al: A 16-year neonatal/pediatric extracorporeal membrane oxygenation transport experience. Pediatrics 2002;109:189-193.

93. Saker DM, Walsh-Sukys M, Spector M, et al: Cardiac recovery and survival after neonatal myocardial infarction. Pediatr Cardiol 1997;18:139-142.

94. Goodwin DA, Lally KP, Null DM Jr: Extracorporeal membrane oxygenation support for cardiac dysfunction from tricyclic antidepressant overdose. Crit Care Med 1993;21:625-627.

95. Ryan CA, Perreault T, Johnston-Hodgson A, et al: Extracorporeal membrane oxygenation in infants with congenital diaphragmatic hernia and cardiac malformations. J Pediatr Surg 1994;29:878-881.

96. Goldman AP, Kerr SJ, Butt W, et al: Extracorporeal support for intractable cardiorespiratory failure due to meningococcal disease. Lancet 1997;349:466-469.

97. Kolovos NS, Schuerer DJ, Moler FW, et al: Extracorporeal life support for pulmonary hemorrhage in children: A case series. Crit Care Med 2002;30:577-580.

98. Meyer DM, Jessen ME: Results of extracorporeal membrane oxygenation in children with sepsis. The Extracorporeal Life Support Organization. Ann Thorac Surg 1997;63:756-764.

99. Pizarro C, Davis DA, Healy RM, et al: Is there a role for extracorporeal life support after stage I Norwood? Eur J Cardiothorac Surg 2001;19:294-301.

100. Paris JJ, Schreiber MD, Statter M, et al: Beyond autonomy: Physicians' refusal to use life-prolonging extracorporeal membrane oxygenation. N Engl J Med 1993;329:354-357.

101. Fuhrman BP, Hernan LJ, Rotta AT, et al: Pathophysiology of cardiac extracorporeal membrane oxygenation. Artif Organs 1999;23:966-969.

102. del Nido PJ, Armitage JM, Fricker FJ, et al: Extracorporeal membrane oxygenation support as a bridge to pediatric heart transplantation. Circulation 1994;90(5 Pt 2):II-66-II-69.

103. Koenig PR, Ralston MA, Kimball TR, et al: Balloon atrial septostomy for left ventricular decompression in patients receiving extracorporeal membrane oxygenation for myocardial failure. J Pediatr 1993;122:S95-S99.

104. Koenig PR, Ralston MA, Kimball TR, et al: Balloon atrial septostomy for left ventricular decompression in patients receiving extracorporeal membrane oxygenation for myocardial failure. J Pediatr 1993;122:S95-S99.

105. Seib PM, Faulkner SC, Erickson CC, et al: Blade and balloon atrial septostomy for left heart decompression in patients with severe ventricular dysfunction on extracorporeal membrane oxygenation. Cathet Cardiovasc Interv 1999;46:179-186.

106. Edmunds LH: Pulseless cardiopulmonary bypass. J Thorac Cardiovasc Surg 1982;84:800-804.

107. Bavaria JE, Ratcliff MB, Gupta KB, et al: Changes in left ventricular systolic wall stress during biventricular circulatory assistance. Ann Thorac Surg 1988;45:526-532.

108. Martin GR, Short BL: Doppler echocardiographic evaluation of cardiac performance in infants on prolonged extracorporeal membrane oxygenation. Am J Cardiol 1988;62:929-934.

109. Sell LL, Cullen ML, Lerner GR, et al: Hypertension during extracorporeal membrane oxygenation: Cause, effect, and management. Surgery 1987;102:724-730.

110. Martin GR, Chauvin L, Short BL: Effects of hydralazine on cardiac performance in infants receiving extracorporeal membrane oxygenation. J Pediatr 1991;118:944-948.

111. Martin GR, Short BL, Abbott C, et al: Cardiac stun in infants undergoing extracorporeal membrane oxygenation. J Thorac Cardiovasc Surg 1991;101 607-611.

112. Rosenberg EM, Cook LN: Electromechanical dissociation in newborns treated with extracorporeal membrane oxygenation: An extreme form of cardiac stun syndrome. Crit Care Med 1991;19:780-784.

113. Secker-Walker JS, Edmonds JF, Spratt EH, et al: The source of coronary perfusion during partial bypass for extracorporeal membrane oxygenation. Ann Thorac Surg 1976;21:138-143.

114. Walther FJ, van de Bor M, Gangitano ES, et al: Left and right ventricular output in newborn infants undergoing extracorporeal membrane oxygenation. Crit Care Med 1990;18:148-151.

115. Kurian MS, Reynolds ER, Humes RA, et al: Cardiac tamponade caused by serous pericardial effusion in patients on extracorporeal membrane oxygenation. J Pediatr Surg 1999;34:1311-1314.

116. Zwischenberger JB, Cilley RE, Hirschl RB, et al: Life-threatening intrathoracic complications during treatment with extracorporeal membrane oxygenation. J Pediatr Surg 1988;23:599-604.

117. Kececioglu D, Galal O, Halees Z, et al: Transesophageal echocardiography in children with cardiac assist. Thorac Cardiovasc Surg 1994;42:21-24.

118. Ettedgui JA, Fricker FJ, Park SC, et al: Cardiac catheterization in children on extracorporeal membrane oxygenation. Cardiol Young 1996;6:59-61.

119. desJardins SE, Crowley DC, Beekman RH, et al: Utility of cardiac catheterization in pediatric cardiac patients on ECMO. Cathet Cardiovasc Interv 1999;46:62-67.

120. Booth KL, Roth SJ, Perry SB, et al: Cardiac catheterization of patients supported by extracorporeal membrane oxygenation. J Am Coll Cardiol 2002;40:1681-1686.

121. Black MD, Coles JG, Williams WG, et al: Determinants of success in pediatric cardiac patients undergoing extracorporeal membrane oxygenation. Ann Thorac Surg 1995;60:133-138.

122. Walters HL, Hakimi M, Rice MD, et al: Pediatric cardiac surgical ECMO: Multivariate analysis of risk factors for hospital death. Ann Thorac Surg 1995;60:329-336.

123. Brown KL, Shekerdemian LS, Penny DJ: Transcatheter closure of a patent arterial duct in a patient on veno-arterial extracorporeal membrane oxygenation. Intensive Care Med 2002;28:501-503.

124. Hoskote A, Bohn D, VanArsdell G, et al: Extracorporeal life support in functional single ventricle following palliative surgery (Abstract). Pediatr Crit Care Med 2003;4:A119.

125. Darling EM, Kaemmer D, Lawson DS, et al: Use of ECMO without the oxygenator to provide ventricular support after Norwood stage I procedures. Ann Thorac Surg 2001;71:735-736.

126. Jaggers JJ, Forbess JM, Shah AS, et al: Extracorporeal membrane oxygenation for infant postcardiotomy support: Significance of shunt management. Ann Thorac Surg 2000;69:1476-1483.

127. Van Heijst AF, van der Staak FH, Hopman JC, et al: Ductus arteriosus with left-to-right shunt during venoarterial extracorporeal membrane oxygenation: Effects on cerebral oxygenation and hemodynamics. Pediatr Crit Care Med 2003;4:94-99.

128. Nelson DP, Schwartz S, Chang AC: Single ventricle physiology before and after Norwood operation. Cardiol Young 2004; 14 Suppl 1:52-60.

129. Saito A, Miyamura H, Kanazawa H, et al: Extracorporeal membrane oxygenation for severe heart failure after Fontan operation. Ann Thorac Surg 1993;55:153-155.

130. Koul B, Willen H, Sjoberg T, et al: Pulmonary sequelae of prolonged total venoarterial bypass: Evaluation with a new experimental model. Ann Thorac Surg 1991;51:794-799.

131. Shen I, Levy FH, Benak AM, et al: Left ventricular dysfunction during extracorporeal membrane oxygenation in a hypoxemic swine model. Ann Thorac Surg 2001;71:868-871.

132. McGowan FX, Ikegami M, del Nido PJ, et al: Cardiopulmonary bypass significantly reduces surfactant activity in children. J Thorac Cardiovasc Surg 1993;106:968-977.

133. Bui KC, Walther FJ, David-Cu R, et al: Phospholipid and surfactant protein A concentration in tracheal aspirates from infants requiring extracorporeal membrane oxygenation. J Pediatr 1992;121:271-274.

134. Coraim FJ, Coraim HP, Ebermann R, et al: Acute respiratory failure after cardiac surgery: Clinical experiences with the application of continuous arteriovenous hemofiltration. Crit Care Med 1986;14:714-718.

135. Kossel H, Bartsch H, Philippi W, et al: Pulmonary embolism and myocardial hypoxia during extracorporeal membrane oxygenation. J Pediatr Surg 1999;34:485-487.

136. Biehl DA, Stewart DL, Forti NH, et al: Timing of intracranial hemorrhage during extracorporeal life support. ASAIO J 1996; 42:938-941.

137. Fukuda S, Aoyama M, Yamada Y, et al: Comparison of venoarterial versus venovenous access in the cerebral circulation of newborns undergoing extracorporeal membrane oxygenation. Pediatr Surg Int 1999;15:78-84.

138. Gannon CM, Kornhauser MS, Gross GW, et al: When combined, early bedside head ultrasound and electroencephalography predict abnormal computerized tomography or magnetic

resonance brain imaging obtained after extracorporeal membrane oxygenation treatment. J Perinatol 2001;21:451-455.

139. Korinthenberg R, Kachel W, Koelfen W, et al: Neurological findings in newborn infants after extracorporeal membrane oxygenation, with special reference to EEG. Dev Med Child Neurol 1993;35:249-257.

140. Gazzolo D, Masetti P, Meli M, et al: Elevated S100B protein as an early indicator of intracranial hemorrhage in infants subjected to extracorporeal membrane oxygenation. Acta Paediatr 2002;91:218-221.

141. Golej J, Trittenwein G: Early detection of neurologic injury and issues of rehabilitation after pediatric cardiac extracorporeal membrane oxygenation. Artif Organs 1999;23:1020-1025.

142. Mild therapeutic hypothermia to improve the neurologic outcome after cardiac arrest. The Hypothermia after Cardiac Arrest Study Group. N Engl J Med 2002;346:549-556.

143. McLaughlin JF, Loeser JD, Roberts TS: Acquired hydrocephalus associated with superior vena cava syndrome in infants. Childs Nerv Syst 1997;13:59-63.

144. Tobias JD: Controlled hypotension in children: A critical review of available agents. Paediatr Drugs 2002;4:439-453.

145. Sorof JM, Stromberg D, Brewer ED, et al: Early initiation of peritoneal dialysis after surgical repair of congenital heart disease. Pediatr Nephrol 1999;13:641-645.

146. Pettignano R, Heard M, Davis R, et al: Total enteral nutrition versus total parenteral nutrition during pediatric extracorporeal membrane oxygenation. Crit Care Med 1998;26:358-363.

147. Duke T, Butt W, South M, et al: The DCO2 measured by gastric tonometry predicts survival in children receiving extracorporeal life support. Chest 1997;111:174-179.

148. Sell LL, Cullen ML, Whittlesey GC, et al: Hemorrhagic complications during extracorporeal membrane oxygenation: Prevention and treatment. J Pediatr Surg 1986;21:1087-1091.

149. Dela Cruz TV, Stewart DL, Winston SJ, et al: Risk factors for intracranial hemorrhage in the extracorporeal membrane oxygenation patient. J Perinatol 1997;17:18-23.

150. Horwitz JR, Cofer BR, Warner BH, et al: A Multi-center trial of e-amino caproic acid (Amicar) in the prevention of bleeding in infants on ECMO. J Pediatr Surg 1998;33:1610-1613.

151. Biswas AK, Lewis L, Sommerauer JF: Aprotonin in the management of life-threatening bleeding during extracorporeal life support. Perfusion 2000;15:211-216.

152. Zavadil DP, Stammers AH, Willett LD, et al: Hematological abnormalities in neonatal patients treated with extracorporeal membrane oxygenation. J Extra Corpor Technol 1998;30:83-90.

153. O'Neill JM, Schutze GE, Heulitt MJ, et al: Nosocomial infections during extracorporeal membrane oxygenation. Intensive Care Med 2001;27:1247-1253.

154. Fridriksson JH, Helmrath MA, Wessel JJ, et al: Hypercalcemia associated with extracorporeal life support in neonates. J Pediatr Surg 2001;36:493-497.

155. Melione JN, Moler FW, Custer JR, et al: Hemodynamic instability after the initiation of extracorporeal membrane oxygenation: Role of ionized calcium. Crit Care Med 1991;19:1247-1251.

156. Bolton DT: Hyperkalemia, donor blood and cardiac arrest associated with ECMO priming. Anaesthesia 2000;55:825-826.

157. Sell LL, Cullen ML, Whittlesey GC, et al: Experience with renal failure during extracorporeal membrane oxygenation: Treatment with continuous hemofiltration. J Pediatr Surg 1987;22:600-602.

158. Hirther M, Simoni J, Dickson M: Elevated levels of endotoxin, oxygen-derived free radicals, and cytokines during extracorporeal membrane oxygenation. J Pediatr Surg 1992;27:1199-1202.

159. Heiss KF, Ettit B, Hirschl RB, et al: Renal insufficiency and volume overload in neonatal ECMO managed by continuous ultrafiltration. ASAIO Trans 1987;33:557-560.

160. Mulla H, Lawson G, von Anrep C, et al: In vitro evaluation of sedative drug losses during extracorporeal membrane oxygenation. Perfusion 2000;15:21-26.

161. Marcus B, Atkinson JB, Wong PC, et al: Successful use of transesophageal echocardiography during extracorporeal membrane oxygenation in infants after cardiac operations. J Thorac Cardiovasc Surg 1995;109:846-848.

162. Vermes E, Houel R, Simon M, et al: Doppler tissue imaging to predict myocardial recovery during mechanical circulatory support. Ann Thorac Surg 2000;70:2149-2151.

163. Meehan JJ, Haney BM, Snyder CL, et al: Outcome after recannulation and a second course of extracorporeal membrane oxygenation. J Pediatr Surg 2002;3:845-850.

164. Milting H, Kassner A, Arusoglu L, et al: Structural and biochemical effects of mechanical unloading of terminal failing heart. In Proceedings of the Third Mechanical Circulatory Support Meeting: Today's Facts and Future Trends. Bad Oeyenhausen, Germany, December 2002.

165. Birks EJ: Myocardial recovery: Harefield approach. In Proceedings of the Third Mechanical Circulatory Support Meeting: Today's Facts and Future Trends. Bad Oeyenhausen, Germany, December 2002.

166. Loebe M, Hennig E, Muller J, et al: Long-term mechanical circulatory support as a bridge to transplantation, for recovery from cardiomyopathy, and for permanent replacement. Eur J Cardiothorac Surg 1997;(11 Suppl):S18-S24.

167. Frazier OH, Macris MT, Myers TJ, et al: Improved survival after extended bridge to cardiac transplantation. Ann Thorac Surg 1994;57:1416-1422.

168. Matta M, Stetson SJ, Perez-Verdia A, et al: Molecular remodelling of dystrophin in patients with end-stage cardiomyopathies and reversal in patients on assistance-device therapy. Lancet 2002;359:936-941.

169. Sodian R, Loebe M, Schmitt C, et al: Decreased plasma concentration of brain natriuretic peptide as a potential indicator of cardiac recovery in patients supported by mechanical circulatory assist systems. J Am Coll Cardiol 2001;38:1942-1949.

170. Law YM, Keller BB, Feingold BM, et al: Usefulness of plasma B-type natriuretic peptide to identify ventricular dysfunction in pediatric and adult patients with congenital heart disease. Am J Cardiol 2005;95:474-478.

171. Chang AC, McKenzie ED: Mechanical cardiopulmonary support in children and young adults: Extracorporeal membrane oxygenation, ventricular assist devices, and long-term support devices. Pediatr Cardiol 2005;26:2-28.

CHAPTER 46

Short-Term Mechanical Cardiopulmonary Support Devices

Raja Joshi
Brian W. Duncan

The provision of mechanical circulatory support when other forms of treatment fail has become increasingly common in the therapeutic approach to patients with cardiac disease. For adults in the acute setting, left ventricular failure resulting from coronary artery disease has been managed with intra-aortic balloon pump (IABP) and left ventricular assist device (VAD) insertion. In children, isolated left ventricular failure is relatively rare, however, whereas right ventricular failure, pulmonary hypertension, and hypoxemia often contribute significantly to circulatory failure that arises secondary to congenital heart disease. Because of these physiologic differences, isolated support of the left ventricle by IABP or left VAD has more limited application in children. Extracorporeal membrane oxygenation (ECMO) provides biventricular cardiopulmonary support and has emerged as the most commonly used form of mechanical circulatory assistance in children in whom conventional medical treatment has failed.[1,2]

This chapter focuses on the support device options that are available for the provision of mechanical circulatory support for children in the acute intensive care setting. Because of its preeminent role for this purpose, ECMO is the focus of this chapter. Centrifugal VADs also are useful for acute support, however, and the pediatric VAD experience is reviewed briefly (see Chapter 47). Finally, although IABP has a more limited role in children, the use of this modality for pediatric circulatory support is reviewed (see Chapter 40). The medical issues regarding acute mechanical cardiopulmonary support are discussed elsewhere in Chapter 45 in more detail.

EXTRACORPOREAL MEMBRANE OXYGENATION SUPPORT FOR THE ACUTELY FAILING PEDIATRIC CIRCULATION

Technical Aspects and Patient Management

For children with cardiac disease, technical considerations related to the circuit are similar to technical concerns encountered in the support of respiratory failure—with some important modifications. Most patients with cardiac disease require a venoarterial mode for full cardiopulmonary support; however, several reports have described the successful use of venovenous ECMO for pediatric cardiac patients.[2,3] Because a substantial amount

of morbidity in congenital heart disease is due to hypoxia, pulmonary hypertension, and right ventricular failure, venovenous ECMO currently may be an underused modality in pediatric cardiac patients. Although it does not provide cardiac pump support, venovenous ECMO still may provide substantial circulatory support owing to improved right ventricular function resulting from the elimination of hypoxia and unloading of the right ventricle.

Most centers use a standard ECMO circuit that employs a membrane oxygenator, roller pump, and heat exchanger (Fig. 46-1). **Membrane oxygenators** continue to be used by most centers; however, the use of hollow-fiber oxygenators has become more common.[4-6] Hollow-fiber oxygenators are highly efficient in terms of gas exchange and are easy to prime, which is especially advantageous when ECMO is used to resuscitate patients after cardiac arrest.[7,8] Long-term use of hollow-fiber oxygenators is limited by leakage of plasma into the gas phase, which may require more frequent replacement compared with membrane oxygenators.[7]

Roller pumps are used widely in ECMO circuits; however, centrifugal pumps also may be employed effectively (Fig. 46-2). New electronic systems may provide a more accurate approach to pump servoregulation and may be used more widely in the future.[9] **Centrifugal pumps** maintain venous inflow independent of gravity drainage, making a bladder box unnecessary and allowing the patient to be positioned at any height relative to the pump. This feature of the centrifugal pump is particularly useful in larger patients to maintain adequate venous return at higher flows.[10-13]

The approach to **cannulation** and ventricular decompression should be flexible and based on the setting in which the need for ECMO arises. Transthoracic cannulation of the right atrial appendage and the ascending aorta is most appropriate for cases that require intraoperative support for failure to wean from cardiopulmonary bypass. In the immediate postoperative period, chest cannulation provides the most expeditious route for the institution of support, especially in patients who experience cardiac arrest. Adequate venous drainage and excellent arterial perfusion are ensured by chest cannulation; however, significant hemorrhage remains the chief disadvantage, making peripheral cannulation sites preferable in most other settings. In addition, the risk of

PEDIATRIC ECLS CIRCUIT (ROLLER PUMP)

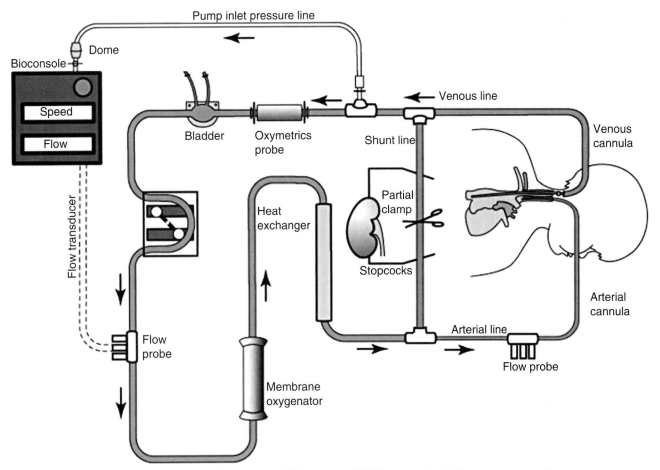

FIGURE 46-1 ■ Standard extracorporeal life support (ECLS) circuit. The ECLS circuit is seen with roller pump, membrane oxygenator, and heat exchanger. Venous return is maintained by gravity siphon in roller pump circuits, which requires attention to positioning to ensure that the pump is dependent relative to the patient. Interruptions of blood return to a roller pump must be avoided to prevent excessively negative pressures in the inflow tubing; this has been achieved by incorporating a "bladder box" into the inflow portion of the circuit. The bladder box is a servoregulatory mechanism that comprises a distensible bladder that compresses a spring-loaded mechanical switching device, which turns the pump off if venous inflow is inadvertently interrupted.

mediastinitis is increased significantly with transthoracic cannulation, which is a potent source of morbidity and which may make cardiac transplantation nearly impossible if recovery does not occur. Cannulation of the right internal jugular vein and the common carotid artery provides excellent venous drainage and perfusion and is the preferred cannulation site in neonates and children weighing less than approximately 15 kg. Cannulation of the femoral vessels provides adequate venous drainage and perfusion for larger children. A second venous drainage cannula placed in the right internal jugular vein may be added if venous drainage through the femoral route alone is inadequate. The risk of lower extremity ischemia can be minimized by placing a perfusion cannula in the distal femoral artery from a side arm brought off of the arterial limb of the circuit.[2,14] Venous congestion of the lower extremity may be prevented by placement of a "saphenous sump" catheter at the time of femoral venous cannulation.[10]

Left ventricular distention must be avoided during ECMO support and can be detected with echocardiography and left atrial pressure monitoring. If left ventricular distention occurs, ECMO flows should be increased, which minimizes pulmonary blood flow, decreasing pulmonary venous return to the left heart. This maneuver relieves left ventricular distention in most cases; however, if unsuccessful, venting of the left atrium should be performed by direct cannulation, or by balloon atrial septostomy performed in the cardiac catheterization laboratory or, preferably, at the patient's bedside under echocardiographic guidance.[15,16]

The status of the patient's anticoagulation is monitored by the whole blood activated clotting time. Achieving an activated clotting time of 180 to 200 seconds with a

PEDIATRIC ECLS CIRCUIT (CENTRIFUGAL PUMP)

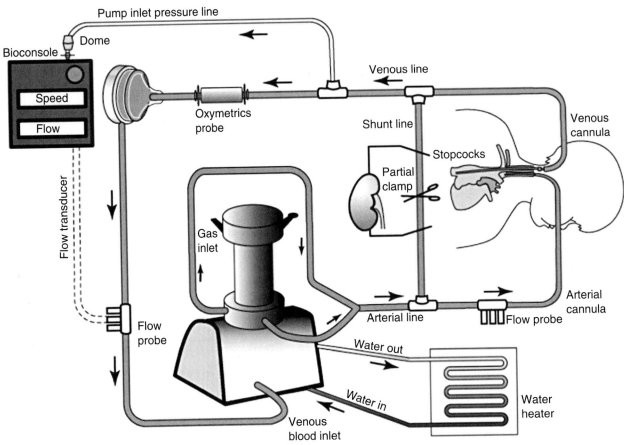

FIGURE 46-2 ■ **Extracorporeal life support (ECLS) circuit with centrifugal pump.** The ECLS circuit configured with a centrifugal pump and hollow-fiber oxygenator. Centrifugal pumps maintain venous inflow independent of gravity drainage, making a bladder box unnecessary and allowing the patient to be positioned at any height relative to the pump. This feature of the centrifugal pump is particularly useful in larger patients to maintain adequate venous return at higher flows. An additional advantage of the centrifugal pump is that, in contrast to the roller pump, occlusion of arterial outflow does not generate excessive arterial line pressure, reducing the risk of "blow-out" of the arterial limb of the circuit if distal occlusion occurs. The chief disadvantage of the centrifugal pump is the high negative pressure that may be generated on the venous side of the circuit, potentially leading to cavitation and hemolysis.

continuous heparin infusion maintains the circuit with a minimal risk of important thrombosis.[2,5,11,12,14,17,18] Platelets are maintained at greater than 100,000/mm³ and in patients requiring postoperative support, in whom bleeding is a critical problem, they are maintained at greater than 150,000/dL. Clotting factors are supplied with infusions of fresh frozen plasma or cryoprecipitate to maintain fibrinogen levels greater than 100 mg/dL. Heparin-bonded hollow-fiber oxygenators and heparin-bonded tubing have been used in an attempt to decrease the amount of systemic heparin that is required.[4] Administration of aminocaproic acid (Amicar) may be another useful adjunct to diminish the risk of postoperative hemorrhage.[2,19]

Other management points are as follows. ECMO flow rates generally are maintained in the range of 80 to 150 cc/kg/min until patients are considered ready for weaning. During support, inotropes are reduced, and small doses of dopamine and a vasodilator, such as milrinone, are used to improve systemic perfusion and to encourage ventricular ejection. Moderate levels of ventilatory support are maintained to ensure that coronary arterial blood, which is primarily derived from the left ventricle during ECMO, is fully saturated.[20,21]

Weaning is performed under echocardiographic guidance to assess ventricular filling and function. At the time of weaning, flows are turned down gradually over several hours until flows of 25 to 40 cc/kg/min are achieved, while ventilatory support and inotrope dosages are increased to appropriate levels. Arterial and venous lines are clamped, maintaining full anticoagulation, and then flushed every 15 to 20 minutes until the patient is stable off ECMO. A useful modification of the weaning strategy for patients with borderline hemodynamics is to extend the weaning period to 48 to 72 hours with gradual reduction in flow over that period. Fragile patients who fail with more rapid weaning may benefit from this approach by gradually accommodating to lower levels of support. Decannulation is performed at the patient's bedside in most cases.

Clinical Experience

A report of the cardiac ECMO experience from Children's Hospital, Boston, described 67 patients supported over a 10-year period.[2] The diagnostic categories included complex cyanotic lesions in more than half of these patients either with increased pulmonary blood flow (33% of the total patients) or decreased pulmonary blood flow (25% of the total patients). In a report by Walters and colleagues[22] of a large series of postcardiotomy patients, complete atrioventricular canal (20%), complex single-ventricle anatomy (17%), and tetralogy of Fallot (14%) were the most common diagnoses. Meliones and coworkers,[23] in their 1991 review of Extracorporeal Life Support Organization registry data, found left-to-right shunt (24%), cyanosis with decreased pulmonary blood flow (22%), and cyanosis with increased pulmonary blood flow (17%) to be the most common diagnostic groups for pediatric cardiac support. ECMO is more useful than VAD for the support of most children with complex cyanotic heart disease in which hypoxia, pulmonary hypertension, or biventricular failure contributes significantly to the pathophysiology necessitating mechanical circulatory support. Because of the presence of an oxygenator in the circuit, ECMO more directly addresses the underlying pathophysiology and provides greater flexibility than VAD in these instances.[2]

Indications for support differ depending on whether ECMO is required for preoperative or postcardiotomy support. Indications for ECMO before surgery are most commonly hypoxia and pulmonary hypertension.[3,24] Postoperative support most commonly is initiated for failure to wean from cardiopulmonary bypass, persistent low cardiac output, or cardiac arrest occurring in the intensive care unit (ICU) after cardiac surgery.[10-14,17,18,22,25-27] As use of ECMO for pediatric cardiac patients has increased, the clinical features defined as **contraindications** for the institution of support have evolved. There is universal agreement that certain conditions, including incurable malignancy, advanced multisystem organ failure, extreme prematurity, and severe central nervous system damage, constitute absolute contraindications.[2,11,22,26] Patients who are not transplantation candidates should be critically evaluated prior to support because any patient placed on ECMO ultimately may require cardiac transplantation for recovery.[11]

Many conditions previously considered absolute contraindications for ECMO support now are successfully treated and at most should be considered to be relative contraindications. Patients with shunted single-ventricle physiology, including patients with hypoplastic left heart syndrome after neonatal palliation, often were denied support in the past; however, most centers now believe that the ability to provide ECMO support is a necessary adjunct for the management of these complex cases.[2,22,27] In general, establishing rigid contraindications for mechanical support besides the above-mentioned features should be avoided, with each case evaluated on its own merits. In addition to patients with shunted single-ventricle physiology, patients experiencing pre-support cardiac arrest, patients undergoing palliative cardiac operations, and cardiac patients with coexisting congenital diaphragmatic hernia have been supported successfully, and these conditions should not be considered absolute contraindications for ECMO.

Weaning rates of 45% to 80% and hospital survival rates of 22% to 70% have been reported.[2,5,10-14,17,18,22,25-29] Reviewing **risk factors** for death from centers reporting large experiences with pediatric cardiac ECMO reveals numerous unifying concepts. Several studies identified the development of renal failure as an adverse prognostic indicator.[2,5,11,22,23] Severe hemorrhage measured directly as the volume of blood lost or the need for excessive transfusion of blood products was a risk factor for death in many studies,[2,13,22,23] whereas the presence of residual cardiac lesions after surgical repair represented a significant risk factor in some reports.[5,22] Other risk factors that have been identified include significant infectious complications, pre-support cardiac arrest, and high inotropic dosages while on support.

Lack of return of ventricular function within 48 to 72 hours was identified as a risk factor in patients supported after cardiac surgery, which has important implications for consideration of cardiac transplantation in these children.[2] Postcardiotomy patients without return of ventricular function within 48 to 72 hours of support should be considered for transplantation or termination of support if there are contraindications to transplantation. Delaying this decision while awaiting return of function beyond this period does not seem to be justified. Because of the scarcity of organ donors in the pediatric population, early identification of patients in whom return of ventricular function is unlikely optimizes the chances of successful organ procurement.

Cardiac failure, multisystem organ failure, and severe neurologic lesions are the most common **causes of death** for pediatric cardiac ECMO patients.[2,12,23,27,28] Attempts to improve results achieved with pediatric cardiac ECMO should address issues related to optimization of ventricular function and avoidance of extended periods of low cardiac output. Prompt institution of ECMO achieves both of these goals by optimally preserving myocardial, central nervous system, and visceral perfusion. Allowing patients to continue in a low cardiac output state on increasing doses of vasoconstrictive agents before ECMO may lead to established end-organ damage, which may not be reversible. When ECMO is initiated, meticulous patient management is required to limit infectious complications, which may contribute to an ongoing clinical picture of sepsis that commonly progresses to multisystem organ failure. For salvage of continuing severe cardiac dysfunction, an early and aggressive approach to cardiac transplantation may be the only lifesaving therapy available.

Special Topics in Pediatric Cardiac Extracorporeal Membrane Oxygenation

Cardiac arrest is a common indication for pediatric cardiac ECMO, constituting nearly 25% of all indications for ECMO in these patients.[2] Several groups have developed systems that allow the expeditious institution of ECMO for children with cardiac disease who experience cardiac arrest refractory to conventional resuscitation measures.[8,30,31]

One such system uses a modified ECMO circuit, an organized team of personnel to perform cannulation, and a streamlined priming process.[30] The "rapid resuscitation" ECMO circuit is maintained vacuum and carbon dioxide-primed in the ICU and is portable with a battery power supply allowing it to be set up quickly in any location throughout the hospital. If standard cardiopulmonary resuscitation (CPR) is unsuccessful within 10 minutes of cardiac arrest, the circuit is moved to the patient's bedside, and crystalloid priming is initiated while cannulation is proceeding. If cannulation is completed before the availability of blood products, ECMO is initiated with a crystalloid-primed circuit, and blood products are added when available. The excess crystalloid volume is removed as blood is added to the circuit using exchange transfusions by hand and performing ultrafiltration after the hemodynamics have stabilized. Establishing a normal cardiac output with ECMO is the most critical factor for successful resuscitation of these children, even if the hematocrit is low at the time support is instituted as a result of the use of a crystalloid-primed circuit.

This approach was used for 11 pediatric patients who had a cardiac arrest; 9 of these children were postoperative cardiac surgical patients, 1 child had cardiac arrest before surgery, and 1 child had cardiac arrest in the cardiac catheterization laboratory.[30] All patients were undergoing CPR at the time of ECMO cannulation. The median duration of CPR for these 11 patients was 55 minutes (range 15 to 103 minutes) compared with a median duration of CPR of 90 minutes (range 45 to 200 minutes) for 7 historical controls rescued with ECMO before the use of the rapid resuscitation system. All but 1 of the 11 rapid resuscitation patients could be weaned from ECMO, with 7 patients (64%) surviving to hospital discharge compared with 2 survivors (29%) of the 7 historical controls.

Jacobs and coworkers[8] reported results for a particularly innovative rapid resuscitation system that uses a hollow-fiber oxygenator to facilitate priming. The circuit employs a centrifugal pump and short lengths of quarter-inch tubing and is heparin bonded throughout.

This system is fully portable and requires a priming volume of 250 mL. The use of the centrifugal pump eliminates the need for gravity drainage, which results in shorter tubing lengths and greater portability. The simplicity of the circuit facilitates priming and minimizes trauma to blood elements, whereas the heparin bonding results in less blood loss. The authors reported their results with this system in 23 children with cardiac disease, most of whom were supported after cardiac surgery. All patients had support instituted with a crystalloid-primed circuit. The simplicity of this system and avoidance of the blood priming step enabled setup time to be only 5 minutes. The duration of CPR was only 12 minutes for the four patients in this series who had cardiac arrest before cannulation. Using this system, the overall survival in this series was 48% with all four of the cardiac arrest patients surviving to hospital discharge.

These reports support the concept that pediatric cardiac patients who experience cardiac arrest are often salvageable and warrant an aggressive approach with prompt institution of ECMO if conventional resuscitative measures fail. Rapid institution of circulatory support with modified ECMO systems can be lifesaving with preservation of end-organ function in these patients.

Indications for the institution of ECMO in patients with **myocarditis** should be based on the clinical response to ICU management. Most patients who are considered for ECMO support are receiving high-dose inotrope infusions with endotracheal intubation and muscle paralysis. If evidence of a low cardiac output state persists despite routine measures, clinically manifest as oliguria, poor cutaneous perfusion, and hypotension, ECMO should be strongly considered. The need for escalating inotrope doses accompanied by widened QRS complexes or significant ventricular ectopy, or both, is an especially lethal combination that suggests mechanical circulatory support is required because of the tendency of these patients to develop sudden and intractable ventricular fibrillation.

The survival rate for children who require mechanical circulatory support for myocarditis is relatively good in most reports.[10,32-37] A recent multi-institution review of 15 patients with viral myocarditis supported by ECMO (12 patients) or VADs (3 patients) showed an overall survival rate of 80%.[38] In this experience, ECMO was believed to be a better choice than VAD for acute support in these children because of the option of peripheral cannulation, maintaining an intact chest cavity. Nine of the 15 patients were weaned from support with 7 survivors (78%), whereas the remaining 6 patients were successfully bridged to transplantation with 5 survivors (83%). An especially important finding was that all non-transplanted survivors are currently alive with normal ventricular function. Historically, it was believed that a significant percentage of children with acute myocarditis would be expected to develop dilated cardiomyopathy with the ultimate need for cardiac transplantation.[39] This study suggests that children with acute, fulminant myocarditis have an overall favorable outcome and a significant degree of disease reversibility if successfully supported during the acute phase of illness.

The reasons for better long-term outcomes and a decreased incidence of progression to dilated cardiomyopathy in patients most severely affected with myocarditis remain unexplained; however, mechanical circulatory support may contribute to the improved long-term outcomes in these children. In patients with dilated cardiomyopathy, prolonged mechanical circulatory support may result in ultimate recovery of ventricular function owing to favorable influences on the neurohormonal cardiovascular milieu and unloading of the left ventricle resulting in normalization of ventricular geometry through "reverse remodeling."[40] The institution of mechanical circulatory support in patients with acute fulminant myocarditis can have a favorable impact on these same factors, resulting in ventricular recovery over a much shorter time course—a process that has been described as "rapid reverse remodeling."[38] In these most severe cases of myocarditis, mechanical circulatory support provides the ultimate form of physiologic rest similar to simple bed rest and oxygen used to support less severe cases. It is compelling to speculate that normalization of ventricular geometry and function by the early institution of support may help to prevent the development of dilated cardiomyopathy.

Based on these results, the optimal approach for children presenting with acute fulminant myocarditis may be to provide mechanical circulatory support, even if required for prolonged periods, in anticipation of eventual ventricular recovery. Previous reports have documented full return of ventricular function in young adults with myocarditis after weeks or months of mechanical support.[41,42] Pulsatile paracorporeal or implantable VAD systems, which allow extended periods of support, have been used successfully in pediatric patients in Europe and have shown the feasibility of this approach.[43,44] Prolonged mechanical circulatory support in a larger number of pediatric patients with fulminant myocarditis may reveal that the capability of supporting these children for weeks or months would allow return of native ventricular function, avoiding transplantation in virtually all of these children.

ECMO support may be used in pediatric **cardiac transplantation** patients as a bridge to transplantation; as perioperative support, especially in the presence of elevated pulmonary vascular resistance; and during rejection episodes. The use of ECMO as a bridge to pediatric cardiac transplantation is especially well summarized in two reviews.[35,36] del Nido and colleagues[36] reported the University of Pittsburgh experience in which 14 patients were placed on ECMO as a bridge to transplantation. This group consisted of postcardiotomy patients with profound ventricular dysfunction, patients with dilated cardiomyopathy, and patients with acute myocarditis. Nine of these 14 patients (64%) were successfully transplanted after an average of 109 hours of ECMO support on the cardiac transplantation list, with 6 patients surviving to hospital discharge. Frazier and associates[35] reviewed the experience at Arkansas Children's Hospital using ECMO as a bridge to cardiac transplantation in 17 patients. Fifteen of these 17 patients were successfully bridged to transplantation (12 patients) or recovered spontaneously (3 patients), whereas 2 patients died while awaiting transplantation on ECMO support. The duration of ECMO support often was quite prolonged in this experience, with a median duration of 269 hours (range 35 to 1078 hours). Meticulous management led to low infection rates despite prolonged periods of support with only one patient developing significant infection requiring removal from the transplantation list. Both of these studies emphasize the need for aggressive treatment of left ventricular distention with atrial septostomy or direct venting because these patients are most prone to develop left-sided distention due to their severe degree of ventricular impairment. Untreated, left-sided distention in these patients may lead to pulmonary edema and hemorrhage, precluding cardiac transplantation should a donor organ become available. Other management techniques used by these successful programs include rigorous patient selection before bridging is initiated and consideration of donors over a broad size range to increase the potential donor pool.

The use of ECMO for postoperative support at the time of cardiac transplantation in children is most often for the treatment of pulmonary hypertension or graft dysfunction in the early postoperative period. Galantowicz[5] reported a multicenter analysis with a 40% success rate in salvaging children who required ECMO in the immediate postoperative period after cardiac transplantation. Other reports with smaller numbers have shown similar results.[2,46] Severe, acute rejection episodes after cardiac transplantation are characterized by rapid deterioration with ECMO providing temporary, lifesaving support until antirejection therapy becomes effective.[45,46]

CENTRIFUGAL VENTRICULAR ASSIST DEVICE SUPPORT FOR THE ACUTELY FAILING PEDIATRIC CIRCULATION

Technical Aspects and Patient Management

The discussion on VAD support is brief because Chapter 47 is devoted to this topic. Historically, centrifugal pump VAD has been the mainstay of pediatric VAD technology. The Bio-Pump (Medtronic BioMedicus, Minneapolis, MN) employs a constrained vortex design to provide flow with power provided by a rotating magnet on the drive console translated to an opposing magnet on a cone-shaped impeller in the pump head.

The impeller produces negative pressure at the apical inlet of the pump head housing and ejects blood tangentially through the outlet cannula at the base of the pump. There are no valves in the system and no obligatory volume displacement by the pump, which results in nonpulsatile flow that is preload and afterload sensitive. The VAD circuit based on this pump is simple and does not contain reservoirs or an oxygenator, allowing priming volumes of 100 mL or less compared with ECMO priming volumes, which often are greater than 300 mL.[2,8] Relatively short tubing segments are used to connect the venous drainage cannula to the pump inlet and the aortic cannula to the pump outlet. Circuit monitors include inlet and outlet pressure monitors and an in-line arterial flow probe.[47]

The Bio-Pump is suitable for use as a right VAD, left VAD, or biventricular VAD; however, most pediatric usage has been configured as a left VAD.[47-49] Biventricular support requires four cannulation sites, which, because of size constraints, is especially cumbersome in infants, in whom biventricular support is most easily provided by ECMO. For left VAD support, the left atrium is cannulated through the appendage or anterior to the right pulmonary veins, whereas arterial cannulation is achieved via the ascending aorta. Single ventricle patients, such as patients with hypoplastic left heart syndrome after the Norwood procedure, can be supported with a VAD instituted via right atrial and aortic cannulation. Because pulmonary and systemic blood flow are provided by VAD, this is analogous to biventricular VAD for two-ventricle patients or ECMO with the patient's own lungs serving as the oxygenator.[50] In the presence of shunt-dependent pulmonary blood flow, increased flow rates 150% of normal cardiac output may be necessary to provide adequate systemic perfusion.[47] As discussed previously, a major safety advantage of the centrifugal pump is that distal occlusion does not result in high positive pressure and the potential for circuit "blow-out." In addition, because venous return is ensured by negative pressure at the pump inlet, the device may be placed at any height in relation to the patient; however, careful monitoring of inlet pressure is essential to avoid excessively negative pressures that might lead to cavitation and hemolysis. Maintaining inlet pressures greater than −20 mm Hg minimizes hemolysis with this system.[47]

Clinical Experience
Reports using the Bio-Pump predominately as a left VAD have shown survival rates of 40% to 70%.[2,51-54] The experience at The Royal Children's Hospital in Melbourne in the period between 1988 and 1998 consisted of 53 children with an average age of 3.5 months and an average weight of 4 kg.[47] Postoperative support for the Norwood procedure, for the arterial switch operation, for aortic root procedures, and for operations performed to treat anomalous coronary artery from the pulmonary artery constituted the largest diagnostic categories.

Of these patients, 38 (72%) were weaned from VAD support, and 24 (46%) survived to hospital discharge with all but 1 patient who survived to discharge surviving during the first year of follow-up. This sharp decline in hazard function at the point of hospital discharge has been reported previously during the long-term follow-up of ECMO-supported and VAD-supported pediatric cardiac patients.[55,56] The authors found that the Bio-Pump left VAD was particularly useful for patients who required support after operations for anomalous left coronary artery from the pulmonary artery, with all five of the patients in this category surviving. Similarly, for patients with transposition of the great arteries, intact ventricular septum, and a deconditioned left ventricle because of late presentation for the arterial switch operation, short-term left VAD was highly successful in supporting the circulation until left ventricular recovery occurred. Finally, the authors successfully used a left VAD after cardiac transplantation when ischemic time was prolonged or configured the device as a right VAD in cases of pulmonary hypertension and right ventricular failure.

As a result of previous reports suggesting that infants and small children are better managed with ECMO, the Melbourne group analyzed their results using the Bio-Pump in 34 infants weighing 6 kg or less (average age 60 days [range 2 to 258 days]; average weight 3.7 kg [range 1.9 to 5.98 kg]).[57] Sixty-three percent were successfully weaned from VAD support, and 31% of this difficult patient population survived to hospital discharge.

The Boston experience consisted of 32 Bio-Pump VAD runs in 29 patients, most (75%) of which were left VADs, whereas 6 were right VADs, and 2 were biventricular VADs.[2] Two thirds of patients were successfully weaned from support. Forty percent of all patients survived to hospital discharge. These rates of weaning and survival were nearly identical to the rates observed in a concurrent group of ECMO-supported patients. Anomalous coronary artery from the pulmonary artery and cardiomyopathy were the most common diagnoses supported with VAD in this report. In addition, these diagnoses attained the highest rates of survival compared with other diagnostic groups, with 71% and 60% survival rates, respectively. Similar to other reports, hemorrhage was the most common complication seen in VAD-supported patients, whereas central nervous system complications occurred significantly less often than in ECMO-supported patients. This trend, observed during the hospital course of these patients, also was seen in the long-term follow-up of this cohort; the ECMO-supported patients were significantly more likely to show neurologic impairment than were the VAD-supported patients.[55,56] Selection issues exist in that the ECMO-supported patients tended to be younger with a higher percentage of newborns; however, the greater complexity of the ECMO circuit may have contributed as well.[2] The presence of an oxygenator and longer tubing lengths may have provided the substrate for cerebral embolic events, whereas the generally higher level of anticoagulation compared with that employed for VAD may have caused a higher incidence of intracranial hemorrhage. In addition to these clinical reports, numerous other studies exist that have described the utility of centrifugal VAD to support the entire spectrum of pediatric cardiac disease.[5,28,49,51-54,58-60]

INTRA-AORTIC BALLOON PUMP SUPPORT FOR THE ACUTELY FAILING PEDIATRIC CIRCULATION

Technical Aspects and Patient Management

Although part of the standard armamentarium for treating myocardial failure secondary to acquired cardiovascular disease in adults, the use of IABP to treat cardiac failure in children has been limited. The reasons for this are discussed subsequently; however, with current technology, IABP is perhaps an underused modality, especially in the acute management of cardiac failure in older children and adolescents. The first reported series of IABP use in children was from Toronto in 1980.[61] Since then, Primary Children's Medical Center in Salt Lake City has been the dominant force in the development of pediatric IABP in the laboratory and clinical settings.[62-67]

Figure 46-3 shows the impact of balloon counterpulsation on the aortic pressure curve with the primary effects of reduction of systolic pressure and augmentation of diastolic pressure. The physiologic results of these alterations in aortic pressure include a decrease in left ventricular afterload and improved coronary arterial blood flow. The full range of physiologic effects from

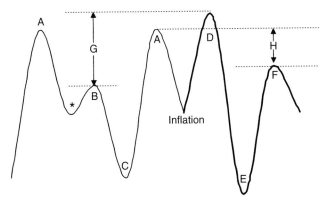

FIGURE 46-3 ■ Impact of balloon counterpulsation on the aortic pressure curve. The impact of balloon counterpulsation on the aortic pressure curve with the primary effects of reduction of systolic pressure and augmentation of diastolic pressure. An arterial line tracing is depicted without an intra-aortic balloon pump *(thin line)* and with an intra-aortic balloon pump **(thick line)**. **A,** Unassisted systolic pressure. **B,** Unassisted diastolic pressure. **C,** Unassisted aortic end-diastolic pressure. **D,** Assisted diastolic pressure. **E,** Assisted aortic end-diastolic pressure. **F,** Assisted systolic pressure. **G,** Diastolic augmentation. **H,** Reduction in systolic pressure. Optimal balloon timing occurs when inflation begins at the dicrotic notch (*).

TABLE 46-1

Physiologic Effects of the Intra-aortic Balloon Pump
Aortic Pressure
↓ SBP
↑ DBP
Left Ventricular Pressure
↓ LVESP
↓ LVEDP
Ventricular Loading
↓ Preload
↓ Afterload
Blood Flow in Vascular Beds
↑ Coronary blood flow
↑ Renal blood flow
Cardiac
↑ CO
↓ PAP
↓ LVEDV
↓ Stroke work
↓ Wall tension

CO, cardiac output; DBP, diastolic blood pressure; LVEDP, left ventricular end-diastolic pressure; LVEDV, left ventricular end-diastolic volume; LVESP, left ventricular end-systolic pressure; PAP, pulmonary artery pressure; SBP, systolic blood pressure.

IABP is shown in Table 46-1. Although the benefit of IABP in the treatment of ischemic heart disease in adults has been well established, anatomic and physiologic differences that exist in congenital heart disease have resulted in less benefit and higher complication rates for IABP therapy in children (Table 46-2). Vascular access remains a problem for pediatric IABP; to minimize ischemic complications, Hawkins and coworkers[67,68] advocated introduction of the balloon through a polytetrafluoroethylene (PTFE) side-arm graft anastomosed to the femoral artery. Direct cannulation of the ascending aorta[69] or external iliac artery[70] also may provide access for the device; however, the lack of a method for percutaneous insertion has been a limitation for IABP use in infants and small children. Balloon timing also has been a problem in pediatrics because of higher heart rates, which may be difficult for the device to track. Minich and associates[63] described the use of M-mode echocardiography to image simultaneously the aortic

TABLE 46-2

Limitations of the Intra-aortic Balloon Pump for Pediatric Use
Limited access through small femoral vessels
Decreased effectiveness of counterpulsation due to compliance of the pediatric aorta
Difficulty with device triggering and timing at high heart rates
Low incidence of ischemic heart disease
Greater incidence of right ventricular and biventricular failure

valve and the balloon, which allowed balloon inflation and deflation to be performed with precision at the time of closing and opening of the aortic valve. Although providing balloon timing with a high degree of accuracy, this approach does not lend itself easily to continuous monitoring and may be too complex for widespread application. IABP effectively treats left ventricular failure resulting from ischemic causes; however, a final limitation for pediatric IABP arises from its inability to treat right ventricular failure, hypoxemia, and pulmonary hypertension, which commonly cause cardiorespiratory failure in children.[1,2,71]

Currently available balloons for pediatric use have volumes of 2.5, 5, 7, 12, and 20 cc with corresponding balloon diameters ranging from 6 to 12 mm and balloon lengths ranging from 10.7 to 19.4 cm (Datascope Corp, Fairfield, NJ). The selection of the appropriate balloon size is determined from the child's estimated stroke volume and should be approximately 40% to 60% of the normal stroke volume.[67,68]

Clinical Experience

The Royal Liverpool Children's Hospital reported their pediatric IABP experience, which consisted of 14 children whose average age was 3 years (range 7 days to 13 years).[69] The indications for support included deterioration in the ICU (n=7), failure to wean from cardiopulmonary bypass (n=5), and prophylactic insertion in the operating room in two patients with poor left ventricular function. Insertion was performed via the ascending aorta in the five smallest patients (average weight 4.5 kg), whereas the remainder had insertion via the femoral artery either directly by cut-down (n=6) or by placement of a PTFE side-arm graft (n=3). Ten of the 14 patients (71%) were weaned from IABP with 8 (57%) long-term survivors. The authors stated that increased aortic compliance in children does not lessen significantly the benefits of counterpulsation. In this series, supersystemic diastolic augmentation as seen in adult IABP use did not occur even at maximal augmentation; however, there was still an increase in the diastolic pressure-time index leading to increased myocardial oxygen supply, whereas the tension-time index was decreased, resulting in decreased myocardial oxygen demand. Generally, the clinical impact of these changes allowed lowering of inotropic dosage to decrease myocardial oxygen demand further while improving systemic perfusion.[69]

Pinkney and colleagues[67] reported 29 children supported with IABP at Primary Children's Medical Center over a 12-year period. The median age was 4 years (range 51 days to 18.5 years); 16 (55%) cases were postoperative cardiac surgical patients, 7 (24%) cases were a bridge to transplantation, and 6 (21%) were nonsurgical cases. All insertions were via the common femoral artery through a side-arm graft of 3.5- to 4-mm PTFE with anticoagulation achieved by using intravenous heparin to maintain a partial thromboplastin time of

40 to 60 seconds. Because of their small size, pediatric balloons do not contain a central pressure monitoring lumen. The authors previously had shown timing errors when based on tracings from a radial arterial line, which made the adjustment of timing for optimal counterpulsation particularly difficult in children.[63] For these reasons, the authors used M-mode echocardiography to determine optimal IABP timing as described earlier. Weaning in this series occurred over 24 to 48 hours by decreasing the inflation frequency progressively from 1:1, then 1:2, and then 1:3, followed by balloon removal. The authors reported no episodes of limb ischemia or other significant complications that required balloon removal. The overall survival rate in this group was 62% with no difference in survival between infants and older children.

DEVICE SELECTION FOR THE ACUTELY FAILING PEDIATRIC CIRCULATION

Table 46-3 summarizes the advantages and disadvantages of each of these modalities. Perhaps the biggest advantage for ECMO in acute pediatric circulatory support is the familiarity that most pediatric centers have with this modality. Although VAD is simpler than ECMO and IABP is simpler still, instituting support ultimately may be easier for ECMO via peripheral cannulation than it is for VAD, which requires sternotomy, or IABP, which often requires a side-arm graft. In addition, if M-mode echocardiography is employed for device timing, maintenance and monitoring of IABP may become more cumbersome. Unloading of the left ventricle is best accomplished by direct cannulation with left VAD, although IABP also substantially unloads the left ventricle. ECMO may provide the same benefit if flows are increased to minimize left heart return, whereas direct cannulation of the left atrium during ECMO support is another alternative to provide left ventricular decompression. Only ECMO with an oxygenator in the circuit treats pulmonary hypertension and hypoxemia; conditions that are complicated by these features should not be treated with VAD or IABP. Finally, biventricular

TABLE 46-3

Summary of Advantages and Disadvantages for IABP, VAD, and ECMO			
	IABP	VAD	ECMO
Experience in pediatric centers	–	–	+++
Simplicity of circuit	+++	++	
Ease of device institution	+	+	++
Left ventricular decompression	++	+++	+
Treatment of pulmonary hypertension/hypoxia	–	–	+++
Biventricular support in neonates	–	+	+++

support may be instituted with either ECMO or biventricular VAD; however, because of size constraints, newborns and small infants who require biventricular support are best treated with ECMO because of the need for only two cannulation sites as opposed to the four cannulation sites required for biventricular VAD.

CURRENT STATUS AND FUTURE TRENDS

These acute cardiopulmonary support devices will continue to undergo technologic modifications to lessen the need for anticoagulation and decrease potential complications. Future application of these existing devices will become more common, even for indications that have not had large clinical experiences to date, such as sepsis.[72] Lastly, the need for more long-term cardiopulmonary support devices in pediatric patients will continue to grow, and these more long-term devices will need to be part of the already complex decision-making process in the acute setting.[73]

Key Concepts

■ For adults in the acute setting, left ventricular failure resulting from coronary artery disease has been managed with IABP and left VAD insertion. In children, isolated left ventricular failure is relatively rare, however, whereas right ventricular failure, pulmonary hypertension, and hypoxemia often contribute significantly to circulatory failure that arises secondary to congenital heart disease. Because of these physiologic differences, isolated support of the left ventricle by IABP or left VAD has more limited application in children.

■ Centrifugal pumps maintain venous inflow independent of gravity drainage, making a bladder box unnecessary and allowing the patient to be positioned at any height relative to the pump. An additional advantage of the centrifugal pump is that, in contrast to the roller pump, occlusion of arterial outflow does not generate excessive arterial line pressure, reducing the risk of "blow-out" of the arterial limb of the circuit if distal occlusion occurs.

■ Lack of return of ventricular function within 48 to 72 hours was identified as a risk factor in patients supported after cardiac surgery, which has important implications for consideration of cardiac transplantation in these children. Postcardiotomy patients without return of ventricular function within 48 to 72 hours of support should be considered for transplantation or termination of support if there are contraindications to transplantation.

■ Indications for the institution of ECMO in patients with myocarditis should be based on the clinical response to ICU management. The need for escalating inotrope doses accompanied by widened QRS complexes or significant ventricular ectopy or both is

an especially lethal combination that suggests mechanical circulatory support is required because of the tendency of these patients to develop sudden and intractable ventricular fibrillation.

■ ECMO support may be used in pediatric cardiac transplantation patients as a bridge to transplantation; as perioperative support, especially in the presence of elevated pulmonary vascular resistance; and during rejection episodes.

■ With current technology, IABP is perhaps an underused modality, especially in the acute management of cardiac failure in older children and adolescents.

■ Perhaps the biggest advantage for ECMO in acute pediatric circulatory support is the familiarity that most pediatric centers have with this modality. Although VAD is simpler than ECMO and IABP is simpler still, instituting support ultimately may be easier for ECMO via peripheral cannulation than it is for VAD, which requires sternotomy, or IABP, which often requires a side-arm graft.

REFERENCES

1. Duncan BW: Mechanical circulatory support for infants and children with cardiac disease. Ann Thorac Surg 2002;73:1670.
2. Duncan BW, Hraska V, Jonas RA, et al: Mechanical circulatory support in children with cardiac disease. J Thorac Cardiovasc Surg 1999;117:529.
3. Trittenwein G, Furst G, Golej J, et al: Preoperative ECMO in congenital cyanotic heart disease using the AREC system. Ann Thorac Surg 1997;63:1298.
4. del Nido PJ: Extracorporeal membrane oxygenation for cardiac support in children. Ann Thorac Surg 1996;61:336.
5. Langley SM, Sheppard SB, Tsang VT, et al: When is extracorporeal life support worthwhile following repair of congenital heart disease in children? Eur J Cardiothorac Surg 1998;13:520.
6. Saito A, Miyamura H, Kanazawa H, et al: Extracorporeal membrane oxygenation for severe heart failure after Fontan operation. Ann Thorac Surg 1993;55:153.
7. Willms DC, Atkins PJ, Dembitsky WP, et al: Analysis of clinical trends in a program of emergent ECLS for cardiovascular collapse. ASAIO J 1997;43:65.
8. Jacobs JP, Ojito JW, McConaghey TW, et al: Rapid cardiopulmonary support for children with complex congenital heart disease. Ann Thorac Surg 2000;70:742.
9. Hirschl RB: Devices. In Zwischenberger JB, Bartlett RH (eds): ECMO: Extracorporeal Cardiopulmonary Support in Critical Care. Ann Arbor, Mich, Extracorporeal Life Support Organization, 1995, pp 150-190.
10. Black MD, Coles JG, Williams WG, et al: Determinants of success in pediatric cardiac patients undergoing extracorporeal membrane oxygenation. Ann Thorac Surg 1995;60:133.
11. Dalton HJ, Siewers RD, Fuhrman BP, et al: Extracorporeal membrane oxygenation for cardiac rescue in children with severe myocardial dysfunction. Crit Care Med 1993;21:1020.
12. Kanter KR, Pennington DG, Weber TR, et al: Extracorporeal membrane oxygenation for postoperative cardiac support in children. J Thorac Cardiovasc Surg 1987;93:27.
13. Klein MD, Shaheen KW, Whittlesey GC, et al: Extracorporeal membrane oxygenation for the circulatory support of children after repair of congenital heart disease. J Thorac Cardiovasc Surg 1990;100:498.

14. Delius RE, Bove EL, Meliones JN, et al: Use of extracorporeal life support in patients with congenital heart disease. Crit Care Med 1992;20:1216.

15. O'Connor TA, Downing GJ, Ewing LL, et al: Echocardiographically guided balloon atrial septostomy during extracorporeal membrane oxygenation (ECMO). Pediatr Cardiol 1993;14:167.

16. Koenig PR, Ralston MA, Kimball TR, et al: Balloon atrial septostomy for left ventricular decompression in patients receiving extracorporeal membrane oxygenation for myocardial failure. J Pediatr 1993; 122:S95.

17. Anderson HL, Attori RJ, Custer JR, et al: Extracorporeal membrane oxygenation for pediatric cardiopulmonary failure. J Thorac Cardiovasc Surg 1990;99:1011.

18. Raithel RC, Pennington DG, Boegner E, et al: Extracorporeal membrane oxygenation in children after cardiac surgery. Circulation 1992;86(Suppl II):II-305.

19. Wilson JM, Bower LK, Fackler JC, et al: Aminocaproic acid decreases the incidence of intracranial hemorrhage and other hemorrhagic complications of ECMO. J Pediatr Surg 1993; 28:536.

20. Kinsella JP, Gerstmann DR, Rosenberg AA: The effect of extracorporeal membrane oxygenation on coronary perfusion and regional blood flow distribution. Pediatr Res 1992;31:80.

21. Secker-Walker JS, Edmonds JF, Spratt EH, et al: The source of coronary perfusion during partial bypass for extracorporeal membrane oxygenation (ECMO). Ann Thorac Surg 1976;21:138.

22. Walters HL, Hakimi M, Rice MD, et al: Pediatric cardiac surgical ECMO: Multivariate analysis of risk factors for hospital death. Ann Thorac Surg 1995;60:329.

23. Meliones JN, Custer JR, Snedecor S, et al: Extracorporeal life support for cardiac assist in pediatric patients. Circulation 1991; 84(Suppl III):168.

24. Hunkeler NM, Canter CE, Donze A, et al: Extracorporeal life support in cyanotic congenital heart disease before cardiovascular operation. Am J Cardiol 1992;69:790.

25. Rogers AJ, Trento A, Siewers RD, et al: Extracorporeal membrane oxygenation for postcardiotomy cardiogenic shock in children. Ann Thorac Surg 1989;47:903.

26. Weinhaus L, Canter C, Noetzel M, et al: Extracorporeal membrane oxygenation for circulatory support after repair of congenital heart defects. Ann Thorac Surg 1989;48:206.

27. Ziomek S, Harrell JE, Fasules JW, et al: Extracorporeal membrane oxygenation for cardiac failure after congenital heart operation. Ann Thorac Surg 1992;54:861.

28. Ferrazzi P, Glauber M, DiDomenico A, et al: Assisted circulation for myocardial recovery after repair of congenital heart disease. Eur J Cardiothorac Surg 1991;5:419.

29. Trento A, Thompson A, Siewers RD, et al: Extracorporeal membrane oxygenation in children. J Thorac Cardiovasc Surg 1988; 96:542.

30. Duncan BW, Ibrahim AE, Hraska V, et al: Use of rapid-deployment extracorporeal membrane oxygenation for the resuscitation of pediatric patients with heart disease after cardiac arrest. J Thorac Cardiovasc Surg 1998;116:305.

31. del Nido PJ, Dalton HJ, Thompson AE, et al: Extracorporeal membrane oxygenator rescue in children during cardiac arrest after cardiac surgery. Circulation 1992;86(Suppl II):II-300.

32. Cofer BR, Warner BW, Stallion A, et al: Extracorporeal membrane oxygenation in the management of cardiac failure secondary to myocarditis. J Pediatr Surg 1993;28:669.

33. Grundl PD, Miller SA, del Nido PJ, et al: Successful treatment of acute myocarditis using extracorporeal membrane oxygenation. Crit Care Med 1993;21:302.

34. Kawahito K, Murata S, Yasu T, et al: Usefulness of extracorporeal membrane oxygenation for treatment of fulminant myocarditis and circulatory collapse. Am J Cardiol 1998;82:910.

35. Frazier EA, Faulkner SC, Seib PM, et al: Prolonged extracorporeal life support for bridging to transplant. Perfusion 1997;12:93.

36. del Nido PJ, Armitage JM, Fricker FJ, et al: Extracorporeal membrane oxygenation support as a bridge to pediatric heart transplantation. Circulation 1994;90:II-66.

37. Martin J, Sarai K, Schindler M, et al: Medos HIA-VAD biventricular assist device for bridge to recovery in fulminant myocarditis. Ann Thorac Surg 1997;63:1145.

38. Duncan BW, Bohn DJ, Atz AM, et al: Mechanical circulatory support for the treatment of children with acute fulminant myocarditis. J Thorac Cardiovasc Surg 2001;122:440.

39. Greenwood RD, Nadas AS, Fyler DC: The clinical course of primary myocardial disease in infants and children. Am Heart J 1976;5:549.

40. Levin GR, Oz MC, Chen JM, et al: Reversal of chronic ventricular dilation in patients with end-stage cardiomyopathy by prolonged mechanical unloading. Circulation 1995;91:2717.

41. Holman WL, Bourge RC, Kirklin JK: Circulatory support for seventy days with resolution of acute heart failure. J Thorac Cardiovasc Surg 1991;102:932.

42. Levin HR, Oz MC, Catanese KA, et al: Transient normalization of systolic and diastolic function after support with a left ventricular assist device in a patient with dilated cardiomyopathy. J Heart Lung Transplant 1996;15:840.

43. Konertz W, Hotz H, Schneider M, et al: Clinical experience with the MEDOS HIA-VAD system in infants and children. Ann Thorac Surg 1997;63:1138.

44. Stiller B, Dahnert I, Weng Y, et al: Children may survive severe myocarditis with prolonged use of biventricular assist devices. Heart 1999;82:237.

45. Galantowicz ME, Stolar CJH: Extracorporeal membrane oxygenation for perioperative support in pediatric heart transplantation. J Thorac Cardiovasc Surg 1991;102:148.

46. Delius RE, Zwischenberger JB, Cilley R, et al: Prolonged extracorporeal life support of pediatric and adolescent cardiac transplant patients. Ann Thorac Surg 1990;50:791.

47. Karl TR, Horton SB: Centrifugal pump ventricular assist device in pediatric cardiac surgery. In Duncan BW (ed): Mechanical Support for Cardiac and Respiratory Failure in Pediatric Cardiac Patients. New York, Marcel Dekker, 2001, pp 21-47.

48. Pennington DG, Swartz MT: Circulatory support in infants and children. Ann Thorac Surg 1993;55:233.

49. Karl TR: Extracorporeal circulatory support in infants and children. Semin Thorac Cardiovasc Surg 1994;6:154.

50. Darling EM, Kaemmer D, Lawson DS, et al: Use of ECMO without the oxygenator to provide ventricular support after Norwood Stage I procedures. Ann Thorac Surg 2001;71:735.

51. Ashton RC, Oz MC, Michler RE, et al: Left ventricular assist device options in pediatric patients. ASAIO J 1995;41:M277.

52. Costa RJ, Chard RB, Nunn GR, et al: Ventricular assist devices in pediatric cardiac surgery. Ann Thorac Surg 1995;60:S536.

53. Karl TR, Sano S, Horton S, et al: Centrifugal pump left heart assist in pediatric cardiac operations: Indication, technique, and results. J Thorac Cardiovasc Surg 1991;102:624.

54. Scheinin SA, Radovancevic B, Parnis SM, et al: Mechanical circulatory support in children. Eur J Cardiothorac Surg 1994;8:537.

55. Ibrahim AE, Duncan BW, Blume ED, et al: Long-term follow-up of pediatric cardiac patients requiring mechanical circulatory support. Ann Thorac Surg 2000;69:186.

56. Ibrahim AE, Duncan BW: Long-term follow-up of children with cardiac disease requiring mechanical circulatory support. In Duncan BW (ed): Mechanical Circulatory Support for Cardiac and Respiratory Failure in Pediatric Cardiac Patients. New York, Marcel Dekker, 2001, pp 205-220.

57. Thuys CA, Mullaly RJ, Horton SB, et al: Centrifugal ventricular assist in children under 6 kg. Eur J Cardiothorac Surg 1998;13:130.

58. Kesler KA, Pruitt AL, Turrentine MW, et al: Temporary left-sided mechanical cardiac support during acute myocarditis. J Heart Lung Transplant 1994;13:268.

59. Khan A, Gazzaniga AB: Mechanical circulatory assistance in paediatric patients with cardiac failure. Cardiovasc Surg 1996;4:43.

60. Chang AC, Hanley FL, Weindling SN, et al: Left heart support with a ventricular assist device in an infant with acute myocarditis. Crit Care Med 1992;20:712.

61. Pollock JC, Charlton MC, Williams WG, et al: Intra-aortic balloon pumping in children. Ann Thorac Surg 1980;29:522.

62. Veasy LG, Blalock RC, Orth JL, et al: Intra-aortic balloon pumping in infants and children. Circulation 1983;68:1095.

63. Minich LL, Tani LY, McGough EC, et al: A novel approach to pediatric intra-aortic balloon pump timing using M-mode echocardiography. Am J Cardiol 1997;80:367.

64. Minich LL, Tani LY, Pantalos GM, et al: Neonatal piglet model of intraaortic balloon pumping: Improved efficacy using echocardiographic timing. Ann Thorac Surg 1998;66:1527.

65. Minich LL, Tani LY, Hawkins JA, et al: Intra-aortic balloon pumping in children with dilated cardiomyopathy as a bridge to transplantation. J Heart Lung Transplant 2001;20:750.

66. Pantalos GM, Minich LL, Tani LY, et al: Estimation of timing errors for the intra-aortic balloon pump use in pediatric patients. ASAIO J 1999;45:166.

67. Pinkney KA, Minich LL, Tani LY, et al: Current results with intra-aortic balloon pumping in infants and children. Ann Thorac Surg 2002;73:887.

68. Hawkins JA, Minich LL: Intra-aortic balloon counterpulsation for children with cardiac disease. In Duncan BW (ed): Mechanical Support for Cardiac and Respiratory Failure in Pediatric Cardiac Patients. New York, Marcel Dekker, 2001, pp 49-60.

69. Akomea-Agyin C, Kejriwal NK, Franks R, et al: Intra-aortic balloon pumping in children. Ann Thorac Surg 1999;67:1415.

70. del Nido PJ, Swan PR, Benson LN, et al: Successful use of intra-aortic balloon pumping in a 2-kilogram infant. Ann Thorac Surg 1988;46:574.

71. Duncan BW: Extracorporeal membrane oxygenation versus ventricular assist device support for children with cardiac disease. In Duncan BW (ed): Mechanical Circulatory Support for Cardiac and Respiratory Failure in Pediatric Cardiac Patients. New York, Marcel Dekker, 2001, pp 61-74.

72. Pathan N, Hemingway CA, Alizadeh AA, et al: Role of interleukin 6 in myocardial dysfunction of meningococcus septic shock. Lancet 2004;363:203-209.

73. Chang AC, McKenzie ED: Mechanical cardiopulmonary support in children and young adults: Extracorporeal membrane oxygenation, ventricular assist devices, and long term support devices. Pediatr Cardiol 2005;26:2-28.

CHAPTER 47

Ventricular Assist Device Support in Pediatric Patients

Tom R. Karl
Stephen B. Horton

Despite improvements in operative techniques, management of cardiopulmonary bypass (CPB), and myocardial protection, myocardial dysfunction remains a problem after some complex pediatric cardiac procedures. The deleterious effects of CPB and myocardial ischemia are most pronounced in infants, especially neonates, because of the immaturity of tissues and organs and the obligatory dilution of blood volume with nonnative fluids. Paradoxically, the increasing ability to separate very sick infants from CPB may increase the incidence of postoperative low cardiac output problems in the intensive care unit (ICU). Chapter 46 focused on extracorporeal membrane oxygenation (ECMO) and other miscellaneous acute support devices; this chapter discusses ventricular assist devices (VADs) and their use as an acute cardiopulmonary support therapy. Additional medical management issues are discussed in Chapter 45.

The impaired myocardium in children after cardiac surgery may be characterized by decreased contractility, abnormal diastolic relaxation, and reduced responsiveness to inotropic and lusitropic pharmacologic stimulation.[2] A common feature of heart failure in children with biventricular hearts is primary involvement of the left ventricle. DeBakey[1] reported the first successful use of a VAD in 1971. His basic concept comprised drainage of left or right heart blood into a pumping chamber with ejection into the aorta (LVAD) or pulmonary artery (RVAD). The ensuing three decades have brought steady refinements in VAD indications and techniques. The increasingly favorable results in adults have made VAD an accepted treatment to sustain patients with myocardial failure until either recovery of native heart function or transplantation.

In the 1990s, new VAD systems came into clinical use, with many being suitable for patients weighing at least 20 kg. The experience with VAD support for smaller children (<20 kg) is limited, however. This situation is partly due to technical considerations, including the fact that relatively low flows may create a diathesis for thromboembolism when adult-sized systems are applied in small children.[3] There is a long-standing perception that children with complex congenital heart disease are unsuitable for univentricular support without the use of an oxygenator. ECMO has been the main form of pediatric circulatory support in many units worldwide, even when the oxygenator is superfluous from a physiologic

point of view. Most of the world experience with extracorporeal life support for cardiac failure in children has been with ECMO, as detailed in the annual Extracorporeal Life Support Organization reports.[4] Experiences suggest, however, that VAD may be an equally useful (and in some cases better) form of circulatory support.[5-8] This chapter discusses the indications, techniques, and outcomes for short-term circulatory support in children, primarily via a centrifugal pump VAD.[1a,3,5-12,19]

CENTRIFUGAL PUMP VENTRICULAR ASSIST DEVICE

Indications and Contraindications

As with any other labor-intensive, invasive, and potentially hazardous therapy, mechanical circulatory assistance requires a careful prospective definition of the indications for its use, projected duration, and desired end point. Postoperative support has been the most common indication for VAD in the institutions with a large experience in VAD usage. Most VAD patients so treated had undergone palliative or reparative open heart operations or cardiac transplantation and could not be weaned from CPB, despite optimization of blood volume, ventilation, acid-base status, and vasoactive/inotropic/lusitropic drug support. A subset of patients had refractory low cardiac output or a sudden cardiac arrest in the ICU after satisfactory primary separation from CPB and required institution of VAD support in the ICU. Low cardiac output not related to surgery (myocarditis, cardiomyopathy) was the primary indication in a small but growing number of pediatric patients.

To select patients intelligently for VAD support, a great deal of judgment on the part of the surgeon, cardiac intensivist, anesthesiologist, and perfusionist is required. This judgment is especially important when deciding exactly when extracorporeal support is justified in a given patient because the devices themselves are not free of complications. In most published series, the strongest correlate of failure of postoperative extracorporeal support has been the presence of a residual cardiac defect. Our own experience supports this finding.[11] Ideally, technical failure of the operation should have been ruled out before beginning VAD support, although in practice this may be quite difficult. Toward this end, there is a role for intraoperative assessment with transesophageal echocardiography with direct cardiac chamber pressure and saturation measurements or a cardiac catheterization even while on VAD support. In addition, one must ask whether there is a potential for recovery and, if not, whether transplantation is a realistic option. Finally, one must consider which type of support (usually ECMO versus VAD) is best for a given patient.

There are numerous relative contraindications to the use of VADs, including multiorgan system failure, severe coagulopathy, intracranial hemorrhage, neurologic impairment, uncontrolled sepsis, prolonged cardiac arrest, and a univentricular circulation. In practice, although all may be relevant, most of these features are difficult or impossible to assess accurately in a child who needs placement of a VAD, especially in an intraoperative or ICU setting. There is the issue of the improbable good outcome after VAD support in a highly compromised child with several relative contraindications. Addressing the sepsis issue, we had supported a patient with essentially untreated endocarditis (with evidence of cerebral embolism) after emergency aortic valve replacement, with a prolonged but complete recovery. Most surgeons involved with circulatory support in children could cite similar cases, and it might be suggested that pediatric patients generally have a greater potential for recovery (without sequelae) than do adults. In institutions capable of offering circulatory support, almost any child accepted for open heart surgery would be a candidate for support should the need arise.

There is now considerable experience with the use of mechanical support (extracorporeal life support [ECLS]) after **cardiac arrest**. Because neurologic outcome is a primary concern, the pre-arrest neurologic condition and the duration of the arrest and resuscitation (ischemia time) largely determine the outcome of post-arrest mechanical circulatory support. Recovery of cardiac function can occur well beyond the point of severe brain damage, but the upper limits are unknown. We have initiated VAD and ECMO support during prolonged (>1 hour) cardiac arrests with good-quality long-term survival. In the Pittsburgh experience, 11 of 17 patients with cardiac arrest (6 of 11 who had >15 minutes of cardiac massage) survived to discharge after ECMO support.[12] The results at Children's Hospital of Philadelphia have been similar; 7 of the 11 patients placed on ECMO after a cardiac arrest and listed for transplantation either were weaned successfully from ECMO ($n = 2$) or survived to transplantation ($n = 5$).[13] A review of the Extracorporeal Life Support Organization registry during the period between 1989 and 1995 revealed that 13% (839 of 6335) of patients supported with ECMO had had a pre-ECMO cardiac arrest.[14] Overall survival for these children was 60.8% versus 81.6% for children who did not require cardiopulmonary resuscitation before ECMO ($P < .001$). Analysis of 112 survivors of post-arrest ECMO showed that 63% had no neurologic impairment, and 4% were graded as

severely impaired.[14] Aharon and coworkers[15] noted that cardiopulmonary arrest before ECMO affected outcome adversely only when the cardiopulmonary resuscitation time was prolonged (>45 minutes). At University of California, San Francisco (UCSF), we have now supported 15 postoperative infants (median age 24 days; median weight 3.7 kg) with a rescue circuit (centrifugal pump plus hollow-fiber oxygenator). Twelve of 15 patients (0.8; confidence limit [CL] = 0.55 to 0.93) were weaned from ECLS, and hospital survival was 0.67 (CL = 0.42 to 0.85). Of patients whose indication for rapid-deployment ECLS was cardiac arrest, survival was 4 of 6 compared with 1 of 12 for historical controls from our center supported with non-rapid deployment roller pump ECMO during the period between 1990 and 2001 ($p = .02$). The age and weight at cannulation, sex, cardiac diagnosis, indication, interval from surgery to ECLS, CPB time, intraoperative myocardial ischemia time, diagnosis of sepsis or mediastinitis, need for arteriovenous hemofiltration or dialysis, and duration of ECLS were not significantly associated with survival probability. The issue of acceptable resuscitation times for children needs to be re-evaluated in the era of circulatory support.

Patients with acute **fulminant myocarditis** may benefit greatly from mechanical circulatory assistance to promote myocardial recovery. Support with VAD may be preferable to ECMO in such cases because it more completely unloads the left ventricle, which may lead to rapid reverse remodeling of the left ventricle.[16] VAD can decrease wall stress in the left ventricle to a greater extent than can ECMO, unless the latter is used with an accessory left ventricular cannula, which usually requires transthoracic cannulation.[17-20] The possibility of recovery, combined with the scarcity of donor organs, has led to prolonged circulatory support of several weeks; some children with acute myocarditis may recover (without transplantation) after prolonged VAD support.[21] For longer term support, neither centrifugal pump VAD nor ECMO can be considered particularly suitable, however, although in many units a better system is not yet available. Hetzer and coworkers[22] have reported successful support in children of all ages using a pneumatic paracorporeal VAD for 98 days. See also Chapters 7 and 45.

Cardiomyopathy may be an indication for VAD when decompensation and low cardiac output signs dominate the clinical picture. Although recovery of adequate native heart function is possible in rare instances, most patients require a VAD as a bridge to transplantation. Although ECMO has the advantage of allowing emergency extrathoracic or peripheral cannulation in the ICU, it has the disadvantage of not fully unloading the poorly ejecting left heart, unless atrial septostomy (or septectomy) is performed or a second cannula is placed in the left atrium. This procedure may be critical in preserving pulmonary function in patients awaiting transplantation. In contrast, VAD unloads the left heart more completely, as also described previously for myocarditis.

The general aims of postoperative centrifugal pump VAD support are recovery and weaning from support within 5 days, although there may be an option for a bridge to transplantation in select cases, with or without interim conversion to a pulsatile paracorporeal support system designed for longer term use (see later and see Chapters 48 and 49).[12,21,23-25] For patients weighing less than 20 kg, two weeks would be considered to be the maximal realistic projected duration of support with a VAD. Patients supported specifically for bridging (as opposed to recovery) should meet institutional criteria for transplantation prospectively.[21] Issues such as size, blood group, pulmonary vascular resistance, HLA status, multiorgan function, and donor availability should be taken into consideration.

VAD support in a patient with a **univentricular circulation** is currently controversial, but centers have supported such patients successfully with VAD and ECMO after the Norwood operation for hypoplastic left heart syndrome and after bidirectional cavopulmonary shunts performed for complex univentricular variants.[26,27] In such cases, higher than normal flows (approximately 150% of calculated) may be required because the assist device provides pulmonary and systemic output. Patency of the shunt open is mandatory. In some units, VAD support is employed routinely after the Norwood operation, to ensure an adequate cardiac output (aorta plus shunt) during the early postoperative period.[28] Results of this strategy have been good, and the physiology rationale is sound, although most teams would reserve this level of support for patients with a demonstrated hemodynamic instability.

Technical Aspects of the Centrifugal Ventricular Assist Device Circuit

The important component of the centrifugal pump head is an impeller consisting of rotating cones or vanes, which create a constrained vortex. The impeller is coupled electromagnetically to the drive unit so that the operator can set the rotational speed of the pump. Rotation creates subatmospheric pressure at the tip of the cone, establishing suction in the venous cannula. Positive pressure is created at the outlet (arterial cannula) (Fig. 47-1). Because there are neither valves nor diaphragms, the flow is nonpulsatile.

The centrifugal pump output (flow) depends on preload and afterload and the rotational speed of the pump. A reduction in preload from inlet obstruction, hypovolemia, or any other cause decreases pump output for a given number of revolutions per minute. Continued rotation of the pump creates a more negative inlet pressure. Care must be taken to keep the inlet pressure greater than −20 mm Hg, or excessive hemolysis can occur. Conversely a significant reduction in afterload automatically results in an increase in flow without any change in revolutions per minute. Because there is no indirect way to determine flow from the

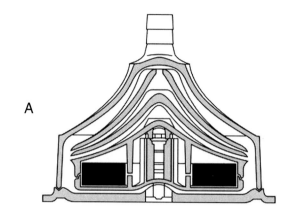

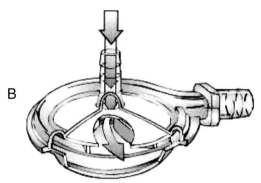

FIGURE 47-1 ■ BioMedicus (BioMedicus, Eden Prairie, MN) centrifugal pump head and Jostra Rotaflow (Jostra Medizintechnik AG, Hirrlingen, Germany) centrifugal pump head. **A,** BioMedicus centrifugal pump head, cutaway view. The important component is an impeller consisting of rotating cones or vanes, which create a constrained vortex. The impeller is coupled electromagnetically to the drive unit so that the operator can set the rotational speed of the pump. Rotation creates subatmospheric pressure at the tip of the cone, establishing suction in the venous cannula. Positive pressure is created at the outlet at the base of the cone, which connects to the arterial limb of the circuit. **B,** Jostra Rotaflow centrifugal pump head. The rotor is suspended and driven by a radial magnetic field that stabilizes the impeller and allows it to be spun on a single blood-flushed pivot bearing. (**B** courtesy of Jostra Medizintechnik AG, Hirrlingen, Germany.)

rotational speed of the pump, a flowmeter is necessary. The most efficient (and least hemolytic) settings for a centrifugal pump occur at the lowest pump speed for a given flow. In this respect, the centrifugal pump allows fine-tuning of the peripheral circulation before and during weaning because it is responsive (flow at a given pressure) to the patient's intravascular volume and resistance.

Although such technical problems are not encountered frequently in roller pumps, which generate constant flow at a given speed, the latter have a greater potential for hemolysis relating to other factors. In vitro studies suggest that hemolysis is less significant in a properly managed centrifugal pump circuit than in a roller pump circuit.[29] The risks of tubing rupture and air embolism also are increased with the roller pump. The perfusion group at the Royal Children's Hospital

(RCH) compared two commercially available centrifugal pumps (BioMedicus, Eden Prairie, MN, and Jostra Rotaflow, Jostra Medizintechnik AG, Hirrlingen, Germany) with a standard roller pump in an in vitro circuit over 6 days. After only 24 hours, there was a significant increase in hemolysis in the roller pump compared with either centrifugal pump. Differences between the Jostra and BioMedicus pump were evident only after 6 days, with the former device faring better.[29-31]

The UCSF VAD circuit consists of a centrifugal pump head (see Fig. 47-1A) (BioMedicus, Eden Prairie, MN) mounted on a flexible drive cable. We employ inlet and outlet pressure monitoring and an in-line arterial flow probe. The tubing length can be minimized by mounting the pump head directly onto the patient's bed. We usually employ heparin-bonded circuits, although this is not considered essential (see later). The battery backup makes the pump convenient for transport of the patient and device during a period of assist. More recently at the RCH, the Jostra Rotaflow pump head (not yet Food and Drug Administration approved in the United States) has been used for VAD and ECMO (see Fig. 47-1B). In the Rotaflow pump, the rotor is suspended and driven by a radial magnetic field that stabilizes the impeller and allows it to be spun on a single blood-flushed pivot bearing. The pump may have advantages in terms of durability and hydraulic efficiency, which could render it superior to previously employed centrifugal devices for children.

Biventricular assist is possible with two centrifugal pumps, and we have (rarely) employed right atrial/pulmonary arterial plus left atrial/aortic cannulation, using two pump heads adjusted for approximately 100% to 70% flow ratio. This setup is technically cumbersome in a small child, however, and we normally prefer ECMO in such a situation.

Since 2001, we also have employed a rapid deployment rescue circuit at UCSF for ECLS. The circuit consists of a heparin-bonded (Carmeda) Medtronic Minimax hollow-fiber oxygenator and a BioMedicus centrifugal pump, using $\frac{1}{4}$-inch tubing and an integral heat exchanger. There is no bridge or reservoir, and the circuit is kept primed in the ICU. Initial support can be established with this system during resuscitation, with conversion to VAD as indicated for weaning or longer term support, depending on anatomy and cannulation setup. This circuit combines some of the advantages of VAD and ECMO and increases flexibility and options for support.

Instituting Centrifugal Ventricular Assist Device Support

The most common scenario in our experience has been intraoperative placement of a VAD for patients who could not be weaned from CPB. In this circumstance, cannulation is usually transmediastinal, using the left atrial appendage or left atrial body (at the right superior pulmonary vein junction) for drainage and the ascending aorta for arterial return. For children with a univentricular circulation, the right atrial appendage and ascending aorta can be used, as can the cervical vessels, because in such patients there is a common circulation. We employ standard or heparin-bonded CPB cannulae designed to carry 150 mL/kg/min flow. Cannulae are secured with purse-string sutures and tourniquets as for CPB. The tourniquets are held fast with vascular clips and left inside the mediastinum. Marelli and colleagues[32] reported a simplified technique for VAD cannulation employing a limited anterior thoracotomy for transmediastinal cannulation. If VAD is instituted for a postoperative cardiac arrest (i.e., outside the operating room), ECMO or CPB may be required initially, but in some cases we have been able to place asystolic postoperative patients undergoing open cardiac massage directly onto left VAD, with a successful outcome.

For VAD support, flow is begun at minimum and quickly increased to 150 mL/kg/min. If the patient remains stable, flow is reduced to 70% of calculated output. We attempt to maintain a left atrial pressure of 3 to 4 mm Hg, allowing for some ejection if possible. This strategy may reduce the risks of stasis and thrombus formation. Heparin can be reversed with protamine, and hemostasis can be secured as for other CPB cases. Administration of protamine to patients supported with a heparin-bonded circuit may neutralize some of the advantages of Carmeda coating, however, and could result in a significantly greater heparin requirement or the potential for thrombus formation during VAD support.[17] When hemostasis has been secured, the skin is closed, with cannulae exiting at either side of the wound. Alternately a polytetrafluoroethylene membrane is sutured to the skin edges, leaving the sternum open.

For some patients, it is not clear that univentricular support with a VAD would be adequate. When global right ventricular and left ventricular failure is present, ECMO or biventricular VAD probably will be required. The same can be said for patients with severe pulmonary hypertension or pulmonary dysfunction complicating their clinical picture. The decrease in left atrial pressure usually seen with left VAD may improve pulmonary hypertension and right ventricular dysfunction dramatically in borderline cases, especially with concurrent use of inhaled nitric oxide. Right ventricular function is sensitive to left ventricular function in numerous ways. By unloading the left ventricle with VAD, right ventricular filling is improved, and the decrease in chamber size and septal shift may improve tricuspid valve function as well.[33] Each case must be assessed individually, and the simplest effective level of support (i.e., VAD rather than ECMO) whenever possible should be considered.

To assess the prospects for VAD rather than ECMO intraoperatively, a venous cannula is placed in the left atrium, then the right atrial or caval cannula used for CPB is clamped. This system is used to assess the effect of partial left heart bypass. Right atrial and pulmonary arterial pressure and right ventricular function are observed at 150 mL/kg/min pump flow. If all are satisfactory (right atrial pressure <12 mm Hg, pulmonary artery systolic pressure less than half of systemic pressure, and no right ventricular dilation), the patient is ventilated normally, while gas exchange in the oxygenator is temporarily interrupted. If PCO_2, PO_2, acid-base status, and hemodynamic profile remain acceptable, the patient is recannulated for VAD. Otherwise, conversion to ECMO (or possibly biventricular VAD) would be a preferred strategy. For univentricular patients, a similar strategy can be employed, looking at common atrial pressure and oxygen saturation. A great deal of judgment is required on the part of the entire surgical team, owing to the extreme patient variability.

Managing the Ventricular Assist Device Patient

During VAD support, patients are sedated and fully ventilated. Inotropes are minimized to the level required to maintain optimal right heart function, based on central venous pressures, oxygenation, and echocardiographic assessment. Arterial pressure, VAD inlet/outlet pressure, right and left atrial pressures, total flow, and activated clotting time are recorded hourly. Leukocyte reduced blood is used for replacement as required. When postoperative bleeding subsides, systemic heparin anticoagulation is begun (approximately 20 IU/kg/hr), keeping the activated clotting time around 160 to 180 seconds.

Two different systems are commercially available for activated clotting time measurement, employing either diatomaceous earth (Hemochron; International Technidyne Corporation, Edison, NJ) or kaolin (Hemotec; Medtronic, Inc, Parker, CO). We have found the Hemotec method advantageous because it requires only 0.2 mL of blood per sample to yield reproducible results. We have found that the Hemochron activated clotting time was, on average, 1.1 times that obtained with Hemotec equipment. It should be kept in mind that neonates and infants have variable responses to heparin. Cyanotic patients are prone to multiple factor and platelet abnormalities, and all baseline deficits can be made worse by a long period on CPB, which typifies postoperative VAD cases.

With surface coating, the centrifugal pump system theoretically can be operated without heparin or at reduced doses, particularly in situations of high flow in larger patients, over a short time span. Clots may form, however, in surface-coated circuits with or without anticoagulation, and this risk of thrombosis must be weighed constantly against the risk of bleeding.[34]

Inhaled nitric oxide (see earlier), an effective treatment for pulmonary hypertension, is useful for support of the right heart during low cardiac output states requiring support with a left VAD. Even if pulmonary arterial pressure is normal, some patients may benefit hemodynamically, with improved left atrial filling.

A secondary benefit may be an improvement in ventilation-perfusion mismatch in select patients with pulmonary dysfunction. Normothermia is maintained during VAD with a heating/cooling blanket and the heat generated by the centrifugal pump head itself. Peritoneal dialysis or hemofiltration or both are used as required for metabolic support and fluid removal. Vasodilators, parenteral nutrition, and antibiotics also are administered. In general, the measures used for metabolic support are much the same as the measures required for other critically ill cardiac patients not being supported with VAD.

Plasma free hemoglobin is monitored at least daily and should remain less than 60 mg/dL. Elevated hemoglobin, especially in conjunction with noise or vibrations in the pump head, may be an indication that mechanical failure is imminent. In this case, the pump head can be changed easily with only a brief period off VAD support. Generally the pump head can be used safely for 5 days. Occasionally, we have replaced a pump head earlier in the presence of signs of imminent failure (see later). The median centrifugal pump head life in our patients has been 71.5 hours (range 0.5 to 480) hours (BioMedicus).

Numerous technical problems relating to centrifugal pump VAD in children may be encountered. Some common issues are outlined in Table 47-1. In addition, a more thorough discussion of medical issues in mechanical support can be found elsewhere in this text (see Chapter 45).

Weaning the Ventricular Assist Device Patient

In patients with improving ventricular function on VAD, one generally notes the appearance of a pulsatile systemic arterial pressure trace as the first sign. Echocardiographic assessment is helpful at this point to evaluate further the ventricular contractility and the response to volume loading. A Starling response suggests that weaning can proceed. We employ gradual flow reduction as the left ventricle begins to eject, down to a total flow of 150 mL/min; this is considered the minimum safe flow from the point of view of risk of circuit thrombosis. Temporary augmentation of heparin may be required at very low flows, and the cannulae may be flushed with heparin (5 IU/mL saline) to test the hemodynamics with pump support discontinued. All of the normal postoperative management strategies for a given lesion are useful during weaning to test the patient's ability to contribute to cardiac output at decreasing levels of support. Oxygenation and carbon dioxide clearance are autogenous, removing an important variable from the formula, which can be especially critical in shunt-dependent univentricular patients. Decannulation is performed in the ICU or operating room, with concurrent sternal closure whenever possible. The question of when transplantation is a better option than continued extracorporeal support in a postoperative patient continues to challenge judgment. It would

TABLE 47-1

Common Technical Problems Related to the Centrifugal Pump Ventricular Assist Device and Possible Solutions	
Problem	Comments and Possible Solutions
1. High Arterial Outlet Pressure	
a. Acute	
(1) Cannula position has changed	(1) Adjust cannula position
(2) Thrombus partly obstructing cannula	(2) Recannulate, adjust ACT as required
(3) LV ejection above support provided by pump (equivalent of increased vascular resistance)	(3) Consider weaning with flow reduction. Vasodilator therapy
b. Chronic	
(1) Flow too high for selected cannula	(1) Recannulate with larger cannula
2. Low (Subatmospheric) Inlet Pressure	
a. Acute	
(1) Cannula position has changed	(1) Adjust cannula position
(2) Thrombus partially obstructing cannula	(2) Recannulate, adjust ACT as required
(3) Atrial wall collapsed around cannula	(3) Reduce flow temporarily (by decreasing rpm), then slowly return to normal flow
(4) Hypovolemia	(4) Infuse volume expander
b. Chronic	
(1) Flow too high for selected cannula	(1) Recannulate with larger cannula
(2) Failing right ventricle, poor LA filling	(2) Pulmonary vasodilators, inotropes. Consider right VAD or ECMO
3. Inability to Achieve Nominal flow	
(1) Any combination of circumstances outlined in 1 and 2 above	(1) See 1 and 2
(2) Cardiac tamponade	(2) Exploration, hemostasis, drainage
4. Excessive Hemolysis	
(1) Low inlet pressure (<−20 mm Hg)	(1) See 2a and 2b
(2) Thrombus in pump head (especially if pump head is noisy)	(2) Change pump head, adjust ACT as required
(3) Venous cannula too small (especially if inlet pressure is low)	(3) Recannulate with larger cannula
5. Inconsistent ACT Readings	
(1) Incorrect preparation of kaolin suspension	(1) Kaolin suspension should be mixed just before use
(2) Incorrect preparation of cuvettes	(2) Cuvettes should be stored at 2°C to 25°C and warmed to 37°C just before use
(3) Sensor contaminated with blood	(3) Clean sensor with H_2O_2. Check to see that blood has actually clotted when ACT reading is made.
(4) Concurrent platelet infusion	(4) Increase heparin dosage by 10% during platelet infusion
(5) Ongoing variation in heparin metabolism	(5) Adjust heparin dose
6. Air in VAD Circuit	
(1) Air entrainment around insertion site (if inlet pressure is very low)	(1) Reduce support to increase filling pressure in left atrium. Infuse volume expander, revise cannulation suture to obtain a seal. Positioning the outlet at 5 o'clock creates a bubble trap to sequester gross air, although small bubbles still can embolize.
(2) Open or faulty tap or connector in system	(2) Change or close connectors or taps. De-air (venous side)
(3) Crack in pump housing	(3) Change pump head
(4) Acute inlet obstruction with very low pressure	(4) See 2a. Under these circumstances, gas can be drawn out of solution in venous limb of circuit
7. Noisy Pump Head	
(1) Thrombus in pump head	(1) Thrombus on wall of cone or bearing causes cone to spin eccentrically. Hemolysis often occurs concurrently. Pump head should be changed.

ACT, activated clotting time; ECMO, extracorporeal membrane oxygenation; LA, left atrial; LV, left ventricular; VAD, ventricular assist device.

be fair to say that at present most cardiac extracorporeal support in children is performed with a view toward myocardial recovery. The usefulness of centrifugal pump VAD and ECMO as a bridge to transplantation depends heavily on the immediate availability of suitable donor hearts, which remains problematic in many parts of the world. In the case of bridge to transplantation, we generally have used the same aortic cannula, but added bicaval venous cannulation to convert to standard CPB for the operation.

OUTCOME OF CENTRIFUGAL VENTRICULAR ASSIST DEVICE SUPPORT IN CHILDREN

A detailed analysis of the initial RCH experience (1989-1998) has been reported previously.[26] We supported 53 infants and children with centrifugal pump VAD, representing approximately 1.2% of our CPB cases during that time period. The median age was 3.5 months (range 2 days to 19 years), and the median weight was 4 kg (range 1.9 to 70 kg). The diagnoses and operative procedures spanned the spectrum of congenital and acquired heart disease in children. Operations preceding VAD support included the Norwood procedure,[10] mitral valve replacement,[2] aortic root procedures,[8] arterial switch operation (ASO),[8] repair of supra-aortic stenosis,[3] heart or heart/lung transplantation,[3] anomalous origin of the left coronary artery from the pulmonary artery (ALCAPA) repair,[5] and cavopulmonary connection.[3] Of the 53 children supported, 38 were weaned from VAD (0.72; CL = 0.57 to 0.83), and 24 ultimately were discharged from the hospital (0.46; CL = 0.31 to 0.61). The results have been sustained to date, with 95 patients supported. The overall weaning probability for the series is now 0.66 (CL = 0.56 to 0.75), with a discharge probability of 0.4 (CL = 0.32 to 0.51).

As in other published series, post-weaning deaths generally reflected continued cardiac problems rather than morbidity specifically attributable to the VAD. Age, weight, timing of support (intraoperative versus postoperative), cyanosis, and presence of a mechanical valve were not associated with incremental risk ($P > .05$ for all). The need for dialysis or ultrafiltration has been identified as risk factors for death in other published series.[35] In our experience, dialysis and ultrafiltration were used routinely (as needed) during VAD and ECMO, however, and have not emerged as independent risk factors. Taking initiation of VAD as day zero, the Kaplan-Meier survival at 1 year for all VAD patients was 0.44 (CL = 0.31 to 0.58), suggesting a sharp decline in hazard function at the point of hospital discharge.

The median support time was 75 hours (range 19 to 428 hours) for patients who could be weaned from VAD. For patients ultimately not able to be weaned, it was 79.5 hours (range 2 to 114 hours). For patients discharged, the median support time was 71.5 hours (range 38 to 144 hours), and for patients not discharged, the median time was 88 hours (range 2 to 428 hours). Analyzed in various ways, VAD support times were similar for survivors and nonsurvivors ($P = .69$). The interpretation of support time data is confounded by the fact that VAD was electively terminated in some children who showed no signs of ventricular recovery after 72 hours in the absence of a realistic transplantation option.

The VAD group of particular interest consists of children weighing less than 6 kg, whose options for support are perhaps more limited and who have

presented the greatest technical challenge. It has been suggested that many of these patients are suitable only for ECMO.[10] We analyzed a subset of 34 of our patients, ages 2 to 258 days (median 60 days) and weights 1.9 to 5.9 kg (median 3.7 kg). Twenty-four patients could not be weaned from CPB, and 10 required support in the ICU for postoperative refractory low cardiac output. Weaning and decannulation were performed in 22 of 34 cases (0.63; CL = 0.45 to 0.78), similar to the patients weighing more than 6 kg ($P = .07$). One-year Kaplan-Meier survival was 0.31 (CL = 0.17 to 0.47), with most deaths being due to irreversible cardiac disease. Within the group weighing less than 6 kg, the parameters of age, weight, VAD duration, CPB duration, cross-clamp duration, and the presence of univentricular anatomy failed to prove useful in predicting hospital discharge ($P > .05$).[36] The smallest surviving patient in this series was a 19-day-old, 1.9-kg infant with Taussig-Bing anomaly and aortic arch obstruction, who was placed on VAD postoperatively, during a prolonged cardiac arrest, and survived with no neurologic sequelae.

Complications were frequent in VAD patients of all ages, as has been the case in most reported series. The term *complication,* at least as it relates to ECLS, might bear redefinition, given the patient population. From the initial cohort of 53 VAD patients, bleeding requiring exploration occurred in 15 patients. Three patients had sepsis with clinical signs and positive blood cultures, whereas positive blood cultures without clinical signs were found in another five. Transient neurologic defects were noted in three survivors, and two have had persistent mild neurologic complications. There have been no permanent renal sequelae. Mechanical complications also were frequent (20 patients), but usually were manageable with appropriate surveillance and action. Included were pump head failure, cracked connectors, kinked cannulae, and air or clots in the circuit. Only four patients required an emergency circuit change as the primary intervention. The true incidence of all complications is underestimated because assessment was incomplete in the nonsurvivors.

Results of postoperative VAD and ECMO in children have been remarkably similar across numerous published series, suggesting that the patient population supported may exert more influence than the technique of support.[23,24,35,37-39] At least for postoperative use, a common feature is that patients who are likely to recover tend to do so within the first few days. Beyond 2 weeks, complications of VAD, such as sepsis and multiorgan system failure, may become major limitations.

Results with short-term VADs reflect a policy of expanding the indications to include nearly all cardiac surgical patients who are not expected to survive without support. Whether this strategy is appropriate or not is a decision to be made by each team in the context of local resources and philosophy. To most surgeons, a 30% to 40% long-term survival probability would justify the effort and expense immediately, especially if the child might have minimal or no disability. Improvements in the technical aspects, safety, and efficacy of centrifugal pump VAD may be obscured to a degree by the liberalization of indications for its use.

Ventricular Assist Device Support in Specific Situations

Short-term circulatory support has been particularly effective for postoperative patients with ALCAPA, transposition of the great arteries (TGA) after ASO, and donor heart dysfunction after transplantation. The unifying principle in these cases is undoubtedly the presence of two relatively normal ventricles, with the left ventricle being temporarily (but critically) impaired. Our patients with ALCAPA and TGA as a group had a 0.91 (CL = 0.59 to 1) overall survival probability (P = .002). Conversely, patients whose cardiac abnormalities bear a poor prognosis without VAD (left heart obstructive syndromes, complex univentricular hearts) also may do poorly after VAD support.

In the uncommon lesion of **anomalous left coronary artery from the pulmonary artery**, the entire left coronary system arises from the pulmonary artery. The basic pathophysiology is considered to be retrograde flow from the left coronary artery into the pulmonary artery, which may increase as the pulmonary vascular resistance decreases postnatally.[36,40] The result is a variable degree of myocardial ischemia, sometimes leading to extensive subendocardial or transmural infarction, with the classic ECG findings including prominent Q waves in leads I and avL. Despite its rarity, ALCAPA is the most common cause of myocardial infarction in children.[36] There is a tendency to develop papillary muscle dysfunction, which causes mitral insufficiency, exacerbated further by left ventricular dilation and loss of wall thickness (Fig. 47-2). The result may be

severe low cardiac output syndrome, and the only effective treatment is surgery with postoperative myocardial support and recovery if needed.

Our preferred surgical option is direct implantation of the anomalous left coronary into the aorta (Fig. 47-3), although other techniques are available.[39,41,42] The ischemic time required for this repair exacerbates the compromised preoperative condition and occasionally renders an infant unable to be weaned from CPB or causes severe postoperative low cardiac output, despite the rational use of myocardial protection strategies, modified ultrafiltration, and excellent surgical technique. Such patients are usually good candidates for centrifugal pump left VAD support because recovery can be expected within a few days.

In ALCAPA patients, recovery of left ventricular function in the long-term is good, and the need for perioperative VAD does not predict a poor late functional status.[40] The mechanism of recovery seems to be reperfusion of areas of dysfunctional but viable myocardium, as in salvage of "hibernating" myocardium after revascularization of ischemic myocardium in adults. Typically, there is an early return of myocyte contractile function, and augmented β-adrenergic responsiveness during VAD support. Some extracardiac factors implicated in the progression of myocardial dysfunction, such as cytokine-mediated toxicity, unfavorable neurohormonal stimulation, and excessive hemodynamic loading conditions, are undoubtedly ameliorated as well. Because these mechanisms all have the potential to depress contractile function and promote myocyte loss through either ischemia or apoptosis, they also represent potential contributors to contractile improvement during and after VAD support.[43] Shivalkar and colleagues[44] reported results of myocardial biopsies in patients undergoing ALCAPA repair. They noted a variable degree of fibrosis and loss of contractile material in myocytes. Glycogen stores were present, however, and the mitochondrial membranes and nuclei were preserved. The findings were consistent with hypoperfusion rather than cell death. All of the hearts studied were normokinetic within 3 years of repair.[44]

Our experience now comprises 26 patients with ALCAPA, with an age range of 6 weeks to 10 years (median 9 months). There were no perioperative deaths, but five patients required VAD support for 48 to 96 hours (median 72 hours). Long-term clinical outcome and left ventricular function have been good, despite severe left ventricular dysfunction at presentation. At late follow-up (Fig. 47-4), the VAD patients are virtually indistinguishable from the remainder of the cohort in terms of ventricular and mitral valve function and clinical status.[36]

Timing is crucial for the safe conduct of the ASO for **transposition of the great arteries**. In neonates with TGA and intact ventricular septum, a regression of muscle mass of the left ventricle occurs over the first month of postnatal life, as the pulmonary vascular

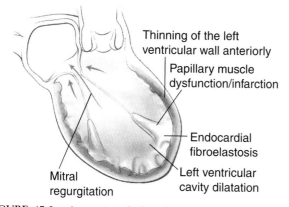

Thinning of the left ventricular wall anteriorly

Papillary muscle dysfunction/infarction

Endocardial fibroelastosis

Left ventricular cavity dilatation

Mitral regurgitation

FIGURE 47-2 ■ Anatomic and physiologic derangements seen with anomalous origin of the left coronary artery from the pulmonary artery. As a result of myocardial ischemia from decreased coronary circulation, anatomic changes occur and require time for recovery. A ventricular assist device is ideal for this to occur after surgical correction of the coronary supply. (See also Color Section)

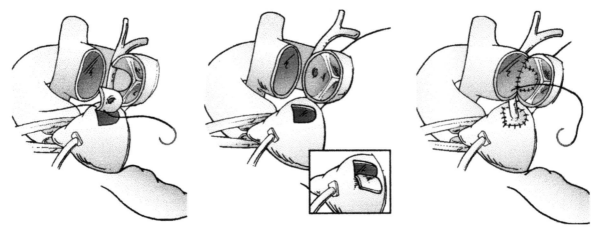

FIGURE 47-3 ■ Surgery for anomalous origin of the left coronary artery from the pulmonary artery. Repair of the lesion resembles the coronary translocation used for the arterial switch operation. The pulmonary artery is transected above the pulmonary valve, and the coronary button is fashioned and directly reimplanted into the aorta.

resistance decreases. The consequence is a potential for a deconditioned left ventricle that does not function adequately when placed acutely in the systemic circuit after an ASO. Since the early days of the ASO experience, it has been appreciated that the risk of operation increases after the second week of life, unless left ventricular pressure is maintained at systemic levels by a large ventricular septal defect, ductus arteriosus, or left ventricular outflow tract obstruction. It also has been appreciated that in postnatal life, myocardial growth is characterized by an early hyperplastic phase of myocyte and capillaries, followed by myocyte hypertrophy. Pressure overload induces hyperplasia, hypertrophy, and angiogenesis in neonates, but only myocyte hypertrophy later in life. The capacity for and rapidity of left ventricular hypertrophy may decrease with increasing age.

Based on the previous information, a two-stage approach has been employed (historically) in many pediatric units for infants with TGA and intact ventricular septum presenting beyond 2 to 3 weeks of age.[45] This approach consists of a primary pulmonary artery band plus modified Blalock-Taussig shunt, to induce left ventricular hypertrophy while maintaining oxygenation. The ASO usually can be performed after a brief period of left ventricular conditioning, usually 2 weeks or less. During this time, left ventricular wall thickness and ventricular mass are seen to increase, based on echocardiographic studies. We prefer an alternate approach and have elected to perform a one-stage ASO for all infants presenting in the first 8 weeks of life, regardless of left ventricular mass, pressure, or geometry.[46] If necessary, left VAD is used selectively as a means of rapid left ventricular conditioning postoperatively because it is clear that there is potential for a rapid increase in left ventricular mass in neonates up to this age. This approach may be less suitable for older children, who are likely to require a longer period of left ventricular conditioning than can be provided safely with a centrifugal pump VAD.

In the RCH experience, 25 children had a one-stage ASO (for TGA and intact ventricular septum) after 3 weeks of age.[46] Four patients required postoperative VAD support for rapid left ventricular conditioning. There were two perioperative deaths, one related to a coronary artery technical problem and the other to extracardiac problems of prematurity. For this cohort, the results compare favorably with a two-stage ASO, even if VAD should be required. We also have used VAD support in older patients undergoing the double-switch operation (Senning plus ASO) for discordant TGA in the presence of a deconditioned left ventricle and in children with complex TGA whose main cause of left ventricular dysfunction was a poor preoperative condition or a long ischemic time (see also Chapter 42).

FIGURE 47-4 ■ Left ventricle recovery after surgery for anomalous origin of the left coronary artery from the pulmonary artery. The y axis is the fractional shortening obtained on echocardiography. Normal range shortening fraction is observed after 1 year but not at 3 months after surgical correction.

In any patient undergoing ASO, a technical problem with a coronary anastomosis must be ruled out as the primary cause of left ventricular failure; otherwise, VAD support would not be helpful. Appearance of the heart and ECG are useful in this regard, but a great deal of judgment is required in deciding whether to use VAD or revise the original repair, with the possibility of an additional ischemic insult. Toward this end, in the current era, echocardiographers are helpful with their abilities to image and assess flow in the proximal coronaries, sometimes beyond the first bifurcation.

Since the 1990s, the proliferation of cardiac transplantation candidates and transplantation teams has led to a generalized shortage of donor organs. Likewise, the use of pretransplantation mechanical support has increased the urgency in many cases, especially since the outcome in such patients is potentially as good as in patients with less advanced cardiac failure. In most centers, the magnitude of the problem increases inversely with the size of the patient. Consequently the criteria for donor acceptability have been relaxed to the point that many units accept hearts with projected ischemic times greater than 6 hours or hearts with compromised ventricular function in the donor. Although reversibility of **donor heart dysfunction** is predicted in such cases, it may appear in delayed fashion, preventing weaning from CPB. Short-term centrifugal left VAD support is ideal in such cases, especially if pulmonary vascular resistance is low. Inhaled nitric oxide, milrinone, and other types of pharmacologic support have been useful as well. The problem is compounded greatly in patients with elevated pulmonary vascular resistance. Although post-transplantation right ventricular heart dysfunction may improve with inhaled nitric oxide therapy and time, it can become critical in the immediate post-transplantation period. Right ventricular centrifugal assist (isolated or as biventricular VAD) has been used successfully for right ventricular failure after cardiac transplantation in such cases.[33]

SUPPORT WITH VENTRICULAR ASSIST DEVICE VERSUS EXTRACORPOREAL MEMBRANE OXYGENATION

Some patients are supportable only with ECMO (or biventricular VAD or VAD with hollow-fiber oxygenator) because of severe right heart failure, pulmonary problems, or complexity of the cardiac anatomy. In many children, even children with complex congenital heart disease, either type of system may work well, however. It is difficult to predict the degree of improvement in right ventricular function that would occur with left ventricular unloading, but in some cases this effect can be impressive, especially in combination with pulmonary vasodilator therapy.

Previous institutional experience with neonatal ECMO for isolated pulmonary problems will have a strong influence on the choice of support systems owing to availability of equipment and trained personnel. During the same time frame as our previously reported RCH VAD experience, 40 children with cardiac or combined cardiopulmonary failure (not related to surgery) were supported with centrifugal pump ECMO.[21] Of the ECMO patients, 19 were weaned, 3 were bridged to transplantation, and 19 eventually were discharged. The weaning probability was better with VAD (0.71 versus 0.48; $P = .014$), although the hospital discharge probability was similar with VAD and ECMO (0.46 versus 0.48; $P = 1.0$). In interpreting these results, one must consider that most of the VAD patients could have been supported with ECMO, but the reverse generally would not apply.

Simplicity

VAD is straightforward in concept and design and requires little technical attention after insertion. Only a few minutes are required to set up and prime the circuit, providing an advantage in the setting of cardiac arrest. ECMO is more complex to set up, prime, and debubble. With ECMO, support can be established in some patients with peripheral closed chest cannulation, which is generally not possible with VAD in small children. In biventricular hearts, the potential for complete left ventricular support with ECMO may be limited without the addition of a left ventricular vent, which complicates the system considerably.

Cost

The cost differential varies considerably from institution to institution, depending on many factors. For the use of VAD, the child's ICU nurse can look after the patient and the support system, with the help of the intensivist, surgeon, and perfusionist as required. The additional hospital costs relate more to the equipment employed than to additional personnel. For ECMO, most units employ two nurses per patient (an ECMO specialist and the patient's regular ICU nurse) during support or perhaps even maintain a perfusionist or other technical specialist in the hospital at all times. In either case, a perfusionist, cardiac surgeon, and intensivist must be available for assistance in troubleshooting the system and for patient management problems. In most centers, the cost of ECMO, including baseline cost of the disposable equipment used in the circuit and personnel, is several times that of centrifugal pump VAD for an equivalent patient.

Oxygenation

ECMO potentially provides pulmonary and cardiac support, although during periods of cardiac ejection the coronaries may be perfused with blood, having a hemoglobin saturation closer to the left atrial level than to that of the oxygenator outlet. There is a potential for myocardial ischemia if pulmonary function is severely impaired. Patients supported with VAD are totally dependent on the lungs for gas exchange, but Po_2 tends to remain uniform throughout the arterial circulation, barring residual intracardiac shunts at the ventricular level in patients with significant cardiac ejection. If an interatrial communication is present, however, significant right-to-left shunting (as a result of the lower left atrial pressure) can cause uniform and significant arterial desaturation in patients on VAD support.

Anticoagulation

Centrifugal pump VAD requires little anticoagulation, especially at higher flows. One can administer protamine and completely reverse anticoagulation before closure of the chest after intraoperative placement. By comparison, ECMO requires a higher level of anticoagulation, even with a surface modified circuit. Also, the presence of the oxygenator results in more platelet damage, platelet consumption, and hemolysis, even when the centrifugal pump is used. The data from the pre-Carmeda (heparin-bonded) era at the RCH suggest that there was a lower blood and platelet transfusion requirement for VAD than for ECMO ($P < .06$). The exact safe level of anticoagulation for either circuit may be difficult to establish, and an approach based on individual patient and circuit factors is required.

The Carmeda process involves covalent attachment of fragmented heparin molecules to the circuit components, including oxygenator, tubing, pump head, cannulae, and all connectors.[48] The bioactive surface covalently binds the polysaccharide containing the active sequence of heparin, through end-point attachment, which is said to provide a more uniform degree of thromboresistance. There is a need for continuous movement of blood over the surfaces of the circuit for the heparin-bonding process to be effective. Theoretically, there is a risk of increased thrombogenicity in patients with anti–thrombin III deficiency. Heparin-coated circuits may reduce the heparin requirements for VAD and ECMO, but in small children, the prospects for either type of support without heparin are still poor.[49,50] Accumulating experience at the RCH and elsewhere suggests that postoperative bleeding is less with the surface-coated system for cardiac ECLS. The indications for ECMO and VAD ultimately may be extended to patients with hemorrhage, coagulopathy, and acute respiratory distress syndrome from trauma.[51] We have supported two children with severe intrapulmonary hemorrhage successfully using Carmeda components and minimal heparinization. This system is attractive for intraoperative conversion of CPB to ECMO or VAD. Even with a fully bonded circuit and moderate heparin doses, however, the problem of thrombus formation in the tubing and pump head has not been eliminated.[52]

The heparin-bonded circuit may have an added advantage of improved biocompatibility.[53-55] Studies in humans suggest that serum concentrations of various inflammatory mediators during support are reduced with heparin-bonded circuits (using low-dose heparin) compared with nonbonded circuits with higher dose heparin. Also, in animals, CPB-induced pulmonary injury seems to be less severe with heparin-bonded than non–heparin-bonded circuits.[54] Heparin coating reduces complement activation during CPB,[56,57] and there is a tendency toward reduced thrombin activation and granular release by neutrophils.[57-59] The clinical significance of these findings perhaps has not been fully shown, especially relating to VAD and ECMO.

Previously the main disadvantage of commercially available heparin-bonded oxygenators for ECMO was that heparin could not be bonded to the silicone polymers used in membranes, so hollow-fiber oxygenators were required. The subsequent generation of surface-coating techniques (Bioline) can be used to coat many surfaces by first laying down a polypeptide coat, then attaching heparin. Microporous hollow-fiber oxygenators are subject to serum leakage with prolonged use and are less suitable for long-term support. Nonmicroporous hollow-fiber oxygenators are now commercially available (Quadrox$_D$ hollow-fiber oxygenator; Jostra Medizintechnik AG, Hirrlingen, Germany) and have been used for long-term support without plasma leakage.[30] In clinical practice, we have employed heparin-bonded oxygenators (Medtronic-Carmeda) for 8 days, although the median time span is closer to 48 hours. This is in contrast to the Avecor non–heparin-bonded membrane, which has a median ECMO life of approximately 5 days, and the Jostra Quadrox$_D$, which has a median life of 149.4 hours, with no plasma leakage and no requirement for an oxygenator replacement because of device failure. The current ECMO protocol at the University of California at San Francisco is to employ Carmeda circuits for all patients requiring intraoperative or early postoperative support, patients who have significant bleeding or coagulopathy for other reasons, or patients who will require surgical procedures on ECMO. Other patients can be supported with an Avecor membrane oxygenator. Detailed analysis will be possible after more patients worldwide have been supported with heparin-bonded circuits, although based on data from Australia, the Jostra Quadrox$_D$ system seems promising.

Long-Term Functional Outcome

Ibrahim and coworkers[47] assessed the long-term outcome (median follow-up 42 months) of 35 children who survived either VAD or ECMO support. They found that 80% of the patients enjoyed good or excellent general health with a New York Heart Association class I or II cardiac status in 90%. Neurologic impairment was more common in the ECMO group, however, than in VAD patients (62% versus 20%), reflecting a combination of factors in ECMO patients, including younger age, complex cyanotic lesions, hypothermic circulatory arrest, the greater complexity of the ECMO circuit, and the need for augmented anticoagulation during ECMO.

CURRENT STATUS AND FUTURE TRENDS

Neither the centrifugal pump VAD nor ECMO system is suitable for long-term support in children. One limiting factor for both systems is the development of sepsis. Another major limitation has been the inability to wean most pediatric patients from ventilator support during centrifugal pump VAD support, mobilize them, and make them independent of ICU care. This experience compares unfavorably with that in adults, in whom patient extubation and mobilization often can be accomplished using numerous devices. Long-term support is possible in the latter group, either via recovery or bridge to transplantation, and some patients can be discharged from the hospital before (or as an alternative to) transplantation.[21,61] To date, this degree of mobilization has not been possible with small children, even with implantable devices designed for long-term support. The usefulness of centrifugal pump VAD as a bridge to transplantation depends on the immediate availability of suitable donor hearts, a major problem in many parts of the world.

The future of centrifugal pump VAD might be considered uncertain in light of advances with paracorporeal or totally implantable pulsatile and nonpulsatile systems (Table 47-2; see also Chapters 48 to 50). The importance of pulsatile flow has been debated for many years. With the centrifugal support system, there is some evidence that arterial endogenous nitric oxide production diminishes when vessels are exposed to nonpulsatile flow.[62] The real issue is suitability for safe longer term support, however. Good results have been obtained in pulsatile and nonpulsatile modes. Examples of systems that may be suitable for older children, or in some cases infants, include the Berlin Heart (Berlin Heart AG, Berlin, Germany) and the MEDOS/HIA (Medos Medizintechnik, AG, Hirrlingen, Germany) assist (both in clinical use in Europe); the Toyoba and Zeon pumps (in clinical use in Japan); the Thoratec VAD (in clinical use worldwide, including some limited application in patients weighing <20 kg); the University of Pittsburgh mini-centrifugal pump (not yet in clinical use); the Pierce-Donachy pediatric system (not yet in clinical use); and axial flow pumps including the MicroMed DeBakey VAD, Jarvik 2000, Heartmate II, and Hemopump.[21,24,32,63-71] A key feature with most of these devices is the potential to wean patients from ventilator support, mobilize them, and, in some cases, discharge them from the hospital. Improvement in the function of multiple organ systems has been well documented, improving the chances for recovery and transplantation.[66,67,72] After transplantation, the long-term outcome has not been affected adversely by the need for VAD before transplantation.[32] Likewise, age and body weight have not influenced outcome within the group.[73] These devices will play an important role in establishment of long-term support for recovery or for bridge to transplantation. Also, many devices are available for children weighing more than 50 to 60 kg (flow >2.5 to 3 L/min), who from a technical point of view could be considered similar to adults.

For short-term postoperative support, the role of most of the above-mentioned devices is controversial.[22,66] The costs involved at the time of this writing for the clinically available systems are substantially greater than for the centrifugal pump VAD for the driving system and for the disposable equipment required per ventricle per patient. We believe that for most cardiac surgical units, especially units not actively involved with transplantation, the simplicity, availability, cost-effectiveness, and good outcome (in selected cases) would ensure the place of the centrifugal pump VAD and ECMO in the surgical armamentarium for the foreseeable future.[74,75] Myocardial changes at the molecular and cellular levels during support, particularly in neonates, warrant future investigations.[76,77]

Key Concepts

■ The impaired myocardium in children after cardiac surgery may be characterized by decreased contractility, abnormal diastolic relaxation, and reduced responsiveness to inotropic and lusitropic pharmacologic stimulation. A common feature of heart failure in children with biventricular hearts is primary involvement of the left ventricle.

■ The experience with VAD support for smaller children (<20 kg) is limited, however. This situation is partly due to technical considerations, including the fact that relatively low flows may create a diathesis for thromboembolism when adult-sized systems are applied in small children. There is a long-standing perception that children with complex congenital heart disease are unsuitable for univentricular support without the use of an oxygenator.

■ Most VAD patients so treated in the postoperative period had undergone palliative or reparative open heart operations or cardiac transplantation and could not be weaned from CPB, despite optimization of blood volume, ventilation, acid-base status, and vasoactive/inotropic/lusitropic drug support. A subset of patients had refractory low cardiac output or a sudden cardiac arrest in the ICU after satisfactory primary separation from CPB and required institution of VAD support in the ICU. Low cardiac output not related to surgery (myocarditis, cardiomyopathy) was the primary indication in a small but growing number of pediatric patients.

■ Ideally, technical failure of the operation should have been ruled out before beginning VAD support, although in practice this may be quite difficult.

TABLE 47-2

Support Systems That Have Had Clinical Applications in Children

Device	Technical Features	Type of Support	Pediatric Application	Availability	Anticoagulation
Intra-aortic balloon pump (Datascope; Paramus, NJ)	Thoracic aortic occlusion in diastole maintains proximal perfusion pressure, with afterload reduction in systole as balloon deflates. Transfemoral or transaortic insertion	Left heart assist for patients with borderline cardiac output, who do not have severe LV dysfunction	Limited, due to size constraints. Most effective with M-mode echocardiography timing. Has been used in infants and older children. Short-term assist	Worldwide	Various (antiplatelet, heparin, dextran)
Hemopump (DLP; Medtronic, Grand Rapids, MI)	Axial flow pump, transaortic valve positioning required, external console, percutaneous drive cable. 14F, 21F, and 24F pumps	Nonpulsatile, left-sided, maximal flow 3.5 L/min. Short-term assist	Limited due to requirements of insertion technique. Short-term assist	Europe (investigated in the U.S.)	Systemic heparinization
Centrifugal pump (BioMedicus, Eden Prairie, MN)	Constrained vortex pump, external power console and pump	Left, right, or biventricular VAD, nonpulsatile, short-term assist	Suitable for patients of all weights and ages. Short-term assist	Worldwide	Systemic heparinization (see text)
ECMO (various devices in use)	External pump (roller or centrifugal) and power supply, with membrane (or hollow-fiber) oxygenator, in closed circuit	Nonpulsatile support of heart and lungs. May require left heart venting for adequate support	Suitable for patients of all weights and ages. Short-term assist	Worldwide (in various formats)	Systemic heparinization (see text)
Berlin Heart and Medos/HIA Heart assist system	Pneumatic paracorporeal VAD, with compressible polyurethane ventricles and inlet/outlet valves	Pulsatile support as left, right, or biventricular VAD	Suitable for all patients, including neonates. May be suitable for long-term support	Europe	Systemic heparinization

ECMO, extracorporeal membrane oxygenation; IV, left ventricular; VAD, ventricular assist device.

Toward this end, there is a role for intraoperative assessment with transesophageal echocardiography with direct cardiac chamber pressure and saturation measurements or a cardiac catheterization even while on VAD support.

■ There are numerous relative contraindications to the use of VADs, including multiorgan system failure, severe coagulopathy, intracranial hemorrhage, neurologic impairment, uncontrolled sepsis, prolonged cardiac arrest, and a univentricular circulation. In practice, although all may be relevant, most of these features are difficult or impossible to assess accurately in a child who needs placement of a VAD, especially in an intraoperative or ICU setting.

■ Patients with acute fulminant myocarditis may benefit greatly from mechanical circulatory assistance to promote myocardial recovery. Support with VAD may be preferable to ECMO in such cases because it more completely unloads the left ventricle, which may lead to rapid reverse remodeling of the left ventricle.

■ Cardiomyopathy may be an indication for VAD when decompensation and low cardiac output signs dominate the clinical picture. Although recovery of adequate native heart function is possible in rare instances, most patients require a VAD as a bridge to transplantation.

■ For patients weighing less than 20 kg, two weeks would be considered to be the maximal realistic projected duration of support with a VAD. Patients supported specifically for bridging (as opposed to recovery) should meet institutional criteria for transplantation prospectively.

■ VAD support in a patient with a univentricular circulation is currently controversial, but centers have supported such patients successfully with VAD and ECMO after the Norwood operation for hypoplastic left heart syndrome and after bidirectional cavopulmonary shunts performed for complex univentricular variants. In such cases, higher than normal flows (approximately 150% of calculated) may be required because the assist device provides pulmonary and systemic outputs.

■ The important component of the centrifugal pump head is an impeller consisting of rotating cones or vanes, which create a constrained vortex. The impeller is coupled electromagnetically to the drive unit so that the operator can set the rotational speed of the pump. Rotation creates subatmospheric pressure at the tip of the cone, establishing suction in the venous cannula. Positive pressure is created at the outlet (arterial cannula).

■ The centrifugal pump output (flow) depends on preload and afterload and the rotational speed of the pump. The most efficient (and least hemolytic) settings for a centrifugal pump occur at the lowest pump speed for a given flow. In this respect, the centrifugal pump allows fine-tuning of the peripheral circulation before and during weaning because it is responsive (flow at a given pressure) to the patient's intravascular volume and resistance.

■ The decrease in left atrial pressure usually seen with left VAD may improve pulmonary hypertension and right ventricular dysfunction dramatically in borderline cases, especially with concurrent use of inhaled nitric oxide. Each case must be assessed individually, and the simplest effective level of support (i.e., VAD rather than ECMO) whenever possible should be considered.

■ In patients with improving ventricular function on VAD, one generally notes the appearance of a pulsatile systemic arterial pressure trace as the first sign. Echocardiographic assessment is helpful at this point to evaluate further the ventricular contractility and the response to volume loading. A Starling response suggests that weaning can proceed.

■ Short-term circulatory support has been particularly effective for postoperative patients with ALCAPA, TGA after ASO, and donor heart dysfunction after transplantation. The unifying principle in these cases is undoubtedly the presence of two relatively normal ventricles, with the left ventricle being temporarily (but critically) impaired.

REFERENCES

1. DeBakey ME: Left ventricular bypass for cardiac assistance: Clinical experience. Am J Cardiol 1971;27:3.
1a. Karl TR: Extracorporeal circulatory support in infants and children. Semin Thorac Cardiovasc Surg 1994;6:154-160.
2. Kipla K, Mattiello JA, Jeevanandam V, et al: Myocyte recovery after mechanical circulatory support in humans with end-stage heart failure. Circulation 1998;97:2316-2322.
3. Herwig V, Severin M, Waldenberger FR, Konertz W: MEDOS/HIA-assist system: First experiences with mechanical circulatory assist in infants and children. Int J Artif Organs 1997;20:692-694.
4. Tracy TF Jr, DeLosh T, Bartlett RH: Extracorporeal Life Support Organisation 1994. ASAIO J 1994;40:1017-1019.
5. Karl TR, Horton SB, Mee RBB: Left heart assist for ischaemic postoperative ventricular dysfunction in an infant with anomalous left coronary artery. J Card Surg 1989;4:352-354.
6. Karl TR, Horton SB, Sano S, Mee RBB: Centrifugal pump left heart assist in pediatric cardiac surgery: Indications, technique and results. J Thorac Cardiovasc Surg 1991;102:624-630.
7. Karl TR, Pennington GD: Extracorporeal circulatory support in infants and children. Semin Thorac Cardiovasc Surg 1994;6:154-160.
8. Cochrane AD, Horton A, Butt W, et al: Neonatal and paediatric extracorporeal membrane oxygenation. Australas J Cardiac Thorac Surg 1992;1:17-22.
9. Karl TR: Circulatory support in children. In Hetzer R, Hennig E. Loebe M (eds): Mechanical Circulatory Support. Berlin, Springer, 1997, pp 7-20.
10. Thuys CA, Mullaly RJ, Horton SB, et al: Centrifugal ventricular assist in children under 6 kg. Eur J Cardiothorac Surg 1998;13:130-134.
11. Warnecke H, Berdjis F, Hennig E, et al: Mechanical left ventricular support as a bridge to cardiac transplantation in childhood. Eur J Cardiothorac Surg 1991;5:330-333.
12. Del Nido PJ, Armitage JM, Fricker FJ, et al: Extracorporeal membrane oxygenation as a bridge to pediatric heart transplantation. Circulation 1994;90: II-66-II-69.

13. Kirshbom PM, Bridges ND, Myung RJ, et al: Use of extracorporeal membrane oxygenation in pediatric thoracic organ transplantation. J Thorac Cardiovasc Surg 2002;123:130-136.

14. Doski JJ, Butler TJ, Louder DS, et al: Outcome of infants requiring cardiopulmonary resuscitation before extracorporeal membrane oxygenation. J Pediatr Surg 1997;32:1318-1321.

15. Aharon AS, Drinkwater DC Jr, Churchwell KB, et al: Extracorporeal membrane oxygenation in children after repair of congenital cardiac lesions. Ann Thorac Surg 2001;72:2095-2101.

16. Duncan BW, Bohn DJ, Atz AM, et al: Mechanical circulatory support for the treatment of children with acute fulminant myocarditis. J Thorac Cardiovasc Surg 2001;122:440-448.

17. Eugene J, Ott RA, McColgan SJ, Roohk HV: Vented cardiac assistance: ECMO versus left heart bypass for acute left ventricular failure. ASAIO Trans 1986;32:538-541.

18. Eugene J, McColgan SJ, Roohk HV, Ott RA: Vented ECMO for biventricular failure. ASAIO Trans 1987;33:579-583.

19. Bavaria JE, Ratcliffe MB, Gupta KB, et al: Changes in left ventricular systolic wall stress during biventricular circulatory assistance. Ann Thorac Surg 1988;45:526-532.

20. Ratcliffe MB, Bavaria JE, Wenger RK, et al: Left ventricular mechanics of ejecting, postischemic hearts during left ventricular circulatory assistance. J Thorac Cardiovasc Surg 1991;101:245-255.

21. Loebe M, Hennig E, Muller J, et al: Long-term mechanical circulatory support as a bridge to transplantation, for recovery from cardiomyopathy, and for permanent replacement. Eur J Cardiothorac Surg 1997;11:S18-S24.

22. Hetzer R, Loebe M, Potapov EV, et al: Circulatory support with pneumatic paracorporeal ventricular assist device in infants and children. Ann Thorac Surg 1998;65:1498-1506.

23. Konertz W, Reul H: Mechanical circulatory support in children. Int J Artif Organs 1997;20:657-658.

24. Ashton RC Jr, Oz MC, Michler RE, et al: Left ventricular assist device options in pediatric patients. ASAIO J 1995;41:M277-M280.

25. Konertz W, Hotz H, Schneider M, et al: Clinical expertise with the MEDOS HIA-VAD system in infants and children: A preliminary report. Ann Thorac Surg 1997;63:1138-1144.

26. Karl TR, Horton SB: Centrifugal pump VAD in paediatric cardiac surgery. In Duncan BW (ed): Mechanical Circulatory Support for Paediatric Cardiac Patients. New York, Marcel Dekker, 1999, pp. 21-48.

27. Jaggers JJ, Forbess JM, Shah AS, et al: Extracorporeal membrane oxygenation for infant postcardiotomy support: Significance of shunt management. Ann Thorac Surg 2000;69:1476-1483.

28. Darling EM, Kaemmer D, Lawson DS, et al: Use of ECMO without the oxygenator to provide ventricular support after Norwood stage I procedures. Ann Thorac Surg 2001;71:735-736.

29. Horton SB, Horton AM, Mullaly RJ, et al: Extracorporeal membrane oxygenation life support: A new approach. Perfusion 1993;8:239-247.

30. Horton S, Thuys C, Bennett M, et al: Experience with the Jostra Rotaflow and Quadrox D oxygenator for ECMO. Perfusion 2004;19:17-23.

31. Vitali E, Lanfranconi M, Bruschi G, et al: Left ventricular assist devices as bridge to heart transplantation: The Niguarda experience. J Card Surg 2003;18:107-113.

32. Marelli D, Laks H, Meehan DA, et al: Minimally invasive mechanical cardiac support without extracorporeal membrane oxygenation in children awaiting heart transplantation. Ann Thorac Surg 1999;68:2320-2323.

33. Pavie A, Leger P: Physiology of univentricular versus biventricular support. Ann Thorac Surg 1996;61:347-349.

34. Costa RJ, Chard RB, Nunn GR, Cartmill TB: Ventricular assist devices in pediatric cardiac surgery. Ann Thorac Surg 1995;60:S536-S538.

35. Pennington DG, Swartz MT: Circulatory support in infants and children. Ann Thorac Surg 1993;55:233-237.

36. Karl TR, Cochrane AD, Brizard CP, et al: Coronary anomalies in children. In Buxton B, Frazier OH, Westaby S (eds): Surgery for Ischaemic Heart Disease Surgical Management. London, Mosby, 1997, pp 261-287.

37. Duncan BW, Hraska V, Jonas RA, et al: Mechanical circulatory support in children with cardiac disease. J Thorac Cardiovasc Surg 1999;117:529-542.

38. Kanter KR, Pennington G, Weber TR, et al: Extracorporeal membrane oxygenation for postoperative cardiac support in children. J Thorac Cardiovasc Surg 1987;93:27-35.

39. Rogers AJ, Trento A, Siewers RD, et al: Extracorporeal membrane oxygenation for postcardiotomy shock in children. Ann Thorac Surg 1989;47:903-906.

40. Cochrane AD, Coleman DM, Davis AD, et al: Excellent long term functional outcome after surgery for ALCAPA. J Thorac Cardiovasc Surg 1999;117:332-342.

41. Neches WH, Mathews RA, Park SC, et al: Anomalous origin of the left coronary artery from the pulmonary artery. Circulation 1974;50:582-587.

42. Laborde F, Marchand M, Leca F, et al: Surgical treatment of anomalous origin of the left coronary artery in infancy and childhood. J Thorac Cardiovasc Surg 1981;82:423-428.

43. Horton AM, Butt W: Pump-induced haemolysis: Is the constrained vortex pump better or worse than the roller pump? Perfusion 1992;7:103-108.

44. Shivalkar B, Borgers M, Daenen W, et al: ALCAPA syndrome: An example of chronic myocardial hypoperfusion? J Am Coll Cardiol 1994;23:772-778.

45. Jonas RA, Giglia TM, Sanders SP, et al: Rapid two-stage arterial switch for transposition of the great arteries and intact ventricular septum beyond the neonatal period. Circulation 1989;80:1203-1208.

46. Davis A, Wilkinson JL, Karl TR, Mee RBB: Transposition of the great arteries with intact ventricular septum: Arterial switch repair in patients 21 days of age or older. J Thorac Cardiovasc Surg 1993;106:111-115.

47. Ibrahim AE, Duncan BW, Blume ED, Jonas RA: Long-term follow-up of pediatrics patients requiring mechanical circulatory support. Ann Thorac Surg 2000;69:186-192.

48. Bindslev L, Bohm C, Jolin A, et al: Extracorporeal carbon dioxide removal performed with surface-heparinized equipment in patients with ARDS. Acta Anesth Scand 1991;95:125-130.

49. Muehrcke DD, McCarthy PM, Stewart RW, et al: Extracorporeal membrane oxygenation for postcardiotomy shock. Ann Thorac Surg 1996;61:684-691.

50. Schreurs HH, Wijers MJ, Gu YJ: Heparin-coated bypass circuits: Effects on inflammatory response in pediatric cardiac operations. Ann Thorac Surg 1998;66:166-171.

51. Rossaint R, Slama K, Lewandowski K, et al: Extracorporeal lung assist with heparin-coated systems. Int J Artif Organs 1992;15:29-34.

52. Bianchi JJ, Swartz MT, Raithel SC, et al: Initial clinical experience with centrifugal pumps coated with the Carmeda process. ASAIO J 1992;38:143-146.

53. Fosse E, Moen O, Johnson E, et al: Reduced complement and granulocyte activation with heparin-coated cardiopulmonary bypass. Ann Thorac Surg 1994;58:472-477.

53. Redmond JM, Gillinov AM, Stuart RS, et al: Heparin-coated bypass circuits reduce pulmonary injury. Ann Thorac Surg 1993;56:474-478.

55. Shigemitsu O, Hadama T, Takasaki H, et al: Biocompatibility of a heparin-bonded membrane oxygenator (Carmeda MAXIMA) during the first 90 minutes of cardiopulmonary bypass: Clinical comparison with the conventional system. Artif Organs 1994;18:963-971.

56. Mollnes TE, Videm V, Gotze O, et al: Formation of C5a during cardiopulmonary bypass: Inhibition by precoating with heparin. Ann Thorac Surg 1991;52:92-97.

57. Videm V, Mollnes TE, Garred P, Svennivig JL: Biocompatibility of extracorporeal circulation: In vitro comparison of heparin-coated and uncoated oxygenator circuits. J Thorac Cardiovasc Surg 1991;101:654-660.

58. Borowiec J, Thelin S, Bagge L, et al: Heparin-coated circuits reduce activation of granulocytes during cardiopulmonary bypass: A clinical study. J Thorac Cardiovasc Surg 1992;104: 642-647.

59. Larsson R, Larm O, Olsson P: The search for thromboresistance using immobilized heparin: Blood in contact with natural and artificial surfaces. Ann N Y Acad Sci 1987;516:102-115.

60. Ziomek S, Harrell JE Jr, Fasules JW, et al: Extracorporeal membrane oxygenation for cardiac failure after congenital heart operation. Ann Thorac Surg 1992;54:861-868.

61. Fey O, El-Banayosy A, Arosuglu L, et al: Out-of-hospital experience in patients with implantable mechanical circulatory support: Present and future trends. Eur J Cardiothorac Surg 1997;11: S51-S53.

62. Macha M, Yamazaki K, Gordon LM, et al: The vasoregulatory role of endothelium derived nitric oxide during pulsatile cardiopulmonary bypass. ASAIO J 1996;42:M800-M804.

63. Litwak P, Butler KC, Thomas DC, et al: Development and initial testing of a pediatric centrifugal blood pump. Ann Thorac Surg 1996;61:448-451.

64. Daily BB, Pettitt TW, Sutera SP, Pierce WS: Pierce-Donach pediatric VAD: Progress in development. Ann Thorac Surg 1996;61:437-443.

65. Goldstein DJ: Worldwide experience with the MicroMed DeBakey Ventricular Assist Device as a bridge to transplantation. Circulation 2003;108(Suppl 1):II-272-II-277.

66. Merkle F, Boettcher W, Stiller B, Hetzer R: Pulsatile mechanical cardiac assistance in pediatric patients with the Berlin heart ventricular assist device. J Extracorpor Technol 2003;35:115-120.

67. El-Banayosy NR, Arusoglu L, Kleikamp G, et al: Recovery of organ dysfunction during bridging to heart transplantation in children and adolescents. Int J Artif Organs 2003;26:395-400.

68. Hendry PJ, Masters RG, Davies RA, et al: Mechanical circulatory support for adolescent patients: The Ottawa Heart Institute experience. Can J Cardiol 2003;31:409-412.

69. Frazier OH, Myers TJ, Gregoric ID, et al: Initial clinical experience with the Jarvik 2000 implantable axial-flow left ventricular assist system. Circulation 2002;105:2855-2860.

70. Griffith BP, Kormos RL, Borovetz HS, et al: HeartMate II left ventricular assist system: From concept to first clinical use. Ann Thorac Surg 200171:S116-120.

71. DeBakey ME: A miniature implantable axial flow ventricular assist device. Ann Thorac Surg 1999;68:637-640.

72. Sidiropoulos A, Hotz H, Konertz W: Pediatric circulatory support. J Heart Lung Transplant 1998;17:1172-1176.

73. Reinhartz O, Stiller B, Eilers R, Farrar DJ: Current clinical status of pulsatile pediatric circulatory support. ASAIO J 2002;48: 455-459.

74. Chang AC, McKenzie ED: Mechanical cardiopulmonary support in children: Extracorporeal membrane oxygenation, ventricular assist devices, and long term assist devices. Pediatr Cardiol 2005;26:2-28.

75. Ungerleider RM, Shen I, Yeh T, et al: Routine mechanical ventricular assist following the Norwood procecure: Improved neurological outcome and excellent hospital survival. Ann Thorac Surg 2004;77:18-22.

76. Birks EJ, Felkin LE, Banner NR, et al: Increased toll like receptor 4 in the myocardium of patients requiring left ventricular assist devices. J Heart Lung Transplant 2004;23:228-235.

77. Patten RD, Denofrio D, El-Zaro M, et al: Ventricular assist device therapy normalizes inducible nitric oxide synthase expression and reduces cardiomyocyte apoptosis in the failing human heart. J Am Coll Cardiol 2005;45:1419-1424.

CHAPTER 48

Long-Term Ventricular Assist Devices in Children

Daniel J. DiBardino
Anthony C. Chang
E. Dean McKenzie

Since the early 1950s, when DeBakey introduced the concept of ventricular assist devices (VADs) and then successfully used a left ventricular bypass pump for cardiac assistance in 1966,[1] nearly all published data and previous technical development with longer term assistance for the failing heart involve adult or adolescent patients.[2] The application of mechanical circulatory assist devices in adults has reached a level of sophistication such that physicians are able to tailor device therapy to specific patient requirements.[3] A broad range of diverse options for adult mechanical circulatory assistance has helped to make such tailored applications possible and has translated into improving results. With the exception of extracorporeal membrane oxygenation (ECMO) and more recently a centrifugal VAD support (both in the intensive care unit [ICU]), novel and longer term options for pediatric mechanical circulatory assistance have largely been undeveloped.

Changing pediatric patient demographics have required a refocusing of attention in long-term VADs. Increasing success of palliative and corrective operations for congenital heart disease has translated into a decreasing need for neonatal and infant heart transplantation and a significant increase in the number of children and youth living with previously palliated or corrected congenital heart disease. Pediatric patients who are likely to have progressive heart failure include children with staged palliation for hypoplastic left heart syndrome and other single-ventricle lesions, children born with transposition of the great arteries who underwent prior atrial switch, children with failing Fontan circulation, and children with cardiomyopathy currently facing varying waiting times for cardiac transplantation.

The REMATCH (Randomized Evaluation of Mechanical Assistance for the Treatment of Congestive Heart Failure) trial has shown that with the application of effective long-term mechanical assist devices in adults, significant improvements in overall survival and quality of life have been possible.[4] The plasticity of pediatric organs and of the heart has led many authors to believe that myocardial recovery is not only possible, but also more likely than in adults in a host of heart failure patient subtypes.

Longer term mechanical assistance is the ultimate implementation of this philosophy of maximizing systemic oxygen delivery while improving myocardial oxygen supply-to-demand ratio and providing the most favorable environment for ventricular recovery on a longer basis. This chapter discusses the use of devices for longer term support of the failing heart in the pediatric patient.

INDICATIONS AND CONTRAINDICATIONS FOR LONG-TERM DEVICES

The indication for any form of mechanical circulatory support is cardiogenic shock refractory to medical management that, if left untreated, would lead to irreversible organ injury or death. Often the most difficult decision is determining the appropriate timing for initiation of support. The physician's objective is to determine the trajectory of the child's deterioration, intervening before the development of irreversible end-organ injury, but avoiding unnecessary mechanical support in children who otherwise would recover. Decision making regarding timing of institution of support is rendered more difficult in infants and small children because of the paucity of viable devices capable of longer term support. (See Chapters 49 and 50.)

When the decision is made to apply mechanical circulatory support, the device options must be weighed carefully according to the particular pathophysiology and the anticipated outcome for the patient. Short-term mechanical support is discussed in Chapters 45 to 47. Longer term ventricular assistance becomes necessary when recovery of myocardial failure is not expected in a matter of days, and either delayed recovery or cardiac transplantation is the expected outcome. Currently the use of mechanical circulatory support as destination therapy is not an option in pediatric patients.

LONG-TERM DEVICE OPTIONS IN CHILDREN

The emergence of better long-term mechanical support devices for adults has made it possible for use of such devices in select pediatric patients. The advent of this

This chapter is especially dedicated to Dr. Michael DeBakey, who has been an ardent advocate for children, an often forgotten patient population in heart failure.

newer type of device has provided a better range of equipment for mechanical support in children in the ICU, but longer term mechanical support devices, especially for neonates, are still lacking. The adult experience of ECMO to implantable device conversion has yielded improved survival,[5] and long-term support has had good results.[6] There also is movement toward use of these devices as destination therapy to preclude the need for orthotopic heart transplantation.[7] Because of lack of corporate interest and obvious size constraints, this area of long-term mechanical support has not been developed fully for pediatric patients.

There is rapidly growing clinical experience with the following devices in adults with postcardiotomy failure, acute myocardial infarction and cardiogenic shock, ischemic cardiomyopathy, and myocarditis. The various devices are used as single VADs or biventricular VADs depending on the device and the patient. These devices are used as bridge to recovery, bridge to transplantation, or bridge to the same or other mechanical device as destination therapy. The REMATCH trial in adult patients with severe heart failure who were ineligible for heart transplantation has illustrated significant improvements in quality of life and short-term survival in patients with severe heart failure with use of VADs as destination therapy compared with optimal medical management. In the same study, the most common causes of death were infection and device failure.

There are no widely accepted longer term support devices for smaller pediatric patients with a body surface area of less than 1.2 m². Implantable left VAD systems have been used for bridge to transplantation, bridge to myocardial recovery, or permanent circulatory support only in larger children. These devices, separated into pulsatile and axial types of devices, are briefly described because they will undoubtedly become more commonplace in children in the coming years. The reader will find more detailed discussions in other chapters in this section relating to mechanical support and the atlas of mechanical devices at the end of the book.

Pulsatile Devices

Since the early report of pneumatic paracorporeal VADs in children,[8] pediatric experience with long-term pulsatile devices has been growing. Advantages of pulsatile devices include long-term support capability, ease of use, capability for biventricular support without an oxygenator, mobility to be out of the ICU, need for low-level anticoagulation, and pulsatile flow nature. Disadvantages include a propensity to have thromboembolic complications, difficulty of implantation and explantation, cumulative cost, need for exteriorization of the cannulae, and size limitations especially with the need for biventricular support. Infection also is a serious complication, but immobilization of the driveline or cannulae as close to the exit site as possible with a binder can decrease the incidence of infections.

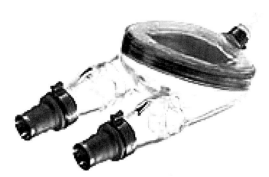

FIGURE 48-1 ■ **Berlin Heart ventricular assist system.** Pulsatile ventricular assist system from the Berlin Heart Institute, Berlin, Germany. This paracorporeal pulsatile device has a pediatric miniaturized version. The polyurethane pumps, with two different valve systems made of either mechanical tilting discs or polyurethane leaflets, have a wide range of stroke volumes of 10 mL, 25 mL, 30 mL, 50 mL, and 60 mL designed for pediatric use, but can go up to 80 mL for adults. (Courtesy of Berlin Heart AG, Berlin, Germany.) (See also Color Section)

German cardiac surgeons have had considerable pediatric experience with longer term circulatory support using two devices currently available only for compassionate use in the United States. The **Berlin Heart VAD** (Berlin Heart AG, Berlin, Germany) is a paracorporeal, pneumatically driven blood pump that incorporates polyurethane trileaflet valves to guard the inflow and outflow in the neonatal and infantile sized models (Fig. 48-1). The Berlin Heart VAD, or EXCOR, has been in use since 1988 and has been available for pediatric patients since 1992 at the Deutsches Herzzenrum, Berlin.[9,10] The pumps, with two different valve systems made of either mechanical tilting discs or polyurethane leaflets, have a wide range of stroke volumes of 10 mL, 25 mL, 30 mL, 50 mL, and 60 mL designed for pediatric use, but can go up to 80 mL for adults. Three membranes provide stability, and the system is heparin-coated. The stationary IKUS driving unit can operate in various modes (synchronous, asynchronous, and independent). A rechargeable battery can supply 5 hours of independent power supply, and its mobile drive unit can transform this into an outpatient device. This device can provide univentricular or biventricular support.

Survival with the Berlin Heart has been reported to be 74% in 66 patients ages 2 days to 18 years for a mean support of 33 days (longest support of 420 days).[11] Early complication of thrombus has been lessened with use of a heparin-coated system. Postoperative care includes use of heparin at 400 to 1200 U/kg/day initially followed by aspirin and dipyridamole without the use of warfarin. Because of its ability to support the heart for this longer duration, this device is well suited for children with myocarditis with longer recovery periods for even biventricular assist.[12]

The **MEDOS-HIA-VAD** (Helmholtz Institute, Aachen, Germany) is a paracorporeal, pneumatically driven blood pump available in 60-mL, 25-mL, and 10-mL stroke volumes and with a similar valve design. In the original description of the pump, the designers elaborate on alternate pump chambers in sizes 10% smaller for complementary right heart bypass should a biventricular configuration become necessary.[13] In 1994, the MEDOS VAD system was developed in Germany, and it is also a pneumatically driven paracorporeal VAD with three left ventricular sizes (10-mL, 25-mL, and 60-mL maximal stroke volumes) and three right ventricular sizes (9-mL, 22.5-mL, and 54-mL maximal stroke volumes)[14,15] and a later modification of a three-leaflet blood pump valve to improve dynamic blood flow of the pump.[16] An animal study of 3-week-old lambs with right ventricular failure showed that this device was successful with a miniaturized pulsatile right VAD.[17] Survival has been reported to be 36.2% in children 16 years old, including an infant with a body surface area of less than 0.3 m².[18]

The **Thoratec Ventricular Assist System** (Thoratec Corp, Berkeley, CA) is a pneumatically powered pulsatile assist device that consists of a flexible, seam-free, segmented sac within a ridged polycarbonate housing (Fig. 48-2). There are Bjork-Shiley concave-convex tilting disc valves in the inlet and outlet portions. The stroke volume is 65 mL with a maximum output of 7 L/min. The inlet portion is cannulation via left atrial or left ventricular apex and the outlet portion is cannulation to the aorta with both of the cannulae exteriorized. Three modes exist for this assist system: fixed rate, synchronous (with wean to 1:3), or fill-to-empty mode. The device is flexible in terms of usage in smaller sized patients.

The pediatric experience is limited and includes a reported series of 176 patients and a survival of 70.7%

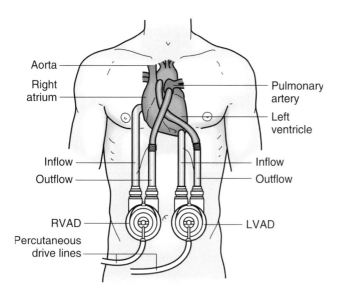

FIGURE 48-2 ■ Thoratec ventricular assist system. Schematic diagram of the Thoratec ventricular assist system for biventricular support (see text for details). LVAD, left ventricular assist device; RVAD, right ventricular assist device. (From Patel H, Pagani FD: *Extracorporeal mechanical circulatory assist*. In Samuels LE and Narula J (eds): *Ventricular Assist Devices and the Artificial Heart. Cardiol Clin* 2003 p. 37, WB Saunders, Philadelphia.)

(longest support of 434 days)[19,20] and a child as small as 17 kg (body surface area 0.7 m²) who had viral cardiomyopathy and was supported for 22 days.[21] These results in children are similar to adult series.[22,23] Neurologic complications in these pediatric patients seem to be higher when cannulation is performed in the left atrium.[24]

Finally, Ashton and associates[25] have reported success with the use of the **BVS-5000** device in four patients 7 to 15 years old with a body surface area of 0.85 to 1.85 m². The size limitations imposed by the devices available in the Untied States and a differential patient population do not allow a direct comparison with the German experience. Neither the Thoratec VAD nor the Abiomed BVS-5000 adult device is practical for use in children with a body surface area of less than 0.8 m². Other than the stated compassionate use exception for the German systems, no paracorporeal, pulsatile VADs are currently available in the United States to provide longer term mechanical circulatory support in small children.

Hypertension while on support with these devices can be treated with numerous agents, including milrinone, calcium channel blockers, angiotensin-converting enzyme inhibitors, β-blockers, α-antagonists, nitroprusside, and nitroglycerin. The anticoagulation regimen is usually heparin or warfarin with antiplatelet therapy.

Rotary/Axial Devices

Axial flow technology may be the most adaptable to miniaturization and intracorporeal application in small children. These devices currently are available only for children ages 5 to 16 years with body surface area of greater than or equal to 0.7 m². The extremely limited experience of axial devices in children is described here. Although the pediatric experience with these axial devices is extremely small and limited to a few adolescents and children, the smaller size holds the best promise for future pediatric use. These devices consist of relatively small axial pumps that involve an impeller within the housing that are almost entirely implantable. Some of these devices can be implanted without cardiopulmonary bypass. The apex of the left ventricle is used as the inflow (to maximize flow conditions), and the ascending aorta is used for the outflow graft secondary to thrombus formation when the graft is placed in the descending aorta.

Advantages of an axial system are the relatively small size, implant/explant procedures that are relatively easy, noiseless system, decreased infection, relatively lower cost, and continuous flow that not only provides unloading throughout the cardiac cycle, but also minimizes stasis and thrombus formation.[26] Disadvantages include the need for a relatively large-sized ventricular apical cannulation and relative size limitation to pediatric patients with a body surface area of greater than 1.5 m².

The **Jarvik-2000** (Jarvik Research, Inc, New York, NY) is an intraventricular assist device that has an ultra-smooth titanium surface and relatively small surface area measuring 25 mm in diameter and 55 mm in length. The device usually is implanted into the left ventricular apex via a left thoracotomy, and the outflow graft is placed into the descending aorta.[27] Blood flow is 2 to 7 L/min and is determined by impeller speed and systemic vascular resistance with the usual setting at 9,000 revolutions per minute (rpm) (range 8,000 to 12,000 rpm). Although there have been more than 30 implantations in humans at the Texas Heart Institute, there has been virtually no pediatric experience to date.[28]

The **MicroMed DeBakey VAD** (MicroMed Technology, Houston, TX) is an axial device with inflow from the left ventricle and outflow to the ascending aorta pushing blood at 7,500 to 12,500 rpm with flow 10 L/min (Fig. 48-3). DeBakey and Noon collaborated with NASA engineer Saucier to use computational fluid dynamics to build this axial flow pump designed to minimize hemolysis and thrombosis.

The adult DeBakey VAD is the prototype of the newer generation of axial VADs. This device was the first long-term axial flow circulatory assist device to be introduced into clinical trials (since November 1998) as a bridge to transplantation and has had the largest clinical experience with more than 350 patients worldwide (Noon GP: personal communication). Because of its relatively small size, it is an attractive potential device in children, and present experience includes patients ages 12 to 76 years and a body surface area of 1.3 m². In Goldstein's reported experience of 150 patients who underwent DeBakey VAD implantation between November 1998 and May 2002, the cumulative support time is 30.4 years, and the mean age was 48 years. The preoperative situation was suboptimal with 25% of patients on intra-aortic balloon pumps, 20% of patients with renal insufficiency, and 40% of patients who were on at least two inotropic agents with a mean cardiac index of 1.8 L/min/m². The mean support time was 75 days. Thrombus formation associated with the MicroMed DeBakey VAD has been

reported and treated with recombinant tissue plasminogen activator.[29]

The advantages of axial devices such as the DeBakey VAD include miniaturization of the device, system ergonomics facilitating ambulation, patient exercise possible with fixed pump speed, and noiseless system. Additional benefits include ease of surgical implantation, rare postoperative infections, reduced surgical bleeding, and end-organ function maintained or improved. Disadvantages include nonpulsatile flow. Other axial devices that may have potential pediatric applications in the future include the Thoratec HeartMate II, the Berlin Heart INCOR I, the SUN Medical Technology Research Corporation IVAP VAD, the University of Pittsburgh Streamliner, the Valvo VAD, and the INTEC axial flow pump.[30]

First Pediatric Implantable Device: DeBakey VAD Child

Because of its small size, the axial VAD holds the most promise for small children as a long-term assist device. The **DeBakey VAD Child**, an implantable assist device intended for long-term left ventricular support in children, marks the first effort to address the ever-increasing population of smaller children with end-stage heart disease. It was approved for use in children (ages 5 to 16 years with a body surface area of 0.7 to 1.2 m²) with end-stage heart failure who need mechanical circulatory support for bridge to transplantation applications under a Humanitarian Device Exemption by the U.S. Food and Drug Administration in February 2004. Contraindications are listed in Table 48-1. These smaller devices have important advantages over the pulsatile devices, particularly in small children (Table 48-2).

Device and Implantation

The DeBakey pediatric device is a modified version of the adult DeBakey VAD. It is an electromagnetically actuated, fully implantable, titanium axial **flow pump** (measuring 30.5 mm × 76.2 mm and weighing 95 g) that is capable of generating 10 L/min of flow (see Fig. 48-3). The pump has several components, including the impeller, flow straightener, flow tube, motor stator, stator housing, and diffuser. The blood inflow is directed to

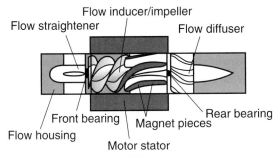

FIGURE 48-3 ■ The DeBakey VAD pump. Schematic diagram illustrates the various internal components of the DeBakey VAD pump. The impeller is the only moving part of the pump and has six blades with eight magnets hermetically sealed in each blade. This impeller is driven by a brushless direct current motor stator that spins the impeller by a changing electromagnetic field. The flow straightener acts as a front-bearing support for the impeller, whereas the diffuser contains the rear bearing and slows the high tangential velocity blood by redirecting the blood axially. All of these components are hermetically sealed in a titanium flow tube. (From MicroMed Technology, Houston, TX.)

TABLE 48-1

Contraindications for Use
Patients <5 years old
Patients with right ventricular failure unresolved by medical therapy
Patients with a primary coagulopathy or platelet disorder
Patients with an allergy or sensitivity to heparin
Prior surgery where apical cannulation, pump replacement, or graft anastomosis is not feasible

TABLE 48-2

Advantages and Disadvantages of Pulsatile Versus Axial Devices		
	Pulsatile	Axial
Pulsatile flow	Yes	Possible
Design	Complicated	Simple
Noise	Yes	No
Size	Large	Small
Valves	Yes	No
Moving parts	Several	One
Compliance chamber	Yes	No
Blood-to-device interface	Large	Small
Infection	Low	Lower
Mobility	Limited	Less limited

the impeller via the flow straightener, then exits the pump via the diffuser.

The inflow component of the DeBakey VAD Child pump consists of a titanium L-shaped **inflow cannula** (modified from the adult model) that is inserted directly into the left ventricular apex via a sewing ring from a midline sternotomy using cardiopulmonary bypass (Fig. 48-4). The inflow cannula should be placed carefully so as not to direct it toward the septum or free wall. The 12-mm Vascutek Gelweave **outflow graft,** with its proximal part covered by a protector, passes through an ultrasonic **flow transducer** (reduced in size for children) that provides real-time measurement of blood flow through the pump and is anastomosed to the ascending aorta via a longitudinal arteriotomy. The intracorporeal components of the device are designed to allow application in children with a body surface area of 0.7 m², whereas the adult device is approved for use in patients with a body surface area of a minimum of 1.2 m². At the end of the implantation, the entire device is carefully de-aired to avoid air embolization. The driveline is tunneled across the midline with the use of a trocar. The implanted pump is connected to the **controller** via a percutaneous cable and a controller connector (Fig. 48-5). Inotropic support for the right ventricle and appropriate intravascular volume are maintained as the patient is weaned from cardiopulmonary bypass.

The controller is a microprocessor-based computer that serves as the brains of the system and maintains the pump speed at 7,500 to 12,500 rpm. It also displays the pump status and alarm messages and sounds audible alarms. The **clinical data acquisition system** (CDAS) is a bedside monitoring device that allows setting of operating parameters (e.g., pump speed, alarm values, and patient data) and viewing of pump information (e.g., flow, power, speed) and stores information onto a memory device. The CDAS also powers the VAD during implantation and recovery and is used to set up the pump operation in the operating room during implantation.

The **VADPAK,** an ergonomically designed battery pack that includes two batteries and the controller, weighs only 5 lbs and powers the pump for 5 to 8 hours, which allows for untethered mobility for extended periods. This portability allows for discharge of the patient from the hospital and greatly improves quality of life and the potential for rehabilitation. The VADPAK also contains an external port for CDAS and patient home support system connection. The controller alternatively can be connected to a power source via the CDAS or the **patient home support system (PHSS),** which also is used to recharge batteries while the patient is resting. A charge PAK is a backup charger that charges two batteries at a time, with each battery lasting 2.5 to 4 hours.

Postoperative Care and Complications

Postoperative care after implantation of the DeBakey VAD Child is provided in the cardiac ICU with an important emphasis on medical management of any **right ventricular dysfunction** because the right ventricular output "preloads" the VAD. Medical management of right ventricular dysfunction includes diuretics; inotropic agents, such as isoproterenol and milrinone; and measures to lower pulmonary vascular resistance, such as use of inhaled nitric oxide (see Chapter 16). A right VAD may be considered if right ventricular dysfunction is refractory to medical therapy. Mixed venous oxygen saturation via a right atrial or pulmonary arterial line may be useful for adjusting pump speed and flow. Extubation is performed when the cardiopulmonary status is stable. Troubleshooting of diagnostic, emergency, and fail-safe alarms is beyond the scope of this chapter.

The flow across the DeBakey VAD Child pump varies with pump speed, whereas the flow across the circulatory system is determined by the preload and afterload. The forward flow across the pump is optimized by maximizing preload and minimizing afterload, while altering pump speed as little as possible. Small increments in afterload or small decreases in preload may result in diminished pump flow; if there is **inadequate ventricular filling** secondary to hypovolemia, bleeding, or right ventricular failure, increasing the pump speed would not increase flow. The key to managing pump speed is to provide the best flow at the lowest pump speed. For each patient on the DeBakey VAD, there is an optimal operating range: Lower flow leads to underperfusion, whereas higher flow can result in ventricular suction. The latter phenomenon can be shown by dual peaks in the flow waveform. In addition, even though the axial flow is a continuous flow VAD, the flow may be pulsatile depending on the native ventricular contractility.[31] In other words, the pressure changes resulting from contractions of the unloaded left ventricle and the partially recovered right ventricle can provide a physiologically pulsatile flow. Lastly, postimplantation **systemic hypertension** can be treated with vasodilators such as milrinone.

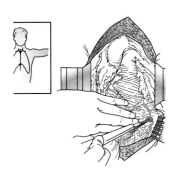

The DeBakey VAD® is implanted through a median sternotomy from the top of the sternum to just below the xiphoid process. A pump pocket is fashioned in the rectus sheath, and the fit is confirmed with the use of a dummy pump.

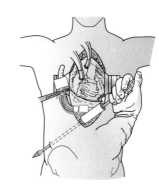

The percutaneous cable is tunneled to exit just above the patient's right iliac crest.

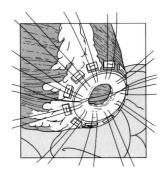

The heart is then elevated and the sewing ring is applied to the apex of the left ventricle.

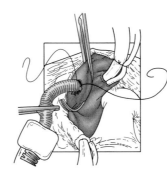

Anastamosis is performed from the outflow graft to the ascending aorta.

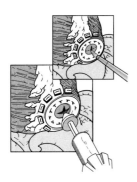

A cruciate incision is made with a #11 blade and the coring device is used to remove a uniform plug from the base of the left ventricle.

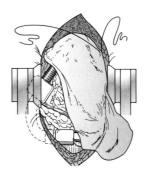

The heart and pump are covered with a Gore-Tex® patch to minimize adhesions and facilitate access to the heart when it is time for the patient's transplant.

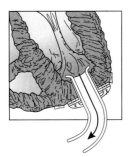

The inflow cannula is placed into the left ventricle and a TEE is used to check for proper placement to avoid positioning too close to the septal or ventricular wall.

The chest is then closed with sternal wires and suture.

FIGURE 48-4 ■ **The steps of the DeBakey VAD implantation surgery are illustrated in these figures and the accompanying text.** TEE, transesophageal echocardiogram. (From MicroMed Technology, Houston, TX.)

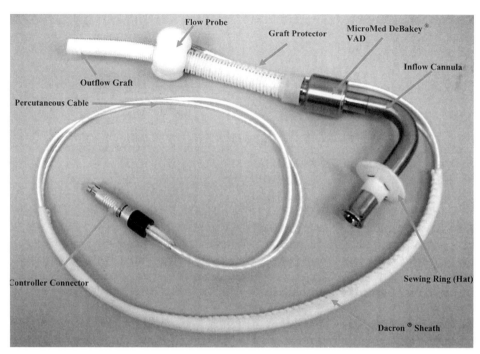

FIGURE 48-5 ■ The DeBakey pump assembly. The various parts of the pump assembly are shown and labeled (see text for details). (From MicroMed Technology, Houston, TX.) (See also Color Section)

The DeBakey VAD Child is a continuous-flow device and alters its flow and output depending on the patient's preload and afterload. One potential problem is due to the ventricular chamber collapsing around the inflow cannula and is termed **ventricular collapse or suction**, which can be recognized by a negative deflection of the flow waveforms visible on the CDAS unit (Fig. 48-6). This phenomenon can be caused by decreased fluid volume, speed of the VAD being set too high, or patient positioning; it rarely can be due to suboptimal inflow cannula positioning (too close to septum or ventricular free wall). Therapeutic maneuvers include fluid resuscitation, repositioning the patient, and contacting the support team. The other primary disadvantage of valveless axial flow technology is physiologically significant **aortic insufficiency** as a consequence of pump failure. This event may require emergent surgical ligation of the outflow graft or immediate device replacement. Currently the components are not replaceable individually, which means the pump may not be replaced without complete removal of the inflow and outflow cannulae. Future application of this device in children would require the pump to be easily replaceable akin to pacemaker generators.

Bleeding issues require meticulous hemostasis and timely re-exploration as needed. If volume replacement does not augment pump flow, potential sources of bleeding need to be ruled out. The large experience with the adult DeBakey VAD model also has revealed a low incidence of **thromboembolic** or **pump thrombus** complications. Most of these patients go on to have a successful outcome with both of these problems, but they underscore the importance of an effective anticoagulation protocol, which includes heparin therapy initially for several days and a combination of warfarin (Coumadin) (with target international normalized ratio of 2 to 3) and antiplatelet therapy with aspirin after the initial few days (Table 48-3). Patients show a triphasic platelet function pattern, and platelet function tests reflect the efficiency of antiaggregation therapy and should be followed.[32] An increase in current (≥ 1.5 amp) and power (≥ 15 W) with decreased flow may suggest a thromboembolic complication and warrant change in therapy, usually with clopidogrel or tissue plasminogen activator. Embolic events also can result in stroke or pulmonary or other noncerebral organ infarction, including limb ischemia or other vascular obstruction. Lastly, continuous flow provided by the adult DeBakey VAD has been shown to provide adequate end-organ perfusion without significant **hemolysis** (Fig. 48-7) because mean plasma-free hemoglobin and serum haptoglobin have not been elevated. To minimize hemolysis, ventricular suction should be avoided, and the pump should be run at the lowest speed that produces an adequate hemodynamic profile.

Neurologic complications are the most common and feared complications during any form of mechanical circulatory assistance and are not unique to longer term support with axial devices. Neurologic dysfunction can be due to preexisting hypoxic injury or hypoxic events during VAD implantation, including cerebral hypoperfusion, hemorrhage, or even drug-related side effects.

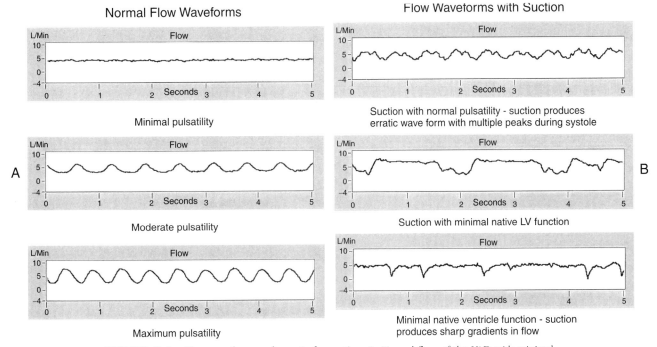

FIGURE 48-6 ■ **Flow waveforms and ventricular suction. A,** Normal flow of the VAD with minimal, moderate, and maximal pulsatilities. **B,** Ventricular suction waveforms with normal pulsatility and with minimal native left ventricular (LV) function. Note the negative deflections. (From MicroMed Technology, Houston, TX.)

Renal function also should be monitored closely for parenchymal dysfunction or infarction or both. In addition, the ability to close the chest provides an important barrier to **infection**; the DeBakey VAD rarely has infectious issues relating to the device itself. Lastly, there is no information on the **inflammatory cascade** consequences of the DeBakey VAD.

As an outpatient, the DeBakey VAD user needs to monitor anticoagulation closely and to optimize fluid intake. In the event of ventricular fibrillation, defibrillation can be performed only when the patient is untethered to the patient home support system unit. Cardiopulmonary resuscitation also can be performed, and the pump does not need to be stopped during cardiopulmonary resuscitation. The system ergonomics facilitate ambulation, but rehabilitation and nutrition are essential issues to ensure timely recovery.

CURRENT STATUS AND FUTURE TRENDS

With the approval for use of the DeBakey VAD Child system under a Humanitarian Device Exemption, we have performed three human implantations since 2004 at Texas Children's Hospital (with the longest support period being 84 days and the smallest patient being 0.6 m²).

The system is presently the subject of a multicenter clinical trial in the United States as a bridge to transplantation in adults with end-stage heart disease.[33]

Reports specifically addressing the outcomes for longer term VAD implantation in pediatric patients do not exist, and what is known must be extrapolated from scattered experiences, such as those from Germany and of older children requiring VAD support in the United States. The indication for assistance is an important predictor of outcome, and the indications for longer term VAD support (cardiomyopathy, bridge to transplantation, or bridge to recovery) will likely translate into lower overall morbidity and mortality than in patients requiring acute ECMO or VAD support. Compared with application of ECMO circuits and centrifugal VADs, longer term devices have additional concerns regarding durability, portability, biocompatibility, and ease of use over time. Because of unpredictable waiting time on the transplantation list and highly varying recovery times, paracorporeal and especially intracorporeal devices are a safer, more easily managed option. These devices generally allow for extubation and mobilization and have shown superior longevity with regard to circuit components.

The need to care effectively for the increasing population of children with heart failure finally is being addressed by industry and government; this is most

TABLE 48-3

Anticoagulation Guidance Document for the DeBakey Ventricular Assist Device*

Baseline

Baseline coagulation workup before implantation includes routine laboratory tests (prothrombin time [INR], activated PTT, D dimer, platelet count, and HIT antiplatelet factor 4 antibody)

Hypercoagulability baseline is recommended, including TEG (if available), proteins C and S levels, factor V Leiden, and anticardiolipin antibodies

Predisposition to hemolysis should be sought where indicated (e.g., hemoglobinopathies)

Postimplant

Anticoagulation:[†] Begin 72 hr postoperatively if chest tube drainage is 30 mL/hr × 4 hr. If chest tubes out earlier, may start anticoagulation earlier: 0 ASA 81 mg daily

Aggrenox (25 mg ASA + 200 mg dipyridamole) po bid

Unfractionated intravenous heparin (no bolus)

Start 750 mg/hr

Titrate to target PTT of 1.5-2 × control

Warfarin 2-5 mg po daily

Titrate to INR 2.5-3.5

If hypercoagulable > 1 wk postoperatively by clinical course, history, or laboratory tests (e.g., TEG), consider clopidogrel 75 mg PO every other day, adjusting dosage to obtain monitored target of –50% inhibition on platelet function monitoring

Monitoring

Postimplant monitoring

PTT every 4-6 hr until therapeutic range, then daily while stable on unfractionated heparin

INR target: 2.5-3.5

INR every day while in hospital

INR every Monday, Wednesday, and Friday after discharge (local hospital, not home test)

Longer intervals for destination trial when INRs stable to be established later

Designated anticoagulation teams (Coumadin clinics) encouraged. Goal: INR within target range 75% of the time. Committee will review INR reports from clinical sites monthly and will contact investigators when INRs are out of range >50% of the time

Platelet monitoring: strongly recommend monitoring platelet function and effect of the antiplatelet regimen with TEG, platelet aggregometry, or PFA 100

Additional Considerations

Malnutrition: typical in chronic heart failure and contributes to abnormal coagulation

Nutrition should be aggressively addressed early, or preemptively

Anticoagulation regimens

Individualize based on above principles and guide by careful monitoring, including the activity of antiplatelet drugs

DeBakey VAD in children: While there is no significant experience using implantable VADs in children, the same general principles are believed to apply with appropriate modifications to fit the special needs of children (size, age, compliance)

*Prepared in cooperation with the MicroMed Anticoagulation Advisory Committee.

†Some Committee members suggest beginning the anticoagulation earlier than 72 hours if the chest tube drainage is low.

ASA, acetylsalicylic acid; HIT, heparin-induced thrombocytopenia; INR, international normalized ratio; PTT, partial thromboplastin time; TEG, thromboelastography; VAD, ventricular assist device.

From MicroMed Technology, Houston, TX.

clearly shown by the development of the DeBakey VAD Child and by the National Heart, Lung and Blood Institute request for development of novel devices to support the circulation of children with heart failure, for which it has committed $25 million in funding. As newer devices become available for smaller patients and are subjected to clinical trial for appropriate indications, a better expectation for the outcome of pediatric long-term mechanical circulatory assistance will be defined. It is crucial that the physician and family members maintain realistic outcome expectations for such heroic measures in critically ill children. As better device options are on the horizon and the number

of pediatric patients requiring VAD support increases, the science of long-term mechanical circulatory support, such as microbiology of the device-circulatory interface, cellular changes in cardiac remodeling and recovery, and end-organ perfusion of pulsatile flow in pediatric patients, will likely be refined in the coming decades.[34]

Key Concepts

■ With the exception of ECMO and a centrifugal VAD support (both in the ICU), novel and longer term options for pediatric mechanical circulatory assistance have largely been undeveloped.

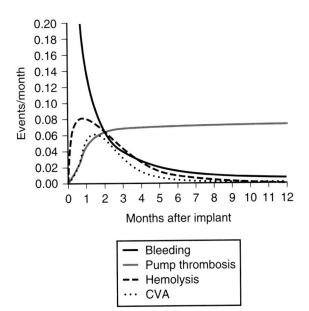

FIGURE 48-7 ■ The hazard function for the DeBakey VAD. The hazard function for four postoperative problems is graphed. Although bleeding is the predominant postoperative complication early on, thromboembolism, infection, and malfunction become important issues later in the postoperative period. (From Goldstein DJ: *Worldwide experience with the MicroMed DeBakey ventricular assist device as a bridge to transplantation. Circulation* 2003;108(Suppl II):II-272-II-277.)

■ Pediatric patients who are likely to have progressive heart failure include children with staged palliation for hypoplastic left heart syndrome and other single-ventricle lesions, children born with transposition of the great arteries who underwent prior atrial switch, children with failing Fontan circulation, and children with cardiomyopathy currently facing varying waiting times for cardiac transplantation.

■ Advantages of pulsatile devices include long-term support capability, ease of use, capability for biventricular support without an oxygenator, mobility to be out of the ICU, need for low-level anticoagulation, and pulsatile flow nature. Disadvantages include a propensity to have thromboembolic complications, difficulty of implantation and explantation, cumulative cost, need for exteriorization of the cannulae, and size limitations especially with the need for biventricular support.

■ The Berlin Heart VAD (Berlin Heart Institute, Berlin, Germany) is a paracorporeal, pneumatically driven blood pump that incorporates polyurethane trileaflet valves to guard the inflow and outflow in the neonatal and infantile sized models.

■ The Thoratec Ventricular Assist System (Thoratec Corp, Berkeley, CA) is a pneumatically powered pulsatile assist device that consists of a flexible, seam-free, segmented sac within a ridged polycarbonate housing.

■ Although the pediatric experience with axial devices is extremely small and limited to a few adolescents and children, the smaller size holds the best promise for future pediatric use.

■ Advantages of an axial system are the relatively small size, implant/explant procedures that are relatively easy, noiseless system, decreased infection, relatively lower cost, and continuous flow that not only provides unloading throughout the cardiac cycle, but also minimizes stasis and thrombus formation. Disadvantages include the need for a relatively large-sized ventricular apical cannulation and relative size limitation to pediatric patients with a body surface area of greater than 1.5 m².

■ The adult DeBakey VAD is the prototype of the newer generation of axial VADs. This device was the first long-term axial flow circulatory assist device to be introduced into clinical trials (since November 1998) as a bridge to transplantation and has had the largest clinical experience with more than 300 patients worldwide.

■ The advantages of axial devices such as the DeBakey VAD include miniaturization of the device, system ergonomics facilitating ambulation, patient exercise possible with fixed pump speed, and noiseless system. Additional benefits include ease of surgical implantation, rare postoperative infections, reduced surgical bleeding, and end-organ function maintained or improved. Disadvantages include nonpulsatile flow.

■ The DeBakey VAD Child, an implantable assist device intended for long-term left ventricular support in children, marks the first effort to address the ever-increasing population of smaller children with end-stage heart disease. It was approved for use in children (ages 5 to 16 years with a body surface area of 0.7 to 1.2 m²) with end-stage heart failure who need mechanical circulatory support for bridge to transplantation applications under a Humanitarian Device Exemption by the U.S. Food and Drug Administration in February 2004.

■ Postoperative care after implantation of the DeBakey VAD Child is provided in the cardiac ICU with an important emphasis on medical management of any right ventricular dysfunction because the right ventricular output "preloads" the VAD.

■ The flow across the DeBakey VAD Child pump varies with pump speed, whereas the flow across the circulatory system is determined by the preload and afterload. The forward flow across the pump is optimized by maximizing preload and minimizing afterload, while altering pump speed as little as possible.

■ The key to managing pump speed is to provide the best flow at the lowest pump speed. For each patient on the DeBakey VAD, there is an optimal operating range: Lower flow leads to underperfusion, whereas higher flow can result in ventricular suction. The latter phenomenon can be shown by dual peaks in the flow waveform.

■ Even though the axial flow is a continuous-flow VAD, the flow may be pulsatile depending on the native ventricular contractility. In other words, the pressure changes resulting from contractions of the unloaded left ventricle, and the partially recovered right ventricle can provide a physiologically pulsatile flow.

■ Because of unpredictable waiting time on the transplantation list and highly varying recovery times, paracorporeal and especially intracorporeal devices are a safer, more easily managed option. These devices generally allow for extubation and mobilization and have shown superior longevity with regard to circuit components.

■ As better device options are on the horizon and the number of pediatric patients requiring VAD support increases, the science of long-term mechanical circulatory support, such as microbiology of the device-circulatory interface, cellular changes in cardiac remodeling and recovery, and end-organ perfusion of pulsatile flow in pediatric patients, will likely be refined in the coming decades.

REFERENCES

1. DeBakey ME: Left ventricular bypass pump for cardiac assistance: Clinical experience. Am J Cardiol 1971;27:3-11.
2. DeBakey ME: The odyssey of the artificial heart. Artif Organs 2000;24:405-411.
3. Digiorgi PL, Rao V, Naka Y, Oz MC: Which patient, which pump? J Heart Lung Transplant 2003;22:221-235.
4. Rose EA, Gelijns AC, Moskowitz AJ, et al: Long-term use of a left ventricular assist device for end-stage heart failure. N Engl J Med 2001;345:1435-1443.
5. Smedira NG, Blackstone EH: Postcardiotomy mechanical support: Risk factors and outcomes. Ann Thorac Surg 2001;71 (3 Suppl):S60-S66.
6. El-Banayosy A, Minami K, Arusoglu L, et al: Long-term mechanical circulatory support. Thorac Cardiovasc Surg 1997;45:127-130.
7. Goldstein DJ, Oz MC, Rose EA: Implantable left ventricular assist devices. N Engl J Med 1998;339:1522-1533.
8. Matsuda H, Taenaka Y, Ohkubo N, et al: Use of paracorporeal pneumatic ventricular assist device for postoperative cardiogenic shock in two children with complex cardiac lesions. Artif Organs 1988;12:423-430.
9. Loebe M, Hennig E, Muller J, et al: Long-term mechanical circulatory support as a bridge to transplantation, for recovery from cardiomyopathy, and for permanent replacement. Eur J Cardiothorac Surg 1997;11(Suppl):S18-S24.
10. Ishino K, Loebe M, Uhlemann F, et al: Circulatory support with paracorporeal pneumatic ventricular assist device (VAD) in infants and children. Eur J Cardiothorac Surg 1997;11:965-972.
11. Hetzer R: Personal communication (May, 2005).
12. Stiller B, Dhanert I, Weng YG, et al: Children may survive severe myocarditis with prolonged use of biventricular assist devices. Heart 1999;82:237-240.
13. Konertz W, Hotz H, Schneider M, et al: Clinical experience with the MEDOS HIA-VAD system in infants and children: A preliminary report. Ann Thorac Surg 1997;63:1138-1144.
14. Herwig V, Severin M, Waldenberger FR, et al: Medos/HIA assist system: First experiences with mechanical circulatory assist in infants and children. Int J Artif Organs 1997;20:692-694.
15. Busch U, Waldenberger FR, Redlin M, et al: Successful treatment of postoperative right ventricular heart failure with the HIA-Medos assist system in a two year-old girl. Pediatr Cardiol 1999;20:161-163.
16. Reul H: The MEDOS/HIA system: Development, results, perspectives. Thorac Cardiovasc Surg 1999;47(Suppl 2):311-315.
17. Shum-Tim D, Duncan BW, Hraska V, et al: Evaluation of a pulsatile pediatric ventricular assist device in an acute right heart failure model. Ann Thorac Surg 1997;64:1374-1380.
18. Weyand M, Keceicioglu D, Kehl HG, et al: Neonatal mechanical bridging to total orthotopic heart transplantation. Ann Thorac Surg 1998;66:519-522.
19. Farrar D: Personal communication (May, 2005).
20. Reinhartz O, Stiller B, Eilers R, et al: Current clinical status of pulsatile pediatric circulatory support. ASAIO J 2002;48:455-459.
21. Copeland JG, Arabia FA, Smith RG: Bridge to transplantation with a Thoratec left ventricular assist device in a 17-kg child. Ann Thorac Surg 2001;71:1003-1004.
22. Farrar DJ, Hill JD, Pennington DG, et al: Preoperative and postoperative comparison of patients with univentricular and biventricular support with the Thoratec ventricular assist device as a bridge to transplantation. J Thorac Cardiovasc Surg 1997;113:202-209.
23. McBride LR, Naunheim KS, Fiore AC, et al: Clinical experience with 111 Thoratec ventricular assist devices. Ann Thorac Surg 1999;67:1233-1239.
24. Reinhartz O, Keith FM, El Banayosy A, et al: Multicenter experience with the Thoratec ventricular assist device in children and adolescents. J Heart Lung Transplant 2001;20:439-448.
25. Ashton RC, Oz MC, Michler RE, et al: Left ventricular assist device options in pediatric patients. ASAIO J 1995;41:M277-M280.
26. Frazier OH, Myers TJ, Gregoric ID, et al: Initial clinical experience with the Jarvik 2000 implantable axial flow left ventricular assist system. Circulation 2002;105:2855-2860.
27. Kaplon RJ, Oz MC, Kwiatkowski PA, et al: Miniature axial flow pump for ventricular assistance in children and small adults. J Thorac Cardiovasc Surg 1996;111:13-18.
28. Kaplon RJ, Oz MC, Kwiatkowski PA, et al: Miniature axial flow pump for ventricular assistance in children and small adults. J Thorac Cardiovasc Surg 1996;111:13-18.
29. Rothenburger M, Wilhelm MJ, Hammel D, et al: Treatment of thrombus formation associated with the MicroMed DeBakey VAD can be treated with recombinant tissue plasminogen activator. Circulation 2002;106(Suppl I):I-189-I-192.
30. Song X, Throckmorton AL, Untaroiu A, et al: Axial flow blood pumps. ASAIO J 2003;49:355-364.
31. Potapov EV, Loebe M, Nasseri BA, et al: Pulsatile flow in patients with a novel nonpulsatile implantable ventricular assist device. Circulation 2000;102(19 Suppl 3):III-183-III-187.
32. Bonaros N, Mueller MR, Salat A, et al: Extensive coagulation monitoring in patients after implantation of the MicroMed DeBakey continuous axial pump. ASAIO J 2004;50:424-431.
33. Chang AC: The Pediatric DeBakey VAD experience, Presented at the Third Annual DeBakey VAD Investigators Meeting. May, 2005, Boston, Massachusetts.
34. DeBakey ME: Personal communication (June, 2005).

CHAPTER 49

The Adult Experience with Long-Term Ventricular Assist Devices

Branislav Radovancevic
Bojan Vrtovec
George P. Noon

Despite medical and surgical advances (e.g., β-blockers, spironolactone, biventricular pacing, implantable defibrillators, mitral valve repair, and infarct exclusion surgery) and significantly improved survival,[1] advanced heart failure in adults continues to be associated with high morbidity and mortality.[2] The only definitive treatment is cardiac transplantation, but transplantation is limited in its usefulness because only the sickest patients accrue a survival benefit,[3] and because there is a constant shortage of donor organs.

One approach to this problem has been the development of long-term ventricular assist device (VAD) technologies, including the left ventricular assist device (LVAD) and the total artificial heart (TAH).[4] In the case of LVADs, obstacles to their use in children remain (see Chapters 45 to 48), but most obstacles to their use in adults have been overcome. Considerable experience has been gained by the long-term application of LVADs in adult patients who have reversible heart failure after myocardial infarction or open heart surgery or who are awaiting heart transplantation. In the case of the TAH, experience has been confined to adult patients awaiting heart transplantation or to patients receiving a TAH as destination therapy. This chapter discusses the cumulative experience with long-term mechanical circulatory support devices in adults. (See also other chapters in this section and the atlas at the end of the text.)

INDICATIONS AND MANAGEMENT FOR LONG-TERM ASSIST DEVICES

The principal indication for long-term implantation of a VAD is end-stage heart failure marked by the heart's inability to supply adequate oxygenated blood to bodily tissues. Eligible patients are often on the transplantation waiting list. The three potential goals of treatment that have emerged from the clinical experience with long-term mechanical circulatory support are bridging to transplantation, bridging to recovery, and destination therapy.

Indications and Contraindications
Successful mechanical circulatory support requires careful patient selection and timing of device implantation. Table 49-1 lists established guidelines for screening

candidates for VAD implantation in adults.[5] Certain preoperative risk factors have been shown to influence post-transplantation survival of LVAD recipients.[6-9] Post-transplantation survival was decreased significantly in HeartMate LVAD (Thoratec Corp, Pleasanton, CA) recipients whose creatinine levels were greater than 2 mg/dL before device implantation (50% versus 94%; $P < .01$),[6] adversely affected in Thoratec VAD (Thoratec Corp, Pleasanton, CA) recipients whose blood urea nitrogen levels were increased and who previously had cardiac surgery,[7] and significantly better in LVAD recipients with no preexisting severe liver failure.[8] Preoperative cardiac

TABLE 49-1

Indications for and Contraindications to Ventricular Assist Device Implantation
Indications
Cardiac index <2 L/min/m²
Pulmonary capillary wedge pressure >20 mm Hg
Systolic blood pressure <80 mm Hg
Maximal medical therapy (inotropic drugs, intra-aortic balloon pump support, or both)
Contraindications
Age >70 years
Chronic renal failure
Chronic obstructive pulmonary disease
Recent pulmonary embolism
Irreversible pulmonary hypertension
Severe right heart failure
Cardiac arrest
HIV positivity
Severe hepatic disease
Cerebrovascular disease
Active systemic infection
Severe blood dyscrasia
Unresolved malignancy
Diffuse, severe peripheral vascular disease
Long-term high-dose steroid therapy
Uncorrected aortic insufficiency (for most, but not all, devices)

Adapted from Frazier OH, Short HD, Wampler RK, et al: Mechanical circulatory support in the transplant population. In Frazier OH (ed): Support and Replacement of the Failing Heart. Philadelphia, Lippincott-Raven, 1996, pp 147-167.)

function, as assessed by cardiac index, left ventricular ejection fraction, and pulmonary capillary wedge pressure, apparently does not correlate with survival.[8]

A common finding in the above-cited studies was that renal and liver dysfunction was more detrimental to outcome than preoperative cardiac function. This finding has led to the conclusion that delaying VAD implantation in patients with borderline cardiac function may result in severe end-organ damage and consequently poorer survival. The general consensus is that timely VAD implantation before renal or liver function deteriorates is crucial for post-transplantation survival. The finding that prolonged VAD support can lead to complete reversal of kidney and liver dysfunction is supported by this idea.[10]

Perioperative Medical Management

Perioperative mortality remains a serious concern in LVAD recipients.[9,11] Preoperative treatment should focus on optimizing the patient's health to improve survival. **Perioperative bleeding** diathesis often accompanies the implantation of an LVAD, and perioperative hemorrhagic complications occur in an estimated 44% of cases.[11] Platelet, coagulant, and fibrinolytic activities have been shown to be greater during HeartMate LVAD implantation and activation than during coronary artery bypass graft surgery.[12] The use of antifibrinolytics, such as aprotinin and aminocaproic acid, is now accepted postimplantation therapy for these patients.[13] Other measures besides antifibrinolytics also have been used successfully to control bleeding during LVAD implantation (Table 49-2). At present, the use of erythropoietin to avoid unnecessary blood transfusions in transplantation candidates is recommended.[14]

Some **thromboembolic and hemolytic** complications are attributable to the blood-contacting surfaces found in some VADs and to the shearing forces of blood flow.[15] Sodium warfarin, heparin, aspirin, or dipyridamole may be used as anticoagulation therapy depending on the specific device used. Some VADs have been engineered to dampen the coagulation cascade. All blood-contacting surfaces of the HeartMate LVAD except for valves are made of textured polyurethane or titanium surfaces that have been engineered to trap and anchor blood components firmly[16]; this allows creation of a stable biologic neointima similar to the lining of natural blood vessels that prevents blood from contacting the artificial materials. The valves are 25-mm porcine xenografts. The neointima and xenograft valves reduce activation of the coagulation cascade to a level that makes all anticoagulation except aspirin unnecessary.

Infectious complications occur frequently in patients supported by LVADs that have percutaneous drivelines (e.g., HeartMate or Novacor [Baxter Health Care Corp, Novacor Division, Oakland, CA]).[17] In one combined registry, the infectious complication rate of 584 patients bridged to transplantation was 28.5%.[18] In another study, the complication rate in patients supported for long periods (mean ± SD, 106 ± 97 days; range, 7 to 504 days) was greater than 40%.[19] As the waiting time for a heart transplantation probably will continue to increase, so too will periods of VAD support and consequently the risk of infection. Infection prophylaxis is similar to that for other cardiac surgery patients, although additional emphasis should be placed on early removal of intravenous catheters and weaning from ventilatory support.

Right ventricular failure, one of the most common causes of death in LVAD recipients, requires special consideration.[20,21] Reactive pulmonary hypertension may be reduced or prevented by avoiding unnecessary blood transfusions; routinely administering isoproterenol; and maintaining an optimal acid-base balance, good oxygenation (Po_2 >100 mm Hg), and adequate ventilation (Pco_2 < 35 mm Hg).[22] Nitric oxide has proved useful in treating and preventing pulmonary hypertension.[23] If these measures fail, early implantation of a right VAD is recommended.[24]

Perioperative **renal dysfunction** resulting from preoperative hypoperfusion and the use of cardiopulmonary bypass is common. Timely LVAD implantation (i.e., before the onset of irreversible end-organ failure) can lead to functional recovery and improved post-transplantation survival. Renal function may be preserved

TABLE 49-2

Non-antifibrolytic Measures Used to Control Bleeding During Left Ventricular Assist Device Implantation
Discontinuation of antithrombotic therapy Correction of thrombocytopenia Use of a centrifugal pump for cardiopulmonary bypass Use of preclot pump conduits and graft-pump connections Thermoregulation

TABLE 49-3

Factors in the Selection of Appropriate Ventricular Assist Devices
Degree of support needed Planned duration of support Univentricular versus biventricular failure Device size Patient mobility Invasiveness of implantation procedure FDA approval status
FDA, Food and Drug Administration.

further by postoperative optimization of heart function and infusion of low-dose dopamine, mannitol, or both.[25]

Numerous VADs are now used clinically. Appropriate device selection is important in avoiding complications (Table 49-3).[26] When a VAD is used as a bridge to transplantation, it is recommended that a less invasive device be used to stabilize the patient and make the patient a better candidate for implantation of a larger or more permanent device.[27] In patients with severe fluid overload, or anasarca, cardiopulmonary bypass may pose too high a risk because of the possibility that further tissue fluid overload may lead to other complications, such as pulmonary edema, pulmonary hypertension, and right heart dysfunction. Hemofiltration may be used to reduce fluid overload and third spacing.

LEFT VENTRICULAR ASSIST DEVICES

In terms of the type of flow produced, there are two main categories of LVADs: pulsatile and nonpulsatile. Pulsatile pumps mimic the rhythm of the native heart, whereas nonpulsatile pumps produce a nonphysiologic, continuous blood flow attributable to the axial rotation of a single moving part (impeller). All of the pulsatile pumps provide adequate support, but some continue to be plagued by complications such as bleeding, infection, and device or equipment malfunction. Although the nonpulsatile pumps are much smaller than the pulsatile pumps, both types of devices are used primarily in adults. The U.S. Food and Drug Administration (FDA) approved a smaller version of the MicroMed DeBakey VAD (MicroMed Technology, Inc, Houston, TX) for use in children.

Pulsatile Left Ventricular Assist Devices

The **Thoratec VAD** is a paracorporeal system that can be used to provide left or right ventricular support or both.[28] Positioned externally on the abdominal wall, the pump consists of an air chamber and a blood sac separated by a polyurethane diaphragm. The pump is powered pneumatically by an immovable console or a portable battery-powered unit. For left ventricular support, inflow and outflow cannulae are placed through either the left atrium or the left ventricular apex. For right ventricular support, the inflow cannula is placed in the right atrium or right ventricle, and the outflow cannula is placed in the pulmonary artery. Both cannulae are connected to the externally placed pump (see also atlas).

More than 1,400 patients have been treated with the Thoratec LVAD, mainly as a bridge to transplantation or as postcardiotomy support. Consistent improvements in hemodynamics and end-organ perfusion during left ventricular support have been noted.[29] Evidence also suggests that the Thoratec LVAD is an effective bridge

to recovery.[30] Many patients with nonischemic cardiomyopathy have been weaned successfully from left ventricular support with the Thoratec VAD. Use of the Thoratec VAD as a bridge to recovery in patients with acute cardiomyopathies and myocarditis has been shown to result in long-term survival equivalent to survival after cardiac transplantation. Although the factors affecting long-term myocardial recovery and the optimal weaning method are unclear, the evidence so far suggests that recovery may be possible in many LVAD- supported patients.

Although the Thoratec LVAD poses a risk of thromboembolism and may limit patient mobility because of its extracorporeal placement, it still represents an important means of long-term LVAD support. It is especially applicable in patients whose abdominal cavity is too small to accommodate an intracorporeal device or who require biventricular support.

The **HeartMate VE LVAD** (Fig. 49-1) requires external venting via its percutaneous driveline. As mentioned previously, the pump contains a flexible, textured, polyurethane diaphragm and sintered titanium surfaces engineered to trap and anchor blood components firmly, which prevents blood from contacting artificial materials, reducing coagulation activation and the need

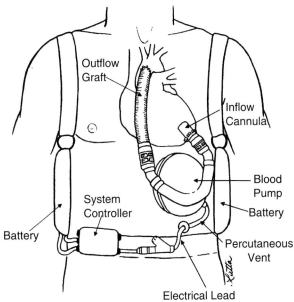

FIGURE 49-1 ■ HeartMate vented electric (VE) left ventricular assist device. The device requires external venting via its percutaneous driveline. The pump contains a flexible, textured, polyurethane diaphragm and sintered titanium surfaces engineered to trap and anchor blood components firmly. The device is implanted through a median sternotomy. The inflow cannula is placed in the left ventricular apex; the outflow graft is passed over the diaphragm to the ascending aorta, where it is anastomosed end-to-side at the aortic root. (From Frazier OH, Rose EA, Oz MC, et al: *Multicenter clinical evaluation of the HeartMate vented electric left ventricular assist system in patients awaiting heart transplantation. J Thorac Cardiovasc Surg* 2001;122:1188.)

for anticoagulants.[31] Wearable external components include batteries and a controller that allow full ambulation and exercise rehabilitation.

In a prospective, multicenter clinical trial, 280 patients with advanced heart failure unresponsive to conventional therapy were treated with the HeartMate VE LVAD for periods of 691 days (mean 112 days).[32] These patients were compared with a historical control group of 48 non–LVAD-supported patients. Despite its association with frequent major adverse events (i.e., bleeding, infection, neurologic dysfunction, and thromboembolic events), LVAD treatment improved liver and kidney function and led to significantly better survival to transplantation (71% versus 33% in controls) and at 1 year after transplantation (84% versus 63%).

The REMATCH (Randomized Evaluation of Mechanical Assistance for the Treatment of Congestive Heart Failure) trial compared survival in patients with end-stage heart failure ineligible for heart transplantation who received LVAD therapy ($n = 68$) versus optimal medical therapy ($n = 61$).[33] One-year survival was 52% for the LVAD group and 25% for the medical group. Two-year survival was 23% and 8%. Serious adverse events, including infection, bleeding, and device malfunction, were problems, however, in the LVAD-treated group. These data suggest that the HeartMate VE LVAD provides adequate hemodynamic support, with an acceptably low incidence of adverse events, and improves survival.

The **Novacor LVAD** is an electrically powered device that is implanted in the left subrectus position within the abdominal wall.[34] Inflow and outflow cannulae are placed in the left ventricular apex and ascending aorta. The pump is powered by an external controller and power source connected to it by a single percutaneous lead through the right abdominal wall. There is also a wearable, battery-powered configuration that can be used for 4 to 6 hours.

The Novacor LVAD has been implanted in more than 1,100 patients worldwide.[35] It has provided effective long-term left ventricular support as a bridge to transplantation and bridge to recovery. Since modification of the pump's inflow conduit in 1998, median support duration has increased from 93 to 202 days, with the longest period of support exceeding 4 years. Neurologic complications (stroke, delirium) and embolic events have been problems, although the incidence of embolic events has decreased by 50% since modification of the inflow conduit.[36]

Nonpulsatile Left Ventricular Assist Devices

The **Jarvik 2000** (Jarvik Heart, Inc, New York, NY) is an implantable LVAD that provides axial flow by means of a single, rotating impeller (Fig. 49-2). The system consists of a blood pump, outflow graft, percutaneous power cable, pump-speed controller, and direct-current

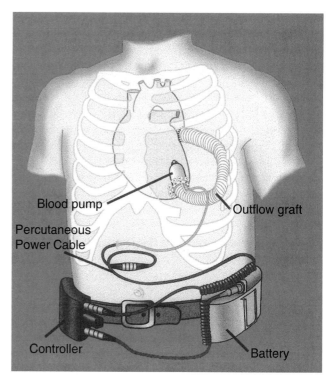

FIGURE 49-2 ■ Jarvik 2000 system and its components. The system consists of a blood pump, outflow graft, percutaneous power cable, pump-speed controller, and direct-current power supply. A brushless direct-current motor rotates the impeller at 8,000 to 12,000 rpm, generating an average flow rate of 3 to 6 L/min. The pump is implanted within the left ventricle through a left thoracotomy or sternotomy. The outflow graft may be placed on the ascending or descending aorta. A percutaneous power cable is connected to the controller, which controls and monitors pump speed. Continuous power is provided by rechargeable lithium-ion or lead-acid batteries. (From Myers TJ, Robertson K, Pool T, et al: *Continuous flow pumps and total artificial hearts: Management issues.* Ann Thorac Surg 2003;75 (Suppl 6):S80.)

power supply. A brushless direct-current motor rotates the impeller at 8,000 to 12,000 revolutions per minute (rpm), generating an average flow rate of 3 to 6 L/min.[37]

The Jarvik 2000 has been evaluated clinically as a bridge to transplantation and as destination therapy in 26 patients.[38] Twenty patients have received it as a bridge to transplantation, and four have received it as destination therapy. The average duration of support is 67.1 days. The device significantly improves hemodynamics, as shown by a 70.6% increase in average cardiac index, a 44% decrease in pulmonary capillary wedge pressure, and a significant decrease in systemic vascular resistance by 48 hours after implantation. In the bridge-to-transplantation experience, 13 patients have received transplants, 7 have died during support, and 2 continue to be supported by the device. The deaths were due to acute myocardial infarction in two cases and multiorgan failure in five cases. Similar results have been seen in patients who received the device as destination therapy.

Although further clinical studies are warranted to define long-term outcomes better, it seems that the Jarvik 2000 can provide safe and effective left ventricular support, and that it can be used in select patients as a bridge to transplantation or as destination therapy. The patients most likely to benefit from this device are apparently patients who require true left ventricular assistance rather than total capture of left ventricular output.

The **MicroMed DeBakey VAD** is an electromagnetically actuated axial flow pump that provides flows of 10 L/min at a rotor speed of 12,500 rpm.[39] A titanium inflow cannula connects the pump to the apex of the left ventricle, and a vascular graft that functions as an outflow conduit connects the pump to the ascending aorta. Pump operation is monitored and can be adjusted from a bedside monitoring unit. The pump is powered via a percutaneous cable that connects to an external controller and either electrical or battery power source. The pump's duration when powered by two 12-volt direct-current batteries is 4 to 8 hours.

The pump is implanted through a median sternotomy or left thoracotomy using cardiopulmonary bypass. A small preperitoneal pocket is formed under the left costal margin to house the pump. The left ventricular apex is cored out, and a ring is sewn to the apex. The inflow cannula is secured to the apical ring, and the outflow graft is anastomosed to the ascending or descending thoracic aorta.

The device has been implanted in more than 350 patients worldwide and has provided a cumulative support time exceeding 79 patient years. (Michael DeBakey: personal communication, June, 2005)[40] The most common etiology of heart failure in this population is ischemia, followed by dilated cardiomyopathy. Bridging to transplantation with the MicroMed DeBakey LVAD has been achieved in 50% to 66% of cases. The adverse events seen are similar to events that occur with other LVADs and include reoperation for bleeding, hemolysis, thromboembolic events, and device thrombus or infection. Device infection and pump failure are rare. An outcome-limiting factor seems to be the development of pump thrombus, which has occurred in less than 15% of patients. This situation is being addressed by standardizing anticoagulation.

In clinical trials, the MicroMed DeBakey VAD has provided adequate circulatory support in a wide range of patients with advanced heart failure, regardless of patient size, even in the outpatient setting.[41,42] The quality of life of patients supported with this type of VAD may improve further with the use of a physiologic responsive controller that would simulate the Frank-Starling mechanism and allow pump speed to increase or decrease automatically in response to the patient's level of activity.[41]

TOTAL ARTIFICIAL HEART

The **AbioCor total artificial heart (TAH)** (ABIOMED Inc, Danvers, MA) is designed to fit totally inside the body and operate without penetrating the skin. The AbioCor's internal components consist of a thoracic unit, an internal transcutaneous energy transfer coil, a controller, and a battery. The thoracic unit consists of two artificial ventricles, four valves, and a motor-driven hydraulic system that shuttles blood from side to side. A right-to-left flow-balancing mechanism compensates for the natural right-to-left flow imbalance. A transcutaneous energy transfer (TET) system powers the implanted system and recharges the AbioCor's internal battery. Hemodynamic and power-related data are displayed on a computer console that communicates with the thoracic unit via radiofrequency communication.[43]

In an ongoing feasibility trial that plans to enroll 15 patients, the AbioCor has been implanted in 12 patients with severe, irreversible biventricular failure.[44] All of these recipients were adults with inotrope-dependent biventricular failure, a predicted 30-day mortality of greater than 70%, and no other therapeutic options, including transplantation. The AbioCor thoracic unit is implanted in an orthotopic position after excision of the ventricles. Two patients have died during the implantation procedure. Four late deaths have been recorded, one as a result of multisystem organ failure and three as a result of cerebrovascular accidents. Autopsy revealed thrombus on the atrial struts of the three patients who had cerebrovascular accidents. Although significant morbidity has been observed, primarily in relation to the severity of the pre-existing illness, three patients recovered to the point of being able to take multiple trips outside of the hospital. Two patients were discharged from the hospital, one of them being discharged home for more than 7 months.

The results of the ongoing feasibility study indicate that the AbioCor may be an effective novel therapy for select patients with end-stage heart failure. Although the device itself seems to be reliable and effective in providing adequate end-organ perfusion, the long-term clinical outcomes of the AbioCor recipients remain limited mainly because of the high risk of stroke. Further studies are needed to define better the background of device thrombus formation and the potential adjuvant therapeutic approaches to prevent thromboembolic complications and improve the long-term outcome of this patient cohort.

REVERSE REMODELING AS AN EMERGING TREATMENT GOAL

Myocardial recovery after long-term ventricular support with pulsatile and nonpulsatile LVADs has been reported. The progression of ventricular dysfunction is accompanied by changes in all components of the myocardium, including cardiomyocytes, fibroblasts, the extracellular matrix, and coronary vasculature. These changes lead to alterations in ventricular geometry (i.e., myocardial remodeling). It has been suggested that heart failure progression is caused by neurohormonal activation, resulting in overexpression of biologically active molecules capable of exerting toxic effects on the heart and circulation.[45] Many of these potentially toxic molecules have been identified, including norepinephrine, angiotensin II, aldosterone, endothelin, and tumor necrosis factor-α (TNF-α).[46] Increasing clinical evidence suggests, however, that the neurohormonal explanation of disease progression in heart failure is incomplete, and that left ventricular remodeling may not simply be an end-organ response, but rather a pathophysiologic mechanism leading to progression.[47] Potential treatments for the prevention and reversal of heart failure progression should be aimed at neurohormonal modulation and at reversing the left ventricular remodeling process.

There is substantial evidence that medical therapy can modulate neurohormonal response beneficially and attenuate left ventricular remodeling.[26] Renin-angiotensin system inhibitors and β-adrenergic receptor blockers are extremely beneficial as neurohormonal modulators in advanced heart failure patients, substantially reducing mortality.[27] The optimal dose of these therapeutic agents is frequently unattainable in these patients, however, mainly because of low systemic arterial pressures and compromised kidney function. The efficiency of neurohormonal blockade seems to lessen over time, suggesting the need for alternative long-term treatment modalities, including LVADs.[48]

Besides improving clinical symptoms, LVADs apparently have proved useful in preventing or reversing heart failure by inducing neuroendocrine modulation and reverse remodeling. In terms of neurohormonal modulation, LVAD support can decrease dramatically plasma levels of epinephrine, norepinephrine, angiotensin II, and arginine vasopressin[49]; attenuate serum levels of interleukin-6 and interleukin-8[50]; and decrease TNF-α content in the failing myocardium.[51] In terms of reverse remodeling, long-term LVAD support has been shown to decrease significantly collagen content and myocyte size[52] and improve myocyte contractility and myocardial response to β-adrenergic stimulation.[53] Together, these findings show that the function of failing human ventricular myocytes can improve with LVAD unloading and improvement in neurohormonal status.

In 1994, the first data showing measurable clinical recovery after prolonged LVAD support in a patient with end-stage heart failure were reported.[31] Since then, numerous studies have shown that prolonged LVAD support can improve symptoms of heart failure significantly and, in some cases, lead to complete cardiac recovery.[54-56]

Depending on the degree of irreversible myocardial damage at the time of LVAD implantation, however, the potential for complete recovery may not extend to all patients with heart failure.[57] Appropriate patient selection plays a major role in determining the outcome after LVAD implantation,[58] but appropriate medical management after implantation is equally important. The improved hemodynamics and end-organ function resulting from increased perfusion open a window of opportunity through which medical therapy (particularly with renin-angiotensin system inhibitors and β-adrenergic receptor blockers) can be optimized. In this light, LVAD therapy in patients with end-stage heart failure should not be viewed merely as an alternative to medical treatment, but also as an adjunct whose synergy helps create an optimal environment for cardiac recovery.

CURRENT STATUS AND FUTURE TRENDS

The clinical experience in adults with advanced heart failure indicates that long-term mechanical circulatory support with VADs is a viable alternative to optimal medical treatment. LVADs may be used as a bridge to transplantation and, at least in the case of the HeartMate VE LVAD, as destination therapy. Emerging evidence of neurohormonal modulation and reverse remodeling in patients whose LVADs have been removed also suggests that LVADs might be used as a bridge to recovery. Early results of an ongoing FDA-sponsored feasibility trial suggest that the AbioCor TAH would be useful in select patients with end-stage heart failure who are ineligible for transplantation. Further advances, such as integrated data acquisition systems,[59] surgical techniques,[60] physiologic research,[61] and immunological alterations[62] can ensure the future successes of these complex biologic engineering devices.[63]

Key Concepts

■ The three potential goals of treatment from the clinical experience with long-term mechanical circulatory support are bridging to transplantation, bridging to recovery, and destination therapy.

■ Renal and liver dysfunction was more detrimental to outcome than preoperative cardiac function. This finding has led to the conclusion that delaying VAD implantation in patients with borderline cardiac function may result in severe end-organ damage and consequently poorer survival.

■ Perioperative bleeding diathesis often accompanies the implantation of an LVAD, and perioperative hemorrhagic complications occur in an estimated 44% of cases.

■ Some thromboembolic and hemolytic complications are attributable to the blood-contacting surfaces found in some VADs and to the shearing forces of blood flow. Sodium warfarin, heparin, aspirin, or dipyridamole may be used as anticoagulation therapy depending on the specific device used.

■ Pulsatile pumps mimic the rhythm of the native heart, whereas nonpulsatile pumps produce a non-physiologic, continuous blood flow attributable to the axial rotation of a single moving part (impeller).

■ Use of the Thoratec VAD as a bridge to recovery in patients with acute cardiomyopathies and myocarditis has been shown to result in long-term survival equivalent to survival after cardiac transplantation. Although the factors affecting long-term myocardial recovery and the optimal weaning method are unclear, the evidence so far suggests that recovery may be possible in many LVAD-supported patients.

■ Although the Thoratec LVAD poses a risk of thromboembolism and may limit patient mobility because of its extracorporeal placement, it still represents an important means of long-term LVAD support. It is especially applicable in patients whose abdominal cavity is too small to accommodate an intracorporeal device or who require biventricular support.

■ The REMATCH trial compared survival in patients with end-stage heart failure ineligible for heart transplantation who received LVAD therapy ($n = 68$) versus optimal medical therapy ($n = 61$). One-year survival was 52% for the LVAD group and 25% for the medical group. Two-year survival was 23% and 8%. Serious adverse events, including infection, bleeding, and device malfunction, were problems in the LVAD-treated group.

■ Although further clinical studies are warranted to define long-term outcomes better, it seems that the Jarvik 2000 can provide safe and effective left ventricular support, and that it can be used in select patients as a bridge to transplantation or as destination therapy.

■ In clinical trials, the MicroMed DeBakey VAD has provided adequate circulatory support in a wide range of patients with advanced heart failure, regardless of patient size, even in the outpatient setting.

■ Although the device itself seems to be reliable and effective in providing adequate end-organ perfusion, the long-term clinical outcomes of the AbioCor recipients remain limited mainly because of the high risk of stroke.

■ Besides improving clinical symptoms, LVADs apparently have proved useful in preventing or reversing heart failure by inducing neuroendocrine modulation and reverse remodeling. In terms of neurohormonal modulation, LVAD support can decrease dramatically plasma levels of epinephrine, norepinephrine, angiotensin II, and arginine vasopressin; attenuate serum levels of interleukin-6 and interleukin-8; and decrease TNF-α content in the failing myocardium.

■ In terms of reverse remodeling, long-term LVAD support has been shown to decrease significantly collagen content and myocyte size and improve myocyte contractility and myocardial response to β-adrenergic stimulation.

REFERENCES

1. Jessup M, Brozena SC: Support devices for end stage heart failure. Cardiol Clin 2003;21:135-139.
2. Young JB: Refractory heart failure. Curr Cardiol Rep 1999;1:67-81.
3. Deng MC, De Meester JM, Smits JM, et al: Effect of receiving a heart transplant: Analysis of a national cohort entered on to a waiting list, stratified by heart failure severity. Comparative Outcome and Clinical Profiles in Transplantation (COCPIT) Study Group. BMJ 2000;321:540-545.
4. Frazier OH, Fuqua JM Jr, Helman DN: Clinical left heart assist devices: A historical perspective. In Goldstein DJ, Oz MC (eds): Cardiac Assist Devices. Armonk, NY, Futura Publishing, 2000, pp 3-13.
5. Frazier OH, Short HD, Wampler RK, et al: Mechanical circulatory support in the transplant population. In Frazier OH (ed): Support and Replacement of the Failing Heart. Philadelphia, Lippincott-Raven, 1996, pp 147-167.
6. Nishimura M, Radovancevic B, Odegaard P, et al: Patients with renal dysfunction before left ventricular assist system (LVAS) implantation are poor transplant candidates and permanent LVAS may be indicated. J Heart Lung Transplant 1997;16:94.
7. Farrar DJ, Thoratec Ventricular Assist Device Principal Investigators: Preoperative predictors of survival in patients with Thoratec ventricular assist devices as a bridge to transplantation. J Heart Lung Transplant 1994;13:93-101.
8. Reinhartz O, Farrar DJ, Hershon JH, et al: Importance of preoperative liver function as a predictor of survival in patients supported with Thoratec ventricular assist devices as a bridge to transplantation. J Thorac Cardiovasc Surg 1998;116:633-640.
9. Richartz BM, Radovancevic B, Frazier OH, et al: Low serum cholesterol levels predict high perioperative mortality in patients supported by a left-ventricular assist system. Cardiology 1998;89:184-188.
10. Burnett CM, Sweeney MS, Frazier OH, et al: Improved multiorgan function in heart transplant candidates requiring prolonged univentricular support. Ann Thorac Surg 1993;55:65-71.
11. Frazier OH, Rose EA, McCarthy P, et al: Improved mortality and rehabilitation of transplant candidates treated with a long-term implantable left ventricular assist system. Ann Surg 1995;222:327-328.
12. Livingston ER, Fisher BA, Bibidakis EJ, et al: Increased activation of the coagulation and fibrinolytic systems leads to hemorrhagic complications during left ventricular assist implantation. Circulation 1996;94(Suppl II):II-227-II-234.
13. Goldstein DJ, Seldomridge JA, Chen JM, et al: Use of aprotinin in LVAD recipients reduces blood loss, blood use, and perioperative mortality. Ann Thorac Surg 1995;59:1063-1068.
14. Radovancevic R, Riggs SA, Radovancevic B, et al: Evaluation of two protocols for administration of recombinant human erythropoietin in left ventricular assist device patients awaiting heart transplantation (Abstract 3756). Blood 1998;92(10 Suppl 1, Pt 2):179b.
15. Oz MC, Argenziano M, Catanese KA, et al: Bridge experience with long-term implantable left ventricular assist devices. Circulation 1997;95:1844-1852.
16. Frazier OH, Baldwin RT, Eskin SG, Duncan JM: Immunochemical identification of human endothelial cells on the lining of a ventricular assist device. Tex Heart Inst J 1993;20:78-82.

17. Argenziano M, Catanese KA, Moazami N, et al: The influence of infection on survival and successful transplantation in patients with left ventricular assist devices. J Heart Lung Transplant 1997;16:822-831.

18. Mehta SM, Aufiero TX, Pae WE Jr, et al: Combined registry for the clinical use of mechanical ventricular assist pumps and the total artificial heart in conjunction with heart transplantation: Sixth official report—1994. J Heart Lung Transplant 1995;14:585-593.

19. Wasler A, Springer E, Radovancevic B, et al: A comparison between intraperitoneal and extraperitoneal left ventricular assist system placement. ASAIO J 1996;42:M573-M576.

20. McCarthy PM, Smedira NO, Vargo RL, et al: One hundred patients with the HeartMate left ventricular assist device: Evolving concepts and technology. J Thorac Cardiovasc Surg 1998;115:904-912.

21. Deng MC, Loebe M, El-Banayousy A, et al: Mechanical circulatory support for advanced heart failure: Effect of patient selection on outcome. Circulation 2001;103:231-237.

22. Booth JV, Wheeldon DR, Ghosh S: Anesthetic management, including cardiopulmonary bypass. In Cooper DK, Miller LW, Patterson GA (eds): The Transplantation and Replacement of Thoracic Organs. UK: Kluwer Academic Publishers, 1996, pp 195-197.

23. Beck JR, Mongero LB, Kroslowitz RM, et al: Inhaled nitric oxide improves hemodynamics in patients with acute pulmonary hypertension after high-risk cardiac surgery. Perfusion 1999;14:37-42.

24. Nakatani T, Radovancevic B, Frazier OH: Right heart assist for acute for right ventricular failure after orthotopic heart transplantation. ASAIO Trans 1987;33:695-698.

25. Cooper DKC, Lidsky NM: Immediate postoperative care and potential complications. In Cooper DK, Miller LW, Patterson GA (eds): The Transplantation and Replacement of Thoracic Organs. UK: Kluwer Academic Publishers, 1996, pp 221-227.

26. Bozkurt B: Medical and surgical therapy for cardiac remodeling. Curr Opin Cardiol 1999;14:196-205.

27. Cowie MR: Best practice: Evidence from the clinical trials. Heart 2002;88 (Suppl 2):II-2-II-4.

28. Farrar DJ: The Thoratec ventricular assist device: A paracorporeal pump for treating acute and chronic heart failure. Semin Thorac Cardiovasc Surg 2000;12:243-250.

29. Holman WL, Davies JE, Rayburn BK, et al: Treatment of end-stage heart disease with outpatient ventricular assist devices. Ann Thorac Surg 2002;73:1489-1493.

30. Farrar DJ, Holman WR, McBride LR, et al: Long-term follow-up of Thoratec ventricular assist device bridge-to-recovery patients successfully removed from support after recovery of ventricular function. J Heart Lung Transplant 2002;21:516-521.

31. Frazier OH: First use of an untethered, vented electric left ventricular assist device for long-term support. Circulation 1994;89:2908-2914.

32. Frazier OH, Rose EA, Oz MC, et al: Multicenter clinical evaluation of the HeartMate vented electric left ventricular assist system in patients awaiting heart transplantation. J Thorac Cardiovasc Surg 2001;122:1186-1195.

33. Rose EA, Gelijns AC, Moskowitz AJ, et al: Long-term mechanical left ventricular assistance for end-stage heart failure. N Engl J Med 2001;345:1435-1443.

34. Robbins RC, Kown MH, Portner PM, Oyer PE: The totally implantable Novacor left ventricular assist system. Ann Thorac Surg 2001;71(3 Suppl):S162-S165.

35. Dagenais F, Portner PM, Robbins RC, Oyer PE: The Novacor left ventricular assist system: Clinical experience from the Novacor registry. J Card Surg 2001;16:267-271.

36. Thomas CE, Jichici D, Petrucci R, et al: Neurologic complications of the Novacor left ventricular assist device. Ann Thorac Surg 2001;72:1311-1315.

37. Westaby S, Banning AP, Saito S, et al: Circulatory support for long-term treatment of heart failure: Experience with an intraventricular continuous flow pump. Circulation 2002;105:2588-2591.

38. Frazier OH, Myers TJ, Westaby S, Gregoric ID: Use of the Jarvik 2000 left ventricular assist system as a bridge to heart transplantation or as destination therapy for patients with chronic heart failure. Ann Surg 2003;237:631-636.

39. Wieselthaler GM, Schima H, Hiesmayr M, et al: First clinical experience with the DeBakey VAD continuous-axial-flow pump for bridge to transplantation. Circulation 2000;101:356-359.

40. Michael DeBakey: Personal communication, June, 2005.

41. Noon GP, Morley DL, Irwin S, et al: Clinical experience with the MicroMed DeBakey ventricular assist device. Ann Thorac Surg 2001;71(3 Suppl):S133-S138.

42. Salzberg S, Lachat M, Zund G, et al: Left ventricular assist device as a bridge to transplantation: Lessons learned with the MicroMed DeBakey axial blood flow pump. Eur J Cardiothorac Surg 2003;24:113-118.

43. Samuels LE, Dowling R: Total artificial heart: Destination therapy. Cardiol Clin 2003;21:115-118.

44. Dowling RD, Gray LA Jr, Etoch SW, et al: The AbioCor implantable replacement heart. Ann Thorac Surg 2003;75(6 Suppl):S93-S99.

45. Goldstein S, Ali AS, Sabbah H: Ventricular remodeling: Mechanisms and prevention. Cardiol Clin 1998;16:623-632.

46. Mann DL: Mechanisms and models in heart failure: A combinatorial approach. Circulation 1999;100:999-1008.

47. Cohn JN, Ferrari R, Sharpe N: Cardiac remodeling—concepts and clinical implications: A consensus paper from an international forum on cardiac remodeling. On behalf of an international forum on cardiac remodeling. J Am Coll Cardiol 2000;35:569-582.

48. McMurray J, Pfeffer MA: New therapeutic options in congestive heart failure: Part I. Circulation 2002;105:2099-2106.

49. James KJ, McCarthy PM, Thomas JD, et al: Effect of the implantable left ventricular assist device on neuroendocrine activation in heart failure. Circulation 1995;92(9 Suppl):II-191-II-195.

50. Goldstein DJ, Moazami N, Seldomridge JA, et al: Circulatory resuscitation with left ventricular assist device support reduces interleukins 6 and 8 levels. Ann Thorac Surg 1997;63:971-974.

51. Torre-Amione G, Stetson SJ, Youker KA, et al: Decreased expression of tumor necrosis factor-alpha in failing human myocardium after mechanical circulatory support: A potential mechanism for cardiac recovery. Circulation 1999;100:1189-1193.

52. Bruckner BA, Stetson SJ, Perez-Verdia A, et al: Regression of fibrosis and hypertrophy in failing myocardium following mechanical circulatory support. J Heart Lung Transplant 2001;20:457-464.

53. Dipla K, Mattiello JA, Jeevanandam V, et al: Myocyte recovery after mechanical circulatory support in humans with end-stage heart failure. Circulation 1998;97:2316-2322.

54. Frazier OH, Myers TJ: Left ventricular assist system as a bridge to myocardial recovery. Ann Thorac Surg 1999;68:734-741.

55. Hetzer R, Muller JH, Weng Y, et al: Bridging-to-recovery. Ann Thorac Surg 2001;71:S109-S113.

56. Westaby S, Coats AJ: Mechanical bridge to myocardial recovery. Eur Heart J 1998;19:541-547.

57. Mancini DM, Beniaminovitz A, Levin H, et al: Low incidence of myocardial recovery after left ventricular assist device implantation in patients with chronic heart failure. Circulation 1998;98:2383-2389.

58. Williams MR, Oz MC: Indications and patient selection for mechanical ventricular assistance. Ann Thorac Surg 2001;1:S86-S91.

59. Koenig SC, Woolard C, Drew G, et al: Integrated data acquisition system for medical device testing and physiology research in compliance with good laboratory practice. Biomed Instrum Technol 2004;38:229-240.

60. Dowling RD, Ghaly AS, Gray LA: Creation of a diaphragm patch to facilitate placement of the AbioCor implantable replacement heart. Ann Thorac Surg 2004;77:1849-1850.

61. Kung RT, Zhang H. Vascular tone estimation in patients implanted with the AbioCor implantable replacement heart. Artif Organs 2004;28:543-547.

62. Akgul A, Youker KA, Noon GP, et al: Quantitative changes in mast cell populations after left ventricular assist device implantation. ASAIOJ 2005;51:275-280.

63. DeBakey ME: Development of mechanical heart devices. Ann Thorac Surg 2005;79:S2228-S2231.

CHAPTER 50

Future of Mechanical Support Devices in Children and Young Adults

Matthew T. Harting
O. H. Frazier

More than 40 years after the initial use of ventricular assist devices (VADs),[1] physicians are expanding the scope of these devices for the treatment of severe heart failure in adults. In the 1990s, smaller, better designed pumps[2-8] with improved power sources[9-11] and antithrombogenic materials were introduced.[12,13] Mechanical circulatory support also has benefited from improved surgical technique,[4,14] better understanding of cardiovascular physiology,[15,16] and advances in adjuvant medical management.[17-19] More than 4000 adults now have received left VADs worldwide. Having evolved from rescue therapy to temporary maintenance therapy (bridging to transplantation), the role of the VAD is progressing rapidly toward destination therapy, starting with long-term support and myocardial recovery.

Cardiopulmonary support in infants and children has had limited success with the use of extracorporeal membrane oxygenation (ECMO),[21-22] and cardiac support with VADs is limited, not only by size but also by availability.[23] Other chapters have explored the current uses of mechanical support devices thoroughly, including indications, possible consequences, and principles of supportive care in children with heart failure. Such devices have been used to manage pediatric heart failure resulting from a wide variety of etiologies, including congenital anatomic variations, myocarditis, cardiomyopathy, respiratory failure, dysrhythmias, and postcardiotomy support. Mechanical circulatory support for the treatment of heart failure has lagged far behind in pediatric patients.

In 2003, the Division of Heart and Vascular Diseases at the National Heart, Lung and Blood Institute (NHLBI) released a request for research proposals focused on the development of "novel circulatory assist devices including left and right ventricular assist devices, extracorporeal gas exchange systems, and other bioengineered systems for infants and children with congenital and acquired cardiovascular disease."[24] The agency called for innovations that can overcome physiologic and bioengineering barriers to the use of assist systems in infants and small children; such innovations are certain to promote the application of ventricular assistance to the care of these critically ill children.

This chapter addresses the current obstacles posed by ventricular assistance in the pediatric population—not only obstacles seen in adults and likely to be transposed to children, but also issues unique to infants, children, and young adults. The discussion focuses on emerging solutions to these challenges and describes the promising future of mechanical circulatory support in this age group.

BRIDGING TO TRANSPLANTATION, DESTINATION THERAPY, AND MYOCARDIAL RECOVERY

With the goal of long-term assistance, the NHLBI originally began funding research into mechanical circulatory support in the early 1970s. The resulting VADs (including the **HeartMate** [Thoratec Corp, Pleasanton, CA], **Thoratec** [Thoratec Corp, Pleasanton, CA], and **Novacor** [Baxter Health Care Corp, Novacor Division, Oakland, CA] devices) initially gained U.S. Food and Drug Administration approvals for use as bridges to transplantation.[25] In this important and lifesaving capacity, ventricular assistance has been used with growing success for more than two decades in adults. As the waiting time for transplantation has lengthened, particularly for larger patients, additional experience with long-term implants has been acquired.

Goldman and colleagues[20] assessed the effectiveness of mechanical assist devices as bridges to transplantation in children with end-stage cardiomyopathy. Of the 22 children (ages 1.2 to 17 years) who were supported by a VAD (*n* = 9) or ECMO (*n* = 13), 77% were successfully bridged to transplantation and discharged from the hospital. Overall, the ECMO recipients fared better, all but one of them (92%) surviving to undergo transplantation and discharge. Of the nine children who received a paracorporeal VAD, six later underwent transplantation, and five (55%) were discharged from the hospital. The authors concluded that bridging to transplantation was successful and could minimize the mortality of children awaiting transplantation; ECMO was an effective form of support, but its advantage was limited to infants, for whom donor organs were more readily obtainable and shorter durations of support were required.

In adults, bridging to transplantation was the first successful step in expanding the indications for mechanical circulatory support toward the inclusion of destination therapy. Since being introduced as bridges to transplantation in the 1980s, the HeartMate and Novacor implantable pumps have improved survival and transplantation outcomes. As of April 2004, according to the Thoratec Corporation, 353 HeartMate patients have been supported for 1 year, and 54 patients have been supported for more than 2 years with implantable pumps as bridges to transplantation. The longest cumulative support duration has been 4.6 years, and the mean support duration has been 110 days.

In 1993, the NHLBI accepted a proposal for the REMATCH (Randomized Evaluation of Mechanical Assistance for the Treatment of Congestive Heart Failure) trial.[27] This prospective multicenter study evaluated ventricular assistance as destination therapy versus optimal medical management in 129 adults with end-stage heart failure.[5] On survival analysis, compared with the medical group, the VAD recipients had a 48% lower risk of death from any cause (relative risk, 0.52; 95% confidence interval, 0.34 to 0.78; $P = .001$). The Kaplan-Meier estimates of survival at 1 year were 52% in the device group and 25% in the medical group ($P = .002$) and were 23% versus 8% at 2 years ($P = .09$). There was a striking difference between the median survival of the device group (408 days) versus the medical group (150 days). The quality of life was significantly better with VAD therapy than with medical therapy. In the VAD patients, however, serious adverse events (rate ratio, 2.35; 95% confidence interval, 1.86 to 2.95)—predominately infection, bleeding, and device malfunction—were associated with this intervention.

Overall, the REMATCH study established new standards for survival and quality of life. It showed that ventricular assistance is superior to medical therapy in these seriously ill patients. More important, it precisely defined modes of failure, such as inflow-valve disruption, bearing wear, and infection, all of which could be corrected or modified. By defining these failure modes, REMATCH also served as a phase I study that resulted in improved device effectiveness. In response to the above-named complications, the HeartMate I (the device used in this trial) underwent appropriate modifications, which should improve significantly the results obtained with this technology. The trial also revealed target areas for future improvements in VAD design and management.

In the early 1990s, clinical, functional, and anatomic improvements in the native heart function of chronic heart failure patients supported by longer term implanted VADs led to speculations about the possibility of VAD removal with myocardial recovery and survival in select patients. In 1995, Hetzer and colleagues[28] removed a malfunctioning pump from such a patient, who retained good cardiac function without pump support or transplantation. Since that time, numerous patients have undergone pump removal followed by sustained improvement in cardiac function.[29-31] Further research has revealed improved hemodynamic, anatomic, histologic,

and biochemical markers in many patients.[32] Some patients have required pump explantation because of device-related patient complications and have maintained improved cardiac function.[33] On the basis of these observations, the Berlin Heart Institute[34] and the Harefield Hospital in London have initiated limited, prospective studies to help clarify the clinical implications of myocardial recovery. Such studies remain impossible in the United States because of regulatory issues.

The possible therapeutic benefits of destination therapy and myocardial recovery during VAD assistance, as opposed to bridging to transplantation, may be particularly important in children. In all patients except perhaps adults in their 60s, transplantation—even when successful—results statistically not only in premature death, but also in a potential for decreased myocardial function. Effective implantable left VAD therapy could offer, however, not only long-term survival, but also the potential for sustained myocardial recovery and a normal life span.

COMPLICATIONS AND SOLUTIONS: NOVEL DEVICES AND THEORIES

Introducing any artificial device into the human body is fraught with possible complications, especially if that device is anastomosed to the circulatory system and designed to augment the flow of blood. Numerous complications are related to the need for a lengthy implant procedure, often in desperately ill patients, and the physiologic alterations created by a VAD. Thrombosis, hemorrhage, infection, device failure, and power loss have occurred.[18,35-40] Although complication rates have decreased substantially over the years, major challenges remain.

Thrombotic and embolic complications related to the blood-biomaterial interface and altered circulatory physiology have been encountered in patients with long-term VADs; these complications are related primarily to the presence of passive flow in an inflow cannula with the degree of stasis that is unavoidable in this type of operational device. Thromboembolic complications have been minimized by the HeartMate I technology. Even with continuous-flow pumps, the altered rheology resulting from the negative pressure generated in the inflow cannula has resulted in inflow occlusion from pseudo-neointima buildup.[41] These complications may be minimized by eliminating or minimizing the length of the inflow cannulae when possible. Reduced blood flow, increased blood viscosity, and inadequate anticoagulation also contribute to thromboembolic complications.

With the goal of eliminating the necessity of venting the pump or implanting a compliance chamber, our laboratories began to study implantable continuous-flow pumps in the early 1980s. The first such pump to be used clinically was the external Biomedicus (Medtronic

Inc., Eden Prairie, MN) device. In April 1988, we initiated clinical use of the intracorporeal **Hemopump** (Nimbus, Inc, Rancho Cordova, CA). Shortly afterward, we implanted this pump in a 7-year-old child dying of post-transplantation rejection. The Hemopump supported this patient for 4 days. For 2 days, there was no cardiac activity at all. After 4 days, however, the rejection was reversed, and cardiac function was reinstated. Implantable, long-term nonpulsatile devices seem to offer hope for the long-term support of infants, children, and young adults. In current devices, the requirement for

blood-immersed bearings is a source of concern, however, because such bearings ultimately fail.

Continuous flow throughout the cardiac cycle, converting diastolic flow from passive to active, is being studied by means of computer-aided design, computational fluid dynamics, and flow simulation studies (Fig. 50-1A).[42,43] These studies are generating new insights that should clarify the hemodynamic ramifications of this form of ventricular assistance. Computer modeling also helps device designers incorporate features that maximize efficiency and minimize complications.

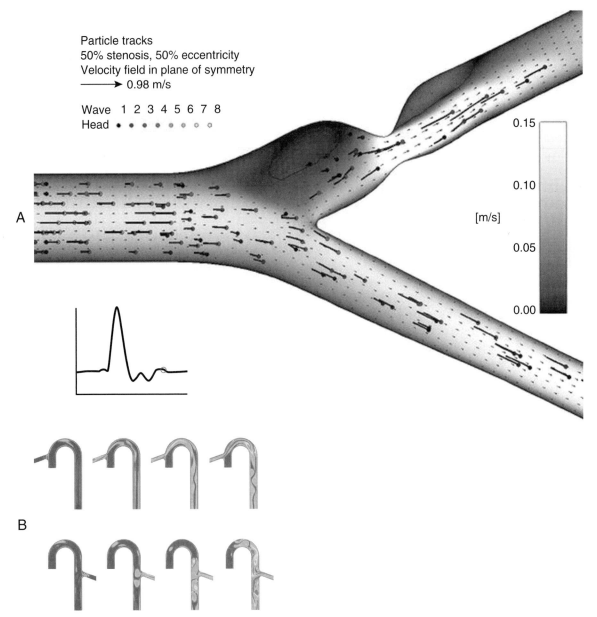

FIGURE 50-1 ■ **Computer-aided flow designs. A,** Continuous flow throughout the cardiac cycle, converting diastolic flow from passive to active, is being studied by means of computer-aided design, computational fluid dynamics, and flow simulation studies. **B,** Computer-aided design studies, comparing flows in ascending *(top)* versus descending *(bottom)* aortic anastomoses. The flow rate increases from left to right. (**A** courtesy of Ralph Metcalfe, University of Houston. For more information, see http://celsius.ifdt.uh.edu/3d/particle/index.html.) (See also Color Section)

Computer modeling of outflow-graft anastomosis to the ascending versus the descending aorta has shown that descending aortic anastomosis may increase stagnation in the ascending aorta (Fig. 50-1B). This stagnation may increase the risk of thrombosis if care is not taken to allow periodic opening of the aortic valve. Computer simulation may play a major role in the future of ventricular assistance.

In addition, novel bioengineered materials are reducing thrombogenic complications in device recipients. The blood-contacting surfaces of VADs have been modified to facilitate the formation of a smooth pseudointima, which is likely to decrease thromboembolic complications.[4,12] Portner and associates[12] found that, compared with conventional conduits, the new Vascutek Gelweave conduit (Vascutek, Ltd, Renfrewshire, Scotland, UK) increases mural flow and neointimal adhesion, reducing the risk of embolic cerebrovascular accidents by 50%.

Medical management of VAD recipients also is improving. Thromboembolic complications are being minimized with platelet inhibitors,[44] recombinant tissue plasminogen activator,[41] and other pharmaceutical therapies. Continued biomedical engineering and clinical testing of innovative blood-contacting materials, grafts, and pharmaceutical agents should decrease further the incidence of thromboembolic complications.

Infection has been a major problem in patients supported by long-term, implantable pulsatile VADs.[45-47] Infection is related to the presence of a large foreign object, the lengthy implant operation, and the need for a percutaneous driveline. In addition, VADs are implanted only in patients who are facing imminent death and who have suffered the ravages of chronic heart failure, including cachexia. This physiologic milieu also increases the likelihood of infectious complications.[35] In pulsatile devices, infection may be reduced by including an implantable compliance chamber and a transcutaneously powered system. This was the original goal of the NHLBI research in the 1970s. The proposal, however, required the compliance chamber to be functional without venting for 2 years; this goal was impossible to achieve. The same technology has been used successfully, however, in the **Arrow LionHeart** (Arrow International, Reading, PA) (Fig. 50-2). With weekly venting of the compliance chamber, this controlled compliance system allows for an operational left VAD without skin-penetrating components. To date, this technology has been implanted in only a few patients, but it seems to reduce infection.[48-50]

Implantable continuous-flow pumps offer decided advantages, particularly for pediatric patients. The miniaturization achieved by this technology, the lack of necessity for a pump pocket, and the elimination of the trauma caused by a pulsatile foreign body should decrease infectious complications. These pumps first were used clinically in 1999.

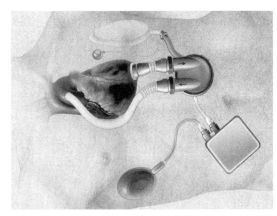

FIGURE 50-2 ■ The Arrow LionHeart Left Ventricular Assist System (Arrow International, Reading, PA). This electrically powered, totally implantable pump consists of inlet and outlet cannulae, a compliance chamber, and a transcutaneously powered motor. (From Frazier OH: *Mechanical circulatory support: New advances, new pumps, new ideas. Semin Thorac Cardiovasc Surg* 2002;14:178-186.)

Currently the two most widely used pumps, the MicroMed DeBakey VAD (MicroMed Technology, Houston, TX) and the Jarvik 2000 FlowMaker LVAD (Jarvik Heart, Inc, New York, NY), have had a marked absence of serious infectious complications, even during long-term use (4 years). Simply miniaturizing the currently available pumps would not meet all of the physiologic challenges that face pediatric patients, however. The increased thrombogenicity and hemolysis in the smaller pumps and the reduced flow must be addressed before widespread use of this technology is undertaken. The NHLBI-funded study now under way should allow a systematic approach to these problems.

The **Jarvik 2000** device is a miniature (90-g), continuous-flow VAD with diminutive blood-contacting surfaces, a simple design, and a single moving part—the rotor (Fig. 50-3). As of late 2003, the Jarvik 2000 had been

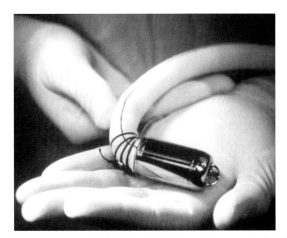

FIGURE 50-3 ■ The Jarvik 2000 (Jarvik Heart, Inc, New York, NY). This device is a miniature (90-g), continuous-flow VAD with diminutive blood-contacting surfaces, a simple design, and a single moving part. (From Frazier OH: *Mechanical circulatory support: New advances, new pumps, new ideas. Semin Thorac Cardiovasc Surg* 2002;14:178-186.)

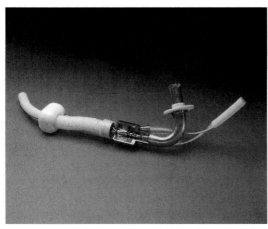

FIGURE 50-4 ■ Cutaway view of the MicroMed DeBakey VAD (MicroMed Technology, Houston, TX). (Courtesy of MicroMed Technology, Inc., Houston, TX.) (See also Color Section)

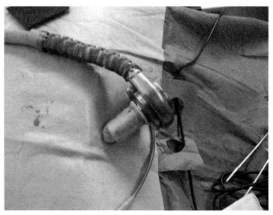

FIGURE 50-5 ■ The HeartWare (HeartWare, Inc, Miramar, FL). This device is a novel miniaturized passive magnetic-levitation centrifugal ventricular assist device. (See also Color Section)

implanted with outstanding results in 40 patients at the Texas Heart Institute. Although clinical studies are just beginning, this pump's perioperative morbidity and mortality data appear superior to the data of many other left VADs. The reliability of this pump is outstanding, as there has not been even a single instance of mechanical failure.

More extensive clinical experience has been achieved with the **MicroMed DeBakey VAD** (Fig. 50-4), which, as of May 2005, had been implanted as a bridge to transplantation in more than 350 patients worldwide.[51] This VAD has been used successfully as a bridge to transplantation and has been used on a compassionate-need basis in pediatric patients. At Texas Children's Hospital, a pediatric version of this pump was used in an effort to sustain a 6-year-old child until a donor heart became available. This was the first use of such an implantable pump.

The pumps in current clinical use all require a bearing; elimination of the bearing may allow even longer support with these pumps. Many pumps without bearings are being investigated, and the smallest and most efficient of these is the **HeartWare** (HeartWare, Inc, Miramar, FL), a miniaturized, passive, magnetic-levitation centrifugal VAD (Fig. 50-5). With its miniature inlet cannula, this device ideally can be implanted through the diaphragmatic surface of the heart on the left and the right sides. This pump is ideally suited for long-term implantable right ventricular support. A functional implantable right ventricular assist pump not only would broaden the number of patients who could benefit from right ventricular support, particularly in the pediatric population, but also would allow increased flow to a similarly implanted left-sided pump and avoid the septal shift seen in long-term implanted continuous-flow left VADs.[15]

Although biventricular support is currently available for smaller children with the external Thoratec pump[52,53] or the Berlin heart,[34] the results have been discouraging,

with a high incidence of complications, particularly in cases of congenital heart disease. In addition, these pumps can be used only as a bridge to recovery or eventual transplantation, and the patient generally is confined to the hospital. A workable pump that would allow excision of the heart, with physiologic and anatomic replacements, would be a great boon, particularly in cases of congenital heart disease. Problems related to size and long-term reliability have plagued the total artificial heart. One pump that shows considerable promise is the **AbioCor Total Artificial Heart** (TAH) (ABIOMED, Danvers, MA) (Fig. 50-6), which was first implanted clinically in July 2001. Initial experience with the AbioCor has been encouraging, and this device represents an important breakthrough for adults with irreparable heart failure.[25]

The mechanics of a pulsatile, biventricular implantable pump severely limit the application of such a device in children. In contrast, a biventricular cardiac replacement system consisting of continuous-flow pumps on the right and left sides and an interatrial shunt to allow physiologic balancing could be made small enough even for children. Our laboratories have implanted such a pump, which appears to be functional in the acute

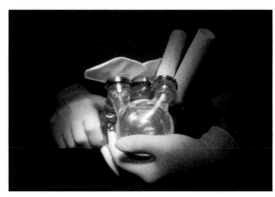

FIGURE 50-6 ■ The AbioCor Total Artificial Heart (ABIOMED, Danvers, MA). (From Frazier OH: *Mechanical circulatory support: New advances, new pumps, new ideas. Semin Thorac Cardiovasc Surg* 2002;14:178-186.)

setting in sheep. An electric total artificial heart developed at Pennsylvania State University and acquired by ABIOMED[25] may be particularly promising for children. ABIOMED is designing a new, smaller version of this pump for use in children and adolescents, and clinical trials are expected to begin in the near future.

CURRENT STATUS AND FUTURE TRENDS

For patients with end-stage heart failure refractory to optimal medical management, heart transplantation is the definitive therapy. Nevertheless, the supply of donor hearts is extremely limited, and the remaining gap is increasingly being filled by mechanical circulatory support devices.[53] In pediatric patients, this option is limited by the large size of current VADs and total artificial hearts. As this technology continues to advance, however, the development of miniaturized devices will improve the survival and quality of life of pediatric patients. When devices that are safe, effective, and anatomically suitable for use in children become available, these devices should play a crucial role in the management of pediatric patients with heart failure.[54]

Key Concepts

■ More than 40 years after the initial use of VADs, physicians are expanding the scope of these devices for the treatment of severe heart failure in adults. In the 1990s, smaller, better designed pumps with improved power sources and antithrombogenic materials were introduced.

■ Having evolved from rescue therapy to temporary maintenance therapy (bridging to transplantation), the role of the VAD is progressing rapidly toward destination therapy, starting with long-term support and myocardial recovery.

■ In the early 1990s, clinical, functional, and anatomic improvements in the native heart function of chronic heart failure patients supported by longer term implanted VADs led to speculations about the possibility of VAD removal with myocardial recovery and survival in select patients.

■ Thrombotic and embolic complications related to the blood-biomaterial interface and altered circulatory physiology have been encountered in patients with long-term VADs; these complications are related primarily to the presence of passive flow in an inflow cannula with the degree of stasis that is unavoidable in this type of operational device.

■ Implantable, long-term nonpulsatile devices seem to offer hope for the long-term support of infants, children, and young adults. In current devices, the requirement for blood-immersed bearings is a source of concern, however, because such bearings ultimately fail.

■ Implantable continuous-flow pumps offer decided advantages, particularly for pediatric patients. The miniaturization achieved by this technology, the lack of necessity for a pump pocket, and the elimination of the trauma caused by a pulsatile foreign body should decrease infectious complications.

■ Simply miniaturizing the currently available pumps would not meet all of the physiologic challenges that face pediatric patients, however. The increased thrombogenicity and hemolysis in the smaller pumps and the reduced flow must be addressed before widespread use of this technology is undertaken.

■ The mechanics of a pulsatile, biventricular implantable pump severely limit the application of such a device in children. In contrast, a biventricular cardiac replacement system consisting of continuous-flow pumps on the right and left sides and an interatrial shunt to allow physiologic balancing could be made small enough even for children.

REFERENCES

1. DeBakey ME, Liotta D, Hall CW: Left heart bypass using an implantable blood pump. In: Mechanical Devices to Assist the Failing Heart. Proceedings of a conference sponsored by The Committee on Trauma, September 9-10, 1964. Washington, DC, National Academy of Sciences–National Research Council, 1966, p 223.
2. Okamoto E, Hashimoto T, Mitamura Y: Design of a miniature implantable left ventricular assist device using CAD/CAM technology. J Artif Organs 2003;6:162-167.
3. Liotta D: Novel left ventricular assist system: An electrocardiogram-synchronized LVAS that avoids cardiac cannulation. Tex Heart Inst J 2003;30:194-201.
4. Strauch JT, Spielvogel D, Haldenwang PL, et al: Recent improvements in outcome with the Novacor left ventricular assist device. J Heart Lung Transplant 2003;22:674-680.
5. Rose EA, Gelijns AC, Moskowitz AJ, et al: Long-term use of a left ventricular assist device for end-stage heart failure. N Engl J Med 2001;345:1435-1443.
6. Locke DH, Swanson ES, Walton JF 2nd, et al: Testing of a centrifugal blood pump with a high efficiency hybrid magnetic bearing. ASAIO J 2003;49:737-743.
7. Pacella JJ, Goldstein AH, Magovern GJ, et al: Modified fabrication techniques lead to improved centrifugal blood pump performance. ASAIO J 1994;40:M767-M772.
8. Masuzawa T, Ezoe S, Kato T, et al: Magnetically suspended centrifugal blood pump with an axially levitated motor. Artif Organs 2003;27:631-638.
9. Ozeki T, Chinzei T, Abe Y, et al: Preliminary study of a new type of energy transmission system for artificial hearts. J Artif Organs 2003;6:14-19.
10. Tamez D, Myers TJ, Inman RW, et al: Clinical evaluation of the HeartPak: A new pneumatic portable driver for use with the HeartMate Implantable Pneumatic Left Ventricular Assist System. ASAIO J 1997;43:M797-M801.
11. Mussivand T, Hum A, Diguer M, et al: A transcutaneous energy and information transfer system for implanted medical devices. ASAIO J 1995;41:M253-M258.
12. Portner PM, Jansen PGM, Oyer PE, et al: Improved outcomes with an implantable left ventricular assist system: A multicenter study. Ann Thorac Surg 2001;71:205-209.

13. Murray SF, Calabrese SJ, Malanoski SB, et al: Selection and evaluation of blood and tribologically compatible journal bearing materials. ASAIO J 1997;43:M603-M608.

14. Macris MP, Parnis SM, Frazier OH, et al: Development of an implantable ventricular assist system. Ann Thorac Surg 1997;63:367-370.

15. Letsou GV, Myers TJ, Gregoric ID, et al: Continuous axial-flow left ventricular assist device (Jarvik 2000) maintains kidney and liver perfusion for up to 6 months. Ann Thorac Surg 2003;76:1167-1170.

16. Giridharan GA, Skliar M: Control strategy for maintaining physiological perfusion with rotary blood pumps. Artif Organs 2003;27: 639-648.

17. Goldstein DJ, Beauford RB: Left ventricular assist devices and bleeding: Adding insult to injury. Ann Thorac Surg 2003;75 (6 Suppl):S42-S47.

18. Fries D, Innerhofer P, Streif W, et al: Coagulation monitoring and management of anticoagulation during cardiac assist device support. Ann Thorac Surg 2003;76:1593-1597.

19. Potapov EV, Pasic M, Bauer M, et al: Activated recombinant factor VII for control of diffuse bleeding after implantation of ventricular assist device. Ann Thorac Surg 2002;74:2182-2183.

20. Goldman AP, Cassidy J, de Leval M, et al: The waiting game: Bridging to paediatric heart transplantation. Lancet 2003;362: 1967-1970.

21. Taghavi S, Ankersmit J, Zuckermann A, et al: A retrospective analysis of extracorporeal membrane oxygenation versus right ventricular assist device in acute great failure after heart transplantation. Transplant Proc 2003;35:2805-2807.

22. Wolfson PJ: The development and use of extracorporeal membrane oxygenation in neonates. Ann Thorac Surg 2003;76:S2224-S2229.

23. Reinhartz O, Copeland JG, Farrar DJ, et al: Thoratec ventricular assist devices in children with less than 1.3 m² of body surface area. ASAIO J 2003;49:727-730.

24. http://grants2.nih.gov/grants/guide/notice-files/NOT-HL-03-004.html. Accessed May 13, 2004.

25. Frazier OH: Mechanical circulatory support: New advances, new pumps, new ideas. Semin Thorac Cardiovasc Surg 2002;14:178-186.

26. Frazier OH, Bricker JT, Macris MP, Cooley DA: Use of a left ventricular assist device as a bridge to transplantation in a pediatric patient. Tex Heart Inst J 1989;16:46-50.

27. Rose EA, Moskowitz AJ, Packer M, et al: The REMATCH Trial: Rationale, design, and end points. Ann Thorac Surg 1999;67: 723-730.

28. Hetzer R, Muller J, Weng Y, et al: Cardiac recovery in dilated cardiomyopathy by unloading with a left ventricular assist device. Ann Thorac Surg 1999;68:742-749.

29. Frazier OH: First use of an untethered, vented electric left ventricular assist device for long-term support. Circulation 1994;89:2908-2914.

30. Frazier OH, Macris MP, Myers TJ, et al: Improved survival after extended bridge to cardiac transplantation. Ann Thorac Surg 1994;57:1416-1422.

31. Maybaum S, Frazier OH, Starling R, et al: Low rate of cardiac recovery despite cellular recovery during LVAD support: Results from the LVAD Working Group. 24th Annual Meeting and Scientific Sessions, the International Society for Heart and Lung Transplantation, San Francisco. April 22, 2004. Abstract available at: http://www.abstracts2view.com/ishlt/.

32. Frazier OH, Harting MT: Recovery of cardiac function through mechanical unloading: An overview of reverse remodeling. Cardiol Spec Edn 2003;9:39-41.

33. Frazier OH, Rose EA, Oz MC, et al: Multicenter clinical evaluation of the HeartMate vented electric left ventricular assist system in patients awaiting heart transplantation. J Thorac Cardiovasc Surg 2001;122:1186-1195.

34. Loebe M, Muller J, Hetzer R: Ventricular assistance for recovery of cardiac failure. Curr Opin Cardiol 1999;14:234-248.

35. Hampton CR, Verrier ED: Systemic consequences of ventricular assist devices: Alterations of coagulation, immune function, inflammation, and the neuroendocrine system. Artif Organs 2002;26:902-908.

36. Morgan JA, Park Y, Oz MC, et al: Device related infections while on left ventricular assist device support do not adversely impact bridging to transplant or posttransplant survival. ASAIO J 2003;49: 748-750.

37. Poston RS, Husain S, Sorce D, et al: LVAD bloodstream infections: Therapeutic rationale for transplantation after LVAD infection. J Heart Lung Transplant 2003;22:914-921.

38. Nabavi DG, Stockmann J, Schmid C, et al: Doppler microembolic load predicts risk of thromboembolic complications in Novacor patients. J Thorac Cardiovasc Surg 2003;126:160-167.

39. Rose AG, Connelly JH, Park SJ, et al: Total left ventricular outflow tract obstruction due to left ventricular assist device-induced subaortic thrombosis in 2 patients with aortic valve prosthesis. J Heart Lung Transplant 2003;22:594-599.

40. Kasirajan V, Smedira NG, Perl J 2nd, McCarthy PM: Cerebral embolism associated with left ventricular assist device support and successful therapy with intraarterial urokinase. Ann Thorac Surg 1999;67:1148-1150.

41. Rothenburger M, Wilhelm MJ, Hammel D, et al: Treatment of thrombus formation associated with the MicroMed DeBakey VAD using recombinant tissue plasminogen activator. Circulation 2002;106(12 Suppl 1):1189-1192.

42. Apel J, Neudel F, Reul H: Computational fluid dynamics and experimental validation of a microaxial blood pump. ASAIO J 2001;47:552-558.

43. Veres JP, Golding LA, Smith WA, et al: Flow analysis of the Cleveland Clinic centrifugal pump. ASAIO J 1997;43:M778-M781.

44. Schmid C, Weyand M, Hanmel D, et al: Effect of platelet inhibitors on thromboembolism after implantation of a Novacor 100: Preliminary results. Thorac Cardiovasc Surg 1998;46:260-262.

45. Grossi P, Dalla Gasperina D, Pagani F, et al: Infectious complications in patients with the Novacor left ventricular assist system. Transplant Proc 2001;33:1969-1971.

46. Mehta SM, Aufiero TX, Pae WE, et al: Combined registry for the clinical use of mechanical ventricular assist pumps and the total artificial heart in conjunction with heart transplantation—Sixth Official Report—1994. J Heart Lung Transplant 1995;14:585-593.

47. Holman WL, Murrah CP, Ferguson ER, et al: Infections during extended circulatory support: University of Alabama at Birmingham experience 1989 to 1994. Ann Thorac Surg 1996;61:366-371.

48. Delgado RM: The future of mechanical circulatory support. Curr Opin Cardiol 2003;18:199-209.

49. Mehta SM, Pae WE Jr, Rosenberg G, et al: The LionHeart LVD-2000: A completely implanted left ventricular assist device for chronic circulatory support. Ann Thorac Surg 2001;71:S156-S161.

50. El-Banayosy A, Arusoglu L, Kizner L, et al: Preliminary experience with the LionHeart left ventricular assist device in patients with end-stage heart failure. Ann Thorac Surg 2003;75:1469-1475.

51. DeBakey ME: Personal communication (May, 2005)

52. Reinhartz O, Copeland JG, Garrar DJ, et al: Thoratec ventricular assist devices in children with less than 1.3 m² of body surface area. ASAIO J 2003;49:727-730.

53. Reddy SL, Hasan A, Hamilton LR, et al: Mechanical versus medical bridge to transplantation in children: What is the best timing for mechanical bridge? Eur J Cardiothorac Surg 2004;25:605-609.

54. Chang AC, McKenzie ED: Mechanical cardiopulmonary support in children and young adults: Extracorporeal membrane oxygenation, ventricular assist devices, and long-term support devices. Pediatr Cardiol 2005;26:2-28.

APPENDIX I
Drug Formulary in Heart Failure

Ra-id Abdulla
Anthony C. Chang
Brady S. Moffett

DIURETICS

Drug	Pharmacology/Mechanism	Route	Dose	Schedule/Administration	Indications	Monitoring Parameters	Comments
Acetazolamide (Diamox)	Carbonic anhydrase inhibitor resulting in increased diuresis and increased excretion of sodium bicarbonate	IV, PO	Children: 5 mg/kg/dose Adults: 250-375 mg/dose Max: 1 g/day	qd-qod	Fluid overload/metabolic alkalosis	HR&R, BP, CO, UO, Na^+, K^+, bicarbonate, SCr/BUN	*Side effects:* GI irritation, paresthesias, sedation, hypokalemia, acidosis, reduced urate secretion, aplastic anemia, polyuria, renal calculi *Contraindications:* hepatic failure, severe renal failure, sulfonamide hypersensitivity
Bumetanide (Bumex)	Loop diuretic that prevents reabsorption of Na^+, K^+, and Cl^- at ascending loop of Henle, resulting in diuresis	IV, PO	>6 mo: 0.015-0.1 mg/kg/dose Adults: 0.5-1 mg/dose Max: 10 mg/day	qd-bid (administer less often in younger patients)	Fluid overload	HR&R, BP, UO, Na^+, K^+, Cl^-, SCr/BUN	*Side effects:* hypotension, dizziness, weakness, vertigo, nausea, muscle cramps, hypoglycemia, increased SCr, hyperuricemia, hypokalemia, hypocalcemia, hyponatremia, hypochloremia, hypercalciuria, metabolic alkalosis *Caution:* renal dysfunction, sulfonamide hypersensitivity
Chlorothiazide (Diuril)	Thiazide diuretic that inhibits renal tubular reabsorption of Na^+ in the distal tubule, resulting in increased diuresis	IV	Infants <6 mo: 2-8 mg/kg/day Infants >6 mo: 4 mg/kg/day	Divided qd-bid	Fluid overload	HR&R, BP, CO, UO, Na^+, K^+, Cl^-, SCr/BUN	*Side effects:* hypokalemia, hypercalcemia, hypochloremia, alkalosis, hypotension, dizziness, vertigo, hyperlipidemia, cholestasis, muscle weakness, paresthesias, prerenal azotemia, hyperuricemia, hyperglycemia, blood dyscrasias *Caution:* hepatic failure, renal dysfunction, sulfonamide hypersensitivity
		PO	Infants <6 mo: 20-40 mg/kg/day Infants >6 mo: 20 mg/kg/day Adults: 250-1000 mg/dose Max: 2 g/day	Divided qd-bid			

Continued

Drug	Action	Route	Dose	Schedule	Indication	Monitor	Side effects / Caution
Ethacrynic acid (Edecrin)	Loop diuretic that prevents reabsorption of Na+, K+, and Cl− at ascending loop of Henle, resulting in diuresis	IV, PO	Children: 1 mg/kg/dose Max: 3 mg/kg/day Adults: 0.5-1 mg/kg/dose Max: 100 mg/dose	q8-24h q8-24h	Fluid overload	HR&R, BP, CO, UO, Na+, K+, Cl−, SCr/BUN	*Side effects:* hypovolemia, hypokalemia, hypochloremic alkalosis, prerenal azotemia, hyperuricemia, ototoxicity, abnormal LFTs, agranulocytosis thrombocytopenia, anorexia, or dysphagia, GI bleeding, GI irritation, rash, hypotension, vertigo, hyponatremia, hyperglycemia, hepatotoxicity, ototoxicity, tinnitus, hematuria, hypomagnesemia *Caution:* renal dysfunction
Furosemide (Lasix, Frusemide)	Loop diuretic that prevents reabsorption of Na+, K+, and Cl− at ascending loop of Henle, resulting in diuresis	IV, PO IV	Neonates and children: 0.5-2 mg/kg/dose Max: 6 mg/kg/day Adults: 20-80 mg/dose 0.05-0.4 mg/kg/hr	q6-24h Continuous infusion	Fluid overload	HR&R, BP, CO, UO, Na+, K+, Cl−, SCr/BUN	*Side effects:* hypovolemia, hypokalemia, hypochloremia, hypocalcemia, hypochloremic metabolic alkalosis; hyperuricemia, dermatitis, hyperglycemia, azotemia, anemia, ototoxicity; hypotension, dizziness, vertigo, headache, photosensitivity, agranulocytosis, hepatitis, anorexia, pancreatitis, interstitial nephritis, hypercalciuria *Caution:* prolonged use may cause nephrocalcinosis; renal or hepatic failure
Hydrochloro-thiazide (Hydrodiuril)	Thiazide diuretic that inhibits renal tubular reabsorption of Na+ in the distal tubule, resulting in increased diuresis	PO	Infants <6 mo: 2-4 mg/kg/day Max: 37.5 mg/day Infants and children >6 mo: 2 mg/kg/day Max: 200 mg/day Adults: 25-100 mg/day Max: 200 mg/day	Divided bid	Fluid overload	HR&R, BP, CO, UO, Na+, K+, Cl−, SCr/BUN	*Side effects:* drowsiness, vertigo, headache, hypokalemia, hyperlipidemia, hypochloremic metabolic alkalosis, nausea, muscle cramps, pancreatitis, agranulocytosis, hemolytic anemia, hepatitis, paresthesia, prerenal azotemia, hyperuricemia, hyperglycemia, blood changes, allergic reaction *Caution:* sulfonamide cross-sensitivity
Metolazone (Zaroxolyn)	Thiazide diuretic that inhibits renal tubular reabsorption of Na+ in the distal tubule, resulting in increased diuresis	PO	Children: 0.2-0.4 mg/kg/day Adults: 2.5-10 mg/dose Max: 20 mg/day	Divided qd-bid	Fluid overload	HR&R, BP, CO, UO, Na+, K+, Cl−, SCr/BUN	*Side effects:* hepatic dysfunction, calcium retention, GI upset, orthostatic hypotension, hypokalemia, hypochloremic metabolic alkalosis, hyperglycemia, hypomagnesemia, hyperuricemia, tinnitus *Caution:* hepatic disease, sulfonamide cross-sensitivity

Drug	Pharmacology/ Mechanism	Route	Dose	Schedule/ Administration	Indications	Monitoring Parameters	Comments
Spironolactone (Aldactone)	Potassium-sparing diuretic. Blockade of aldosterone action on the collecting duct, resulting in diuresis	PO	Neonates: 1-3 mg/kg/day Children: 1-3.3 mg/kg/day Adults: 25-200 mg/day Max: 200 mg/day	Divided qd-qid	Fluid overload	HR&R, BP, CO, UO, Na$^+$, K$^+$, Cl$^-$, SCr/BUN	*Side effects:* hyperkalemia, GI irritation, rash, gynecomastia, hyperchloremic metabolic acidosis, amenorrhea, anorexia, agranulocytosis, hyponatremia *Contraindication:* renal failure *Caution:* hyperkalemia may occur when used with K$^+$ supplements or medications that increase K$^+$
INOTROPIC AGENTS							
Calcium chloride (27% elemental Ca)	Enhances contractility through regulation of action potential	IV (central)	Infants/children: 5-20 mg/kg Adults: 250-500 mg/dose Max: 1 g	Slow push (<100 mg/min)	Hypocalcemia/ inotropy	HR&R, ionized calcium, BP, CO	*Side effects:* hypotension, bradycardia, hypercalcemia *Caution:* extravasation can lead to tissue necrosis (treated with hyaluronidase), may precipitate arrhythmia in digitalized patient
Calcium gluconate (9% elemental Ca)	Enhances contractility through regulation of action potential	IV (central)	Neonates: 200-800 mg/kg/ day Infants/children: 200-500 mg/kg/ day Adults: 5-15 g/day Max: 1 g/dose or 15 g/day	Divided q6h or as continuous infusion	Hypocalcemia/ inotropy	HR&R, ionized calcium, BP, CO	*Side effects:* hypotension, bradycardia, hypercalcemia *Caution:* extravasation can lead to tissue necrosis (treated with hyaluronidase), may precipitate arrhythmia in digitalized patient
		PO	Infants: 400-800 mg/kg/ day Children: 200-500 mg/kg/ day Adults: 2-10 g/day Max: 3 g/dose	Divided q6h			

Drug	Action	Route	Dose	Administration	Indication	Monitoring	Side effects/Contraindications
Digoxin (Lanoxin, Lanoxicaps)	Inhibition of Na⁺, K⁺ pump resulting in increased Ca intracellular influx. Results in increased inotropy	IV (maintenance doses divided bid)	Premature neonates: TLD 15 µg/kg (3-4 µg/kg) Infants <6 mo: TLD 20 µg/kg (6-8 µg/kg) Children >6 mo: TLD 20-40 µg/kg (4-12 µg/kg)	TLD protocol TLD protocol TLD protocol	Heart failure/to increase contractility/atrial arrhythmias	HR&R, BP, CO, Na⁺, K⁺. Serum digoxin levels are not routinely recommended	*Side effects:* (commonly associated with toxicity) sinus bradycardia, AV block, fatigue, headache, nausea, anorexia, neuralgias, blurred vision, photophobia *Caution:* renal failure, hypothyroidism. Cardioversion or calcium infusion may cause VF in patients receiving digoxin (lidocaine can be given) *Contraindications:* ventricular arrhythmia, AV block, IHSS, constrictive pericarditis
		IV (maintenance dose qd)	Adults: TLD 0.5-1 mg (0.125-0.5 mg)	TLD protocol			
		PO (maintenance doses divided bid)	Premature neonates: TLD 20 µg/kg (5 µg/kg) Infants <6 mo: TLD 30 µg/kg (8-10 µg/kg) Children >6 mo: TLD 20-50 µg/kg (5-15 µg/kg)	TLD protocol TLD protocol TLD protocol			
		PO (maintenance dose qd)	Adults: TLD 0.75-1.5mg (0.125-0.5mg)	TLD protocol			
Dobutamine (Dobutrex)	Stimulates β₁-adrenergic receptors, resulting in increased myocardial contractility. Stimulates β₂-receptors, resulting in mild peripheral vasodilation	IV	2-20 µg/kg/min	Continuous infusion	Increase inotropy	HR&R, BP, CO, renal function	*Side effects:* ventricular arrhythmias, hypertrophic cardiomyopathy, tachycardia, hypertension, angina, palpitations, headache *Contraindications:* IHSS, tachycardia, arrhythmias, hypertension

Continued

Drug	Pharmacology/ Mechanism	Route	Dose	Schedule/ Administration	Indications	Monitoring Parameters	Comments
Dopamine (Intropin)	A precursor to epinephrine, causes endogenous release of catecholamines and stimulates dopaminergic receptors. Dopaminergic receptor agonism with renal vasodilation. β_1-Receptor agonism with increased inotropy. α_1-Receptor agonism with peripheral vasoconstriction	IV	2-5 μg/kg/min (dopaminergic agonism) 5-15 μg/kg/min (β-agonism) 15-20 μg/kg/min (α-agonism)	Continuous infusion	Renal perfusion, inotropy, hypotension	HR&R, BP, CO, renal function, UO	*Side effects:* tachyarrhythmias, premature beats, hypertension, headache, nausea
Epinephrine (Adrenalin)	β_1-Receptor agonism with increased inotropy. α_1-Receptor agonism with peripheral vasoconstriction	IV (1:10,000 concentration)	Neonates/children: 0.01-0.03 mg/kg Max: 1 mg Adults: 1-5 mg 0.01-1 μg/kg/min	Rapid push Continuous infusion	Hypotension/ bradycardia/ decreased CO	HR&R, BP, CO, renal function, UO	*Side effects:* tachyarrhythmias, hypertension, headache, nervousness, nausea, vomiting, decrease renal flow *Caution:* hyperthyroidism, hypertension, arrhythmias *Contraindication:* coronary artery disease
Isoproterenol (Isuprel)	β_1-Receptor, β_2-receptor agonism resulting in increased inotropy and peripheral arterial vasodilation	IV	0.05-2 μg/kg/min	Continuous infusion	Heart failure (especially right heart failure)/ bradycardia/ decreased CO	HR&R, BP, CO, renal function, UO	*Side effects:* tachyarrhythmias, hypotension, headache, nausea, vomiting *Caution:* hyperthyroidism, history of tachyarrhythmias, diabetes *Contraindications:* myocardial ischemia, narrow-angle glaucoma, preexisting ventricular arrhythmias
Norepinephrine (Levophed)	Stimulates α_1-receptors (predominantly) and β_1-receptors, resulting in increased contractility and heart rate	IV	0.01-2 μg/kg/min	Continuous infusion	Hypotension/ septic shock	HR&R, BP, CO, renal function, UO	*Side effects:* arrhythmias, hypertension, angina, headache, vomiting, uterine contractions, respiratory distress, diaphoresis *Caution:* hypertension, arrhythmia, occlusive vascular disease *Contraindications:* pheochromocytoma, severe hypertension, tachyarrhythmias, severe coronary artery disease

Drug	Action	Route	Dose	Administration	Indication	Monitor	Side effects / Caution / Contraindications
Phenylephrine	Pure α_1-agonist, resulting in peripheral vasoconstriction	IV	Bolus: 5-20 µg/kg; 0.1-0.5 µg/kg/min	Push; Continuous infusion	Hypotension	HR&R, BP, CO, UO	*Side effects:* tremors, hypertension, angina, bradycardia. *Caution:* hypertension, hyperthyroidism, arrhythmia, hyperglycemia. *Contraindications:* pheochromocytoma, severe hypertension, tachyarrhythmias, coronary artery disease

PHOSPHODIESTERASE INHIBITORS

Drug	Action	Route	Dose	Administration	Indication	Monitor	Side effects / Caution / Contraindications
Amrinone (Inocor)	Myocardial cAMP phosphodiesterase inhibitor, resulting in increased contractility. Pulmonary and systemic vasodilator	IV	Load: 0.75-1 mg/kg (may repeat twice if needed) Max total load: 3 mg/kg; 3-10 µg/kg/min	Over 5 min; Continuous infusion	Decreased contractility/afterload reduction	HR&R, platelet count, BP, CO	*Side effects:* hypotension, arrhythmia, thrombocytopenia, GI effects. *Caution:* hypertrophic cardiomyopathy, hypotension, valvular obstructive disease
Milrinone (Primacor)	Myocardial cAMP phosphodiesterase inhibitor, resulting in increased contractility. Pulmonary and systemic vasodilator	IV	Load: 25-50 µg/kg; 0.25-1 µg/kg/min	Over 10 min; Continuous infusion	Decreased contractility/afterload reduction	HR&R, BP, CO, renal function, UO	*Side effects:* arrhythmia, headache, hypotension. *Caution:* renal dysfunction, fluid status. *Contraindications:* severe pulmonary or aortic obstructive disease

VASODILATORS AND ANGIOTENSIN-CONVERTING ENZYME INHIBITORS

Drug	Action	Route	Dose	Administration	Indication	Monitor	Side effects / Caution / Contraindications
Captopril (Capoten)	Short-acting inhibitor of ACE	PO	Neonates: 0.1-0.4 mg/kg/day; Infants/children: 0.15-0.3 mg/kg/dose (titrate to max of 2 mg/kg/dose); Adults: 6.25-50 mg/dose (titrate to max of 150 mg/dose)	tid; tid; tid	Heart failure/hypertension	HR&R, BP, renal function, K+	*Side effects:* hypotension, rash, proteinuria, neutropenia, tachycardia, cough, diminution of taste, hyperkalemia. *Caution:* collagen vascular disease, renal dysfunction, renal artery stenosis. Administer 1 hr before meals. Potassium-sparing agents (spironolactone) potentiate hyperkalemic effect
Diazoxide (Hyperstat)	Arteriolar vasodilator	IV	1-3 mg/kg Max: 150 mg/dose	Rapid push PRN until BP controlled	Hypertension/hypertensive crisis	HR&R, BP, CO	*Side effects:* hyponatremia, salt and water retention, arrhythmia, hypotension, GI disturbances, ketoacidosis, rash, hyperuricemia, hyperglycemia, flushing, tachycardia, dizziness, phlebitis. *Caution:* diabetes mellitus, renal or hepatic disease. *Contraindications:* coarctation of the aorta, AV shunts, dissecting aortic aneurysm

Continued

Drug	Pharmacology/Mechanism	Route	Dose	Schedule/Administration	Indications	Monitoring Parameters	Comments
Enalapril/enalaprilat (Vasotec)	ACE inhibitor	PO (enalapril) IV (enalaprilat)	Infants/children: 0.1 mg/kg/day (titrate to max of 0.5 mg/kg/day) Adults: 2.5-5 mg/day Max: 40 mg/day 5-10 µg/kg/dose	Divided qd-bid q6-24h	Heart failure/hypertension	HR&R, BP, renal function, K+	*Side effects:* hypotension, rash, proteinuria, neutropenia, tachycardia, cough, diminution of taste, hyperkalemia. *Caution:* collagen vascular disease, renal dysfunction, renal artery stenosis. Administer 1 hr before meals. Potassium-sparing agents (spironolactone) potentiate hyperkalemic effect
Hydralazine (Apresoline)	Direct arteriolar vasodilator with little venous effect	IV PO	Children: 0.1-0.2 mg/kg/dose Max: 20 mg/dose Adults: 10-40 mg Children: 0.75-1 mg/kg/day (titrate to effect) Max: 25 mg/dose Adults: 10-50 mg/dose Max: 300 mg/day	q4-6h Divided bid-qid	Hypertension/afterload reduction	HR&R, BP, CO	*Side effects:* SLE-like syndrome (reversible), palpitations, flushing, rash, hematologic changes, hypotension, reflex tachycardia, headache, anorexia, nausea. *Caution:* severe renal failure and cardiac disease, CVA. *Contraindications:* coronary artery disease, dissecting aortic aneurysm, mitral valve rheumatic heart disease
Nifedipine (Adalat, Procardia)	Dihydropyridine calcium channel blocker. Results in peripheral vasodilation	PO	Children: 0.25-0.5 mg/kg/dose Max: 10 mg/dose Adults: 10-30 mg/dose Max: 180 mg/day	q6-8h tid	Hypertension/hypertrophic cardiomyopathy	HR&R, BP, CO	*Side effects:* hypotension, flushing, tachycardia, headache, dizziness, nausea, palpitations, bone marrow suppression, arthralgia, shortness of breath. *Caution:* heart failure, aortic stenosis. Profound hypotension, MI, and death have been reported in adults when immediate-release nifedipine (orally and sublingually) is used for acute reduction of blood pressure. The manufacturer does not recommend use of immediate-release capsules for acute reduction of BP. For sublingual administration, puncture capsule and express fluid sublingually

Drug	Action	Route	Dose	Frequency	Indication	Monitoring	Side effects / Caution / Contraindications
Nitroglycerin (Tridil, Nitro-Bid)	Direct arteriovenous vasodilator, with greater venous effects than arterial	IV	0.25-5 µg/kg/min	Continuous infusion	Hypertension/acute decompensated heart failure/coronary insufficiency	HR&R, BP, CO	*Side effects:* flushing, headache, hypotension, tachycardia, nausea, perspiration, tolerance, increased ICP *Caution:* hypovolemia, renal impairment, increased ICP *Contraindications:* glaucoma, severe anemia
Nitroprusside (Nipride, Nitropress)	Arteriolar and venous vasodilator	IV	0.3-10 µg/kg/min (monitor cyanide and thiocyanate if >48 hr or if >2 µg/kg/min)	Continuous infusion	Hypertension/acute decompensated heart failure	HR&R, BP, CO. Monitor for S/S of cyanide and thiocyanate toxicities	*Side effects:* profound hypotension, metabolic acidosis, weakness, psychosis, headache, increased ICP, thyroid suppression, nausea, sweating, cyanide and thiocyanate toxicities (acidosis/methemoglobinemia and seizures) *Caution:* renal failure more susceptible to cyanide toxicity *Contraindications:* reduced cerebral perfusion, coarctation of the aorta, AV shunts
Prazosin (Minipress)	α_1-Antagonist, resulting in peripheral vasodilation	PO	Children: 25-150 µg/kg/day (5 µg/kg test dose) Max: 15 mg/day Adults: 1 mg/dose Max: 20 mg/day	Divided qid	Hypertension/afterload reduction	HR&R, BP, CO	*Side effects:* orthostatic hypotension, syncope, tachycardia, dizziness, headache, fluid retention, nausea, dry mouth, nasal congestion, urinary frequency *Caution:* first-dose phenomenon: orthostasis, syncope, usually within 90 min of first dose
β-BLOCKERS Atenolol (Tenormin)	Antagonism of β_1-receptors and β_2-receptors (only at higher doses)	PO	Children: 1-2 mg/kg/day Max: 2 mg/kg/dose Adults: 25-100 mg/day Max: 200 mg/day	qd qd	Hypertension, antiarrhythmic agent	HR&R, BP, S/S of heart failure, CO	*Side effects:* hypotension, hypoglycemia, headache, fatigue, reduced cardiac output, dizziness, rash, bradycardia *Caution:* reactive airway disease, renal dysfunction, hypotension, abrupt withdrawal *Contraindications:* decompensated heart failure or cardiogenic shock, sinus bradycardia, heart block with concurrent use of verapamil

Continued

Drug	Pharmacology/ Mechanism	Route	Dose	Schedule/ Administration	Indications	Monitoring Parameters	Comments
Carvedilol (Coreg)	Antagonism of β_1-receptors, β_2-receptors, and α_1-receptors	PO	Children: starting at 0.025 mg/kg/dose (titrate to 0.5 mg/kg/dose) Adults: highest starting dose 3.125 mg bid. Titrate up as tolerated every other week Max: 50 mg bid	Divided bid	Heart failure	HR&R, BP, S/S of heart failure, CO	*Side effects:* hypotension, hypoglycemia, headache, fatigue, reduced cardiac output, dizziness, rash, bradycardia *Caution:* reactive airway disease, diabetes, hypotension *Contraindications:* decompensated heart failure or cardiogenic shock, sinus bradycardia, heart block with concurrent use of verapamil
Metoprolol (Lopressor, Toprol-XL)	Antagonism of β_1-receptors and β_2-receptors	PO	Children: 0.1–0.2 mg/kg/dose. Titrate up as tolerated Max: 100 mg/day Adults: 12.5 mg/day Titrate up as tolerated Max: 450 mg/day	bid (extended-release formulations may be dosed once daily)	Heart failure	HR&R, BP, S/S of heart failure, CO	*Side effects:* hypoglycemia, hypotension, nausea, vomiting, abdominal pain, CNS symptoms (depression, weakness, dizziness). bronchospasm, heart block, bradycardia, negative inotropic effect *Caution:* reactive airway disease, diabetes, hypotension *Contraindications:* decompensated heart failure or cardiogenic shock, sinus bradycardia, heart block with concurrent use of verapamil
Propranolol (Inderal)	β Blockade and antiarrhythmic	PO	0.5–1.0 mg/kg/day Max: 16 mg/kg/ or 60 mg/day Adults: 10-40 mg/dose Max: 320 mg/day	tid-qid	Heart failure	HR&R, BP, S/S of heart failure, CO	*Side effects:* hypotension, hypoglycemia, headache, fatigue, reduced cardiac output, dizziness, rash, bradycardia *Caution:* reactive airway disease, diabetes, hypotension *Contraindications:* decompensated heart failure or cardiogenic shock, sinus bradycardia, heart block with concurrent use of verapamil

ANTIDYSRHYTHMIC AGENTS

Drug		Route	Dose		Indication	Monitor	Side effects / Cautions
Amiodarone (Cordarone)	Class III antiarrhythmic agent that inhibits adrenergic stimulation, prolongs action potential and refractory period, and decreases AV conduction and sinus node function	PO	Children: < 1 year: 600-800 mg/1.73 m²/24 hrs × 4-14 days, then reduce to 200-400 mg/1.73 m²/24 hrs > 1 year: 10-15 mg/kg/24 hrs × 4-14 days, then reduce to 5 mg/kg/24 hrs	qd or divided bid	Supraventricular and ventricular tachycardia	HR&R, BP, CO, level (1–2.5 mg/L), hepatic and thyroid function (Note: Levels do not correlate with efficacy or toxicity)	*Side effects:* hypotension, nausea, vomiting, abdominal pain, pulmonary fibrosis, CNS symptoms (depression, weakness, dizziness), hypothyroidism, corneal deposits, photosensitivity, heart block, bradycardia, negative inotropic effect. *Caution:* reactive airway disease, diabetes, hypotension, calcium channel blockade, hyperthyroidism or hypothyroidism. *Contraindications:* sinus bradycardia, AV block, cardiogenic shock
			Adults: loading dose 800-1600 mg/day, then 600-800 mg/day Maintenance dose 200-400 mg/day	qd or divided bid			
		IV	Children: loading dose 5 mg/kg Max: 150 mg Maintenance dose 10-20 mg/kg/day or 5-15 µg/kg/min	Over 15-30 min / Continuous infusion			
			Adults: loading dose 150 mg followed by 360 mg over 6 hr Maintenance dose 0.5 mg/min	Over 10 min / Continuous infusion			
Lidocaine	Class Ib antiarrhythmic agent that suppresses automaticity of conduction tissue	IV	Children and adults: 1 mg/kg slow push, then 20-50 µg/kg/min	Continuous infusion	Ventricular tachycardia or premature beats	HR&R, BP, level (1.5-5 µg/mL)	*Side effects:* bradycardia, hypotension, drowsiness, seizures, nausea, vomiting. *Caution:* renal or hepatic dysfunction, hypovolemia. *Contraindications:* AV block
Procainamide (Procan SR)	Class Ia antiarrhythmic agent that decreases myocardial excitability and conduction velocity	PO	Neonates and children: 15-50 mg/kg/day Max: 4 g/day Adults: 250-500 mg/dose	Divided q3-6h / q3-6h	Supraventricular and ventricular tachycardia	HR&R, BP, CO, level (4-10 µg/mL and N acetyl metabolite NAPA 6-20 µg/mL)	*Side effects:* chest pain, palpitations, SLE-like syndrome, hypoglycemia, hypotension, nausea, vomiting, abdominal pain, CNS symptoms (depression, weakness, dizziness), bronchospasm, heart block, bradycardia, negative inotropic effect. *Caution:* AV block, hypotension, renal or hepatic dysfunction (Note: These are immediate and sustained release forms of oral procainamide)

Continued

Drug	Pharmacology/ Mechanism	Route	Dose	Schedule/ Administration	Indications	Monitoring Parameters	Comments
		IV	Neonates and infants: 3-10 mg/kg over 30-60 min, then 20-80 µg/kg/min Children: 3-15 mg/kg over 30-60 min, then 20-80 µg/kg/min Adults: 50-100 mg/dose load, then 1-6 mg/min	Continuous infusion			*Contraindications:* sinus bradycardia, AV block, SLE, long QT syndrome, cardiogenic shock
Sotalol (Betapace)	Class II and class III (cardiac action potential duration prolongation) antiarrhythmic agent	PO	Infants: (based on BSA- consult with pharmacy) Children > 2 years: 30-60 mg/M² /dose Adults: 80 mg bid Can increase to 240-320 mg/day	tid Divided bid	Supraventricular and ventricular tachycardia	HR&R, BP, S/S of heart failure, CO, QTc (discontinue if > 550 msec)	*Side effects:* chest pain, palpitations, hypoglycemia, hypotension, torsade de pointes, nausea, vomiting, abdominal pain, CNS symptoms (depression, weakness, dizziness), bronchospasm, heart block, bradycardia, negative inotropic effect *Caution:* reactive airway disease, diabetes, hypotension, calcium channel blockade *Contraindications:* sinus bradycardia, AV block, long QT syndrome, cardiogenic shock

TRANSPLANTATION MEDICATIONS

Drug	Pharmacology/ Mechanism	Route	Dose	Schedule/ Administration	Indications	Monitoring Parameters	Comments
Azathioprine (Imuran)	Immunosuppressant agent that antagonizes purine metabolism and inhibit synthesis of DNA, RNA, and proteins	IV/PO	Children: 3-5 mg/kg/day, then 1-3 mg/kg/day as maintenance Adults: 3-5 mg/kg/day, then 1-3 mg/kg/day as maintenance	qd Over 30-60 min	Immunosuppression for transplantation	CBC, bilirubin, alkaline phosphatase, BUN, creatinine	*Side effects:* fever, rash, stomatitis, alopecia, nausea/vomiting, leukopenia, thrombocytopenia, anemia, hepatotoxicity, arthralgia *Caution:* liver disease, renal dysfunction *Contraindications:* hypersensitivity, pregnancy
Cyclosporine (Neoral Gengraf)	Immunosuppressant agent that inhibits production and release of interleukin-2 and inhibits interleukin-2-induced activation of resting T lymphocytes; a calcineurin inhibitor	PO IV	15-20 mg/kg/dose, then reduce to 4-10 mg/kg/day 2-10 mg/kg/day until patient able to tolerate oral medication	Divided bid or qd (first dose pre-transplan-tation) Continuous infusion or q8-24h	Immunosuppression for transplantation	BUN, creatinine, electrolytes, trough levels (100-300 ng/mL for cardiac transplantation)	*Side effects:* seizures (associated with steroid use, electrolyte imbalance, and hypertension), hypertension, headaches, hirsutism, increased triglycerides, nausea, diarrhea, tremor, renal dysfunction *Caution:* renal dysfunction *Contraindications:* rheumatoid arthritis, renal dysfunction, arthritis, renal dysfunction, hypertension

Drug	Action	Route	Dose	Administration	Indication	Monitoring	Comments
Mycophenolate mofetil (Cell Cept)	Inhibitor of de novo pathway of purine biosynthesis		Children: 20 mg/kg/dose then 30-50 mg/kg/day or 600 mg/m² /dose Max: 2000 mg/24 hrs Adults: 2000-3000 mg/24 hrs	bid	Immunosuppression for transplantation	CBC, BUN, creatinine, electrolytes	*Side effects:* hypertension, chest pain, dizziness, headache, rash, diarrhea, hypercholesterolemia, abdominal pain, leukopenia, anemia, thrombocytopenia, renal dysfunction. *Caution:* renal dysfunction, gastrointestinal disease, neutropenia *Contraindication:* hypersensitivity
Sirolimus (Rapamune)	Immunosuppressant agent that suppresses cellular immunity (inhibits T lymphocyte activation and proliferation in response to antigenic and cytokine stimulation)	PO	Children: loading dose 3 mg/m² followed by maintenance dose of 1 mg/m² /day Adults: loading dose is 6 mg, maintenance dose is 2 mg/day	qd	Immunosuppression for transplantation	BUN, creatinine, electrolytes, trough levels (9-17 ng/mL)	*Side effects:* chest pain, hypertension, peripheral edema, fever, acne, hypercholesterolemia, neurotoxicity (arthralgia, weakness, tremor), abdominal pain, anemia, dyspnea *Caution:* administering with cyclosporine, hepatic or renal dysfunction, hypercholesterolemia *Contraindication:* hypersensitivity
Tacrolimus (Prograf, FK506)	Immunosuppressant agent that suppresses cellular immunity (inhibits T lymphocyte activation); a calcineurin inhibitor	PO	Children and adults: 3-4 times the IV dose or 0.05-0.4 mg/kg/day	Divided bid	Immunosuppression for transplantation, graft-versus-host disease	BUN, creatinine, electrolytes, trough levels (5-15 ng/mL for cardiac transplantation)	*Side effects:* chest pain, hypertension, diabetes, neurotoxicity (dizziness, headaches, insomnia, tremor), rash, electrolyte imbalance, nephrotoxicity, abdominal pain, ascites, anemia, cough *Caution:* administering with cyclosporine, hepatic or renal dysfunction *Contraindication:* hypersensitivity
		IV	0.03-0.15 mg/kg/day	Continuous infusion			
MISCELLANEOUS							
Levosimendan (Simdax)†	Enhances binding of Ca^{2+} to troponin C, which increases myocardial contractility without impairing diastolic function	IV	Load: 6-24 μg/kg	Over 10 min	Heart failure/decreased CO	HR&R, BP, CO, renal function, UO	*Side effects:* nausea, headache
			0.05-0.2 μg/kg/min	Continuous infusion			

Continued

Drug	Pharmacology/ Mechanism	Route	Dose	Schedule/ Administration	Indications	Monitoring Parameters	Comments
Nesiritide (Natrecor)[†]	Recombinant BNP, resulting in afterload reduction and diuresis	IV	Bolus: 2 mcg/kg 0.005-0.04 mcg/kg/min Titrate up by 0.005 mcg/kg/min as tolerated.	Continuous infusion	Acute decompensated heart failure	HR&R, BP, CO, UO, endogenous BNP	*Side effects:* arrhythmias, hypotension, increased serum creatinine *Caution:* renal insufficiency, greater risk of hypotension when administered with ACE inhibitors *Contraindications:* significant valvular stenosis, restrictive or obstructive cardiomyopathy, constrictive pericarditis, pericardial tamponade, suspected low cardiac filling

*TLD protocol: total loading dose (TLD) administered in 3 divided doses:
First dose: 1/2 TLD
Second dose: 1/4 TLD 8 hr after first dose
Third dose: 1/4 TLD 8 hr after second dose
†Limited information available with this agent in children.

ACE, angiotensin-converting enzyme; AV, atrioventricular; BNP, B-type natriuretic peptide; BP, blood pressure; BUN, blood urea nitrogen; CNS, central nervous system; CBC, complete blood count; CO, cardiac output; CVA, cerebrovascular accident; ET, through endotracheal tube; GI, gastrointestinal tract; HR&R, heart rate and rhythm; ICP, intracranial pressure; IHSS, idiopathic hypertrophic subaortic stenosis; LFTs, liver function tests; MI, myocardial infarction; NSAIDs, nonsteroidal anti-inflammatory drugs; PRN, as needed; SCr, serum creatinine; SLE, systemic lupus erythematosus; S/S, signs and symptoms; UO, urine output

References:
Abdulla R, Young S, Barnes S: The pediatric cardiology pharmacopoeia. Pediatr Cardiol 1997;18:162-183;
Barnes S, Shields B, Bonney W, Abdulla R: The pediatric cardiology pharmacopoeia: 2004 update. Pediatr Cardiol 2004;25:620;
Gunn VL, Nechyba C: The Harriet Lane Handbook, 16th ed. St Louis, Mosby-Year Book, 2000, pp 575-889;
Micromedex Healthcare Series (electronic version). Greenwood Village, Colo, Thomson Micromedex. Available at: http://www.thomsonhc.com. Accessed February 16, 2004;
Siberry GK, Iannone R: The Harriet Lane Handbook, 15th ed. St Louis, Mosby-Year Book, 2000;
Taketomo CK, Hodding JH, Kraus DM: Pediatric Dosage Handbook, 9th ed. Hudson, NY, Lexi-Comp, 2002, pp 28-1128.

Selected Clinical Trials in Adult Heart Failure Therapy

Anthony C. Chang
Frank Smart

Clinical Trial	Study Specifics	Findings/Results
BEST Beta-Blocker Evaluation Survival Trial Anderson JL, et al: J Card Fail 2003;9:266	2,708 patients in NYHA III and IV with LVEF <35% randomized to bucindolol versus placebo	There was no significant decrease in mortality, sudden death, or death due to pump failure with bucindolol Bucindolol did not reduce death or CHF hospitalization and was associated with early hazard in class IV patients
BNP Breathing Not Properly McCullough PA, et al: Circulation 2002;106:416	1,538 patients presenting with dyspnea and had BNP measured	BNP had a sensitivity of 90% and a specificity of 73% when using a cutoff of 100 pg/mL
CHARM Candesartan in Heart failure Assessment of Reduction in Mortality and morbidity Pfeffer MA, et al: Lancet 2003;362:759	7,061 patients in NYHA II-IV randomized to candesartan or placebo	Candesartan reduced cardiovascular deaths and admission for CHF In patients with LVEF >40%, there is no significant reduction in mortality, but in patients with LVEF <40%, there is a 14% or 23% reduction in admission for CHF or death with candesartan
CIBIS-II Cardiac Insufficiency BIsoprolol Study–II Lancet 1999;353:9.	2,647 patients in NYHA III and IV with LVEF ≤35% randomized to bisoprolol or placebo	Bisoprolol showed a mortality benefit with lower all-cause mortality (11.8% versus 17.3%) and a lower incidence of sudden death (3.6% versus 6.3%) versus placebo Treatment withdrawal was associated with a significant increase in mortality
COMET Carvedilol Or Metoprolol European Trial Poole-Wilson PA, et al: Lancet 2003;362:7	3,029 patients in NYHA II-IV with LVEF <35% randomized to carvedilol or metoprolol	Carvedilol reduced cardiovascular mortality, sudden death, death caused by stroke, or fatal/nonfatal myocardial infarction All-cause mortality in carvedilol cohort was lower (34% versus 40% for metoprolol)
COMPANION Comparison of Medical Therapy, Pacing, and Defibrillation in Chronic Heart Failure Salukhe TV, et al: Int J Cardiol 2003;87:119	1,634 patients in NYHA III and IV with LVEF <35% and QRS duration >120 msec randomized to a three-arm study	CRT in combination with an ICD led to a 43% reduction in composite end point of all-cause mortality and hospitalization Although no therapy had a mortality of 19%, CRT alone led to a mortality of 15%, whereas combined devices (CRT + ICD) had a mortality of 11%
COPERNICUS Carvedilol Prospectively Randomized CUmulative Survival Packer M, et al: N Engl J Med 2001;106:2194	2,289 patients in NYHA IV with LVEF <25% randomized to carvedilol or placebo	Carvedilol reduced combined risk of death or hospitalization for a cardiovascular reason by 27% and reduced days in the hospital for heart failure by 40%

Continued

Clinical Trial	Study Specifics	Findings/Results
DIG Digitalis Investigation Group Rich MW, et al: J Am Coll Cardiol 2001;38:806	7,788 patients in CHF with LVEF ≤45% randomized to digoxin or placebo	Digoxin was beneficial in reducing all-cause admissions, CHF admissions, and CHF-related deaths, but higher digoxin serum levels (>1.2 ng/mL) were associated with higher absolute mortality The strongest predictors of death were glomerular filtration rate, male gender, NYHA III or IV, and older age
ELITE-II Losartan Heart Failure Survival Study Pitt B, et al: Lancet 2000;355:1582	3,152 patients in NYHA II-IV with LVEF <40% randomized to losartan or captopril	No significant difference between two groups in all-cause mortality or sudden death There were significantly fewer patients in the losartan group due to discontinued study treatment because of adverse effects
EPHESUS Eplerenone Post-acute myocardial infarction Heart failure Efficacy and SUrvival Study Pitt B, et al: Cardiovasc Drugs Ther 2001;15:79	6,632 patients within 14 days of AMI with LVEF <40% randomized to eplerenone or placebo	Eplerenone had a 15% reduction in all-cause death and a 21% reduction in sudden death
LIDO Levosimendan Infusion versus DObutamine Study Follath F, et al: Lancet 2002;360:196	203 patients in NYHA III and IV randomized to levosimendan or dobutamine infusion	Primary hemodynamic end point (≥30% increase in cardiac output and ≥25% decrease in pulmonary artery wedge pressure) reached in more levosimendan patients (28% versus 15% in dobutamine group) Levosimendan group had a lower mortality at 1 and 6 months compared with the dobutamine group (7.8% versus 17% and 26% versus 38%)
MADIT II Multicenter Automatic Defibrillator Implantation – Trial II Moss AJ, et al: Circulation 2004;110:3760	720 patients with CAD and LVEF ≤30% randomized to ICD therapy or none	Prophylactic ICD therapy was associated with significantly improved survival in patients with ischemic cardiomyopathy (30% reduction) without requiring screening for ventricular arrhythmias or inducibility by electrophysiologic study
MDC Metoprolol in Dilated Cardiomyopathy Trial Waagstein F, et al: Lancet 1993;342:1441	383 patients with idiopathic dilated cardiomyopathy and LVEF <40% randomized to metoprolol or placebo	34% fewer patients needed transplantation or died with metoprolol Change in LVEF from baseline was greater with metoprolol compared with placebo
MERIT-HF MEtoprolol Randomized Intervention Trial in Heart Failure Lancet 1999;353:2001	3,991 patients in NYHA II-IV with LVEF ≤40% randomized to metoprolol CR/XL or placebo	All-cause mortality was lower in the treated group (7.2%) versus the placebo group (11%) There were fewer sudden deaths and deaths from worsening heart failure in the metoprolol group

Continued

Clinical Trial	Study Specifics	Findings/Results
MIRACLE Multicenter InSync RAndomized CLinical Evaluation Abraham WT, et al: N Engl J Med 2002;346:1845	453 patients in NYHA III or IV with LVEF ≤35% and QRS interval of ≥130 msec randomized to CRT or control	CRT group had improvement in 6-minute walk test, functional class, QOL, time on treadmill, and ejection fraction Fewer patients in CRT group required hospitalization or intravenous medications for CHF
MOCHA Multicenter Oral Carvedilol Heart failure Assessment trial Bristow MR, et al: Circulation 1996;94:2807	345 patients with mild-to-moderate CHF randomized to low-, medium-, or high-dose carvedilol and placebo	Carvedilol was associated with dose-related improvements in left ventricular function and survival (6%, 6.7%, and 1.1% with increasing doses of carvedilol compared with 15.5% in the placebo group) Carvedilol group had a 73% reduction in all-cause mortality and lower hospitalization rate (58% to 64%)
MUSTIC MUltisite STimulation In Cardiomyopathies Linde C, et al: J Am Coll Cardiol 2002;40:111	131 patients in NYHA III or IV and left ventricular systolic dysfunction and QRS interval of ≥150 msec on/off biventricular pacing	Biventricular pacing increased 6-minute walk distance, QOL, NYHA class, and ejection fraction in patients with sinus rhythm or atrial fibrillation
OPTIME-CHF Outcomes of a Prospective Trial of Intravenous Milrinone for Exacerbation of Chronic Heart Failure Cuffe SM, et al: JAMA 2002;287:1541	952 patients with CHF randomized to 48-hour infusion of milrinone or placebo	No difference between groups in in-hospital mortality, 60-day mortality, or incidence of death or re-admissions Sustained hypotension requiring intervention and new atrial arrhythmias occurred more frequently with milrinone
RALES Randomized ALdactone Evaluation Study Pitt B, et al: N Engl J Med 1999;341:709	1,663 patients in NYHA III or IV with LVEF <35% randomized to spironolactone and placebo	Spironolactone group had a lower mortality (35%) versus placebo group (46%) and a 35% decrease in hospitalization rate Spironolactone group had improvement based on NYHA class
REMATCH Randomized Evaluation of Mechanical Assistance for the Treatment of Congestive Heart failure Rose EA, et al: N Engl J Med 2001;345:1435	129 patients in end-stage CHF who are ineligible for OHT were randomized to LVAD therapy or maximal medical therapy	Survival rates were 52% and 23% at 1 and 2 years for LVAD patients versus 25% and 8% for medical management patients The frequency of adverse events was 2.35 higher in the device group, with infection in LVAD patients causing substantial morbidity and mortality
RENEWAL (RECOVER and RENAISSANCE) Randomized EtaNErcept Worldwide evALuation Mann DL, et al: Circulation 2004;109:1594	2,038 patients in NYHA II-IV with LVEF ≤30% randomized to different doses of etanercept or placebo	1,113 patients in RECOVER and 925 patients in RENAISSANCE studies showed no proven benefit for the tumor necrosis factor antagonist

Continued

Clinical Trial	Study Specifics	Findings/Results
RESOLVD Randomized Evaluation of Strategies for Left Ventricular Dysfunction McKelvie RS, et al: Circulation 1999;100:1056	768 patients in NYHA II-IV with LVEF ≤40% and 6-minute walk test <500 m randomized to candesartan/enalapril	Blood pressure decreased with combination therapy, but BNP and aldosterone were decreased compared with monotherapy There were no differences among groups with regard to 6-minute walk test, NYHA class, or QOL
RUSSLAN Moiseyev VS, et al: Eur Heart J 2002;23:1422	504 patients with post AMI left ventricular failure in NYHA III and IV randomized to levosimendan at various doses or placebo	Levosimendan at 0.1 to 0.2 µg/kg/min versus placebo reduced risk of worsening CHF and lowered mortality at 14 days and 180 days (11.7% versus 19.6% and 22.6% versus 31.4%) Hypotension and ischemia were observed at higher doses of levosimendan
SOLVD Studies Of Left Ventricular Dysfunction SOLVD investigators: N Engl J Med 1992;325:293	4,228 patients with CHF with LVEF ≤35% randomized to enalapril or placebo	There was a 16% reduction in mortality in the enalapril group with the greatest reduction (22%) in patients with progressive heart failure Fewer patients treated with enalapril died or were hospitalized for worsening heart failure (18% versus 34%)
USCS US Carvedilol Study Packer M, et al: N Engl J Med 1996;334:1349	1,094 patients with CHF with LVEF ≤35% randomized to carvedilol or placebo	There was a 65% reduction in all-cause death in the carvedilol group versus placebo There was a 27% reduction in risk of hospitalization from cardiac cause and a 38% reduction in combined risk of hospitalization or death
Val-HeFT Valsartan Heart Failure Trial Cohn J, et al: Circulation 2003;108:1306	5,010 patients in NYHA II-IV with LVEF <40% randomized to valsartan or placebo	There was an 8% reduction in all-cause hospitalizations Among patients not treated with ACE inhibitors, all-cause mortality and combined mortality and morbidity were reduced with valsartan Mean aldosterone level was lower with valsartan group (decreased by 17%) versus placebo (increased by 12%)
VALIANT VALsartan In Acute myocardial iNfarcTion Trial Pfeffer MA, et al: N Engl J Med 2003;349:1893	14,703 patients who had AMI within 10 days randomized to valsartan, captopril, and combination	Compared with captopril, valsartan showed no differences in death from cardiovascular causes or hospitalizations from CHF Combining valsartan with captopril increased the rate of adverse events without improving survival
VEST VESnarinone Trial Deswal A, et al: Chest 2001;120:453	1,046 patients with CHF randomized to two different doses of vesnarinone or placebo	Placebo patients showed increasing circulating levels of TNF, interleukin-6, and soluble TNF receptors, but vesnarinone did not show measurable anticytokine effects
V-HeFT II Vasodilator-Heart Failure Trial II Cohn JN, et al: N Engl J Med 1991;325:303	804 men with chronic CHF with LVEF <45% randomized to enalapril or hydralazine and isosorbide dinitrate	Mortality (2-year) was significantly lower in the enalapril group (18%) versus the hydralazine/isosorbide dinitrate group (25%) Improved ejection fraction and exercise capacity with hydralazine/isosorbide dinitrate group

Continued

Clinical Trial	Study Specifics	Findings/Results
VMAC Vasodilatation in the Management of Acute Congestive heart failure VMAC investigators: JAMA 2002;287:1531	489 patients with decompensated CHF randomized to intravenous nesiritide, intravenous nitroglycerin, or placebo	Pulmonary capillary wedge pressure lower at 3 and 24 hours (−5.8 mm Hg and −8.2 mm Hg versus baseline) compared with nitroglycerin and placebo Self-reported dyspnea was less with nesiritide compared with nitroglycerin or placebo

ACE, angiotensin-converting enzyme; AMI, acute myocardial infarction; BNP, B-type natriuretic peptide; CAD, coronary artery disease; CHF, congestive heart failure; CRT, cardiac resynchronization therapy; ICD, implantable cardioverter defibrillator; LVAD, left ventricular assist device; LVEF, left ventricular ejection fraction; NYHA, New York Heart Association; OHT, orthotopic heart transplantation; QOL, quality of life; TNF, tumor necrosis factor.

Atlas of Circulatory Support Devices

Wei Wang
Matthias Loebe
Anthony C. Chang

INTRODUCTION

Since the first circulatory support device described by DeBakey,[1] momentous progress has been made in the last few decades. Mechanical circulatory support for the failing heart in myriad of forms has entered the clinical area worldwide.[2-5] Currently, mechanical circulatory support has attained an increasingly important role in the treatment of heart failure in children and young adolescents.[6,7] The present strategy of mechanical circulatory support is not only as a bridge to recovery or transplantation, but also as a destination therapy.[9]

This is an atlas of acute and long-term mechanical devices used to support the failing heart with either limited experiences or potential applications in children and young adults. Intra-aortic balloon pump, extracorporeal membrane oxygenation, and centrifugal ventricular assist devices (VADs) all are amply discussed in the main text and are not presented separately in this atlas. Simplistic support devices (e.g., the Acorn cardiac support device and the Myosplint device) also have been discussed adequately in appropriate chapters and are not addressed in this atlas. Finally, devices that are no longer available (e.g., the LionHeart) or that are still under development (e.g., the Levitronix Centrimag) are not included here.

For each device, a brief history of development and the mechanism of the device are discussed. This discussion is followed by a summary of the clinical experience (including pediatric experience, if any) and selected references. For each device, accompanying tables provide available information. Because of the rapid evolution of these devices, this atlas is meant to serve as basic compendium of mechanical devices with relatively large experiences rather than an encyclopedic reference of mechanical devices.

These devices are categorized by three classifications: duration, type, and position. Duration is **short-term** if the device is meant for intensive care unit use and usually for less than 1 month. **Long-term** devices usually are meant for longer duration of use (>1 month).

The type of device is classified as pulsatile, rotary, total artificial heart (TAH), or miscellaneous. A **pulsatile** pump provides an ejection and filling phase; a rotary device can provide pulsatile flow if the native ventricle ejects with sufficient force. These pulsatile pumps can be driven by air (pneumatic) or fluid (hydraulic). Various **rotary** devices usually are characterized by lower priming volume and less blood trauma. Rotary pumps are classified into axial, centrifugal, and diagonal, depending on the impeller geometry. The axial pumps, the smallest of the rotary pumps, have the inflow and outflow of the pump along the axis of the pump. The centrifugal pump, with its inflow and outflow at right angles, has an impeller that creates a centrifugal force to drive the blood. Lastly, the diagonal type of rotary pump is a hybrid of the other two types of rotary pumps. The **total artificial heart** features two pulsatile ventricles for biventricular support. Devices that cannot be classified as pulsatile, rotary, or TAH are categorized as miscellaneous.

The positions of these devices are categorized as follows. A device is considered **fully implantable** if all of the device is in the thoracic or abdominal cavity. A device is considered **partially implantable** if there are parts outside the body, and these devices are divided further into thoracic and abdominal types. **Paracorporeal** devices have trancutaneous cannulas with the device affixed to the body, whereas **extracorporeal** devices have components distant from the body.

REFERENCES

1. DeBakey ME: The odyssey of the artificial heart. Artif Organs 2000;24:4-11.

This atlas is dedicated to Dr. Michael DeBakey for his encouragement and wisdom. The authors also thank Dr. Seema Mital for her critical review of the atlas.

2. Frazier OH: Mechanical circulatory support: New advances, new pumps, and new ideas. Semin Thorac Cardiovasc Surg 2002;14: 178-186.
3. Song X, Throckmorton AL, Untaroiu A, et al: Axial flow blood pumps. ASAIO J 2003;49:355-364.
4. Wheeldon DR: Mechanical circulatory support: State of the art and future perspectives. Perfusion 2003;18:159-169.
5. Delgado RM: The future of mechanical circulatory support. Curr Opin Cardiol 2003;18:199-209.
6. Reinhartz O, Stiller B, Eilers R, et al: Current clinical status of pulsatile pediatric circulatory support. ASAIO J 2002;48:455-459.
7. Throckmorton AL, Allaire PE, Gutgesell HP, et al: Pediatric circulatory support systems. ASAIO J 2002;48:216-221.
8. Chang AC, McKenzie ED: Mechanical cardiopulmonary support in children and young adults: Extracorporeal membrane oxygenation, ventricular assist devices, and long-term support devices. Pediatr Cardiol 2005;26:2-28.
9. Raman J, Jeevanadam V: Destination therapy with ventricular assist devices. Cardiology 2004;101:104-110.

ABIOCOR TOTAL ARTIFICIAL HEART

Device Classification

TABLE A1-1

Classification		
Category	Group	Sub-group
Duration	Long-term	
Type	Total artificial heart	Hydraulic
Position	Fully implantable	Orthotopic

History of Development

In 1985, the National Heart, Lung and Blood Institute supported a study to develop long-term mechanical circulatory devices. In 1988, it awarded contracts to four research groups to develop the artificial heart. One of these groups, ABIOMED, developed the AbioCor implantable replacement heart.[1] The AbioCor is the first completely self-contained TAH. The AbioCor II, the next-generation implantable replacement heart, which is smaller with a 5-year reliability, incorporates the technologic assets of the AbioCor and the Penn State Heart.

Mechanism of Device

The AbioCor TAH is designed for long-term, tether-free use in adult patients with end-stage heart disease as a destination therapy. It is made of titanium and Angioflex, which is AbioMed's proprietary polyurethane plastic, and is the first completely self-contained TAH for patients with biventricular failure, with no wires or tubes protruding through the skin (Fig. A1-1).[2]

The pumping unit, weighing about 2 pounds consists of two artificial ventricles, which are actuated by a compact unidirectional centrifugal hydraulic pump, mounted between the two ventricles (Fig. A1-2). A cylindrical rotary valve alternately directs the hydraulic fluid to the right ventricle and left ventricle, which results in alternate left systole and right systole. Cardiac output is determined by the right atrial pressure, so the device can respond in a Starling-like manner.[3] Balance between left and right blood flow is achieved using a hydraulic balancing chamber attached to the left inflow port and to the right pumping chamber, by way of a shunt.[4] This shunt allows regulation of the right output according to left input pressure. Power to the AbioCor is achieved with an energy-transfer device called a transcutaneous energy transmission system. When the external coil is put over the implanted one, power moves through the skin to the internal coil without any wires.[5] On January 24, 2002, the plastic cage in the AbioCor was removed because of fears it may cause blood clotting in users.

AbioCor: Representative Anatomic Positions

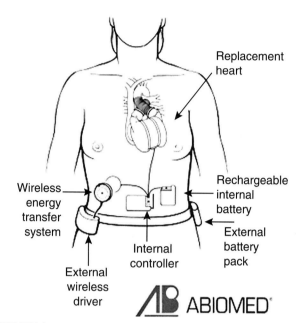

FIGURE A1-1 ■ Schematic diagram of the AbioCor TAH system. (Website: www.texasheartinstitute.org).

Components

Besides the pump mechanism itself, other important parts and the specifications (e.g., cannulas or consoles) are presented (Fig. A1-3).

Clinical Experience

On July 2, 2001, the first implant of the AbioCor was performed in a 59-year-old man[7]; he died on November 30, 2001, after uncontrollable bleeding that led to multiorgan failure.[8] On September 13, 2001, a 71-year-old man was the second patient and the first successfully discharged patient to receive the AbioCor TAH.

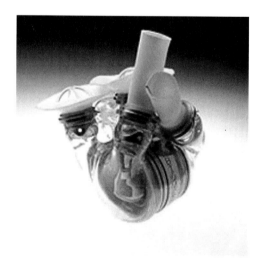

FIGURE A1-2 ■ The AbioCor TAH pumping unit. (Website: www.texasheartinstitute.org.)

TABLE A1-2

Components		
Pump	Stroke volume (mL)	~80
	Beats/min	~75-150
	Flow rate (L/min)	≤10
	Valves	Four tri-leaflet polymeric valves
Cannula	Position	Orthotopic
	Inflow	Left and right atrium
	Outflow	Aorta and main pulmonary artery
Console	Internal	Implanted in the abdominal area; monitors and controls the pumping speed of the artificial heart
	External	Bedside; can be remote monitored
Others	Internal parts	Rechargeable battery Controller Power transfer coil
	External parts	Power transfer coil Battery pack

Data from references 2 and 6.

TABLE A1-3

Total Clinical Experience	
Total cases (as of January 2004)	11
Duration of use	> 450 days
Patient age range	51-79 yr
Patient weight range	NA
Weaning rate	NA
Discharge rate	29%

NA, not available.
Data from references 9 and 10.

TABLE A1-4

Complications	
Complications	**Percentage**
Bleeding	29% (2/7)
Respiratory dysfunction	14% (1/7)
Renal dysfunction	29% (2/7)
Hepatic dysfunction	29% (2/7)
Thromboembolism	58% (4/7)
Neurologic dysfunction	43% (3/7)
Multisystem organ failure	14% (1/7)

Data from reference 9.

The clinical experience from publications, registries, or data from the companies are collected. Data such as total cases, duration of use, patient age and weight range, and weaning and discharge rates are presented if available.

Complications
The complications are listed with relative percentages.

Contact Information
Company: ABIOMED, Inc
Address: 22 Cherry Hill Drive, Danvers, MA 01923, USA
Contact: Telephone: 978-777-5410; fax: 978-777-8411

Website: www.abiomed.com
Physician: Dr. O.H. Frazier, Texas Heart Institute, Houston, Texas

REFERENCES

1. Frazier OH: Ventricular assist devices and total artificial hearts: A historical perspective. Cardiol Clin 2003;21:1-15.
2. AbioCor totally implantable artificial heart: How will it impact hospitals? Health Devices 2002;31:332-341.
3. Yu LS, Finnegan M, Vaughan S, et al: A compact and noise free electrohydraulic total artificial heart. ASAIO J 1993;39: M386-M391.
4. Kung RT, Yu LS, Ochs B, et al: An atrial hydraulic shunt in a total artificial heart: A balance mechanism for the bronchial shunt. ASAIO J 1993;39:M213-M217.
5. Dowling RD, Etoch SW, Stevens KA, et al: Current status of the AbioCor implantable replacement heart. Ann Thorac Surg 2001; 71(3 Suppl):S147-S149.
6. Dowling RD, Etoch SW, Stevens K, et al: Initial experience with the AbioCor implantable replacement heart at the University of Louisville. ASAIO J 2000;46:579-581.
7. SoRelle R: Cardiovascular news: Totally contained AbioCor artificial heart implanted July 3, 2001. Circulation 2001;104:E9005-E9006.
8. SoRelle R: First AbioCor trial patient dies. Circulation 2001;104: E9050-E9060.
9. Dowling RD, Gray LA Jr, Etoch SW, et al: The AbioCor implantable replacement heart. Ann Thorac Surg 2003;75(6 Suppl):S93-S99.
10. Frazier OH, Dowling RD, Gray LA, et al: The total artificial heart: Where we stand. Cardiology 2004;101:117-121.

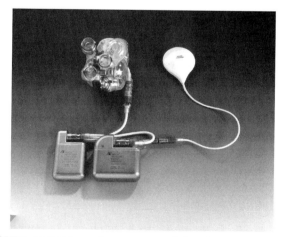

FIGURE A1-3 ■ Internal components of the AbioCor TAH. (From Dowling RD, Gray LA Jr, Etoch SW, et al: The AbioCor implantable replacement heart. Ann Thorac Surg 2003;75[6 Suppl]:S93-S99.)

ABIOMED BVS 5000

Device Classification

TABLE A2-1

Classification		
Category	**Group**	**Sub-group**
Duration	Short-term	
Type	Pulsatile	Pneumatic
Position	Extracorporeal	

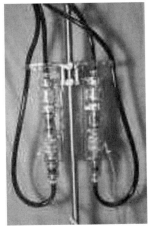

FIGURE A2-2 ■ The Abiomed BVS 5000 pump. (Website: www.abiomed.com.)

History of Development

The AbioMed BVS 5000 was developed in the 1980s. Animal experiments and later clinical implantation of this device were performed at the Texas Heart Institute.[1] The AbioMed BVS 5000 was the first heart support device to be approved by the U.S. Food and Drug Administration (FDA) for the support of postcardiotomy patients.

Mechanism of Device

The Abiomed BVS 5000 is an automated pulsatile VAD designed to provide temporary univentricular or biventricular support. The system consists of an extracorporeal, dual-chamber, pneumatically powered pulsatile pump and a pneumatic drive console (Figs. A2-1 and A2-2).

The pump is placed at the bedside; blood drains from the patient's left or right atrium into the top of the pump and returns to the patient's aorta or pulmonary artery from the bottom of the pump. The left and right sides are triggered independently of each other. The atrial and ventricular chambers contain a smooth-surfaced polyurethane bladder (volume 100 mL). The atrial chamber fills passively from the patient throughout pump systole and diastole. This dual-chamber design produces continuous flow from the patient to the pump and pulsatile flow from the pump back to the patient.

Vascular access is achieved with 32F, 36F, and 42F, wire-reinforced cannulas.[1] The arterial cannula incorporates a 14-mm woven Dacron graft in place of the lighthouse tip. The cannulas are externalized subcostally through tunnels from the pericardial space through the skin. A pneumatic drive console can operate one or two blood pumps, which can provide support to one or both ventricles, without intensive bedside management. The Abiomed BVS 5000 can be operated in two control modes—full-flow operating mode and weaning mode.

Components

TABLE A2-2

Components		
Pump	Stroke volume (mL)	82
	Beats/min	≤80
	Flow rate (L/min)	~0.5-6
	Valves	Two polyurethane tri-leaflet valves
	Position	~0-25 cm below the level of the patient's atria
Cannula	Inflow	Left atrium or left ventricular apex and right atrium
	Outflow	Aorta or main pulmonary artery
Console	Electromagnetic console (Fig. A2-3)	
Others	Internal parts	
	External parts	Foot pump (backup power source) Backup battery

Clinical Experience

In 1987, the Abiomed BVS 5000 was first used in a 50-year-old man for postcardiotomy support.[2] The Abiomed BVS 5000 is the first circulatory assist device to receive pre-market approval from the FDA in November 1992.[3] In one registry, most patients (>50%) are postcardiotomy patients. The mean duration of support was 5 days for postcardiotomy patients and slightly more than 8 days

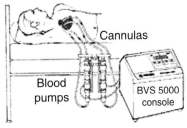

FIGURE A2-1 ■ Schematic diagram of Abiomed BVS 5000. (Website: www.abiomed.com.)

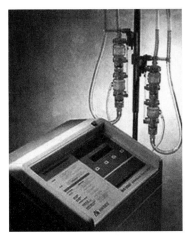

FIGURE A2-3 ■ The console and the pump of the Abiomed BVS 5000. (Website: www.texasheartinstitute.org.)

for cardiomyopathy patients. Of patients, 50% have been weaned, and 7% have been transplanted. The overall survival rate is 34%.[4] Reported in 1990, the first pediatric case was a 9-year-old girl with cardiomyopathy who required biventricular support until a donor heart became available.[5]

TABLE A2-3

Total Clinical Experience	
Total cases	>5000
Duration of use	≤63 days
Patient age range	8-80 yr
Patient weight range	20-83 kg
Weaning rate	49-83%
Discharge rate	27-50%

Data from references 3-12.

Complications

TABLE A2-4

Complications	
Complications	Percentage
Bleeding	40-75%
Infection	9-28%
Renal dysfunction	32-52%
Respiratory dysfunction	50-54%
Neurologic dysfunction	18-26%
Multisystem organ failure	9-41%
Mechanical problem	6-13%

Data from references 4 and 8-16.

Contact Information
Company: ABIOMED, Inc
Address: 22 Cherry Hill Drive, Danvers, MA 01923, USA
Contact: Telephone: 978-777-5410; fax: 978-777-8411
Website: www.abiomed.com
Physician: Many

REFERENCES

1. Jett GK: ABIOMED BVS 5000: Experience and potential advantages. Ann Thorac Surg 1996;61:301-304.
2. von Segesser LK, Leskosek B, Redha F, et al: Performance characteristics of a disposable ventricle assist device. Thorac Cardiovasc Surg 1988;36:146-150.
3. Wassenberg PAJ: The Abiomed BVS 5000 biventricular support system. Perfusion 2000;15:369-371.
4. Jett GK, Lazzara RR: Extracorporeal support: The ABIOMED BVS-5000. In Goldstein DJ, Oz MC (eds): Cardiac Assist Devices. New York, Futura, 2000, pp 235-250.
5. Champsaur G, Ninet J, Vigneron M, et al: Use of the Abiomed BVS System 5000 as a bridge to cardiac transplantation. J Thorac Cardiovasc Surg 1990;100:122-128.
6. Moazami N, McCarthy PM: Temporary circulatory support. In Cohn LH, Edmunds LH (eds): Cardiac Surgery in the Adult, 2nd edition. New York, McGraw-Hill, 2003, pp 495-520.
7. Sadeghi AM, Marelli D, Talamo M, et al: Short-term bridge to transplant using the BVS 5000 in a 22-kg child. Ann Thorac Surg 2000;70:2151-2153.
8. Minami K, Posival H, el-Bynayosy A, et al: Mechanical ventricular support using pulsatile Abiomed BVS 5000 and centrifugal Biomedicus-pump in postcardiotomy shock. Int J Artif Organs 1994;17:492-498.
9. Ashton RC Jr, Oz MC, Michler RE, et al: Left ventricular assist device options in pediatric patients. ASAIO J 1995;41:M277-M280.
10. Krofer R, El-Banayosy A, Ausogul L, et al: Temporary pulsatile ventricular assist devices and biventricular assist devices. Ann Thorac Surg 1999;68:678.
11. Guyton RA, Schonberger JP, Everts PA, et al: Postcardiotomy shock: Clinical evaluation of the BVS 5000 Biventricular Support System. Ann Thorac Surg 1993;56:346-356.
12. Samuels LE, Holmes EC, Thomas MP, et al: Management of acute cardiac failure with mechanical assist: Experience with the ABIOMED BVS 5000. Ann Thorac Surg 2001;71(3 Suppl):S67-S72.
13. Smedira NG, Blackstone EH: Postcardiotomy mechanical support: Risk factors and outcomes. Ann Thorac Surg 2001;71:S61.
14. Dekkers RJ, FitzGerald DJ, Couper GS: Five-year clinical experience with Abiomed BVS 5000 as a ventricular assist device for cardiac failure. Perfusion 2001;16:13-18.
15. Castells E, Calbet JM, Saura E, et al: Acute myocardial infarction with cardiogenic shock: Treatment with mechanical circulatory assistance and heart transplantation. Transplant Proc 2003;35:1940-1941.
16. Potapov EV, Weng Y, Hausmann H, et al: New approach in treatment of acute cardiogenic shock requiring mechanical circulatory support. Ann Thorac Surg 2003;76:2112-2114.

BERLIN HEART VENTRICULAR ASSIST DEVICE

Other names for the Berlin Heart VAD include Berlin Heart and Berlin Heart EXCOR.

Device Classification

TABLE A3-1

Classification		
Category	Group	Sub-group
Duration	Long-term	
Type	Pulsatile	Pneumatic
Position	Paracorporeal	

History of Development

The artificial heart experience began in Berlin in the early 1960s.[1] After in vivo and in vitro experiences, the transplantation program at the German Heart Institute in Berlin started in 1986.[2] In 1992, the Berlin Heart became the first commercially available pulsatile assist device for small children.[3,4] All blood-contacting surfaces inside the pump have been heparin coated since 1994.

Mechanism of Device

The Berlin Heart EXCOR comprises a family of pneumatically actuated pulsatile ventricles that were designed to provide univentricular or biventricular support for patients of various sizes from neonates to adults (Figs. A3-1 and A3-2).[3,4] This system consists of a paracorporeal air-driven blood pump, cannulas for the connection of the pump to the heart chambers and the great vessels (Figs. A3-3 and A3-4), and electropneumatic driving systems (Fig. A3-5).

Within the semi-rigid polyurethane housing, the blood chamber and the air chamber are separated by a three-layer flexible polyurethane membrane. The two diaphragm layers facing the air chamber serve as driving membranes; the layer facing the blood chamber is moved by the two driving membranes.[5] A set of arterial and atrial silicone cannulas is available with inner diameters ranging from 3.2 to 12.7 mm. Today the system can be implanted in patients of various sizes.[3-7] Three control modes can be chosen during support.

Components

TABLE A3-2

Components		
Pump	Stroke volume (mL)	10, 25, 30, 50, 60, and 80
	Beats/min	≤140
	Flow rate (L/min)	
	Valves	Two tri-leaflet polyurethane valves (all types)
		Metal tilting disc (50, 60, 80)
	Position	Externally on the skin of the upper abdomen
Cannula	Outflow	Aorta or main pulmonary artery
	Inflow	Left atrium or left ventricular apex for left VAD; right atrium for right VAD
Console	Stationary applications	Heimes HD 7 IKUS stationary driving unit (Fig. A3-6)
	Mobile unit	EXCOR drive system (Fig. A3-7)
Others	Internal parts	
	External parts	Rechargeable battery

Clinical Experience

This paracorporeal pulsatile device has been in use since 1986. The early complication of thrombus has been lessened with the use of a heparin-coated system. As of January 2004, more than 900 adult patients with heart failure have been supported with the Berlin Heart EXCOR in more than 10 countries worldwide.[11] The survival rate of these patients ranged from one third to one half.

Since 1990, 95 pediatric patients have been supported with the Berlin Heart EXCOR. The survival rate of the 57 patients in Deutsches Herzzentrum Berlin was 54%. The main cause of death was multiple organ failure (18/26) (Elff M, Metayer K: private communication). The survival rate in patients weighing less than 10 kg was significantly lower than others.[11]

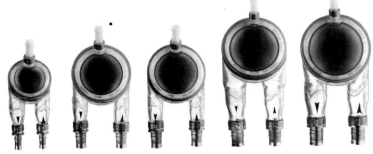

FIGURE A3-1 ■ Berlin Heart pumps of different sizes with tilting-disc or polyurethane and tri-leaflet valves. (From Drews T, Loebe M, Hennig E, et al: The 'Berlin Heart' assist device. Perfusion 2000; 15:387-396.)

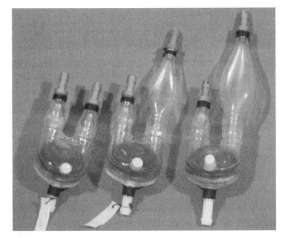

FIGURE A3-2 ■ Berlin Heart pediatric pumps (with stroke volume of 10 mL) with elastic venous reservoirs. (From Drews T, Loebe M, Hennig E, et al: The 'Berlin Heart' assist device. Perfusion 2000;15:387-396.)

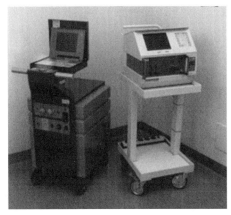

FIGURE A3-5 ■ The IKUS 2000 driver *(left)* and the lighter Heimes HD-7 driver *(right).* (From Hetzer R, Loebe M, Potapov EV, et al: Circulatory support with pneumatic paracorporeal ventricular assist device in infants and children. Ann Thorac Surg 1998;66:1498-1506.)

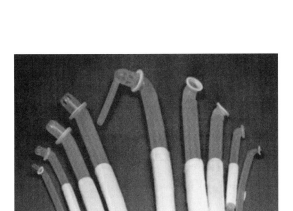

FIGURE A3-3 ■ Atrial and arterial cannulas for the Berlin Heart EXCOR with flat metal-tip, "press-button" type of pediatric arterial cannula. *Far right,* Sewing ring; *middle,* transmitral atrial cannula; *far left,* small infant-type atrial cannula. (From Drews T, Loebe M, Hennig E, et al: The 'Berlin Heart' assist device. Perfusion 2000; 15:387-396.)

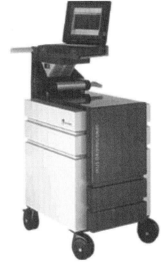

FIGURE A3-6 ■ The IKUS driver. (Website: www.berlinheart.com.)

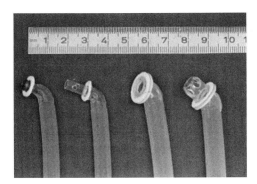

FIGURE A3-4 ■ Pediatric cannulas close-up with flat metal-tip, "press-button" type of arterial cannula. *Far left,* Sewing ring; *center left,* small infant-type atrial cannula; *center right and right,* pair of cannula tips for small children. (From Hetzer R, Loebe M, Potapov EV, et al: Circulatory support with pneumatic paracorporeal ventricular assist device in infants and children. Ann Thorac Surg 1998;66: 1498-1506.)

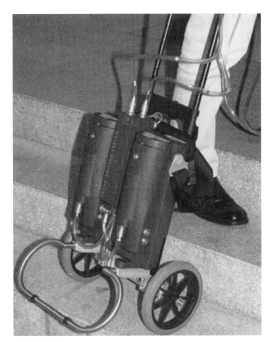

FIGURE A3-7 ■ The wearable EXCOR drive unit. The unit can be carried on a cart or in a shoulder pack.

TABLE A3-3

Total Clinical Experience	
Total cases	945
Duration of use	≤1100 days in an adult and ≤420 days in a child
Patient age range	2 days-72 yr
Patient weight range	≥2.2 kg
Weaning rate	48-64%
Discharge rate	36-51%

Data from references 4-10.

Complications

TABLE A3-4

Complications	
Complications	Percentage
Bleeding	25-46%
Infection	0-28%
Thromboembolism	18-22%
Neurologic dysfunction	7-15%
Multiple organ failure	~31%
Mechanical dysfunction	<5%

Data from references 4-10.

Contact Information
Company: Mediport Kardiotechnik
Address: Wiesenweg 10, 12247 Berlin, Germany
Contact: Telephone: 49(0)30-8187-2600; fax: 49(0)30-8187-2601

Website: www.berlinheart.com
Physician: Dr. Roland Hetzer, German Heart Center, Berlin, Germany

REFERENCES

1. Bucherl ES: The artificial heart research program in Berlin, Germany. J Heart Transplant 1985;4:510-517.
2. Goullon A, Ries D: Experience with the Berlin Heart Assist Device. Artif Organs 1994;18:490-493.
3. Drews T, Loebe M, Hennig E, et al: The 'Berlin Heart' assist device. Perfusion 2000;15:387-396.
4. Hetzer R, Loebe M, Potapov EV, et al: Circulatory support with pneumatic paracorporeal ventricular assist device in infants and children. Ann Thorac Surg 1998;66:1498-1506.
5. Merkle F, Boettcher W, Stiller B, et al: Pulsatile mechanical cardiac assistance in pediatric patients with the Berlin heart ventricular assist device. J Extra Corpor Technol 2003;35:115-120.
6. Loebe M, Hennig E, Muller J, et al: Long-term mechanical circulatory support as a bridge to transplantation, for recovery from cardiomyopathy, and for permanent replacement. Eur J Cardiothorac Surg 1997;11(Suppl):S18-S24.
7. Schiessler A, Warnecke H, Friedel N, et al: Clinical use of the Berlin Biventricular Assist Device as a bridge to transplantation. ASAIO Trans 1990;36:M706-M708.
8. Reinhartz O, Stiller B, Eilers R, et al: Current clinical status of pulsatile pediatric circulatory support. ASAIO J 2002;48:455-459.
9. Hetzer R, Loebe M, Weng Y, et al: Pulsatile pediatric ventricular assist devices: Current results for bridge to transplantation. Semin Thorac Cardiovasc Surg Pediatr Card Surg Annu 1999;2:157-176.
10. Ishino K, Loebe M, Uhlemann F, et al: Circulatory support with paracorporeal pneumatic ventricular assist device (VAD) in infants and children. Eur J Cardiothorac Surg 1997;11:965-972.
11. Reinhartz O, Stiller B, Eilrs R, et al: Current clinical status of pulsatile pediatric circulatory support. ASAIO J 2002;48:455-459.

BERLIN HEART INCOR

Device Classification

TABLE A4-1

Classification		
Category	Group	Sub-group
Duration	Long-term	
Type	Rotary	Axial
Position	Partially implantable	Intrathoracic

History of Development

The Berlin Heart EXCOR (see previous section) has been developed and clinically applied at the Deutsches Herzzentrum Berlin in Germany. The INCOR has been developed and distributed by the Berlin Heart group in the era of axial pump development. On April 3, 2003, this device received the European Conformity Mark certification.

Mechanism of Device

The Berlin Heart INCOR is 200 g in weight, 114 mm in length, and 30 mm in diameter. It is the first axial device with a magnetically suspended impeller system, with neither friction nor heat generated by the device. There are also theoretical advantages of minimal wear and thrombus formation (Fig. A4-1).

The INCOR consists of an inducer region with guide vanes, impeller section, and stationary diffuser to enhance the fluid's pressure increase. The impeller region is magnetically levitated by passive radial and axially active bearings.[1] All components that come into contact with blood are made of titanium (pump) with heparin coating or silicone (cannulas). In the long-term, INCOR is capable of bridging to transplantation and recovery. Continued development will aim at reducing the system's size and improving system control (Fig. A4-2).

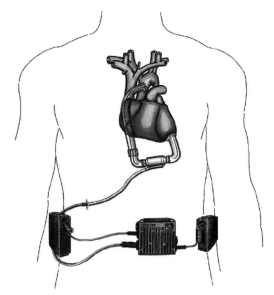

FIGURE A4-2 ■ The schematic of INCOR implanted in a patient. (From Wheeldon DR: Mechanical circulatory support: State of the art and future perspectives. Perfusion 2003;18:233-243.)

Components

TABLE A4-2

Components		
Pump	Revolutions/min	7500-10,000
	Flow rate (L/min)	5 (against 100 mm Hg)
	Position	Left thoracic cavity
Cannula	Inflow	Left ventricular apex
	Outflow	Aorta
Console	Control pump, magnetic bearing, and power supply	
	Generates and stores messages and signals	
	Connectors for pump, batteries power supply and laptop	
Others	Internal parts	
	External parts	Accumulator batteries
		Power supply unit
		Battery charger

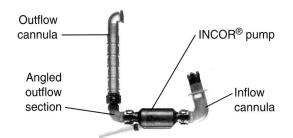

FIGURE A4-1 ■ The Berlin Heart INCOR. (Website: www.berlin-heart.com.)

Clinical Experience

In June 2002, the first patient, a 41-year-old man who had coronary heart disease and serious myocardial insufficiency for many years, received an INCOR.[2] Currently, 90 patients have been implanted in Europe and China; 32 of them are still ongoing, and 35 died. The average length of treatment with this system is 120 days (Metayer K, Elff M: Private communication).

TABLE A4-3

Total Clinical Experience	
Total cases (as of March 2004)	>100
Duration of use (as of August 2004)	>2 yr
Patient age range	39-65 yr
Patient weight range	≥50 kg
Weaning rate	39%
Discharge rate	46.7%

Data from Metayer K, Elff M: Private communication.

Complications

TABLE A4-4

Complications	
Complications	Percentage
Bleeding	10%
Thromboembolism	10%
Neurologic dysfunction	20%
Right ventricular failure	13.3%

Data from Metayer K, Elff M: Private communication.

Contact Information

Company: Mediport Kardiotechnik
Address: Wiesenweg 10, 12247 Berlin, Germany
Contact: Telephone: 49(0)30-8187-2600; fax: 49(0)30-8187-2601
Website: www.berlinheart.com
Physician: Dr. Roland Hetzer, German Heart Center, Berlin, Germany

REFERENCES

1. Muller J, Weng YG, Goettel P, et al: The first implantations in patients of the INCOR I axial flow pump with magnetic bearing. In Program and Abstracts of the 10th Congress of the International Society for Rotary Blood Pumps, Osaka, Japan, September 12, 2002.
2. Chang AC, McKenzie ED: Perioperative care of the pediatric patient on mechanical support. In The First International Conference on Heart Failure in Children and Young Adults: From Molecular Mechanisms to Medical and Surgical Strategies, Houston, December, 2003.

CARDIOWEST TOTAL ARTIFICIAL HEART

Other names for the CardioWest TAH include Jarvik-7, Symbion, and Syncardia TAH.

Device Classification

TABLE A5-1

Classification		
Category	Group	Sub-group
Duration	Long-term	
Type	Total artificial heart	Pneumatic
Position	Fully implantable	Intrathoracic

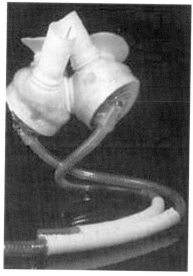

FIGURE A5-2 ■ CardioWest TAH. (Website: www.syncardia.com.)

History of Development

CardioWest TAH, formerly known as Jarvik-7 TAH and then Symbion, originally was designed by Kolff, Olsen, and Jarvik (Fig. A5-1). After 20 years of development and research, Jarvik-7 became the first TAH implant intended to provide permanent support.[1]

The current version differs little from the original Jarvik-7 except that it has a smaller maximum stroke volume (70 mL) and an average flow of less than 8 L/min.[2,3] Two additional minor changes were made from the Jarvik-7. First, drivelines of the CardioWest prosthesis are covered with Dacron velour to allow tissue ingrowth and to avoid penetrating infection along the lines. Second, a drop of silicone oil is placed on the air drive side of the diaphragm.[4] Today the CardioWest TAH is used in select centers as a bridge to transplantation and is the first FDA-approved temporary TAH.

Mechanism of Device

The CardioWest TAH is a pneumatic biventricular pulsatile pump that is implanted in the orthotopic position (Figs. A5-2 and A5-3). The two polyurethane ventricles and adjacent intraventricular space displace a total of 750 mL.[4] The TAH is attached via Dacron cuffs to the atria at the level of the atrioventricular valves, whereas the outflow cannulas are attached to the aorta and pulmonary artery by means of Dacron grafts. Each ventricle has a semi-rigid, polyurethane polyester (Biomer) outer shell (Ethicon, Somerville, NJ) and a four-layer flexible polyurethane polyester diaphragm. The diaphragm

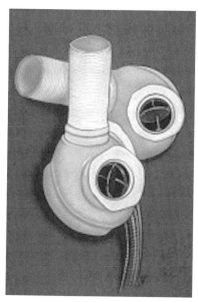

FIGURE A5-1 ■ Jarvik-7 TAH. (Website: www.texasheartinstitute.org.)

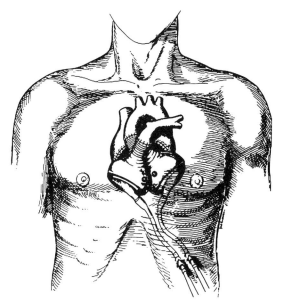

FIGURE A5-3 ■ Schematic of the CardioWest TAH. (From Arabia FA, Copeland JG, Smith RG, et al: CardioWest total artificial heart: A retrospective controlled study. Artif Organs 1999;23:204-207.)

was the interface used to transmit the air pressure and turn it into a pumping action for the blood. It retracts during diastole and is displaced forward by compressed air during systole to propel blood out of the prosthetic ventricle. One-way blood flow is achieved by Medtronic-Hall tilting-disc valves located in the inflow and outflow tracts.[3,5]

A driveline covered with double velour-covered Silastic passes from each ventricle transcutaneously to a console that pulses pressurized air and monitors pump function. The pneumatic drive system uses compressed air to flex the diaphragm, which pumps the blood. This pressure is modulated so that over the course of a cycle the air pressure applied to the ventricles rapidly decreases. The drive console provides adjustments of the pump rate, systolic duration, and pumping pressure.[6] The left ventricle never fills completely; the device adjusts automatically for the volume difference pumped between the two ventricles up to the filling volume limit (70 mL).[4]

Components

TABLE A5-2

Components		
Pump	Stroke volume (mL)	70
	Beats/min	40-120
	Flow rate (L/min)	≤10 (usually 6-8)
	Valves	Four Medtronic-Hall tilting-disc valves
	Position	Orthotopic
Cannula	Inflow	Left and right atria
	Outflow	Aorta and main pulmonary artery
Console	An air-driven console	
	A laptop	
Others	Internal parts	
	External parts	A rechargeable battery

Clinical Experience

In 1982, DeVries first applied the Jarvik-7 TAH to a 61-year-old man as destination therapy; the patient was supported for 112 days, and his death was unrelated to the device.[4] Since 1985, this device has been used for bridge to transplantation. Until 1991, the Jarvik-7 (renamed the Symbion) TAH supported 170 transplant candidates, 66% of whom eventually underwent successful transplantation. Sepsis and multiorgan failure were the primary causes of death during the support period.[7]

In 1991, the Jarvik-7 TAH was renamed CardioWest TAH. This device was approved for clinical investigation by the FDA in 1993.[3] Currently, the CardioWest TAH is used exclusively as a bridge to transplant. More than

400 patients have been supported with this device. Most of them successfully bridged to cardiac transplantation. Copeland and associates[8] reported that almost 90% of patients supported with CardioWest TAH were successfully discharged after transplantation.

TABLE A5-3

Total Clinical Experience	
Total cases	>175
Duration of use	≤620 days
Patient age range	11-64 yr
Patient weight range	NA
Weaning rate	69-96%
Discharge rate	43-92%

NA, not available.
Data from references 3, 4, 8, and 9.

Complications

TABLE A5-4

Complications	
Complications	Percentage
Bleeding	25-41%
Infection	22-89%
Renal dysfunction	29-57%
Liver dysfunction	27-41%
Thromboembolism	4-10%
Neurologic dysfunction	12-62%
Multisystem organ failure	4-9%
Mechanical dysfunction	8-26%

Data from references 3 and 8-11.

Contact Information
Company: CardioWest Technologies, Inc
Address: 1501 North Campbell Avenue, Tucson, AZ, 85721, USA
Contact: Telephone: 520-694-5200
Website: www.cardiowest.org
Physician: Dr. Jack Copeland, University of Arizona, Tucson, Arizona

REFERENCES

1. DeVries WC, Anderson JL, Joyce LD, et al: Clinical use of the total artificial heart. N Engl J Med 1984;310:273-278.
2. Arabia FA, Smith RG, Rose DS, et al: Success rates of long-term circulatory assist devices used currently for bridge to heart transplantation. ASAIO J 1996;42:M542-M546.
3. Copeland JG, Pavie A, Duveau D, et al: Bridge to transplantation with the CardioWest total artificial heart: The international experience 1993 to 1995. J Heart Lung Transplant 1996;15:94-99.
4. Leprince P, Bonnet N, Rama A, et al: Bridge to transplantation with the Jarvik-7 (CardioWest) total artificial heart: A single-center 15-year experience. J Heart Lung Transplant 2003;22:1296-1303.

5. Wheeldon DR: Mechanical circulatory support: State of the art and future perspectives. Perfusion 2003;18:233-243.

6. Arabia FA, Copeland JG, Smith RG, et al: Infections with the CardioWest total artificial heart. ASAIO J 1998;44: M336-M339.

7. Jonnson KE, Prieto M, Joyce LD, et al: Summary of the clinical use of the Symbion total artificial heart: A registry report. Ann Surg 1995;222:327-336.

8. Copeland JG, Smith RG, Arabia FA, et al: The CardioWest total artificial heart as a bridge to transplantation. Semin Thorac Cardiovasc Surg 2000;12:238-242.

9. Arabia FA, Copeland JG, Smith RG, et al: CardioWest total artificial heart: A retrospective controlled study. Artif Organs 1999;23: 204-207.

10. Copeland JG, Arabia FA, Smith RG, et al: Arizona experience with CardioWest Total Artificial Heart bridge to transplantation. Ann Thorac Surg 1999;68:756-760.

11. Copeland JG 3rd, Arabia FA, Banchy ME, et al: The CardioWest total artificial heart bridge to transplantation: 1993 to 1996 national trial. Ann Thorac Surg 1998;66:1662-1669.

DEBAKEY VENTRICULAR ASSIST DEVICE

Device Classification

TABLE A6-1

Classification		
Category	**Group**	**Sub-group**
Duration	Long-term	
Type	Rotary	Axial
Position	Partially implantable	Intra-abdominal

History of Development

The concept of the MicroMed DeBakey VAD was developed in 1987 and was a collaboration between Baylor College of Medicine with DeBakey and Noon, MicroMed Corporation, and the National Aeronautics and Space Administration with Saucier. MicroMed Corporation received the license for the technology in June 1996 and since then has been developing the device for commercial use.[1] The DeBakey VAD Child, the first pediatric implantable VAD and a modified version of the adult DeBakey VAD, is the first miniaturized heart pump for children and received Human Device Exemption from the FDA in February 2004.

Mechanism of Device

The MicroMed DeBakey VAD is a miniaturized (3.5 cm in diameter, 7.62 cm in length), electromagnetically actuated, implantable titanium axial flow pump weighing 93 g, designed for long-term circulation support for patients with end-stage heart failure (Fig. A6-1).[2,3] The internal pump system consists of a titanium inflow cannula and apical ring, the pump housing unit, and a Vascutec gel-weaved vascular graft that exits the pump as an outflow conduit and connects to the aorta (Fig. A6-2).

The pump housing contains a brushless direct current (DC) motor stator surrounding the flow path. The pump head consists of a flow straightener that is stationary and that supports the rotor and front ruby sapphire bearing. The impeller is the only moving part and features a sophisticated miniature rotor and a stationary diffuser that supports the rotor and rear bearing. The pump is connected to the controller via

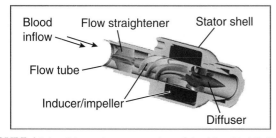

FIGURE A6-1 ■ Schematic cutaway view of the MicroMed DeBakey VAD. (Website: www.micromedtech.com.)

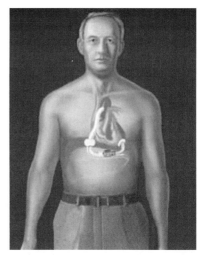

FIGURE A6-2 ■ The implanted MicroMed DeBakey VAD. (Website: www.micromedtech.com.)

a percutaneous cable, which includes the flow probe's wire that is passed through the skin well above the right iliac crest. The controller, consisting of the controller module, battery packs, and battery charger, is designed to operate the pump.[4] On December 18, 2002, Carmeda BioActive surface was added to the DeBakey VAD, but later was discontinued. The device is now commercially available in Europe and approved by the FDA for the U.S. pivotal trial.[5]

Components

TABLE A6-2

Components		
Pump	Revolutions/min	10,000
	Flow rate (L/min)	≤10 (against 100 mm Hg)
	Position	Abdominal wall
Cannula	Inflow	Left ventricular apex
	Outflow	Ascending or descending aorta
Console	DeBakey VAD Data Acquisition System (Fig. A6-3) Patient Home Support System (10 lb) (Fig. A6-4) VADPAK carrying case (5 lb) (Fig. A6-5)	
Others	Internal parts	Ultrasonic flow probe
	External parts	Batteries

Clinical Experience

The DeBakey VAD was the first long-term axial flow circulatory assist device to be introduced into clinical trials and has had the largest clinical experience worldwide. On November 13, 1998, a 44-year-old man was implanted with the DeBakey VAD.[6] At present, more than 300

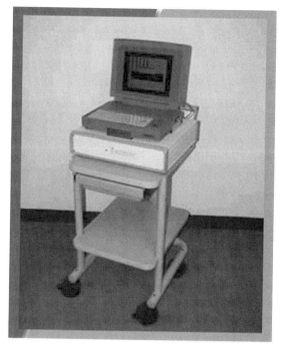

FIGURE A6-3 ■ DeBakey VAD clinical data acquisition system. (Website: www.micromedtech.com.)

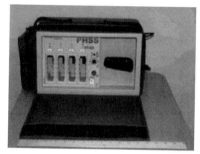

FIGURE A6-4 ■ Patient home support system. (Website: www.micromedtech.com.)

patients have received an implant as a bridge to transplantation, and a few have received an implant as destination therapy. The mean support time was 75 ± 81 days, and 45% of patients have died.[5] The DeBakey VAD Child, the first pediatric implantable VAD, was first implanted in a child in October 2003 at Texas Children's Hospital. There have been six DeBakey VAD Child implantations to date.

TABLE A6-3

Total Clinical Experience	
Total cases (up to April 2005)	315
Duration of use	≤492 days
Patient age range	6-76 yr
Patient weight range	NA
Weaning rate	35-66%
Discharge rate	NA

NA, not available.
Data from references 5-9.

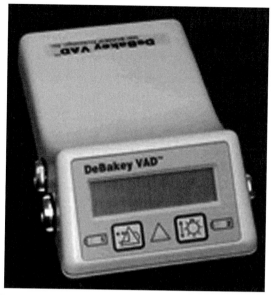

FIGURE A6-5 ■ Portable VADPAK carrying case. (Website: www.micromedtech.com.)

Complications

TABLE A6-4

Complications	
Complications	**Percentage**
Bleeding	32%
Infection	3.3%
Hemolysis	12%
Thromboembolism	11.3%
Mechanical dysfunction	2.7%

Data from reference 5.

Contact Information

Company: MicroMed Technology, Inc
Address: 8965 Interchange Drive, Houston, TX 77054, USA
Contact: Telephone: (713) 838-9210; fax: (713) 838-9214
Website: www.micromedtech.com
Physicians: Drs. Michael DeBakey, George Noon, and Mathias Loebe, Methodist Hospital, Houston, Texas

REFERENCES

1. Noon GP, Morley D, Irwin S, et al: The DeBakey ventricular assist device. In Goldstein DJ, Oz MC (eds): Cardiac Assist Devices. New York, Futura, 2000, pp 375-386.
2. DeBakey ME: A miniature implantable axial flow ventricular assist device. Ann Thorac Surg 1999;68:637-640.
3. Noon GP, Morley D, Irwin S, et al: Development and clinical application of the MicroMed DeBakey VAD. Curr Opin Cardiol 2000;15:166-171.
4. Westaby S: The new rotary blood pumps: An alternative to cardiac transplantation? In Franco KL, Verrier ED (eds): Advanced Therapy in Cardiac Surgery, 2nd ed. BC Decker, London, 2003, pp 499-513.

5. Goldstein DJ: Worldwide experience with the MicroMed DeBakey ventricular assist device as a bridge to transplantation. Circulation 2003;108(Suppl II):II-272-II-277.

6. Wieselthaler G, Schima H, Hiesmayr M, et al: First clinical experience with the DeBakey VAD continuous axial flow pump for bridge to transplantation. Circulation 2000;101:356-359.

7. Gardy KL, Mattea A, Irmaza S, et al: Improvement in quality of life outcomes 2 weeks after left ventricular assist device implantation. J Heart Transplant 2001;20:657-669.

8. Vitali E, Lanfranconi M, Ribera E, et al: Successful experience in bridging patients to heart transplantation with the MicroMed DeBakey ventricular assist device. Ann Thorac Surg 2003;75:1200-1204.

9. Noon GP, Morley DL, Irwin S, et al: Clinical experience with the MicroMed DeBakey ventricular assist device. Ann Thorac Surg 2001;71(3 Suppl):S133-S138.

10. Morales DL, DiBardino DJ, McKenzie ED, et al: Lessons learned from the first application of the DeBakey VAD Child: An intracorporeal ventricular assist device for children. J Heart Lung Transplant 2005;24:331-337.

HEARTMATE LEFT VENTRICULAR ASSIST DEVICE

Other names for the HeartMate Left VAD include HeartMate IP, HeartMate VE, HeartMate XVE, and TCI LVAD.

Device Classification

TABLE A7-1

Classification		
Category	Group	Sub-group
Duration	Long-term	
Type	Pulsatile	Pneumatic/electric
Position	Partial implantable	Intra-abdominal

History of Development

The Heartmate Left VAD was developed and tested by Thermo Cardiosystems, Inc. (Woburn, MA) and the Texas Heart Institute in the 1960s.[1] Since then, this pump has been acquired by Thoratec (Pleasanton, CA). In 1988, it was the first device approved by the FDA for use as a long-term bridge to heart transplantation and more recently for destination therapy.[2,3]

Mechanism of Device

The HeartMate Left VAD is a pulsatile diaphragm pump that is designed to perform substantially all or part of the pumping function of the left ventricle of the natural heart for patients with cardiovascular disease (Fig. A7-1). Two systems have been commercialized for patients requiring cardiac support: an implantable pneumatic left VAD (HeartMate IP), which is powered by an external, electrically driven air pump, and an electric left VAD (HeartMate VE), which is driven by an implanted electric motor and powered by a lightweight battery pack worn by the patient.[1]

The HeartMate pump is a flattened titanium cylinder about 2 inches thick and 4 inches in diameter. The pump

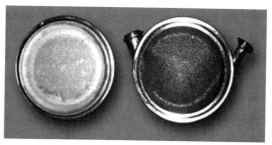

FIGURE A7-2 ■ The two chambers in the HeartMate Left VAD. (Website: www.cts.usc.edu.)

has two chambers—the blood chamber and the air chamber. A flexible diaphragm separates these two chambers (Fig. A7-2). The blood chamber is pressurized by a pusher plate to supply the body with blood. Valves located on either side of the device's pumping chamber keep blood flowing in only one direction.[4] In addition, the HeartMate does not require systemic anticoagulation because of the special design of blood-contacting surfaces.

The system can operate in three modes—automatic mode, fixed-rate mode, and external (synchronous) mode. In the automatic mode, the left VAD pumps at a responsive rate determined by the hemodynamic requirements of the patient. In the fixed-rate mode, the left VAD pumps at a preset beat rate.

In recent years, the HeartMate XVE system, an enhanced version of the HeartMate VE, has been developed, and it was approved in November 2002 for use for destination therapy (Fig. A7-3).

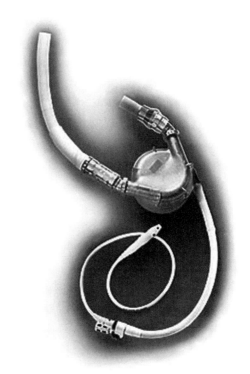

FIGURE A7-3 ■ HeartMate XVE.

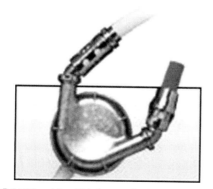

FIGURE A7-1 ■ HeartMate IP left VAD. (Website: www.thoratec.com.)

Components

TABLE A7-2

Components		
Pump	Stroke volume (mL)	83
	Beats/min	≤140
	Flow rate (L/min)	≤12
	Valves	Two 25-mm porcine valves
	Position	Abdominal wall
Cannula	Inflow	Left ventricular apex
	Outflow	Ascending aorta
Console	A microprocessor-based drive console (Figs. A7-4 and A7-5)	
Others	Internal parts	
	External parts	Power base unit Portable battery pack

TABLE A7-3

Total Clinical Experience	
Total cases	>3600
Duration of use	≤884 days
Patient age range	8-78 yr
Patient weight range	NA
Weaning rate	67-76%
Discharge rate	56-65%

NA, not available.
Data from references 8-11.

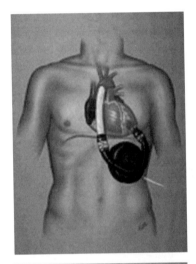

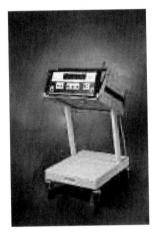

FIGURE A7-4 ■ Console of HeartMate IP. (Website: www.texasheartinstitute.org.)

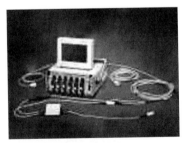

FIGURE A7-5 ■ Console of HeartMate VE. (Website: www.texasheartinstitute.org.)

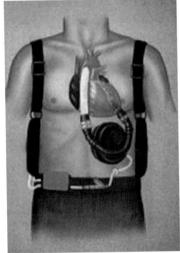

FIGURE A7-6 ■ Implanted HeartMate IP *(top)* and VE *(bottom)*.

Clinical Experience

In 1986, Frazier and colleagues[5] first implanted the HeartMate as a bridge to transplantation, and the electrically powered HeartMate was first used as a bridge to transplantation in 1991.[6] In 1994, after the completion of a 9-year clinical trial, the HeartMate IP left VAD became the first commercially available, FDA-approved, left VAD for use as a bridge to transplantation in the United States. In the same year, the HeartMate IP received the European Conformity Mark, and the HeartMate VE received the same status in August 1995 and FDA commercial approval in 1998. In August 1998, the HeartMate IP received Canadian approval, permitting the sale of the air-driven and electric versions throughout Canada. To date, more than 3600 patients worldwide have been supported with the HeartMate left VAD (Fig. A7-6). As of January 2004, 85 patients younger than 18 years old have been implanted with HeartMate left VAD, and the survival rate is 71% (Farrar DJ: Private communication).

Complications

TABLE A7-4

Complications

Complications	Percentage
Bleeding	10-35.2%
Infection	5-40%
Renal, hepatic dysfunction	30-60%
Thromboembolism	2-6%
Neurologic dysfunction	5.2-25%
Mechanical dysfunction	1-77%

Data from references 8-11.

Contact Information

Company: Thoratec Corporation
Address: 6035 Stoneridge Drive, Pleasanton, CA 94588, USA

Contact: Toll-free telephone: 1-800-528-2577; telephone: 925-847-8600; fax: 925-847-8574
Website: www.thoratec.com
Physicians: Dr. David Farrar, Thoratec, Pleasanton, California, *or* Dr. Ronald Hill, University of California San Francisco, San Francisco, California

REFERENCES

1. Goldstein DJ: Thermo cardiosystems ventricular assist devices. In Goldstein DJ, Oz MC (eds): Cardiac Assist Device. New York, Futura, 2000, pp 307-321.
2. McCarthy PM, Smedira NO, Vargo RL, et al: One hundred patients with the HeartMate left ventricular assist device: Evolving concepts and technology. J Thorac Cardiovasc Surg 1998;115: 904-912.
3. Frazier OH, Myers TJ, Padovancevic B: The HeartMate left ventricular assist systems: Overview and 12 year experience. Texas Heart Inst J 1998;25:265-271.
4. Frazier OH: The development of an implantable portable electrically powered left ventricular assist device. Semin Thorac Cardiovasc Surg 1994;6:181-187.
5. Frazier OH, Pose EA, Macmanus Q, et al: Multicenter clinical evaluation of the HeartMate 1000 IP left ventricular assist device. Ann Thorac Surg 1992;53:1080-1090.
6. Frazier OH: First use of an untethered, vented electric left ventricular assist device for long-term support. Circulation 1994;89: 2908-2914.
7. Pagani FD, Aaronson KD: Mechanical devices for temporary cardiac support. In Franco KL, Verrier ED (eds): Advanced Therapy in Cardiac Surgery, 2nd ed. BC Decker, London, 2003, pp 460-483.
8. Long JW: Advanced mechanical circulatory support with the HeartMate left ventricular assist device in the year 2000. Ann Thorac Surg 2001;71(3 Suppl):S176-S182.
9. Rose EA, Gelijns AC, Moskowitz AJ, et al: Long-term use of a left ventricular assist device for end-stage heart failure. N Engl J Med 2001;345:1435-1443.
10. Frazier OH, Rose EA, Oz MC, et al, HeartMate LVAS investigators: Left ventricular assist system: Multicenter clinical evaluation of the HeartMate vented electric left ventricular assist system in patients awaiting heart transplantation. J Thorac Cardiovasc Surg 2001;122:1186-1195.
11. El-Banayosy A, Korfer R: Long-term implantable left ventricular assist devices: Out-of-hospital program. Cardiol Clin 2003;21: 57-65.

IMPELLA RECOVER SYSTEM

Device Classification

TABLE A8-1

Classification		
Category	Group	Sub-group
Duration	Short-term	
Type	Rotary	Axial
Position	Partially implantable	Intrathoracic

History of Development

In 1991, the device-related research was initiated at the Helmholtz Institute in Aachen, Germany, and resulted in a first European Conformity Mark–labeled product for intraoperative use in 1999. Current developments, including a 12F (diameter 4 mm) percutaneous catheter–based pump (Recover LP 2.5), are geared toward further miniaturization of the device and devices suitable for prolonged support of patients.[1]

Mechanism of Device

The Impella device includes two independent intracardiac axial pumps designed for left or right ventricular assistance. The left-side pump (Recover 100) is a 9F catheter-mounted, 6.4-mm axial pump that can be placed in either the femoral artery via the percutaneous approach or the aorta via the transthoracic route. Blood is pumped from the left ventricle into the descending aorta at flows of 5 L/minute.

The right VAD (Recover 600) comprises the same axial pump mounted in a cage designed to be implanted into the right atrium. A polytetrafluoroethylene 8-mm graft connects the output to the pulmonary artery, and the pumps can deliver 6 L/minute (Fig. A8-1).[2,3] The right-side Impella pump is introduced via the right atrium and pumps the blood forward from the atrium into the pulmonary artery with the inflatable ring balloon on the tip to stabilize the pump. The left-side Impella pump is positioned across the aortic valve and aspirates the blood from the left ventricle and pumps it in the ascending aorta. Both pumps are designed for short-term ventricular support in the intensive care unit (Figs. A8-2 and A8-3). The console serves as the interface between the pump and the user.[4]

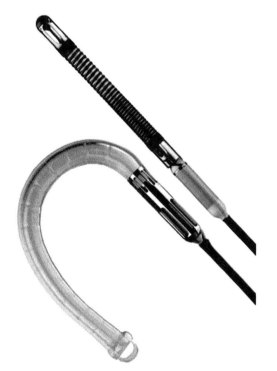

FIGURE A8-1 ■ The Impella intracardiac micropumps with the left-side pump *(upper)* and the right-side pump *(lower)*. (From Song X, Throckmorton AL, Untarqiu A, et al: Axial flow blood pumps. ASAIO J 2003;49:355-364.)

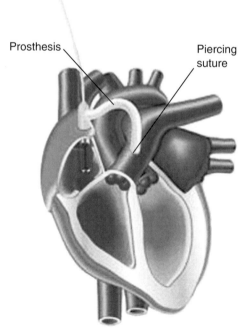

FIGURE A8-2 ■ Impella system for right ventricular assist (Recover 600). (Website: www.impella.com.)

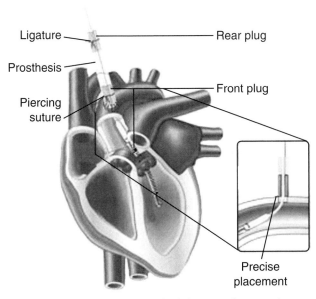

FIGURE A8-3 ■ Impella system for left ventricular assist (Recover 100). (Website: www.medgadget.com.)

Clinical Experience

To date, the Impella recover assist system has been implanted more than 140 times in 34 clinics in eight different countries. Most of them were supported by an Impella left VAD exclusively, and others were supported by either an Impella right VAD or biventricular support. The combination of a long-term left VAD with an Impella right VAD also has been used under clinical conditions in the case of transient right ventricular failure.[4-6]

Complications

TABLE A8-4

Complications	
Complications	Percentage
Hemolysis	37.5%
Infection	19%
Multisystem organ failure	19%
Mechanical dysfunction	19%
Data from reference 6.	

Contact Information

Company: Impella CardioSystems AG
Address: Neuenhofer Weg 3, 52074 Aachen, Nordrhein-Westfalen, Germany
Contact: Telephone: ++49 241 8860-0; fax: ++49 241 8860-111
Website: www.impella.com
Physician: Dr. Ettore Vitali, Niguarda Ca'Granda Hospital, Milan, Italy

Components

TABLE A8-2

Components		
Pump	Revolutions/min	30,000
	Flow rate (L/min)	5-6
	Position	Intracardiac
Cannula	Inflow	Left ventricle (left VAD) or right atrium (right VAD)
	Outflow	Aorta (left VAD) or main pulmonary artery (right VAD)
Console	Impella mobile console	
Others	Internal parts	
	External parts	Impella power supply Impella purger

TABLE A8-3

Total Clinical Experience	
Total cases	>140
Duration of use	≤18 days
Patient age range	43-75 yr
Patient weight range	NA
Weaning rate	55-68%
Discharge rate	35-37%
NA, not available.	
Data from references 5 and 6.	

REFERENCES

1. Siess T, Nix C, Menzler F: From a lab type to a product: A retrospective view on Impella's assist technology. Artif Organs 2001;25:414-421.
2. Isgro F, Kiessling AH, Rehn E, et al: Intracardiac left ventricular support in beating heart, multi-vessel revascularization. J Card Surg 2003;18:240-244.
3. Meyns B, Stolinski J, Leunens V, et al: Left ventricular support by catheter-mounted axial flow pump reduces infarct size. J Am Coll Cardiol 2003;41:1087-1095.
4. Vercaemst L, Vandezande E, Janssens P, et al: Impella: A miniaturized cardiac support system in an era of minimal invasive cardiac surgery. J Extra Corpor Technol 2002;34:92-100.
5. Colombo T, Garatti A, Bruschi G, et al: First successful bridge to recovery with the Impella Recover 100 left ventricular assist device for fulminant acute myocarditis. Ital Heart J 2003;4:642-645.
6. Meyns B, Dens J, Sergeant P, et al: Initial experiences with the Impella device in patients with cardiogenic shock: Impella support for cardiogenic shock. Thorac Cardiovasc Surg 2003;51:312-317.

JARVIK 2000 FLOWMAKER

Device Classification

TABLE A9-1

Classification		
Category	Group	Sub-group
Duration	Long-term	
Type	Rotary	Axial
Position	Partial implantable	Intrathoracic

History of Development

Jarvik 2000 was developed under the cooperation of Jarvik Heart, Inc., and the Texas Heart Institute. The project began in 1989 through the collaboration of Frazier and Jarvik.[1]

Mechanism of Device

The Jarvik 2000, an intraventricular assist device, has an ultrasmooth titanium surface and is 2.5 cm in diameter and 5.5 cm in length with a weight of 85 g.[2] The system consists of a blood pump, 16-mm outflow graft, percutaneous power cable, pump-speed controller, and DC power supply; a fully implantable version also is available. A totally implantable version has two power leads that exit from the blood pump and are connected to the internal power and control unit. In this model, primary and secondary transcutaneous energy transmission system coils are placed in different places (Figs. A9-1 and A9-2).[3]

The pump is a valveless, electrically powered axial flow pump that fits directly into the left ventricle. The impeller, the only moving part in the pump, is a neodymium-iron-boron magnet, which is housed inside a welded titanium shell. On the impeller's outer surface are two titanium hydrodynamic blades. The impeller is

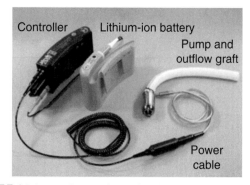

FIGURE A9-1 ▪ Jarvik 2000 FlowMaker. (From Frazier OH, Myers TJ, Westaby S, et al: Clinical experience with an implantable, intracardiac, continuous flow circulatory support device: Physiologic implications and their relationship to patient selection. Ann Thorac Surg 2004;77: 133-142.)

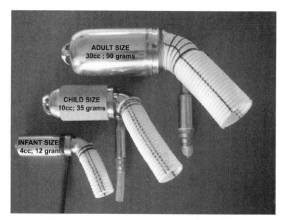

FIGURE A9-2 ▪ Totally implantable version of the Jarvik 2000. (From Frazier OH, Myers TJ, Jarvik RK, et al: Research and development of an implantable, axial-flow left ventricular assist device: The Jarvik 2000 heart. Ann Thorac Surg 2001;71(3 Suppl):S125-S132.)

supported by ceramic bearings. A brushless DC motor contained within the housing creates the electromagnetic force necessary to rotate the impeller. A small cable, which exits the body through the abdominal wall, delivers power to the impeller. The pump speed, controlled by an analogue system controller, can be adjusted manually from 8000 to 12000 revolutions/minute in increments of 1000. The control unit monitors the pump function and the remaining power in the batteries.[4-7]

Components

TABLE A9-2

Components		
Pump	Revolutions/min	8000-12,000
	Flow rate (L/min)	≤7
	Position	Intraventricular
Cannula	Inflow	Left ventricular apex
	Outflow	Descending aorta
Console	Analogue system controller	
Others	Internal parts	
	External parts	Battery pack

Clinical Experience

In April 2000, the Texas Heart Institute was granted permission by the FDA to evaluate the Jarvik 2000 as a bridge to transplantation in five patients. On June 28, 2002, the first patient, a 52-year-old woman, received a Jarvik 2000 for bridging to transplantation.[8] Patients have been sustained for more than 200 days with this device. This device also is used as a permanent implanted device for patients with cardiac failure.[9] To date, several patients have been supported for more than 2 years, and one patient is doing well after more than 3 years of support.

TABLE A9-3

Total Clinical Experience	
Total cases	<100
Duration of use	>200 days
Patient age range	21-72 yr
Patient weight range	NA
Weaning rate	59-70%
Discharge rate	54-70%

NA, not available.
Data from references 1, 4, 8, 10, and 11.

Complications

TABLE A9-4

Complications	
Complications	**Percentage**
Bleeding	5%
Infection	16%
Thromboembolism	0-10%
Neurologic dysfunction	5%
Multisystem organ failure	10%
Mechanical dysfunction	≤30%

Data from references 1, 4, 8, 10, 11.

Contact Information
Company: Jarvik Research, Inc
Address: 333 W. 52nd Street, New York, NY, USA
Contact: Not available
Website: www.jarvikheart.com
Physician: Dr. OH Frazier, Texas Heart Institute, Houston, Texas

REFERENCES

1. Cooley DA: Initial clinical experience with the Jarvik 2000 implantable axial-flow left ventricular assist system. Circulation 2002;105:2808-2809.
2. Song X, Throckmorton AL, Untaroiu A, et al: Axial flow blood pumps. ASAIO J 2003;49:355-364.
3. Frazier OH, Myers TJ, Westaby S, et al: Clinical experience with an implantable, intracardiac, continuous flow circulatory support device: Physiologic implications and their relationship to patient selection. Ann Thorac Surg 2004;77:133-142.
4. Frazier OH, Myers TJ, Jarvik RK, et al: Research and development of an implantable, axial-flow left ventricular assist device: The Jarvik 2000 heart. Ann Thorac Surg 2001;71(3 Suppl):S125-S132.
5. Macris MP, Parmis SM, Frazier OH, et al: Development of an implantable ventricular assist system. Ann Thorac Surg 1997;63:367-370.
6. Parnis SM, Conger JL, Fuqua JM, et al: Progress in the development of a transcutaneously powered axial flow blood pump ventricular assist system. ASAIO J 1997;43:M576-M580.
7. Westaby S, Katsumata T, Houel R, et al: Jarvik 2000 heart potential for bridge to myocyte recovery. Circulation 1998;98:1568-1574.
8. Frazier OH, Myers TJ, Gregoric ID, et al: Initial clinical experience with the Jarvik 2000 implantable axial-flow left ventricular assist system. Circulation 2002;105:2855-2860.
9. Saito S, Robson D, Freeland A, et al: First permanent implant of the Jarvik 2000 Heart. Lancet 2000;356:900-903.
10. Frazier OH, Myers TJ, Westaby S, et al: Use of the Jarvik 2000 left ventricular assist system as a bridge to heart transplantation or as destination therapy for patients with chronic heart failure. Ann Surg 2003;237:631-636.
11. Siegenthaler MP, Martin J, Pernice K, et al: The Jarvik 2000 is associated with less infections than the HeartMate left ventricular assist device. Eur J Cardiothorac Surg 2003;23:748-754.

MEDOS HIA VENTRICULAR ASSIST DEVICE

Device Classification

TABLE A10-1

Classification		
Category	Group	Sub-group
Duration	Long-term	
Type	Pulsatile	Pneumatic
Position	Paracorporeal	

History of Development

The design of the MEDOS HIA VAD was initiated in 1982 at the Helmholtz Institute. Over a 10-year development period, an optimal configuration was achieved. In 1990, this device entered a commercial phase. After the first clinical implants in 1994, European Conformity Mark was obtained in 1997.[1,2]

Mechanism of Device

The MEDOS HIA VAD system consists of a pulsatile pneumatic blood pump, a driving system, and corresponding cannulas (Fig. A10-1). The pump is manufactured in various sizes of 10 mL, 25 mL, 60 mL, and 80 mL for left VADs and 9 mL, 22.5 mL, 54 mL, and 72 mL for right VADs (Fig. A10-2). The device is suitable for patients ranging from neonates to adults in need of univentricular or biventricular support. The pump is made of clear polyurethane and consists of a semirigid outer chamber within which a seamless double-layered blood sac is mounted. Unidirectional blood flow is achieved via two valves mounted externally to the pump chamber (Fig. A10-3).[2-4]

To match the anatomic conditions, MEDOS offers venous cannulas in various sizes (14F to 58F) and angular

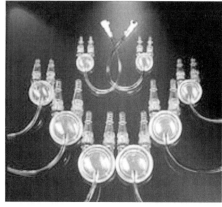

FIGURE A10-2 ■ Available sets of ventricles for left and right MEDOS HIA VAD heart support. (From Thuaudet S: The Medos ventricular assist device system. Perfusion 2000;15:337-343.)

positions. The apex-cannula, as an alternative to the venous cannula, can be applied directly to the apex of the heart and is provided in various sizes (6 mm, 8 mm, 12 mm, and 15 mm). Pneumatic supply is provided by a driver, mounted on a support console, which also enables patient monitoring. The MEDOS VAD console (Fig. A10-4) supports the use of any size of pump, configured in univentricular or biventricular mode. Fixed rate and ECG trigger modes are available, and the operator has control over the systolic and diastolic pneumatic drive pressures, the percentage systole, and the alarm windows. An automatic operating mode is under development.[2]

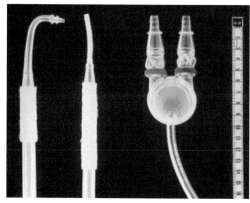

FIGURE A10-1 ■ The MEDOS HIA VAD with a 10-mL artificial ventricle (*right*) with atrial (*left*) and aortic (*middle*) conduits. (From Weyand M, Kececioglu D, Kehl HG, et al: Neonatal mechanical bridging to total orthotopic heart transplantation. Ann Thorac Surg 1998;66:519-522.)

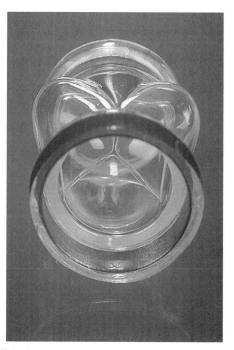

FIGURE A10-3 ■ Polyurethane tri-leaflet valve in MEDOS HIA VAD. (Website: www.medos-ag.com.)

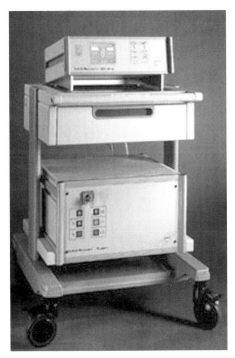

FIGURE A10-4 ■ Drive unit with interactive touch screen monitor. (From Konertz W, Hotz H, Schneider M, et al: Clinical experience with the Medos HIA-VAD system in infants and children: A preliminary report. Ann Thorac Surg 1997;63:1138-1144.)

Clinical Experience

The MEDOS HIA VAD system has been in clinical use since February 1994.[4-6] Most patients supported with the MEDOS device were bridged to transplantation. The overall survival rate of postcardiotomy patients is about 70% and of patients with cardiogenic shock is about 40%.[2]

From 1994 to 2001, 64 children ages 3 days to 16 years received MEDOS devices in Europe. Duration of support was 1 to 97 days (median 5.5 days), with an overall survival rate of 36.2%. Survival was similar for all pump sizes (9/10 mL, 37.5%; 22/25 mL, 34.8%; 54/60 mL, 37.5%).[6]

TABLE A10-3

Total Clinical Experience	
Total cases	>400 (including ~75 children)
Duration of use	≤144 days
Patient age range	3 days-76 yr
Patient weight range	3.1-135 kg
Weaning rate	36-70%
Discharge rate	33-66%

Data from references 2, 3, 5, and 6.

Complications

TABLE A10-4

Complications	
Complications	**Percentage**
Bleeding	33-66%
Infection	19-50%
Renal dysfunction	32-66%
Hepatic dysfunction	~50%
Thromboembolism	~66%
Neurologic dysfunction	~33%
Multisystem organ failure	5-10%

Data from references 2, 3, 5, and 6.

Contact Information

Company: MEDOS Medizintechnik AG
Address: Obere Steinfurt 8-10 D-52222 Stolberg, Germany
Contact: Telephone: +49 (0) 24 02-96 64-10; fax: +49 (0) 24 02-96 64-60
Website: www.medos-ag.com
Physician: Not available

Components

TABLE A10-2

Components		
Pump	Stroke volume (mL)	10, 25, 60, and 80 (left VAD) 9, 22.5, 54, and 72 (right VAD)
	Beats/min	60-180 (9/10 mL VAD); 60-150 (22.5/25 mL VAD); 60-120 (54/60 mL VAD); 60-100 (72/80 mL VAD)
	Flow rate (L/min)	≤8
	Valves	Two polyurethane tri-leaflet valves
	Position	On the abdominal wall
Cannula	Inflow	Left atrium (left VAD) or right atrium (right VAD)
	Outflow	Aorta (left VAD) or main pulmonary artery (right VAD)
Console	Medos VAD supply system	Touching screen monitor
		Main processor
	Medos VAD driving system	Battery
		Compressor units
Others	Internal parts External parts	

REFERENCES

1. Knierbein B, Rosarius N, Reul H, et al: New methods for the development of pneumatic displacement pumps for cardiac assist. Int J Artif Organs 1990;13:751-759.
2. Thuaudet S: The Medos ventricular assist device system. Perfusion 2000;15:337-343.

3. Reul H: The Medos/HIA system: Development, results, perspectives. Thorac Cardiovasc Surg 1999;47(Suppl 2):311-315.

4. Weyand M, Kececioglu D, Kehl HG, et al: Neonatal mechanical bridging to total orthotopic heart transplantation. Ann Thorac Surg 1998;66:519-522.

5. Konertz W, Hotz H, Schneider M, et al: Clinical experience with the Medos HIA-VAD system in infants and children: A preliminary report. Ann Thorac Surg 1997;63:1138-1144.

6. Reinhartz O, Stiller B, Eilrs R, et al: Current clinical status of pulsatile pediatric circulatory support. ASAIO J 2002;48:455-459.

NOVACOR LEFT VENTRICULAR ASSIST SYSTEM

Device Classification

TABLE A11-1

Classification		
Category	Group	Sub-group
Duration	Long-term	
Type	Pulsatile	Electromechanical
Position	Partial implantable	Intra-abdominal

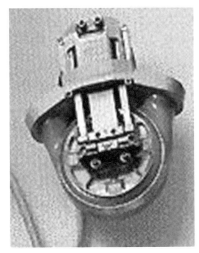

FIGURE A11-1 ■ Novacor left ventricular assist system. (Website: www.worldheart.com.)

History of Development

The Novacor system, invented by Portner, has been under development since 1970.[1] It was first used clinically in 1984 and evolved to the current wearable model first used clinically in 1993.[2,3] The Novacor left ventricular assist system has been marketed in Europe since 1994 as a bridge to transplantation and a long-term alternative to other medical therapies, such as long-term drug treatment and heart transplantation. Now the system is commercially approved in the United States, Canada, and Japan. Since 1998, a gelatin-sealed, knitted polyester graft with integral wall reinforcement has replaced the low-porosity, woven polyester to use for inflow conduit.[4] Novocor II, a smaller, bearingless VAD, is under development with animal implants expected by the end of 2005.

Mechanism of Device

The Novacor left ventricular assist system is an electromechanically driven pump, about the size of a human heart, designed for patients with left ventricular failure (Fig. A11-1).[4] It consists of an electric pump, an extracorporeal controller, and a rechargeable battery pack.

The pump incorporates a dual pusher plate, sac-type blood pump with a 70-mL stroke volume, and a smooth polyurethane blood contact surface. Modular porcine-valved conduits provide directional flow control. Actuation of the pusher plates is accomplished via a decoupled solenoid actuator and two titanium beam springs connected to the pusher plates. The pump-drive unit is implanted in a pocket created below the diaphragm and unloads the left ventricle via an apical cannula, returning blood to the ascending aorta. The system is operated and monitored by an electronic controller and powered by primary and reserve battery packs, which are worn on a belt around the individual's waist or carried in a shoulder bag. The controller and batteries are connected to the implanted pump by a percutaneous cable (Fig. A11-2). The system is capable of running in four

modes: fixed rate, ECG trigger, full rate trigger, and fill-to-empty. Apart from the fixed rate, all other modes are responsive to the recipient's changing heartbeat and circulatory demands. Portable power packs provide for 7 hours of tether-free operation.[5-7]

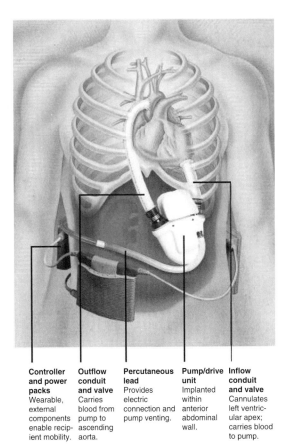

Controller and power packs	Outflow conduit and valve	Percutaneous lead	Pump/drive unit	Inflow conduit and valve
Wearable, external components enable recipient mobility.	Carries blood from pump to ascending aorta.	Provides electric connection and pump venting.	Implanted within anterior abdominal wall.	Cannulates left ventricular apex; carries blood to pump.

FIGURE A11-2 ■ Novacor left ventricular assist system with wearable controller and batteries. (Website: www.worldheart.com.)

Components

TABLE A11-2

Components		
Pump	Stroke volume (mL)	70
	Beats/min	≤120
	Flow rate (L/min)	≤8.5
	Valves	Modular porcine-valve
	Position	Abdominal wall
Cannula	Inflow	Left ventricular apex
	Outflow	Ascending aorta
Console	Small electronic compact controller	
Others	Internal parts	
	External parts	Wearable controller
		Portable power packs

Clinical Experience

The first use of the Novacor left ventricular assist system was in 1984 at Stanford University in the first successful bridge to transplantation.[8] This device has had vast experience with more than 1450 implants, with the longest use of 4.8 years (total support of 443 years). Most applications are as a bridge to transplantation, with approximately a 60% success rate. The outcomes have improved with time.[3,9] Similar to the HeartMate, there has been experience with patients going home with this device, but there has been a higher incidence of neurologic complications.[10,11]

TABLE A11-3

Total Clinical Experience	
Total cases	>1500
Duration of use	≤6 yr
Patient age range	13-75 yr
Patient weight range	44-142 kg
Weaning rate	52-89%
Discharge rate	30-69%

Data from references 3, and 9-17.

Complications

TABLE A11-4

Complications	
Complications	**Percentage**
Bleeding	12-70%
Infection	20-59%
Right heart failure	9-24.5%
Renal dysfunction	17-41%
Thromboembolism	12-31%
Neurologic dysfunction	6-39%
Multisystem organ failure	11-17%
Mechanical dysfunction	0.7%

Data from references 3, and 9-18.

Contact Information

Company: World Heart Corporation
Address: 1 Laser Street, Ottawa, Ontario, Canada, K2E 7V1
Contact: Telephone: (613) 226-4278; fax: (613) 723-8522
Website: www.worldheart.com
Physician: Not available

REFERENCES

1. Wheeldon DR, Jansen PGM, Porter PM: The Novacor electrical implantable left ventricular assist system. Perfusion 2000;15: 355-361.
2. Robbins RC, Kown MH, Portner PM, et al: The totally implantable Novacor left ventricular assist system. Ann Thorac Surg 2001;71: S162-S165.
3. Dagenais F, Portner PM, Robbins RC, et al: The Novacor left ventricular assist system: Clinical experience from the Novacor registry. J Card Surg 2001;16:267-271.
4. de Vivo F, De Santo LS, Maiello C, et al: Novacor left ventricular assist device: Present experience. Int J Artif Organs 1999;22:11-13.
5. Loisance D, Deleuze PH, Mazzucotelli JP, et al: The initial experience with the wearable Baxter Novacor ventricular assist system. J Thorac Cardiovasc Surg 1994;108:176-177.
6. Shinn JA: Novacor left ventricular assist system. AACN Clin Issues Crit Care Nurs 1991;2:575-586.
7. Jacquet L, Dion R, Noirhomme P, et al: Successful bridge to retransplantation with the wearable Novacor left ventricular assist system. J Heart Lung Transplant 1996;15:620-622.
8. Portner PM, Oyer PE, McGregor CGA, et al: First human use of an electrically powered implantable ventricular assist system (Abstract). Artif Organs 1985;9:36.
9. Strauch JT, Spielvogel D, Haldenwang PL, et al: Recent improvements in outcome with the Novacor left ventricular assist device. J Heart Lung Transplant 2003;22:674-680.
10. Pasque MK, Rogers JG: Adverse events in the use of HeartMate vented electric and Novacor left ventricular assist devices: Comparing apples and oranges. J Thorac Cardiovasc Surg 2002; 124:1063-1067.
11. Thomas CE, Jichici D, Petrucci R, et al: Neurologic complications of the Novacor left ventricular assist device. Ann Thorac Surg 2001;72:1311-1315.
12. Grossi P, Dalla GD, Pagani F, et al: Infectious complications in patients with the Novacor left ventricular assist system. Transplant Proc 2001;33:1969-1971.
13. El-Banayosy A, Deng M, Loisance DY, et al: The European experience of Novacor left ventricular assist (LVAS) therapy as a bridge to transplant: A retrospective multi-centre study. Eur J Cardiothorac Surg 1999;15:835-841.
14. Murali S: Mechanical circulatory support with the Novacor LVAS: World-wide clinical results. Thorac Cardiovasc Surg 1999;47 (Suppl 2):321-325.
15. Starnes VA, Shumway NE: Heart transplantation: Stanford experience. Clin Transpl 1987;1:7-11.
16. Schmid C, Weyand M, Nabavi DG, et al: Cerebral and systemic embolization during left ventricular support with the Novacor N100 device. Ann Thorac Surg 1998;65:1703-1710.
17. McCarthy PM, Portner PM, Tobler HG, et al: Clinical experience with the Novacor ventricular assist system: Bridge to transplantation and the transition to permanent application. J Thorac Cardiovasc Surg 1991;102:578-586.
18. El-Banayosy A, Korfer R: Long-term implantable left ventricular assist devices: Out-of-hospital program. Cardiol Clin 2003;21: 57-65.

TANDEMHEART PERCUTANEOUS VENTRICULAR ASSIST DEVICE

Device Classification

TABLE A12-1

Classification		
Category	Group	Sub-group
Duration	Short-term	
Type	Rotary	Centrifugal
Position	Paracorporeal	

History of Development

Since October 2000, cardiologists at the University of Pittsburgh Medical Center's Cardiovascular Institute have been involved in a phase I study of the TandemHeart percutaneous VAD that provides circulatory support for a damaged heart, allowing the heart to rest and strengthen.

Mechanism of Device

The TandemHeart percutaneous VAD is intended for short-term circulatory support. It is dual-chambered with an upper housing and a lower housing assembly (Fig. A12-1). The upper housing provides a conduit for inflow and outflow of blood. The lower housing assembly provides communication with the controller; the means for rotating the impeller of the VAD; and an anticoagulation infusion line integral to the pump to provide a hydrodynamic bearing, cooling of the bearing, and local anticoagulation.

The inflow cannula is introduced via the femoral vein through the interatrial septum into the left atrium.

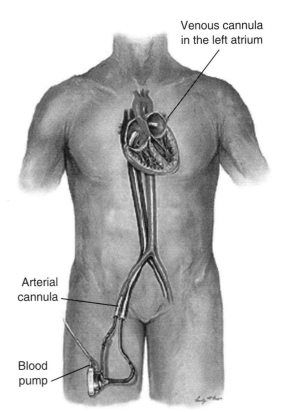

FIGURE A12-2 ■ Schematic of TandemHeart percutaneous VAD and associated blood circuit components. (Website: texasheartinstitute.org.)

Blood is returned into the femoral artery (Fig. A12-2).[1,2] The controller is a microprocessor-based electromechanical drive and infusion system. The controller generates the signals to drive the VAD, which turns the impeller and serves to infuse the anticoagulant solution.

Components

TABLE A12-2

Components		
Pump	Priming volume (mL)	7
	Revolutions/min	7500
	Flow rate (L/min)	≤4
	Position	Near the leg
Cannula	Inflow	Left atrium
	Outflow	Femoral artery
Console	Microprocessor-based electromechanical drive	
	Backup control unit	
Others	None	

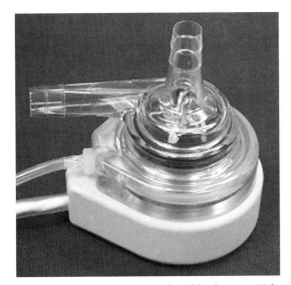

FIGURE A12-1 ■ TandemHeart centrifugal blood pump. (Website: www.texasheartinstitute.org.)

Clinical Experience

The clinical experience so far is limited. In May 2000, the TandemHeart percutaneous VAD was introduced in clinical use (Fig. A12-3). Currently, this device is a European Conformity Mark product. Thiele and

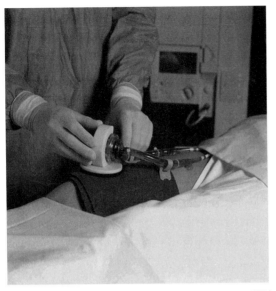

FIGURE A12-3 ■ TandemHeart percutaneous VAD in use. (Website: www.newsbureau.upmc.com.)

associates[2] reported 18 patients supported by the TandemHeart percutaneous VAD. In this group of patients, mean duration of support was 4 ± 3 days, and the mean flow of the VAD was 3.2 ± 0.6 L/minute. Fourteen patients were weaned successfully, and 10 patients were discharged.

TABLE A12-3

Total Clinical Experience	
Total cases (up to September 2004)	100
Duration of use	≤14 days
Patient age range	44-89 yr
Patient weight range	NA
Weaning rate	77.7-100%
Discharge rate	55.5-100%

NA, not available.
Data from references 1 and 2.

Complications

TABLE A12-4

Complications	
Complications	Percentage
Bleeding	27.7%
Limb ischemia	11.1%
Neurologic dysfunction	5.5%

Data from references 1 and 2.

Contact Information

Company: Cardiac Assist Technologies, Inc. (Pittsburgh, PA)
Address: 200 Meiling Hall, 370 West 9th Avenue, Columbus, OH 43210, USA
Contact: Toll-free telephone: 800-373-7421; telephone: 412-963-7770; fax: 412-963-0800
Website: www.cardiacassist.com
Physician: Not available

REFERENCES

1. Vranckx P, Foley DP, de Feijter PJ, et al: Clinical introduction of the Tandemheart, a percutaneous left ventricular assist device, for circulatory support during high-risk percutaneous coronary intervention. Int J Cardiovasc Interv 2003;5:35-39.
2. Thiele H, Lauer B, Hambrecht R, et al: Reversal of cardiogenic shock by percutaneous left atrial-to-femoral arterial bypass assistance. Circulation 2001;104:2917-2922.

THORATEC INTRACORPOREAL VENTRICULAR ASSIST DEVICE

Device Classification

TABLE A13-1

Classification		
Category	Group	Sub-group
Duration	Long-term	
Type	Pulsatile	Pneumatic
Position	Partial implantable	Intra-abdominal

History of Development

To fulfill the need for a versatile intracorporeal VAD that can benefit a diverse patient population, an implantable version of the Thoratec VAD was developed in 1999.[1]

Mechanism of Device

The Thoratec intracorporeal VAD is an intracorporeal centrifugal-type device that is designed as a long-term implantable assist device with ongoing clinical trials (Fig. A13-1). It uses the same blood sac, actuation diaphragm, and unidirectional blood valves as the Thoratec VAD. This intracorporeal VAD, weighing 339 g, has a smooth-contoured, polished titanium alloy housing and a small-diameter flexible pneumatic line.

The pumping chamber is separated from the air chamber by a polyurethane actuation diaphragm. The diaphragm serves as a volume limiter and safety chamber. The blood-contacting geometry of the valve housings, the components that connect the cannula to the VAD, is identical for the two pumps. The only difference is the Thoratec VAD valve housings are constructed of stainless steel, whereas the intracorporeal VAD valve housings are constructed of titanium alloy. The cannulas for the intracorporeal VAD have the same internal dimensions and blood-contacting material as the cannulas used with the Thoratec VAD. The lengths of the cannulas are reduced to accommodate the intracorporeal placement of the intracorporeal VAD.[1-3] Preperitoneal or intraperitoneal position is used for left ventricular, right ventricular, or biventricular support. A separate pocket and one percutaneous pneumatic driveline are used for each intracorporeal VAD. The pneumatic line tunnel route is adjusted to maximize the length for tissue ingrowth.

Components

TABLE A13-2

Components		
Pump	Stroke volume (mL)	65
	Beats/min	NA
	Flow rate (L/min)	≤7.2
	Valves	Two Bjork-Shiley concave-convex, tilting-disc valves
	Position	Preperitoneal or intraperitoneal (Fig. A13-2)
Cannula	Inflow	Left ventricular apex for left VAD Right atrium for right VAD
	Outflow	Aorta and/or main pulmonary artery
Console	Dual-drive console	
	TLC-II	Portable VAD system (see Thoratec VAD) Docking station (see Thoratec VAD)
Others	Internal parts External parts	
NA, not available.		

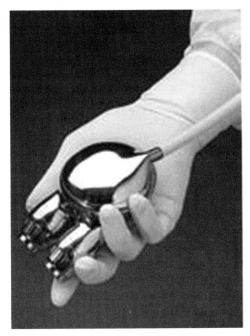

FIGURE A13-1 ■ Thoratec intracorporeal VAD. (Website: www.thoratec.com.)

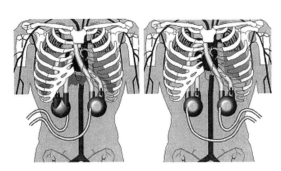

FIGURE A13-2 ■ Preperitoneal or intraperitoneal position for left, right, or biventricular support. (From Reichenbach SH, Farrar DJ, Hill JD: A versatile intracorporeal ventricular assist device based on the Thoratec VAD system. Ann Thorac Surg 2001;71(3 Suppl):S171-S175.)

Clinical Experience

On October 5, 2001, a 63-year-old German man became the first patient to be supported with the intracorporeal VAD. As of 2004, more than 25 patients have been supported with the Thoratec intracorporeal VAD with good results.

TABLE A13-3

Total Clinical Experience	
Total cases	>25
Duration of use	≤298 days
Patient age range	16-71 yr
Patient weight range	42-103 kg
Weaning rate	14% (3/22) (9 transplants)
Discharge rate	77% (17/22)

Complications

TABLE A13-4

Complications	
Complications	**Percentage**
Bleeding	32% (7/22)
Infection	27% (6/22)
Renal dysfunction	18% (4/22)
Hepatic dysfunction	14% (3/22)
Thromboembolism	0%
Neurologic dysfunction	5% (1/22)
Multisystem organ failure	14% (3/22)
Mechanical dysfunction	0%

Contact Information

Company: Thoratec Corporation

Address: 6035 Stoneridge Drive, Pleasanton, CA 94588, USA

Contact: Toll-free telephone: 1-800-528-2577; telephone: 925-847-8600; fax: 925-847-8574

Website: www.thoratec.com

Physician: Dr. David Farrar, Thoratec, Pleasanton, California, *or* Dr. Ronald Hill, University of California San Francisco, San Francisco, California

REFERENCES

1. el-Banayosy A, Minami K, Arusoglu L, et al: Long-term mechanical circulatory support. Thorac Cardiovasc Surg 1997;45:127-130.
2. Reichenbach SH, Farrar DJ, Hill JD: A versatile intracorporeal ventricular assist device based on the Thoratec VAD system. Ann Thorac Surg 2001;71(3 Suppl):S171-S175.
3. Farrar DJ, Reichenbach SH, Rossi SA, et al: Development of an intracorporeal Thoratec ventricular assist device for univentricular or biventricular support. ASAIO J 2000;46:351-353.

THORATEC VENTRICULAR ASSIST DEVICE

Another name for the Thoratec VAD is the Pierce-Donachy VAD.

Device Classification

TABLE A14-1

Classification		
Category	Group	Sub-group
Duration	Long-term	
Type	Pulsatile	Pneumatic
Position	Paracorporeal	

FIGURE A14-2 ■ Thoratec VAD. (Website: texasheartinstitute.org.)

History of Development

In 1970, a multidisciplinary group was established at the Pennsylvania State University to develop a left ventricular assist pump for use in patients with potentially reversible left ventricular failure.[1] In 1976, approval for clinical use was obtained,[2,3] and in 1996, the Thoratec VAD system received pre-marketing approval by the FDA for use as a bridge to cardiac transplantation. It also has received approval for use as a bridge to cardiac recovery. Currently, the Thoratec VAD system is the only device approved by the FDA that can provide left ventricular, right ventricular, or biventricular support for bridge to heart transplantation and recovery (Fig. A14-1).

Mechanism of Device

The Thoratec VAD is a pneumatic pulsatile system designed for univentricular or biventricular support. The system consists of a pulsatile pump, a series of cannulas for atrial or arterial connections, and a pneumatic drive console. The Thoratec VAD can be used for univentricular or biventricular support. In left ventricular support, the left VAD inflow cannula is inserted into the left ventricular apex or left atrium, and outflow graft is sutured to the ascending aorta. For right ventricular support, the right VAD withdraws blood from the right atrium and ejects outflow to the main pulmonary artery.

The pump consists of a seamless blood sac contained within a rigid polycarbonate housing (Fig. A14-2). The blood sac, composed of Thoratec's Thoralon, a proprietary polyurethane multipolymer, is compressed by air from the pneumatic driver to eject blood from the sac. A fill switch detects when the VAD is full of blood and automatically signals the console to eject blood from the pump. The pneumatic drive console provides alternating positive and negative air pressure to empty and fill the blood pump. The valves within the inflow and outflow conduits ensure unidirectional blood flow.

The Thoratec VAD can be operated in three control modes—asynchronous (fix rate), volume (full-to-empty

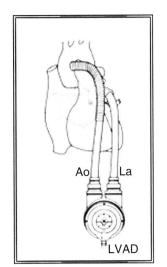
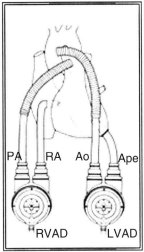
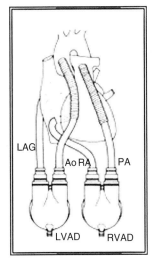

FIGURE A14-1 ■ The Thoratec VAD can be used for univentricular or biventricular support. (Website: www.thoratec.com.)

variable rate), and synchronous mode.[3,4] Volume mode is preferred because it maximizes support of the cardiac output. A briefcase-sized portable device unit, the Thoratec TLC-II portable VAD device, has been developed.

Components

TABLE A14-2

Components		
Pump	Stroke volume (mL)	65
	Beats/min	20-110
	Flow rate (L/min)	1.3-7.2
	Valves	Two Bjork-Shikey tilting-disc valves
	Position	Externally on the skin of the upper abdomen
Cannula	Inflow	Left atrium or left ventricular apex (left VAD)
		Right atrium (right VAD)
	Outflow	Aorta (left VAD) or main pulmonary artery (right VAD)
Console	Dual-drive console	Model 2600 or 2601 (Fig. A14-3)
	TLC-II	Portable VAD system (9.8 kg) (Fig. A14-4)
		Docking station (Fig. A14-5)
Other components	Internal parts	Flow sensor
	External parts	Auxiliary battery

Clinical Experience

The Thoratec VAD was first used clinically in 1977 for postcardiotomy support,[4] in 1982 in a pediatric patient, and in 1984 as a bridge to cardiac transplantation.[5]

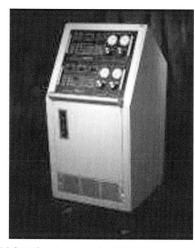

FIGURE A14-3 ■ Thoratec console. (Website: www.thoratec.com.)

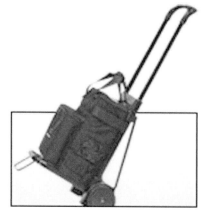

FIGURE A14-4 ■ TLC-II portable VAD driver. (Website: www. thoratec.com.)

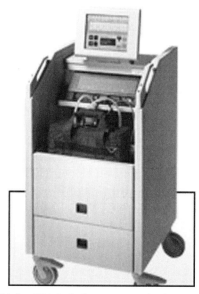

FIGURE A14-5 ■ TLC-II docking station. (Website: www.thoratec. com.)

As of January 2004, more than 2500 patients have been implanted with this device. The longest duration is more than 1.5 years. Currently, the Thoratec VAD system has been used in almost 200 medical centers worldwide. The total survival rate for 1 year is 25% to 61%.[6-13] As of January 2005, Thoratec VADs have been

TABLE A14-3

Total Clinical Experience	
Total cases	3835 devices in 2511 patients
Duration of use	≤566 days
Patient age range	6-77 yr
Patient weight range	17-144 kg
Weaning rate	37-72%
Discharge rate	21-66%

Data from references 6-10.

implanted in 177 pediatric patients worldwide, and the survival rate is about 70%. Results are comparable with results in adult patients and are independent of age or body size (Farrar DJ: Private communication).

Complications

TABLE A14-4

Complications	
Complications	Percentage
Bleeding	26-45%
Infection	13-52%
Renal dysfunction	13-36%
Thromboembolism	4-8%
Neurologic dysfunction	11-27%
Multisystem organ failure	5-25%
Mechanical dysfunction	7-13%

Data from references 6-13.

Contact Information

Company: Thoratec Corporation

Address: 6035 Stoneridge Drive, Pleasanton, CA 94588, USA

Contact: Toll-free telephone: 1-800-528-2577; telephone: 925-847-8600; fax: 925-847-8574

Website: www.thoratec.com

Physician: Dr. David Farrar, Thoratec, Pleasanton, California, *or* Dr. Ronald Hill, University of California San Francisco, San Francisco, California

REFERENCES

1. Pierce WS, Brighton JA, O'Bannon W, et al: Complete left ventricular bypass with a paracorporeal pump: Design and evaluation. Ann Surg 1974;180:418.

2. Pierce WS, Donachy JH, Landis DL, et al: Prolonged mechanical support of the left ventricle. Circulation 1978;58(Suppl I):I-133-I-146.

3. Olsen EK, Shaffer LJ, Pae WE, et al: Biventricular mechanical assistance in the postcardiotomy patient. Trans Am Soc Artif Intern Organs 1980;26:29-32.

4. Hill JD, Farrar DJ, Hershon JJ, et al: Use of a prosthetic ventricle as a bridge to cardiac transplantation for postinfarction cardiogenic shock. N Engl J Med 1986;314:626-628.

5. Farrar DJ, Hill JD, Gray LA, et al: Heterotopic prosthetic ventricles as a bridge to cardiac transplantation: A multicenter study in 29 patients. N Engl J Med 1988;318:333-340.

6. Pennington DG, McBride LR, Swartz MT, et al: Use of the Pierce-Donachy ventricular assist device in patients with cardiogenic shock after cardiac operations. Ann Thorac Surg 1989;47: 130-135.

7. Reinhartz O, Keith FM, El-Banayosy A, et al: Multicenter experience with the Thoratec ventricular assist device in children and adolescents. J Heart Lung Transplant 2001;20:439-448.

8. Reinhartz O, Copeland JG, Farrar DJ: Thoratec ventricular assist devices in children with less than 1.3 m² of body surface area. ASAIO J 2003;49:727-730.

9. Reichenbach SH, Farrar DJ, Hill JD: A versatile intracorporeal ventricular assist device based on the thoratec VAD system. Ann Thorac Surg 2001;71:S171-S175.

10. Korfer R, El-Banayosy A, Arusoglu L, et al: Single-center experience with the Thoratec ventricular assist device. J Thorac Cardiovasc Surg 2000;119:596-600.

11. Farrar DJ, Hill JD: Univentricular and biventricular assist devices. Ann Thorac Surg 1993;55:276.

12. McBride LR, Naunheim KS, Fiore AC, et al: Clinical experience with 111 Thoratec ventricular assist devices. Ann Thorac Surg 1999;67:1233.

13. Goldstein DJ, Oz MC: Mechanical support for postcardiotomy cardiogenic shock. Semin Thorac Cardiovasc Surg 2000;12:220.

TOYOBO TYPE VENTRICULAR SYSTEM

Device Classification

TABLE A15-1

Classification		
Category	Group	Sub-group
Duration	Long-term	
Type	Pulsatile	Pneumatic
Position	Paracorporeal	

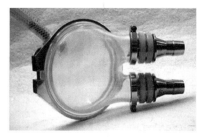

FIGURE A15-1 ■ Toyobo pump. (Website: www.schulli.de.)

History of Development

The Toyobo-NCVC type VAD was developed at the National Cardiovascular Center in Osaka, Japan, in the early 1980s.[1] On January 13, 1990, this device was approved for commercial release by the Japanese government.

Mechanism of Device

The Toyobo pump is a paracorporeal pneumatic diaphragm device made of Toyobo series segmented polyether polyurethane without a seam (Fig. A15-1). Unidirectional blood flow is achieved by two Bjork-Shiley valves located in the inlet and outlet tracts. Two sizes of pumps have been developed (20 mL and 70 mL) and the maximum output is 7 L/minute and 2.4 L/minute.

The two types of control drive unit are the standard type with two regular and two backup drives and the compact type with one regular driver and one backup driver. The main part of the control device unit consists of an automatic blood flow control system and an automatic ECG synchronization system.[2-4]

Components

TABLE A15-2

Components		
Pump	Stroke volume (mL)	20, 70
	Beats/min	80-100
	Flow rate (L/min)	2.4, 7
	Valves	Two Bjork-Shiley valves
	Position	Paracorporeal
Cannula	Inflow	Left atrium
	Outflow	Ascending aorta
Console	Blood flow control system	
	ECG synchronization system	
Other components	Internal parts	
	External parts	

Clinical Experience

Between 1982 and 2000, 362 patients were implanted with the Toyobo pneumatic extracorporeal ventricular assist system (Yosuke K: Private communication). The data before 1994 showed 124 patients supported by this device. The duration of ventricular assist system application ranged from 1 hour to 192 days; the mean was 14.3 days.[2-4] The Toyobo pump has been implanted in 7 children ranging in age from 9 months to 10 years. Three children were weaned from VAD, but none were long-term survivors.[4]

TABLE A15-3

Total Clinical Experience	
Total cases	362
Duration of use	≤390 days
Patient age range	9 mo-82 yr
Patient weight range	NA
Weaning rate	47.6-52.2%
Discharge rate	22.8-25%

NA, not available.
Data from references 2-4 and Yosuke K: Private communication.

Complications

TABLE A15-4

Complications	
Complications	Percentage
Bleeding	50%
Infection	NA
Respiratory dysfunction	17.7%
Renal dysfunction	NA
Thromboembolism	21.5-25%
Neurologic dysfunction	50%
Multisystem organ failure	24.8-50%
Mechanical dysfunction	~25%

NA, not available.
Data from references 2-4.

Contact Information

Company: Toyobo Co., Ltd

Address: 3-9-3 Honjo-Nishi Kita-Ku, Osaka, 531-8510, Japan

Contact: Telephone: 81-6-6372-2331; fax: 81-6-6375-0669

Website: www.nipro.co.jp (Japanese)

Physician: Not available

REFERENCES

1. Taenaka Y, Takano H, Nakatani T, et al: Ventricular assist device (VAD) for children: In vitro and in vivo evaluation. Trans Am Soc Artif Intern Organs 1984;30:155-158.

2. Masai T, Shimazaki Y, Kadoba K, et al: Clinical experience with long-term use of the Toyobo left ventricular assist system. ASAIO J 1995;41:M522-M525.

3. Takano H, Taenaka Y, Noda H, et al: Multi-institutional studies of the National Cardiovascular Center Ventricular Assist System: Use in 92 patients. ASAIO Trans 1989;35:541-544.

4. Takano H, Nakatani T: Ventricular assist systems: Experience in Japan with Toyobo pump and Zeon pump. Ann Thorac Surg 1996;61:317-322.

Glossary of Heart Failure

Jeffrey Kim
Anthony C. Chang

A

Actin Cytoskeletal protein composed of two helical strands that, along with tropomyosin and troponin complex, constitute the thin filament of the sarcomere.

Adenylate cyclase Enzyme that catalyzes the formation of cAMP from ATP, which, on activation, leads to increased intracellular calcium and an increased inotropic state of the myocardium.

Afterload Interaction of all the factors that contribute to total myocardial wall stress or tension during systolic ejection, or the force that resists myofibril shortening. Indices of afterload include aortic pressure, total peripheral resistance, arterial elastance, and myocardial peak wall stress.

Aldosterone Steroid hormone that is secreted by the zona glomerulosa of the adrenal cortex in response to changes in fluid and electrolyte balance and blood pressure, which acts directly on the kidney to decrease sodium ion excretion (leading to the retention of water) and increase potassium and hydrogen ion excretion.

American Heart Association/American College of Cardiology classification A more current classification scheme for adults with heart failure that is based on the evolution and progression of heart failure (stages A-D).

Angiotensin II Effector polypeptide of the RAS with important vasoconstrictive properties, resulting in renal and extrarenal effects, such as vasoconstriction of efferent arterioles of the glomerulus and increased sodium reabsorption of the proximal tubular epithelium.

Angiotensin-converting enzyme (ACE) Enzyme that acts on angiotensin I (by cleaving two amino acids from the C-terminal end) to form angiotensin II (site of action for the drug class ACE inhibitors).

Angiotensin-converting enzyme (ACE) inhibitors Class of drugs that acts by inhibiting the conversion of angiotensin I to angiotensin II and by preventing the degradation of bradykinin.

Angiotensin receptor blocker (ARB) Class of drugs that ameliorates the effects of the RAS in heart failure by blocking angiotensin II receptors AT_1 and AT_2 (losartan and candesartan).

Apoptosis The regulated process in which cells undergo programmed cell death with cell shrinkage and condensation of cytoplasm and nuclear materials that yields orderly fragmentation of DNA.

Area-length method Common method of measuring left ventricular volume by using a manually traced endocardial outline and calculated axial length and diameter.

Arginine vasopressin (*see vasopressin*)

Arrhythmogenic right ventricular dysplasia (ARVD) A genetic, progressive disorder of the myocardium resulting in fibrosis and fatty infiltration of the right ventricular free wall, leading to cardiomyopathy and arrhythmias (incidence 1 in 5000).

Arterial elastances (Ea) The ratio of end-systolic pressure and stroke volume (Pes/SV) as a measure of arterial load and as represented by the slope of the line joining the end-diastolic and end-systolic points.

Atrial natriuretic peptide (ANP) (see also *natriuretic peptides*) Cyclic 28-amino acid polypeptide with natriuretic properties, which is synthesized predominantly from the atria and is secreted in response to tension and stretch of the atrial wall.

Axial device Category of assist devices that involves an axial pump mechanism (DeBakey VAD and Jarvik 2000).

B

Barth syndrome An X-linked recessive disorder consisting of neutropenia, cardiomyopathy, muscle weakness, and failure to thrive.

Batista procedure (partial left ventricular ventriculectomy) Surgical resection of the left ventricle between the anterior and posterior papillary muscles (along with a mitral valve repair or replacement) initially used for cardiomyopathy related to Chagas disease.

Bradykinin (*see kinins*)

Braking effect The phenomenon in which decreased clinical responsiveness to diuretics with time is observed, most likely secondary to sodium retention.

Bridge-to-bridge The concept of using a mechanical support device to support the failed myocardium and transitioning the first device to another device that is more suited for longer term support.

Bridge-to-transplantation The concept of using a mechanical support device to support the failed myocardium until a donor heart becomes available for a longer term heart replacement.

Please see other appendices for specific drugs, adult clinical trials, and mechanical assist devices.

B-type natriuretic peptide (BNP) Cardiac neurohormone produced from the cardiac ventricles during states of systolic or diastolic dysfunction and along with ANP, forms a counter-regulatory system against the RAS with its effects of natriuresis and vasodilation.

C

Calcium-sensitizing agents New class of drug that works by binding to troponin C and increasing myocardial calcium sensitivity during systole, increasing contractility without increasing cAMP or intracellular calcium.

Calcium-triggered calcium release The phenomenon in which a small calcium inward current via the L-type calcium channels triggers calcium release from the sarcoplasmic reticulum.

Calmodulin Calcium storage protein with four binding sites in the cytoplasm.

Calsequestrin High-capacity, low-affinity calcium binding protein found in the sarcoplasmic reticulum that acts as a calcium sink.

Carbonic anhydrase inhibitors Agents that produce an alkaline diuresis by inhibiting membrane-bound and cytoplasmic carbonic anhydrase and by blocking sodium bicarbonate reabsorption, increasing excretion of sodium, potassium, bicarbonate, and water.

Cardiac resynchronization therapy (CRT) Pacing therapy that attempts to re-establish the synchronous contraction between the left ventricular free wall and the interventricular septum so that left ventricular efficiency is maximized.

Centrifugal pump A rotary pump that works via a constrained vortex and is able to maintain venous inflow independent of gravity drainage.

Chamber stiffness Ability of the ventricular chamber to distend under pressure, constituting an important part of passive relaxation during diastole (can be derived from the EDPVR [slope dP/dV]).

Cheyne-Stokes respiration–central sleep apnea (CSR-CSA) A periodic breathing disorder common in heart failure patients, characterized by apnea and hypopnea alternating with ventilatory periods.

Chymase Alternate pathway for production of angiotensin II in tissue that is independent of the converting enzyme.

Compliance The inverse of stiffness that is calculated by the change in volume for a given change in pressure (dV/dP).

Conductance catheter Catheters integrated with high-fidelity pressure sensors that generate real-time, pressure-volume loops for assessing myocardial performance.

Constrictive pericarditis A disease of the pericardium that results in restricted cardiac filling and cardiac compression from a diseased or scarred pericardium.

Contractility Intrinsic ability of the myofibers of the heart to generate force (not synonymous with systolic function).

CorCap A unique polyester knit, netlike device that is positioned around the cardiac ventricles and is anchored to the atrioventricular groove as a passive ventricular constraint support device.

Costamere Site of interconnection between various cytoskeletal networks linking sarcomere and sarcolemma, which functions as an anchor site for stabilization of the sarcolemma and for integration of pathways involved in mechanical force transduction.

Coupling Interaction, such as that of the G protein and the adrenergic receptor, that links an activated receptor to a specific biologic response.

Coxsackie-adenoviral receptor (CAR) Transmembrane protein with immunoglobulin-like domains that binds coxsackievirus and adenovirus and allows internalization of the virus genome.

C-type natriuretic peptide (CNP) The third member of the natriuretic family, which acts not centrally as the other two natriuretic hormones, but locally in the vasculature as a vasodilatory agent.

Cycle efficiency The relationship between the mechanical work done by a ventricle to the maximal work possible for given changes in pressure and volume.

Cytokines Biologic mediators that provide a molecular infrastructure for immune modulation of cardiac function.

D

Danon disease An X-linked dominant disorder resulting from a deficiency of LAMP-2 (lysosomes-associated membrane protein 2) characterized by intracytoplasmic vacuoles in cardiac and skeletal muscle cells, leading to cardiomyopathy, skeletal myopathy, and varying degrees of mental retardation.

Deflecting accelerating factor (DAF) Factor that acts as a coreceptor to enhance the binding efficiency of coxsackievirus B onto the DAF-CAR complex to permit the uncoating of the viral genome and to facilitate internalization.

Desensitization A decreased affinity of the adrenergic receptors for circulating catecholamines.

Desmin Intermediate filament protein of the cytoskeleton that is associated with Z lines and contributes to myofibril integrity and force transmission.

Destination therapy Term usually used to refer to mechanical support devices that are meant to be an alternative therapy (versus bridge) to orthotopic heart transplantation.

Dilated cardiomyopathy A heterogeneous group of myocardial disorders that result in ventricular dilation and impaired systolic contractile function.

Doppler tissue imaging (DTI) Novel method of assessing quantitative longitudinal and radial ventricular function by measuring pulse-wave Doppler velocities directly from underlying myocardium.

Dor procedure An endoventricular circular patch plasty repair of the left ventricle (to exclude the areas that are akinetic or dyskinetic) with associated coronary grafting or surgical ventricular restoration used for patients with left ventricular dysfunction after an infarction with resultant akinesis or dyskinesis.

Double-switch operation An anatomic surgical correction for congenitally corrected transposition of the great arteries (ccTGA) (atrial switch with an arterial switch for ccTGA without pulmonary stenosis and a Rastelli repair with an atrial switch operation for ccTGA with pulmonary stenosis or atresia).

Dynamic cardiomyoplasty Procedure that entails the training of skeletal (latissimus dorsi) muscle to contract in concert with ventricular muscle (via electrical pacing) to assist or boost its function.

Dystrophin Sarcomeric protein associated with a transmembrane glycoprotein complex, which connects the actin-myosin complex with the extracellular matrix of the cardiomyocyte, the disruption of which results in myocardial dysfunction.

E

Ejection fraction (EF) Change in ventricular volume during the cardiac cycle usually measured by the modified Simpson biplane method and calculated by the equation: EF (%) = ([LVEDV − LVESV] / LVEDV) × 100.

Elastance (*see end-systolic and arterial elastances*)

End-diastolic pressure-volume relationship (EDPVR) The nonlinear relationship of pressure and volume during ventricular diastole, which represents an index of diastolic function, or ventricular compliance, with the assumption that the ventricle exhibits elastic behavior.

Endocardial fibroelastosis (EFE) Cardiomyopathy that is characterized by excessive endocardial thickening secondary to proliferation of fibrous and elastic components.

Endomyocardial fibrosis (EMF) Cardiomyopathy typified by fibrosis of the endocardium in three main regions (right ventricular and left ventricular apical areas and the mitral valve apparatus) that occurs in patients who have lived in tropical regions.

Endothelin Endothelium-derived vasoactive peptide with vasoconstrictive properties, which is also a potent inducer of cardiac hypertrophy.

Endothelin receptor antagonists Agents that selectively or nonselectively block the endothelin receptors (ET$_A$ and ET$_B$) (darusentan and sitaxsentan).

End-systolic elastance (Ees) An index of systolic contractile function (in units of elastance, mm Hg/mL) represented by the upper left-hand corner of the pressure-volume loop (slope of ESPVR), which is relatively resistant to changes in loading conditions.

End-systolic pressure-volume relationship (ESPVR) A useful measure of ventricular contractility represented by the upper left-hand corner of variable loaded pressure-volume loops (slope Ees).

End-systolic wall stress (σ_{es}) A measurement of ventricular afterload that is used to measure ventricular contractility in the stress-velocity index.

Epinephrine Endogenous catecholamine secreted by the adrenal medulla, which stimulates β_2-receptors, resulting in increased heart rate, increased cardiac contractility, and increased peripheral vasoconstriction.

Epithelial sodium channel inhibitors Also known as potassium-sparing diuretics, agents that directly block the sodium-selective channels.

Extracorporeal life support (ECLS) Broad term that entails all modes of mechanical support (mainly ECMO and VAD) for the failed cardiopulmonary system.

Extracorporeal membrane oxygenation (ECMO) Mode of cardiopulmonary support used primarily in small children with cardiopulmonary failure, which consists of either a roller pump system with a servoregulatory mechanism or a centrifugal pump for controlling circuit flow and a membrane or hollow fiber oxygenator.

F

Fabry disease An X-linked recessive disorder with deficiency of α-galactosidase that leads to hypertrophic cardiomyopathy and mitral insufficiency in affected males.

Force-frequency relationship The intrinsic property of the myocardium to alter contractile force with change in frequency of stimulation (also known as the "treppe" effect).

Force-velocity relationship The ability of the myocyte to shorten more rapidly and to a greater degree when faced with a lighter load.

Frank-Starling relationship Length dependence of the heart function that is manifested by increased contractile force with augmented preload or resting length.

G

G protein The guanine nucleotide regulatory protein, which, by its interaction with adenylate cyclase, allows adrenergic receptors to mediate their biologic activities.

Guyton diagrams Physiologic diagrams with venous return, atrial pressure, and cardiac output.

H

Hemodynamic defense response The homeostatic mechanisms observed in heart failure, which include salt and water retention, vasoconstriction, and cardiac stimulation.

Hydrops fetalis End-stage fetal heart failure manifested by pleural or pericardial effusions, ascites, and generalized skin edema.

Hypereosinophilic syndrome (HES) or Löffler endocarditis Cardiomyopathy similar to EMF, but typified by varying degrees of eosinophilic myocarditis.

I

Impedance Opposition to flow. (see *vascular impedance*).

Inositol triphosphate receptor Specialized calcium release channel in the sarcoplasmic reticulum (similar to the ryanodine receptor), which is increased in myocytes under heart failure conditions.

Intercalated disc The specialized area of interdigitating cell membrane where cardiac myocytes are joined at each end.

Intercellular cell adhesion molecules (ICAM) Molecules that promote leukocyte adherence and transendothelial migration.

Interleukin A cytokine believed to be involved in changes observed with heart failure in the myocyte, particularly in the forms of IL-1 and IL-6.

Intra-aortic balloon pump (IABP) A percutaneously placed device that uses a counterpulsation technique to improve diastolic pressure in the aorta and coronary perfusion (by inflating the balloon during diastole) and reduce afterload (by deflating the balloon during systole).

Isovolumic contraction The phase of the cardiac cycle during which the ventricular volume remains constant and the aortic pressure still exceeds left ventricular pressure; there is an increase in left ventricular pressure without change in left ventricular volume.

Isovolumic relaxation The phase of the cardiac cycle during which the ventricular volume remains constant and the ventricle is relaxed with decrease in pressure while the mitral valve remains closed.

J

JAK-STAT pathway A functional signal-transduction mechanism in the context of interferon signaling.

Janus kinase (JAK) Intracellular receptor–associated tyrosine kinase that plays a role in rapid transduction of signals from the cell surface to the nucleus and together with the signal transducer and activators of transcription (STAT) form the JAK-STAT pathway.

K

Kearns-Sayre syndrome Mitochondrial myopathy that is characterized by ptosis, chronic progressive external ophthalmoplegia, abnormal retinal pigmentation, cardiac conduction defects, and dilated cardiomyopathy.

Kinins Potent vasodilatory peptides that have a broad spectrum of activities, such as diuresis and natriuresis and myocardial protective effects.

L

Lamins A + C Nuclear envelope proteins that form the intermediate filaments.

Left ventricular noncompaction Rare form of dilated cardiomyopathy that is characterized by a developmental arrest in the normal compaction of the ventricular endocardium resulting in prominent trabeculations with deep recesses within the myocardium.

Levosimendan Calcium-sensitizing drug that improves the inotropic state of the heart by increasing the interaction between troponin C and calcium without increasing intracellular calcium.

Löffler endocarditis (see *hypereosinophilic syndrome (HES)*).

L-type calcium channel (also dihydropyridine receptor) Sarcolemmal membrane calcium channel that contributes to the cardiac action potential in ventricular cells, but also triggers the opening of the sarcoplasmic reticulum calcium channels, initiating excitation-contraction.

M

Maze procedure An intraoperative electrophysiologic procedure that reduces the likelihood of postoperative intra-atrial reentrant tachycardia.

Mineralocorticoid/glucocorticoid receptor antagonists Agents that inhibit the reabsorption of sodium in the distal convoluted tubule and collecting duct.

Mitochondrial cardiomyopathy Cardiomyopathy secondary to mitochondrial diseases, most commonly respiratory chain defects.

Myocardial performance index (MPI) (also known as the Tei index) Doppler-derived quantitative measure of global ventricular function that incorporates systolic and diastolic time intervals and measures the ratio of total time in isovolumic activity divided by the time in ventricular ejection.

Myocardial stiffness Resistance of the myocardium to stretch when subjected to stress, expressed as the slope ($d\sigma/d\varepsilon$) of a tangent drawn to the stress-strain relationship at that strain; along with chamber stiffness, constitutes passive relaxation during diastole.

Myocarditis Inflammation of the heart with four distinct clinicopathologic subtypes that include acute myocarditis, fulminant myocarditis, chronic active myocarditis, and chronic persistent myocarditis.

Myosin Thick filament protein that consists of six polypeptides separated into a tail section with long heavy chains and a globular head section with two sets of light chains. The head sections form cross-bridges with actin to result in sarcomere shortening.

Myosin-binding protein C Sarcomere protein that is located in the sarcomere A bands and binds myosin heavy chains and titin in elastic filaments.

Myosplint A transcavitary tensioning device that consists of three rods with wide buttons at either end, which changes the left ventricular shape from globular to bilobular.

N

Natriuretic peptides These agents (ANP, BNP, and urodilatin) cause renal afferent arteriolar dilation and efferent arteriolar constriction, leading to an increase in glomerular filtration while antagonizing intrarenal vasoconstriction.

New York Heart Association (NYHA) classification A functional classification for adults with heart failure that assigns patients to one of four classes (I-IV) depending on the degree of effort needed to elicit symptoms of angina, fatigue, dyspnea, or palpitations.

Nitric oxide Small gaseous molecule that has potent vasodilatory effects via cGMP, but also has negative cardiac effects, including myocardial depression, apoptosis, and β-adrenergic desensitization.

Nitrovasodilators Pharmacologic agents that produce vascular smooth muscle relaxation by mimicking the activity of nitric oxide, activating guanylate cyclase and cGMP.

Norepinephrine Secreted by the adrenal medulla and by sympathetic nerves close to vasculature, which results in intense vasoconstriction and myocyte hypertrophy; also a useful heart failure biomarker.

Nuclear factor κB (NF-κB) Dimeric nuclear transcription factor that is liberated from its inhibitory component on activation to result in activation of cytokines (as seen in chronic heart failure).

O

Osmotic diuretics Agents that act by increasing the osmotic pressure of the glomerular filtrate, which inhibits tubular reabsorption of water and electrolytes.

P

Panel reactive antibodies (PRA) Antibodies detected by testing the recipient's serum against a panel of lymphocytes from numerous donors selected to represent all of the common HLA antigens.

Phosphodiesterase inhibitors Inotropic agents that work independent of β-adrenergic receptors by inhibiting phosphodiesterase and increasing cAMP and intracellular calcium.

Phospholamban Inhibitory regulatory protein of the sarcoplasmic reticulum calcium pump, which when phosphorylated, changes its configuration and detaches from SERCA to allow calcium sequestration to take place.

Platelet-derived growth factor (PDGF) Factor that can stimulate myocardial fibrosis.

Polymerase chain reaction (PCR) The amplification process of specific genomes, which is sensitive and specific.

Pompe disease Genetic deficiency of acid α-1,4-glucosidase (involved in the breakdown of glycogen to glucose), which results in organomegaly and hypertrophic cardiomyopathy.

Post-transplant lymphoproliferative disorders (PTLD) Post-transplant complication that has a bimodal presentation and can be protean, with early-onset disease possessing a less aggressive polymorphic histology and late-onset disease possessing variable histology, but often consistent with aggressive B cell lymphoma.

Potential energy Energy produced during contraction that does not result in stroke work and comprises the triangular area bounded by the ESPVR line, the EDPVR line, and the left border of the pressure-volume loop.

Preload All the factors that contribute to passive ventricular wall stress or tension at the end of diastole; myocardial cell length, which underpins Starling's law.

Pressure-volume area The sum of stroke work and potential energy that is linearly related to myocardial oxygen consumption.

Pressure-volume relationship The interaction between pressure and volume in the ventricle during the cardiac cycle that has provided a foundation for the understanding of ventricular function.

Pulsatile device The category of ventricular assist devices that involves a pneumatic paracorporeal configuration (Berlin Heart VAD, Thoratec Ventricular Assist System, and HeartMate VE LVAD).

R

Receptor down-regulation Decreased density of adrenergic receptors secondary to chronic exposure to catecholamines.

Regurgitant fraction (RF) The difference between the angiographic measurement of stroke volume and that determined by the Fick and thermodilution methods.

Relaxation constant (τ) The rate of left ventricular pressure decay measured during early relaxation; the inverse slope of the linear relationship between the natural log of ventricular diastolic pressure plotted against time.

Remodeling The geometry-altering process in which the heart undergoes chronic maladaptive changes, involving cardiomyocytes, fibroblasts, and the extracellular matrix secondary to excessive circulating catecholamines and mediators, such as renin, angiotensin, and aldosterone.

Renin The proteolytic enzyme synthesized, stored, and secreted from the juxtaglomerular apparatus in the renal cortex to generate angiotensin II (via angiotensinogen and angiotensin I).

Renin-angiotensin system (RAS) Neurohormonal system that is activated in heart failure, which leads to vasoconstriction, decreased diuresis, and sodium retention, ultimately resulting in myocardial fibrosis.

Restrictive cardiomyopathy Cardiomyopathy characterized by restrictive filling with dilated atria and reduced diastolic volume of either or both ventricles with normal or near-normal systolic function and wall thicknesses.

Reverse remodeling The reversal of maladaptive heart failure processes secondary to excessive circulating catecholamines and mediators, such as renin, angiotensin, and aldosterone.

Ross classification A classification system for infants with heart failure that parallels the NYHA classification scheme.

Ross procedure Implantation of the native pulmonary valve in the aortic position and replacement of the pulmonary valve with a homograft.

Ross score A scoring system for infants with heart failure based on time and volume per feeding, respiratory rate and pattern, and cardiac examination.

Rotary devices Category of assist devices that involves centrifugal or axial pump mechanisms (DeBakey VAD and Jarvik 2000).

Ryanodine receptor (also termed calcium release channel) The calcium release channel in the sarcoplasmic reticulum that allows for release of large amounts of calcium into the cytoplasm to initiate the actin-myosin interaction.

S

Sarcoglycan Transmembrane protein that associates with dystrophin and links cytoskeleton to the extracellular matrix.

Sarcolemma The cell membrane of the myocyte, which has deep invaginations called t-tubules that allow for rapid spread of action potentials and inflow of extracellular calcium into the intracellular space.

Sarcomere The fundamental morphologic unit of the contractile apparatus in the myocyte that consists of contractile proteins (myosin, actin, troponin, and tropomyosin) and cytoskeletal proteins (dystrophin, desmin, titin, and others).

Sarcoplasmic reticulum Intracellular membranous network, which, along with the transverse tubules of the sarcolemma, is involved in the excitation-contraction and relaxation processes.

Sarcoplasmic reticulum calcium pump (SERCA) The calcium pump that sequesters calcium during the relaxation of the myocyte and is regulated by its inhibitory subunit, phospholamban.

Sequential nephron hypertrophy (also segmental nephron hypertrophy) Compensatory hypertrophy of the tubular epithelium distal to the site of action of loop diuretics that results in an increased ability for the tubule to reabsorb solutes.

Shortening fraction (SF) The change in left ventricular short-axis diameter calculated by the equation: SF(%) = ([LVEDD − LVESD] / LVEDD) × 100 (normal values range from 28% to 44%).

Signal transducer and activators of transcription (STAT) Unique class of transcription factors that play a role in the transcriptional regulation of multiple genes.

Simpson rule Method of estimating ventricular volume by summed volumes of graduated discs.

Sodium-calcium exchanger (NCX) The main calcium extrusion mechanism in the heart that exchanges sodium for calcium across the cardiac sarcolemma and is reversible (can operate in forward or reverse modes to result in calcium efflux or influx).

Sodium-chloride cotransporter inhibitors Formerly known as thiazide-like diuretics, these agents act by inhibiting the reabsorption of the sodium-chloride cotransporter in the distal convoluted tubule and increase the urinary excretion of sodium and chloride.

Sodium-potassium-chloride cotransporter inhibitors Formerly known as loop diuretics, agents that act by reversibly inhibiting the sodium-potassium-chloride cotransport system in the thick ascending limb of the loop of Henle and increase the excretion of sodium, potassium, chloride, hydrogen, and water.

Starling's equation Equation that describes the forces driving fluid filtration in the lung as: $Q_f = K_f [(P_{mv} − P_{pmv}) − \delta(P_{mv} − P_{pmv})]$ (see text for abbreviations).

Steady-state free procession (SSFP) MRI Commonly used ECG-gated cine MRI technique that results in high contrast between blood and myocardium for assessment of ventricular function.

Strain rate imaging Echocardiographic technique used to measure regional elongation and shortening (deformation) of myocardial tissue segments.

Stress-velocity index Inverse linear relationship between Vcf_c and end-systolic wall stress (σ_{es}) that is independent of preload, normalized for heart rate, and incorporates afterload.

Stroke work The pressure-volume loop area that represents the external work done by the heart.

Systolic function   A factor of contractility, preload, and afterload that can be impaired while the contractility is normal; not synonymous with contractility.

T

Tafazzin   Cytoskeletal protein with unknown function.

Tei index (see *myocardial performance index*)

Thick filaments   Interdigitating myosin molecules that make up the H zone of the sarcomere.

Thin filaments   Monomers of α-actin that are arranged into long intertwined filaments, which, along with the Z line, constitute the I band of the sarcomere.

Titin   Large sarcomere cytoskeletal protein that participates in sarcomere organization and the Z line complex.

Toll-like receptors (TLRs)   Receptors that are homologues of the *Drosophila* toll and are responsible for up-regulating the expression of a variety of inflammatory mediators.

Transforming growth factor (TGF)   Factor that can simulate myocardial fibrosis.

Treppe effect   (see *force-frequency relationship*).

Triiodothyronine (T₃)   Thyroid hormone with a role in regulation of the heart via its many actions, such as up-regulation of β-receptors, increased synthesis of contractile proteins, and stimulation of L-type calcium channels.

Troponin   Heterotrimer that consists of troponins C, I, and T and provides the substrate for the biochemical interaction that initiates actin-myosin interaction. Troponins I and T are intracellular cytoskeletal proteins that are sensitive and specific for acute myocardial injury.

Tropomyosin   A support protein with double-stranded polypeptide chains that stretch along the longitudinal grooves of actin strands.

T-tubules   Deep invaginations of the myocyte cell membrane that allow for rapid spread of action potentials and inflow of extracellular calcium into the intracellular space.

Tumor necrosis factor (TNF)-α   Multifunctional cytokine that has a central role in the systemic inflammatory response and is up-regulated in heart failure with myocardial depressant effects.

Tumor necrosis factor (TNF)-α inhibitors   Pharmacologic agents that block the proinflammatory effects of TNF-α (etanercept and infliximab).

U

Urodilatin   Natriuretic peptide that comes from the renal distal tubular cells.

V

Vascular impedance   Vascular load that varies with the cardiac cycle as a result of the combination of the pulsatile nature of blood flow and pressure, elastic properties of blood vessels, and blood inertia.

Vasopeptidase inhibitors   Agents that inactivate neutral endopeptidases to prolong the biologic half-life of natriuretic peptides (candoxatril and ecadotril).

Vasopressin   Polypeptide that is formed in the supraoptic nuclei of the hypothalamus and is secreted by the posterior pituitary gland in the regulation of fluid balance via its antidiuretic action; also a potent vasoconstrictor.

Vasopressin antagonist   Agents designed to overcome effects of vasopressin by blocking V_{1a} and V_2 receptors (conivaptan and relcovaptan).

Vasopressin V₂ receptor antagonists   New agents that increase free water clearance by inhibiting the action of vasopressin and by down-regulating the aquaporin-2 water channel expression.

Velocity of circumferential fiber shortening (Vcf)   A noninvasive index of contractility (corrected for heart rate is Vcfc) that is calculated using the equation: Vcf = [LVEDD − LVESD] / [LVEDD × LVET] (see text for abbreviations).

Ventricular assist device (VAD)   Mechanical device that provides support (usually via a pneumatic or a rotary mechanism) to the failing ventricle either as an acute support device or as a longer term (>3 weeks) device.

Ventricular interdependence   The concept that volume change of one ventricle affects the other based on mechanisms such as a noncompliant pericardial sac and the series relationship between the right and left ventricles.

Ventriculoarterial coupling (V-A coupling)   Coupling between ventricle and vasculature that reflects the mechanical efficiency of the heart, which is determined by the relationship between arterial and end-systolic elastances (Ea to Ees).

W

Wall stress (σ)   Calculated by: $\sigma = [P \times r] / 2h$, where *P* is chamber pressure, *r* is radius, and *h* is thickness of the chamber wall.

Index

Note: Page numbers followed by f and t refer to figures and tables, respectively.

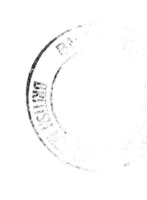